SECOND EDITION

Coding with Modifiers

A Guide to Correct *cpt*® and HCPCS Level II Modifier Usage

Deborah J. Grider

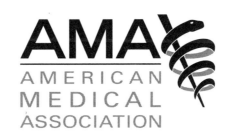

AMA

AMERICAN
MEDICAL
ASSOCIATION

Coding with Modifiers
A Guide to Correct CPT and HCPCS
Level II Modifier Usage, 2nd Edition

© 2006 by the American Medical Association.
All rights reserved.
Printed in the United States of America.

www.ama-assn.org

This book is for information purposes only. It is not intended to constitute legal advice. If legal advice is required, the services of a competent professional should be sought. All comments, opinions, and observations are those of the authors, and do not represent official positions or opinions unless specifically noted. *Coding with Modifiers* is intended to serve as an educational tool to aid in the understanding of CPT coding and modifiers. Please refer to the most current edition of the American Medical Association's *Current Procedural Terminology* containing the complete listing and most current CPT codes, descriptions, and modifiers. This publication does not replace the CPT codebook or other appropriate coding authorities.

Cover illustration: (c) Rob Colvin/Images.com

Additional copies of this book may be ordered by calling 800 621-8335 or from the secure AMA Web site at www.amabookstore.com. Refer to product number OP322006.

ISBN 1-57947-771-2
BP03:06-P-081:3/06

Contents

Chapter 3 — Modifiers 25 to 47 — 59

Chapter 4 — Modifiers 50 to 56 — 101

Chapter 5 — Modifiers 57 to 63 — 149

Chapter 6   Modifiers 66 to 82   191

Chapter 7   Modifiers 90 to 99   233

Chapter 8   HCPCS Level II Modifiers   249

Chapter 9

Ambulatory Surgery Center and Hospital Outpatient Modifiers 315

Chapter 10

Genetic Testing Modifiers and Category II Modifiers   375

Appendix A

HCPCS (Level I) CPT Modifiers   393

Appendix B

HCPCS (Level II) Modifiers   407

Appendix C

Genetic Testing Modifiers   421

Appendix D

Logic Trees   429

Preface

A Current Procedural Terminology (CPT®) code set modifier is a two-digit code reported in addition to the CPT service or procedure code that indicates that the service or procedure was modified in some way. A modifier provides the means by which a rendering physician may indicate that a service or procedure has been performed, or has been altered by some specific circumstances, but not changed in its definition or code. Understanding how and when to use CPT modifiers is vital for proper reporting of medical services and procedures. The lack of modifiers or the improper use of modifiers can result in claims delays or denials.

Modifiers are essential tools in the coding process. The American Medical Association (AMA) developed modifiers to be used with its CPT code set to explain various aspects of coding. Modifiers are used to enhance a code narrative to describe the circumstances of each procedure or service and how it individually applies to the patient. They are essential ingredients to effectively communicate between providers and payers. Modifiers are also used as a method to:

- record a service or procedure that has been modified but not changed in its identification or definition;
- explain special circumstances or conditions of patient care;
- indicate repeat or multiple procedures;
- show cause for higher or lower costs while protecting charge history data;
- report assistant surgeon services; and
- report a professional component of a procedure or service.

The ability of all users to recognize and accept CPT modifiers is important for the implementation of the CPT coding system. While acceptance of CPT modifiers is important, the subsequent step involving interpretation of modifiers in a manner that is consistent with established CPT guidelines is also critical. Modifiers can help the provider code for services more accurately and get paid for the work performed.

Coding with Modifiers: A Guide to Correct CPT and HCPCS Level II Modifier Usage, 2nd edition, introduces the principles of correct CPT and HCPCS modifier usage and prepares the reader to accomplish the following objectives:

- Understand the purpose of modifiers
- Understand the relationship to the reimbursement process
- Understand logic trees related to modifier usage
- Understand how Medicare carriers and intermediaries vary on the use and acceptance of modifiers

Coding with Modifiers is divided into 10 chapters organized by modifier. Each chapter provides step-by-step guidance as to proper and improper use of CPT and HCPCS modifiers through the use of clinical examples. Icons easily identify guidelines specific to the AMA, CMS, and third-party payers. Coding tips, checkpoint exercises, and end-of-chapter exercises are also included to help the reader gain a full understanding of a modifier's correct usage. A mid-term and final examination is located in the back of the book for educators or readers who want to apply and build knowledge related to the material.

The text is designed to be used by community colleges and career college and vocational school programs for training medical assistants, medical insurance specialists, and other health care providers. It can also be used as an independent study training tool for new medical office personnel, physicians, independent billing services personnel, and any others in the health care field who want to learn additional skills.

About the Author

Deborah J. Grider is a Certified Professional Coder (CPC), a Certified Professional Coder—Hospital (CPC-H), a Certified Professional Coder—Payer (CPC-P), and an E/M Specialist (EMS) with the American Academy of Professional Coders, and a Certified Coding Specialist—Physician (CCS-P) with the American Health Information Management Association. Her background includes many years of practical experience in reimbursement issues, procedural and diagnostic coding, and medical practice management.

Ms Grider teaches and consults with private practices, physician networks, and hospital-based educational programs. Under a federal retraining grant, she helped develop and implement a Medical Assisting Program for Methodist Hospital of Indiana. She conducts many seminars throughout the year on coding and reimbursement issues and teaches several insurance courses including the Professional Medical Coder Curriculum of which she is licensed and an approved instructor by the American Academy of Professional Coders.

Ms Grider is a speaker for the American Academy of Professional Coders as well as for other nationally known organizations. Deborah is a national advisory board member for the American Academy of Professional Coders, and currently is President-Elect. Prior to becoming a consultant, Ms Grider worked as a billing manager for 6 years, and a practice manager in a specialty practice for 12 years.

As president of Medical Professionals, Inc, Ms Grider continues to provide consulting and educational services to medical groups, physician practices, and large hospital organizations, and provides coding training education to organizations such as the Indiana State Medical Association and the Kentucky State Medical Association.

Her professional affiliations include the American Academy of Professional Coders; the Central Indiana Chapter of the American Academy of Professional Coders (of which she was the founder and president from 1996–1999 and 2001–2004); AAPC National Advisory Board member; President-Elect of the American Academy of Professional Coders National Advisory Board; member of the American Health Information Management Association (AHIMA); corporate sponsor of the Indiana Medical Group Management Association; member of the American Society of Training Development and the National Association of Female Executives (NAFE); member of the Indianapolis Chamber of Commerce; and member of the Better Business Bureau.

Acknowledgments

As this is my sixth publication for the AMA, I want to specifically thank everyone at AMA who helped turn this book into reality. Specifically, I want to thank Elise Schumacher, Senior Acquisitions Editor, for her confidence and support; and Erin Vorhies, Project Manager, who guided me through the changes and revisions expertly. Thanks also to Grace Kotowicz, Contributing Coding Consultant, who lent her expertise and helped me with the outpatient modifier chapter; and Karen O'Hara, Senior Coding Consultant, who helped me make changes along the way with her positive and constructive comments. Others who contributed to the publication of this book include:

Anthony J. Frankos, Vice President, Business Products
Mary Lou White, Executive Director, Editorial and Operations
Jean Roberts, Director, Production and Manufacturing
Amy Burgess, Marketing Manager
Rosalyn Carlton, Senior Production Coordinator
Ronnie Summers, Senior Print Coordinator

Thanks also to Michelle Yaden, who pored over the material with me, offered suggestions and proofreading changes, and helped relieve my workload. I could not have accomplished this without her.

Lastly, to my husband, Jerry; my son, Jerry, my daughter Robyn; and grandchildren, Tristan, Cassidy, and Delaney, who endured canceled appointments and outings and my late nights spent researching and writing. Without their continued love and support, I could not have completed this project.

CHAPTER 1

Introduction to CPT Modifiers

History and Purpose of CPT Nomenclature

The American Medical Association (AMA) works to promote quality and correct coding of health care services through its maintenance of the Current Procedural Terminology (CPT®) code set. The CPT code set is a listing of descriptive terms, guidelines, and identifying codes for reporting medical services and procedures. The purpose of the CPT code set is to provide a uniform language that accurately describes medical, surgical, and diagnostic services, and thereby serves as an effective means for reliable nationwide communication among physicians, patients, and third parties.

The descriptive terms and identifying codes of the CPT code set serve a wide variety of important functions. This system of terminology is the most widely accepted nomenclature used to report medical procedures and services under public and private health insurance programs. The CPT code set is also used for administrative management purposes such as claims processing and developing guidelines for medical care review.

CPT Development

The AMA first developed and published the CPT code set in 1966. The first edition helped encourage the use of standard terms and descriptors to document procedures in medical records; helped communicate accurate information on procedures and services to agencies concerned with insurance claims; provided the basis for a computer-oriented system to evaluate operative procedures; and contributed basic information for actuarial and statistical purposes.

The first edition of the CPT book (CPT®), published in 1966, contained primarily surgical procedures, with limited sections on medicine, radiology, and laboratory procedures. The second edition was published in 1970 and presented an expanded system of terms and codes to designate diagnostic and therapeutic procedures in surgery, medicine, and the specialties. At that time, a five-digit coding system was introduced, replacing the former four-digit classification. Another significant change was a listing of procedures relating to internal medicine.

In the mid- to late 1970s, the third and fourth editions of the CPT book were introduced. The fourth edition, published in 1977, represented significant updates in medical technology, and a system of periodic updating was introduced to keep pace with the rapidly changing medical environment. In 1983 the CPT code set was adopted as part of the Common Procedure Coding System (HCPCS) developed by the Health Care Financing Administration (HCFA; now the Centers for Medicare and Medicaid Services [CMS]). With this adoption, CMS mandated the use of HCPCS to report services for Part B of the Medicare program and in the Medicaid Management Information System. In July 1987, as part of the Omnibus Budget Reconciliation Act, CMS mandated the use of the CPT code set for reporting outpatient hospital surgical procedures.

Today, in addition to use in federal programs (Medicare and Medicaid), the CPT code set is used extensively throughout the United States as the preferred system of coding and describing health care services.

HIPAA and CPT

The Administrative Simplification Section of the Health Insurance Portability and Accountability Act (HIPAA) of 1996 mandates that the Department of Health and Human Services (HHS) adopt national standards for electronic transmission of health care information. This includes transmissions of codes sets, national provider identifier, national employer identifier, security, and privacy. The Final Rule for transmissions and code sets was issued on August 17, 2000. The rule names the CPT code set (including codes and modifiers) and HCPCS as the procedure code set for:

- Physician services
- Physical and occupational therapy services
- Radiological procedures
- Clinical laboratory tests
- Other medical diagnostic procedures
- Hearing and vision services
- Transportation services including ambulance

The Final Rule also adopted the International Classification of Diseases, Ninth Revision; Clinical Modification (ICD-9-CM) volumes 1 and 2 as the code set for diagnosis codes; ICD-9-CM volume 3 for inpatient hospital services; Current Dental Terminology (CDT) for dental services; and the National Drug Code (NDC) directory for drugs.

All health care plans and providers who transmit information electronically must use the established national standards. This Final Rule was implemented October 16, 2003. The Final Rule mandates the elimination of local codes for the transition to national standard code sets. The information regarding the elimination of local code sets (HCPCS level III) was published in a Program Memorandum by HHS and CMS on January 18, 2002 (Transmittal AB-02-005), which is discussed later in this chapter.

Who Maintains the CPT Code Set Nomenclature?

The AMA's CPT Editorial Panel is responsible for maintaining CPT code sets. This panel is authorized to revise, update, or modify CPT codes. The panel is composed of 17 members as follows:

- 11 members nominated by the AMA
- 2 representatives from the Health Care Professionals Advisory Committee (HCPAC)
- 1 physician nominated from the Blue Cross and Blue Shield Association
- 1 nominated by the Health Insurance Association of America
- 1 nominated by CMS
- 1 nominated by the American Hospital Association (AHA)

The AMA's Board of Trustees appoints the panel members. Seven of the 11 AMA seats on the panel are regular seats, which have a maximum tenure of two 4-year terms, or a total of 8 years for any one individual. The four remaining seats, referred to as rotating seats, have one 4-year term. These rotating seats allow more multidisciplinary input.

The panel's Executive Committee includes a chairman, the vice chairman, and three other members of the panel, as elected by the entire panel. One of the three members-at-large of the executive committee must be a third-party payer representative.

The AMA provides staff support for the CPT Editorial Panel and appoints a staff secretary who records the minutes of the meetings and keeps records.

Supporting the CPT Editorial Panel in its work is the CPT Advisory Committee. Committee members are primarily physicians nominated by the national medical specialty societies represented in the AMA House of Delegates.
The committee's primary objectives are to:

1   Serve as a resource to the CPT Editorial Panel by giving advice on procedure coding and appropriate nomenclature as relevant to the member's specialty;

2   Provide documentation to staff and the CPT Editorial Panel regarding the medical appropriateness of various medical and surgical procedures under consideration for inclusion in the CPT code set;

3   Suggest revisions to the CPT code set (the Advisory Committee meets annually to discuss items of mutual concern and to keep abreast of current issues in coding and nomenclature);

4   Assist in the review and further development of relevant coding issues and in the preparation of technical education material and articles pertaining to the CPT code set;

5   Promote and educate its membership on the use and benefits of the CPT code set.

The HCPAC was formed by the CPT Editorial Panel to allow for participation of organizations representing limited license practitioners and allied health professional in the CPT process. The cochairman of the HCPAC is a voting member of the CPT Editorial Panel.

How Suggestions for Changes to the CPT Code Set Are Reviewed

There are specific procedures for addressing suggestions to revise the CPT code set by adding or deleting a code or modifying existing nomenclature. The AMA staff reviews all correspondence to evaluate coding suggestions. If the AMA staff determines that the panel has previously addressed the question, a member of the staff informs the requestor of the panel's interpretation.

If the staff determines the request is a new issue or significant new information is received on an item that the panel has previously reviewed, the request is referred to the appropriate member of the CPT Advisory Committee. If all advisors agree that no new code or revision is needed, the AMA staff provides information to the requestor on how to use the existing codes to report the procedure. If all advisors concur that a change should be made, or if two or more advisors disagree or give conflicting information, the issue is referred to the CPT Editorial Panel for resolution.

Current medical periodicals and textbooks are used to provide up-to-date information about the procedure or service in addition to the Advisory Committee opinions. Further data are also obtained about the efficacy and clinical utility of procedures from other sources, such as the AMA's Diagnostic and Therapeutic Technology Assessment Program and various other technology assessment panels. The AMA staff prepares agenda material for each CPT Editorial Panel meeting. Topics for the agendas are gathered from several sources: Medical specialty societies, physicians, hospitals, third-party payers, and other interested parties may submit materials for consideration by the Editorial Panel. Panel members receive agenda materials at least 30 days in advance of each meeting, allowing them time to review the material and confer with experts on each subject.

The CPT Editorial Panel meets each quarter and addresses complex problems associated with new and emerging technology as well as the difficulties encountered with outmoded procedures. The panel addresses nearly 350 major topics a year, which typically involve more than 3000 votes on an individual basis. Panel actions may result in one of three outcomes:

- A new code is added or nomenclature is revised and appears in a forthcoming volume of the CPT book;
- An item is tabled to obtain further information; or
- The item is rejected.

Since this is a multi-step process, deadlines are important. The deadlines for change requests and for Advisory Committee comments are based on a schedule that allows at least 3 months of preparation and processing time before the issue is ready for review by the CPT Editorial Panel. The initial step, including staff and specialty advisor review, is completed when all appropriate advisors have been contacted and have responded, and all information requested of a specialty society or an individual requestor has been provided to the AMA staff.

The requestor must have completed and submitted a coding change request form. If the advisors' comments indicate that action by the CPT Editorial Panel is warranted, a second step is taken by the AMA staff to prepare an agenda item that includes a ballot for the request to be acted on by the CPT Editorial Panel. Once the panel has taken action and minutes of the meeting are approved, the AMA staff informs the requestor of the outcome. The requestor may appeal the panel's decision if the appeals process is followed:

- A written request for reconsideration is sent to the AMA staff.
- The reason for the appeal must be included in the request, indicating the reason the requestor believes the panel's actions are incorrect, and response to the panel's stated rationale.
- The information is then referred to the CPT Executive Committee for a decision to reconsider.

The CPT Process

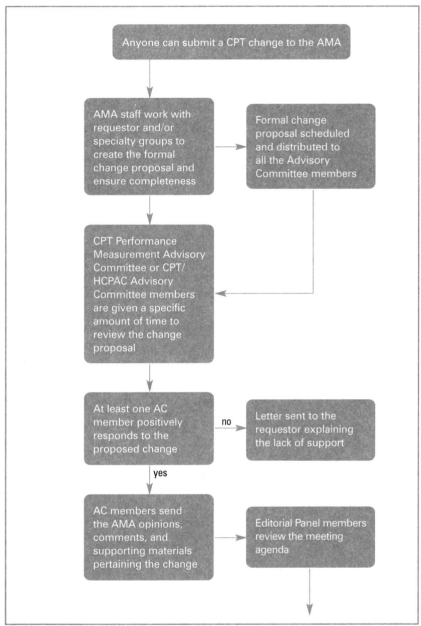

continued

The CPT Process, continued

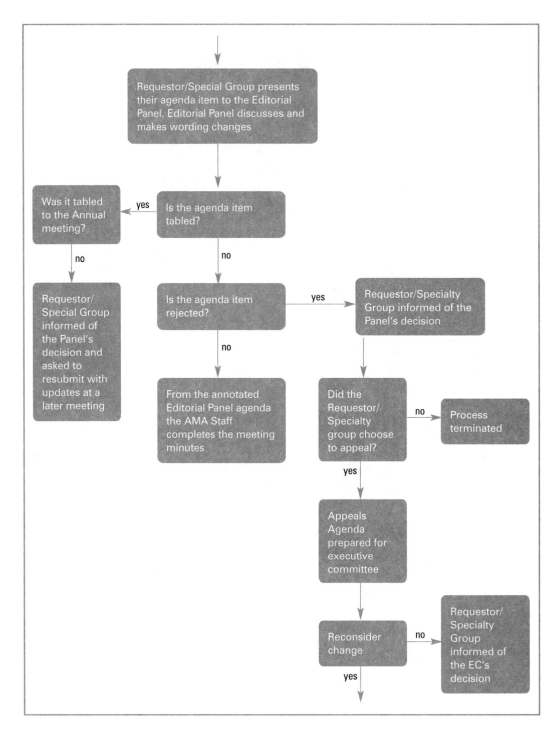

Category I CPT Codes

Category I CPT codes describe a procedure or service identified with a five-digit numeric CPT code and descriptor nomenclature. The inclusion of a descriptor and its associated specific five-digit identifying code number in this category of CPT codes is generally based on the procedure being consistent with contemporary medical practice and being performed by many physicians in a clinical practice in multiple locations.

When developing new and revised codes, the Advisory Committee and the Editorial Panel require that:

- The service/procedure has received approval from the Food and Drug Administration (FDA) for the specific use of devices or drugs;
- The suggested procedure/service is a distinct service performed by many physicians/practitioners across the United States (US);
- The clinical efficacy of the services/procedure is well established and documented in US peer-reviewed literature;
- The suggested service/procedure is neither a fragmentation of an existing procedure/service nor currently reportable by one or more existing codes; and
- The suggested service/procedure is not requested as a means to report extraordinary circumstances related to the performance of a service/procedure already having a specific CPT code.

Category II CPT Codes: Performance Measurement

Category II CPT codes are intended to facilitate data collection by coding certain services and/or test results that are agreed on as contributing to positive health outcomes and quality patient care. This category of CPT codes is a set of tracking codes for performance measurement. These codes may be services that are typically included in an evaluation and management (E/M) service or other component part of a service and are not appropriate for Category I CPT codes. Consequently, the Category II codes do not have relative values associated with them. The use of tracking codes for performance measures will decrease the need for record abstraction and chart review, and minimize administrative burdens on physicians and survey costs for health plans.

CPT Performance Measurement codes are assigned an alphanumeric identifier with the letter "F" in the last field (eg, 4018F). These codes are located in a separate section of the CPT book, following the Medicine section. Introductory language is placed in this code section to explain the purpose of the codes. The use of these codes is optional and is not required for correct coding.

Tracking codes are reviewed by the Performance Measures Advisory Group (PMAG), an advisory group to the CPT Editorial Panel and the CPT Health Care Professionals Advisory Committee (CPT/HCPAC). Requests for Category II codes are then forwarded to the CPT/HCPAC Advisory Committee just as requests for Category I CPT codes are reviewed. The interest of the PMAG is as follows:

- Measurement that is developed and tested by a national organization
- Evidenced-based measurements with established ties to health outcomes

- Measurement that addresses clinical conditions of high prevalence, high risk, or high cost
- Well-established measurements that are currently being used by large segments of the health care industry across the country.

In order to expedite reporting Category II codes, once these codes have been approved by the CPT Editorial Panel, the newly added codes are made available on a semiannual basis via electronic distribution on the AMA Web site (www.ama-assn.org/go/cpt). The AMA's CPT Web site features updates of the Category II codes in July and January in a given CPT nomenclature cycle.

Category III CPT Codes: Emerging Technology

This section of the CPT book contains a temporary set of tracking codes for emerging technologies, services, and procedures. Category III CPT codes are intended to facilitate data collection on and assessment of these services and procedures. These codes are used for data collection purposes to substantiate widespread usage or in the FDA approval process. Category III CPT codes may not conform to the usual CPT coding requirements for a Category I code that:

- Services or procedures be performed by many health care professionals across the country;
- FDA approval be documented or be imminent within a given CPT cycle; and
- The service or procedure has proven clinical efficacy.

The service or procedure must have relevance for research, either ongoing or planned. These codes have an alphanumeric identifier with the letter "T" in the last field (eg, 0078T). These codes are located in a separate section of the CPT book following the Category II code section. Introductory language is placed in this code section to explain the purpose of these codes.

Once approved by the Editorial Panel, the newly added Category III CPT codes are made available on a semiannual (twice a year) basis via electronic distribution on the CPT page of the AMA Web site (www.ama-assn.org). The full set of Category III CPT codes is included in the next published edition for the CPT cycle.

Category III CPT codes are not referred to the AMA/Specialty RVS Update Committee (RUC) for evaluation because no relative value units (RVUs) are assigned. Payment for these services/procedures is based on the policies of payment and not on a yearly fee schedule.

These codes are archived after 5 years if the code has not been accepted for placement in the Category I section of the CPT book, unless it is demonstrated that a Category III code is still needed. These archived codes are not reused.

The HCPCS Coding System

HCPCS is the CMS's Health Care Common Procedure Coding System. Formerly called HCFA, CMS developed this system in 1983 to standardize the coding systems used to process Medicare claims on a national basis. The HCPCS coding system is structured in two levels: CPT nomenclature and national codes. (Level III local codes were eliminated under HIPAA regulations.) Each level has its own unique coding system.

Level I: CPT Nomenclature

Level I is the American Medical Association's CPT nomenclature. CPT nomenclature makes up the majority of the HCPCS coding system. Most of the procedures and services performed by physicians, physician extenders, and other health care professionals, even with respect to Medicare patients, are reported with CPT code sets. The CPT code set nomenclature includes the following:

- Each procedure or service is identified with a five-digit numeric code or a five-character alphanumeric code.
- Two-digit numeric modifiers are used (except for the Physical Status modifiers, Genetic Testing Modifiers, and Performance Measures modifiers).
- Codes are revised and updated on an annual basis.
- Updates and revisions become effective each January.
- Revisions, additions, and deletions are prepared by the AMA's CPT Editorial Panel.

Level II: National Codes

Level II national codes are assigned, updated, and maintained by CMS. Codes in this level identify services and supplies not found in the CPT code set. Examples of HCPCS level II codes are durable medical equipment, ambulance services, medical and surgical supplies, drugs, orthotics, prosthetics, dental procedures, and vision services. HCPCS level II national codes are made up of the following:

- Five-character alphanumeric codes. The first character is a letter A through V (except I)[1] followed by four numeric digits (eg, J3490).
- Alphabetic (eg, RT) and alphanumeric (eg, E2) modifiers.

Codes are updated annually by CMS and are required for reporting most medical services and supplies provided to Medicare and Medicaid patients.

Level III: Local Codes

CMS has taken steps to eliminate local codes and their descriptors developed by Medicare contractors for use by physicians, practitioners, providers, and suppliers. The level III HCPCS codes were alphanumeric codes of five digits, in the W, X, Y, or Z series, that were not representative of HCPCS level I or II codes. HCPCS level III codes also contained two-digit alphabetic modifiers and were represented by WA through ZZ. The elimination of these codes was necessary to prepare for full

---

1. The I codes are reserved for use by the Health Insurance Association of American (HIAA) to fulfill member companies' unique coding needs. The S codes are created and maintained by the Blue Cross Blue Shield Association for its needs. C codes are used for reporting drugs and biologicals for outpatient hospital services.

implementation of HIPAA. These codes were eliminated effective October 16, 2003, because the local codes did not support the objectives of HIPAA, which calls for an efficient coding system that meets uniform standards and requirements. The Consolidation Appropriations Act of 2001 (Public Law 106-554), enacted December 21, 2000, extended the maintenance and use of the official HCPCS level III codes and modifiers until December 31, 2003 (CMS Program Memorandum Transmittal AG-02-005). A copy of the transmittal may be found at www.cms.hhs.gov. The local codes are no longer in use.

Modifiers

The CPT code set nomenclature uses modifiers as an integral part of its structure. A modifier provides a means by which a practitioner can indicate that a service or procedure was altered by specific circumstances, but not changed in its definition or code.

Modifiers are essential tools in the coding process. The AMA developed HCPCS level I modifiers, which are numeric. CMS developed HCPCS level II alphabetic modifiers to be used with codes to explain various circumstances of procedures and/or services. Modifiers are used to enhance a code narrative to describe the circumstances of each procedure or service and how it individually applies to the patient. They are also essential ingredients to effectively communicate between providers and payers. Modifiers do not ensure reimbursement. Some modifiers may increase reimbursement, while some are only informational.

Not only are there dozens of different modifiers, but the rules for using them can vary. For example, a modifier may be used in one way for physician services and in another way for hospital services.

In the CPT code set nomenclature, modifiers may be used in many instances, such as:

- To report only the professional component of a procedure or service
- To report a service mandated by a third-party payer
- To indicate that a service or procedure was performed bilaterally
- To report that multiple procedures were performed at the same session by the same provider
- To report that a portion of a service or procedure was reduced or eliminated at the physician's discretion
- To report assistant surgeon services
- To report that a service or procedure was performed by more than one physician
- To report exclusionary circumstances (Category II)

The following example shows when a modifier would be applicable.

Example 1

A chest X ray, with two views, is performed on a patient with suspected pneumonia. This service was performed in the outpatient radiology department of the hospital. The radiologist is not employed by the hospital.

CPT Code(s) Billed: 71020 26

71020   Radiologic examination, chest, two views, frontal and lateral

Appending modifier 26 in the previous example indicates that the radiologist performed only the professional component (reading the chest X ray and dictating the formal report). Appending modifier 26 at the end of the code does not change the original definition, but it does indicate that the total procedure was not performed by the physician, only the reading of the film(s) and the interpretation and report.

Two surgeons might be required to perform a specific surgical procedure together. When two surgeons work together as primary surgeons and perform distinct part(s) of a procedure, each surgeon should report his or her surgical work by adding modifier 62 to the procedure code and any associated code(s) for that procedure as long as both surgeons continue to work together as primary surgeons. Each surgeon reports the co-surgery once using the same procedure code. If additional procedure(s), including add-on procedure(s), are performed during the same surgical session, separate code(s) may also be reported with modifier 62 added.

NOTE: If a co-surgeon acts as an assistant in the performance of additional procedure(s) during the same surgical session, those services may be reported by using separate procedure code(s) with modifier 80 or 82 added as appropriate.

Example 2

A neurosurgeon and an otolaryngologist work together to perform a transsphenoidal excision of a pituitary neoplasm. Each physician performs a distinct part of the procedure.

CPT Code(s) Billed: 61548 62

61548   Hypophysectomy or excision of pituitary tumor, transnasal or transseptal approach, nonstereotactic

In this example, modifier 62 indicates to the insurance carrier that two surgeons performed specific parts of the procedure, but it does not change the original definition of the code.

When billing the surgical procedure, each surgeon would bill by using the CPT code 61548 with modifier 62.

61548 62   *Neurosurgeon*

61548 62   *Otolaryngologist*

Types of Modifiers Used in the Reimbursement Process

There are two levels of modifiers within the HCPCS coding system:
- HCPCS level I (CPT modifiers)
  - ~ Category II Modifiers
  - ~ Genetic Testing Modifiers

- HCPCS level II (HCPCS modifiers)

HCPCS Level I (CPT Modifiers)

CPT modifiers are two-digit numeric and/or alphanumeric (as in the physical status modifiers in anesthesia, the genetic testing modifiers, and the Category II modifiers) designations that explain to an insurance carrier a change in the description of the code without changing its meaning. The CPT Editorial Panel determines the definition and guidelines for CPT modifier usage on the basis of input from the Advisory Committee. A complete listing of CPT modifiers and their descriptors can be found in Appendix A of this book.

The following are examples of HCPCS level I (CPT modifiers) along with clinical examples.

Example 1

Modifier 24—Unrelated Evaluation and Management Service by the Same Physician During a Postoperative Period

Definition: The physician may need to indicate that an E/M service was performed during a postoperative period for a reason(s) unrelated to the original procedure. This circumstance may be reported by adding the modifier 24 to the appropriate level of E/M service.

A 35-year-old recreational skier injured his right knee, with peripheral longitudinal tears of both medial and lateral menisci, and underwent an arthroscopic meniscus repair using a suture technique. The CPT code used for this procedure is 29883, and the global period in which the physician provides typical follow-up care is usually 90 days with many insurance carriers.

The physician submitted a claim to the insurance carrier with the following CPT code:

29883   Arthroscopy, knee, surgical; with meniscus repair (medial AND lateral)

The patient returned to his orthopedic surgeon 3 weeks later for follow-up and indicated that he had been experiencing pain in the right shoulder. He told the surgeon that he had gone out to his garage to get a hammer and slipped and fell on the garage floor, and he had been experiencing pain in the right shoulder since that time. After an expanded problem-focused history and exam, the physician determined that the patient had sprained his right shoulder, and he provided the appropriate medication and treatment. The physician also examined the knee and determined that it was healing appropriately. The patient was advised to limit activities that would cause further injury.

The physician could bill for an E/M service in this example because the reason for the visit procedure (shoulder pain) was unrelated to the surgical procedure.

99213   Office or other outpatient visit for the evaluation and management of an established patient, which requires at least two of these three key components: an expanded problem focused history; an expanded problem focused examination; medical decision making of low complexity

However, without a modifier, the carrier would consider the visit part of the surgical global (package) procedure and might deny the visit. When modifier 24 is appended to the encounter with an unrelated diagnosis, the claim would be reviewed and in most cases paid by the carrier. The visit should be submitted with the use of modifier 24 (**99213 24**).

Example 2

Modifier 58—Staged or Related Procedure or Service by the Same Physician During the Postoperative Period

A surgeon performed a radical mastectomy on a 56-year-old female patient. The patient indicated that she preferred a permanent prosthesis after the surgical wound healed. The surgeon took the patient back to the operating room during the postoperative global period and inserted a permanent prosthesis.

The physician submitted a claim to the insurance carrier with the following CPT codes:

19200   Mastectomy, radical, including pectoral muscles, axillary lymph nodes

11970 58   Replacement of tissue expander with permanent prosthesis

The surgeon in this case reported the code for the permanent prosthesis insertion 11970 with modifier 58 to indicate that the service was related to the mastectomy (staged to occur at a time after the initial surgery). The original procedure was coded without a modifier.

Physical Status Modifiers

Physical status modifiers are consistent with the American Society of Anesthesiologists ranking of the patient's physical status; they distinguish at various levels of complexity the anesthesia service provided. Table A-2 in Appendix A of this book lists the physical status modifiers used in anesthesia to convey to the carrier the health and condition of a patient who is undergoing surgery in relation to anesthesia.

The following example demonstrates when a physical status modifier might be appropriate.

Example 3

A 72-year-old woman with hypertension, insulin-dependent diabetes, uncontrolled chronic obstructive pulmonary disease, and a history of severe claudication in both lower extremities was scheduled for diagnostic femoral arteriography and venography under general anesthesia.

CPT Code(s) Billed: 01916 P3—Anesthesia for diagnostic arteriography/venography

Notice that adding the physical status modifier P3 does not change the definition of the code, but the modifier explains the complexity or risk involved with anesthesia because the P3 modifier indicates the patient has a severe systemic disease, which puts the patient at higher risk than a patient who is healthy.

Example 4

A 45-year-old patient in good physical condition underwent a lumbar and ventral (incisional) hernia repair under general anesthesia in the outpatient surgery department of a local hospital.

CPT Code(s) Billed: 00752 P1—Anesthesia for hernia repairs in upper abdomen; lumbar and ventral (incisional) hernias and/or wound dehiscence

In this example adding the physical status modifier P1 indicates the patient is a normal healthy patient with less risk.

NOTE: Not all carriers accept the use of physical status modifiers.

The question always arises as to whether CPT modifiers can be used when Medicare, Medicaid, and private health plans are billed. Medicare carriers and fiscal intermediaries vary on the use and acceptance of modifiers listed in the CPT book. Other commercial payers may accept only some CPT modifiers. The same is true for private health care plans and managed care plans. It is important to check with individual payers regarding their billing requirements. A good source of this information is the insurance carriers' provider manual. Another source of reference is the individual carrier's Web site.

HCPCS Level II (HCPCS Modifiers)

The HCPCS modifiers were developed by the Health Care Financing Administration (now Centers for Medicare and Medicaid Services, or CMS) for use in the Medicare program. Many carriers now accept HCPCS modifiers. However, before HCPCS national modifiers (level II) are used, providers should determine whether specific carriers accept these codes. The HCPCS data set is published and updated yearly and may be purchased from various publishers and bookstores across the country. Because HCPCS codes and modifiers may change and some may be added throughout the year, checking the CMS Web site is recommended (www.cms.hhs.gov/providers). The complete listing of HCPCS modifiers is provided in Table B-1 in Appendix B of this book.

Each year, in the US, health care insurers process more than 5 billion claims for payment. For Medicare and other health insurance programs to ensure that claims are processed in a consistent manner, HCPCS level II codes were developed. Level II is a standardized coding system that is used primarily to identify products, supplies, and services not included in the CPT code set. Level II HCPCS codes were established for submitting claims for these services. The development and use of level II HCPCS began in the 1980s. HCPCS level II codes are considered alphanumeric codes because they consist of a single alphabetical letter followed by a numeric four-digit code. In some instances, insurance carriers require that a HCPCS code of either level I or level II be accompanied by a modifier to provide additional information regarding the service, item, and/or procedure by the HCPCS code. Modifiers are used when the information provided by the code descriptor needs to be supplemented to identify any special or unusual circumstances that may apply to the item or service. These modifiers are either alphanumeric or two letters.

Some HCPCS modifiers are located in Appendix A of the CPT book, but a complete listing is found in the HCPCS Manual. It is strongly recommended

---

Level III Modifiers: Local Codes

The CMS eliminated local codes and their descriptors developed by Medicare contractors for use by physicians, practitioners, providers, and suppliers. These codes were officially eliminated effective October 16, 2002, and providers were given 12 months to prepare their systems for the discontinued use of the codes. They were eliminated because the local codes did not support the objectives of HIPAA, which calls for an efficient coding system that meets uniform standards and requirements.

Level III modifiers were phased out December 31, 2003. These modifiers and their guidelines were unique to each Medicare Part B contracted carrier, sometimes referred to a fiscal intermediary who defines usage of a local modifier. Some examples of local modifiers are W, X, Y, and Z. They are not covered in this text.

that an updated HCPCS coding manual be purchased each year for coding, since codes are added and deleted yearly. HCPCS modifiers are discussed in more detail in Chapter 8 of this book.

Many carriers accept a combination of CPT and HCPCS modifiers. For example, in coding radiology services, there is a professional component and a technical component, which are components of the CPT code, unless indicated in the code definition. These modifiers split out the service provided by the physician (professional, 26) and the facility, which includes the technician, supplies, equipment, and so on (technical, TC).

When the provider bills the global component technical and professional, a modifier is not required. Modifier TC is a HCPCS modifier and modifier 26 is a CPT modifier.

Why Use Modifiers?

As discussed earlier, modifiers explain to the insurance carrier that the description of the code is the same, but something about the procedure or service was changed without changing the definition of the CPT code set. Some modifiers impact reimbursement, while others are informational and help get the claim paid without costly delays. Modifiers can be appended to a CPT code, further defining the service and, therefore, increasing the likelihood of getting paid accurately.

Using a modifier—CPT or a HCPCS modifier—does not guarantee reimbursement. In some cases, the provider might be asked to provide a report and/or documentation to support the service(s) billed. The report or documentation should be complete, describing in detail the complexity of the patient's problems and/or physical findings, with any therapeutic or diagnostic procedures. An accurate diagnosis and any associated conditions and/or signs and symptoms should be evident to the carrier.

If the medical record documentation does not support the modifier billed by the provider, the provider risks denial of the claim and possible penalties for submitting an incorrect claim. It is not necessary to become an expert in coding modifiers; however, it is important to understand how to use modifiers correctly along with which modifiers should be appended to the claim appropriately. Each modifier will be explored individually with correct usage, documentation requirements, carrier guidelines, clinical examples, and tips in this text.

Surgical Procedures

When surgical procedures are billed, every procedure is connected to a "global period," which is 0 to 90 days and defined by each carrier individually.

The global period includes preoperative management, the surgical procedure, certain types of anesthesia, and all typical follow-up care up to and including the global period, sometimes referred to as "global days."

If the patient requires care related to the surgery, routine follow-up care, dressing changes, and so on, during the required postoperative period, the provider cannot bill additional charges. They are included in the procedure. However, when the service or procedure performed by the same practitioner and/or group is unrelated or is significantly separately identifiable, a modifier would indicate that the service is not included in the procedure and/or service.

Example 1

A 30-year-old man, who was an established patient, came in for a follow-up office visit for a 3-month history of fatigue, weight loss, and intermittent fever, and showing diffuse adenopathy and splenomegaly. A detailed history was taken, including complaints and possible exposures such as sexual, travels abroad, etc. Comprehensive examination including lymphatic and abdominal examination was performed. Medical decision making of moderate complexity included discussion of possible diagnosis, possible diagnostic testing needed, and importance of follow-up. During the encounter, the patient mentioned he had a lesion on the right arm. The physician evaluated the 2.3-cm lesion, determined it was benign, and excised it.

Two separate encounters occurred during the visit: The patient came in with multiple medical problems that needed to be addressed, including fatigue, weight loss, intermittent fever, and diffuse adenopathy and splenomegaly. The physician also evaluated a lesion, determining that it was benign but needed to be removed. The E/M service and the lesion removal both are significantly and separately identifiable, and both services may be reported on the same day. Here is the correct way to submit the claim:

99214 25   *Office visit*

11403   *Benign lesion excision*

The descriptions of the codes selected are as follows:

99214   Office or other outpatient visit for the evaluation and management of an established patient, which requires at least two of these three key components: a detailed history; a detailed examination; medical decision making of moderate complexity

11403   Excision, benign lesion including margins, except skin tag (unless listed elsewhere), trunk, arms or legs; excised diameter 2.1 to 3.0 cm

CPT modifier 25 is appended only to the E/M service when the physician needs to indicate that an evaluation and management service was performed, and it is a significant, separately identifiable evaluation and management service performed on the same day as another procedure or service. The physician may need to indicate that on the day a procedure or service identified by a CPT code was performed, the patient's condition required a significant, separately identifiable E/M service above and beyond the other service provided or beyond the usual preoperative and postoperative care associated with the procedure that was performed. A significant, separately identifiable service is defined or substantiated by documentation that satisfies the relevant criteria for the respective E/M service to be reported.

Without modifier 25 (Significant, Separately Identifiable Evaluation and Management Service by the Same Physician on the Same Day of the Procedure or Other Service), the claim would most likely be denied on the basis of the initial claim submitted, even with a different diagnosis. Modifier 25 will be discussed in further detail in Chapter 3.

Modifiers and Reimbursement

Coding has become an integral part of any hospital or medical practice. It is complex and constantly changing, and there are stiff penalties for incorrect coding. Accurate coding is the antidote to the decline in the reimbursement rate.

Unfortunately, using modifiers does not always mean payers will recognize or accept them. Reimbursement policy has been developed through consideration of the AMA's CPT code set and instructions with many insurance carriers. Many payers develop their own payment policies that differ with CPT guidelines. It is always beneficial to discuss modifier usage with the payer to determine if the individual carrier has developed a separate policy from CPT guidelines prior to submitting claims.

The CMS uses resource-based relative value units (RBRVS) and recommendations from the National Correct Coding Initiative (NCCI). With rare exception, reimbursement policy may also be developed on the basis of input from external provider consultants, contract language, and benefits.

RBRVS Payment Rules and Policies

The RBRVS payment system required the development of national payment policies and their uniform implementation by the Medicare carriers. Under customary, prevailing, and reasonable payment, each Medicare carrier established its own policies, including issues such as which services were included in the payment for a surgical procedure. As with the elimination of specialty differentials and customary charges, there was no transition period for standardizing carrier payment policies under the RBRVS payment system. Standardization of payment policies became effective January 1, 1992.

One of the most significant standardization provisions included in the Omnibus Budget Reconciliation Act of 1989 (OBRA 89) was the requirement that CMS adopt a uniform coding system for Medicare. In the June 1991 Notice of Proposed Rulemaking, CMS stated that the AMA's CPT code set would serve as that uniform system. The CPT code set includes more than 8000 codes to describe physicians' services, including codes for E/M services that became effective

January 1, 1992. These codes are used to describe visit and consultation services and were developed for use under Medicare's RBRVS-based payment system.

In addition to the five-digit CPT codes, CMS recognizes other alphanumeric codes for some nonphysician services and supplier services, such as ambulance services. Together, the CPT code set and the alphanumeric codes compose the HCPCS.

Besides coding, CMS established a multitude of national policies as part of the revisions to the payment system, including uniform national policies on payment for the following:

- Global surgical packages
- Assistants-at-surgery
- "Incident-to" services
- Supplies and drugs
- Technical component–only services
- Diagnostic tests
- Nonphysicians' services
- Several other aspects of Medicare Part B

It is important for physicians to understand that the carriers are required to implement these policies in a nationally uniform manner. Carriers do not have an option to develop a different policy for their local area.

CMS sets national guidelines, but individual insurance carriers may interpret guidelines for their own organization or regional office. CPT and/or HCPCS modifiers accepted for use by one insurance company may not be accepted by another company. Also, interpretation of a modifier may differ. It is recommended that local carrier guidelines be reviewed before a modifier is used.

Nonrecognition of modifiers is an important issue and significantly impacts physician reimbursement and administrative burden for physicians. Because of the publication of the modifier list, physicians justifiably presume that the modifiers will be recognized and they will be reimbursed for medically necessary and appropriate services. When claims are not paid appropriately, the physician is forced to endure time-consuming, costly, and often futile efforts through the appeals process.

Third-party payers define their own policy for the acceptance of modifiers, and the coder and/or practitioner must review each carrier's acceptance of a particular modifier.

Modifiers to the CPT procedure codes are used to describe special circumstances under which the basic service was provided. With implementation of the Medicare RBRVS, the use of modifiers was standardized to establish national payment policies.

The instructional notes pertaining to reporting five-digit modifiers have been deleted from the CPT code set to coincide with the CMS-1500 claim form reporting instructions, as this was in conflict with the previous instructions included in the CPT code set regarding the use of a separate five-digit modifier.

According to the National Uniform Claim Committee, the new electronic claim format for the CMS-1500 claim form, in compliance with the regulations that apply to HIPAA, will not accommodate a five-digit modifier. The current field length of the electronic format that holds a modifier is limited to two characters.

The Proper Use of Modifiers: Step by Step

To appropriately code with modifiers, the health care organization should include commonly used modifiers on charge tickets, superbills, or encounter forms. Even though they may be listed appropriately, not all practitioners will use them correctly without guidance and training. Careful documentation is the key to supporting the use of modifiers. Every claim with modifiers should be reviewed to make sure the documentation, if requested by the insurance carrier, will support the claim. Practitioners should take a preventive, proactive approach rather than waiting until a claim is denied to take action. Below is a checklist of steps to take when coding modifiers:

- Review CPT (AMA) guidelines.
- Review individual carrier guidelines.
- Refer to the practitioner's or facility's patient medical record and/or visit note before appending modifiers.
- Use only two digits when appending modifiers (unless instructed otherwise by an individual carrier); with implementation of standard code sets with HIPAA, five-digit modifiers are no longer accepted.
- Provide training for physicians, staff, clinicians, etc, and update training regularly.
- Take a proactive approach and find the errors in modifier application before the claim is submitted to the insurance carrier.

Tips for Using Coding Modifiers Correctly

- Always have the most recent edition of the CPT book on hand.
- Have your billing staff regularly attend coding workshops.
- Remember that modifiers are often used differently for physician services and hospital outpatient services.
- Learn as much as you can about using coding modifiers so you can help your billing staff with coding questions.
- Keep up to date on coding changes and modifier interpretations.
- Obtain the National Correct Coding Initiative (NCCI) regarding policy on correct modifier usage for government payers and other commercial payers who follow the NCCI.
- Communicate with the individual payer regarding policy and use of modifiers.

- Understand that insurance carrier interpretations are not always the same as those given in the CPT book.
- Review the National Correct Coding Initiative (NCCI) each quarter for correct modifier usage for each CPT code that your organization uses.

The CMS accepts the use of CPT modifiers, but not all private insurance carriers recognize modifiers. Different interpretations of application of a modifier may be defined by each individual carrier. Practitioners' offices should develop a system of tracking denials based on the use of modifiers.

Chapter 1 Review

- Level I (CPT) modifiers are two-digit extenders that are appended to a CPT code.
- Modifiers explain to a carrier that the descriptor of the CPT code has not changed, but has been modified to explain unusual circumstances.
- Modifiers appended to the CPT code designate the need for additional consideration.
- Some modifiers are informational, while others impact proper reimbursement.
- To support coding with modifiers, the practitioner's documentation must clearly support the circumstance.
- HCPCS modifiers are used by some carriers to designate specific information, such as RT for right and LT for left.
- HCPCS level I and level II modifiers may not be recognized by all insurance carriers.
- Understanding modifiers, updating code manuals, and ongoing training are the keys to correct coding with modifiers.

Test Your Knowledge

1 _____ CPT modifiers are published by:
    a. Centers for Medicare and Medicaid Services
    b. Centers for Disease Control and Prevention
    c. American Medical Association
    d. local fiscal intermediary

2 _____ Modifiers are:
    a. two-digit extenders
    b. numeric only
    c. used only to track diseases
    d. none of the above

3 _____ HCPCS modifiers are level:
    a. 2
    b. 1
    c. 3
    d. 4

4 _____ Level 1 modifiers are published by:
    a. Centers for Medicare and Medicaid Services
    b. American Medical Association
    c. Centers for Disease Control and Prevention
    d. fiscal intermediary

5 _____ These modifiers were introduced in 2006 to indicate:
    a. genetic testing
    b. physical status
    c. performance measures inclusion/exclusions
    d. none of the above

6 _____ Modifiers explain:
    a. that a code has changed in its definition
    b. that a code has not changed in its definition, but has been modified
    c. that reimbursement should be higher
    d. b and c

7 _____ What is the antidote to an incorrect reimbursement rate?
    a. modifiers
    b. unbundling
    c. billing claims during the global period
    d. accurate coding

8 _____ To append a modifier to a claim, you should:
    a. review CPT guidelines only
    b. review CPT and carrier guidelines for interpretation
    c. bill without regard to carrier rules
    d. none of the above

9 _____ Level II modifiers are:
   a. published by the AMA
   b. published by Centers for Medicare and Medicaid Services
   c. published by each individual state
   d. a and b

10 _____ CPT modifiers are:
   a. level I modifiers
   b. level II modifiers
   c. level III modifiers
   d. level IV modifiers

CHAPTER 2

Modifiers 21 to 24 and the Physical Status Modifiers

Modifier 21: Prolonged Evaluation and Management Services

Definition

When the face-to-face or floor/unit service(s) provided is prolonged or otherwise greater than that usually required for the highest level of evaluation and management service within a given category, it may be identified by adding modifier 21 to the evaluation and management code number. A report may also be appropriate.

AMA Guidelines

Modifier 21 was added to the CPT® code set in 1992 and revised in 1994. This modifier reports services that take more time or are greater than the highest-level evaluation and management (E/M) code in a particular category. This modifier is used with codes such as 99205, 99215, 99223, 99233, 99245, and 99255.

Modifier 21 is used only with E/M services at the highest level within a given category, with the exception of critical care services that are time-based E/M codes. This modifier means that the physician's service(s) has exceeded the highest level of E/M service.

In certain specialties, modifier 21 may be reported more frequently than in other specialties because of the nature of the problems seen by that specialist. However, the documentation provided by any physician must indicate the prolonged or otherwise greater services provided at the encounter when modifier 21 is appended to the highest level of service in a given category.

For example, a physician sees a new patient in the office with severe chronic obstructive pulmonary disease, congestive heart failure, and hypertension. The physician performs the three key components found in CPT code 99205, which are:

- Comprehensive history
- Comprehensive examination
- Medical decision making of high complexity

In addition, the physician spends a total of 30 additional minutes performing repeated evaluations to stabilize the patient's condition so that the patient may be sent home instead of being admitted to the hospital. Diagnostic tests are also performed at the visit.

The actual performance of diagnostic tests/studies for which specific CPT codes are available are reported in addition to the level of E/M service provided. The time spent performing diagnostic test procedures, which have specified CPT codes, is not included in the time associated with an E/M code.

To report the modifier 21 with 99205, the physician's work must meet at a minimum "a comprehensive history, a comprehensive examination, and medical decision making of high complexity."

CMS Guidelines

Modifier 21 is used when the time spent with the patient is 30 minutes or less beyond the time stated in the code description. If the time spent is more than 30 minutes beyond the stated time, the Prolonged Service codes 99354-99357 are reported in addition to the E/M code.

Third-Party Payer Guidelines

While some third-party payers recognize the use of modifier 21, other payers ignore this modifier. Many third-party payers require the provider to attach the office or hospital documentation, which should indicate the additional time spent with the patient and the reason for the additional time.

Modifier 21 can only be used with the E/M section of the CPT book. It is recommended that time spent in addition to the E/M service be documented in the medical record along with the reason for the additional time spent to validate the use of modifier 21. If lesser E/M levels are selected, prolonged services codes 99354 and/or 99355 must be used.

Modifier 21 cannot be used with all E/M codes. The E/M CPT codes that are time based would not require modifier 21 because the additional work performed for these codes can sometimes be reflected in other codes for the additional time spent with the patient. For example, CPT codes 99291 and 99292 for critical care are time-based codes, and modifier 21 would not be necessary because 99291 is reported for the first 30 to 74 minutes and 99292 is reported for each additional 30 minutes. There is no limit in reporting 99292 as long as the time and work are documented completely in the medical record.

Example 1

An office visit was made for the initial outpatient evaluation of a 69-year-old man with severe chronic obstructive pulmonary disease, congestive heart failure, and hypertension. A comprehensive history was taken, including extensive review of the patient's medical record from other physicians as to prior treatment, tests, and details needed to seek old records. A comprehensive examination including neurologic examination was performed. A lengthy problem list with plans for new diagnostic testing was developed. Medical decision making of high complexity included a lengthy discussion with the patient about the severity of his multisystem illness, prognosis without adequate treatment, and follow-up. Counseling included smoking, diet, and medication compliance. The physician spent an additional 29 minutes counseling the patient.

CPT Code(s) Billed: 99205 21

Example 2

An initial office evaluation was performed of a 65-year-old woman with exertional chest pain, intermittent claudication, syncope, and a murmur of aortic stenosis. The physician performed a comprehensive history and comprehensive physical examination including supine and upright blood pressures, vascular system in neck and extremities, heart, and neurological system. Medical decision making was of high complexity and involved ordering appropriate diagnostic procedures (electrocardiogram, two-dimensional and Doppler echocardiography for estimated degree of stenosis and function of ventricle, chest X ray to check for cardiac hypertrophy and valvular and/or aortic root calcification) and decision making regarding hospitalization for cardiac catheterization and coronary angiography and possible head-up tilt table testing. Alternative approaches to diagnosis and therapy were explained to the patient. The physician spent an additional 30 minutes with the patient discussing alternative treatment and therapy.

CPT Code(s) Billed: 99205 21

Example 3

A return office visit was made by a 68-year-old man with previous prosthetic valve replacement, diabetes, and morbid obesity who now presented with new-onset dyspnea and fluid retention. The physician performed a comprehensive history and comprehensive physical examination, including heart, lungs, abdomen, venous system in the neck and legs while lying, sitting, and standing, skin, and soft tissue of the legs. Fluid restriction, diet, and therapeutic goals were discussed with the patient. Medical decision making was of high complexity and involved ordering a chest X ray and echocardiogram to assess valvular function, lab work to evaluate control of diabetes and renal function, and initiating appropriate medical therapy. The physician spent an additional 29 minutes with the patient discussing options and diabetes control.

CPT Code(s) Billed: 99215 21

Example 4

A 78-year-old woman with left lower-lobe pneumonia and a history of coronary artery disease, congestive heart failure, osteoarthritis, and gout was admitted to the hospital. After performing a comprehensive history and physical examination with high complexity decision making, the physician spent an additional 30 minutes reviewing the patient's medical records and discussing treatment alternatives with the patient.

CPT Code(s) Billed: 99223 21

Example 5

An outpatient consultation was performed for a 74-year-old man with a history of coronary artery disease and diabetes undergoing a preoperative evaluation for elective hip replacement. Comprehensive history included cardiopulmonary system, blood sugar control, medications, and previous complication with anesthesia. A comprehensive examination was performed, including heart, lungs, extremities, and skin. Medical decision making of high complexity included recommendations for preoperative lab tests and medications and possible postoperative complications. The physician spent an additional 30 minutes in discussion with the patient about nutrition and blood sugar control and the importance of compliance and follow-up.

CPT Code(s) Billed: 99245 21

Example 6

An initial hospital consultation was performed for a 50-year-old man with a history of previous myocardial infarction who now presented with acute pulmonary edema and hypotension. After a comprehensive history and examination, with high complexity decision making, the physician spent an additional 29 minutes reviewing records, explaining treatment options to the patient, discussing findings with the patient's cardiologist, and scheduling diagnostic testing.

CPT Code(s) Billed: 99255 21

Example 7

An 83-year-old male new patient had previously been followed up at home by a recently retired physician for multi-infarct dementia, diabetes mellitus, and osteoarthritis of the back, hip, and knee. He had a temperature of 101.5°F, cough, chest congestion, rapid respirations, marked decline in mental alertness, and cloudy urine. Oral intake had dropped sharply during the preceding 2 days. His family did not want him to be hospitalized, but wanted to take all available measures to help him recover at home. The physician spent an additional 30 minutes discussing treatment options with the patient and his family and arranging ongoing nursing care for the patient.

CPT Code(s) Billed: 99345 21

Prolonged Service Code Sets vs Modifier 21

AMA Guidelines

In CPT nomenclature for 1994, the prolonged services codes were modified to allow a physician to report services involving direct (face-to-face) patient contact that is beyond the usual service in either the inpatient or outpatient setting. The difference between modifier 21 and prolonged physician service with direct (face-to-face) patient contact is that the time the physician spent with the patient was continuous and the services exceeded the highest level of service in that category.

The prolonged physician services with direct (face-to-face) patient contact can be intermittent and can be reported with any level of E/M service. These codes are intended for use in unusual circumstances only and should not be applied just because the physician's time exceeds the time it normally takes for the E/M service.

Prolonged services are grouped into two main categories:

- Prolonged Physician Services With Direct Face-to-Face Contact (99354-99357)
- Prolonged Physician Services Without Direct Face-to-Face Contact (99358-99359)

The code series 99354 to 99357 is used when a physician provides prolonged service involving direct (face-to-face) patient contact or service care that is beyond the usual service (ie, beyond the typical time) in either the inpatient or outpatient setting. The term *face-to-face* refers only to patient face-to-face contact.

CPT codes 99354 and 99355 are used to report prolonged physician services with direct face-to-face contact in the office or other outpatient settings. CPT codes 99356 and 99357 are used to report prolonged physician services with direct face-to-face contact in the inpatient hospital setting.

These codes are time based and reported for the total time spent by a physician providing prolonged services on a given date. It is not necessary for the time spent by the physician providing the prolonged service to be continuous. Prolonged services of less than 30 minutes in total duration on a given date are not reported.

These codes are all "add-on" codes in the CPT code set nomenclature. They are reported separately in addition to the E/M services at any level when the physician and/or practitioner spends an additional 30 minutes or more with the patient, over and above the usual time spent for the E/M service. Codes 99354 and 99356 are used only one time per date of service. Codes 99355 and 99357 are used to report each additional 30 minutes.

Codes 99358 and 99359 are used to report prolonged services without direct (face-to-face) patient contact in either the outpatient or inpatient setting. The total time spent providing these services on a given date is reported, even if the time spent by the physician is not continuous. Prolonged services of less than 30 minutes in total duration on a given date are not reported.

The following codes are considered "add-on" codes in the CPT code set and are reported in addition to the E/M code(s) in either the inpatient or outpatient setting:

+99354   Prolonged physician service in the office or other outpatient setting requiring direct (face-to-face) patient contact beyond the usual service (eg, prolonged care and treatment of an acute asthmatic patient in an outpatient setting); first hour (list separately in addition to code for office or other outpatient Evaluation and Management service)

+99355   Prolonged physician service in the office or other outpatient setting requiring direct (face-to-face) patient contact beyond the usual service (eg, prolonged care and treatment of an acute asthmatic patient in an outpatient setting); each additional 30 minutes (list separately in addition to code for prolonged physician service)

+99356   Prolonged physician service in the inpatient setting, requiring direct (face-to-face) patient contact beyond the usual service (eg, maternal fetal monitoring for high risk delivery or other physiological monitoring, prolonged care of an acutely ill inpatient); first hour (list separately in addition to code for inpatient Evaluation and Management service)

+99357   Prolonged physician service in the inpatient setting, requiring direct (face-to-face) patient contact beyond the usual service (eg, maternal fetal monitoring for high-risk delivery or other physiological monitoring, prolonged care of an acutely ill inpatient); each additional 30 minutes (list separately in addition to code for prolonged physician service)

Prolonged Service codes can be used at any level and are different from modifier 21 as they can be used with an E/M service at all levels.

Codes 99358 and 99359 are used for prolonged E/M services before and/or after direct (face-to-face) patient care, which includes reviewing of extensive records and/or tests and communication with other health care professionals and/or the patient or family. CPT code 99358 is for the first hour and 99359 is for each additional 30 minutes beyond the first hour.

+99358   Prolonged evaluation and management service before and/or after direct (face-to-face) patient care (eg, review of extensive records and tests, communication with other professionals and/or the patient/family); first hour (list separately in addition to code(s) for other physician service(s) and/or inpatient or outpatient Evaluation and Management service)

+99359   Prolonged evaluation and management service before and/or after direct (face-to-face) patient care (eg, review of extensive records and tests, communication with other professionals and/or the patient/family); each additional 30 minutes (list separately in addition to code for prolonged physician service)

The difference between the two codes is that with the non-face-to-face encounter, the service may not involve face-to-face contact during the encounter.

Threshold Times for Codes 99354 and 99355

If the total direct face-to-face time equals or exceeds the threshold time for code 99354, but is less than the threshold time for code 99355, the physician should bill the visit and code 99354. Only one unit of code 99354 may be billed per patient per day. If the total direct face-to-face time equals or exceeds the threshold time for code 99355 by no more than 29 minutes, the physician should bill the visit code 99354 and one unit of code 99355. One additional unit of code

99355 is billed for each additional increment of 30 minutes of extended duration. Threshold times are given in the table that follows.

Prolonged Services

Total Duration of Prolonged Services	Code(s)
Less than 30 minutes (less than 1/2 hour)	Not reported separately
30–74 minutes (1/2 hour–1 hour, 14 minutes)	99354 × 1
75–104 minutes (1 hour, 15 minutes–1 hour, 44 minutes)	99354 × 1 and 99355 × 1
105–134 minutes (1 hour, 45 minutes–2 hours, 14 minutes)	99354 × 1 and 99355 × 2
135–164 minutes (2 hours, 14 minutes–2 hours, 44 minutes)	99354 × 1 and 99355 × 3
165–194 minutes (2 hours, 45 minutes–3 hours, 14 minutes)	99354 × 1 and 99355 × 4

Threshold Times for Codes 99356 and 99357

If the total direct face-to-face time equals or exceeds the threshold time for code 99356, but is less than the threshold time for code 99357, the physician should bill the visit and code 99356. Only one unit for 99356 should be coded per patient per day. If the total direct face-to-face time equals or exceeds the threshold time for code 99356 by no more than 29 minutes, the physician bills the visit code 99356 and one unit of code 99357. One additional unit of code 99357 is billed for each additional increment of 30 minutes of extended duration. Threshold times are given in the table that follows to determine whether the prolonged services codes 99356 and/or 99357 can be billed with the inpatient and consultation codes.

Prolonged Services

Total Duration of Prolonged Services	Code(s)
Less than 30 minutes (less than 1/2 hour)	Not reported separately
30–74 minutes (1/2 hour–1 hour, 14 minutes)	99356 × 1
75–104 minutes (1 hour, 15 minutes–1 hour, 44 minutes)	99356 × 1 and 99357 × 1
105–134 minutes (1 hour, 45 minutes–2 hours, 14 minutes)	99356 × 1 and 99357 × 2
135–164 minutes (2 hours, 14 minutes–2 hours, 44 minutes)	99356 × 1 and 99357 × 3
165–194 minutes (2 hours, 45 minutes–3 hours, 14 minutes)	99356 × 1 and 99357 × 4

AMA CODING TIP

Note that 99354 and 99356 (Prolonged Service codes) are add-on codes and are preceded by a ✚ symbol. They cannot be used alone and must be used in conjunction with an E/M CPT code. CPT code(s) 99355 and 99357 are for each additional 30 minutes beyond the first hour and must be used in conjunction with 99354 and 99356. Code selection is based on whether the patient is seen in an outpatient or inpatient setting.

CMS Guidelines

The Medicare Carriers Manual (15511-15511.3) states that prolonged services without *face-to-face service* (codes 99358 and 99359) are not covered because they do not require direct face-to-face patient contact. Payment for these services is included in the payment for direct face-to-face services for which physicians bill. The physician cannot bill the patient for these services, since they are Medicare-covered services and payment is included in the payment for other billable services.[1]

Medicare Guidelines

The Medicare Carriers Manual (15511-15511.3) states that prolonged services (codes 99354 and 99355) require companion codes when billed on the same day by the same physician as the companion E/M services. The services are allowed when the criteria for prolonged services are met.

The companion codes for 99354 are 99201-99205, 99212-99215, 99241-99245, 99301-99345, and 99347-99350. The companion codes for 99355 are 99354 and one of the E/M codes required for 99354. The companion codes for 99356 are 99221-99223, 99231-99233, and 99251-99255. The companion codes for 99357 are 99356 and one of the E/M codes required for 99357.

Medicare will not pay prolonged services codes 99354-99358 unless they are accompanied by one of the above companion codes. Only the duration of face-to-face contact between the patient and physician, whether continuous or not, beyond the typical time of the visit can be billed by using prolonged services. For example, if the patient spends the time with the office or clinical staff, the time cannot be billed as prolonged services.

In the case of prolonged hospital services, time spent waiting for test results, for changes in the patient's condition, for end of a therapy, or for use of facilities cannot be billed to CMS as prolonged services.

CMS does not require documentation to accompany the bill for prolonged services unless the physician has been targeted for medical review. To support billing for prolonged services, the medical record must document the duration and content of the E/M code billed and that the physician has personally furnished at least 30 minutes of direct service after the typical time of the E/M service had been exceeded by at least 30 minutes.

Prolonged services codes can be billed only if the total duration of all physician direct face-to-face service (including the visit) equals or exceeds the threshold time for the E/M service the physician provided (typical time plus 30 minutes). If the total duration of direct face-to-face time does not equal or exceed the threshold time for the level of E/M service the physician provided, the physician may not bill for prolonged services.

---

1. CMS Carriers Manual, available at http://www.cms.hhs.gov/physicians.

Example 1

A patient was seen in the endocrinologist's office for follow up of her diabetes. The patient's blood sugar was unusually high and the physician documented a level three (99213) established patient E/M visit. The physician spent an additional 45 minutes counseling the patient on diet and exercise as she also is 50 pounds overweight, which is affecting her blood sugar control. The physician documented a total duration of time for the encounter as 60 minutes with the patient and documented a brief note stating the reason for the counseling with the patient. The patient encounter was reported as follows:

> *99213—Office or other outpatient visit for the evaluation and of an established patient, which requires at least two of these three key components: an expanded problem focused history; an expanded problem focused examination; and medical decision making of low complexity.*

> *99354—Prolonged physician service in the office or other outpatient setting requiring direct (face-to-face) patient contact beyond the usual service (eg, prolonged care and treatment of an acute asthmatic patient in an outpatient setting); first hour (list separately in addition to code for office or other outpatient Evaluation and Management service)*

Example 2

A new patient with symptoms of chest pain and shortness of breath saw a cardiologist for evaluation. The physician documented a detailed history and examination with medical decision-making of low complexity. The physician ordered diagnostic tests to rule out cardiac problems but suspected gastroesophogeal reflux as the problem. The patient was a smoker and also had a weight problem with a Body Mass Index of 36.2. The physician spent an additional 15 minutes counseling the patient on smoking cessation along with diet and exercise. The additional time is documented in the medical record.

Based on guidelines for using prolonged services, may the physician report the E/M service with prolonged services?

The answer to the question is no. The physician must spend an additional 30 minutes over and above the average time for the E/M service level. These time elements, though not the controlling factor for the E/M service unless counseling and/or coordination of care dominates at least 50% of the visit, are found under each CPT code in the Evaluation and Management section in which key components are required. Codes in the Evaluation and Management section of the CPT codebook that are time based would not apply to prolonged services.

When reviewing the level of service the physician should select for the new patient office visit, the physician selects 99203. The claim should be reported as follows:

99203—New patient evaluation and management service, office or other outpatient.

Documentation Requirements

Documentation in the patient's progress notes must support billing for prolonged services no matter what insurance carrier is billed. Documentation does not need to be submitted with the claim but must be available upon request for most carriers. The patient's medical record must document the duration and content of the E/M code billed and that the physician has personally furnished at least 30 minutes of direct service after the typical time of the E/M service had been exceeded by at least 30 minutes.

Review of Modifier 21

1 Use modifier 21 only with E/M services.

2 Use this modifier with the highest level in each given E/M service category.

3 Do not use modifier 21 with time-based codes (eg, critical care services).

4 Do not use modifier 21 with any other sections of the CPT book.

5 If using prolonged E/M services, do not use modifier 21.

Modifier 22: Unusual Procedural Services

Definition

When the service(s) provided is greater than that usually required for the listed procedure, it may be identified by adding modifier 22 to the usual procedure number. A report may also be appropriate.

In 1992, modifier 22 was revised adding "procedural" to the descriptor. This indicates that modifier 22 may be used with any procedure, but is not used with the E/M codes.

This modifier may be used in the following sections of the CPT code set:
- Anesthesia
- Surgery
- Radiology
- Laboratory and Pathology
- Medicine

AMA Guidelines

This modifier should be used only when additional work factors requiring the physician's technical skill involve significantly increasing physician work, time, and complexity of the procedure normally performed. The procedure and/or service may be surgical or nonsurgical. The reimbursement for a procedure already takes into account that sometimes the procedure will be simpler and other times more difficult than normal. However, there are times when a procedure will be significantly more difficult.

In some circumstances, surgeons perform services or procedures that entail greater physician work than described by the CPT code descriptor. In many cases, there are not additional or add-on codes to describe the increased complexity of the service. In these cases, modifier 22 should be appended to the CPT code(s).

Modifier 22 is appropriate in reporting unusual operative cases, such as:

- Trauma extensive enough to complicate the particular procedure and that cannot be billed with additional procedures
- Significant scarring requiring extra time and work
- Extra work resulting from morbid obesity
- Increased time resulting from extra work by the physician

CMS Guidelines

The CMS Medicare Carrier Manual (MCM15028) indicates that for modifier 22 the relative value units for services represent the average work effort and practice expenses required to provide a service. For any given procedure code, there could typically be a range of work effort or practice expense required to provide the service. Thus, the payment for a service may be increased or decreased only under very unusual circumstances based on review of medical records and other documentation.

When modifier 22 is used with a procedure, CMS requires submission of documentation to support the unusual circumstances of the procedure. This modifier does affect reimbursement of the procedure. CMS requires the following information when submitting the claim:

- A concise statement about how the service differs from the usual; and
- An operative report submitted with the claim.

Because of the extenuating circumstances, an increase in reimbursement usually is indicated.

Third-Party Payer Guidelines

Carriers continue to have authority to increase payment for unusual circumstances on the basis of review of medical records and other documentation. Modifier 22 would likely place a claim in manual review. This translates into a longer waiting period for the organization to receive payment for the claim. Many insurance carriers will not consider claims that use modifier 22 without the documentation and a separate statement written by the physician explaining the unusual amount of work required. Modifier 22 may also be considered for other situations on a case-by-case basis.

Invalid uses of modifier 22 include the following:

- When there is also a "reoperation" code used with the primary procedure code (eg, if the patient has had previous coronary artery bypass grafting [CABG] and is now undergoing a new CABG, code 33530 is billed in addition to the primary procedure)
- If the cause of the complication results from the surgeon's choice of approach (eg, open vs laparoscopic)
- To describe an average amount of lysis or division of adhesions between organs and adjacent structures (routine lysis of adhesions is considered an integral and inclusive part of the procedure)

Modifier 22 produces an automatic review or audit by payers, so supporting documentation must be sent with the claim. In addition, modifier 22 may not be honored for extra payment if it is used too frequently. It is to be used for unusual services only. If the claim is approved, many carriers may allow an additional 20% to 50% of the allowable rate for the procedure performed, depending on the circumstances. The physician's documentation should be thorough. If it does not indicate the nature or difficulty of the additional work, insurance carriers may not automatically increase the reimbursement for the claim. Modifier 22 indicates an automatic manual review.

Information to Be Submitted for Manual Review

A letter requesting consideration of the claim should accompany all documentation, indicating the payment increase the provider is requesting and what percentage it is over the usual fee. Copies of operative reports, radiology reports, pathology reports, and so on should be included.

The report should be complete, clear, concise, and easily understood. The report must show the complex nature of the procedure and/or service and describe the rationale for the additional physician work for the service. Simple medical explanations and terminology should be used, since the encounter may not be reviewed by a physician. The normal time to complete the procedure and/or service should be compared to the actual time it took to complete the unusual procedure and/or service. Diagnoses that explain the complication should be included if available.

Correct Coding Initiative Guidelines

Chapter 1 of the National Correct Coding Initiative states, "Routine use of the modifier is inappropriate as this practice would suggest cases routinely have unusual circumstances. When an unusual or extensive service is provided, it is more appropriate to utilize the 22 modifier than to report a separate code that does not accurately describe the service provided."[2] Local Part B carriers may also have authoritative written guidelines for using modifier 22.

---

2. Source: National Correct Coding Initiative (NCCI) Guidelines.

Appending Modifier 22 to a Procedure or Service

The following factors should be considered before the decision is made to append modifier 22:

- The surgeon's documentation should be thorough. If it does not indicate the nature of the difficulty or the extra work performed, carriers will not automatically increase the fee.
- The documentation should be submitted with the claim because modifier 22 claims may spur an automatic manual review.
- The additional time and work must be significant. Many coding specialists say that unless 25% more work was performed, modifier 22 should not be appended. For CMS and many other third-party payers, if the physician's operative time is increased by 50% or more, modifier 22 should be appended. A second diagnosis code may be warranted to account for the unusual circumstances.
- Any additional fees should be charged up-front to payers, which are unlikely to raise fees on their own just because modifier 22 is appended.
- When claims are submitted with modifier 22 appended to the procedure, the insurance carrier(s) requires submission of documentation to validate any additional fees charged for the service.

Example 1: Surgical Procedure

In a patient undergoing laparoscopic oophorectomy, significant omental adhesions were noted upon entrance into the abdomen. A small clear space allowed placement of a right-lower-quadrant 10-mm trocar. An offset scope was used through this port to lyse adhesions to free the omentum from the anterior abdominal wall, allowing inspection of the pelvis. This required approximately 20 to 30 minutes of additional surgical time. Inspection of the pelvis revealed complete distortion of the normal anatomical relationships. The uterus was deviated to the left. The left round ligament could not be visualized. The sigmoid colon was densely adherent to the left pelvic sidewall. The left fallopian tube remnant could not be identified. The right adnexa demonstrated an irregular enlarged ovary with cystic enlargement consistent with an endometrioma. A second left-lower-quadrant trocar was placed. With a combination of electrodissection, sharp blunt dissection, and hydrodissection, the multiple dense adhesions were lysed. Relative anatomical relationships were restored. The dissection involved releasing the dense adhesions of the sigmoid colon to the peritoneum with mobilization of the sigmoid to identify the infundibula pelvic vessels and the course of the left ureter. The left pelvic sidewall was opened and the left round ligament was identified. The total additional operative time to restore anatomy so as to identify vital anatomical structures before proceeding with oophorectomy was 1 hour of surgical work.

CPT Code(s) Billed: 58661 22—Laparoscopy, surgical; with removal of adnexal structures (partial or total oophorectomy and/or salpingectomy)

Rationale for Using Modifier 22

In this example, there are two reasons why modifier 22 would be appropriate. The first is the extensive lysis of adhesions requiring 20 to 30 additional minutes of surgical time. The second reason is that the physician spent an additional hour to reverse the distortion of the anatomy before proceeding with the intended oophorectomy.

Example 2: Surgical Procedure

A physician performed a laminotomy with decompression of the nerve root with a partial facetectomy, foraminotomy, and excision of a herniated disk. During the surgery the physician encountered excessive bleeding (hemorrhage) that was difficult to control. This required an additional 60 minutes to complete the surgery.

CPT Code(s) Billed: 63020 22—Laminotomy (hemilaminectomy), with decompression of nerve root(s), including partial facetectomy, foraminotomy and/or excision of herniated intervertebral disk; one interspace, cervical

Rationale for Using Modifier 22

The patient experienced excessive hemorrhaging, control of which required an additional 60 minutes of surgical time.

Example 3: Anesthesia

A 72-year-old woman initially underwent left cemented total hip arthroplasty 1 year previously. After recovery from the first total hip replacement, the patient suffered two left hip dislocations. Radiographic studies revealed a loosening of the femoral component. The surgical plan included removal and replacement of the femoral component and assessment, and possible replacement of the acetabular components to prevent further dislocations. During the surgery, the patient went into cardiac arrest, and it took the anesthesiologist 45 minutes to stabilize the patient before the procedure could be continued. The procedure was then completed and the patient was taken to the recovery room in critical condition. She was closely monitored and moved to the critical care unit after 2 hours. The circumstances of the case prolonged the surgery by 45 minutes. The anesthesia code was submitted with modifier 22 along with the documentation.

CPT Code(s) Billed: 01215 22—Anesthesia for open procedures involving hip joint; revision of total hip arthroplasty

The patient went into cardiac arrest and had to be stabilized by the anesthesiologist before the procedure could be completed. This additional work of stabilization required an additional 45 minutes over and above the usual procedure time, so modifier 22 is appropriate.

Example 4: Cardiac Catheterization

A 68-year-old man was hospitalized with unstable angina. He had been treated in the past with coronary bypass surgery. A cardiac catheterization and coronary and graft angiograms were ordered. The cardiologist performed retrograde left heart catheterization, left ventriculography, selective coronary angiography, and vein graft angiography. In addition, the cardiologist injected the internal mammary artery to determine whether it would be a suitable arterial conduit for a second bypass operation. Because the patient was morbidly obese, 50 minutes additional time were required to perform the procedure. The physician determined that the patient's diagnoses were arteriosclerotic heart disease of native coronary arteries, arteriosclerotic heart disease of autologous venous grafts, and left ventricular hypertrophy.

CPT Code(s) Billed: 93510 22, 93539, 93543, 93545, 93555, and 93556

Rationale for Using Modifier 22
Since the patient was morbidly obese, it took an additional 50 minutes over and above the typical time to perform the cardiac catheterization. It would be appropriate to submit the claim with modifier 22.

Modifier 22 Coding Tips

The following should be kept in mind when modifier 22 is used:

1 The physician's documentation should be thorough. If it does not indicate the nature of the difficulty or the extra work performed, carriers will not automatically increase the fee.

2 The documentation should be submitted with the claim because modifier 22 claims may spur an automatic manual review.

3 The additional time and work must be significant. Many insurance carriers say that, unless 25% more work was performed, modifier 22 should not be appended.

4 For some third-party payers, if the physician's operative time is increased by 50% or more, modifier 22 should be appended.[3] A second diagnosis code may be required to warrant the unusual circumstances.

5 Any additional fees should be charged up-front to payers, which are unlikely to raise fees on their own just because modifier 22 is appended.

---

3. Source: Medicare Carrier's Manual, available at www.cms.hhs.gov/physicians.

6   Where possible, diagnoses with appropriate International Classification of Diseases, Ninth Revision, Clinical Modification (ICD-9-CM) code(s) that further describe the circumstance warranting the use of this modifier should be included.

7   Normal time to complete a procedure and the actual time to complete the procedure should be compared by using modifier 22. For a surgical procedure that typically requires 1 to 2 hours to perform, reimbursement from payers will be the same whether the procedure takes 1 or 2 hours. This is because reimbursement averages out across patients over time. The use of the unusual services modifier would be inappropriate if the procedure took 2 hours, just as use of the reduced service modifier would not be appropriate if the procedure took 1 hour.

8   If a claim is submitted with modifier 22 appended to the CPT code, many carriers including CMS will pay the normal reimbursement as if modifier 22 was not appended.

9   Modifier 22 should not be overused. Abuse of this modifier will attract unwanted scrutiny by an insurance carrier. Repeated misuse could trigger a carrier audit.

Modifier 23: Unusual Anesthesia

Definition

Occasionally, a procedure that usually requires either no anesthesia or local anesthesia must be done under general anesthesia because of unusual circumstances. This circumstance may be reported by adding the modifier 23 to the procedure code of the basic service.

Anesthesia administration service may be reported by means of the CPT codes in the Anesthesia section of the CPT book (codes 00100-01999), the appropriate anesthesia modifier (P1-P6), and qualifying circumstances codes (99100-99140) if appropriate. However, some insurance carriers do not accept anesthesia codes and instead require the use of codes from the Surgery section of the CPT book for reporting anesthesia services. It is important to develop an understanding of CPT coding guidelines as well as payer-specific guidelines for reporting anesthesia services.

AMA Guidelines

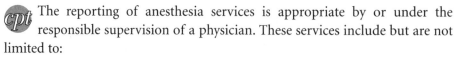 The reporting of anesthesia services is appropriate by or under the responsible supervision of a physician. These services include but are not limited to:

- General, regional supplementation of local anesthesia
- Other supportive services to afford the patient the anesthesia care deemed optimal by the anesthesiologist during any procedure

Also included are:
- Usual preoperative and postoperative visits
- Anesthesia care during the procedure
- Administration of fluids and/or blood
- Usual monitoring services (eg, electrocardiogram, temperature, blood pressure, oximetry, capnography, and mass spectrometry)

Unusual forms of monitoring (eg, intra-arterial, central venous, and Swan-Ganz) are not included.

To report moderate (conscious) sedation (with or without analgesia) provided by the physician also performing the service for which conscious sedation is being provided, see codes 99143-99145 in the CPT codebook.[4]

In 2006, the codes for conscious sedation changed along with the category and guidelines. Moderate conscious sedation is described as a drug-induced depression of consciousness during which patients respond purposefully to verbal commands, either alone or accompanied by light tactile stimulation. No interventions are required to maintain a patent airway, and spontaneous ventilation is adequate. Cardiovascular function is usually maintained.

CMS Guidelines

 The CMS guidelines state that anesthesia services typically include:

- Preoperative and postoperative visits by the anesthesiologist
- Anesthesia care during the procedure
- Administration and management of fluids and/or blood and the usual monitoring of services (eg, heart rate, temperature, blood pressure, and oxygen saturation levels) during the surgical procedure
- Placement of intravenous lines necessary for fluid and medication administration
- Placement of an endotracheal or orotracheal airway for ventilator management
- Intraoperative interpretation of laboratory tests that are performed perioperatively

In cases where unusual circumstances occur, additional information might be necessary to support the administration of general anesthesia when local or no anesthesia is typically required. The following should be submitted with the claim for payment:
- Surgeon's operative note, including:
    - ~ surgical time
    - ~ medications administered
- Anesthesia record, including:
    - ~ anesthesia time
    - ~ monitors placed

4. Source: *CPT* *2006*; Anesthesia Guidelines.

AMA CODING TIP

Local anesthesia administered by the surgeon is not coded in the anesthesia section of CPT, and the surgeon should not append modifier 23 to the surgical procedure.

~ medication administered by anesthesia
~ documentation of monitored readings

In addition to providing anesthesia care, anesthesiologists may perform medically necessary surgical and medical services. These include:

- Swan-Ganz catheter insertion (CPT code 93503)
- Central venous pressure line insertion (CPT codes 36555-36571)
- Intra-arterial line insertion (CPT codes 36620-36625)

Reporting Anesthesia Services

The anesthesia procedure is first assigned a number of base units based on the complexity of the procedure. This information is available in the Medicare Part B Anesthesia manual on the CMS Web site (www.cms.hhs.gov). For example, a hernia repair is assigned 46 units, while a liver transplant is assigned 30 base units.

The amount of time the procedure requires is calculated according to time units. Billable time starts when the anesthesia provider begins preparation of the patient for anesthesia in the operating room or equivalent area, and ends when the patient is safely placed under postanesthetic supervision and care. The amount of time assigned per unit varies throughout the United States from 6- to 15-minute increments.

Physical status and/or qualifying circumstances that affect the risk of the procedure are documented through the use of modifiers to the procedure (CPT) code. Each modifier is also assigned a unit value. Modifiers such as physical status, age, and emergency factors may be added to the procedure code. The total number of units is then multiplied by a conversion value to create a total charge for the procedure.

AMA Guidelines

The guidelines in the Surgery section of the CPT book for listed surgical procedures indicate that the following anesthesia services are always included in a given CPT surgical code in addition to the operation per se: local infiltration, metacarpal/metatarsal/digital block, or topical anesthesia. Certain codes in the CPT code set nomenclature represent services performed with the patient under general anesthesia. It would not be appropriate to append modifier 23 to these services, which normally require general anesthesia.

Procedures that generally do not require general anesthesia because of the extent of the services or circumstances may be reported with modifier 23.

The condition of some patients may support necessity to perform general anesthesia. For example, patients with tremors or patients who have mental incapacities may require the use of general anesthesia instead of local anesthesia because of extenuating circumstances.

Modifier 23 is appended when a procedure that usually requires no anesthesia or local anesthesia must be done under general anesthesia.

Anesthesia services must be provided by or under the medical supervision of a physician to be reported. Certain procedures that generally do not require general anesthesia may, in some cases, require general anesthesia because of the extent of the service (eg, 11044, Debridement, skin, subcutaneous tissue, muscle, and bone).

There are several HCPCS anesthesia claims modifiers that will be discussed in Chapter 8 of this text.

CMS Guidelines

Documentation must be submitted to support the unusual anesthesia. The documentation must indicate in detail the reason the case is unusual, and submit documentation with the claim.

Example 1

A 4-year-old patient with Down syndrome was diagnosed with acute lymphoblastic leukemia after presenting with fatigue, fever, and weight loss. Significant history included surgical repair of a ventricular septal defect at 2 years of age. The patient was extremely anxious, and the parents requested that the child be anesthetized for cerebrospinal fluid testing and administration of intrathecal methotrexate.

CPT Code(s) Billed: 00635 23—Anesthesia for procedures in lumbar region; diagnostic or therapeutic lumbar puncture

Rationale for Using Modifier 23

Since the child had Down syndrome and was anxious, there was a possibility that local anesthesia might not be effective and/or might increase the child's anxiety. The anesthesiologist agreed with the parents and anesthetized the patient with the general method.

Example 2

An 85-year-old man with a history of chronic obstructive pulmonary disease (COPD), hypertension, and 40 pack-years of smoking with a 3-cm peripheral nodule in the right upper lobe was scheduled for a diagnostic thoracoscopy and biopsy by means of a left lateral position. The patient was nervous and uncooperative, so general anesthesia with double-lumen endotracheal tube and arterial blood pressure monitoring was performed.

CPT Code(s) Billed: 00528 23—Anesthesia for closed chest procedures; mediastinoscopy and diagnostic thoracoscopy not utilizing one lung ventilation

Rationale for Using Modifier 23

Since the documentation indicated that the patient was anxious and uncooperative, the anesthesiologist determined that general anesthesia was indicated.

Example 3

A 69-year-old man with COPD, hypertension, and severe back and radicular pain secondary to possible herniated lumbar disks presented for lumbar myelography of the L3/L4, L4/L5, and L5/S1 disks in the prone position. Since the patient was extremely anxious and agitated and in a great deal of pain, the physician elected to perform the procedure under general anesthesia instead of local anesthesia, which would normally have been used.

CPT Code(s) Billed: 01905 23—Anesthesia for myelography, diskography, vertebroplasty

Rationale for Using Modifier 23

The patient was anxious and agitated and in a great deal of pain, which supports the use of general anesthesia to perform the procedure, so modifier 23 was appended to the claim.

Insurance companies will want to know why the anesthesia was required. Therefore, when the unusual anesthesia modifier is submitted, a report should be included that focuses on the circumstances that necessitated the general anesthetic. Most insurance carriers will require documentation to support the use of general anesthesia when local is the accepted method.

Review of Modifier 23

Modifier 23 is:
- Used for procedures that would normally not require general anesthesia
- Not applicable for local anesthesia
- Not applicable for moderate conscious sedation

Physical Status Modifiers

Many anesthesia services are provided under difficult circumstances and/or when the patient's physical status is impaired. This adds to the complexity of the anesthesia service provided and may be reported by using physical status modifiers and/or qualifying circumstance codes. When these modifiers or codes are reported, additional American Society of Anesthesiologists units may be allowed and combined with the base unit value for the anesthesia service performed. More information regarding the American Society of Anesthesiologists may be found on their Web site at www.asahq.org.

AMA Guidelines

cpt All anesthesia services are reported by means of the five-digit anesthesia modifier procedure code (00100-01999) plus the addition of a physical status modifier. The physical status modifiers are located in the Anesthesia

Guidelines of the CPT book. They are identified with the letter "P" followed by a single digit, 1 to 6. The physical status modifiers, which reflect the American Society of Anesthesiologists ranking of physical status, are as follows:

- P1—A normal healthy patient
- P2—A patient with mild systemic disease
- P3—A patient with severe systemic disease
- P4—A patient with severe systemic disease that is a constant threat to life
- P5—A moribund patient who is not expected to survive without the operation
- P6—A declared brain-dead patient whose organs are being removed for donor purposes

Physical status is included in the CPT code set nomenclature to distinguish between various levels of complexity of the anesthesia service provided. In addition to the physical status modifiers, other modifiers may be appropriate when procedural services are coded and are reported in addition the anesthesia procedure code. If the anesthesiologist performs other additional procedures, each is reported separately.

Physical status modifiers are appended directly to all anesthesia codes (eg, 01810, Anesthesia for all procedures on nerves, muscles, tendons, fascia, and bursae of forearm, wrist, and hand) and reflect the level of complexity associated with the anesthesia service provided. They do not apply to conscious sedation services.

Third-Party Payer Guidelines

Many carriers will pay 1 to 3 additional base units, respectively, for physical status modifiers P3 to P5. These patients are at a higher risk for the anesthesiologist than those rated P1 or P2, so the payment should be increased accordingly on these cases. The carrier should not need to see a specific diagnosis code to substantiate the physical status modifier billed as long as the preoperative assessment documentation supports the modifier. The insurance carrier should be consulted before the modifier is appended. Some carriers still do not recognize the physical status modifier(s).

Example 1

A 68-year-old man with progressive coronary artery disease was prepared for coronary artery bypass. On the basis of the anatomy, a direct coronary artery bypass surgery without pump oxygenator was selected for the surgical procedure.

CPT Code(s) Billed: 00566 P3

Rationale for Using Physical Status Modifier

Since the patient had progressive coronary artery disease, which is systemic, the term progressive supports the rationale for the severity. Physical status modifier P3 is appropriate to indicate a higher risk.

Example 2

A 90-year-old female with mild hypertension underwent anesthesia for a therapeutic bronchoscopy. An anesthesiologist administered the anesthesia, while the pulmonologist performed the bronchoscopy, removing a tumor from the right upper lobe.

CPT Code(s) Billed: 00520 P2

In addition to the physical status modifier a qualifying circumstances CPT code should be reported to identify that the patient is of extreme age. The appropriate coding should be reported as follows:

CPT Code(s) Billed: 00520 P2, 99100

Rationale for Using Modifier P2

P2 identifies anesthesia on a patient with mild systemic disease as indicated in the note (mild hypertension), and the add-on code 99100 identifies this patient is of extreme age, which according to CPT guidelines is either under 1 year old or over 70, which puts the patient at higher risk.

The qualifying circumstances CPT codes include the following codes, which are add-on codes reported in addition to the anesthesia code for the primary procedure and if the circumstance warrants additional information to support the procedure or service:

+99100   Anesthesia for patient of extreme age, under 1 year and over 70 (List separately in addition to code for primary anesthesia procedure)

+99116   Anesthesia complicated by utilization of total body hypothermia (List separately in addition to code for primary anesthesia procedure)

+99135   Anesthesia complicated by utilization of controlled hypotension (List separately in addition to code for primary anesthesia procedure)

+99140   Anesthesia complicated by emergency conditions (specify) (List separately in addition to code for primary anesthesia procedure)

An emergency is defined as existing when delay in treatment of the patient would lead to a significant increase in the threat to life or body part.

Review of the Physical Status Modifier

1   Modifiers P1 through P6 should not be used with CMS claims. CMS does not recognize physical status modifiers.

2   Many third-party insurance carriers recognize the use of physical status modifiers P3 through P6 and will increase payment for procedures provided.

3   Physical status modifiers are appended to the anesthesia procedure code only.

4   Physical status modifiers are located in the Anesthesia guidelines in the CPT book.

Modifier 24: Unrelated Evaluation and Management Service by the Same Physician During a Postoperative Period

Definition

The physician may need to indicate that an E/M service was performed during a postoperative period for a reason(s) unrelated to the original procedure. This circumstance may be reported by adding the modifier 24 to the appropriate level of E/M service.

AMA Guidelines

Modifier 24 was added to the CPT code set nomenclature in 1992. This modifier is used to indicate an E/M service unrelated to the surgical procedure that was performed during a postoperative period. Modifier 24 is appropriate when a physician provides a surgical service related to one problem and, during the postoperative period or follow-up care for the surgery, provides an E/M service unrelated to the problem requiring the surgery. The diagnosis code selection is critical when indicating the reason for the additional E/M service.

This modifier is only used with E/M services in the CPT book. It is not used in any other section of the CPT book. This modifier will not change the reimbursement (increase or decrease), but it will get the claim paid in most cases without a denial.

The key with using modifier 24 is that the same physician is providing an E/M service that is during the postoperative period (which can be 10 to 90 days). During that period of time all E/M services for typical postoperative follow-up care, including hospital visits, office or any other E/M service, are included in the postoperative care for the particular problem that was an initial indication for the surgery.

Insurance carriers have edit tools in their computer systems that often will automatically deny a claim for an E/M service if the claim is submitted by the

CMS CODING TIP

Modifier 24 is intended for use with services that are unrelated to the surgery. It is not to be used for the medical management of a patient by the surgeon after surgery. A different diagnosis is typically required.

THIRD-PARTY PAYER CODING TIP

For surgical procedures that have "0" global days, modifier 24 is not to be used.

same provider during the postoperative period. However, when a patient has a problem that is treated by the physician who performed the surgery, and a different reason or diagnosis is evident, it is appropriate to report the E/M service with modifier 24 to report the performance of the unrelated service. Appending modifier 24 will allow the carrier to pay the claim appropriately.

CMS Guidelines

The Medicare Carrier's Manual (MCM 4822 and 4824) indicates that an E/M service(s) submitted with modifier 24 must be sufficiently documented to establish that the visit was unrelated to the surgery. The diagnosis must support that the claim is unrelated to the initial procedure.

For 99291 or 99292 (critical care) to be paid for services furnished during the preoperative or postoperative period, with modifier 24, documentation must be submitted to support that the critical care was unrelated to the specific anatomic injury or general surgical procedure performed. An ICD-9-CM code in the range 800.0 through 959.9 (except 930-939), which clearly indicates that the critical care was unrelated to the surgery, is acceptable documentation.

Modifier 24 is recognized for an unrelated E/M service during the postoperative period unless:

- The care is for immunotherapy management furnished by the transplant surgeon
- The care is for critical care for a burn or trauma patient
- The documentation demonstrates that the visit occurred during a subsequent hospitalization and the diagnosis supports the fact that it is unrelated to the original surgery

Third-Party Payer Guidelines

Many times, the insurance carriers will request documentation when modifier 24 is used. If documentation is requested, the physician must indicate that the reason was unrelated to the original procedure. If documentation is not submitted with the initial claim, the insurance carrier can suspend (hold) the claim until the supporting documentation is received.[5]

Example 1

A patient had a cholecystectomy and returned to the general surgeon for his 2-week follow-up visit. At that time, the patient complained of a sore throat and throbbing headache. Examination showed a streptococcal throat infection, which was unrelated to the postoperative follow-up, and the physician prescribed medication for the infection in addition to the routine postoperative evaluation.

---

5. Source: Cigna Health; Anthem Blue Cross/Blue Shield.

CPT Code(s) Billed: 99212 24—Office or other outpatient visit for the evaluation and management of an established patient, which requires at least two of these three key components: a problem-focused history; a problem-focused examination; straightforward medical decision making.

Rationale for Using Modifier 24

The streptococcal throat infection was unrelated to the cholecystectomy, and the claim would be submitted with a different diagnosis.

Example 2

A 65-year-old diabetic man who was pacemaker dependent was noted to have episodic failure of the pacemaker. Noninvasive telemetry was performed and a low impedance was detected. The patient was taken to the catheterization laboratory after receiving mild sedation. A temporary transvenous pacemaker was inserted through the contralateral internal jugular vein and its pacing parameters were tested. The original pacemaker site was prepared and, under local anesthesia, the pacemaker and lead were carefully dissected free of scar tissue. The lead was disconnected from the pacemaker and visually inspected. Its electrical integrity was evaluated with a pacing system analyzer. A focal defect in external insulation was noted and repaired with a piece of tubular insulation, adhesive, and suture material. The electrical integrity was confirmed by means of the pacing system analyzer. The temporary lead was withdrawn and the pacemaker and repaired lead were carefully reinserted into the pocket, which was closed in layers. The entire procedure was performed with automated cuff blood pressure, pulse oximeter, and electrocardiogram monitoring.

The patient returned 4 weeks later for routine follow-up with complaints of lethargy and weakness. His blood glucose level had been ranging between 280 and 350 mg/dL for the past week. The physician performed an expanded problem-focused examination and determined that the patient's insulin dosage needed to be adjusted in addition to counseling on diet and exercise.

Routine follow-up for the pacemaker was also performed.

CPT Code(s) Billed: 99213 24—Office or other outpatient visit for the evaluation and management of an established patient, which requires at least two of these three key components: an expanded problem-focused history; an expanded problem-focused examination; medical decision making of low complexity.

Rationale for Using Modifier 24

The patient was returning to the cardiologist for a recheck on the pacemaker and indicated that other health problems existed unrelated to the surgical procedure. The physician performed an E/M service to address these unrelated problems. Many carriers append a 90-day global period for a pacemaker insertion.

Example 3

A patient underwent a pericardiotomy for removal of a clot and returned 6 weeks later for a surgical follow-up visit to the cardiovascular surgeon. The patient was feeling fatigued and lethargic and had a migraine-type headache. After a detailed history and examination was performed, the physician determined that the patient's blood pressure was exceptionally higher than normal and adjusted the patient's medication. The physician asked that the patient keep a record of the blood pressure reading for the next 3 days and contact the office daily with the results.

CPT Code(s) Billed: 99214 24—Office or other outpatient visit for the evaluation and management of an established patient, which requires at least two of these three key components: a detailed history; a detailed examination; medical decision making of moderate complexity.

Rationale for Using Modifier 24

Since the increased blood pressure did not appear to be related to the surgery, and the physician felt it necessary to perform a detailed history and examination to determine the problem, modifier 24 would be appropriate as long as there was evidence in the documentation and/or diagnosis to support that the encounter was unrelated to the surgery. This surgery typically carries a 90-day global period with many insurance carriers.

Example 4

An established patient who underwent an anterior cruciate ligament reconstruction on the right knee 4 weeks prior visited the orthopedic surgeon complaining of pain in the left knee. He indicated the right knee was healing well and he was doing well since starting physical therapy. After an expanded problem-focused history and examination, the physician diagnosed the patient with fluid on the left knee and recommended an anti-inflammatory drug to see if it would help. The physician discussed arthrocentesis with the patient and suggested if the patient's left knee was not better in 3 weeks, it would be wise to move forward with the procedure. The complexity of the decision making was moderate.

CPT Code(s) Billed: 99213 24—Office or other outpatient visit for the evaluation and management of an established patient, which requires at least two of these three key components: an expanded problem focused history; an expanded problem focused examination; medical decision making of low complexity.

Rationale for Using Modifier 24

The procedure initially performed, 29887, has a 90-day global period. The use of modifier 24 appended to the evaluation and management service, along with the appropriate diagnosis, will justify how the evaluation and management service is not related to the procedure on the right knee.

Test Your Knowledge

True or False

1 _____ Modifier 24 is used in Evaluation and Management, Surgery, and Anesthesia.

2 _____ When a claim is submitted with modifier 22, the carrier often will require the documentation to support the additional work.

3 _____ The definition of modifier 23 is prolonged services.

4 _____ When billing with modifier 24, the service must be related to the E/M service.

5 _____ Modifier 21 does not affect payment.

6 _____ Physical status modifiers are used to indicate unusual procedures.

7 _____ Modifier 24 can be used when visiting the patient after surgery in the hospital.

8 _____ Modifier 21 can be used on all sections of the CPT book.

9 _____ Modifier 23 is used for anesthesia services normally performed under local or regional anesthesia and when general anesthesia is necessary.

10 _____ The meaning of modifier 22 is that the procedure and/or service is greater than is usually required for the procedure.

Select the Appropriate Modifier for Each Case Scenario

11 _____ A patient presented during the postoperative period with pain in the upper arm because of a fall. The patient was visiting the orthopedic surgeon 10 days after a meniscectomy with ligament repair of the right knee. The carrier's global period for this procedure is 60 days. The physician examined the patient's arm and determined that it was sprained, prescribed pain medication, and put the arm in a sling. During the visit, the physician examined the patient's right knee and determined that it was healing nicely and it was time for the patient to begin physical therapy.

12 _____ A 58-year-old man with prostatic carcinoma was scheduled for a radical prostatectomy under general anesthesia. Blood loss was estimated to be 1500 to 2500 mL, and patient donated 2 units of autologous blood.

13 _____ A 27-year-old male victim of a drug-related shooting presented to the emergency department with a low-velocity handgun wound to the left side of the neck in zone II. The patient was neurologically and hemodynamically stable with a moderate

hematoma over the left midneck area, which was nonexpanding and pulsatile. Anterior and lateral neck X rays showed the bullet to be embedded in the vertebral body. The patient was given antibiotics and taken to the operating room, where he was electively intubated and prepared for neck exploration. The neck was explored through a left sternomastoid incision along the sternocleidomastoid muscle. The carotid sheath was opened, and the internal jugular and common carotid arteries were uninjured. The phrenic nerve was identified and was intact. There were several bleeding muscular branches, which were coagulated. The esophagus and trachea were then mobilized. There was no evidence of trauma to the laryngotracheal area of the esophagus. The bullet track appeared to traverse posterior to the esophagus into the vertebral body. There was a massive amount of hemorrhage from the area, which took an additional 1 hour and 40 minutes to control. The left lateral portion of the thyroid gland was exposed and found to be uninjured. The left superior laryngeal nerve appeared to be intact. The wound was irrigated, closed suction drains were placed and brought out interiorly and laterally to the skin, and the fascia over the sternocleidomastoid was closed with interrupted 2-0 polyglactin sutures. Skin staples were applied, and the procedure was terminated.

14 _____ A 78-year-old woman with left-lower-lobe pneumonia and a history of coronary artery disease, congestive heart failure, osteoarthritis, and gout had undergone CABG 10 days earlier. The patient was admitted to the hospital by the surgeon because she was experiencing a high fever with an altered state of consciousness, which was unrelated to the procedure. The global period indicated by the insurance company was 90 days.

15 _____ A 30-year-old male, established patient was seen in the office because of a 3-month history of fatigue, weight loss, and intermittent fever and presented with diffuse adenopathy and splenomegaly. Comprehensive history included complaints and possible exposure such as sexual, travels abroad, etc. A comprehensive examination was performed, which includes lymphatic and abdominal examination. Medical decision making of high complexity included discussion of possible diagnosis, possible diagnostic tests needed, and importance of follow-up. The physician spent an additional 40 minutes discussing the importance of the patient's taking oral medications for his diabetes and monitoring his blood pressure regularly, as it has been running extremely high.

CHAPTER 3

Modifiers 25 to 47

Modifier 25: Significant, Separately Identifiable Evaluation and Management Service by the Same Physician on the Same Day of the Procedure or Other Service

Definition (Revised, 2006)

The physician may need to indicate that on the day a procedure or service identified by a CPT code was performed, the patient's condition required a significant, separately identifiable evaluation and management (E/M) service above and beyond the other service provided or beyond the usual preoperative and postoperative care associated with the procedure that was performed. A significant, separately identifiable E/M service is defined or substantiated by documentation that satisfies the relevant criteria for the respective E/M service to be reported (see **Evaluation and Management Services Guidelines** for instructions on determining level of E/M service). The E/M service may be prompted by the symptom or condition for which the procedure and/or service was provided. As such, different diagnoses are not required for reporting of the E/M service. **Note:** This modifier is not used to report an E/M service that resulted in a decision to perform surgery (see modifier 57).

AMA Guidelines

cpt Modifier 25 is used to indicate that a significant, separately identifiable E/M service was performed by the same physician on the day of a procedure. The CPT® guidelines do not require different diagnoses for an E/M service and the procedure or service performed to be reported separately. The E/M service must meet the key components (ie, history, examination, medical decision making) of that E/M service including medical record documentation. New language was added in 2006 that states: "A significant, separately identifiable E/M service is defined or substantiated by documentation that satisfies the relevant criteria for the respective E/M service to be reported (see Evaluation and Management Services Guidelines for instructions on determining level of E/M service)."

Modifier 25 is critical to appropriate communication about what happened in a patient encounter on a given date. The appropriate use of this modifier, by physicians and payers alike, will enable accurate identification of distinct services and aid information collection and accurate and timely payments.

Modifier 25 was added to the CPT code set nomenclature in 1992 to help the Centers for Medicare and Medicaid Services (CMS) implement a national payment policy and to help reduce the documentation burden on physicians. The American Medical Association (AMA) further revised modifier 25 in 1999 to indicate that it is not necessary to have a diagnosis for the E/M service described that is different from the procedure and/or other service provided. The same diagnosis may accurately describe the nature or reason for the encounter and the procedure. The revision in 1999 helps to identify an E/M service that goes "above and beyond" the other service provided or beyond the usual preoperative and postoperative care associated with the procedure performed.

To use modifier 25 correctly, the chosen level of E/M service needs to be supported by adequate documentation for the appropriate level of service, as well as referenced by a diagnosis code. The E/M service can occur at the same visit when a surgical procedure is performed. Modifier 25 is not restricted to any particular level of E/M service. For example, modifier 21 is used only with the highest level of E/M code. Because of differences in payment policies, some payers do not recognize the modifier 25.

From a coding perspective, it is essential that the appropriate modifiers be used to describe the services provided. The CPT codes for procedures do include the evaluation services necessary before the performance of the procedure (eg, assessing the site and condition of the problem area, explaining the procedure, obtaining informed consent); however, when significant and identifiable (ie, key components or counseling) E/M services are performed, these services are not included in the descriptor for the procedure or service performed. It is important to note that the diagnosis reported with both the procedure or service and E/M service need ***not*** be different, if the same diagnosis accurately describes the reasons for the encounter and the procedure.

CMS Guidelines

CMS recognizes the use of modifier 25 with E/M services within the range of CPT codes 99201-99499, 92002-92014, and Health Care Common Procedure Coding System (HCPCS) level II codes G0101-G0175.

CMS Guidelines for the Appropriate Use of Modifier 25

Modifier 25 should be used only when a significant, separately identifiable E/M visit is rendered on the same day as a minor surgical procedure. Payment for preoperative and postoperative visits is included in the payment for the procedure. For minor procedures where the decision to perform the procedure is typically made immediately before the service (eg, whether sutures are needed to close a wound, whether to remove a mole or wart), the E/M visit is considered to be a routine preoperative service and should not be billed in addition to the minor procedure.

The policy applies only to minor surgeries and endoscopies for which a global period of 0 to 10 days applies.

What does significant, separately identifiable mean to CMS? The patient's medical record documentation is expected to be clearly evident that the E/M service performed and billed was "above and beyond" the usual preoperative and postoperative care associated with the procedure performed on the same day. The need to perform an independent evaluation and management service may be prompted by a symptom, complaint, condition, problem, or circumstance that may or may not be related to the procedure or other service. Different diagnoses are not required for reporting purposes. The record, however, should document an important, notable, distinct correlation with signs and symptoms to make a diagnostic classification or demonstrate a distinct problem.

For example, a pulmonologist examines a new patient on Tuesday and schedules a bronchoscopy for Thursday of that week. The physician will bill an

E/M service on Tuesday, documenting the key components (history, examination, medical decision making) without modifier 25. The sole purpose of the patient encounter on Thursday is the bronchoscopy, and since the physician already evaluated the patient on Tuesday and surgery was indicated, only the bronchoscopy will be billed on Thursday.

If the global period concept does not apply to the minor surgery or procedure, separate payment is made for the service and visit on the same day. In circumstances where the physician provides an E/M service that is beyond the usual preoperative and postoperative work for the service, the visit may be billed with a modifier 25 (eg, examination performed before suturing a forehead laceration to assess the patient's condition). A modifier is not necessary if the visit was performed the day before a minor surgery because the global period for minor procedures does not include the day before the surgery.

The global surgery periods are 0, 10, and 90 days for CMS and many other third-party payers. Review Table 3-1.

TABLE 3-1 **CMS Global Surgical Days**	
Global Period	**Definition**
000	Endoscopic and minor surgeries with related preoperative and postoperative relative values on the day of the procedure only included in the fee schedule payment amount. Evaluation and management services on the day of the procedure generally are not payable. **Preoperative:** E/M services are not payable on the same day as the surgery. **Postoperative:** E/M services are payable on the day following surgery.
010	Minor surgical procedure with preoperative relative values on the day of the procedure and a postoperative relative value during a 10-day postoperative period is included in the fee schedule amount. E/M services on the day of the procedure during this 10-day postoperative period generally are not payable. **Preoperative:** E/M services are not payable on the same day as the surgery. **Postoperative:** E/M services are not payable up to 10 days after the surgery unless the E/M service is unrelated to the original procedure (modifier 24).
090	Major surgical procedure with a 90-day postoperative period is included in the fee schedule amount. **Preoperative:** E/M services are not payable 1 day prior to and on the same day as the surgery. **Postoperative:** E/M services are not payable up to 90 days following the surgery unless the E/M service is unrelated to the original procedure (modifier 24).

The Medicare Fee Schedule Database (MFSDB) provides postoperative periods that apply for surgical procedures. The CMS rules for surgical global days include:

1 Codes with "090" days are major surgical procedures.

2 Codes with "000" or "010" are endoscopies or minor surgical procedures.

3 Codes with "ZZZ" are add-on codes always reported with another procedure or service.

CMS Rules: Minor Surgeries and Endoscopies

E/M visits by the same physician on the same day as a minor surgery or endoscopy are included in the payment for the procedure, unless a significant, separately identifiable service is also performed. An example of this would be a physician performing a full neurological exam on a patient who had been in a car accident and suturing a wound of the scalp from the patient hitting the windshield.

Billing for an E/M visit would not be considered if the physician only identified the need for sutures and confirmed allergy and immunization status. The confirmation of the allergy and immunization status would be incidental and would not support an E/M service with the procedure, since the status is only mentioned and the patient is not being treated for the condition at the visit.

What does this mean? The key is recognizing when the extra work is "significant." One way to determine if the work goes beyond the usual pre- and postoperative work is to ask the following questions:

1 Does the complaint or problem stand alone as a billable service?

2 Did the physician perform and document the key components of an E/M service for the complaint or problem?

3 Is there a different diagnosis for a significant portion of the visit? Or if the diagnosis is the same, was extra work that went above and beyond the usual pre- and postoperative work associated with the procedure code?

If the answer to all of the questions is yes, it may be possible to report the appropriate E/M service based on documented key components with a minor surgical procedure, or in the instance of split care (preventive and problematic E/M services), on the same day.

Third-Party Payer Guidelines

Unfortunately, not all third-party payers recognize the use of modifier 25. Some insurance carriers "rebundle" the E/M service into the other procedure and/or service on the same day. The AMA, as one of its priorities, encourages consistency in the use of CPT codes, guidelines, and conventions, as well as advocating the adoption of these standards. Acceptance of the CPT code set, guidelines, and conventions does not imply standardized payment for documented and reported services. CPT coding guidelines only aid the users in applying CPT codes correctly and do not dictate the circumstances for payment and the amount of payment.

Many third-party payers deny modifier 25 on the same day as another procedure and/or service for the purpose of bundling. Examples include:

- Preventive medicine services with problem-oriented E/M services
- Surgical services such as removal of a foreign body with an E/M service
- Destruction of benign or premalignant lesions with an E/M service
- Diagnostic services such as an endoscopy or colonoscopy with an E/M service

It is recommended that the person coding the claim know the payer rules for the use of modifier 25. Some insurance carriers also fail to recognize the additional physician and nonphysician professional work involved with providing multiple services on the same date. Instead of rewarding the practitioner for providing the necessary patient care efficiently and consistently with current medical guidelines and standards at the same visit, some insurance carriers penalize the practitioner. To have the patient come back for a subsequent visit for necessary care, when the treatment could have been provided at the original visit, jeopardizes quality patient care and safety and threatens the patient-physician relationship.

According to the most recent AMA survey of health plans and other payers on acceptance of CPT modifiers, more than 80% of the respondents using the resource-based relative value system payment method reported the acceptance of modifier 25.

As the only national health insurance program, CMS has the ability of instituting national payment policies and geographically adjusted reimbursement levels. Even though the AMA was successful in having CPT designated as the national standard code set under HIPAA, CPT guidelines were not named as a national standard for implementing CPT. Naming CPT guidelines as a national standard would have helped to resolve issues of ignoring modifiers by bundling.

Even if the CPT guidelines related to modifiers were accepted by all payers, it is likely that payment policies regarding bundling, reduced reimbursement, and various payment amounts would still exist. All payers are free to set payment policy and payment rates. Only CMS currently is relatively standard in terms of its interpretation of CPT modifiers with reimbursement.

Modifier 25 and the Preventive Medicine Codes

When a significant problem is encountered while a preventive medicine E/M service is performed, requiring additional work to perform the key components of an E/M service, the appropriate office outpatient code also should be

> **THIRD-PARTY PAYER CODING TIP**
>
> Some third-party payers will not pay for an E/M service on the same day as a procedure and/or service deemed "minor" by the carrier.

reported for that service, with modifier 25 appended. Modifier 25 allows for separate payment for these visits without requiring documentation when the claim is submitted. However, insurance carrier interpretations vary on the use of this modifier and the requirements for documentation.

Modifier 25 and Critical Care Services

The CPT surgical package includes typical postoperative care. Critical care services are not typical postoperative care, and the services can be used postoperatively if illness or injury and the treatment being provided meet the critical care requirements as stated in the CPT Critical Care Services guidelines.

Critical Care and CMS[1]

Preoperative and postoperative critical care may be paid in addition to a global fee if the patient is critically ill and requires the constant attendance of the physician, and the critical care is unrelated to the specific anatomic injury or general surgical procedure performed. Such patients are potentially unstable or have conditions that could pose a significant threat to life or of prolonged impairment.

In order for these services to be paid for CMS, two reporting requirements must be met. Codes 99291 and 99292, and modifier 25 (preoperative) or modifier 24 (postoperative) must be used, and documentation that the critical care was unrelated to the specific anatomic injury or general surgical procedure performed must be submitted. An ICD-9-CM code in the range of 800.0 through 959.9 (except 930-939), which clearly indicates that the critical care was unrelated to the surgery, is acceptable documentation.

Example 1

A 65-year-old patient was admitted to the hospital in the morning for chest pains and shortness of breath. The physician performed and documented a comprehensive history and examination with moderately complex decision making. The patient had a history of heart disease, and her last myocardial infarction was 6 months prior. The patient's physician was called to the hospital in the evening because the patient had just suffered another myocardial infarction. The patient was transferred to the critical care unit where the physician spent 1 hour and 45 minutes stabilizing her after the heart attack. It was expected the patient would remain critical for several days due to her history.

1. Source: Medicare Carrier's Manual, available at www.cms.hhs.gov/physicians.

In this example, the patient was admitted in the morning and the heart attack occurred in the evening. Since the diagnosis for the morning admission would be chest pain and shortness of breath with the history of a past MI, an E/M service for the admission would be appropriate. However, since the patient's condition changed significantly in the evening and resulted in the myocardial infarction, it also would be appropriate to report critical care services with modifier 25.

> *CPT Code(s) Billed:* *99222 25—Initial hospital care, per day, for the evaluation and management of a patient, which requires these three key components: a comprehensive history; a comprehensive examination; and medical decision making of moderate complexity.*
>
> *99291—Critical care, evaluation and management of the critically ill or critically injured patient; first 30-74 minutes*
>
> *99292 × 2—each additional 30 minutes*

24.	A DATE(S) OF SERVICE From MM DD YY	To MM DD YY	B Place of Service	C Type of Service	D PROCEDURES, SERVICES, OR SUPPLIES (Explain Unusual Circumstances) CPT/HCPCS | MODIFIER	E DIAGNOSIS CODE	F $ CHARGES	G DAYS OR UNITS	H EPSDT Family Plan	I EMG	J COB	K RESERVED FOR LOCAL USE
1					99222 | 25							
2					99291 |							
3					99292 |			2				
4												
5												
6												

25. FEDERAL TAX I.D. NUMBER SSN EIN	26. PATIENT'S ACCOUNT NO.	27. ACCEPT ASSIGNMENT? (For govt. claims, see back) YES NO	28. TOTAL CHARGE $	29. AMOUNT PAID $	30. BALANCE DUE $

General-Use Guidelines for Modifier 25

Modifier 25 should be used with E/M codes only and not appended to the surgical procedure code(s). The global surgery policy does not apply to services of other physicians who may be rendering services during the preoperative or postoperative period unless the physician is a member of the same group and/or same specialty as the operating physician.

- A good standard for determining whether modifier 25 should be used is this: If documentation in the patient's clinical record shows that extra preoperative and/or postoperative work beyond what is usually performed with that service was done, then it is proper to use modifier 25 to indicate that extra work.

- To document the extra work performed, the clinical record should clearly indicate that extra or unusual work.
- The physician must determine whether the E/M service being billed is distinct from the surgical service.

Example 2

A 30-year-old established patient saw her gynecologist for her annual well-woman examination. The physician performed and documented a comprehensive review of systems along with an interval past medical, family, and social history. A comprehensive GU examination was performed and a Pap smear was obtained. Counseling on diet, exercise, and prevention was provided, and appropriate labs were ordered. During the encounter, the patient asked for renewal of her allergy medication.

The services for this patient would only be considered preventive.

CPT Codes(s) Billed: *99395—Periodic comprehensive preventive medicine reevaluation and management of an individual including an age and gender appropriate history, examination, counseling/anticipatory guidance/risk factor reduction interventions, and the ordering of appropriate immunization(s), laboratory/diagnostic procedures, established patient; 18-39 years*

Rationale for Not Using Modifier 25

Since the request for allergy medication is considered "incidental" to the visit, and the key components of a problem-oriented E/M service were not performed, a problematic E/M service would not be warranted.

Example 3

A 45-year-old male patient visited his family physician for his annual visit. The physician performed and documented a comprehensive review of systems along with an interval medical, family, and social history. A comprehensive multi-system examination is performed. Counseling on diet, exercise, and prevention is provided along with appropriate labs ordered. During the encounter the patient complained of bilateral knee pain with tenderness and swelling. The physician discovered during the exam that both knees were swollen. The patient was given a nonsteroidal anti-inflammatory drug prescription and was asked to follow up in 2 weeks.

CPT Codes(s) Billed: 99396—Periodic comprehensive preventive medicine reevaluation and management of an individual including an age and gender appropriate history, examination, counseling/anticipatory guidance/risk factor reduction interventions, and the ordering of appropriate immunization(s), laboratory/diagnostic procedures, established patient; 40–64 years

99212 25—Office or other outpatient visit for the evaluation and management of an established patient, which requires at least two of these three key components: a problem focused history; a problem focused examination; straightforward medical decision making.

Rationale for Using Modifier 25

Because the extra physician work is significant and the physician spent more time obtaining a history and examining a problem-focused area, and providing straightforward medical decision making for the knee problem, it would be appropriate to provide split care (preventive and problem-oriented) at the same visit. Both the preventive and problem-oriented E/M codes could be reported with modifier 25 appended. The extent of the problem-oriented E/M service is based on the amount of additional work the physician provides along with the systems examined. Because the patient encounter was focused on one body system and key components of a problem-oriented E/M service were performed, a problem-focused E/M service would be appropriate. The diagnosis code for the knee pain would be linked to the problem-oriented visit with a "V" code for the preventive visit to support the services billed.

Considerations When Deciding to Use Modifier 25

The phrase "the patient's condition required" is extremely important. This gives the insurance carrier information that it was medically necessary for the patient to have the service on the same day that another procedure or service was performed. In addition, the phrase "a significant, separately identifiable E/M service above and beyond" the other service provided indicates that the additional service was clearly different from the other procedure or service that was performed.

Example 4

An established patient presented to his family physician's office with a 2.0-cm laceration of the right index finger. After the physician sutured the finger, the patient asked the physician to evaluate swelling of the left leg and ankle. An expanded problem-focused history and physical examination with low medical decision making were performed for this problem.

CPT Code(s) Billed: *12001—Simple repair of superficial wounds of scalp, neck, axillae, external genitalia, trunk and/or extremities (including hands and feet); 2.5 cm or less*

99213 25—Office or other outpatient visit for the evaluation and management of an established patient, which requires at least two of these three key components: an expanded problem-focused history; an expanded problem-focused examination; medical decision making of low complexity

Diagnosis Code(s): *719.07—Effusion of joint*

883.0—Open wound of finger(s) without mention of complication

Rationale for Using Modifier 25

Since the patient presented to the physician with two problems that were separately identifiable and significant, the swelling of the left leg and ankle and a laceration, a surgical procedure and a separate E/M service were performed and documented indicating both problems. The evaluation of the laceration is considered inclusive or part of the preoperative evaluation and is included in the surgical procedure code 12001. The appropriate diagnosis code would be appended to both encounters. The diagnosis code for the open wound can be appended to the E/M code when the claim is submitted.

Example 5

An established patient sustained a severe laceration to the scalp. The physician performed a comprehensive history and examination to determine whether the patient sustained neurological damage before suturing the laceration. The physician performed and documented a 3.0-cm intermediate repair to the scalp.

CPT Code(s) Billed: *99215 25—Office or other outpatient visit for the evaluation and management of an established patient, which requires at least two of these three key components: a comprehensive history;*

a comprehensive examination; medical decision making of high complexity.

12032—Layer closure of wounds of scalp, axillae, trunk and/or extremities (excluding hands and feet); 2.6 cm to 7.5 cm

Diagnosis Code(s):   873.0—Open wound of scalp, without mention of complication

Rationale for Using Modifier 25

The exam is not considered to be a routine preoperative service, and a visit can be billed in addition to the closure of the laceration. The reason for this is that the physician had to evaluate the patient for other injuries and/or complication of the patient's injury. Modifier 25 must be added to the E/M service to report both services. The diagnosis is the same with both services because there was no indication in the documentation that the physician found any other injuries or conditions related to the laceration, but because the evaluation went beyond the usual preoperative workup, it is appropriate to report an E/M service with modifier 25.

Example 6

A 75-year-old man with benign hypertension had recurrent nasal bleeding. He had significant blood loss and was bleeding out of both nostrils and the mouth. He had a complex anterior pack placed (30906) and was still bleeding. The patient's previous pack was removed, and a pack was placed in both the nasopharynx and nasal cavity. The patient required both anterior and posterior packing. The patient also complained of painful respirations and mild fatigue, and was on a β-blocker/thiazide regimen. An expanded problem-focused history including compliance, diet, and stress issues was documented. An expanded problem-focused exam including vital signs, chest and heart exam, and check for edema was performed. Medical decision making of moderate complexity, including counseling about medication and alternatives, a plan for appropriate lab work, and a review of possible medication side effects, was documented.

CPT Code(s) Billed: 30906—Control nasal hemorrhage, posterior, with posterior nasal packs and/or cautery, any method; subsequent

99213 25—Office or other outpatient visit for the evaluation and management of an established patient, which requires at least two of these three key components: an expanded problem-focused history; an expanded problem-focused examination; medical decision making of low complexity.

Diagnosis Code(s):   786.52—Painful respiration

780.79—Other malaise and fatigue

401.1—Essential hypertension, benign

784.7—Epistaxis

Rationale for Using Modifier 25

The evaluation of the patient for hypertension along with other signs and symptoms was a medically necessary, significant, and separately identifiable service performed on the same day as control of the nosebleed. The hypertension was exacerbating the nosebleed and could be related to the epistaxis, but management of the hypertension was a separate service from actually packing the nose. The diagnosis code for the treatment of the nasal hemorrhage (30906) would be appended with diagnosis code 784.7 (epitaxis), which clearly identifies the service as significant from the E/M service.

Example 7

A patient with an acute exacerbation of extrinsic asthma went to the emergency department. The physician performed a detailed history and examination, and decided that the patient needed a nebulizer treatment after reviewing the patient's medical history and treatment options. The treatment was performed by the physician, and the patient was stabilized and released from the emergency department several hours later.

CPT Code(s) Billed: *99284 25—Emergency department visit for the evaluation and management of a patient, which requires these three key components: a detailed history; a detailed examination; and medical decision making of moderate complexity*

94640—Pressurized or nonpressurized inhalation treatment for acute airway obstruction or for sputum induction for diagnostic purposes (eg, with an aerosol generator, nebulizer, metered dose inhaler or intermittent positive pressure breathing (IPPB) device)

Diagnosis Code(s): *493.02—Extrinsic asthma, with (acute) exacerbation*

Rationale for Using Modifier 25

Using modifier 25 lets the insurance carrier know that the physician performed both an E/M service and a procedure on the same day. The reason for billing both the E/M service and the procedure is that the physician had to evaluate the patient before making a decision regarding treatment options, which involved significantly more work to identify the problem and to formulate a treatment plan.

Example 8

Improper Use of Modifier 25

A 66-year-old woman presented with complaints of growing skin lesions on her neck and axillary areas. She had a family history of similar lesions. The tags on her neck were irritated by her collars and caught in her necklaces, and the tags in the axillae itched in warm weather and with exercise. On examination, there were 12 pedunculated papules on the sides of the neck, 3 to 5 mm, and 11 tags, 2 to 6 mm, in the axillary areas, all typical of skin tags. Because the tags were symptomatic, removal was recommended. The procedure was described and informed consent was obtained. After the area was cleansed with alcohol, each tag was anesthetized with 1% lidocaine. The bases of the tags were electrodessicated and the larger tags were removed by scissors excision. Aluminum chloride was applied topically as needed for hemostasis. The larger sites were covered with topical bacitracin zinc/polymyxin B and bandages.

CPT Code(s) Billed: *99212 25—Office or other outpatient visit for the evaluation and management of an established patient, which requires at least two of these three key components: a problem-focused history; a problem-focused examination; straightforward medical decision making*

11200—Removal of skin tags, multiple fibrocutaneous tags, any area; up to and including 15 lesions

11201—Removal of skin tags, multiple fibrocutaneous tags, any area; each additional ten lesions (list separately in addition to code for primary procedure)

Diagnosis Code(s): *701.9—Unspecified hypertrophic and atrophic condition of skin*

Correct Reporting: ***11200—Removal of skin tags, multiple fibrocutaneous tags, any area; up to and including 15 lesions***

11201—Removal of skin tags, multiple fibrocutaneous tags, any area; each additional ten lesions (list separately in addition to code for primary procedure)

Diagnosis Code(s): ***701.9—Unspecified hypertrophic and atrophic condition of skin***

Rationale for Improper Use of Modifier 25

Even though it could be argued that an evaluation of the problem was necessary to perform the skin tag removal, many payers consider the office visit as part of the preoperative workup for the surgical service, and therefore it is not separately

AMA CODING TIP

Modifier 25 is not meant to be used with E/M services associated with procedures, only for E/M services above and beyond the usual preoperative and postoperative care associated with the procedure performed. If the intraoperative portion of a procedure is unusually prolonged or difficult and involves an unusual amount of intraoperative work, then modifier 22 should be used with the pertinent procedure code.

CMS CODING TIP

Medicare will not reimburse separately for providing an initial hospital service (99221-99223) that prompted the physician to perform the procedure.

reimbursable. The use of modifier 25 is inappropriate because the E/M service did not go beyond the usual preoperative service.

Insurance carrier standards have been in place since modifier 25 was created. While it has been rare in the industry that this modifier is reviewed before payment is made, the practice is becoming more and more common. Payers who are not reviewing on a prepayment basis may audit on a postpayment basis (eg, Medicare). The Office of the Inspector General has even targeted this modifier for investigation of overuse and abuse in a special fraud alert.

Example 9

Improper Use of Modifier 25

Ms Smith scheduled an appointment to remove a lesion from her right leg. The physician looked at the lesion, which appeared benign, and infiltrated the lesion with 1% xylocaine. The lesion was removed and a simple closure was performed. The lesion measured 1.0 cm in diameter, including margins. The physician decided to send the specimen to pathology, and the report indicated the lesion was benign.

CPT Code(s) Billed: 99212 25—Office or other outpatient visit for the evaluation and management of an established patient, which requires at least two of these three key components: a problem-focused history; a problem-focused examination; straightforward medical decision making

11401—Excision, benign lesion including margins, except skin tag (unless listed elsewhere), trunk, arms or legs; excised diameter 0.6 to 1.0 cm

Rationale for Improper Use of Modifier 25

Since the patient's sole purpose of the visit was the lesion removal, and the examination was limited to looking at the lesion and deciding to remove it, an E/M service would not be appropriate. The evaluation prior to removing the lesion is considered part of the preoperative workup and is not significantly and separately identifiable.

The National Correct Coding Initiative and Modifier 25

The National Correct Coding Initiative (NCCI) was developed by CMS to promote national correct coding methodologies and to control improper coding that leads to inappropriate payment in Part B claims. The coding policies developed are based on coding conventions defined in the AMA's CPT book, national and local policies and edits, coding guidelines developed by national societies, analysis of standard medical and surgical practice, and review of current coding practice.

Modifier 25 may be appended to an E/M service code reported with another procedure on the same day of the service or procedure. When a provider performs a significant and separately identifiable E/M service beyond the usual preprocedure, intraprocedure, and postprocedure physician work, the E/M may be reported with modifier 25 appended. The E/M service and the procedure(s) may be related to the same diagnosis or different diagnoses. The NCCI edits are published quarterly; a subscription may be purchased from numerous vendors, or the edits may be accessed on the CMS Web site at www.cms.hhs.gov/physicians.

CMS also will not reimburse for an E/M service in addition to the procedure when the service results in the decision to perform a minor surgical procedure on the same date. CMS's definition of a minor surgical procedure is a procedure with a 10-day global period.

Procedures with a global surgical indicator of "XXX" are not covered by these rules. Many of the "XXX" procedures are performed by physicians and have inherent preprocedure, intraprocedure, and postprocedure work performed at the same time. This work should never be reported with a separate E/M code. However, according to NCCI, "with most 'XXX' procedures, the physician may, however, perform a significant and separately identifiable E/M service on the same day of service which may be reported by appending modifier 25 to the E/M code. The E/M service may be related to the same diagnosis necessitating performance of a procedure with an 'XXX,' but cannot include any of the work inherent to the 'XXX' procedure, supervision of others performing the procedure or time for interpreting the result of the 'XXX' procedure. Appending modifier 25 to a significant, separately identifiable E/M service when performed on the same date of an 'XXX' procedure is correct coding."

Example 10

A patient presented with complaints of left knee pain. The physician evaluated the knee and determined that the patient would benefit from arthrocentesis. The physician gave the patient an injection and scheduled a follow-up visit for 1 month.

In this example it would not be appropriate to bill the E/M service because the focus of the visit is related to the knee pain, which precipitated the arthrocentesis.

Correct Reporting: ***20610—Arthrocentesis, aspiration and/or injection; major joint or bursa (eg, shoulder, hip, knee joint, subacromial bursa)***

In the following example, it is appropriate to bill modifier 25 with an E/M service with the same problem addressed.

Example 11

An established patient visited her internist in follow-up for hypertension and diabetes. The patient also complained of left knee pain, which started to bother her while working in the garden. The physician performed a problem-focused history and examination, evaluated the patient's hypertension, determined that the blood pressure was higher than it should be, and adjusted medications. The patient's blood glucose level was normal and the diabetes was well controlled with the current insulin regimen. During the encounter, the physician also evaluated the knee and determined that the patient would benefit from arthrocentesis. The physician gave the patient an injection and scheduled a follow-up visit for 1 month.

CPT Code(s) Billed: *99212 25—Office or other outpatient visit for the evaluation and management of an established patient, which requires at least two of these three key components: a problem-focused history; a problem-focused examination; straightforward medical decision making*

20610—Arthrocentesis, aspiration and/or injection; major joint or bursa (eg, shoulder, hip, knee joint, subacromial bursa)

Correct Reporting: 99212 25, 20610

In the second encounter, the physician is evaluating the knee before performing the procedure (arthrocentesis), but is also evaluating other problems (hypertension and diabetes), and billing an office visit and procedure on the same day with a modifier 25 appended to the E/M service would be appropriate.

Split Billing with Modifier 25

Modifier 25 was revised in the 1995 CPT book to include use for symptoms that are encountered during a preventive medicine visit. Thus, if during a preventive medicine visit a significant amount of additional work is required of a physician to perform the key requirements of a problem-oriented E/M visit, the preventive medicine visit and appropriate office or outpatient "sick" visit are coded to indicate that a significant, separately identifiable E/M service was performed in addition to the preventive medicine visit. If the problem is not significant (does not require additional work), only the preventive medicine visit is coded (99381-99397). Many carriers, when two E/M service(s) are billed during the same patient encounter (well visit and problematic visit), will pay for no more than the preventive visit.

Example 12

If the preventive visit is $150 and the typical visit for a code 99201 is $65, the bill is split. To split the bill, many carriers require the physician to bill the problem visit at the normal fee and subtract the charge from the preventive fee.

| Typical Preventive Visit Charge for 99383 | $150.00 |
| Typical Visit Charge for 99201 | $ 65.00 |

Split Billing
Preventive Visit:	$ 85.00
Problem Visit:	$ 65.00
Total charge:	**$150.00**

Example 13

A 9-year-old boy presented for the first time to the office for health supervision and evaluation. His complete medical, family, social, religious, and cultural history was reviewed. A complete review of systems was done. A complete physical examination was performed. Speech and blood pressure were checked. Growth, development, and behavior were assessed. Immunizations were reviewed. Anticipatory guidance was given to the child regarding good health habits and self-care. Anticipatory guidance was given to the parents about good parenting practices. Risk factors were identified and interventions discussed. Medically appropriate lab tests were ordered. During the encounter, the patient's mother indicated that the patient was having respiratory difficulties, ear pain, fever, cough, and inability to sleep at night. A problem-focused history including labored breathing, characteristics of pain, and the respiratory system was completed. The problem-focused examination included ears, nose, throat, chest, and hydration status. Medical decision making was of low complexity, and the physician discussed tonsillectomy and adenoidectomy with the patient's mother, who indicated that the patient had had this problem five or six times since age 5 years. The diagnosis for the problematic visit was chronic tonsillitis and adenoiditis. Antibiotics were prescribed, and the patient was scheduled to return in 3 weeks for reevaluation.

Correct Reporting: *99383—Initial comprehensive preventive medicine evaluation and management of an individual including an age and gender appropriate history, examination, counseling/anticipatory guidance/ risk factor reduction interventions, and the ordering of appropriate immunization(s), laboratory/ diagnostic procedures, new patient; late childhood (age 5 through 11 years)*

99201 25—Office or other outpatient visit for the evaluation and management of a new patient, which requires these three key components: a problem-focused history; a problem-focused examination; and straightforward medical decision making

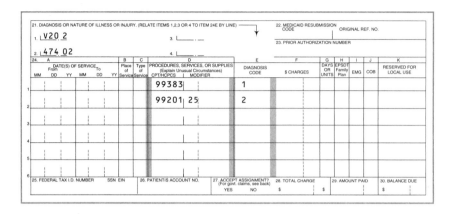

Two diagnoses are required to identify the preventive visit and the problem:

- V20.2 Routine infant or child health check
- 474.02 Chronic tonsillitis and adenoiditis

Rationale for Split Billing

Since both a preventive (routine well) visit and a significant problem were addressed, both can be separately identified according to the CPT guidelines. The guidelines state that preventive medicine E/M services can be reported with problem-oriented E/M services (99201-99215) if the abnormality encountered or the preexisting condition addressed during the preventive medicine examination requires significant additional work to perform key components of a problem-oriented E/M service. Modifier 25 is appended to the E/M code to indicate that a separately identifiable E/M service was provided.

Review of Modifier 25

1 Modifier 25 may be used with emergency department E/M services 99281-99285 when services lead to the decision to provide a diagnostic/therapeutic medical or surgical service on the same date.

2 Use modifier 25 only when the E/M service is significantly and separately identifiable from the procedure or other service performed on the same day. When the only service provided is the procedure, an E/M code with modifier 25 may not be appropriate.

3 Make sure the diagnosis code is correctly linked to the procedure and/or E/M service.

4 When billing preventive medicine services and problem-oriented E/M services on the same day with modifier 25, make sure that the problem is

significant and requires additional work to perform the key components of a problem-oriented E/M service.

5   When billing for osteopathic manipulative treatment, make sure that the E/M service can be identified on the same date as the treatment. Osteopathic manipulative treatment (98925-98929) services are considered to be procedures, so make sure the service goes above and beyond any preservice or postservice work associated with osteopathic manipulative treatment when provided.

6   When billing for chiropractic manipulative treatment, make sure that the E/M service can be identified on the same date as the treatment. Chiropractic manipulative treatment (98940-98943) services are considered to be procedures, and a premanipulative patient assessment is included. Make sure the service goes above and beyond any preservice or postservice work associated with chiropractic manipulative treatment when provided.

7   When billing Medicare, make sure modifier 25 is appended if the decision for surgery is made on the same day as a minor procedure (global period, 0–10 days) or a diagnostic procedure.

8   Append modifier 25 only to the E/M service.

9   No documentation is required to be submitted before payment, unless there are special circumstances related to the patient encounter.

10 Prepayment and/or postpayment review may be required by Medicare and/or third-party payers.

11 The Office of the Inspector General has targeted this modifier for overutilization under a special fraud alert.

Modifier 25 Usage Checklist

Ask yourself the following questions before billing an E/M visit on the same day as a procedure and/or other service with modifier 25:

1   Why is the patient being seen? Are there signs, symptoms, and/or conditions the physician must address before deciding to perform a procedure or service?
    ~ If the answer is yes, an E/M service might be medically necessary with modifier 25.

2   Was the physician's evaluation and management of the presenting problem significant and beyond the normal preoperative and postoperative work?
    ~ If the answer is yes, then an E/M service may be billed with modifier 25.
    ~ If the answer is no, it would not be appropriate to bill an E/M.

3 Was the procedure or service scheduled in advance of the patient encounter?

~ If the answer is yes, it would not be medically necessary to bill an E/M service unless the patient has other medical concerns or problems that are addressed.

4 Is there more than one diagnosis present that is being addressed and/or affecting the treatment and outcome?

~ If the answer is yes, it would be appropriate to bill both the procedure and the E/M service with modifier 25.

Checkpoint Exercises 1

Multiple Choice

1 Guidelines for billing an E/M visit and a procedure on the same date of service include:

a. Both services are billable only if the diagnosis for the E/M is different from the diagnosis for the procedure. Modifier 25 is used with the E/M code.

b. Both the E/M service and the procedure are billed when the decision to perform the procedure was made during another visit.

c. Only the procedure may be billed if the decision to perform the procedure was made during the same encounter as the E/M visit.

d. The procedure and the E/M visit may both be billed with the same diagnosis code and during the same encounter, if the decision to perform the procedure was made at the time of the encounter and the service is significantly and separately identifiable. Modifier 25 is appended to the E/M code.

2 Mr Jones visited his cardiologist in the hospital because of increasing signs and symptoms of heart failure. After completing a detailed history and examination for this established patient, the cardiologist adjusted the patient's medication. In the course of the examination, the cardiologist discovered that the patient's pacemaker, placed 1 year ago, was malfunctioning. An analysis of the patient's dual-chamber pacemaker was evaluated in the EP lab by the same physician. The pacemaker was reprogrammed, and the patient was asked to return in 2 weeks for follow up. How should the service be reported?

a. 99214 25, 93732

b. 93732

c. 99214

d. 99203 25, 93732

3   A new patient visited the emergency department of the local hospital complaining of abdominal pain and constipation that has gotten progressively worse over the past 3 hours. There was no evidence in the patient's medical history of alcohol or drug dependence. Bowel sounds were present, and the abdomen was rotund. There was tenderness on palpation in the right lower quadrant, but the liver was not enlarged, and there was no organomegaly. All other systems examined were negative. The physician performed and documented a comprehensive history and examination, and ordered a radiologic examination, single view of the abdomen. The medical decision making was moderate. How should the physician report the service?

   a. 74000

   b. 99214 25, 74000

   c. 99284 25, 74000

   d. None of the above is correct.

4   An orthopedist was asked to evaluate in consultation a new patient with complaints of left shoulder pain that had been occurring for the past 3 months. The pain had been increasing in intensity and had limited the patient's activities. The patient is an active tennis player and anxious to return to his game. The physician performed a detailed history and examination with moderately complex decision making. He also performed a complete X ray of the left shoulder in which two views were taken. The procedure was performed in the office. The shoulder appeared normal. The diagnosis documented was joint inflammation, and the physician administered a cortisone injection. How should the procedure be reported?

   a. 99243 25, 73030, 20610

   b. 99253 25, 73030, 20610

   c. 73030, 20610

   d. 20610

5   Mrs Thomas, who was new to the area, brought her son in to visit a new pediatrician for his 6-month well-baby checkup. The physician performed and documented a comprehensive review of systems and an interval past, family, and social history, and he counseled the patient's mother on feeding, growth patterns, and social skills. The mother stated her baby had been pulling at his ears for 3 days and had a low-grade fever off and on. She had been treating the baby with children's Tylenol, and the baby showed some improvement. The physician documented the patient's diagnosis as acute otitis media along with an upper respiratory infection. How should the service be reported?

   a. 99381

   b. 99213

   c. 99381 25, 99212 25

   d. 99381, 99212 25

Modifier 26: Professional Component

Definition

Certain procedures are a combination of a physician component and a technical component. When the physician component is reported separately, the service may be identified by adding the modifier 26 to the usual procedure number.

AMA Guidelines

Reporting the technical and professional components of a procedure is a complex process. CPT codes are intended to represent physicians and other practitioners' services; the CPT code set nomenclature does not contain a coding convention to designate the technical component of a procedure or service. CPT coding guidelines do not specifically address billing the technical component of a procedure or service.

CPT coding does provide modifier 26 for separately reporting the professional component (practitioner or physician) of a procedure or service. Certain procedures are a combination of the physician's professional component and a technical component (total procedure) in the CPT code set. Modifier 26 is used to identify the professional component of a service or procedure that is being reported separately.

Diagnostic services are performed for both inpatients and outpatients. Outpatient services are provided in various locations, such as physician offices, diagnostic centers, and hospital outpatient departments. Third-party payers require that submitted claims clearly define whether a complete, technical, or professional service was rendered for the physician to receive appropriate reimbursement.

Many CPT codes are global, meaning the technical and professional components encompass the total procedure. If the radiologist owns the equipment, interprets the test, and pays the technologist, modifiers TC and 26 do not apply and the procedure is reported without a modifier. If the physician provides only the interpretation and report for a diagnostic study and does not own the equipment, modifier 26 is appended to the appropriate CPT code for the interpretation (professional component). In addition, the facility providing the equipment, technician, and supplies may also report the appropriate procedure code with modifier TC.

CPT codes that do not have a technical component are not applicable. For example, CPT code 76140 (Consultation on X-ray examination made elsewhere, written report) is a CPT code that only has the professional component.

CMS Guidelines

A complete service, as defined by CMS, is one in which the physician provides the entire service, including equipment, supplies, technical personnel, and the physician's professional services. The complete service can then be divided into a technical and a professional component. The HCPCS level II modifier TC was developed by CMS to identify the technical component versus the professional component, even though facilities are not always required to use HCPCS modifier TC for reporting purposes. CMS recognizes the use of modifier 26 when the professional component is billed on the claim.

The technical component includes providing the equipment, supplies, technical personnel, and costs attendant on the performance of the procedure other than the professional services.

The professional component includes the physician's work in providing the services (eg, reading films, interpreting diagnostic tests), and interpretation and written report provided by the physician performing the service.

In some instances, a separate CPT code has been developed to describe the professional component. In others, modifier 26 is required to identify the services as a professional component. Generally, the physician reports only the professional component of services when that service is provided in a setting where the physician does not own the equipment (such as a hospital outpatient department).

Third-Party Payer Guidelines

Many third-party payers have established modifier and/or specific reporting policies for reporting the technical component. Many carriers recognize the TC modifier for reporting the technical component. Some carriers have developed their own guidelines for reporting the professional and technical component(s) separately. When the technical component is reported, reporting requirements of the individual insurance carrier policies in the provider's area should be taken into consideration, because reimbursement policies vary among insurance companies.

Example 1

A 66-year-old woman complained of urinary frequency and urgency, with residual urine volume of 120 mL. The physician decided to perform a cystometrogram as a diagnostic measure to identify the cause. The patient was sent to the outpatient department of the hospital for the test. The physician will interpret the diagnostic test and render a report.

CPT Code(s) Billed: 51725—Simple cystometrogram (CMG) (eg, spinal manometer)

CPT code 51725 includes all supplies, equipment, and the technician's work, including interpretation of the results. If the physician only interprets the results and dictates a report, modifier 26 would be appended to the claim. The outpatient hospital department will append a HCPCS level II modifier TC (technical component) to the same procedure code to report the supplies, equipment, facility, and technician's work.

THIRD-PARTY PAYER CODING TIP

Most third-party payers recognize the use of this modifier for CPT codes that have a professional and a technical component. They will pay the physician for his or her professional services with modifier 26 and the facility with HCPCS level II modifier TC.

CMS CODING TIP

The Medicare fee schedule lists codes that have a professional and a technical component and can be found on the CMS Web site at www.cms.hhs.gov.

AMA CODING TIP

Modifier 26 is not appended to the cardiac catheterization injection procedure codes 93539-93545 since these are performed solely by the physician.

24. A DATE(S) OF SERVICE From To MM DD YY MM DD YY	B Place of Service	C Type of Service	D PROCEDURES, SERVICES, OR SUPPLIES (Explain Unusual Circumstances) CPT/HCPCS I MODIFIER	E DIAGNOSIS CODE	F $ CHARGES	G DAYS OR UNITS	H EPSDT Family Plan	I EMG	J COB	K RESERVED FOR LOCAL USE
1			51725 |26							
2										
3										
4										
5										
6										
25. FEDERAL TAX I.D. NUMBER SSN EIN		26. PATIENTIS ACCOUNT NO.	27. ACCEPT ASSIGNMENT? (For govt. claims, see back) YES NO	28. TOTAL CHARGE $	29. AMOUNT PAID $	30. BALANCE DUE $				

The physician will bill 51725 26 to indicate that he or she interpreted the
study and wrote the report.

24. A DATE(S) OF SERVICE From To MM DD YY MM DD YY	B Place of Service	C Type of Service	D PROCEDURES, SERVICES, OR SUPPLIES (Explain Unusual Circumstances) CPT/HCPCS I MODIFIER	E DIAGNOSIS CODE	F $ CHARGES	G DAYS OR UNITS	H EPSDT Family Plan	I EMG	J COB	K RESERVED FOR LOCAL USE
1			51725 |TC							
2										
3										
4										
5										
6										
25. FEDERAL TAX I.D. NUMBER SSN EIN		26. PATIENTIS ACCOUNT NO.	27. ACCEPT ASSIGNMENT? (For govt. claims, see back) YES NO	28. TOTAL CHARGE $	29. AMOUNT PAID $	30. BALANCE DUE $				

The outpatient hospital department where the diagnostic procedure was
performed will bill the claim with modifier TC to indicate that it performed
only the technical component.

Rationale for Using Modifier 26

In this example, the hospital outpatient department is providing the technical
component of the service and would be billed by using the same CPT code with
modifier TC, and the physician who interprets and reports will submit the claim
with modifier 26.

Example 2

A 5-year-old boy with an implanted programmable cerebrospinal fluid
valve and shunt system was referred by a pediatrician for recent onset
of constant complaints of headache. His history included implantation
of the shunt 3 years earlier for hydrocephalus. After reviewing
the patient chart and previous films and evaluating the patient in the
office, the surgeon decided to decrease the shunt pressure. The surgeon ordered a radiograph to determine the current setting of the
shunt valve. After reviewing the results of the radiograph, the physician reprogrammed the shunt from 120 mm H_2O to 80 mm H_2O in the
radiology department. After the pressure setting was confirmed, the
patient was released from the radiology department. The surgeon dictated a written interpretation report, and a follow-up telephone call to
the boy's family several days later found that a headache had not

occurred since the reprogramming. The written report was sent to the referring pediatrician.

CPT Code(s) Billed by the Surgeon: 62252 26

CPT Code(s) Billed by the Radiology Department: 62252 TC

Rationale for Using Modifier 26

The surgeon is providing the professional component only and is performing the service in a hospital radiology department, which is not owned by the surgeon. The HCPCS level II modifier TC is used by the facility to report the facility portion of the procedure, which includes the equipment, a technician to perform the procedure, film if used, and the room in which the procedure is performed.

Example 3

A radiologist read and rendered a written report for a posteroanterior and lateral chest X ray in his own facility.

CPT Code(s) Billed: 71020

Rationale for Not Using Modifier 26

Since the physician did not append modifier 26 to the claim, it is assumed that the X ray was taken in a setting where the global procedure would apply, where the technical and professional components are provided by the physician.

Example 4

A patient with possible occlusive disease underwent magnetic resonance angiography (MRA) of the lower extremity in the radiology department of the hospital. MRA is widely used to visualize lower-extremity arterial circulation in patients with occlusive disease. The femoropopliteal artery was readily identified and characterized in terms of stenosis. The radiologist read the MRA and dictated a report that was sent to the ordering physician. Since the radiologist was contracted by the hospital and did not own the equipment and supplies and did not employ the technicians, the physician billed only the professional component.

CPT Code(s) Billed by the Radiologist: 73725 26

CPT Code(s) Billed by the Radiology Department: 73725 TC

Rationale for Using Modifier 26

Since the procedure was performed in the hospital radiology department and the physician is not employed by the hospital, modifier 26 would be correct to append to the radiologist's claim.

Pathology Services for CMS

Billing for anatomical and surgical pathology services (both technical and professional components) must comply with the contractual arrangements between the facility and the pathologist and with Medicare, Medicaid, and other third-party payer requirements. This information may be accessed on the CMS Web site at www.cms.hhs.gov.

Hospitals and other health care facilities have the following three options for billing of pathology services, depending on the physician's contractual relationship:

- **Bill technical component only.** Hospitals and other health care facilities billing the technical component of Anatomical, Surgical, Cytology, and Interpretative Pathology services must either perform the technical services, be responsible for providing the services, refer the technical services under arrangement, or refer the technical services and meet the guidelines as outlined in the Billing Referred Testing Policy.
- **Do not bill either component.** Facilities may choose not to bill either the technical or the professional component if the pathologist is not employed by the facility, and a contractual agreement exists permitting the pathologist to bill both components.
- **Bill globally.** The facility must bill globally (technical and professional component) when the pathologist is employed by the facility and/or a contractual agreement exists permitting the facility to bill globally. Both components are billed on a HCFA-1500 with the applicable CPT codes(s) and no modifiers.

CMS Guidelines for Independent Laboratory Billing for the Technical Component of Physician Pathology Services to Hospital Patients

Before the final physician fee schedule regulation was published on November 2, 1999, CMS stated that it would implement a policy to pay only hospitals for the technical component of physician pathology services furnished to hospital inpatients. Before this proposal, any independent laboratory could bill the carrier under the physician fee schedule for the technical component of physician pathology services to a hospital inpatient.

The regulation, which went into effect on or after January 2001, states that the Medicare carrier can continue to pay the technical component of the pathology services when an independent laboratory furnishes services to an inpatient or outpatient of a covered hospital (a hospital that had an arrangement with an independent laboratory) under which the laboratory furnished the technical component of physician pathology services.

Example 5

A pathologist performed a level II gross and microscopic examination of an appendix. The pathologist was independent, under contract with an independent laboratory, and he was providing only the professional component of the procedure.

CPT Code(s) Billed: 88302 26—Level II-Surgical pathology, gross and microscopic examination

Rationale for Using Modifier 26

This examination may be ordered as a gross and microscopic pathology exam or a gross and microscopic tissue exam. The tissue is harvested in the course of a surgery and sent for routine lab evaluation. Since the pathologist is an independent physician and provided only interpretation and report, a modifier 26 would be applicable.

Example 6

A 48-year-old man with hypertension and a history of cigarette smoking described occasional exertional chest discomfort that was thought to be possible, but not definite, angina pectoris. His resting electrocardiogram demonstrated left ventricular hypertrophy with QRS widening and secondary repolarization changes. A treadmill stress echocardiogram was requested to evaluate for inducible myocardial ischemia and to aid in risk stratification.

The cardiologist reviewed the referral information (eg, request for the procedure) and relevant clinical data with the patient to clarify the indications for the procedure and determine the clinical questions that needed to be answered. A sequence of baseline tomographic images from apical and precordial windows was recorded on videotape and into computer memory by means of cine-loop format. The physician verified the suitability of the baseline images and considered the need for border enhancement with echocardiographic contrast material.

The patient then underwent conventional treadmill exercise by means of a symptom-limited protocol. Immediately on completion of treadmill exercise, the patient was again imaged and a sequence of poststress tomographic images was recorded from apical and precordial windows, again using both videotape and digital recording techniques. The patient tolerated the procedure well.

CPT Code(s) Billed by the Cardiologist: 93350 26—Echocardiography, transthoracic, real-time with image documentation

*(2D), with or without M-mode recording, during rest
and cardiovascular stress test using treadmill, bicycle
exercise and/or pharmacologically induced stress,
with interpretation and report*

Rationale for Using Modifier 26

Since the physician is providing only the interpretation and report and the equipment, supplies, and technical support are owned by the outpatient hospital facility, only the professional component is billed by the physician.

Review of Modifier 26

1 Modifier 26 is appended to the procedure code when the professional component is provided by the physician.

2 The physician providing the total global component including the equipment, supplies, technical support, and the interpretation and report will not use a modifier to report the procedure since he or she is providing the global component.

3 The technical component includes the equipment, supplies, technician(s), and facility.

4 Modifier 26 may be used in Surgery, Radiology, Pathology and Laboratory, and Medicine sections of the CPT book.

Checkpoint Exercises 2

True or False

1 _____ Deb, a 42-year-old established patient, saw her physician for a physical examination. During the exam, the physician noted a mass in the right breast and performed a needle biopsy. Modifier 25 can be billed for the E/M service and the breast biopsy on the same date.

2 _____ Modifier 26 is used for the technical component only.

3 _____ Modifier 25 is appended to the surgical procedure.

4 _____ When appending modifier 25, it is not necessary to submit documentation with the claim to the insurance carrier.

5 _____ Modifier 26 must include a written interpretation and report provided by the physician providing the service.

Modifier 27: Multiple Outpatient Hospital E/M Encounters on the Same Date

Definition

For hospital outpatient reporting purposes, utilization of hospital resources related to separate and distinct E/M encounters performed in multiple outpatient hospital settings on the same date may be reported by adding the modifier 27 to each appropriate level outpatient and/or emergency department E/M code(s). This modifier provides a means of reporting circumstances involving evaluation and management services provided by physician(s) in more than one (multiple) outpatient hospital setting(s) (eg, hospital emergency department, clinic). **Note:** This modifier is not to be used for physician reporting of multiple E/M services performed by the same physician on the same date. For physician reporting of all outpatient evaluation and management services provided by the same physician on the same date and performed in multiple outpatient setting(s) (eg, hospital emergency department, clinic), see Evaluation and Management, Emergency Department, or Preventive Medicine Services codes.

Modifier 27 was created in 2001 and is used to identify multiple outpatient hospital E/M encounters on the same date. This modifier is not to be used by physician practices. It was created exclusively for hospital outpatient departments. The CPT book defines modifier 27 as multiple outpatient hospital E/M encounters on the same date.

This modifier may be used with the E/M section of the CPT book.

Modifier 27 is discussed in more detail in Chapter 9, Ambulatory Surgery Center and Hospital Outpatient Modifiers.

Modifier 32: Mandated Services

Definition

Services related to mandated consultation and/or related services (eg, PRO, third-party payer, governmental, legislative, or regulatory requirement) may be identified by adding the modifier 32 to the basic procedure.

AMA Guidelines

cpt Modifier 32 was revised in 2000 to include examples of other parties that may request the performance of a mandated consultative service. For example, hospitals are required by federal COBRA/EMTALA (Consolidated Omnibus Budget Reconciliation Act, Emergency Medical Treatment and Active Labor Act) laws to provide at least a medical screening examination to determine the presence or absence of an emergency medical condition or active labor in any patient who presents to the facility.

CMS Guidelines

Using modifier 32 with claims submitted to CMS has no effect on reimbursement even when a second and/or third opinion might be required before a therapeutic service or operative procedure.

Third-Party Payer Guidelines

Some third-party payers require the patient to undergo certain mandated services, such as second or third opinions, before a procedure and/or therapeutic service. In these instances, when the patient is scheduled for this type of service, the procedure code for the service provided (ie, consultation) is reported with modifier 32 appended to the code.

Modifier 32 is informational and, when used, many insurance carriers allow 100% of the allowed amount of the reimbursement without deductibles or co-payments. The one exception is Medicare, which has no effect on payment or reimbursement. It is common for insurance companies to require a second opinion for certain surgical procedures that the carrier considers overutilized before performance of the procedure.

When a patient and/or family member requests a second opinion, this does not constitute or validate use of modifier 32. A third-party payer, government carrier, and/or workers' compensation insurer may request a second opinion, a medical evaluation, or the service to be provided by a physician and/or practitioner for E/M services, procedures, and diagnostic and/or therapeutic services, wherein the modifier 32 would be appropriate.

In workers' compensation cases, it is common for the insurance carrier paying for the patient's medical care to ask for a second opinion or an independent medical evaluation of the patient's condition. The physician providing the opinion could bill a consultation using 99241-99245 with modifier 32 appended in an office or other outpatient setting, or 99251-99255 with modifier 32 in an inpatient setting. The confirmatory consultation codes (99271-99275) were deleted from CPT in 2006.

Example 1: E/M Service

A 40-year-old man sustained a work-related back injury without subsequent surgical repair/reconstruction. He participated in an acute therapy program but continued to exhibit pain, weakness, fatigue, stiffness, and possible psychosocial limitations. Potential to return to work was undetermined. The workers' compensation carrier requested an evaluation of the patient's current condition and prognosis from an orthopedic surgeon for a second opinion. The physician performed a comprehensive history and examination with moderate-complexity decision making.

CPT Code(s) Billed: 99244 32—Office or other outpatient consultation for a new or established patient, which requires these three key components: a comprehensive

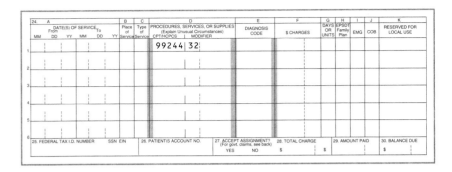

*history; a comprehensive examination; and medical
decision making of moderate complexity*

Rationale for Using Modifier 32

Because the insurance carrier was requesting a second opinion as a confirmatory consultation regarding the patient's current condition and prognosis, the physician can bill the E/M service with modifier 32 and should be reimbursed at 100% of the allowed amount for the service.

Example 2: Radiology

A 29-year-old construction worker presented for assessment of upper-extremity vasculature because of crush injury. The workers' compensation insurance carrier requested a second computed tomographic scan to determine the extent of the patient's injury before approving more surgery, which was recommended.

CPT Code(s) Billed: 73206 32—Computed tomographic angiography, upper extremity, without contrast material(s), followed by contrast material(s) and further sections, including image post-processing

Rationale for Using Modifier 32

Because the insurance carrier was requesting a second opinion from a diagnostic perspective regarding the patient's current condition related to the injury, the physician can bill the procedure with modifier 32 and should be reimbursed at 100% of the allowed amount for the service.

Example 3: Pathology and Laboratory

A clinical laboratory was asked to perform a drug test under court order to confirm alcohol or drug consumption in a person who was arrested while driving under the influence, causing an accident.

CPT Code(s) Billed: 80102 32—Drug confirmation, each procedure

Rationale for Using Modifier 32

Because the court ordered the drug test, the use of modifier 32 would be appropriate for the drug confirmation.

Example 4: Medicine

A physician was asked to render an opinion before cataract surgery for a patient by a third-party payer. The ophthalmologist performed a comprehensive evaluation and determined that the patient did have cataracts and the surgery was medically necessary. The physician performed a complete visual system examination, including history, general medical observation, external and ophthalmoscopic examination, gross visual fields, and basic sensorimotor examination consisting of biomicroscopy, examination with mydriasis (dilation of the pupils), and tonometry. Near visual acuity testing, keratometry, tear testing, corneal staining, corneal sensitivity, fundus examination, and exophthalmometry were also performed. The services were performed on two different dates.

CPT Code(s) Billed: *92004 32—Ophthalmological services: medical examination and evaluation with initiation of diagnostic and treatment program; comprehensive, new patient, one or more visits*

Diagnosis Code: *366.17—Total or mature senile cataract*

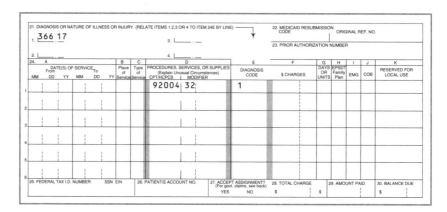

Rationale for Using Modifier 32

Because the insurance carrier was requesting a second opinion from the physician to determine whether surgery was medically necessary, the physician can bill the procedure with modifier 32 and should be reimbursed at 100% of the allowed amount for the service. The ophthalmological procedure code was selected over the confirmatory consultation code because the services provided were more specific to the services and examination rendered during a visit related to the ocular system.

Review of Modifier 32

1 Use modifier 32 when the insurance carrier or other governmental agency requests a procedure and/or service be performed.

2 This modifier may be used with all sections of the CPT book.

3   Modifier 32 is not to be used when the patient and/or family requests a second opinion.

4   Modifier 32 is used commonly by workers' compensation carriers to evaluate a patient's condition.

5   Modifier 32 is typically reimbursed at 100% of the allowed amount by most insurance carriers except Medicare.

AMA CODING TIP

Codes from the anesthesia section (00100-01999) would not be used with modifier 47.

Modifier 47: Anesthesia by Surgeon

Definition

Regional or general anesthesia provided by the surgeon may be reported by adding the modifier 47 to the basic service. (This does not include local anesthesia.) **Note:** Modifier 47 would not be used as a modifier for the anesthesia procedures.

If a physician personally performs the regional or general anesthesia for a surgical procedure that he or she also performs, modifier 47 would be appended to the surgical code and no codes from the anesthesia section would be used.

AMA Guidelines

Local anesthesia is not included because it is included in the typical surgical package in the Surgery guidelines of the CPT book. The surgical package according to the CPT guidelines includes:

- Local infiltration, metacarpal/metatarsal/digital block, or topical anesthesia
- Subsequent to the decision for surgery, one related E/M encounter on the date immediately prior to or on the date of procedure (including history and physical)
- Immediate postoperative care, including dictating operative notes, talking with the family and other physicians
- Writing orders
- Evaluating the patient in the postanesthesia recovery area
- Typical postoperative follow-up care

This modifier is not to be used if the surgeon is monitoring general anesthesia performed by an anesthesiologist, certified registered nurse anesthetist, resident, or intern.

CMS Guidelines

CMS, including Medicare and many state Medicaid programs, does not recognize modifier 47 and does not cover anesthesia services provided by the surgeon/physician separately.

Third-Party Payer Guidelines

Many third-party payers and managed care plans do allow additional reimbursement for the use of modifier 47 appended to the surgical CPT code when more than local anesthesia is used.

Example 1

The surgeon initiated a regional nerve block before performing a repair of the flexor tendon. The physician monitored the patient and block while performing a flexor tendon repair of the forearm.

CPT Code(s) Billed: 25260 47—Repair, tendon or muscle, flexor, forearm and/or wrist; primary, single, each tendon or muscle

64450—Injection, anesthetic agent; other peripheral nerve or branch

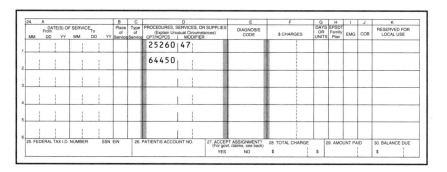

Rationale for Using Modifier 47

Since the surgeon performed the nerve block to repair the flexor tendon of the forearm, modifier 47 would be appended to the surgical code 25260 to indicate that the anesthesia is performed by the surgeon. The surgeon may also report the injection for the anesthetic agent, 64450.

Example 2

A 30-year-old patient had pain and clicking with forearm rotation due to an unstable distal ulna. Soft-tissue reconstruction was performed for stabilization. The surgeon administered a regional Bier block.

CPT Code(s) Billed: 25337 47—Reconstruction for stabilization of unstable distal ulna or distal radioulnar joint, secondary by soft tissue stabilization (eg, tendon transfer, tendon graft or weave, or tenodesis) with or without open reduction of distal radioulnar joint

64450—Injection, anesthetic agent; other peripheral nerve or branch

Rationale for Using Modifier 47

In both examples, the surgeon administered a Bier block, which is more extensive than local anesthesia, and it would be appropriate to submit the claim with the surgical procedure and modifier 47 along with the anesthetic injection for the Bier block.

Moderate (Conscious) Sedation

CPT codes 99141 and 99142 for conscious sedation were deleted in 2006. The category was renamed, and new guidelines have been established. New codes 99143-99145 may be used by the surgeon when reporting moderate conscious sedation as long as the conscious sedation is not included in the procedure or service. When the CPT code is preceded by a "bulls eye" ⊙, moderate conscious sedation is included in the procedure (see appendix G of the CPT codebook), and may not be reported separately.

Modifier 47 is not recognized for use with moderate conscious sedation.

However, keep in mind that many payers, including CMS, have bundled moderate conscious sedation into the procedure and/or service, and it may not be reported separately. It is important to check with the individual payer before submitting a claim with a moderate conscious sedation CPT code.

CMS has bundled moderate (conscious) sedation into the NCCI edits, and it may not be reported when submitting a claim to Medicare.

General Payment Rule[2]

> The fee schedule amount for physician anesthesia services furnished on or after January 1, 1992 is, with the exceptions noted, based on allowable base and time units multiplied by an anesthesia conversion factor specific to that locality. The base unit for each anesthesia procedure is listed in subsection K, Exhibit 1. The way in which time units are calculated is described in subsection G. Do not allow separate payment for the anesthesia service performed by the physician who also furnishes the medical or surgical service. In that case, payment for the anesthesia service is made through the payment for the medical or surgical service. For example, do not allow separate payment for the surgeon's performance of a local or surgical anesthesia if the surgeon also performs the surgical procedure. Similarly, separate payment is not allowed for the psychiatrist's performance of the anesthesia service associated with the electroconvulsive therapy if the psychiatrist performs the electroconvulsive therapy.

When anesthesia is provided by the physician performing the primary service, the anesthesia services are included in the primary procedure (CMS

---

2. Source: Fee Schedule for Physicians' Service, available at www.cms.hhs.gov/manuals/.

Anesthesia Rules), and the operating physician should not report G0347-G0354 (90760-90775 in 2006) for administration of anesthetic agents. If it is medically necessary for a separate provider (anesthesiologist/anesthetist) to provide the anesthesia services (eg, monitored anesthesia care), a separate service may be reported.

To report moderate (conscious) sedation with or without analgesia (conscious sedation) provided by a physician also performing the service for which conscious sedation is being provided, see codes 99143-99145.

⊘**99143**   Moderate sedation services (other than those services described by codes 00100-01999) provided by the same physician performing the diagnostic or therapeutic service that the sedation supports, requiring the presence of an independent trained observer to assist in the monitoring of the patient's level of consciousness and physiological status; under 5 years of age, first 30 minutes intra-service time

⊘**99144**   age 5 years or older, first 30 minutes intra-service time

+**99145**   each additional 15 minutes intra-service time (List separately in addition to code for primary service)

(Use 99145 in conjunction with 99143, 99144)

When a second physician, other than the health care professional performing the diagnostic or therapeutic services, provides moderate (conscious) sedation in the facility setting (eg, hospital, outpatient hospital/ambulatory surgery center, skilled nursing facility), the second physician reports the associated moderate sedation procedure/service 99148-99150; when these services are performed by the second physician in the non-facility setting (eg, physician office, freestanding imaging center), codes 99148-99150 would not be reported.

⊘**99148**   Moderate sedation services (other than those services described by codes 00100-01999), provided by a physician other than the health care professional performing the diagnostic or therapeutic service that the sedation supports; under 5 years of age, first 30 minutes intra-service time

⊘**99149**   age 5 years or older, first 30 minutes intra-service time

+**99150**   each additional 15 minutes intra-service time (List separately in addition to code for primary service)

(Use 99148 in conjunction with 99149, 99150)

Moderate sedation does not include minimal sedation (anxiolysis), deep sedation, or monitored anesthesia care (00100-01999).

Review of Modifier 47

1 Anesthesia must be administered by the surgeon performing the procedure.

2 The anesthesiologist would not use this modifier.

3 This modifier should be appended only to the surgical procedure (not applicable for anesthesia).

4 Do not report modifier 47 when the physician reports moderate (conscious) sedation.

Test Your Knowledge

Multiple Choice

1 Modifier 25 is:
a. used when a surgical procedure is billed.
b. used when a significant, separately identifiable E/M service is performed on the same day as a procedure or service.
c. used when billing for anesthesia.
d. not used with E/M services.

2 If a patient requests a second opinion, modifier 32 may be used.
a. True
b. False

3 Modifier 47 can be used:
a. when billing for general anesthesia.
b. when an anesthesiologist is involved in the service and/or procedure.
c. when a surgeon performs anesthesia service that is not considered local or general anesthesia.
d. None of the above.

4 Modifier 26 indicates to the insurance carrier that:
a. the professional component of the procedure was performed.
b. the technical component of the procedure was performed.
c. the global component was performed.
d. a and b.

5 Split billing can be used with what modifier?
a. Modifier 32
b. Modifier 47
c. Modifier 25
d. Modifier 26

Select the Appropriate Modifier

6 _____ A patient was sent to the hospital radiology department for posteroanterior and lateral chest X rays after getting into a fight at school. The physician performed the procedure and dictated an interpretation and report.

7 _____ A patient visited her physician's office with complaints of chest pain and shortness of breath. During the visit, the physician determined that the patient had a small lesion on the left leg that looked suspicious and removed the lesion the same day.

8 _____ A 58-year-old patient underwent diagnostic coronary angiography by a transfemoral approach on the day preceding the discovery of a pulsatile groin hematoma (3×4 cm in diameter by physical examination). Objective confirmation/ultrasound-guided compression of an iatrogenic pseudoaneurysm was undertaken. Doppler ultrasound (duplex) scanning revealed a unilocular pseudoaneurysm with a patent femoral puncture site. The available coagulation studies and the peripheral pulses in the ipsilateral lower extremity were assessed. The compression site was anesthetized and the transducer was applied at a variety of angles. The angle that produced compression without disturbing the native arterial flow was pursued. Under continuous ultrasound visualization, the neck of the pseudoaneurysm was compressed until the pseudoaneurysm was obliterated. The distal circulation and pulses were then reevaluated. The cardiologist performed the service in the outpatient surgery department of the hospital. A written interpretation and report was dictated by the cardiologist.

9 _____ Injection procedure for pyelography was performed by a surgeon through a pyelostomy tube. The surgeon used a Bier block as the anesthesia and performed the anesthesia services himself.

10 _____ A court ordered a patient to undergo drug testing to determine whether early release from a juvenile detention facility would be indicated. The court asked the laboratory to perform the test and render the results to the court.

11 _____ A patient was admitted to the hospital, and a combined right and retrograde left hearth catheterization was performed. What modifier would the physician append to CPT code 93526 in the outpatient surgery center of a hospital?

12 _____ A patient was seen by her primary care physician for her annual checkup, and the physician performed a comprehensive preventive medical evaluation based on the age of the patient. During the exam, the physician discovered the patient's blood pressure was 150/110, which was unusually high. After completing the preventive medicine examination, the physician decided to perform an additional exam along with prescribing medication for elevated blood pressure. What modifier may be appended to the problem-oriented visit?

13 _____ A physician in a farm community saw a 40-year-old female patient in the ER who had severe abdominal pain. The physician determined the patient had a ruptured appendix and needed surgery on an emergency basis. The anesthesiologist could not be reached, and the physician decided to perform the open procedure personally administering general anesthesia. What modifier would the physician append to indicate he performed the anesthesia?

14 _____ A patient was diagnosed with endometriosis by her GYN physician, Dr Dogood. He had been treating her for more than a year with medication that did not appear to be alleviating the problem. The physician recommended a hysterectomy with removal of the uterus, tubes, and ovaries. When the physician's office contacted the insurance company for pre-authorization, they were informed a second opinion was required. The insurance company scheduled an appointment with Dr Cutter for the next day. Dr Cutter agreed with Dr Dogood's findings and recommended the same course of treatment. What modifier would Dr Cutter append to the consultation code reported on his claim?

15 _____ When a radiologist reads and interprets X rays performed in the hospital and the radiologist is not employed by the hospital (contracted), which modifier is used for each procedure the radiologist reports?

CHAPTER 4

Modifiers 50 to 56

To understand how to bill claims with the use of surgical modifiers, it is important to understand the National Correct Coding Initiative (NCCI), which states, "Procedures should be reported with the CPT® code set(s) that most comprehensively describe the services performed. Unbundling occurs when multiple procedure codes are billed for a group of procedures that are covered by a single comprehensive code."

Correct coding requires reporting a group of procedures with the appropriate comprehensive code. Examples of unbundling include the following:

1   Fragmenting one service into component parts and coding each component part as if it were a separate service. For example, the correct CPT code to use for upper gastrointestinal endoscopy with biopsy of stomach is CPT code 43239. Separating the service into two component parts, using CPT code 43235 for upper gastrointestinal endoscopy and CPT code 43600 for biopsy of the stomach, is inappropriate.

2   Reporting separate codes for related services when one comprehensive code includes all related services.

3   Breaking out bilateral procedures when one code is appropriate.

4   Downcoding a service to use an additional code when one higher level, more comprehensive code is appropriate.

5   Separating a surgical approach from a major surgical service.

Modifier 50: Bilateral Procedure

Definition

Unless otherwise identified in the listings, bilateral procedures that are performed at the same operative session should be identified by adding the modifier 50 to the appropriate five-digit code.

AMA Guidelines

Modifier 50 was revised in 1999. This modifier is used to report bilateral procedures that are performed at the same operative session. The use of modifier 50 is applicable only to services and/or procedures performed on identical anatomical sites, aspects, or organs. In 1991, many of the bilateral codes were deleted from the CPT code set nomenclature. This was done to standardize how bilateral procedures are reported. Bilateral procedures are procedures typically performed on both sides of the body (mirror image) during the same operative session. The intent of this modifier is to be appended to the appropriate unilateral code as a one-line entry on the claim form indicating that the procedure was performed bilaterally.

Unless otherwise identified in the listings, bilateral procedures that are performed at the same operative session should be identified by the appropriate

THIRD-PARTY PAYER CODING TIP

A few insurance carriers still require a two-line item listed on the CMS-1500 claim form to indicate that the procedure is performed bilaterally.

AMA CODING TIP

Although the CPT Editorial Panel intends that the code be listed only once, check with your local third-party payers to determine what is their preferred way for providers to report bilateral procedures.

five-digit code describing the first procedure. Procedures performed bilaterally are identified by adding modifier 50 to the procedure code. This modifier is used to report bilateral procedures that are performed at the same operative session by the same physician. For example, if bilateral inguinal hernias on a 2-year-old were performed, code 49500 would be reported with modifier 50 (49500 50).

> *CPT Code(s) Billed: 49500—Repair initial inguinal hernia, age 6 months to under 5 years, with or without hydrocelectomy; reducible*

The intent of the CPT Editorial Panel is for all modifiers to be appended to the appropriate code as a one-line entry. To report the unilateral code with modifier 50 appended to the CPT code as a one-line entry on the claim form indicates that the procedure was performed bilaterally.

Some third-party payers have requested that providers repeat a code and append modifier 50 to the code on the second line of the claim form. The following examples show two different ways to report modifier 50.

Example 1 illustrates listing the CPT code with modifier 50 as a one-line item, which is what CMS and most insurance carriers require.

Example 1

Example 2 illustrates a two-line item for submitting a claim with modifier 50. Modifier 50 is appended to the second line item.

Example 2

When a procedure code is appended with modifier 50, the units box on the claim form should indicate that "1" unit of service was provided, since one procedure was performed bilaterally. Payers should be asked about their preferred method of reporting bilateral procedures.

This modifier does affect payment, sometimes reducing the second procedure's value by up to 50%.

Many CPT code descriptors are intended for use unilaterally. However, there are many CPT code descriptors that indicate the procedure is inherently bilateral. When the definition of a CPT code indicates unilateral and/or bilateral, the procedure can be performed either way and would not indicate usage of modifier 50. Therefore, it is not appropriate to append modifier 50 when a procedure is performed bilaterally if the code descriptor indicates unilateral or bilateral.

For example, if a physician removes impacted cerumen from both ears, the CPT code selection would be 69210 Removal impacted cerumen (separate procedure), one or both ears. Modifier 50 would not be appended to code 69210 because the code descriptor indicates that the procedure may be performed on one or both ears.

If the procedure is performed unilaterally and the code descriptor indicates that the procedure is bilateral, then the appropriate code would be reported with modifier 52, Reduced services, appended. (Modifier 52 is discussed in more detail later in this chapter.)

Review the following examples of bilateral CPT code sets:
- 69210 Removal impacted cerumen (separate procedure), one or both ears
- 55300 Vasotomy for vasograms, seminal vesiculograms, or epididymograms, unilateral or bilateral
- 27158 Osteotomy, pelvis, bilateral (eg, congenital malformation)
- 30801 Cautery and/or ablation, mucosa of inferior turbinates, unilateral or bilateral, any method; superficial
- 40843 Vestibuloplasty; posterior, bilateral
- 35549 Bypass graft, with vein; aortoiliofemoral, bilateral

Some CPT codes were developed for unilateral and bilateral procedures:
- 35548 Bypass graft, with vein; aortoiliofemoral, unilateral
- 35549 Bypass graft, with vein; aortoiliofemoral, bilateral

In the previous example, it would not be appropriate to append modifier 50 to CPT code 35548 because there is a code to report the bilateral procedure.

CMS Guidelines

The bilateral modifier is used to indicate cases in which a procedure normally performed on only one side of the body was performed on both sides of the body. The CPT descriptors for some procedures specify that the procedure is bilateral. In such cases, the bilateral modifier is not used for increased payment. Harvard research on multiple surgical procedures found similar results for the physician work required for bilateral procedures. Medicare has maintained the policy of approving 150% of the global amount when the bilateral modifier is used. If additional procedures are performed on the same day as the bilateral surgery, they should be reported with modifier 51. The multiple surgery rules apply, with the highest valued procedure paid at 100% and the second through fifth procedures paid at 50%. All others beyond the fifth are paid on a by-report basis. The multiple surgery reduction rule will be discussed later in this chapter.

When identical procedures are performed by two different physicians on opposite sides of the body or when bilateral procedures requiring two surgical teams working during the same surgical session are performed, the following rules apply:

- The surgery is considered co-surgery (see modifier 62) if the CPT descriptor designates the procedure as bilateral (eg, 27395). The CMS payment rules allow 125% of the procedure's payment amount divided equally between the two surgeons.
- If CPT does not designate the procedure as bilateral, CMS payment rules first calculate 150% of the payment amount for the procedure. Then the co-surgery rule is applied: split 125% of that amount between the two surgeons.[1]

Third-Party Payer Guidelines

When these claims are submitted to the carrier, most insurance carriers will pay for the first procedure at 100% of the allowed amount or usual and customary amount, and the second procedure will be reduced to one half of the allowed amount or usual and customary. Many third-party payers will approve 150% of the global amount when the bilateral modifier is used. When additional procedures are performed on the same day at the same operative session as the bilateral procedure, they should be reported with modifier 51. Many insurance carriers follow the multiple surgery rule, with the highest-valued procedure paid at 100% and the second through fifth procedures paid at 50%.

Many insurance carriers will not accept modifier 50 when radiology procedures are performed bilaterally. Some carriers allow the use of HCPCS level II modifiers LT (left) and RT (right) to indicate right and left identical anatomy. It is a good idea to verify with the individual insurance carrier when modifier 50 is applicable to the code(s) submitted.

CMS also allows in some instances the HCPCS modifiers LT and RT instead of modifier 50 when the code description does not indicate a bilateral procedure.

Example 3

A 46-year-old female presented with failure and persisting sepsis of a secondary total knee implantation after a treated infected primary total knee arthroplasty affecting both the right and left knees. The implants were removed and the infection was treated. A knee arthrodesis (fusion) was subsequently performed on both knees.

This example should be reported using modifier 50, but many carriers including CMS allow using RT or LT.

---

1. Source: Medicare Carriers Manual, available at www.cms.hhs.gov/physicians.

CPT Code(s) Billed: 27580 50—Arthrodesis, knee, any technique

24.	A DATE(S) OF SERVICE From To		B Place of Service	C Type of Service	D PROCEDURES, SERVICES, OR SUPPLIES (Explain Unusual Circumstances) CPT/HCPCS | MODIFIER	E DIAGNOSIS CODE	F $ CHARGES	G DAYS OR UNITS	H EPSDT Family Plan	I EMG	J COB	K RESERVED FOR LOCAL USE
	MM DD YY MM DD YY				27580 | 50							
1												
2												
3												
4												
5												
6												
25. FEDERAL TAX I.D. NUMBER SSN EIN			26. PATIENT¡S ACCOUNT NO.		27. ACCEPT ASSIGNMENT? (For govt. claims, see back) YES NO	28. TOTAL CHARGE $		29. AMOUNT PAID $		30. BALANCE DUE $		

CPT Code(s) Billed: 27580 RT—Arthrodesis, knee, any technique

          27580 LT—Arthrodesis, knee, any technique

24.	A DATE(S) OF SERVICE From To		B Place of Service	C Type of Service	D PROCEDURES, SERVICES, OR SUPPLIES (Explain Unusual Circumstances) CPT/HCPCS | MODIFIER	E DIAGNOSIS CODE	F $ CHARGES	G DAYS OR UNITS	H EPSDT Family Plan	I EMG	J COB	K RESERVED FOR LOCAL USE
	MM DD YY MM DD YY				27580 | RT							
1					27580 | LT							
2												
3												
4												
5												
6												
25. FEDERAL TAX I.D. NUMBER SSN EIN			26. PATIENT¡S ACCOUNT NO.		27. ACCEPT ASSIGNMENT? (For govt. claims, see back) YES NO	28. TOTAL CHARGE $		29. AMOUNT PAID $		30. BALANCE DUE $		

Example 4

The surgeon performed a carpal tunnel release at the median nerve (neuroplasty) on the right and left wrist during the same operative session in a 40-year-old woman with carpal tunnel syndrome.

CPT Code(s) Billed: 64721 50—Neuroplasty and/or transposition;
                       median nerve at carpal tunnel

Diagnosis Code: 354.0—Carpal tunnel syndrome

21. DIAGNOSIS OR NATURE OF ILLNESS OR INJURY. (RELATE ITEMS 1,2,3 OR 4 TO ITEM 24E BY LINE)				22. MEDICAID RESUBMISSION CODE ORIGINAL REF. NO.								
1. 354.0 3.				23. PRIOR AUTHORIZATION NUMBER								
2. 4.												
24.	A DATE(S) OF SERVICE From To		B Place of Service	C Type of Service	D PROCEDURES, SERVICES, OR SUPPLIES (Explain Unusual Circumstances) CPT/HCPCS | MODIFIER	E DIAGNOSIS CODE	F $ CHARGES	G DAYS OR UNITS	H EPSDT Family Plan	I EMG	J COB	K RESERVED FOR LOCAL USE
	MM DD YY MM DD YY				64721 | 50	1						
1												
2												
3												
4												
5												
6												
25. FEDERAL TAX I.D. NUMBER SSN EIN			26. PATIENT¡S ACCOUNT NO.		27. ACCEPT ASSIGNMENT? (For govt. claims, see back) YES NO	28. TOTAL CHARGE $		29. AMOUNT PAID $		30. BALANCE DUE $		

Rationale for Using Modifier 50

Since the same surgical procedure was performed on the right and left wrists during the same operative session, it is correct to append modifier 50.

Example 5

A 25-year-old police officer with 4 diopters of myopia was intolerant of contact lenses and sought surgical correction to improve his vision in both eyes. Radial incisions were made in the anterior surface of the central cornea to alter the shape of the cornea and its refractive properties. The patient required frequent postoperative evaluation and care for more than 4 months. The patient's insurance company agreed to pay for the surgery if performed bilaterally.

CPT Code(s) Billed: 65771 50—Radial keratotomy

Rationale for Using Modifier 50

Since the radial keratotomy was performed on both right and left eyes during the same operative session, modifier 50 would apply.

Example 6

A 30-year-old skier sustained a complete tear of the anterior cruciate ligament, tear of the medial collateral ligament, and injury to the posterior lateral capsular ligaments of both knees. In both knees, the anterior cruciate ligament was reconstructed through a mini-arthrotomy approach followed by an open repair of the posterior lateral corner of the knee and extra-articular anterior-lateral tenodesis.

CPT Code(s) Billed: 27429 50—Ligamentous reconstruction (augmentation), knee; intra-articular (open) and extra-articular

Rationale for Using Modifier 50

The surgical procedure was performed on both the left and right knees during the same operative session, which supports using modifier 50.

Example 7

A 9-year-old boy with cerebral palsy, spastic diplegia, and a progressive gait disturbance underwent bilateral multiple hamstring tendon lengthening to the patella on both legs.

CPT Code(s) Billed: 27395—Lengthening of hamstring tendon; multiple tendons, bilateral

NCCI CODING TIP

Breaking out bilateral procedures and coding them individually when the description of the code indicates "bilateral" violates the National Correct Coding Initiative.

Rationale for Not Using Modifier 50

In this example, the code description indicates bilateral in the description, which includes both sides of the body. Modifier 50 would not be applicable in this case.

Review of Modifier 50

1 Do not use modifier 50 when the code descriptor indicates bilateral.

2 Do not use modifier 50 when the code descriptor indicates unilateral or bilateral.

3 Use modifier 50 to describe procedures performed on both sides of the body (mirror image) at the same operative session.

4 Check with the insurance carrier to determine whether the carrier wants a one- or two-line item listed on the claim form.

5 Use modifier 50 for surgery procedures.

6 Determine which carriers will accept modifier 50. When radiology procedures are billed, it is recommended to determine which carriers accept HCPCS level II RT and LT designations.

7 When a procedure descriptor indicates a bilateral procedure and is performed unilaterally, use modifier 52, Reduced services.

Modifier 51: Multiple Procedures

Definition

When multiple procedures, other than E/M services, are performed at the same session by the same provider, the primary procedure or service may be reported as listed. The additional procedure(s) or service(s) may be identified by appending modifier 51 to the additional procedure or service code(s). **Note:** This modifier should not be appended to designated "add-on" codes (see Appendix D of the CPT book).

AMA Guidelines

cpt When multiple procedures other than the evaluation and management (E/M) services are performed on the same day or at the same session, by the same provider, the primary procedure or services may be reported as listed. Any additional, or lesser procedure(s) or service(s) may be identified by adding the modifier 51 to the secondary procedure or service code(s). This modifier may be used to report multiple medical procedures performed at the same session, as well as a combination of medical and surgical procedures, or several surgical procedures performed at the same operative session by the same physician.

If possible, list procedures in ranking order from the one requiring the most physician work to the procedure requiring the least physician work.

NOTE: The software in many third-party payer systems automatically ranks the procedures. However, some insurers' systems do not have this capacity.

Also, if multiple medical procedures are performed at the same session or if a combination of medical and surgical procedures are performed, modifier 51 is used to indicate this to third-party payers. This modifier is used to identify the secondary procedure or when multiple procedures are performed during a single operative session. The procedures may be through the same operative incision or a different anatomical site. This modifier is not appended to "add-on" codes.

To understand modifier 51, first it is important to understand when not to use modifier 51 and the associated reporting rules.

Historically, insurance carriers and providers have used modifier 51 (multiple procedures) in varying ways. To alleviate confusion about the intent of the modifier, it was revised in CPT nomenclature in 1997 and again in 1999. During development of the revised instructions, the CPT Editorial Panel learned that some payers were appending modifier 51 to procedures performed and reported by another physician at the same session. Therefore, the language "by the same provider" was added to the descriptor. The complete descriptor now reads as follows:

- The modifier is only appended to secondary procedure codes when multiple procedures are performed at the same session.
- When multiple procedures, other than E/M services, are performed at the same session by the same provider, the primary procedure or service may be reported as listed. The additional procedure(s) or service(s) may be identified by appending the modifier 51 to the additional procedure or service code(s).
- This modifier may be used to report multiple medical procedures performed at the same session, as well as a combination of medical and surgical procedures, or several surgical procedures performed at the same operative session.

Modifier 51 has three applications, namely to identify:
- Multiple, related surgical procedures performed at the same session
- Surgical procedures performed in combination, whether through the same or another incision or involving the same or different anatomy
- A combination of medical and surgical procedures performed at the same session

Modifier 51 should not be appended to report an E/M service and a procedure performed on the same day (modifier 25, appended to the E/M code, serves this purpose), or "add-on" codes. All add-on codes found in the CPT code set nomenclature are exempt from the multiple procedure concept. They are exempt from the use of modifier 51, as these procedures are not reported as stand-alone codes. These additional or supplemental procedures are designated as "add-on" codes. Add-on codes in the CPT code set can be readily identified by add-on code symbol (✚) and the specific descriptor nomenclature, which includes phrases such as "each additional" or "List separately in addition to primary procedure."

Add-on codes describe services that are additional or supplemental procedures, done in conjunction with the more comprehensive (primary) portion of a surgery, and are exempt from the multiple procedure concept and should not be reported with modifier 51. (A complete list of add-on codes can be found in Appendix D of the CPT book.)

CMS Guidelines

CMS considers multiple surgeries as more than one procedure performed by a single physician or physicians in the same group practice on the same patient at the same operative session or on the same day for which separate payment is allowed. Co-surgeons, assistant surgeons, or a surgical team may participate in performing multiple surgeries on the same patient on the same day if the procedure allows them.

Multiple procedures are distinguished from procedures that are components of or incidental to the primary procedure. Incidental procedures or components of a procedure are not separately reportable.

Major surgical procedures are determined based on the Medicare Fee Schedule Database (MFSDB) approved amount, which is not necessarily the submitted amount by the provider.

The Medicare Resource-Based Relative Value Scale reimbursement system has assigned a specific relative value to each add-on code, prompting these codes to be exempt from the usual payment reduction associated with the use of modifier 51. Distinctive language in the code descriptors for add-on CPT codes includes such terminology as "List separately in addition to primary procedure" or "each additional" (as noted with lesions, vertebral segments, etc).

CMS also designates procedure codes that are modifier 51 exempt. Based on the CMS list of procedure codes eligible for modifier 51, these additional procedures, as long as they are not considered incidental or bundled, are subject to multiple procedure fee reduction to reflect their secondary nature.

There may be times when two or more physicians are performing distinctly different unrelated surgeries at the same operative session or on the same day. When this occurs, the payment adjustment rules for multiple surgeries do not apply. In this case each surgeon will report the procedure individually performed without modifier 51.

Third-Party Payer Guidelines

Many third-party payers follow the CMS rules for reimbursement when modifier 51 is used and multiple procedures are performed during the same operative session by the same physician and also follow the multiple surgery reduction rule(s) listed below.

Reimbursement Policy

Reimbursement policy has been developed through consideration of the American Medical Association (AMA) CPT coding descriptions and instructions, CMS Resource-Based Relative Value Units and recommendations, CMS reimbursement policies, and the NCCI.

Medicare payment policy is based on the lesser of the actual charge or 100% of the payment schedule for the procedure with the highest payment, while payment for the second through fifth surgical procedures is based on the lesser of the actual charge or 50% of the payment schedule. Surgical procedures beyond the fifth are priced by carriers on a "by-report" basis. The payment adjustment rules do not apply if two or more surgeons of different specialties (eg, multiple trauma cases) each perform distinctly different surgeries on the same patient on the same day. CMS has clarified that payment adjustment rules for multiple surgery, co-surgery, and team surgery do not apply to trauma surgery situations when multiple physicians from different specialties provide different surgical procedures. Modifier 51 is used only if one of the same surgeons individually performs multiple surgeries.

Under CMS's previous policy, carriers based payment for the second procedure on the lesser of the actual charge or 50% of the payment schedule amount; the third, fourth, and fifth procedures were each based on 25%; any subsequent procedures were paid on a by-report basis.

A good way to understand which code should be ranked first is to review the RVUs (relative value units) for a procedure or service. These values are modified and adjusted each calendar year.

Example 1

A patient was diagnosed with a bladder tumor and surgery was indicated. The surgeon performed a cystourethroscopy with fulgeration and resected the 10-cm tumor. The physician also performed a cystourethroscopy inserting an indwelling urethral stent.

CPT Code(s) Billed: *52240—Cystourethroscopy, with fulguration (including cryosurgery or laser surgery) and/or resection of; large bladder tumor*

52282 51—Cystourethroscopy, with insertion of urethral stent

In 2006, CPT code 52240 had a RVU of 13.71 and code 52282 had a RVU of 9.08. Since code 52240 had the higher RVU, the procedure had more value than code 52282 and should be reported without modifier 51.

Multiple Endoscopic Procedures

Special rules apply to multiple endoscopic procedures and to some dermatologic procedures. In the case of multiple endoscopic procedures, the full value of the higher-valued endoscopy will be recognized, plus the difference between the next highest endoscopy and the base endoscopy. CMS provides the following example:

In the course of performing a fiberoptic colonoscopy (CPT code 45378), a physician performs a biopsy on a lesion (code 45380) and removes a polyp (code 45385) from a different part of the colon. The physician bills for codes 45380 and 45385. The value of code 45380 and code 45385 both have the value of the diagnostic colonoscopy (45378) built in.

45378	$295.45
45380	$320.45
45385	$450.25

Rather than recognizing 100% for the highest valued procedure (45385) and 50% for the next (45380), the carrier pays the full value of the higher valued endoscopy (45385) plus the difference between the next highest endoscopy (45380) and the base endoscopy (45378). In this example, 45385 is paid at 100% ($450.25) and the difference between 45380 and 45378 is paid, which is $25.00. The total expected reimbursement is $475.25.

CMS Payment Rules

In situations when two unrelated endoscopies are performed, the special endoscopy rules are applied to each series, followed by the multiple surgery rules of 100% and 50%. In the case of two unrelated endoscopic procedures (eg, 46606 and 43217), the usual multiple surgery rules apply. When two related endoscopies and a third unrelated endoscopy (eg, 43215, 43217, and 45305) are performed in the same operative session, the special endoscopic rules apply only to the related endoscopies. To determine payment for the unrelated endoscopy, the multiple surgery rules are applied. The total payment for the related endoscopies are considered one service and the unrelated endoscopy as another service.[2]

For some dermatology services, the CPT descriptors contain language such as "additional lesion" to indicate that multiple surgical procedures have been performed (eg, 11201 and 17003). In addition, these codes are add-on codes and do not require modifier 51. The multiple procedures rules do not apply because the relative value units for these codes have been adjusted to reflect the multiple nature of the procedure. These services are paid according to the unit. A 50% reduction in value for the second procedure applies to dermatologic codes in the following series: 11400, 11600, 17260, 17270, 17280. If dermatologic procedures are billed with other procedures, the multiple surgery rules apply.[3]

Multiple Surgery Reduction Rule

Many carriers, including CMS, follow the multiple surgery reduction rules that determine how multiple surgery reductions apply:

1   The primary (highest fee schedule allowable) procedure will always be allowed at 100%.

2   Base payment for each ranked procedure will be based on the lower of the billed amounts:
    a. 100% of the fee schedule amount for the highest valued procedure
    b. 50% of the fee schedule amount for the second-highest valued procedure
    c. 25% of the fee schedule amount for the third- through fifth-highest valued procedures

3   There may be instances in which two or more physicians each perform distinctly different, unrelated surgeries on the same patient on the same day, for example, in some multiple trauma cases. When this occurs, CPT modifier 51 is not used and the multiple procedure payment reductions do not apply unless one of the surgeons individually performs multiple surgeries.

4   If any of the multiple surgeries are bilateral or co-surgeries, the allowed amount for the procedure is determined, this amount is ranked with the

---

2. Source: Medicare Carrier's Manual, available at www.cms.hhs.gov/physicians.
3. Source: Medicare Carrier's Manual, available at www.cms.hhs.gov/physicians.

remaining procedures, and finally, the appropriate multiple surgery payment reductions are applied.

5   The multiple endoscopy payment rules apply if the procedure is billed with another endoscopy in the same family (ie, another endoscopy that has the same base procedure). For purposes of this item, the term "endoscopy" also includes arthroscopy procedures. If an endoscopy procedure is performed on the same day as another endoscopy procedure within the same family, the payment for the procedure with the highest relative value units is 100% of the maximum allowed fee and the maximum allowed fee for every other procedure in that family is reduced by the value of the base code for that family of procedures. No separate payment is made for the base procedure when other endoscopy procedures in the same family are performed on the same day.

Add-on Codes

Some procedures listed in the Surgery section of the CPT book are commonly carried out in addition to the primary procedure. These additional procedures are listed as "add-on" codes with the ✚ symbol and are listed in Appendix D of the CPT book. Add-on codes can be identified with descriptors such as "each additional" or "list separately in addition to the primary procedure." An add-on code may not be used alone, as these codes describe procedures that would not be performed unless some other procedure was also performed (ie, they are "added on" to another procedure). The multiple procedure modifier 51 is not appended to add-on codes. These codes are exempt from the multiple procedure concept.

Example 2

A 66-year-old woman presented with complaints of growing skin lesions on her neck and axillary areas. She had a family history of similar lesions. The tags on her neck were irritated by her collars and caught in her necklaces, and the tags in the axillae itched in warm weather and with exercise. On examination, there were 12 pedunculated papules on the sides of the neck, 3 to 5 mm, and 11 tags, 2 to 6 mm, in the axillary areas; all were typical of the diagnosis of skin tags. Because the tags were symptomatic, removal was recommended. The procedure was described and informed consent was obtained. After the area was cleansed with alcohol, each tag was anesthetized with 1% lidocaine.

The bases of the tags were electrodessicated and the larger tags were removed by scissors excision. Aluminum chloride was applied as needed topically for hemostasis. The larger sites were covered with topical bacitracin zinc/polymyxin B and bandages. The procedure performed was removal of 22 skin tags.

CPT Code(s) Billed: 11200, 11201

Rationale for Not Using Modifier 51

Modifier 51 would not be appended to code 11201 because it is an add-on code, and therefore is exempt from the multiple procedure concept and use of modifier 51.

Example 3

A 74-year-old mechanic was admitted to the burn center with burns of both legs, lower back, and abdomen after his gasoline-saturated clothing was ignited from a spark. The burns involved 40% of body surface area. During the first operative session, the patient underwent surgical preparation of the burn tissue from the left lower leg beginning at the ankle and extending to the popliteal area. After excision and hemostasis, allografts were obtained from the skin bank. Approximately 300 cm² of allograft was then grafted to the excised surface and secured with 60 interrupted absorbable sutures. The graft was dressed with a low-adherent dressing, reinforced with absorbent dressing, and secured with net dressing.

CPT Code(s) Billed: 15300—Allograft skin for temporary wound closure, trunk, arms, legs; first 100 sq cm or less, or one percent of body area of infants and children

15301—Each additional 100 sq cm, or each additional one percent of body area of infants and children, or part thereof (List separately in addition to code for primary procedure)

The add-on code is also listed to report the complete operation. Modifier 51 is not appended to either code.

CPT Code(s) Billed: 15300, 15301 × 2

The units column of the claim form indicates the number of times the add-on code is billed. Since the descriptor of code 15301 is for each additional 100 cm², it would be billed twice because an additional 200 cm² is reported.

Rationale for Not Using Modifier 51

Because CPT code 15301 is an add-on code and is identified in CPT with a ✚ symbol, the multiple surgical reduction rule does not apply. Some of the listed procedures in the CPT book are commonly carried out in addition to the primary procedure performed. All add-on codes found in CPT are exempt from the multiple procedure concept.

Modifier 51 Exempt

Codes in CPT with the symbol ⊘ indicate that the procedure is modifier 51 exempt. These surgical procedures have been determined to be exempt because the work values have already been reduced. The codes that are exempt from modifier 51 are located in Appendix E of the CPT book.

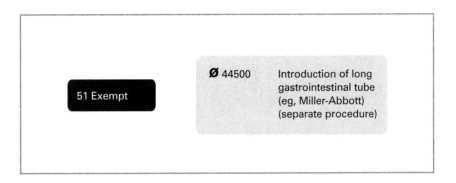

Example 4

A middle-aged patient presented with progressive, painful restriction of the hallux metatarsophalangeal joint. The patient had been treated conservatively without success. The patient underwent a distal first metatarsal cheilectomy. This included removal of bone at the distal first metatarsal, proximal phalanx, debridement of the metatarsophalangeal joint, and capsular. During the same operative session, the surgeon corrected a hammertoe on the third toe.

CPT Code(s) Billed for Primary Procedure: 28289—Hallux rigidus correction with cheilectomy, debridement and capsular release of the first metatarsophalangeal joint

CPT Code(s) Billed for Secondary Procedure: 28285 51—Correction, hammertoe (eg, interphalangeal fusion, partial or total phalangectomy)

Rationale for Using Modifier 51

Modifier 51 is appropriate because both procedures involve the same area, the same foot (same anatomy), during the same operative session.

Reporting Twin Births with Modifiers

The method most preferred for reporting delivery of twins is to append the global obstetric care code and appending modifier 22. For example if a physician, or a physician in the same group, provides the routine obstetric care including antepartum, vaginal delivery, and postpartum care, the global code of 59400 is utilized. Code 59610 also may be used to report a global service in which antepartum care, vaginal delivery after a previous cesarean delivery, and postpartum care are provided. However, some payers mandate that the physician report an E/M code for each antepartum visit and postpartum visit, and report the delivery separately.

An alternative method of reporting vaginal delivery of twins is with code 59400 or 59610 for the first twin and 59409 or 59612 with modifier 51 appended for the second twin.

If both twins are delivered via cesarean delivery, then report code 59510, Routine obstetric care including antepartum care, cesarean delivery, and postpartum care, since only one cesarean delivery is performed.

If the cesarean delivery is significantly more difficult, then append modifier 22 to the code 59510. Keep in mind that when reporting modifier 22 with the cesarean delivery, a copy of the operative report should be submitted to the third-party payer with the claim.

If one twin is delivered vaginally and the other by cesarean delivery, and the global obstetric care is provided by the same physician or group, then report the global CPT code 59510 or 59618 for the cesarean delivery, and 59409 or 59612 for the vaginal delivery with modifier 51 appended.

Example 5

Dr Smith provided the antepartum care to Mrs Martin, who was expecting twins. This was her first pregnancy and she had been doing well. The patient went into labor at 7pm. Dr Smith was called, and the patient was admitted to labor and delivery at the birthing center in the hospital. The patient vaginally delivered a 6 lb 4 oz female at 10:30pm and delivered a 6 lb 2 oz baby boy at 11:10pm. Both babies appeared healthy and were transferred to the nursery. Mrs Martin was in good condition when transferred to recovery.

There are two ways of reporting this patient encounter. Reporting depends on the preference of the insurance carrier:

CPT Code(s) Billed: 59400 22—Routine obstetric care including ante-partum care, vaginal delivery (with or without episiotomy, and/or forceps) and postpartum care

24.	A					B	C	D		E	F	G	H	I	J	K
	From DATE(S) OF SERVICE To					Place of	Type of	PROCEDURES, SERVICES, OR SUPPLIES (Explain Unusual Circumstances)		DIAGNOSIS		DAYS OR	EPSDT			RESERVED FOR
	MM	DD	YY	MM	DD	YY	Service	Service	CPT/HCPCS	MODIFIER	CODE	$ CHARGES	UNITS	Family Plan	EMG	COB	LOCAL USE
1									59400	22							
2																	
3																	
4																	
5																	
6																	
25. FEDERAL TAX I.D. NUMBER			SSN EIN		26. PATIENTIS ACCOUNT NO.			27. ACCEPT ASSIGNMENT? (For govt. claims, see back) YES NO		28. TOTAL CHARGE $		29. AMOUNT PAID $		30. BALANCE DUE $			

CPT Code(s) Billed: *59400—Routine obstetric care including antepartum care, vaginal delivery (with or without episiotomy, and/or forceps) and postpartum care*

59409 51—Vaginal delivery only (with or without episiotomy and/or forceps)

24.							B	C	D		E	F	G	H	I	J	K
		DATE(S) OF SERVICE					Place of Service	Type of Service	PROCEDURES, SERVICES, OR SUPPLIES (Explain Unusual Circumstances)		DIAGNOSIS CODE	$ CHARGES	DAYS OR UNITS	EPSDT Family Plan	EMG	COB	RESERVED FOR LOCAL USE
	From MM	DD	YY	To MM	DD	YY			CPT/HCPCS	MODIFIER							
1									59400								
2									59409	51							
3																	
4																	
5																	
6																	
25. FEDERAL TAX I.D. NUMBER			SSN EIN			26. PATIENT'S ACCOUNT NO.			27. ACCEPT ASSIGNMENT? (For govt. claims, see back) YES NO		28. TOTAL CHARGE $		29. AMOUNT PAID $		30. BALANCE DUE $		

Anesthesia and Modifier 51

Additional procedural services provided in conjunction with basic anesthesia administration are separately reportable and coded according to standard CPT coding guidelines applicable to the given code and the respective CPT section (eg, Surgery or Medicine sections) in which they are listed. Modifiers may be appended to code(s) for procedural services if applicable and appropriate.

Example 6

In addition to providing basic anesthesia administration service for the operation on a 40-year-old male, a Swan-Ganz catheter was also inserted by the anesthesiologist for monitoring during and after the operation.

At the conclusion of the surgical procedure, the anesthesiologist inserted an epidural catheter into the lumbar spinal region to induce continuous postoperative analgesia for therapeutic pain management.

CPT Code(s) Billed: *93503—Insertion and placement of flow directed catheter (eg, Swan-Ganz) for monitoring purposes*

62319 51—Injection, including catheter placement, continuous infusion or intermittent bolus, not including neurolytic substances, with or without contrast (for either localization or epidurography), of diagnostic or therapeutic substance(s) (including anesthetic, antispasmodic, opioid, steroid, other solution), epidural or subarachnoid; lumbar, sacral (caudal)

CMS CODING TIP

CMS designates which procedure codes are eligible for modifier 51 and subject to multiple-procedure fee reductions. CMS also designates procedure codes that are modifier 51 exempt. Most fiscal intermediaries reimburse modifier 51 based on the CMS list of procedure codes eligible for modifier 51.

Rationale for Using Modifier 51

The anesthesiologist will report the following: the basic anesthesia services as appropriate; the insertion of the Swan-Ganz catheter for monitoring (93503); and the insertion of the lumbar epidural catheter (62319) with modifier 51 appended to the lumbar epidural catheter. Modifier 51 indicates that the physician (ie, the anesthesiologist) performed multiple surgical procedures on the same date. On separate lines, the physician reports the code for insertion of the Swan-Ganz catheter, which is modifier 51 exempt, and the insertion of the lumbar epidural catheter, for which modifier 51 would be applicable. If the anesthesiologist performs other additional procedures, each is separately reportable. When additional procedures performed by the anesthesiologist are reported, it is important to consider the various code symbols and modifier definitions.

Example 7

A carpenter with a 6-week-old median and ulnar nerve injury was referred to a therapist for splinting to improve hand use. He had sustained multiple trauma from an automobile accident and was experiencing decreased strength and coordination of both upper extremities and poor standing tolerance. Through a combination of gross impairment assessment and clinical reasoning, the therapist designed a splint that stabilized the thumb for 3 jaw chuck prehension and facilitated the finger extension required to place the hand around large objects. During the fitting process, the patient was instructed in splint application, uses and frequency of wear, how to check for pressure areas, and care of the splint. The provider also designed a woodworking project requiring the patient to make a series of items that necessitated standing for periods of time and use of upper-extremity coordination. The difficulty of each project required progressively increased strength, coordination, endurance, and standing tolerance.

CPT Code(s) Billed: *97530—Therapeutic activities, direct (one-on-one) patient contact by the provider (use of dynamic activities to improve functional performance), each 15 minutes*

97760 51—Orthotic(s) management and training (including assessment and fitting when not otherwise reported), upper extremity(s), lower extremity(s), and/or trunk, each 15 minutes

Rationale for Using Modifier 51

Two procedures were performed at the same operative session, and neither code is modifier 51 exempt or an add-on code, so modifier 51 would be appropriate.

Review of Modifier 51

1   Use when multiple procedures are performed on the same day at the same operative session.

2   List the major procedure first, with additional lesser procedures secondary with modifier 51.

3   Multiple endoscopy payment rules apply if the procedure is billed with another endoscopy in the same family.

4   Do not append modifier 51 to add-on codes.

5   Do not append modifier 51 to modifier 51-exempt procedure codes.

6   When delivery of twins is billed, one method of reporting is to use the appropriate CPT code with modifier 51 appended to the second procedure (eg, 59400 and 59409 51).

Modifier 52: Reduced Services

Definition

Under certain circumstances a service or procedure is partially reduced or eliminated at the physician's discretion. Under these circumstances the service provided can be identified by its usual procedure number and the addition of the modifier 52, signifying that the service is reduced. This provides a means of reporting reduced services without disturbing the identification of the basic service.

> **NOTE:** For hospital outpatient reporting of a previously scheduled procedure/service that is partially reduced or canceled as a result of extenuating circumstances or those that threaten the well being of the patient prior to or after administration of anesthesia, see modifiers 73 and 74 (see modifiers approved for ASC hospital outpatient use).

AMA Guidelines

Under certain circumstances a service or procedure is partially reduced or eliminated at the physician's election. Under these circumstances the service provided can be identified by its usual procedure code and the addition of modifier 52, signifying that the service is reduced. This provides a means of reporting reduced services without disturbing the identification of the basic service.

Modifier 52 is appended when a service or procedure is partially reduced or eliminated at the physician's discretion, ie, started but discontinued. This circumstance may be reported by adding modifier 52 to the code for the discontinued procedure. This modifier is not used to report the elective cancellation of a procedure before anesthesia induction and/or surgical preparation in the operating suite.

CMS Guidelines

When the procedure or service performed is significantly less than usually required, modifier 52 may be appended to the procedure code. Medicare does not recognize modifier 52 with E/M services. CMS will ignore this modifier if documentation (chart note, operative note) and a statement from the practitioner regarding reduction of service are not appended to the claim.

Even though this modifier may be used with E/M services, it is rare that the provider will provide a reduced E/M service.

Third-Party Payer Guidelines

When a claim is submitted to the insurance carrier, a letter or statement should be attached to the claim to indicate what was different about the procedure. If a surgical procedure is performed, an operative report should accompany the claim.

Example 1: E/M Service

A 28-year-old woman, an established patient, presented to the office for a health evaluation and physical examination. Her interval medical, family, and social history was reviewed. A complete review of systems was documented. A detailed physical examination was performed. The patient refused a pelvic examination, Pap smear, and breast exam. Counseling was provided regarding diet and exercise, substance use, sexual activity, and dental health. Risk factors were identified and interventions were discussed. Medically appropriate lab tests were ordered.

CPT Code(s) Billed: *99395 52—Periodic comprehensive preventive medicine reevaluation and management of an individual including an age and gender appropriate history, examination, counseling/anticipatory guidance/risk factor reduction interventions, and the ordering of appropriate immunization(s), laboratory/diagnostic procedures, established patient; 18-39 years*

V70.0—Routine general medical examination at health care facility

Rationale for Using Modifier 52

Because the patient refused part of the comprehensive examination, modifier 52 would be appended to the CPT code. The preventive medicine CPT code requires a comprehensive examination, which was not performed, since the patient refused part of the exam. Modifier 52 indicates to the insurance carrier that the service was reduced. The physician will need to attach documentation and a letter to the carrier explaining the reduction in service.

Example 2: Surgery

A blind man presented with bilateral upper-extremity amputation at the wrist, requiring tendon transfer and interosseous release to allow abduction and adduction of the radius from the ulna (Krukenberg procedure) on both extremities. At operation, tendons were transferred, but because of vascular malformation, the surgeon was unable to release the interosseous membrane. The skin flaps were rotated as needed, and the arm was placed in a bulky dressing.

CPT Code(s) Billed: 25915 52 50—Krukenberg procedure

Rationale for Using Modifier 52

Because the surgeon was unable to release the interosseous membrane, the procedure was not complete, but it did accomplish some result. The surgeon must submit the operative note, with a statement indicating what part of the procedure was not completed.

Example 3: Radiology

A 27-year-old pregnant woman was at 42 weeks' gestation, 2 weeks past her due date. Evaluation of fetal well-being was needed to facilitate the physician's decision of whether to induce labor. A fetal biophysical profile with nonstress testing was obtained.

The health of the fetus was assessed with ultrasound to monitor movements, tone, and breathing. The amniotic fluid volume could not be checked. The fetal heart rate was monitored electronically in the biophysical profile. A nonstress test was conducted to monitor the fetus' heart rate during a period of 20 minutes to look for accelerations with fetal movement.

CPT Code(s) Billed: 76818 52—Fetal biophysical profile; with non-stress testing

Rationale for Using Modifier 52

Since the amniotic fluid volume was not checked and the total procedure includes the amniotic fluid volume, not all of the procedure was performed and the services should be reported as reduced with modifier 52.

Example 4: Laboratory and Pathology

A surgeon ordered evaluation and report of a fibrinolysin screening panel in a 40-year-old man with massive diffuse postoperative bleeding. The test was ordered as a fibrinolysin screen. The specimen was collected by venipuncture. The method combined automated coagulation instrument, latex agglutination, and automated cell counter. Automated cell counting was not completed. An interpretation and report were sent to the surgeon.

AMA CODING TIP

This modifier is not to be used for a procedure that was discontinued; see modifier 53.

*CPT Code(s) Billed: 85390 52—Fibrinolysins or coagulopathy screen,
interpretation and report*

Rationale for Using Modifier 52

Because automatic cell counting was not performed but is included in the procedure, modifier 52 indicates that services were reduced.

Example 5: Medicine

A 60-year-old man with diabetes presented with calf pain in the right leg. The patient had a left above-the-knee amputation 2 years earlier because of his diabetes. He had begun walking during the past year. He was experiencing pain in the right leg after walking 2 blocks. Pain was relieved with cessation of walking. There were palpable but diminished dorsalis pedal pulses bilaterally. Lower-extremity arterial Doppler and segmental volume plethysmography at rest and after treadmill exercises were performed. The physician evaluated the arteries of the right leg to check blood flow in relation to blockage.

*CPT Code(s) Billed: 93924 52—Noninvasive physiologic studies of lower
extremity arteries, at rest and following treadmill
stress testing, complete bilateral study*

Rationale for Using Modifier 52

Since the left leg was amputated and could not be included in the study, and the CPT code selected is a bilateral study, modifier 52 would indicate the reduction in the procedure. A statement and the report should be submitted with the claim.

Example 6: Laboratory and Pathology

A physician gave a patient three hemocult cards to obtain three separate specimens to test for hemocult blood. The patient returned only one card, indicating he forgot to obtain the specimens on the cards. The physician determined from the single specimen that the hemocult was negative.

*CPT Code(s) Billed: 82270—Blood, occult, by peroxidase activity (eg,
guaiac), qualitative; feces, consecutive collected
specimens with single determination, for colorectal
neoplasm screening (ie, patient was provided three
cards or single triple card for consecutive collection)*

Rationale for Not Using Modifier 52

Code 82270 specifies a single determination for colorectal neoplasm screening. Even though the code descriptor indicates three cards or a single triple card is given to the patient, only one determination is necessary for the procedure.

Review of Modifier 52

1 The use of modifier 52 may or may not affect payment, depending on the insurance carrier.

2 Not all carriers recognize the use of modifier 52.

3 Use modifier 52 when the outcome (result) is less than anticipated.

4 Do not use this modifier if the procedure is discontinued after administration of anesthesia (use modifier 53).

5 Use either modifier 73 or 74 for outpatient hospital or ambulatory surgery center reporting (see Chapter 9).

6 Medicare does not recognize the use of modifier 52 with E/M services.

7 A statement along with an operative or chart note should accompany the claim when it is submitted to Medicare and many other third-party payers.

8 If Medicare does not receive documentation with rationale for coding with modifier 52, the modifier will be ignored as if it were not appended to the code.

9 Check payer guidelines for using modifier 52, as many payers do not recognize this modifier.

Modifier 53: Discontinued Procedure

Definition

Under certain circumstances, the physician may elect to terminate a surgical or diagnostic procedure. Due to extenuating circumstances or those that threaten the well being of the patient, it may be necessary to indicate that a surgical or diagnostic procedure was started but discontinued. This circumstance may be reported by adding the modifier 53 to the code reported by the physician for the discontinued procedure. **Note:** This modifier is not used to report the elective cancellation of a procedure prior to the patient's anesthesia induction and/or surgical preparation in the operating suite. For outpatient hospital/ambulatory surgery center (ASC) reporting of a previously scheduled procedure/service that is partially reduced or canceled as a result of extenuating circumstances or those that threaten the well being of the patient prior to or after administration of anesthesia, see modifiers 73 and 74 (see modifiers approved for ASC hospital outpatient use).

AMA Guidelines

Modifier 53 was added to the CPT code set in 1991, 1997, and revised in 1999. In 1999, the CPT definition for this modifier was editorially revised to clarify its intent for outpatient physician reporting of this circumstance.

Modifier 53 is used for physician reporting purposes. It is used to report circumstances when patients experience unexpected responses (hypotension, crisis, arrhythmia) that cause a procedure to be terminated.

Modifier 53 differs from modifier 52. Modifier 52 describes a procedure that was reduced at the physician's discretion. Modifier 53 indicates that a patient's life-threatening condition requires termination of the procedure. Modifier 53 is not used to report elective cancellation of a procedure before anesthesia induction and/or surgical preparation in the operating suite.

Outpatient hospital ambulatory surgery center (ASC) facility reporting refers to modifiers 73 and 74 in the list of approved modifiers for ASCs. Do not use modifier 53 for reporting ASC facility services.

CMS Guidelines

Since the October 1, 1987, implementation of the Omnibus Budget Reconciliation Act of 1986, certain hospital outpatient surgical procedures have been identified by CMS to be performed in hospitals on an outpatient basis or an approved ASC. Currently ASC procedures are reported by means of CPT codes. Modifier 53 assists to communicate extenuating circumstances to carriers, because ASC policy requires documented narrative regarding how far the procedure had progressed at the point of termination.

Modifier 53 is valid only when attached to a surgical code or medical diagnostic code when the procedure was started but had to be discontinued. Modifier 53 is not valid when used for elective cancellation of a procedure before anesthesia induction and/or surgical preparation in the operating suite.

For outpatient hospital/ASC reporting of a previously scheduled procedure/service that is partially reduced or canceled as a result of extenuating circumstances or those that threaten the well being of the patient before or after administration of anesthesia, use modifier 73 or 74 (modifiers approved for ASC hospital use). More about modifiers 73 and 74 is discussed in Chapter 9.

Modifier 53 is not valid:

- For use with E/M service CPT codes
- When used for elective cancellation of a procedure before the patient's anesthesia induction and/or surgical preparation in the operating suite
- When a laparoscopic or endoscopic procedure is converted to an open procedure. Also, it is not valid when a procedure is changed or converted to a more extensive procedure.

Third-Party Payer Guidelines

Many insurance carriers will cover only one procedure code with modifier 53. Also, if modifier 53 is determined to be valid, many carriers will reimburse at only 25% of the allowance for the primary procedure. Individual payer guidelines should be reviewed before the claim is submitted. However, with some carriers, reimbursement will be reduced according to the service's performed before the procedure was discontinued and priced to a code that reflects the service performed. Documentation in the form of an operative report is required to make a determination of payment.

Example 1

A 72-year-old woman initially underwent left cemented total hip arthroplasty 1 year previously. After recovery, she suffered two left hip dislocations. Radiographic studies disclosed a loosening of the femoral component. The surgical plan included removal and replacement of the femoral component and assessment and possible replacement of the acetabular components to prevent further dislocations. After induction of general anesthesia, the patient's blood pressure dropped suddenly and she went into cardiac arrest. The procedure was immediately discontinued and measures were taken to save the patient.

CPT Code(s) Billed: 27134 53—Revision of total hip arthroplasty; both components, with or without autograft or allograft

24. A					B	C	D	E	F	G	H	I	J	K
DATE(S) OF SERVICE From			To		Place of Service	Type of Service	PROCEDURES, SERVICES, OR SUPPLIES (Explain Unusual Circumstances) CPT/HCPCS | MODIFIER	DIAGNOSIS CODE	$ CHARGES	DAYS OR UNITS	EPSDT Family Plan	EMG	COB	RESERVED FOR LOCAL USE
MM	DD	YY	MM	DD	YY									
1							27134 | 53							
2														
3														
4														
5														
6														
25. FEDERAL TAX I.D. NUMBER SSN EIN							26. PATIENTIS ACCOUNT NO.	27. ACCEPT ASSIGNMENT? (For govt. claims, see back) YES NO	28. TOTAL CHARGE $	29. AMOUNT PAID $			30. BALANCE DUE $	

Rationale for Using Modifier 53

Since the procedure was immediately discontinued because the patient went into cardiac arrest, modifier 53 is appended to the planned procedure.

Example 2

A patient was in the operating room for a diagnostic arthroscopy of the knee. The physician inserted the arthroscope and the patient suddenly went into respiratory distress. The arthroscope was withdrawn and the procedure was terminated.

CPT Code(s) Billed: 29870 53—Arthroscopy, knee, diagnostic, with or without synovial biopsy (separate procedure)

Rationale for Using Modifier 53

Because the patient's medical condition caused the discontinuation of the procedure, modifier 53 would be appended to the surgical procedure code.

CMS CODING TIP

Modifier 53 is valid only when attached to a surgical code or medical diagnostic code when the procedure was started but had to be discontinued. Modifier 53 is not valid when used for elective cancellation of a procedure before anesthesia induction and/or surgical preparation in the operating suite.

Example 3

A 55-year-old woman with progressive exertional dyspnea and a history of hypertension was referred for cardiac blood pool imaging. The resting electrocardiogram was abnormal, suggesting a possible remote myocardial infarction. There was peripheral edema. After the procedure began, the patient became agitated and anxious, and the radiologist decided to discontinue the procedure because of the patient's medical history.

CPT Code(s) Billed: 78472 53—Cardiac blood pool imaging, gated equilibrium; planar, single study at rest or stress (exercise and/or pharmacologic), wall motion study plus ejection fraction, with or without additional quantitative processing

Rationale for Using Modifier 53

Since the procedure was discontinued because of the patient's agitation and anxiety after the procedure was well under way, it would be appropriate to append modifier 53 to the procedure.

Pathology and Laboratory

When this modifier is used for pathology and laboratory procedures, its usage should be verified with the insurance carrier. Many carriers do not accept usage in the Pathology and Laboratory section of CPT. It is rare that modifier 53 would be applicable in this section unless the patient is at risk.

Example 4

A 68-year-old patient scheduled for a duodenal intubation and aspiration was taken into the laboratory where the procedure was to be performed. The patient was given a local anesthetic by the physician and a tube was inserted nasally and positioned in the duodenum. Before the specimen was obtained, the patient experienced severe nausea with vomiting. The physician elected to discontinue the procedure before obtaining the specimen.

CPT Code(s) Billed: 89100 53—Duodenal intubation and aspiration; single specimen (eg, simple bile study or afferent loop culture) plus appropriate test procedure

Rationale for Using Modifier 53

Since the procedure was discontinued because the patient became ill after the procedure had begun and before the specimen was obtained, it would be appropriate to append modifier 53 to the procedure.

Example 5

A 6-year-old girl with a history of tetralogy of Fallot had previously undergone repair, which included patching of her branch pulmonary arteries for pulmonary artery stenosis. She was brought to the catheterization lab with recurrent obstruction of both branch pulmonary arteries for assessment and pulmonary angioplasty. The patient was sedated with intravenous morphine and midazolam. After hemostasis was obtained, complete hemodynamic and angiographic assessment was performed. This confirmed severe stenosis of both proximal branch pulmonary arteries. A 7F end-hole catheter was positioned in the distal left and right pulmonary arteries, and a 0.035-inch Rosen wire was positioned into the left pulmonary artery. The patient exhibited a ventricular arrhythmia on the monitor before the balloon angioplasty was performed. The cardiovascular surgeon decided to discontinue the procedure.

CPT Code(s) Billed: 92997 53—Percutaneous transluminal pulmonary artery balloon angioplasty; single vessel

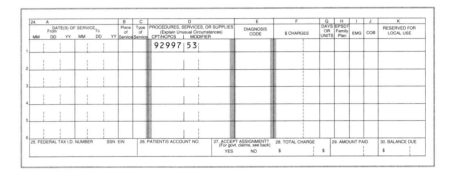

Review of Modifier 53

1   Use modifier 53 when the procedure is discontinued after anesthesia is administered to the patient.

2   Modifier 53 is valid only when attached to a surgical code or medical diagnostic code when the procedure was started but had to be discontinued because of extenuating circumstances.

3   Do not use modifier 53 when a laparoscopic or endoscopic procedure is converted to an open procedure.

4   Many insurance carriers will cover only the primary procedure with modifier 53 even if other procedures are planned.

Checkpoint Exercises 1

Select the appropriate modifier.

1   _____   A patient is scheduled for a colonoscopy for which she was given a bowel prep to be administered at home. At the time of the procedure, the prep was inadequate and the physician was unable to complete the procedure scheduled.

2 _____ A patient underwent a bilateral arthrocentesis of the knee joint in the physician's office.

3 _____ When two or more procedures are performed on the same day by the same physician at the same operative session, what modifier is appended to the secondary procedure(s)?

4 _____ What modifier indicates that a procedure is discontinued before administration of anesthesia?

5 _____ If a patient went into cardiac arrest in the operating room, after the administration of anesthesia, what modifier is appended to the CPT code?

Modifiers 54, 55, and 56

It is important when using modifiers 54, 55, and 56 to understand the definition of each modifier and how to apply them to a specific insurance carrier.

Definitions

- **Modifier 54—Surgical Care Only:** When one physician performed a surgical procedure and another provided preoperative and/or postoperative management, surgical services may be identified by adding the modifier 54 to the usual procedure number.
- **Modifier 55—Postoperative Management Only:** When one physician performed the postoperative management and another physician performed the surgical procedure, the postoperative component may be identified by adding the modifier 55 to the usual procedure number.
- **Modifier 56—Preoperative Management Only:** When one physician performed the preoperative care and evaluation and another physician performed the surgical procedure, the preoperative component may be identified by adding the modifier 56 to the usual procedure number.

The Surgery guidelines in the CPT book state that surgical procedures include the operation per se, in addition to the following:
- local infiltration, metacarpal/metatarsal/digital block, or topical anesthesia;
- subsequent to the decision for surgery, one related E/M encounter on the date immediately prior to or on the date of procedure (including history and physical);
- immediate postoperative care, including dictating operative notes and talking with the family and other physicians;
- writing orders;
- evaluating the patient in the postanesthesia recovery area; and
- typical postoperative follow-up care.

This concept is referred to as a "package" for a surgical procedure or, sometimes, as the "global surgical package" concept. Third-party payer surgical packages often vary from the AMA CPT definition. It is important to check with the third-party payer for its specific definition of a surgical package.

CMS and many third-party payers include in their definition of global physician services the following:

- Preoperative management
- Surgical procedure
- Postoperative management

Defining a Global Surgical Package: Major Surgical Procedures

A global surgical package for major surgical procedures refers to a payment policy of bundling payment for the various services associated with an operation into a single payment covering the operation and these other services, such as postoperative hospital visits. It is common practice among surgeons to bill for such global surgical packages, which generally include the immediate preoperative care, the operation itself, and the normal, typical follow-up care. Medicare carriers were allowed a wide latitude in establishing a global package, resulting in global surgery policies that varied from carrier to carrier and from service to service.

For example, about half of the carriers included preoperative care in their global surgery packages. In addition, carrier policies for the number of days included in postoperative care differed widely, from 0 to 270 days after surgery.

CMS and Global Surgical Policy

Revising Medicare's physician payment system required a nationally standardized definition of what constitutes the preoperative and postoperative time periods, as well as the specific services included in these periods. In the 1991 Final Rule, CMS identified specific services included in the global surgical package when provided by the physician who performs the surgery: preoperative visits the day before the surgery; intraoperative services that normally are a usual and necessary part of a surgical procedure; services provided by the surgeon within 90 days of the surgery that do not require a return trip to the operating room and follow-up visits provided during this time by the surgeon that are related to recovery from the surgery; and postsurgical pain management.

Each component of CMS's global surgical policy—evaluation or consultation, preoperative visits by the surgeon, intraoperative services, and postoperative period—is discussed below in further detail. Physician work relative value units for surgical services were generally based on the Harvard Resource-Based Relative Value Scale study, which included preoperative visits on the day before surgery or the day of surgery; the hospital admission workup; the primary operation; immediate postoperative care, including dictating operative notes and talking with the family and other physicians; writing orders; evaluating the patient in the recovery room; postoperative follow-up on the day of surgery; and postoperative hospital and office visits.

Third-Party Payer Guidelines for Initial Evaluation or Consultation by the Surgeon

The surgeon's initial evaluation or consultation is considered a separate service from the surgery and is paid as a distinct service, even if the decision, based on the evaluation, is not to perform the surgery. Previously, some carriers bundled the initial evaluation or consultation into the global surgery payment if it occurred within the week before the surgery and, in some cases, even within 24 hours of surgery. If the decision to perform a major surgery (surgical procedures with a 90-day global period) is made on the day of or the day before the surgery, separate payment is allowed for the visit at which the decision is made if adequate documentation is submitted with the claim demonstrating that the decision for surgery was made during a specific visit. Modifier 57 (Decision for surgery) is used to indicate that an E/M service resulted in the initial decision to perform the surgery. Modifier 57 is discussed in more detail in Chapter 5.

AMA Guidelines for Preoperative Visits by the Surgeon

According the surgical guidelines in CPT, subsequent to the decision for surgery, one related E/M encounter on the date immediately prior to or on the date of the procedure (including history and physical) is included in the surgical package. The CPT surgical package definition was revised in 2002 to add greater specificity, standardized language, and facilitate correct coding.

CMS Guidelines for Preoperative Visits by the Surgeon

CMS adopted a preoperative period that includes any visits by the surgeon, in or out of the hospital, for 1 day before the surgery. CMS emphasized that preoperative billings are carefully monitored as part of carrier postpayment review of medical necessity and a longer preoperative period may be adopted later.

CMS Guidelines for Intraoperative Services and Complications After Surgery

All intraoperative services that are normally included as a necessary part of a surgical procedure are included in the global package. If a patient develops complications after surgery that require additional medical or surgical services but do not require a return trip to the operating room, Medicare will include these services in the approved amount for the global surgery, with no separate payment made. However, if the complications require the patient's return to the operating room for any reason for care determined to be medically necessary, these services are paid separately from the global surgery amount. Modifier 78 is reported in this instance.

CMS Definition of Operating Room

CMS's definition of an operating room is "a place of service specifically equipped and staffed for the sole purpose of performing procedures. The term 'operating room' includes a cardiac catheterization suite, a laser suite, and an endoscopy suite. It does not include a patient room, a minor treatment room, a recovery room or an intensive care unit (unless the patient's condition was so critical there would be insufficient time for transportation to an operating room)."

Separate payment is allowed for treatment for complications requiring expertise beyond that of the surgeon. Full payment will be made to the physician who provides such treatment. In addition, separate payment is allowed for the following tests when performed during the global period of a major surgery: visual field (92081-92083), fundus photography (92250), and fluorescein angiography (92235).

Postoperative Services by the Surgeon

The CMS global surgery package includes a standard postoperative period of 90 days when no separate payment is made for the surgeon's visits or services.[4] Postoperative services specifically identified by CMS as part of the global package include the following:
- Dressing changes
- Local incisional care
- Removal of operative packs; removal of cutaneous sutures, staples, lines, wires, tubes, drains, casts, and splints
- Insertion, irrigation, and removal of urinary catheters
- Routine peripheral intravenous lines and nasogastric and rectal tubes
- Change and removal of tracheostomy tubes

Exceptions to the postoperative period when separate payment is allowed include the surgeon's E/M services that are unrelated to the diagnosis for which the surgery was performed. These services are paid separately by appending modifier 24 to the appropriate level of E/M service and submitting appropriate documentation.

Services provided by the surgeon for treating the underlying condition and for a subsequent course of treatment that is not part of the normal recovery from the surgery are also paid separately. CMS provides an example of a urologist who performs surgery for prostate cancer and subsequently administers chemotherapy services. The chemotherapy services would not be part of the global surgery package. When these circumstances are reported, modifier 79 should be included. Modifier 79 will be discussed in further detail in Chapter 6.

---

4. Source: Centers for Medicare and Medicaid, Global Surgical Package, Medicare Policy Manual.

Full payment for the procedure (not just the intraoperative services) is allowed for situations when distinctly separate but related procedures are performed during the global period of another surgery (eg, reconstructive and burn surgery) in which the patient is admitted to the hospital for treatment, discharged, and then readmitted for further treatment. When the decision is made prospectively or at the time of the first surgery to perform a second procedure (ie, to stage a procedure), modifier 58 (Staged or related procedure or service by the same physician during the postoperative period) should be reported.

When postoperative care after surgery is provided by a nonsurgeon for an underlying condition or medical complication, it is reported and will be considered as concurrent care and should be reported with the appropriate E/M code. The nonsurgeon should not append modifier 55 when reporting such services.

Postoperative Pain Management

CMS payment for physician services related to patient-controlled analgesia is included in the surgeon's global payment. Pain management, for example, by continuous epidural is paid by reporting CPT code 62319 on the first day of service. This code includes the catheter and injection of the anesthetic substance. Payment will be allowed by CMS for CPT code 01996 for daily management of the epidural drug administration after the day on which the catheter was introduced. Payment is not allowed for both 01996 and 62319 on the same day. The global surgical payment will be reduced if postpayment audits indicate that a surgeon's patients routinely receive pain management services from an anesthesiologist.

Duration of the Global Surgical Period

The CMS preoperative period for major surgeries is the day immediately before the day of surgery, and the postoperative period is, for example, 90 days immediately after the day of surgery. Services provided on the day of surgery but before the surgery are considered preoperative by CMS, while services furnished on the same day but after the surgery are considered postoperative.

Not included in the CMS global surgery fee are the following:
- The initial consultation or evaluation of the problem by the surgeon to determine the need for surgery
- Services of other physicians, except where the surgeon or other physician(s) agree on the transfer of care
- Treatment for any underlying condition or unrelated course of treatment not part of the surgical procedure
- Diagnostic test and procedures, including radiological procedures
- Distinct surgical procedures during the postoperative period that are not complications or reoperations (a new postoperative period begins with the subsequent procedure)

- Treatment for postoperative complications that require a return trip to the operating room, not including a recovery room, intensive care unit, or minor treatment room, unless there would be insufficient time to transport the patient to an operating room because of the patient's condition
- A more extensive procedure performed because the less extensive procedure failed (the second procedure is separately payable)
- A surgical tray (A4550) in the physician's office, for which separate payment may be made if covered by the Medicare contractor
- Critical care services (99291 and 99292) unrelated to the surgery, when a seriously injured or burned patient is critically ill and requires constant attendance by the surgeon.

CMS rules and guidelines apply to minor surgeries and endoscopies:
- Visits by the same physician on the same day as a minor surgery or endoscopy are included in the payment for the procedure, unless a separately identifiable service is also performed. For example, a visit on the same day could be properly billed in addition to a repair of the scalp, if a full neurological examination is made for a patient with head trauma.
- The postoperative period for minor surgeries and endoscopies is either 0 or 10 days. If the period is 10 days, postoperative visits or services related to the procedure that are provided within 10 days of surgery are not separately billable.
- The exception to this rule is a follow-up visit billed after a minor emergency department procedure. The visit may be allowed when the visit is in a physician's office and a physician other than the emergency department physician performs the service. In this instance, the emergency department physician is not required to split the global fee with the physician providing postoperative care. Each physician will bill the services provided with no modifiers.
- If a diagnostic biopsy with a 10-day global period precedes a major surgery on the same day or in the 10-day period, the major surgery is separately payable.
- Services by other physicians are not included in the global fee for a minor procedure.
- If the postoperative period is 0 days, postoperative visits are not included in the payment amount for the surgery. Separate payment is made in this instance.

The following CMS rules and guidelines apply when a physician furnishes less than the full global package:
- There are occasions when more than one physician provides services included in the global package. The physician who performs the surgical procedure may not always furnish the follow-up care. Payment for the postoperative, postdischarge care is split between two or more physicians when the physicians agree on the transfer of care. The sum of the amount

approved for all physicians may not exceed what would have been approved if a single physician had provided all services.

The following CMS guidelines apply in determining the duration of a global period:

- To determine the global period for major surgeries, count 1 day immediately before the day of surgery, the day of the surgery, and the 90 days immediately after the day of surgery. For example, if the date of surgery is January 5, and the last day of the postoperative period is April 5, the global period would be considered January 4 through April 5.
- To determine the global period for minor procedures, count the day of surgery and the appropriate number of days immediately after the date of surgery.

The following CMS guidelines provide coverage and billing requirements for global surgical packages that are split between two or more physicians, services not included in the global surgery fee, and guidance on the proper use of modifiers for services performed during the global period of a procedure:

- Physicians who furnish the entire global package:

    Physicians who perform the surgery and furnish all of the usual preoperative and postoperative work will be paid for the global package by entering the appropriate CPT code only.
- Physicians in a group practice:

    When different physicians in a group practice participate in the care of the patient, the group bills for the entire global package if the physicians reassign benefits to the group. The physician who performs the surgery is shown as the performing physician.
- Physicians who furnish part of a global package:

    Payment for the postoperative, postdischarge care is split between two or more physicians when the physicians agree on the transfer of care. Physicians must add the appropriate CPT code and modifier (54 or 55) to the surgical procedure code.

If a physician other than the surgeon provides preoperative care, modifier 56 should be billed with the surgery code. Services billed with modifier 56 are normally manually priced. Payment is based on the preoperative value of the global surgery fee. The date of service reported will be the date the surgical procedure was performed. Services billed with modifier 56 usually will be suspended for medical review.

NOTE: CMS requires the agreement to be in the form of a letter requesting a transfer of care, or documentation in the discharge summary of the hospital record or ASC record to indicate the transfer.

Modifiers 54, 55, and 56 do not apply to surgical procedures that have a follow-up period (global days) of 0.

For example, the surgical procedure 33400 refers to an aortic valve repair with cardiopulmonary bypass. CMS has a 90-day global period for this procedure. If the surgeon provides the surgical care only, modifier 54 would be applicable and appended to the CPT code.

- CMS in 2006 split this procedure up into three pieces, which equal 100% of the surgical package:

  Preoperative: 9%
  Intraoperative: 84%
  Postoperative: 7%

If the surgeon provided only the surgical portion of the procedure, the reimbursement would be based on 84% of the approved amount.

If a pulmonologist performs a diagnostic bronchoscopy with lavage for a Medicare patient, in the surgery department of the hospital, the global days would not apply. For example, CPT code 31624 is a bronchoscopy with bronchial alveolar lavage. The use of modifiers 54, 55, and 56 would not apply in this example because there are no preoperative or postoperative days, as this procedure has 0 global days for 2006.

> **NOTE:** Split care refers to a situation in which one physician performs a surgical procedure and another physician performs the postoperative care. Another physician rarely will perform the preoperative management.

Third-Party Payer Guidelines

Split care refers to a situation in which one physician performs a surgical procedure and another physician performs the postoperative care. Rarely, another physician will perform the preoperative management. Modifier 56 identifies the preoperative management for the procedure and is rarely accepted by third-party payers. The preoperative services are usually reported by means of the E/M codes. Third-party payer guidelines should be reviewed when modifiers 54, 55, and 56 are used. Many insurance carriers determine their own global days for many surgical procedures. The carrier's global periods should be checked when all surgical procedures are billed, including procedures performed in the office.

Following is a review of modifiers 54, 55, and 56.

Modifier 54: Surgical Care Only

This modifier is to be used when the surgeon provides the surgical care only and does not provide the preoperative and postoperative care. Modifier 54 is appended to the surgical code. The physician is paid a portion of the total procedure (global package).

Example 1

A 67-year-old woman in a rural area saw a general surgeon regarding abdominal pain. She had a history of abdominal surgery, and a strictured segment of small bowel was evident on small bowel follow-through radiographs. The general surgeon assessed the patient, ordered X rays and laboratory testing, and determined that the patient needed surgery. Since the physician did not perform this surgery, the patient was sent to a gastroenterologist. The general surgeon contacted the gastroenterologist and provided all supporting data and test results, and surgery was scheduled. The general surgeon sent a letter to the gastroenterologist requesting that he provide only the surgical portion of the surgery and stating that the general surgeon would provide the postoperative care.

Before the surgery, the gastroenterologist reviewed laboratory and X ray/imaging studies to plan the operative approach, discussed the procedure with the patient, and obtained informed consent. At operation, the small bowel was dissected. The strictured segment was mobilized and resected, and bowel continuity was reestablished. The patient was released from the hospital the next morning in good condition, and her care was transferred back to the general surgeon in her home town.

CPT Code(s) Billed by the Surgeon: 44120 54—Enterectomy, resection of small intestine; single resection and anastomosis

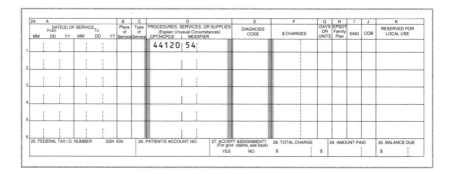

Rationale for Using Modifier 54

In this example, the surgeon only performed the surgery and then transferred care back to the general surgeon, who will provide the postoperative care. The surgeon will bill the appropriate CPT code with modifier 54 for the surgical procedure only. The modifier indicates to the carrier that only the surgical procedure was performed. This procedure has a typical 90-day global period for most carriers.

For 2006, the preoperative is 9%, the intraoperative is 81%, and the postoperative care split is 10%.

Example 2

A 62-year-old man had undergone sphincter implantation for post-prostatectomy incontinence 2 years prior. He subsequently developed edema and erythema of the scrotum, and was seen by a general surgeon. The patient had a low-grade fever but was not systemically toxic. Examination showed some scrotal edema and skin fixation. The sphincter pump was notable, palpated, and apparently fixed to the skin. The general surgeon sent the patient to a urologist in a neighboring city for the surgery. The general surgeon sent a letter with all of the supporting documentation to the urologist, who would see the patient the morning of surgery.

The urologist removed the inflatable urethra bladder neck sphincter and replaced it, inserting a pump reservoir and cuff. The infected tissue was debrided. The patient was released from the recovery room, and care was turned over to the general surgeon in the patient's home town.

> *CPT Code(s) Billed by the Surgeon: 53448 54—Removal and replacement of inflatable urethral/bladder neck sphincter including pump, reservoir, and cuff through an infected field at the same operative session including irrigation and debridement of infected tissue*

Rationale for Using Modifier 54

The surgeon performed only the surgical portion of the procedure and turned over the postoperative care to the general surgeon. This procedure has a typical 90-day global period for many carriers, including CMS. The global split for 2006 is 8% preoperative, 83% intraoperative, and 9% for the postoperative care. This physician can expect to receive 83% of the total global package.

THIRD-PARTY PAYER CODING TIP

Many insurance carriers determine their own global days for many surgical procedures. The carrier's global periods should be checked when all surgical procedures are billed, including procedures performed in the office.

Modifier 55: Postoperative Management Only

Modifier 55 is appended to the surgical procedure code when a physician provides only the postoperative surgical care. Per CMS, if the surgical CPT code has 0 global days, modifier 55 would not apply to the postoperative care. CMS guidelines state, "If the physician is providing medical care unrelated to the surgical procedure, or if the procedure is considered a minor surgical procedure with '0' global days, the global package would not apply."

When the physician is providing the postoperative care, the surgical CPT code is billed with modifier 55. The reimbursement is dependent on the percentage at which the carrier has priced or valued the procedure. When claims for CMS are billed, the global days assigned can be found on the Medicare Physician Fee Schedule Relative Value File. The file is available on the CMS Web site at www.cms.hhs.gov/PhysicianFeeSched/PFSRVF/list.asp. The information can be downloaded and is updated yearly.

For CMS, a written agreement must become part of the patient's file. Modifier 54, 55, or 56 may not be billed unless the written agreement exists. Physicians must bill the appropriate procedure code if the written agreement does not exist.

When postoperative management is billed, the dates of service must reflect the dates care was assumed and relinquished, and the units field on the CMS - 1500 reflects the total number of postoperative care days provided. The postoperative period begins the day after surgery.

Postoperative management claims should not be submitted to the carrier until the physician treating the patient sees the patient for the first time in follow-up. Surgical procedures with a 10-day global period normally allow 10 days or units of postoperative care, whereas those with a 90-day global period allow 90 days or 90 units of postoperative care.

Most carriers will deny claims that exceed the number of allowed units.

Split Care

As an example, two physicians are involved in providing the care of a surgical patient. The surgeon is providing the preoperative care and surgical procedure and the internist is providing the postoperative care. The procedure billed is 43045, *Esophagotomy, thoracic approach, with removal of foreign body*. The allowed amount for the procedure is $450.

Global Split Table

Description	Percentage	Modifier
Preoperative percentage: Surgeon	9%	56
Intraoperative percentage: Surgeon	81%	54
Postoperative percentage: Internist	10%	55
Total value of the procedure:	**100%**	

Sometimes two providers will split the postoperative care. In this case, each physician will bill for the amount of time spent providing postoperative management to the patient.

Example 1

A physician in Philadelphia was managing a patient's postoperative care for procedure code 43045. The patient's wife was transferred to Seattle and the patient moved during the 90-day global period. Another physician took over care within the global surgical period for management of the typical postoperative care.

Postoperative Days

Description	Number of Days	Modifier
Physician 1 in Philadelphia	60	55
Physician 2 in Seattle	30	55
Total value of the procedure	**90**	

Since both physicians are managing the postoperative care, each will bill the number of days that they provided the postoperative management. The reimbursement will be based on the percentage of the postoperative management, which, with this procedure code, is 10% of the total allowable fee for the procedure and will be divided on the basis of the amount of care provided to the patient. The following examples illustrate the billing.

Physician 1

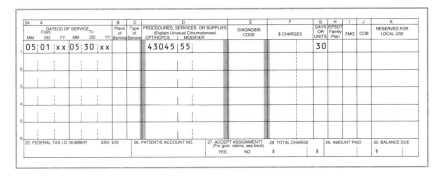

The date of service should equal the units or number of days the postoperative care was provided.

Physician 2

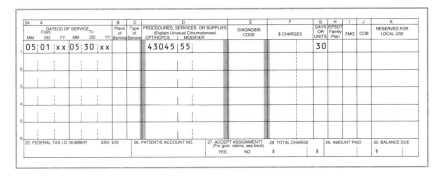

Example 2

A 70-year-old man who had had a previous cerebrovascular accident presented with esophagogastric dysmotility and repeated episodes of pulmonary aspiration. The patient required enteral feedings for long-term nutritional support. A laparoscopic jejunostomy was performed, and the patient was discharged 2 days postoperatively with instructions on wound care and enteral feeding procedures. The postoperative care was turned over to the patient's internist because the hospital where the patient had the procedure was 90 miles from his home. A letter of transfer of care had been established before the procedure was performed. The global period for this procedure is typically 90 days.

CPT Code(s) Billed by the Surgeon: 44186 54—Laparoscopy, surgical; jejunostomy (eg, for decompression or feeding)

CPT Code(s) Billed by the Internist: 44186 55—Laparoscopy, surgical; jejunostomy (eg, for decompression or feeding)

Rationale for Using Modifier 54 and Modifier 55

The surgeon performed only the operation, billed the surgical procedure with modifier 54, and turned the postoperative care over to the internist, who used modifier 55 to identify that only this portion of the service was provided.

Example 3

Eight months after surgery, a 70-year-old woman complained of diminished vision in her operated-on eye. An eye examination showed posterior capsular opacification of sufficient severity to warrant treatment. Laser surgery was performed. The patient was examined postoperatively for signs of complications and released. The patient went home with her daughter, who would care for her during the next few months. Her care was transferred to a general ophthalmologist in the daughter's city. The general ophthalmologist provided the postoperative care of the patient for the 90-day global period.

CPT Code(s) Billed by the Specialist (Surgeon): 66821 54

CPT Code(s) Billed by the General Ophthalmologist: 66821 55—for the postoperative management

66821   Discission of secondary membranous cataract (opacified posterior lens capsule and/or anterior hyaloid); laser surgery (eg, YAG laser) (one or more stages)

Diagnosis Code: 366.53—After-cataract, obscuring vision

21. DIAGNOSIS OR NATURE OF ILLNESS OR INJURY. (RELATE ITEMS 1,2,3 OR 4 TO ITEM 24E BY LINE)									22. MEDICAID RESUBMISSION CODE		ORIGINAL REF. NO.	

1. 366.53   3. └──.──
                                                         23. PRIOR AUTHORIZATION NUMBER
2. └──.──   4. └──.──

24.	A					B	C	D			E	F	G	H	I	J	K
	From DATE(S) OF SERVICE To					Place of Service	Type of Service	PROCEDURES, SERVICES, OR SUPPLIES (Explain Unusual Circumstances) CPT/HCPCS | MODIFIER			DIAGNOSIS CODE	$ CHARGES	DAYS OR UNITS	EPSDT Family Plan	EMG	COB	RESERVED FOR LOCAL USE
	MM	DD	YY	MM	DD	YY											
1	01	11	xx	04	11	xx			66821	55		1		90				
2																		
3																		
4																		
5																		
6																		

25. FEDERAL TAX I.D. NUMBER	SSN EIN	26. PATIENTIS ACCOUNT NO.	27. ACCEPT ASSIGNMENT? (For govt. claims, see back) YES NO	28. TOTAL CHARGE $	29. AMOUNT PAID $	30. BALANCE DUE $

Rationale for Using Modifier 55

Since the general ophthalmologist does not perform surgery but is providing the postoperative care, modifier 55 would be appropriate. Procedure code 66821 has a preoperative value of 10%, intraoperative value of 70%, and postoperative value of 20%. The physician providing the postoperative care can expect to receive 20% of the global procedure.

Modifier 56: Preoperative Management Only

Modifier 56 identifies a situation in which one physician provides the preoperative management and another physician performs the surgery. Another possibility might be that the surgeon provides the preoperative management along with the procedure and another physician assumes the postoperative care. In rural areas, sometimes the preoperative and postoperative management are provided by the patient's physician, and the patient may travel to a larger city for the surgical procedure.

It is important for each physician to have a clear understanding of the role they are to play in the patient care. The surgeon must supply the physician providing the preoperative and/or postoperative care with the appropriate CPT code in order to correctly report the services.

When splitting care, the physician who provides the preoperative care will append modifier 56 to the surgical procedure code. Modifier 56 usually is not used with claims for CMS. Many third-party payers will not accept the use of modifier 56. Modifier 56 is limited to surgical procedures only.

Typically for many payers, services billed with modifier 56 are manually priced. Payment is based on the preoperative value of the global surgery fee. The date of service reported will be the date the surgical procedure was performed. Services billed with modifier 56 will suspend for medical review in many cases.

Example 1

A 55-year-old man complained of a large uncomfortable bulge in his left groin. He had undergone an aortobifemoral bypass graft 20 years earlier.

The current examination showed an 8-cm pulsatile mass under the femoral incision of the previous operation. There was no tenderness or erythema. On a computed tomographic scan, it appeared that the old graft limb had pulled away from the femoral artery, resulting in a false aneurysm. The aortic and right femoral anastomoses of the graft were normal. The physician sent the patient to a hospital in a nearby city because the hospital in their small town did not have the appropriate facilities to perform the procedure. The physician contacted a cardiovascular surgeon to perform the procedures. Results of the preoperative history and physical examination and a written transfer of care were sent to the surgeon. The surgeon reconstructed the anastomosis by means of a short segment of synthetic conduit and provided the postoperative care to the patient.

CPT Code(s) Billed by the Physician: 35141 56

24.	A				B	C	D		E	F	G	H	I	J	K
	DATE(S) OF SERVICE				Place	Type	PROCEDURES, SERVICES, OR SUPPLIES		DIAGNOSIS		DAYS	EPSDT			RESERVED FOR
	From		To		of	of	(Explain Unusual Circumstances)		CODE	$ CHARGES	OR	Family	EMG	COB	LOCAL USE
	MM DD YY	MM DD YY			Service	Service	CPT/HCPCS	MODIFIER			UNITS	Plan			
1							35141	56							
2															
3															
4															
5															
6															
25. FEDERAL TAX I.D. NUMBER		SSN EIN		26. PATIENT'S ACCOUNT NO.			27. ACCEPT ASSIGNMENT? (For govt. claims, see back) YES NO		28. TOTAL CHARGE $		29. AMOUNT PAID $				30. BALANCE DUE $

CPT Code(s) Billed by the Surgeon: 35141 54, 35141 55

35141   Direct repair of aneurysm, pseudoaneurysm, or excision (partial or total) and graft insertion, with or without patch graft; for aneurysm, pseudoaneurysm, and associated occlusive disease, common femoral artery (profunda femoris, superficial femoral)

Rationale for Using Modifier 56

Because the physician who sent the patient to the nearby hospital is providing preoperative management, appending modifier 56 to the surgical code for the physician is appropriate. This is identified as split care since the surgeon is providing the surgery and the postoperative care. Based on the global days concept, this procedure has a 90-day global with the procedure split of preoperative care 9%, intraoperative care (surgery) 84%, and postoperative care at 7%. The surgeon will report the surgical procedure code with modifiers 54 (surgical care only) and 55 for the postoperative care. The physician providing the preoperative should expect to receive 9% of the total value of the procedure code.

Example 2

A 70-year-old, right-handed, male smoker had disabling right arm pain with exercise. The patient's cardiologist found that no pulses were palpable at the right brachial, radial, or ulnar positions. An aortogram revealed a critical stenosis of the distal axillary and brachial arteries.

The cardiologist consulted with a cardiovascular surgeon, who agreed to perform only the surgery and postoperative care, and not the preoperative history and physical examination. The cardiologist performed the preoperative history, physical examination, and appropriate tests. The patient underwent an endarterectomy performed through an axillary and arm incision by the cardiovascular surgeon.

CPT Code(s) Billed by the Cardiologist: 35321 56

CPT Code(s) Billed by the Cardiovascular Surgeon: 35321 54, 55

35321   Thromboendarterectomy, with or without patch graft; axillary-brachial

Rationale for Using Modifier 56

The cardiologist does not perform this type of surgery, so the patient is sent to the cardiovascular surgeon. The cardiovascular surgeon indicates that the preoperative work should be done by the cardiologist, who performs the necessary examination and testing. The cardiologist may expect 9% for the preoperative service, while the surgeon who performed the procedure would receive 84% of the global fee for the surgery and 7% for providing the postoperative care.

Review of Modifiers 54, 55, and 56

1 Check with the insurance carrier to determine whether these modifiers are recognized.

2 Append modifiers 54, 55, and 56 only to the surgical procedures codes.

3 Many third-party payers specify that modifiers 54, 55, and 56 must be appended to surgical procedures that have more than 0 global days.

4 When these modifiers are used for CMS, a request of transfer of care must be available in the patient's records.

5 When providing the postoperative management, make sure the number of days the management was provided is listed in the units column on the claim form and that the dates of service equal the global days.

6 Bill for the postoperative management only after the patient is seen initially in follow-up.

7 Check with insurance carriers for the percentage of reimbursement for the preoperative, intraoperative, and postoperative care.

Checkpoint Exercises 2

Fill in the blanks.

1 Local infiltration, metacarpal/metatarsal/digital block, or topical anesthesia is part of the _____ _____.

2 When a surgeon provides only the surgical care, the applicable CPT code for the procedure is appended with modifier _____.

3 When a physician provides postoperative management of the patient, a request of transfer of care must be available in the _____ _____.

4 The modifier used for preoperative management is _____.

5 The three parts of the global surgical procedure are: _____, _____, and _____.

Test Your Knowledge

True or False

1. _____ The narrative for modifier 52 indicates that fees should be reduced.

2. _____ Modifier 55 is used to indicate only the preoperative management of the patient.

3. _____ Modifier 50 indicates that multiple procedures were performed on the same day.

4. _____ A physician began a surgical procedure and the patient went into respiratory distress. The physician used modifier 53 to indicate that the procedure was discontinued.

5. _____ When a patient's postoperative management is provided by a physician, an E/M service is used instead of a modifier.

6. _____ The modifier for reporting bilateral procedure is modifier 51.

7. _____ Modifier 54 is used to report the postoperative management.

Fill in the Blanks

8. _____ The patient was seen and evaluated by a general surgeon 100 miles away at the nearest hospital. The surgeon performed the surgery. The patient returned home and all follow-up care was rendered by the primary care physician. What modifier should the primary care physician use?

9. _____ A surgeon attempted to excise a deep vascular malformation of the hand. The surgeon was unable to completely excise it secondary to entrapment of other structures, and the procedure was terminated. What modifier should be used?

10. _____ If a patient had multiple procedures during the same operative session, what modifier would be added to the lesser of the two codes?

11. _____ This modifier can be listed as a one-line item or a two-line item, depending on the carrier.

12. _____ A physician excised a 0.6-cm benign lesion on a patient's face and also a 0.7-cm lesion on the nose. What modifier would be appended to the secondary procedure?

13. _____ In the CPT guidelines for multiple repairs, when more than one classification of wound(s) is repaired, what modifier is appended to the second procedure?

14 _____ A 49-year-old male with a body mass index (BMI) of 55 kg/m^2 presented with a history of Type II diabetes controlled with three oral hypoglycemic medications, and hypertension controlled with two medications. Family and diet history confirmed morbid obesity. The patient was taken to the operating room and underwent a laparoscopic gastric restrictive procedure with gastric bypass and Roux-en Y gastroenterostomy. Anesthesia was administered, and during the procedure, the patient went into cardiac arrest. The physician elected to discontinue the procedure and to stabilize the patient. What modifier should be appended to the procedure?

15 _____ A middle-aged, alcoholic patient with bleeding esophageal varices underwent a diagnostic flexible esophagoscopy. The procedure could not be completed due to an obstruction. The procedure is reported with what modifier?

CHAPTER 5

Modifiers 57 to 63

Modifier 57: Decision for Surgery

Definition

An evaluation and management service that resulted in the initial decision to perform the surgery may be identified by adding the modifier 57 to the appropriate level of E/M service.

AMA Guidelines

 Modifier 57 was added to the CPT® code set nomenclature in 1994 and is used when an evaluation and management (E/M) service results in the initial decision to perform a surgical procedure. Modifier 57 allows separate payment for the visit at which the decision to perform the surgery was made, if adequate documentation is available demonstrating that the decision for surgery was made during a specific visit.

CMS Guidelines

CMS defines a major surgery as a procedure with global days of 90 and a minor surgery as a procedure with 0 to 10 days or endoscopies.

Chapter 4 identified the global surgical package for CMS. This package includes preoperative visits after the decision is made to operate beginning with the day before the day of surgery for major procedures and the day of surgery for minor procedures.

Modifier 57 should be appended to an E/M code only when that E/M service represents the initial decision to perform a major surgical procedure.

Modifier 57 should not be used with E/M visits furnished during the global period of minor procedures (0–10 global days) unless the purpose of the visit is a decision for major surgery. No separate documentation is required for the use of this modifier when the claim form is submitted.

One service not included in the global surgical package is the initial consultation or evaluation of the problem by the surgeon to determine the need for a major procedure. Keep in mind that as stated in Chapter 4, CMS's policy only applies to major procedures with 90-day global; the initial evaluation is always included in the allowance for a minor surgical procedure.

Third-Party Payer Guidelines

If a CPT code is submitted with modifier 57, then the E/M service is allowed separately from the procedure code. This applies to all surgery codes for many third-party payers. Office notes are sometimes required when this modifier is billed. Claims may be reviewed to determine whether the E/M service resulted in the decision for surgery.

Because this modifier is informational, there is no increase in fees for its use. Rather, the modifier assists in recouping payment for this visit because many payers will reimburse for the visit at which surgery is decided, but will not pay for other preoperative visits. This modifier should indicate to the payer that additional time and effort were necessary and that all necessary counseling, including risks and outcomes, was provided to the patient. Individual carriers should be consulted to determine the specific definition of what is considered a minor procedure. Many third-party payers have different policies and guidelines for using modifier 57.

Example 1

A physician was consulted to determine whether surgery was necessary for a 72-year-old Medicare patient with severe abdominal pain. The physician services met the criteria necessary to report a consultation, including documented findings, and the consulting physician communicated with the requesting physician. The consulting physician documented a 99244 consultation. The requesting physician agreed with the consultant's findings and requested that the consultant take over the case and discuss his findings with the patient. The patient consented to undergo surgery to repair a perforated ulcer; the operation was performed later that same day. The procedure planned, on the basis of the findings, was 44602 Suture of small intestine (enterorrhaphy) for perforated ulcer, diverticulum, wound, injury or rupture; single perforation. The global period, based on CMS guidelines, was 90 days for this planned procedure.

CPT Code(s) Billed: *99244 57—Office consultation for a new or established patient, which requires these three key components: a comprehensive history; a comprehensive examination; and medical decision making of moderate complexity*

44602—Suture of small intestine (enterorrhaphy) for perforated ulcer, diverticulum, wound, injury, or rupture; single perforation

24.	A DATE(S) OF SERVICE						B Place of Service	C Type of Service	D PROCEDURES, SERVICES, OR SUPPLIES (Explain Unusual Circumstances) CPT/HCPCS | MODIFIER	E DIAGNOSIS CODE	F $ CHARGES	G DAYS OR UNITS	H EPSDT Family Plan	I EMG	J COB	K RESERVED FOR LOCAL USE
	From MM	DD	YY	To MM	DD	YY										
1									99244 | 57							
2									44602							
3																
4																
5																
6																
25. FEDERAL TAX I.D. NUMBER SSN EIN							26. PATIENT'S ACCOUNT NO.		27. ACCEPT ASSIGNMENT? (For govt. claims, see back) YES NO	28. TOTAL CHARGE $		29. AMOUNT PAID $		30. BALANCE DUE $		

Rationale for Using Modifier 57

To code this, the surgeon reports the E/M services (consultation) by means of the appropriate consultation code and appends modifier 57. The surgeon also reports the appropriate code for the surgery (without a modifier) in addition to the E/M service, since both services were performed on the same day. It is incorrect to append modifier 25 to the consultation code for the decision to perform surgery. Appending modifier 57 to the consultation described above indicates to the insurance carrier that the consultation is not part of the global surgical procedure.

Example 2

A patient with coronary artery disease who was well known to the cardiologist was seen for the patient's annual visit. The patient had not seen the cardiologist for the past year. After performing a comprehensive history and detailed examination, the cardiologist determined that the patient would benefit from a valve replacement and scheduled surgery for the following day. The patient was counseled for 15 minutes regarding treatment options, risks, and projected outcomes. The procedure planned was a valvuloplasty, mitral valve, with cardiopulmonary bypass (33425).

CPT Code(s) Billed: *99214 57—Office or other outpatient visit for the evaluation and management of an established patient, which requires at least two of these three key components: a detailed history; a detailed examination; and medical decision making of moderate complexity*

Rationale for Using Modifier 57

Since the decision to perform the major procedure (33425), which has a typical 90-day global period, was made during a regular visit, the E/M service (99214) should not be considered part of the global surgical package. Modifier 57 should be appended to the code for the E/M service.

Example 3

A 67-year-old woman was referred to an ophthalmologist because of complaints of vision problems. Examination showed that a cataract in her right eye had matured to the point of visual impairment. She had difficulty reading and had recently failed a driving test. The physician performed a comprehensive ophthalmic examination and determined, after evaluation and testing, that the patient would benefit from cataract surgery, which was scheduled for the next morning. The cataract surgery was performed and an intraocular lens was implanted. Recovery was monitored and the patient was sent home with an appointment for follow-up.

CPT Code(s) Billed: *92004 57—Ophthalmological services: medical examination and evaluation with initiation of diagnostic and treatment program; comprehensive, new patient, one or more visits*

Surgical Code(s) Billed: *66984—Extracapsular cataract removal with insertion of intraocular lens prosthesis (one stage procedure), manual or mechanical technique (eg, irrigation and aspiration or phacoemulsification)*

Rationale for Using Modifier 57

To code this, the surgeon reports the E/M service by means of the appropriate E/M code and appends modifier 57. The surgeon also reports the appropriate code for the surgery (without a modifier) in addition to the E/M service.

Example 4

A 63-year-old man was referred to a surgeon for evaluation because of painless jaundice and anorexia, 9 kg weight loss, and evidence on a computed tomographic scan of a 2.5 cm mass in the head of the pancreas. There was marked dilation of the extrahepatic and intrahepatic biliary ductal system with no evidence of cholelithiasis or choledo-cholithiasis. There was no evidence of lymphadenopathy or hepatic metastasis. A comprehensive history and examination were performed, and the physician determined that a biopsy of the pancreas was indicated immediately. Surgery was scheduled for the same day. Risks and benefits were explained to the patient, and he was sent to the hospital for admission.

The surgeon performed the procedure the same afternoon. During the surgery, a biopsy of the head of the pancreas (ie, transduodenal core needle) confirmed a diagnosis of carcinoma of the head of the pancreas. There was no evidence of nodal or hepatic metastasis. A modified Whipple procedure was done with preservation of the pyloric sphincter. The patient tolerated the procedure well.

CPT Code(s) Billed: 99205 57—Office or other outpatient visit for the evaluation and management of a new patient, which requires these three key components: a comprehensive history; a comprehensive examination; and medical decision making of high complexity

Surgical Code(s) Billed: 48153—Pancreatectomy, proximal subtotal with near-total duodenectomy, choledochoenterostomy and duodenojejunostomy (pylorus-sparing, Whipple-type procedure); with pancreatojejunostomy

24.	A						B	C	D		E	F	G	H	I	J	K
	From DATE(S) OF SERVICE To						Place of Service	Type of Service	PROCEDURES, SERVICES, OR SUPPLIES (Explain Unusual Circumstances) CPT/HCPCS | MODIFIER		DIAGNOSIS CODE	$ CHARGES	DAYS OR UNITS	EPSDT Family Plan	EMG	COB	RESERVED FOR LOCAL USE
	MM	DD	YY	MM	DD	YY											
1									99205 |57								
2									48153								
3																	
4																	
5																	
6																	
25. FEDERAL TAX I.D. NUMBER				SSN EIN			26. PATIENTIS ACCOUNT NO.		27. ACCEPT ASSIGNMENT? (For govt. claims, see back) YES NO		28. TOTAL CHARGE $		29. AMOUNT PAID $			30. BALANCE DUE $	

The biopsy of the pancreas would not be reported separately, since it was performed at the same time as the therapeutic procedure and is considered included in the therapeutic procedure.

Rationale for Using Modifier 57

The patient was evaluated and the decision to perform the procedure with a 90-day global period was made the same day. This would not be considered part of the global surgical package, and modifier 57 should be appended to the E/M service (99205).

Example 5

A 68-year-old Medicare patient presented to the ED following an auto accident. The ED physician performed a history and examined the patient. The physician then called in a surgeon to consult. The surgeon saw the patient in the ED. He performed a detailed history and a comprehensive exam. Medical decision was of high complexity. During the course of the workup, the physician determined the patient had a ruptured spleen, and the patient was taken to the OR for emergency surgery to repair the spleen (38115). The consultant reported the E/M service with consultation code 99243. The procedure has a 90-day global.

CPT Code(s) Billed: 99243 57—Office consultation for a new or established patient, which requires these three components: a detailed history; a detailed examination; and medical decision making of low complexity

Rationale for using Modifier 57

Because the procedure is a major procedure with a 90-day global for CMS, modifier 57 would be appended to the surgeon's consultation, which was an evaluation to determine if surgery was indicated.

Review of Modifier 57

1   Modifier 57 is used only with an E/M service.

2   For most payers, modifier 57 is appended to the E/M service only when a procedure with a 90-day global period is planned when the decision for surgery is made.

3   For CMS, modifier 57 is used when a surgical procedure with a 90-day global period is planned and performed the same day or the next day.

4   For most payers, modifier 57 is not used when surgery is scheduled for a date in the future (eg, 2 weeks, 3 months).

5   Modifier 57 is not appended to the E/M service for CMS claims when the global surgical procedure has a global period of 0 to 10 days. The global surgical package does not include the day before surgery for minor

surgical procedures (with a global period of less than 90 days) unless the purpose of the visit was the decision for surgery.

6 For most payers, modifier 25 is used when the decision is made on the same day to perform a minor surgical procedure with a global period of 0 to 10 days.

7 Each individual insurance carrier should be consulted regarding the specific criteria for billing the E/M service with modifier 57.

Modifier 58: Staged or Related Procedure or Service by the Same Physician During the Postoperative Period

Definition

The physician may need to indicate that the performance of a procedure or service during the postoperative period was: (a) planned prospectively at the time of the original procedure (staged); (b) more extensive than the original procedure; or (c) for therapy following a diagnostic surgical procedure. This circumstance may be reported by adding the modifier 58 to the staged or related procedure. **Note:** This modifier is not used to report the treatment of a problem that requires a return to the operating room. See modifier 78.

AMA Guidelines

Modifier 58 was added to the CPT code set nomenclature in 1994. This modifier is used to report a staged or related procedure by the same physician during the postoperative period of the first procedure. At times, it may become necessary for a surgeon to perform one procedure and then, during the postoperative period associated with the original procedure, perform a procedure that is "staged" or related. Modifier 58 is appended to the procedure code for a second procedure performed by the initial surgeon or provider during the postoperative period of the original procedure that falls into one of three categories:

- Planned prospectively at the time of the original procedure (staged)
- More extensive than the original procedure
- Therapy following a diagnostic surgical procedure

This circumstance may be reported by adding the modifier 58 to the staged or related procedure. Use this modifier only during the global surgical period for the original procedure.

CMS Guidelines

Modifier 58 is not used to report the treatment of a problem that requires a return to the operating room. Modifiers 78 and 79 are the modifiers used to return to the operating room for either a related or unrelated procedure by the same or a different physician. These modifiers will be reviewed in Chapter 6.

If a diagnostic biopsy precedes the major surgery performed on the same day or in the postoperative period of the biopsy, modifier 58 should be reported with the major surgical procedure code, for which full payment is allowed (eg, mastectomy within 10 days of a needle biopsy). In addition, if a less extensive procedure fails and a more extensive procedure is required, the second procedure should be reported with modifier 58. If the less extensive procedure and the more extensive procedure are performed as staged procedures, the second procedure should be reported with modifier 58.

Third-Party Payer Guidelines

Most third-party payers recognize the use of modifier 58 when it is billed as part of the global surgical package (during the global days). It is important, however, to have a good understanding of the number of global days for the procedure(s) billed.

The National Correct Coding Initiative and Modifier 58

The National Correct Coding Initiative (NCCI) states as follows:

> If a procedure is planned prospectively, because it was more extensive than the original procedure or service during the postoperative period or because it represents therapy after a diagnostic procedure, modifier 58 may be appended to the second procedure during the postoperative period. This may be because it was planned prospectively, because it was more extensive than the original procedure or because it represents therapy after a diagnostic procedural service. When an endoscopic procedure is performed for diagnostic purposes at the time of a more comprehensive therapeutic procedure, and the endoscopic procedure does not represent "scout" endoscopy, modifier 58 may be appropriately used to signify that the endoscopic procedure and the more comprehensive therapeutic procedure are staged or planned procedures.

From the NCCI perspective, this action would result in the allowance and reporting of both services as separate and distinct. A new postoperative period begins with each subsequent procedure.

Example 1

A surgeon performed a radical mastectomy (19200) on a 56-year-old woman. The patient indicated that she preferred a permanent prosthesis after the surgical wound healed. The surgeon took the patient back to the operating room during the postoperative global period and inserted a permanent prosthesis.

THIRD-PARTY PAYER CODING TIP

If the physician does not append modifier 58, a third-party payer could reject the claim because the surgery occurred during the global period associated with the mastectomy. The global period is dependent on the insurance carrier's policy. Most carriers, including Medicare, have a 90-day global period for mastectomies.

24.	A					B	C	D	E	F	G	H	I	J	K
	From DATE(S) OF SERVICE To					Place of Service	Type of Service	PROCEDURES, SERVICES, OR SUPPLIES (Explain Unusual Circumstances) CPT/HCPCS | MODIFIER	DIAGNOSIS CODE	$ CHARGES	DAYS OR UNITS	EPSDT Family Plan	EMG	COB	RESERVED FOR LOCAL USE
	MM	DD	YY	MM	DD	YY										
1									11970 | 58							
2																
3																
4																
5																
6																

25. FEDERAL TAX I.D. NUMBER	SSN EIN	26. PATIENTIS ACCOUNT NO.	27. ACCEPT ASSIGNMENT? (For govt. claims, see back) YES NO	28. TOTAL CHARGE $	29. AMOUNT PAID $	30. BALANCE DUE $

CPT Code(s) Billed: 11970 58—Replacement of tissue expander with permanent prosthesis

Rationale for Using Modifier 58

The surgeon, in this case, reports the code for the permanent prosthesis insertion with modifier 58 to indicate that the service was related to the mastectomy (staged to occur at a time after the initial surgery). If the physician did not append modifier 58, a third-party payer could reject the claim because the surgery occurred during the global period associated with the mastectomy.

Example 2

A surgeon performed a choroidal neovascularization (G0186) on a Medicare patient by means of a photocoagulation technique. Because of the size and location of the lesions, the physician accomplished the procedure in three operative sessions on 3 separate days.

CPT Code(s) Billed: G0186—Destruction of localized lesion choroid (for example, choroidal neovascularization); photocoagulation, feeder vessel technique (one or more sessions)

Rationale for Not Using Modifier 58

Because the code descriptor indicates one or more sessions, modifier 58 would not be applicable. Even if the service takes two sessions to complete the procedure, G0186 is used only once.

Example 3

A diabetic patient with advanced circulatory problems had three gangrenous toes removed from her left foot (28820, 28820 51, 28820 51). During the postoperative period it became necessary to amputate the patient's left foot.

CPT Code(s) Billed: 28805 58—Amputation, foot; transmetatarsal

Rationale for Using Modifier 58

To report this, modifier 58 would be appended to the code for the amputation of the foot. Because there was a possibility, in light of the patient's condition, that amputation might be necessary, this is considered a staged procedure.

Example 4

A patient underwent a colectomy and surgery that required a return to the operating room to stop postoperative bleeding. Surgery was performed to explore for postoperative hemorrhage.

CPT Code(s) Billed: 35840—*Exploration for postoperative hemorrhage, thrombosis or infection; abdomen*

Rationale for Not Using Modifier 58

Since this procedure is a complication of the original procedure (44140), the postoperative hemorrhage would be reported with modifier 78 appended; modifier 58 would not be used. Modifier 78 is appended to procedures that are performed during the postoperative period when a patient was required to return to the operating room for a cause directly related to the performance of the initial operation.

Example 5

A patient with squamous cell carcinoma underwent Mohs micrographic surgery, which was completed in two stages.

CPT Code(s) Billed: 17304—*Chemosurgery (Mohs micrographic technique), including removal of all gross tumor, surgical excision of tissue specimens, mapping, color coding of specimens, microscopic examination of specimens by the surgeon, and complete histopathologic preparation including the first routine stain (eg, hematoxylin and eosin, toluidine blue); first stage, fresh tissue technique, up to 5 specimens*

17305—*Chemosurgery (Mohs micrographic technique) including removal of all gross tumor, surgical excision of tissue specimens, mapping, color coding of specimens, microscopic examination of specimens by the surgeon, and complete histopathologic preparation including the first routine stain (eg, hematoxylin and eosin, toluidine blue); second stage, fixed or fresh tissue, up to 5 specimens*

Rationale for Not Using Modifier 58

Since the description of the procedure indicates that the procedure is staged, modifier 58 should not be appended.

Example 6

A 23-year-old woman had sustained full-thickness burns of her scalp and had undergone primary reconstruction with a split-thickness skin graft. Three weeks after initial treatment, the defect was to be reconstructed with tissue expansion of hair-bearing scalp, and the patient had achieved full expansion. At operation, an incision was made and the tissue expander was removed (separate CPT code, 11971). The residual scalp skin after expansion was designed and tailored to fit the previous skin graft. This skin graft was removed. The flap was rotated and/or advanced into position and the wound was closed.

CPT Code(s) Billed: **15572 58**—*Formation of direct or tubed pedicle, with or without transfer; scalp, arms, or legs*

11971 58 51—*Removal of tissue expander(s) without insertion of prosthesis*

Rationale for Using Modifier 58

Because this procedure is planned after the initial burn debridement, it would be appropriate to bill the skin grafting with modifier 58.

Example 7

On June 20, a 57-year-old female presented to a surgeon after having a routine mammogram, which showed a 1.5-cm ill-defined mass in the left breast, and an ultrasound, in which the mass was found to be heterogeneous and solid. A histological diagnosis was indicated. In order to more accurately discuss her diagnosis and treatment options, the decision was made, with the patient's consent, to perform an image-guided percutaneous needle core breast biopsy the same day. The skin was prepped with an appropriate surgical antiseptic solution. The skin was anesthetized using 1% xylocaine, using a 10-ml disposable syringe and a 1½ inch long 25-gauge hypodermic needle. A small puncture incision was made with a no. 11 scalpel. During the course of the procedure more anesthetic was injected into the deeper portions of the breast to help alleviate discomfort. The biopsy needle was advanced into the breast to the front of the lesion under ultrasound visualization. Meticulous care was taken to assure that the biopsy needle was accurately positioned. After proper position was obtained, multiple cores of tissue were removed. Hemostasis was obtained with manual compression over the biopsy site for 5 to 10 minutes. A dressing was applied. The patient was released in good condition from the outpatient surgery department of the hospital.

The pathology report indicated a malignancy, and the patient was returned to the operating room 5 days later on June 25 for a lumpectomy, followed by accelerated partial breast irradiation to treat the newly diagnosed early-stage cancer. She had no prior history of breast cancer treated by lumpectomy and radiation in the same breast. At the conclusion of the patient's lumpectomy, surgical techniques were employed to maintain a skin spacing distance of 5 to 7 mm between the lumpectomy cavity and the skin surface. The surgeon's clinical judgment, combined with immediate specimen evaluation, indicated that the tissue margins surrounding the lumpectomy cavity were free of cancerous cells, and a sentinel node biopsy or axillary dissection was negative in its findings. Using imaging guidance, a radiotherapy afterloading balloon catheter was placed into the breast for future interstitial radioelement application.

CPT Code(s) Billed, June 20: 19102—Biopsy of breast; percutaneous, needle core, using imaging guidance

76942—Ultrasonic guidance for needle placement (eg, biopsy, aspiration, injection, localization device), imaging supervision and interpretation

CPT Code(s) Billed, June 25: 19160 58—Mastectomy, partial (eg, lumpectomy, tylectomy, quadrantectomy, segmentectomy)

19297 58—Placement of radiotherapy afterloading balloon catheter into the breast for interstitial radioelement application following partial mastectomy, includes imaging guidance; concurrent with partial mastectomy (List separately in addition to code for primary procedure)

Rationale for Using Modifier 58

The first procedure involved a breast biopsy using imaging guidance reported with 19102 and 76942 for the ultrasonic guidance. CPT code 19102 has a 10-day global period. Since the possibility of further surgical intervention was possible because of the suspected malignancy, using modifier 58 with CPT code 19160 indicated that the procedure was a therapeutic procedure following a diagnostic procedure. In addition, code 19297 is reported for the placement of the balloon catheter with modifier 58.

Review of Modifier 58

1 A new postoperative period begins when the next procedure is billed.

2 Modifier 58 is not used for staged procedures when the description of the code indicates "one or more visits or one or more sessions."

3 Modifier 58 is not to be used when treatment of a problem that requires a return to the operating room is reported.

4 Modifier 58 indicates that the procedure was planned prospectively because it was more extensive than the original procedure or represents a therapeutic or diagnostic procedure or service.

5 For most payers, modifier 58 is to be used only when there is a global period appended to the CPT code for all carriers.

Checkpoint Exercises 1

Select the correct modifier.

1 _____ This modifier is used when the procedure is planned during or after the initial procedure or service.

2 _____ This modifier is used when the decision for surgery is made.

3 _____ A 46-year-old woman had a modified radical mastectomy for invasive carcinoma of the right breast. She simultaneously had a transverse rectus abdominus myocutaneous flap reconstruction of the right breast. Two months later, the reconstructed breast was symmetrical but lacked a nipple and areola. A nipple and areola graft on the right breast was planned. The patient was measured in the standing position to determine the location of the nipple and areola on the right breast. With the patient under local anesthesia, a skin flap was elevated at the site selected for the nipple reconstruction and a full-thickness skin graft was taken from the right groin to reconstruct the areola. The right groin donor site was closed primarily.

4 _____ A patient visited her ear, nose, and throat physician with complaints of recurrent acute sinusitis. The physician ordered a computed tomographic scan, which demonstrated opacities in the anterior ethmoid cells, abnormalities in the ipsilateral maxillary sinus, and/or associated anatomic abnormalities of the middle turbinate. Polyps might have been present. Risks and benefits of the procedure were explained to the patient and the surgery was performed the next day. The surgery involved removal of anterior ethmoid cells and polyps, opening of the

OMC, resection of concha bullosa, and discussion of postoperative results and care.

5 _____ This modifier is used when a physician performs an evaluation and makes a decision for surgery performed on the same day for a Medicare patient. The global period for the procedure is 90 days.

Modifier 59: Distinct Procedural Service

Definition

Under certain circumstances, the physician may need to indicate that a procedure or service was distinct or independent from other services performed on the same day. Modifier 59 is used to identify procedures/services that are not normally reported together, but are appropriate under the circumstances. This may represent a different session or patient encounter, different procedure or surgery, different site or organ system, separate incision/excision, separate lesion, or separate injury (or area of injury in extensive injuries) not ordinarily encountered or performed on the same day by the same physician. However, when another already established modifier is appropriate, it should be used rather than modifier 59. Only if no more descriptive modifier is available, and the use of modifier 59 best explains the circumstances, should modifier 59 be used.

AMA Guidelines

cpt In January 1996, CMS introduced the GB modifier. This modifier was created to clearly designate instances when distinct and separate multiple services are provided to a patient on a single date of service. In the 1997 edition of the CPT book, modifier 59 was added to be used for the same purpose. Modifier 59 was intended to clearly designate instances when distinct and separate multiple services are provided to a patient on a single date of service.

Not all multiple procedures performed at the same operative session are the same. They may be within the same incision, within the same field, and/or in different fields.

Under certain circumstances, the physician may need to indicate that a procedure or service was distinct or independent from other services performed on the same day. Modifier 59 is used to identify procedures or services that are not normally reported together, but are appropriate under the circumstances. This may represent any of the following:

- A different session or patient encounter
- A different procedure or surgery
- A different site or organ system
- A separate incision or excision
- A separate lesion
- A separate injury (or area of injury in extensive injuries) not ordinarily encountered or performed on the same day by the same physician

However, when another already established modifier is appropriate, it should be used rather than modifier 59. Only if no more descriptive modifier is available, and the use of modifier 59 best explains the circumstances, should modifier 59 be used.

As the code descriptor indicates, some examples of common uses of the modifier 59 may include separate sessions or patient encounters, different procedures or surgeries, surgery directed to different sites or organ systems, surgery directed to a separate incision/excision or separate lesions, or treatment to separate injuries.

Separate Procedure

Coinciding with the addition of CPT modifier 59, some CPT codes were designated as "separate procedures." Some of the procedures or services listed in the CPT nomenclature that are commonly carried out as an integral component of a total service or procedure have been identified by including the term "separate procedure." The codes designated as separate procedures should not be reported in addition to the code for the total procedure or service of which it is considered an integral component.

However, it is important to consider that when a procedure or service designated as a separate procedure is carried out independently, or considered to be unrelated or distinct from other procedures or services provided at that time, it may be reported by itself or in addition to other procedures or services by appending the modifier 59 to the specific separate procedure code. This indicates that the procedure is not considered a component of another procedure but is a distinct, independent procedure. This may represent a different session or patient encounter, different procedure or surgery, different site or organ system, separate incision/excision, separate lesion, or separate injury (or area of injury in extensive injuries).

Examples of CPT codes with the term "separate procedure" in the code description are as follows:
- 29870—Arthroscopy, knee, diagnostic, with or without synovial biopsy (separate procedure)
- 38780—Retroperitoneal transabdominal lymphadenectomy, extensive, including pelvic, aortic, and renal nodes (separate procedure)
- 44312—Revision of ileostomy; simple (release of superficial scar) (separate procedure)
- 53230—Excision of urethral diverticulum (separate procedure); female
- 60520—Thymectomy, partial or total; transcervical approach (separate procedure)
- 66625—Iridectomy, with corneoscleral or corneal section; peripheral for glaucoma (separate procedure)

CMS and the NCCI Guidelines

Modifier 59 has been established for use when several procedures are performed on different anatomical sites, or at different sessions (on the same day). When certain services are reported together on a patient by the same physician on the same date of service, there may be a perception of "unbundling," when, in fact, the services were performed under circumstances that did not involve this practice at all.

Because carriers cannot identify this simply on the basis of CPT coding on either electronic or paper claims, modifier 59 was established to permit services of such a nature to bypass correct coding edits if the modifier is present. Modifier 59 indicates that the procedure represents a distinct service from others reported on the same date of service. This may represent a different session, different surgery, different site, different lesion, or different injury or area of injury (in extensive injuries).

Another already-established modifier frequently has been defined that describes this situation more specifically. In the event that a more descriptive modifier is available, it should be used in preference to modifier 59.

CPT modifier 59 is appended when distinct and separate multiple services are provided to a patient on a single date of service. CPT modifier 59 was developed explicitly for the purpose of identifying services not typically performed together.

Within the NCCI, there is an assigned modifier indicator. A modifier indicator of "0" indicates that an NCCI-associated modifier cannot be used to bypass the edit. When the code has a modifier indicator of "1," an NCCI-associated modifier may be used to bypass the edit if it meets the criteria under appropriate circumstances. A modifier indicator of "9" in NCCI indicates the edit has been deleted on the same date as it became effective.[1]

Review the NCCI edit in Table 5-1.

It is important to note that NCCI modifiers are used only when the procedures are performed at separate patient encounters, separate anatomic sites, separate organs, separate specimens, or as a distinct service. Most code pair edits should not be reported with NCCI-associated modifiers if the procedure is performed on ipsilateral organ structures unless there is appropriate rationale to bypass the edit. A modifier should not be used to bypass the NCCI edit unless the two procedures are performed at two separate operative sessions or two separate anatomical locations, or as a distinct service, recognized by coding conventions. NCCI-associated CPT modifiers include 25, 58, 59, 78, 79, and 91. HCPCS modifiers include E1-E4, FA, F1-F9, LC, LD, LT, RC, RT, TA, and T1-T9, which are the anatomical modifiers.

Third-Party Payer Guidelines

Even though many carriers follow CMS guidelines and the NCCI, policies vary from carrier to carrier. When a claim is submitted to the carrier, the documentation should be clear as to the separate distinct procedure before modifier 59 is appended to the procedure code. The modifier allows the codes to bypass carrier edits, but often the carrier will suspend the claim and request documentation before payment is rendered.

Modifier 59 is used only if another modifier does not describe the circumstance(s) more accurately.

> **NCCI CODING TIP**
>
> When two corresponding procedures are performed at the same patient encounter and in contiguous structures, it often is not appropriate to append an NCCI-associated modifier to bypass the edit.

---

1. Source: National Correct Coding Initiative, available at www.cms.hhs.gov/physicians.

TABLE 5-1 NCCI Edit Example

Column 1	Column 2	* = In existence prior to 1996	Effective Date	Deletion Date *=no data	Modifier 0=not allowed 1=allowed 9=not applicable
33226	00540		20030101	*	0
33226	33210		20050701	*	1
33226	33211		20050701	*	0
33226	33233		20030101	*	1
33226	33240		20030101	*	1
33226	33241		20030101	*	1
33226	36000		20030101	*	1
33226	36410		20030101	*	1
33226	37202		20030101	*	1
33226	62318		20030101	*	1
33226	62319		20030101	*	1
33226	64415		20030101	*	1
33226	64417		20030101	*	1
33226	64450		20030101	*	1
33226	64470		20030101	*	1
33226	64475		20030101	*	1
33226	69990		20030101	*	0
33226	75860		20040101	*	0
33226	76000		20031001	*	1
33226	76001		20031001	*	1
33226	90780		20030101	20041231	1
33226	G0345		20050101	*	1
33226	G0347		20050101	*	1
33226	G0351		20050701	*	1
33226	G0353		20050701	*	1
33226	G0354		20050701	*	1

Some problems with claims that use modifier 59 may result in delay or denial because:

- The carrier does accept CPT modifier 59 but only on first radiology CPT codes.
- Procedures are bundled regardless of CPT modifier 59 use.
- CPT modifier 59 is recognized, but claims are delayed and the carrier may request medical records, which is a manual process.

The documentation in the medical record should clearly support the separate and distinct procedures, since many carriers may ask for documentation to support the use of modifier 59.

Example 1: From NCCI Book-Surgery

A patient underwent placement of a flow-directed pulmonary artery catheter for hemodynamic monitoring via the subclavian vein (93503). Later in the day, the catheter had to be removed and a central venous catheter was inserted through the femoral vein.

CPT Code(s) Billed: *93503—Insertion and placement of flow directed catheter (eg, Swan-Ganz) for monitoring purposes*

36010 59—Introduction of catheter, superior or inferior vena cava

Rationale for Using Modifier 59

Because the pulmonary artery catheter requires passage through the vena cava, it may appear that the service for the catheter was being "unbundled" if both services are reported on the same day. Accordingly, the central venous catheter code should be reported with modifier 59 (CPT code 36010 59), indicating that this catheter was placed in a different site as a different service on the same day.

Example 2

A surgeon removed a soft tissue tumor from a patient's left wrist in the outpatient surgery department. During the same operative session, the physician also excised a 0.8-cm lesion from the patient's right leg.

THIRD-PARTY PAYER CODING TIP

There has been much controversy among insurance carriers regarding the use of modifier 59. Check each individual carrier for the carrier's policy and interpretation on the use of modifier 59.

NCCI CODING TIP

Modifier 59 is often misused. The two codes in a code pair edit often by definition represent different procedures. The provider cannot use modifier 59 for such an edit on the basis of the two codes being different procedures. However, if the two procedures are performed at separate sites or at separate patient encounters on the same date of service, modifier 59 may be appended. In addition, modifier 59 cannot be used with E/M services (CPT codes 99201-99499) or radiation treatment management (CPT code 77427).

CPT Code(s) Billed: 25077—Radical resection of tumor (eg, malignant neoplasm), soft tissue of forearm and/or wrist area

11401 59—Excision, benign lesion including margins, except skin tag (unless listed elsewhere), trunk, arms or legs; excised diameter 0.6 to 1.0 cm

Rationale for Using Modifier 59

Since both procedures were performed on different anatomic areas and are separate and distinct procedures, modifier 59 would be appropriate. Modifier LT may also be appended to the removal of the soft tissue tumor *(25077 LT)* whereas modifier RT may be appended to the lesion excision *(11401 59 RT)*. Modifiers LT and RT are not mandatory in this example, but are helpful to the insurance carrier to identify which procedure was performed on each side of the body.

Example 3: Surgery

A Medicare patient who was complaining of left knee pain underwent an arthroscopy of the left knee with medial meniscetomy with chondral fragmentation during the same operative session

CPT Code(s) Billed: 29881—Arthroscopy, knee, surgical; with meniscectomy (medial OR lateral, including any meniscal shaving)

Rationale for Not Using Modifier 59

Because code 29874, *Arthroscopy, knee, surgical; for removal of loose body or foreign body (eg, osteochondritis dissecans fragmentation, chondral fragmentation),* is included in the meniscectomy and under the National Correct Coding Initiative, modifier 59 is not allowed to report both procedures within the same compartment, so modifier 59 would not be appropriate. Only code 29881 should be reported in this instance.

Example 4

A 52-year-old male patient underwent a total colonoscopy with hot biopsy destruction of a sessile 3-mm mid sigmoid colon polyp and multiple cold biopsies taken randomly throughout the colon in the outpatient GI lab. The diagnosis in the medical record indicated fecal incontinence, diarrhea, and constipation. The bowel preparation with GoLytely was good. Demerol 50 mg and Versed 3 mg both were given intravenously. The digital examination revealed no masses. The pediatric variable flexion Olympus colonoscope was introduced into the rectum and advanced to the cecum. A picture was taken of the appendiceal orifice and the ileocecal valve. The scope then was carefully extubated. The mucosa looked normal. Random biopsies were taken from the ascending colon, the transverse colon, the descending colon, the sigmoid colon, and the rectum. There was a 3-mm sessile polyp in the mid sigmoid colon that a hot biopsy destroyed. The patient tolerated the procedure well.

CPT Code(s) Billed: *45383—Colonoscopy, flexible, proximal to splenic flexure; with ablation of tumor(s), polyp(s), or other lesion(s) not amenable to removal by hot biopsy forceps, bipolar cautery or snare technique*

45380 59—Colonoscopy, flexible, proximal to splenic flexure; with biopsy, single or multiple

Rationale for Using Modifier 59

Based on the AMA's CPT coding guidelines, if one lesion is biopsied, and a separate lesion is removed, it is appropriate to append modifier 59 to the code reported for the biopsy procedure. In this case, one lesion was destroyed with hot biopsy forceps, and multiple sites unrelated to the hot biopsy site also was biopsied.

Radiology with Modifier 59

Modifier 59 may be used with radiology procedures in CPT. Radiology has both a professional and technical component, as was reviewed in an earlier chapter. Modifier 59 may be used when the service is a distinct and separate procedure.

Example 5

A 70-year-old woman, who was experiencing shortness of breath, underwent a chest X ray single view. Later in the day, the radiologist asked the patient to return for a more extensive study because he discovered infiltrates in the lungs. The patient returned to the radiology department, and a PA and lateral chest X ray were performed for suspected pneumonia.

CPT Code(s) Billed: *71010—Radiologic examination, chest; single view, frontal*

71020 59—Radiologic examination, chest, two views, frontal and lateral

Rationale for Using Modifier 59

Since both procedures were performed at different sessions and the first procedure indicated medical necessity for an additional study, modifier 59 would be appended to the second procedure performed later in the day.

Laboratory Reporting with Modifier 59

Since the introduction of modifier 91, many questions have been raised regarding its use vs modifier 59. Some third-party payers have suggested that modifier 91 can be appended to every laboratory code that is reported more than one time on the same date of service. However, per the CPT coding guidelines, this is not the appropriate method of reporting modifier 91.

For example, if multiple bacterial blood cultures are tested, including isolation and presumptive identification of isolates, then code 87040, *Culture, bacterial; blood, with isolation and presumptive identification of isolates (includes anaerobic culture, if appropriate)*, should be used to identify each culture procedure performed. Modifier 59 should be appended to the additional procedures performed to identify each additional culture performed as a distinct service.

To assist users with the appropriate use of this series of codes, additional instructions for use of modifiers 59 and 91 are given in the microbiology subsection of the CPT book.

The microbiology guidelines state:

> Presumptive identification of microorganisms is defined as identification by colony morphology, growth on selective media, Gram stains, or up to three tests (eg, catalase, oxidase, indole, urease). Definitive identification of microorganisms is defined as an identification to the genus or species level that requires additional tests (eg, biochemical panels, slide cultures). If additional studies involve molecular probes, chromatography, or immunologic techniques, these should be separately coded in addition to definitive identification codes (87140-87158). For multiple specimens/sites, use modifier 59. For repeat laboratory tests performed on the same day, use modifier 91.

Modifier 91 will be discussed further in Chapter 7 of this text.

Example 6: Laboratory and Pathology

A 14-year-old boy presented as an outpatient to the laboratory for aerobic and anaerobic culture of two sites of a single vertical wound to the anterior left foreleg, which was a result of a scooter mishap. The laboratory technologist obtained independent specimens, one from the proximal wound site and one from the distal wound site, for aerobic culture of the drainage material for testing, using the appropriate type of aerobic culturettes. The laboratory technologist also obtained independent specimens by means of anaerobic culturettes, one from the proximal wound site and one from the distal wound site, for anaerobic culture of the drainage material for testing.

CPT Code(s) Billed: *87071—Culture, bacterial; quantitative, aerobic with isolation and presumptive identification of isolates, any source except urine, blood or stool*

87071 59—Culture, bacterial; quantitative, aerobic with isolation and presumptive identification of isolates, any source except urine, blood or stool

87073—Culture, bacterial; quantitative, anaerobic with isolation and presumptive identification of isolates, any source except urine, blood or stool

87073 59—Culture, bacterial; quantitative, anaerobic with isolation and presumptive identification of isolates, any source except urine, blood or stool

Rationale for Using Modifier 59

Because the specimens are taken from two distinct sites (one from the proximal wound site and one from the distal wound site) for aerobic culture of the drainage material, and independent specimens also are obtained from the two sites for anaerobic culture, it would be appropriate to append modifier 59 to both 87071 and 87073 for the testing of multiple specimens from the distinct wound sites.

Example 7: Medicine

Pressure sores that were 20 sq cm on a patient's right ankle and right hip were debrided in the morning but, because of the patient's condition, selective debridement of a 17–sq cm sacral pressure sore was performed at a separate session in the afternoon on that same date by the same provider.

CPT Code(s) Billed: 97597, 97597 59

97597   Removal of devitalized tissue from wound(s); selective debridement, without anesthesia (eg, high pressure waterjet with/without suction, sharp selective debridement with scissors, scalpel and forceps), with or without topical application(s), wound assessment, and instruction(s) for ongoing care, may include use of a whirlpool, per session; total wound(s) surface area less than or equal to 20 square centimeters.

Rationale for Using Modifier 59

In this example, codes 97597 and 97597 59 should be reported to identify procedures that are not normally reported together, but are appropriate under the circumstance, and represent a different session or patient encounter and different site. Since 97597 is per session and two sessions on the same day are medically necessary, it is appropriate to bill 97597 59 for the second session.

Example 8: Medicine

A patient underwent chemotherapy for prostate cancer. Two methods of administration must be used for this patient because of the medicinal agents used.

CPT Code(s) Billed: *96409—Chemotherapy administration; intravenous, push technique, single or initial substance/drug*

96413 59—Chemotherapy administration, intravenous infusion technique; up to one hour, single or initial substance/drug

CMS Guidelines for Use of Modifier 59 With the Medicine Section of the CPT Book

1   Chemotherapy administration codes include codes for the administration of chemotherapeutic agents by multiple routes, the most common being the intravenous route. Separate payment is allowed for chemotherapy administration by push and by infusion technique on the same day, but only one push administration is allowed on a single day. It is recognized that combination chemotherapy is frequently provided by different routes at the same session. Modifier 59 can be appropriately used when two different modes of chemotherapy administration are used. Modifier 59 is used in this situation to indicate that two separate procedures are used to administer chemotherapeutic drug(s), not to indicate that two separate drugs are administered.

2   When the sole purpose of fluid administration (eg, saline, 5% dextrose in water, etc) is to maintain patency of the access device, the infusion is neither diagnostic nor therapeutic; therefore, the injection, infusion, or chemotherapy administration codes are not to be separately reported (CPT codes 90760-90761). In the case of transfusion of blood or blood products, the insertion of a peripheral intravenous line (CPT codes 36000, 36410) is routinely necessary and is not separately reported. Administration of fluid in the course of transfusions to maintain line patency or between units of blood products is, likewise, not to be separately reported. If fluid administration is medically necessary for therapeutic reasons (correct dehydration, prevent nephrotoxicity, etc) in the course of a transfusion or chemotherapy, this could be separately reported with the modifier 59, as the fluid is being administered as medically necessary for a different diagnosis.

3   Biofeedback services involve the use of electromyographic techniques to detect and record muscle activity. CPT codes 95860-95874 (electromyography) should not be reported with biofeedback services based on the use of electromyography during a biofeedback session. If an electromyogram is performed as a separate medically necessary service for diagnosis or follow-up of organic muscle dysfunction, the appropriate electromyography codes (CPT codes 95860-95874) may be reported. Modifier 59 should be added to indicate that the service performed was a separately identifiable diagnostic service. Reporting only an objective electromyographic response to biofeedback is not sufficient to bill the codes referable to diagnostic electromyography.

4   Pulmonary stress testing (CPT code 94620) is a comprehensive stress test with a number of component tests separately defined in the CPT manual. It is inappropriate to separately code venous access, electrocardiogram monitoring, spirometric parameters performed before, during, and after exercise, oximetry, oxygen consumption, carbon dioxide production, rebreathing cardiac output calculations, etc, when performed as part of a progressive pulmonary exercise test. It is also inappropriate to bill for a cardiac stress test and the component codes used to perform a routine pulmonary stress test, when a comprehensive pulmonary stress test was performed. If a standard exercise protocol is used, serial electro-cardiograms are obtained, and a separate report describing a cardiac stress test (professional component) is included in the medical record, both a cardiac and a pulmonary stress test could be reported. Modifier 59 should be reported with the secondary procedure. In addition, if both tests are reported, both tests must satisfy the requirement for medical necessity.

Review of Modifier 59

1   Modifier 59 is used to report distinct and separate procedures performed on the same day.

2   Modifier 59 should be used with caution since this modifier affects reimbursement and tells payers that, under distinct circumstances, it is appropriate to bill procedures as separate and distinct. This modifier is not designed to provide reimbursement for separate procedures that are performed as an integral part of another procedure and is watched closely by carriers.

3   When a procedure is described in the CPT code descriptor as a "separate procedure" but is carried out independently or is unrelated to other services performed at the same session, the CPT code may be reported with modifier 59.

4   Modifier 59 should not be used when another, more descriptive modifier is available.

5   Documentation needs to be specific to the distinct procedure or service and be clearly identified in the medical record.

6   When appropriate, modifier 59 allows the CPT code to bypass edits with the NCCI when claims are edited for unbundling.

Modifier 62: Two Surgeons

Definition

When two surgeons work together as primary surgeons performing distinct part(s) of a procedure, each surgeon should report his/her distinct operative work by adding the modifier 62 to the procedure code and any associated add-on code(s) for that procedure as long as both surgeons continue to work together as primary surgeons. Each surgeon should report the co-surgery once using the same procedure code. If additional procedure(s), including add-on procedure(s), are performed during the same surgical session, separate code(s) may also be reported without the modifier 62 added. **Note:** If a co-surgeon acts as an assistant in the performance of additional procedure(s) during the same surgical session, those services may be reported using separate procedure code(s) with the modifier 80 or modifier 82 added, as appropriate.

AMA Guidelines

Co-surgery may be required because of the complexity of the procedure(s), the patient's condition, or both. The additional surgeon is not acting as an assistant, but is performing a distinct portion of the procedure.

Changes in the 2002 CPT codebook expanded the use of this modifier to include the following:

- Any associated add-on code(s) for that procedure as long as both surgeons continue to work together as primary surgeons
- Additional procedure(s) including add-on procedures performed during the same surgical session

In addition, each surgeon should report the co-surgery once using the same procedure code(s), including if a co-surgeon acts as an assistant in the performance of an additional procedure(s) during the same surgical session. Those services may also be reported by means of separate procedure code(s) with modifier 80 (assistant surgeon) or modifier 82 (assistant surgeon when a qualified resident is not available).

Guidelines for Spine Surgery

Spine surgery commonly requires the use of two surgeons to perform the procedure. To alert users to these changes, introductory notes were added to the guidelines in the CPT book for use of spinal procedures performed by an anterior approach to expose the surgical site. These notes are found in both the musculoskeletal and nervous system sections of the CPT book.

If one surgeon performs an incision and exposes the area requiring surgery, and another surgeon performs the surgery indicated in the code, both surgeons may report the same procedure code with modifier 62 appended. This indicates that only one total procedure listed in the CPT nomenclature was performed by two surgeons.

For example, if one surgeon opens the area of the spine where the decompression will be performed, and another surgeon performs the decompression, to indicate that one procedure was performed, both surgeons would report 63064 62, *Costovertebral approach with decompression of spinal cord or nerve root(s) (eg, herniated intervertebral disk), thoracic; single segment.*

In separate operative reports, both physicians would document their level of involvement in the surgery. Each should include a copy of the operative note when reporting the service to the third-party payer. If one surgeon does not use the modifier 62, the third-party payer may assume that the physician reporting the procedure without the modifier performed the entire procedure, even though the second physician reported the procedure with the modifier 62.

The surgeon who handles the approach and the spine surgeon must discuss in advance what portion of the procedure each is expected to perform on the basis of the complexity of the surgical case. Because of the complexity of the procedure, the approach surgeon is required to act as a co-surgeon, and both serve as primary surgeons. Each may need to perform additional procedures as co-surgeons, and modifier 62 may be appended to each additional procedure performed.

When the approach surgeon opens and closes only, modifier 62 is appended to the distinct primary procedure along with any additional level(s) that require approach work by the approach surgeon.

Modifier 80 is used if the approach surgeon is needed to continue to work as an assistant to the spine surgeon. Modifier 80 will be discussed in more detail in Chapter 6.

Example 1

A 50-year-old man underwent anterior arthrodesis of the cervical spine for degenerative disk disease. This procedure necessitated two surgeons working together. By an anterior cervical approach, the disk was excised and the end plates were prepared for fusion. A transverse incision was made anteriorly over the level of the proposed arthrodesis. The platysma muscle was cut in line with the skin incision. The interval between the sternocleidomastoid and carotid sheath laterally and the trachea and esophagus medially was developed and the prevertebral fascia was cleared from the front of the spine. The disk between the vertebrae to be fused was identified and the level was confirmed by X ray. The longus colli muscles were mobilized along their medial edges. Lateral and longitudinal self-retaining traction devices were inserted. The anterior longitudinal ligament and anterior annulus were removed by sharp dissection. The disk and cartilaginous end plates were removed by curettage. Bone cutting instruments were used to remove the bony end plates and expose the cancellous bone of the vertebral body. With the disk space under distraction, the bone graft was inserted into the disk space. The traction was released and the graft checked for security. Any protruding parts of the graft were trimmed to avoid esophageal compression. A drain was placed in the wound. The platysma muscle, subcutaneous tissue, and skin were sutured. Sterile dressings and a collar were applied. Surgeon A performed the initial incision via the cervical approach, the excision of the disk, and the preparation of the end plates for fusion. Surgeon B removed the anterior longitudinal ligament, the anterior annulus, and the cartilaginous end plates, along with inserting and trimming the bone graft. Surgeon A closed the wound and applied the sterile dressing.

CPT Code(s) Reported by Surgeon A: 22554 62

CPT Code(s) Reported by Surgeon B: 22554 62

22554   Arthrodesis, anterior interbody technique, including minimal diskectomy to prepare interspace (other than for decompression); cervical below C2

24.	A DATE(S) OF SERVICE From To		B Place of Service	C Type of Service	D PROCEDURES, SERVICES, OR SUPPLIES (Explain Unusual Circumstances) CPT/HCPCS	MODIFIER	E DIAGNOSIS CODE	F $ CHARGES	G DAYS OR UNITS	H EPSDT Family Plan	I EMG	J COB	K RESERVED FOR LOCAL USE
	MM DD YY	MM DD YY			22554	62							
1													
2													
3													
4													
5													
6													
25. FEDERAL TAX I.D. NUMBER SSN EIN			26. PATIENTIS ACCOUNT NO.		27. ACCEPT ASSIGNMENT? (For govt. claims, see back) YES NO		28. TOTAL CHARGE $		29. AMOUNT PAID $		30. BALANCE DUE $		

Rationale for Using Modifier 62
Since both surgeons were involved in performing distinct components of the same surgical procedure and were working together, modifier 62 should be used with the surgical procedure 22554. Each surgeon reported the same procedure code with modifier 62. Any instrumentation and/or bone grafting would be reported separately with the appropriate code(s).

NOTE: When bone grafting and/or instrumentation is performed in conjunction with the definitive procedure, modifier 62 should not be appended to the codes for these procedures. This is indicated in the instructions for coding the definitive procedures in the CPT book.

Example 2

A 67-year-old male Medicare patient with chronic obstructive pulmonary disease, coronary artery disease, and a previous myocardial infarction presented with a 5.8-cm aortic aneurysm. Imaging studies indicated that the aneurysm was infrarenal with an adequate neck to allow successful deployment of an endovascular prosthesis. There was also adequate normal aorta below the aneurysm to allow use of a tube graft. The iliac artery anatomy accommodated passage of the device. This procedure was performed by two surgeons acting as co-surgeons.

CPT Code(s) Reported by Surgeon A: 34800 62

CPT Code(s) Reported by Surgeon B: 34800 62

34800	Endovascular repair of infrarenal abdominal aortic aneurysm or dissection; using aorto-aortic tube prosthesis

Rationale for Using Modifier 62

Endovascular repair or dissection of an infrarenal aortic aneurysm can sometimes require the use of two surgeons. In endovascular repair, a small incision is made in the groin over one or both femoral arteries. Under separately reportable fluoroscopy, a synthetic stent graft, contained inside a long plastic holding capsule, is threaded through the arteries to the site of the infrarenal aneurysm. Once the stent is in place, the holding capsule is removed. Typically, when two surgeons perform the procedure, one surgeon will thread the synthetic graft to the site of the aneurysm and one will remove the holding capsule. Since two surgeons were performing distinct parts of the same procedure, modifier 62 would be appended to the procedure code. Both surgeons would report the same procedure with modifier 62.

NOTE: CMS allows the use of modifier 62 with this procedure.

Example 3

A 42-year-old man with a history of posttraumatic degenerative disk disease at L3-4 and L4-5 (internal disk disruption) underwent surgical repair. Surgeon A performed an anterior exposure of the spine with mobilization of the great vessels. Surgeon B performed anterior (minimal) diskectomy and fusion of L3-4 and L4-5 by means of the anterior interbody technique.

CPT Code(s) Reported by Surgeon A: 22558 62, 22585 62

CPT Code(s) Reported by Surgeon B: 22558 62, 22585 62, 20931

22558	Arthrodesis, anterior interbody technique, including minimal diskectomy to prepare interspace (other than for decompression); lumbar
22585	Arthrodesis, anterior interbody technique, including minimal diskectomy to prepare interspace (other than for decompression); each additional interspace (List separately in addition to code for primary procedure)
20931	Allograft for spine surgery only; structural

> **AMA CODING TIP**
>
> Modifier 62 may be used to indicate any surgery requiring the skills of two surgeons who act as co-surgeons and perform distinct components of a single surgical procedure.

NOTE: Surgeon B performed the allograft alone.

CMS Usage of Modifier 62 in Radiology

Modifier usage is limited in the Radiology section of the CPT book when work by two surgeons is coded. The following CPT code(s) allow the usage of modifier 62:

- 77776—Interstitial radiation source application; simple
- 77777—Interstitial radiation source application; intermediate
- 77778—Interstitial radiation source application; complex
- 77782—Remote afterloading high intensity brachytherapy; 5-8 source positions or catheters
- 77783—Remote afterloading high intensity brachytherapy; 9-12 source positions or catheters
- 77784—Remote afterloading high intensity brachytherapy; over 12 source positions or catheters

CMS Guidelines for Use of Modifier 62 With the Radiology Section of the CPT Book

1 Procedures may be paid with modifier 62 (two surgeons who are performing co-surgery) with a Medicare Fee Schedule Database (MFSDB) indicator of 1 if documentation is submitted with the claim.

2 Procedures may be paid with modifier 62 (two surgeons who are performing co-surgery) with a MFSDB indicator of 2 without documentation submitted with the claim.

3 Procedures with a MFSDB indicator of 0 or 9 in the two-surgeon (co-surgery) field may not be billed as co-surgery.

Table 5-2 is an example of the MFSDB; in the column for "TWO SURG," with the indicator of 2 in the co-surgery field, the surgery may be paid without documentation as long as the specialty requirement is met.

Example 4 (Radiology)

A 68-year-old man with cancer of the prostate underwent transperineal permanent palladium 103 implantation of the prostate. The patient was placed in an extended dorsal lithotomy position. A Foley catheter was inserted and the scrotum was retracted onto the anterior abdominal wall. The area was prepared and draped in the usual sterile manner.

Transrectal ultrasound was attached to the fixation device and inserted into the rectum to mimic the preplanning diagram. The template was

TABLE 5-2 CMS Medicare Fee Schedule Database (MFSDB)

HCPCS	Stat	Srg Day	Sos	Pre-op	Intra-op	Post-op	Pctc Ind	Mult Surg	Bila Surg	Asst Surg	Two Surg	Team Surg	Phys Supv
77776	A	090	1	0.00	0.00	0.00		0	0	0	0	0	09
77776 26	A	090	1	0.00	0.00	0.00		0	0	0	2	0	09
77776 TC	A	090	1	0.00	0.00	0.00		0	0	0	0	0	09
77777	A	090	1	0.00	0.00	0.00		0	0	0	0	0	09
77777 26	A	090	1	0.00	0.00	0.00		0	0	0	2	0	09
77777 TC	A	090	1	0.00	0.00	0.00		0	0	0	0	0	09
77778	A	090	1	0.00	0.00	0.00		0	0	0	0	0	09
77778 26	A	090	1	0.00	0.00	0.00		0	0	0	2	0	09
77778 TC	A	090	1	0.00	0.00	0.00		0	0	0	0	0	09
77781	A	090	1	0.00	0.00	0.00		0	0	0	0	0	09
77781 26	A	090	1	0.00	0.00	0.00		0	0	0	0	0	09
77781 TC	A	090	1	0.00	0.00	0.00		0	0	0	0	0	09

then attached. A total of 13 hollow, 18-gauge trocars were inserted by the urologist (Surgeon A). Once that placement was confirmed, a total of 60 palladium 103 seeds were inserted by the radiologist (Surgeon B). There were 25 seeds with an activity of 1.07 mCi and 35 seeds with an activity of 1.34 mCi. The total activity was 73.2 mCi, with an average activity per seed of 1.22 mCi. The patient tolerated the procedure well. There was minimal blood loss.

A postimplant cystogram performed by the urologist showed the seeds to be in excellent position. The patient went to the recovery room in stable condition. Follow-up dosimetry was arranged.

CPT Code(s) Billed by Surgeon A: 77778 26 62
CPT Code(s) Billed by Surgeon B: 77778 26 62

77778   Interstitial radiation source application; complex

Rationale for Using Modifier 62

Modifier 26 indicates that the professional component is reported. Modifier 62 indicates two surgeons. Because this is a Medicare patient, the indicator is approved for two surgeons, and both surgeons worked together as co-surgeons, modifier 62 can be billed on the claim. Each physician will bill with modifier 62.

CMS and Modifier 62

Rules for CMS and modifier 62 may be found in the Medicare Carriers' Manual (MCM), sections 4820-4828 and 15044-15046. Modifier 62 may be billed when two or more surgeons of the same specialty, with or without the same areas of subspecialization, are performing one of the following:

- Parts of a single procedure (eg, two surgeons performing a procedure identified by a single CPT code)
- The same or similar procedures in separate body areas (eg, two surgeons simultaneously applying skin grafts to different parts of the body, or two surgeons repairing different fractures in the same patient)
- Components of a related procedure or procedures generally performed by the same surgeon (eg, two surgeons performing separate components of eye surgery)
- A single procedure (identified by a single CPT code) or components of related procedures performed by two or more surgeons of different specialties (eg, one surgeon performs the abdominal exposure and/or closure for another surgeon who then performs anterior spine surgery)

What co-surgery means in this context is that two surgeons are performing portions of the procedure simultaneously. Documentation of medical necessity is required when reporting co-surgery with modifier 62. A list of procedures in which CMS allows co-surgery can be found in the Medicare Fee Schedule Database (MFSDB) on the CMS website at http://www.cms.hhs.gov.

Two-surgeon (co-surgeon) reimbursement is only available for procedure codes designated by CMS as eligible for modifier 62.

For co-surgeons (modifier 62), the fee schedule amount applicable to the payment for each co-surgeon is 62.5% of the global surgery fee schedule amount based on the MFSDB (MCM, section 15046).

Charges for additional surgical assists (beyond the two co-surgeons) will be reviewed for medical necessity. If medical necessity is established, each eligible assistant at surgery will be reimbursed according to his or her eligible allowance.

If two surgeons (each in a different specialty) are required to perform a specific procedure, each surgeon bills for the procedure with a modifier 62. Co-surgery also refers to surgical procedures involving two surgeons performing the parts of the procedure simultaneously, (ie, heart transplant or bilateral knee replacements). Documentation of the medical necessity for two surgeons is required for certain services identified in the MFSDB. (See MCM, section 4828.C.5.)

If surgeons of different specialties each are performing a different procedure (with specific CPT codes), neither co-surgery nor multiple surgery rules apply even if the procedure(s) are performed through the same incision. If one of the surgeons performs multiple procedures, the multiple procedure rules apply to that surgeon's services (MCM, section 4826 for multiple surgery payment rules).

When reviewing the MFSDB, pay attention to the indicators that identify when two surgeons of different specialties may be reimbursed. Review Table 5-3.

THIRD-PARTY PAYER CODING TIP

Many insurance carriers do not recognize modifier 62. The Medicaid carrier should be consulted before modifier 62 is billed.

TABLE 5-3	**CMS Medicare Fee Schedule Database Indicators**
Indicator	**Description**
0	Co-surgeons not permitted for the procedure.
1	Co-surgeons may be paid if supporting documentation is supplied to establish medical necessity.
2	Co-surgeons permitted. No documentation is required if the two-specialty requirement is met.
9	If a team of surgeons (more than two surgeons of different specialties) is required to perform a specific procedure, each surgeon reports the procedure with modifier 66, team surgery.

Medicare will recognize the use of the modifier 62 with the endovascular repair procedures (34800, 34802, 34804, 34808, 34812, 34813, 34820, 34825, 34826, 34830-34832).

Third-Party Payer Guidelines

Many third-party payers will deny two surgeons of the same specialty as co-surgeons. The insurance carrier should be consulted before the claim is submitted with modifier 62. Some payers reimburse at a lesser reimbursement rate than CMS. Many insurance carriers do not recognize modifier 62. Medicaid carriers should also be consulted before modifier 62 is billed; many Medicaid carriers do not recognize this modifier.

Review of Modifier 62

1   Specific insurance carrier guidelines should be reviewed for acceptance of modifier 62.

2   When modifier 62 is billed, documentation must support medical necessity for two surgeons.

3   Each surgeon should report the co-surgery with the same procedure code.

4   When Medicare claims are billed, the MFSDB indicator should be checked to determine whether two surgeons are allowed for the procedure performed.

5   The MCM, sections 4820-4828 and 15044-15046 should be referred to when claims are submitted with billing for two surgeons for Medicare patients.

6   The multiple procedure reduction rule applies on any additional procedures performed that require the use of modifier 50 or 51 in addition to the primary procedure.

7   Each surgeon must dictate his or her own operative report when billing is submitted for two surgeons, and each submits his or her own claim with modifier 62.

8   When two surgeons of the same specialty are billing with modifier 62, documentation may be required to support the necessity of using surgeons of the same specialty.

9   Modifier 62 should not be used when a surgeon acts as the "assistant surgeon"; modifier 81 or 82 is used.

Modifier 63: Procedure Performed on Infants Less than 4 kg

Definition

Procedures performed on neonates and infants up to a present body weight of 4 kg may involve significantly increased complexity and physician work commonly associated with these patients. This circumstance may be reported by adding the modifier 63 to the procedure number. **Note:** Unless otherwise designated, this modifier may only be appended to procedures/services listed in the 20000-69990 code series. Modifier 63 should not be appended to any CPT codes listed in the **Evaluation and Management Services, Anesthesia, Radiology, Pathology/ Laboratory**, or **Medicine sections.**

AMA Guidelines

Modifier 63 was created in 2003 for procedures performed on neonates and infants up to a present body weight of 4 kg, which may involve significantly increased complexity and physician work commonly associated with these patients. This may be reported by adding the modifier 63 to the procedure number.

This modifier may be used only in the Surgery section of the CPT book (codes 20000-69990).

Modifier 63 is appended only to invasive surgical procedures and reported only for neonates or infants up to a present body weight of 4 kg. With this group of neonates/infants, there is a significant increase in work intensity specifically related to temperature control, obtaining intravenous access (which may be required for upward of 45 minutes), and the operation itself, which is technically more difficult with regard to maintenance of homeostasis.

The procedures with which modifier 63 cannot be reported are generally procedures performed on infants for the correction of congenital abnormalities. It is not appropriate to report the modifier 63 because the additional work that this modifier is intended to represent has been previously identified as an inherent element within the procedures in this list. When appended to a procedure, the modifier 63 indicates the additional difficulty of performing a procedure, which may involve significantly increased complexity and physician work commonly associated with neonates and infants up to a body weight of 4 kg. Since many procedures already include the pediatric status as part of the CPT descriptors, the parenthetical notes that prohibit the use of modifier 63 should be reviewed.

Following are examples of CPT codes for which modifier 63 would be appropriate:

33820	Repair of patent ductus arteriosus; by ligation
44120	Enterectomy, resection of small intestine; single resection and anastomosis
44140	Colectomy, partial; with anastomosis
43220	Esophagoscopy, rigid or flexible; with balloon dilation (less than 30 mm diameter)
43246	Upper gastrointestinal endoscopy including esophagus, stomach, and either the duodenum and/or jejunum as appropriate; with directed placement of percutaneous gastrostomy tube
47000	Biopsy of liver, needle; percutaneous

> **AMA CODING TIP**
>
> The invasive procedure must be in the CPT code range of 20000 to 69990. Modifier 63 is not valid with E/M, anesthesia, radiology, pathology/laboratory, or medicine codes.

Following are examples of CPT codes for which modifier 63 is not appropriate:

30540	Repair choanal atresia; intranasal
30545	Repair choanal atresia; transpalatine
36420	Venipuncture, cutdown; under age 1 year
43313	Esophagoplasty for congenital defect (plastic repair or reconstruction), thoracic approach; without repair of congenital tracheoesophageal fistula
44055	Correction of malrotation by lysis of duodenal bands and/or reduction of midgut volvulus (eg, Ladd procedure)
46070	Incision, anal septum (infant)
49491	Repair, initial inguinal hernia, preterm infant (less than 37 weeks gestation at birth), performed from birth up to 50 weeks postconception age, with or without hydrocelectomy; reducible
54150	Circumcision, using clamp or other device; newborn
63704	Repair of myelomeningocele; less than 5 cm diameter

In each of the previous examples, the CPT book includes cross references after each code stating not to use modifier 63 in conjunction with the code.

Third-Party Payer Guidelines

When the procedure code is valid, modifier 63 may be reviewed and processed in the same manner as modifier 22 for many insurance carriers. Many carriers require the documentation (operative note) submitted with the claim for review.

Example 1

A premature neonate (28 weeks' gestation) was born with patents ductus arteriosus. At the age of 3 weeks (weight, 800 g), medical therapy for the condition had failed, including three cycles of indomethacin and fluid restriction. The oxygen requirements on the ventilator were increasing, and there was evidence of decreasing compliance. There was a loud holosystolic murmur with bounding peripheral pulses. Echocardiography demonstrated a large patent ductus arteriosus.

The patient was accompanied into the operating suite by the attending physician. After the patient was prepared and draped, a posterior lateral incision was made. The patent ductus arteriosus and recurrent laryngeal nerve were identified. The patent ductus arteriosus was the same size as the descending aorta, and blood was seen through the delicate wall.

The vessel was 1 cm long and therefore too short to obtain proximal and distal control. The surrounding tissues were separated from the wall of the ductus next to the aorta. The recurrent nerve was swept medially. The vessel was ligated with a single ligature. A vascular clip was used because the ligature seemed inadequate. The chest cavity was evacuated with a red rubber catheter while the chest was closed. The patient was placed into the incubator and transferred to the neonatal intensive care unit still on the ventilator. A chest X ray was obtained in the neonatal intensive care unit and the family was briefed on the success of the procedure. The oxygen requirements were weaned back to room air during the next 24 hours, and the overall condition of the neonate was improved.

CPT Code(s) Billed: 33820 63—Repair of patent ductus arteriosus; by ligation

Rationale for Using Modifier 63

The patient was 3 weeks old and weighed 800 g, which put the patient at higher risk, so modifier 63 is appropriate.

Example 2

A 3-week-old premature neonate weighing 1500 g developed abdominal distention, intolerance of feeding, and clinical signs of sepsis. The neonate requires intubation and the start of vasopressors for blood pressure control and peripheral and renal perfusion. Plain radiographs revealed necrotizing enterocolitis. Surgical consultation was obtained. The premature infant's status continued to decline. Eight hours after presentation, repeat radiographs showed pneumoperitoneum and surgery was recommended. At laparotomy, necrotizing enterocolitis was seen throughout the small-bowel terminal ileum and right colon. The necrotic bowel was resected, the remaining bowel was irrigated, and a stoma with Hartman pouch was fashioned. The neonate had a difficult postoperative course but was tolerating enteral formula with supplemental hyperalimentation by the second postoperative week.

CPT Code(s) Billed: 44120 63—Enterectomy, resection of small intestine; single resection and anastomosis

Rationale for Using Modifier 63

The patient, who was 3 weeks old, weighed approximately 1500 g, which put the patient at higher risk, so modifier 63 is appropriate.

Review of Modifier 63

1 Modifier 63 is used only for invasive surgical procedures reported in neonates or infants up to 4 kg.

2 Modifier 63 should not be used when the CPT book indicates that modifier 63 is not to be used with a procedure code.

3 This modifier is to be used only in the Surgery section of the CPT book.

4 The invasive procedure must be in the CPT code range of 20000 to 69990. This modifier is not valid with E/M, anesthesia, radiology, pathology/ laboratory, or medicine codes.

5 The invasive procedure is not for a surgery that assumes the patient is a neonate or infant. When a procedure is usually performed on neonates or infants (eg, surgery to correct a congenital abnormality), the relative value units for the code already reflect the additional work.

6 For most insurance carriers, when the procedure code is valid, modifier 63 will be reviewed and processed in the same manner as a modifier 22.

7 Modifiers 63 and 22 will not be valid when used for the same procedure code(s).

8 Documentation may be required to validate the additional work.

Checkpoint Exercises 2

Select the correct modifier.

1 _____ This modifier is used to indicate that the procedure is distinct and separate.

2 _____ Two surgeons work together as primary surgeons performing distinct part(s) of a single reportable procedure.

3 _____ An esophageal dilation using a guidewire (43453) is performed on a 5-week-old neonate who weighs 3.2 kg.

4 _____ When using this modifier, each surgeon must dictate his or her own operative note and submit the claim with the same CPT code.

5 _____ A patient is seen in the outpatient surgery department during a 90-day follow-up period for a second (staged) destruction procedure in regard to infrared coagulation of hemorrhoids (IRC). Select the appropriate code for the second staged procedure. Which modifier would be appended to the CPT code?

Test Your Knowledge

True or False

1 _____ Modifier 58 is used to describe staged or related procedures that are described in the CPT code set with the code descriptor "staged."

2 _____ Modifier 59 can be used to report a separate incision/excision.

3 _____ The CPT modifier that indicates that a decision for surgery was made is modifier 57.

4 _____ If two surgeons perform different procedures on the same day at the same operative session, modifier 62 is appended.

5 _____ Modifier 59 is used to report multiple procedures.

Select the Appropriate Modifier

6 _____ A surgeon performed a liver biopsy (percutaneous needle) on a 6-week-old, 3.5 kg neonate with a 2-week history of cholestasis. The biopsy was performed to differentiate between biliary atresia and other causes of neonatal hepatitis.

7 _____ A patient was admitted to the intensive care unit with possible peritonitis. The patient's internist requested a consultation from a general surgeon. The general surgeon performed a comprehensive history and examination with medical decision making of moderate complexity. After reviewing the patient's records, the physician made a diagnosis of "acute abdomen" and scheduled surgery for the same day. The physician documented the appropriate history and physical examination with recommendations for immediate surgery in the medical record. The attending physician asked the general surgeon to assume care of the patient's acute abdominal problem, including recommended surgery and its associated postoperative follow-up care. Intraoperatively, the general surgeon found that the patient did have generalized peritonitis due to a perforated duodenal ulcer. The surgeon repaired the small intestine perforation by suture.

8 _____ A patient had three lesions removed from the scalp (1.0 cm), the nose (1.0 cm), and the left leg (2.0 cm). All were removed with a scalpel. The physician sent the specimens for pathological examination. The pathology report indicated that the lesions on the scalp and nose were benign and the lesion on the leg was malignant. What modifier is appended to the code for the lesion excision on the leg?

9 _____ A 69-year-old car accident victim was rushed to the emergency department of a local hospital. The emergency department physician determined that the patient had a hip dislocation. An orthopedic surgeon saw the patient and decided to perform the

surgery that evening because the patient was in so much pain. What modifier would be used?

10 _____ A patient had an angioma removed from the face, which created a deep defect. The patient returned to the surgeon 4 weeks later for a repair. The physician repaired the 3.5-cm defect by means of a complex closure. What modifier is appended to the secondary procedure?

11 _____ A patient with a crush injury with open fracture right middle finger distal phalanx and nailbed laceration underwent surgery correction in the outpatient surgery department at the local hospital. The service was reported with procedure codes 26765 and 11760. Which modifier would be appended to the procedure code?

12 _____ An 80-year-old male with advanced congestive heart failure has critical ischemia of both lower extremities. The cardiologist performs a physical exam which is notable for the absence of femoral pulses. An arteriogram performed by a brachial approach reveals complete occlusion of both common and external iliac arteries with reconstitution of the common femorals. At operation an axillo-bifemoral bypass is scheduled for the next morning. What modifier would be reported for this patient encounter?

13 _____ A patient was in the outpatient surgery center with a foreign body in his left heel and had right knee degenerative joint disease. Once prepped and draped, an Esmarch was used as a tourniquet for about 10 minutes. An elliptical incision was made over the foreign body, and it appeared to be an embedded piece of glass within the dermis. It was then excised without difficulty. The underlying sub-Q was exposed. Approximately a 1-cm incision was made. There was no other underlying subcutaneous lesion. It then was irrigated and closed with 3-0 nylon. The tourniquet was released, and hemostasis had been achieved. The right knee was sterilely prepped and injected with 40 mg of Kenalog and 2 cc of Marcaine. A bandage was applied. He tolerated the procedure well. What is the correct modifier for this encounter?

14 _____ Which modifier is reported to indicate the procedure is more difficult for an infant weighting less than 4 kg?

15 _____ A 68-year-old man who was diagnosed with Parkinson's disease had an essential tremor that had become quite severe and was disabling. Intervention failed to give him tremor relief using various oral medications and physical therapy. A two-stage operation was planned for deep brain stimulation (ie, the neurostimulator electrode array is placed and connected to an external generator, which is successful allaying symptomology), and the stimulator generator was subcutaneously placed the next week. What modifier should be used to report this procedure?

CHAPTER 6

Modifiers 66 to 82

Modifier 66: Surgical Team

Definition

Under some circumstances, highly complex procedures (requiring the concomitant services of several physicians, often of different specialties, plus other highly skilled, specially trained personnel, various types of complex equipment) are carried out under the "surgical team" concept. Such circumstances may be identified by each participating physician with the addition of the modifier 66 to the basic procedure number used for reporting services.

AMA Guidelines

With certain CPT® codes, one major procedure is listed without indicating the various components of that service (eg, 33945 Heart transplant, with or without recipient cardiectomy). The code lists one major service that combines the work of several physicians and other specially trained personnel. Generally each physician on a heart transplant team performs the same portion of the surgery each time. Each surgeon reports the same code with the modifier 66. Each surgeon on the team jointly writes a description of each physician's role on the heart transplant team and sends the report to the insurance carrier to indicate each physician's role in the performance of the surgery.

When one surgeon assists another surgeon with a procedure, modifier 80 Assistant surgeon, 81 Minimum assistant surgeon, or 82 Assistant surgeon (when qualified resident surgeon not available) may be more appropriate to report than modifier 66.

When additional services are provided by any of the physicians on the surgical team, this should be indicated in a separate operative note. The physician performing the additional services should provide a written explanation of the additional services to the insurance carrier.

Examples of procedures where modifier 66 may be used include the following:

32851	Lung transplant, single; without cardiopulmonary bypass
32852	Lung transplant, single; with cardiopulmonary bypass
32853	Lung transplant, double (bilateral sequential or en bloc); without cardiopulmonary bypass
32854	Lung transplant, double (bilateral sequential or en bloc); with cardiopulmonary bypass
33935	Heart-lung transplant with recipient cardiectomy-pneumonectomy
33945	Heart transplant, with or without recipient cardiectomy
47135	Liver allotransplantation; orthotopic, partial or whole, from cadaver or living donor, any age

47136	Liver allotransplantation; heterotopic, partial or whole, from cadaver or living donor, any age
48554	Transplantation of pancreatic allograft
48556	Removal of transplanted pancreatic allograft
50360	Renal allotransplantation, implantation of graft; without recipient nephrectomy
50365	Renal allotransplantation, implantation of graft; with recipient nephrectomy

CMS Guidelines

CMS guidelines for surgical teams may be found in section 15046 of the Medicare Carriers' Manual (MCM), which indicates that complex medical procedures, including multistage transplant surgery and coronary bypass, may require a team of physicians. (The MCM can be accessed on the CMS Web site at www.cms.hhs.gov/manuals.) In these situations, each of the physicians performs a unique function requiring special skills integral to the total procedure. Each physician is engaged in a level of activity different from assisting the surgeon in charge of the case. Thus, reimbursement for these services of team physicians is on the basis of the general reasonable charge criteria consistent with reimbursement practices in the service area. That is, the special payment limitation is not applied. (If reimbursement is made on the basis of a single team fee, additional claims would normally be denied.) If there are additional physicians involved in the surgical procedure who are actually assisting the primary surgeon and charges for their services can be identified, the special limitation is applied.

Physicians should determine which procedures performed in their service area require a team approach to surgery. There are some situations where the services of physicians of different medical specialties are necessary during surgery, and where each specialist is required to play an active role in the patient's treatment because of the existence of more than one medical condition requiring diverse, specialized medical services. For example, a patient's cardiac condition may require that a cardiologist be present to monitor the patient's condition during abdominal surgery. In these types of situations, the physician furnishing the concurrent care is functioning at a different level than that of an assistant at surgery, and reimbursement for his or her service may be made on the basis of the general reasonable charge criteria consistent with reimbursement practices in that service area.

For co-surgeons (modifier 62), the fee schedule amount applicable to the payment for each co-surgeon is 62.5% of the global surgery fee schedule amount. Team surgery (modifier 66) is paid for on a "by report" basis.

NOTE: "By report" means that a report including chart notes and operative notes must be submitted to the insurance carrier before the carrier will render payment.

Team surgery involves a single procedure (reported as a single procedure code) that requires more than two surgeons of different specialties and is reported by each surgeon (with the same procedure code) with modifier 66. Payment amounts are determined by carrier medical directors on an individual basis.

Third-Party Payer Guidelines

Modifier 66 refers to surgical treatment that may require several surgeons of different specialties, performing different portions of a procedure(s). Each primary surgeon who is eligible for modifier 66 may be reimbursed the usual reimbursement he or she would receive as a separate surgeon. All applicable reimbursement policies will apply (eg, incidental procedures, modifier 51, and modifier 50, global period). The primary surgeons are eligible for reimbursement as assistant surgeons when they assist each other.

Surgical team (team surgery) is reported by modifier 66 appended to the procedure codes. Modifiers 62 and 66 designate services performed by two surgeons or a surgical team and with most third-party payers will be reviewed on an individual basis.

Modifier 66 is only valid with surgery procedure codes, and in many cases requires medical review; operative records, clearly demonstrating that each surgeon performed components of a procedure in a team fashion, must accompany the claim.

Example 1

A 49-year-old man had end-stage cardiac disease secondary to ischemic cardiomyopathy. His medical history was significant for a strong family history of coronary artery disease and hypertension. The patient had undergone coronary artery bypass grafting 3 years before the current evaluation. He did well until readmitted recently with increasing congestive heart failure, fatigue, and a 9 kg weight loss over 6 months. Transplant evaluation demonstrated a left ventricular ejection fraction of 12%, patent coronary artery bypass grafts, and a pulmonary vascular resistance of 2 Wood units. Evaluation further demonstrated no systemic diseases, good compliance and family support, and no evidence of infection. The patient required dopamine for blood pressure support until an appropriate donor heart became available.

At operation, the pericardial space was remarkably adhered. Patent bypass grafts were demonstrated and dissected free. Close coordination with the donor procurement team was maintained during the entire preoperative and intraoperative procedure to reduce the ischemic time of the transported heart. Once the heart was in the operating room, the patient was placed on cardiopulmonary bypass and a standard cardiectomy procedure was performed with excision of the right and left atria at the level of the ventricles and the aorta and pulmonary artery just proximal to their respective semilunar valves. The heart was then placed in the pericardium and the 4 anastomoses (left atrium, right atrium, pulmonary artery, and aorta) were completed. The patient was weaned from cardiopulmonary bypass, hemostasis was obtained, and he was transferred to the intensive care unit.

The patient required ventilatory support for 1 day and hemodynamic monitoring for 3 to 6 days, following which the patient was transferred to a cardiac recovery floor, where the average stay was 10 to 14 days.

During this time, the patient was intensively monitored for rejection and infection. He required intensive rehabilitation because of his debilitated state before operation.

CPT Code(s) Billed: 33945 66—Heart transplant, with or without recipient cardiectomy

Rationale for Using Modifier 66

Since the procedure is performed by a team of surgeons, modifier 66 would be appended to the procedure. Each surgeon would report the same procedure code with modifier 66.

Example 2

A 44-year-old woman was dyspneic at rest from severe chronic obstructive lung disease and required home oxygen therapy. Her physician decided a lung transplant was necessary. At thoracotomy, the left lung was removed by dividing the left main stem bronchus at the level of the left upper lobe. The two pulmonary veins and single pulmonary artery were divided distally. An allograft left lung was inserted. The recipient left main stem bronchus and pulmonary artery were re-resected to accommodate the transplant. The recipient pulmonary veins were opened into the left atrium. An end-to-end anastomosis of the recipient's respective structures (pulmonary artery, main stem bronchus, and left atrial cuffs) was made to the similar donor structures. Two chest tubes were inserted. Bronchoscopy was performed in the operating room.

CPT Code(s) Billed: 32851 66—Lung transplant, single; without cardiopulmonary bypass

Rationale for Using Modifier 66

Since lung transplantation is performed by a team of surgeons, modifier 66 would be appended to the procedure. Each surgeon would report the same procedure code with modifier 66.

Example 3

A healthy sibling of a patient suffering from chronic renal failure became a kidney donor. A kidney transplant was performed by a surgical team.

CPT Code(s) Billed: 50365 66—Allotransplantation, implantation of graft, with recipient nephrectomy

Rationale for Using Modifier 66

Since kidney transplants are performed by a team of surgeons, modifier 66 would be appended to the procedure. Each surgeon would report the same procedure code with modifier 66. Carriers often must approve these procedures before performance of the procedure, and documentation is often required to support claims submitted with modifier 66.

Review of Modifier 66

1   Modifier 66 is used for procedures that are highly complex and require the skill of several surgeons, often of different specialties, and a highly skilled team of professionals to perform the procedure.

2   The documentation must support the need for team surgery.

3   For most carriers, payment for team surgery will be made by submission of the operative note to the insurance carrier.

4   Claims for a surgical team must contain sufficient documentation to support medical necessity.

5   Modifier 66 should not be used when two surgeons are acting as co-surgeons. When co-surgery conditions are met, use modifier 62.

6   Many insurance carriers require authorization before performance of team surgery.

Repeat Procedures

Repeat procedure modifiers are used when the procedure performed is the exact procedure performed by either the same or a different physician. Review the illustration below:

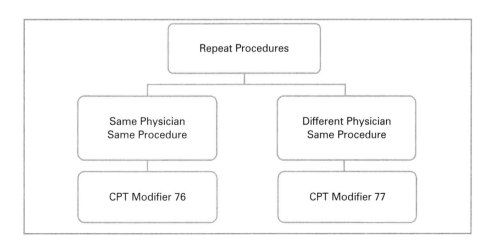

Modifier 76: Repeat Procedure by Same Physician

Definition

The physician may need to indicate that a procedure or service was repeated subsequent to the original procedure or service. This circumstance may be reported by adding the modifier 76 to the repeated procedure/service.

AMA Guidelines

When a procedure or service is repeated by the same physician subsequent to the original service, modifier 76 is used. From a coding perspective, modifier 76 is intended to describe the same procedure or service repeated, rather than the same procedure being performed at multiple sites.

CMS Guidelines

CMS states that the procedure must be performed in an operating room or place equipped specifically for procedures. CMS recognizes the use of modifier 76 for repeat procedures when medical necessity is supported. The services must be identical when modifier 76 is used. An operating room defined by CMS is a place of service specifically equipped and staffed for the sole purpose of performing procedures. This can be a hospital operating room, ambulatory surgery center (ASC), cardiac catheterization suite, laser suite, or endoscopy suite. It does not include a minor treatment room. The laser suite should be a separate, defined area, not used for any other purpose. The patient's room would not be an appropriate place of service unless the patient could not be moved for medical reasons.

CMS examples of repeat procedures include the following:

- Follow-up X rays (after chest tube placement, central venous line placement, new onset of distress, previous setting of fracture, etc)
- Repeat electrocardiograms for evaluation or treatment of arrhythmia or ischemia
- Repeat coronary angiogram or coronary artery bypass after abrupt closure of previously treated vessel

These services should be coded by attaching modifiers 76 or 77 (by same or different provider, respectively) to the appropriate CPT or Health Care Common Procedure Coding System (HCPCS) code. When modifier 76 or 77 is used, the reason for the repeat service should be entered in the narrative field in item 19 (on the CMS-1500 form) or in the electronic notepad for electronic claims.

Reasons may include one of the following statements about the service:

- It was performed for comparative purposes.
- The two services were performed at different times (may indicate actual time).
- It was for follow-up after treatment or intervention.
- It was to repeat a test at different intervals.

Third-Party Payer Guidelines

Third-party payers recognize the use of modifier 76. Documentation supporting the reparation along with the operative note should be provided to the insurance carrier when these services are reported.

Example 1

A physician performed a femoral-popliteal bypass graft in the morning. Later that day, the graft clotted and the same physician repeated the entire procedure.

CPT Code(s) Billed for First Procedure: 35556
CPT Code(s) Billed for Second Procedure: 35556 76

35556   Bypass graft, with vein; femoral-popliteal

Rationale for Using Modifier 76

The physician performed a femoral-popliteal bypass graft in the morning. Later that day, the graft clotted and the entire procedure was repeated. The initial procedure is reported as 35556. The repeat procedure is reported as 35556 76. This alerts the third-party payer that the physician did not accidentally report 35556 twice. Documentation supporting the reparation should be provided to the third-party payer when these services are reported.

If, for example, the patient's operative site bled after the initial surgery and required a return to the operating room to stop the bleeding, the same procedure would not be repeated. Thus, a different code (35860) with modifier 78 would be reported. (35860 Exploration for postoperative hemorrhage, thrombosis or infection; extremity; and 78 Return to the operating room for a related procedure during the postoperative period). Since the same procedure was not repeated, the modifier 76 would not be appropriate to use.

Example 2

A 38-year-old man presented to the emergency department with hypotension and a stab wound of the high right anterolateral chest after an attempted robbery. Diagnostic tests were ordered and reviewed to rule out other injury and to plan the operative approach. The surgeon reviewed and assessed the preexisting medical problems, laboratory studies, and all X rays and other imaging studies; evaluated the pulmonary and cardiac function; and stabilized, prepared, and transported the patient for emergency surgery. The physician communicated with the patient and family, as well as coordinated care with other physicians and health care providers. At operation, through a posterolateral thoracotomy, the hemithorax was explored, blood clot was evacuated, and a bleeding source in the lacerated lung was identified and repaired. The entire thorax and all thoracic and mediastinal structures were also explored to rule out other injury. Chest tubes were placed as appropriate.

AMA CODING TIP

Do not use modifier 76 when the definition of the code indicates a repeat procedure or "redo" (ie, 57511 Cautery of cervix; cryocautery, initial or repeat).

The next morning, the patient was returned to the operating room to repeat the procedure because of another blood clot in the hemithorax. The blood clot was evacuated, and another bleeding source in the lacerated lung was identified and repaired.

CPT Code(s) Billed for First Procedure: 32110
CPT Code(s) Billed for Second Procedure: 32110 76

32110   Thoracotomy, major; with control of traumatic hemorrhage and/or repair of lung tear

Rationale for Using Modifier 76

The physician performed a thoracotomy, with control of traumatic hemorrhage and repair of lung tear, on the first day. The next day, another tear with a clot was discovered that required a return trip to the operating room for the identical procedure. The initial procedure is reported as 32110. The repeat procedure is reported as 32110 76. This alerts the insurance carrier that the physician has not accidentally reported 32110 twice, even if the dates of service are different. With this procedure the typical global period is 90 days, and without modifier 76, the claim would likely be denied. Documentation supporting the reoperation should be provided to the third-party payer when these services are reported.

Example 3

A pulmonologist inserted a chest tube in a patient in the emergency department. A chest X ray was performed before and after placement of the chest tube to verify the position of the chest tube at the same operative session.

CPT Code(s) Billed for First Procedure: 32020, 71020 26
CPT Code(s) Billed for Second Procedure: 71020 76 26

32020   Tube thoracostomy with or without water seal (eg, for abscess, hemothorax, empyema) (separate procedure)

71020   Radiologic examination, chest, two views, frontal and lateral

Rationale for Using Modifier 76

The physician performed a chest tube placement in the emergency department. A chest X ray is typically performed before and after chest tube placement to verify the position of the chest tube. Without modifier 76 appended to the second procedure (71020), the carrier would likely deny the claim as a duplicate bill. Modifier 26 is also

24. A					B	C	D	E	F	G	H	I	J	K
DATE(S) OF SERVICE From MM DD YY		To MM DD YY			Place of Service	Type of Service	PROCEDURES, SERVICES, OR SUPPLIES (Explain Unusual Circumstances) CPT/HCPCS MODIFIER	DIAGNOSIS CODE	$ CHARGES	DAYS OR UNITS	EPSDT Family Plan	EMG	COB	RESERVED FOR LOCAL USE
1							32020							
2							71020 26							
3							71020 76 26							
4														
5														
6														
25. FEDERAL TAX I.D. NUMBER SSN EIN						26. PATIENT'S ACCOUNT NO.		27. ACCEPT ASSIGNMENT? (For govt. claims, see back) YES NO	28. TOTAL CHARGE $	29. AMOUNT PAID $				30. BALANCE DUE $

used because the physician is providing the interpretation and report and not the technical portion of the procedure. The hospital will report 71020 with modifier TC to indicate the technical component for the radiology procedure.

Example 4

A 67-year-old woman with atrial fibrillation underwent intracardiac cardioversion to return to sinus rhythm. After a thorough discussion of the risks and benefits and providing of informed consent, the patient was taken to the procedure room, local anesthesia was administered, and an electrode catheter was placed in a vein and advanced to the right atrium under fluoroscopic guidance. A second electrode catheter was placed in the coronary sinus or pulmonary artery. The patient was then sedated, and synchronized cardioversion was performed. The electrode catheters were then removed, hemostasis was obtained, and the patient was observed until the effect of sedation had cleared. The patient was taken to the recovery room. Two hours later the procedure had to be repeated. The second procedure was successful and the patient was released and sent home the next morning.

CPT Code(s) Billed for First Procedure: 92961
CPT Code(s) Billed for Second Procedure: 92961 76

92961   Cardioversion, elective, electrical conversion of arrhythmia; internal (separate procedure)

Rationale for Using Modifier 76

Since the initial cardioversion did not achieve the desired results, the procedure was repeated on the same day by the same physician. To alert the carrier that reporting of the procedure was not duplicated by the physician, modifier 76 would be appended to the procedure.

Example 5

A 67-year-old woman with a long history of a female urethral syndrome and interstitial cystitis is treated with DMSO. A bladder irrigation was performed in the morning and needed to be repeated in the late afternoon.

CPT Code(s) Billed for the Morning: 51700
CPT Code(s) Billed for the Afternoon: 51700 76

51700   Bladder irrigation, simple, lavage and/or instillation

24. A DATE(S) OF SERVICE From To MM DD YY MM DD YY	B Place of Service	C Type of Service	D PROCEDURES, SERVICES, OR SUPPLIES (Explain Unusual Circumstances) CPT/HCPCS MODIFIER	E DIAGNOSIS CODE	F $ CHARGES	G DAYS OR UNITS	H EPSDT Family Plan	I EMG	J COB	K RESERVED FOR LOCAL USE
1	10 01 XX			51700						
2	10 01 XX			51700 76						
3										
4										
5										
6										
25. FEDERAL TAX I.D. NUMBER SSN EIN			26. PATIENTIS ACCOUNT NO.	27. ACCEPT ASSIGNMENT? (For govt. claims, see back) YES NO	28. TOTAL CHARGE $		29. AMOUNT PAID $		30. BALANCE DUE $	

Rationale for Using Modifier 76

Because the same procedure was repeated in the afternoon, modifier 76 is reported for the procedure performed in the afternoon during the postoperative period.

Review of Modifier 76

1 Modifier 76 should be used for all procedures when the physician repeats the procedure the same day or during the postoperative period.

2 This modifier indicates that the claim is not a duplicate bill, but is the same procedure that was performed earlier.

3 The procedure repeated must be the same procedure (same procedure code) by the same physician.

4 An explanation of medical necessity for the repeat procedure is required by many insurance carriers.

Modifier 77: Repeat Procedure by Another Physician

Definition

The physician may need to indicate that a basic procedure or service performed by another physician had to be repeated. This situation may be reported by adding modifier 77 to the repeated procedure/service.

AMA Guidelines

Modifier 77 is reported when the procedure is repeated by another physician (not by the original physician who performed the first procedure). Modifier guidelines for 76 are the same as for 77 with one exception. Both are repeat procedures, but modifier 77 is used when a procedure is repeated by a different physician than the original physician.

CMS Guidelines

CMS recognizes the use of modifier 77 as with modifier 76. Medical necessity must be supported as to the reason for the repeated procedure. Modifier 77 is to be used when another physician repeats a procedure or service on the same day or for multiple diagnostic testing performed on the same day. Documentation may be required to support medical necessity for repeating a procedure on the same day or during the global surgical period.

Third-Party Payer Guidelines

Documentation may be required to support medical necessity for repeating a procedure on the same day or during the global surgical procedure.

Modifier 77, like modifier 76, is recognized by many commercial and third-party insurance carriers.

Example 1

A physician performed a femoral-popliteal bypass graft in the morning. Later that day, the graft clotted and the entire procedure was repeated. However, the surgeon (Physician A) who performed the surgery in the morning was not available to perform the repeat operation later that day. A second surgeon (Physician B) performed the same procedure later that night.

CPT Code(s) Billed by Physician A: *35556*
CPT Code(s) Billed by Physician B: *35556 77*

35556   Bypass graft, with vein; femoral-popliteal

Physician A

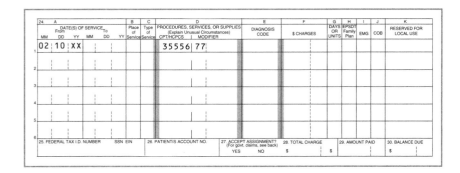

Physician B

Rationale for Using Modifier 77

Physician B is not affected by Physician A's global service. Physician B's performance of a surgical service (35556) will begin a global package related to the repeat surgical procedure. Again, documentation should be provided to the third-party payer to clarify that a repeat procedure was performed by another surgeon.

Example 2

A primary care physician performed a chest X ray on a patient in the physician's office and observed a suspicious mass. He sent the patient to a pulmonologist, who, on the same day, repeated the chest X ray. The pulmonologist also provided the total procedure for the X ray (technical and professional). The rationale for repeating the chest X ray was that the film did not give the pulmonologist a good picture and he wanted to repeat the X ray to confirm the diagnosis.

CPT Code(s) Billed by Primary Care Physician: 71020
CPT Code(s) Billed by Pulmonologist: 71020 77

71020   Radiologic examination, chest, two views, frontal and lateral

Rationale for Using Modifier 77
The pulmonologist is not affected by the primary care physician's performance of the service and/or procedure. Documentation should be provided to the insurance carrier to clarify that a repeat procedure was performed by another physician and was medically necessary.

Example 3

A 30-year-old construction worker got metal shavings in the left eye from welding, so he visited the ophthalmologist in the emergency department of the local hospital. After the physician evaluated the patient, he proceeded to remove an embedded foreign body using a slit lamp. An antibiotic was applied and a patch was placed over the patient's left eye. The patient was instructed to return to his physician in 2 days.

Later in the day the patient was still experiencing pain, so he contacted another ophthalmologist to look at his left eye. The physician examined the patient using a slit lamp, and he discovered another foreign body embedded in the left eye. The procedure was repeated by a different physician and the foreign body was removed, an antibiotic was applied, and the eye was patched again. The patient was instructed to return the next afternoon for follow-up.

CPT Code(s) Billed by Ophthalmologist 1: 65222

24. A DATE(S) OF SERVICE						B Place of Service	C Type of Service	D PROCEDURES, SERVICES, OR SUPPLIES (Explain Unusual Circumstances) CPT/HCPCS | MODIFIER	E DIAGNOSIS CODE	F $ CHARGES	G DAYS OR UNITS	H EPSDT Family Plan	I EMG	J COB	K RESERVED FOR LOCAL USE
From MM	DD	YY	To MM	DD	YY										
1 11	04	XX						65222							
2															
3															
4															
5															
6 25. FEDERAL TAX I.D. NUMBER SSN EIN						26. PATIENTIS ACCOUNT NO.		27. ACCEPT ASSIGNMENT? (For govt. claims, see back) YES NO	28. TOTAL CHARGE $		29. AMOUNT PAID $		30. BALANCE DUE $		

CPT Code(s) Billed by Ophthalmologist 2: 65222 77

65222   Removal of foreign body, external eye; corneal, with slit lamp

Review of Modifier 77

1. Modifier 77 is used when the same procedure is repeated on the same day or during the global days (if applicable) by a different physician.

2. Medical necessity must be supported (rationale) when a repeat procedure is billed by a different physician.

3. Use of this modifier does not guarantee reimbursement from the insurance carrier if medical necessity cannot be supported.

Checkpoint Exercises 1

True or False

1. _____ Modifier 76 can be used when the service is performed on the same day by a different physician.

2. _____ Modifier 66 may be used for all surgeries when more than one surgeon is performing the same procedure at the same operative session.

3. _____ The definition of modifier 76 is "repeat procedure or service by the same physician."

4. _____ When a related procedure is performed by a different physician, modifier 77 is used.

5. _____ CMS recognizes the use of modifiers 76 and 77.

Modifier 78: Return to the Operating Room for a Related Procedure During the Postoperative Period

Definition

The physician may need to indicate that another procedure was performed during the postoperative period of the initial procedure. When this subsequent procedure is related to the first, and requires the use of the operating room, it may be reported by adding the modifier 78 to the related procedure. (For repeat procedures on the same day, see modifier 76.)

AMA Guidelines

Modifier 78 is used when a related procedure is performed during the postoperative period. If postoperative complications do not require a trip to the operating room, this modifier is not applicable. Modifier 78 is not used for procedures that indicate in the code descriptor "subsequent, related or redo."

CMS Guidelines

This modifier is used when the related procedure is performed on the same day or during a global period with more than 0 global days. Payment for reoperations is made only for the intraoperative services. No additional payment is made for preoperative and postoperative care because CMS considers these services to be part of the original global surgery package. The approved amount will be set at the value of the intraoperative service the surgeon performed when an appropriate CPT code exists, for example, 32120 Thoracotomy, major; for postoperative complications. However, when reporting patient encounters for CMS, if no CPT code exists to describe the specific reoperation, the appropriate "unlisted procedures" code from the Surgery section of the CPT book would be used. Payment in these cases is based on up to 50% of the value of the intraoperative service that was originally provided.

This modifier is used to indicate that a subsequent procedure related to the initial procedure was performed during the postoperative period of the initial procedure. This modifier should be reported when complications arising from the surgery require use of the operating room. This circumstance is reported by adding modifier 78 to the related procedure.

With modifier 78, the CPT code that describes the related procedure performed during the return trip should be used. The procedure code for the original procedure should not be used. The key to the use of this modifier is that the repeat procedure is a direct complication of the original procedure. For reimbursement, CMS will consider the value of the intraoperative portion of the service of the code that describes the treatment in processing for payment.

CMS will only consider a procedure for a complication if it is treated in the operating room. When reporting a procedure with modifier 78, a new global period does not begin.

Payment under CMS for a Return Trip to the Operating Room for Treatment of Complications

When a procedure is reported with modifier 78, which indicates a return trip due to a complication, the carrier will pay the value of the intraoperative service of the code that describes the treatment of the complication(s). The value of the procedure may be found in the Medicare Fee Schedule Database (see an excerpt of the Database in Table 6-1).

The CMS fee schedule for the procedure is multiplied by the percent of the intraoperative work and rounded to the nearest cent. For example, procedure

TABLE 6-1 Medicare Fee Schedule Database Excerpt

HCPCS	Short Description	Facility Price	GPCI Work	GPCI PE	GPCI MP	WORK RVU	Non-Facility PE RVU	Facility PE RVU	MP RVU	Non-Facility Total	Facility Total	PCTC	Global	Pre Op	Intra Op	Post Op	Mult Surg	Bilt Surg	Asst Surg	Co Surg	Team Surg	Conv Fact
33915	Remove lung artery emboli	$1,339.13	1.027	1.109	1.867	20.99	9.63	9.63	1.66	32.28	32.28	0	090	0.09	0.84	0.07	2	0	2	1	0	37.8975
33916	Surgery of great vessel	$1,737.91	1.027	1.109	1.867	25.79	11.34	11.34	3.64	40.77	40.77	0	090	0.09	0.84	0.07	2	0	2	1	0	37.8975
33917	Repair pulmonary artery	$1,722.87	1.027	1.109	1.867	24.46	12.18	12.18	3.66	40.3	40.3	0	090	0.09	0.84	0.07	2	0	2	1	0	37.8975
33918	Repair pulmonary atresia	$1,826.69	1.027	1.109	1.867	26.41	12.07	12.07	4.12	42.6	42.6	0	090	0.09	0.84	0.07	2	0	2	1	0	37.8975
33919	Repair pulmonary atresia	$2,707.86	1.027	1.109	1.867	39.94	17.51	17.51	5.9	63.35	63.35	0	090	0.09	0.84	0.07	2	0	2	1	0	37.8975
33920	Repair pulmonary atresia	$2,130.19	1.027	1.109	1.867	31.9	13.82	13.82	4.35	50.07	50.07	0	090	0.09	0.84	0.07	2	0	2	1	0	37.8975
33922	Transect pulmonary artery	$1,588.48	1.027	1.109	1.867	23.48	10.9	10.9	3.06	37.44	37.44	0	090	0.09	0.84	0.07	2	0	2	1	0	37.8975
33924	Remove pulmonary shunt	$349.03	1.027	1.109	1.867	5.49	1.84	1.84	0.82	8.15	8.15	0	ZZZ	0	0	0	0	0	2	1	0	37.8975
33930	Removal of donor heart/lung	$0.00	1.027	1.109	1.867	0	0	0	0	0	0	9	XXX	0	0	0	9	9	9	9	9	37.8975
33933	Prepare donor heart/lung	$0.00	1.027	1.109	1.867	0	0	0	0	0	0	0	XXX	0	0	0	2	0	2	1	0	37.8975
33935	Transplantation, heart/lung	$4,211.51	1.027	1.109	1.867	60.87	28.77	28.77	8.95	98.59	98.59	0	090	0.09	0.84	0.07	2	0	2	1	2	37.8975
33940	Removal of donor heart	$0.00	1.027	1.109	1.867	0	0	0	0	0	0	9	XXX	0	0	0	9	9	9	9	9	37.8975
33944	Prepare donor heart	$0.00	1.027	1.109	1.867	0	0	0	0	0	0	0	XXX	0	0	0	2	0	2	1	0	37.8975
33945	Transplantation of heart	$2,965.40	1.027	1.109	1.867	42.04	21.39	21.39	6.08	69.51	69.51	0	090	0.09	0.84	0.07	2	0	2	1	2	37.8975

code 33935 has an intraoperative percentage of 84%. If the allowed amount for 33935 in Chicago, Illinois, is $4,042.27, then 85% of the fee schedule is $3,436.32.

When a procedure that has a "0" global period is reported with modifier 78, carriers will pay the full value for the procedure, which has no preoperative, intraoperative, or postoperative value. Caution is warranted because the physician's definition of a complication may differ from that of CMS. For example, a retinal detachment repair after cataract surgery is considered an unrelated procedure by Medicare and, thus, repair in the global period by the same surgeon would require modifier 79 to be appended to the procedure. Evacuation of a hyphema after cataract surgery, needling of a bleb after trabeculectomy, and hematoma evacuation after blepharoplasty are all examples of procedures that should be coded with modifier 78.

If the patient is returned to the operating room **after the initial operative session**, but on the same day as the original surgery for one or multiple procedures, append modifier 78 to each procedure performed that requires treatment for the complication. The multiple surgery rules would not apply.

If the patient is returned to the operating room **during the postoperative period**, and multiple procedures are required to treat the complication, the complication rules apply, but the multiple surgery rules would not.

If the patient is returned to the operating room **during the postoperative period of the original surgery but not on the same day of the original procedure**, and bilateral procedures are required as a result of the complication from the original surgery, the complication rules apply. The bilateral surgery rules would not apply.

Third-Party Payer Guidelines

 Insurance carriers and third-party payers recognize the use of modifier 78 if the reason for the return to the operating room is related to the original procedure and not a repeat procedure. Carrier reimbursement is based on the value of the intraoperative portion of the procedure that is performed. Failure to use modifier 78 may result in denial of the procedure within the postoperative period.

Example 1

A partial colectomy was performed on a Medicare patient in the hospital on March 1. The postoperative period for this procedure (code 44140) is 90 days. On March 15, the patient was returned to the operating room for a secondary suture of the abdominal wall. The secondary suture was related to the original surgery.

CPT Code(s) Billed for First Procedure: *44140—Colectomy, partial; with anastomosis*

CPT Code(s) Billed for Second Procedure: *49900 78—Suture, secondary, of abdominal wall for evisceration or dehiscence*

Rationale for Using Modifier 78

Since the suture of the abdominal wall was a complication related to the initial procedure within the global period, using modifier 78 would indicate to the insurance carrier that the procedure is related to the first procedure and, for Medicare should be paid only on the basis of the intraoperative service. The preoperative and postoperative care is not included when modifier 78 is used.

Example 2

A 70-year-old male underwent endoscopic nasal polypectomy and ethmoidectomy as an outpatient. Later that day, the patient experienced increased bleeding with clots, and he presented to the surgeon for treatment. Following unsuccessful manual pressure, packing insertion, and local vasoconstrictors performed in the surgeon's office, the patient was returned to the operating room in the surgery center where the bleeding was controlled with extensive packing and cautery. To control bleeding that was coming from the posterior (back) of the nose (nasopharynx), the physician placed extensive packing into the nasal cavity through the back of the throat. Extensive electrical coagulation was required during the procedure.

CPT Code(s) Billed for the First Procedure: 31237—Nasal/sinus endoscopy, surgical; with biopsy, polypectomy or debridement (separate procedure)

CPT Code(s) Billed for the Second Procedure: 30905 78—Control nasal hemorrhage, posterior, with posterior nasal packs and/or cautery, any method; initial

Rationale for Using Modifier 78

In this instance, the medical documentation reflected that the post-procedure bleeding was attributable to the initial operation. Therefore, a different code describing the procedure would be reported with modifier 78 appended. Because the same procedure is not repeated, modifier 76 would not be appropriate. The second procedure is reported with code 30905.

Review of Modifier 78

1 Modifier 78 is added to the procedure when the subsequent procedure is related to the initial procedure and requires the use of an operating room.

2 If a complication does not require a trip to the operating room, modifier 78 is not applicable.

3 For many carriers, a new postoperative period does not begin when a related procedure is performed and reported with modifier 78.

4 Insurance carriers reimburse on the basis of the intraoperative services provided.

5 An operating room is defined by CMS as a hospital, cardiac catheterization suite, ASC, laser suite, and/or endoscopy suite.

6 For CMS, this modifier should be used for a procedure not performed in an operating room only if the patient's condition was critical and there is no time to transport the patient to the operating room.

Modifier 79: Unrelated Procedure or Service by the Same Physician During the Postoperative Period

Definition

The physician may need to indicate that the performance of a procedure or service during the postoperative period was unrelated to the original procedure. This circumstance may be reported by using the modifier 79. (For repeat procedures on the same day, see modifier 76.)

AMA Guidelines

This modifier is used to indicate that the operating surgeon performed a procedure on a surgical patient during the postoperative period for problems unrelated to the original surgical procedure. The procedure must be performed by the same physician and is reported by appending modifier 79 to the procedure code. Modifier 79 is used to report, for example, a colposcopy performed during the global period of a mastectomy by the same surgeon.

CMS Guidelines

This modifier is used to show that a second procedure by the same physician (or physician of the same specialty in the same surgical group) is unrelated to a prior procedure for which the postoperative period has not been completed. Documentation, such as a different diagnosis (International Classification of Diseases, Ninth Revision, Clinical Modification), will usually be sufficient. Its use does not mandate a return to the operating room, nor is it limited to surgical procedures. Procedures are reimbursed at 100% of the allowable amount. The MCM, section 4824, Adjudication of Claims for Global Surgeries, provides further reference and clarification.

This modifier is often necessary with identical surgical procedures that are not performed on the same day, such as in cataract surgery, where both eyes are treated within a 90-day period. A new global period begins with modifier 79.

Third-Party Payer Guidelines

Many third-party payers recognize the use of modifier 79. Documentation must be supported for medical necessity. A new global period begins with modifier 79.

Example 1

A 70-year-old female Medicare patient complained of vision problems. Examination showed that cataracts in both her right and left eyes have matured to the point of visual impairment. She had difficulty reading and had recently failed a driving test. Cataract surgery was performed and an intraocular lens was implanted in the right eye on April 1. Recovery was monitored and the patient was examined through regularly scheduled postoperative visits. The global period for CMS for this procedure is 90 days. The patient's right eye was healing well and she decided to undergo the surgery on the left eye on May 15 (45 days postoperatively). The patient was admitted to the ASC and a cataract extraction with an intraocular lens implant of the left eye was performed.

CPT Code(s) Billed: *(April 1) 66984 RT—Extracapsular cataract removal with insertion of intraocular lens prosthesis (one stage procedure), manual or mechanical technique (eg, irrigation and aspiration or phacoemulsification)*

(May 15) 66984 LT 79—Extracapsular cataract removal with insertion of intraocular lens prosthesis (one stage procedure), manual or mechanical technique (eg, irrigation and aspiration or phacoemulsification)

CMS CODING TIP

HCPCS code(s) RT and LT identify right and left and help differentiate the right and left sides of the body. They should be used in addition to modifier 79 (when applicable), not in place of it.

CMS CODING TIP

CMS does not allow separate payment for additional procedures with a global fee period furnished during the postoperative period for a previous procedure by the same provider if billed without modifier 58, 78, or 79. These services will be denied without one of these modifiers.

Rationale for Using Modifier 79

Even though this is the exact same procedure on different dates, they are unrelated because they are performed on different sides of the body (right vs. left) and are not related to each other. Modifier 79 would be appropriate since the second surgery is performed during the 90-day global period for the procedure. For Medicare, if the procedure has 0 global days, modifier 79 would not be used.

Example 2

A patient had a repeat femoral-popliteal graft (35556) on June 1. The patient went home, and the incision and graft healed well. However, acute renal failure developed on June 9, a week after the patient went home, and he was hospitalized. The renal failure did not respond to medical treatment. Hemodialysis was indicated, and the same physician inserted a cannula for hemodialysis (36810 Insertion of cannula for hemodialysis, other purpose [separate procedure]; arteriovenous, external [Scribner type]) on June 10.

CPT Code(s) Billed for First Procedure: 35556—Bypass graft, with vein; femoral-popliteal (typical global days 90)

CPT Code(s) Billed for Second Procedure: 36810 79—Insertion of cannula for hemodialysis, other purpose (separate procedure); arteriovenous, external (Scribner type)

Rationale for Using Modifier 79

The physician's services for the insertion of the cannula for hemodialysis are reported as 36810 79, because this service (36810) is unrelated to the femoral-popliteal bypass graft (35556) performed during the previous hospitalization.

If modifier 79 is not appended to this procedure, the third-party payer may not know that this service is unrelated to the femoral-popliteal graft (ie, the computer program used by the third-party payer may not be able to distinguish that this service is not related to the previous surgery and may automatically reject this claim). Again, providing documentation to indicate that this service is unrelated to the first procedure may be helpful compared to clearing up a problem retrospectively.

Example 3

A 75-year-old Medicare patient underwent cataract surgery on May 14 on the right eye. The procedure code selected for the procedure was 66984 RT. On day 15 of the postoperative period, the patient was complaining of pain in the right eye. After examination, the surgeon discovered that the retina had detached, and the patient was returned to the operating room for the repair.

CPT Code(s) Billed for First Procedure: 66984 RT—Extracapsular cataract removal with insertion of intraocular lens prosthesis (one stage procedure), manual or mechanical technique (eg, irrigation and aspiration or phacoemulsification)

CPT Code(s) Billed for Second Procedure: 67107 RT 79—Repair of retinal detachment; scleral buckling (such as lamellar scleral dissection, imbrication or encircling procedure), with or without implant, with or without cryotherapy, photocoagulation, and drainage of subretinal fluid

Rationale for Using Modifier 79 vs Modifier 78

A retinal detachment repair after cataract surgery is considered an unrelated procedure according to CMS, and repair in the global period by the same surgeon would take modifier 79 instead of modifier 78 because the second procedure is not related to or a complication of the initial procedure.

NOTE: For Medicare, a new global period begins with the use of modifier 79.

Example 4

A patient underwent an excision of a deep soft tissue tumor of the neck on March 15. The procedure has a 90-day global. He presented to the same general surgeon on May 19 complaining of a persistent pain across his abdomen. The pain increased in severity and the patient began complaining of nausea. After examination, the patient underwent emergency surgery for a ruptured appendix.

CPT Code(s) Billed: 21556—Excision tumor, soft tissue of neck or thorax; deep, subfascial, intramuscular

44960 79—Appendectomy; for ruptured appendix with abscess or generalized peritonitis

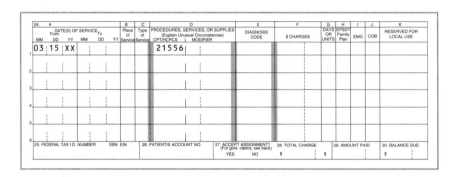

Rationale for Using Modifier 79

Because the two procedures are not related, and the second procedure is performed during the postoperative period of the soft tissue tumor removal of the neck, modifier 79 appended to the appendectomy informs the payer that the two procedures are not related and the appendectomy is not part of the global surgical period.

Review of Modifier 79

1 Modifier 79 is used when the procedure or service is unrelated to a procedure during the postoperative period.

2 Use of modifier 79 is restricted to the same physician.

3 Section 4824 of the MCM provides information on Medicare claims for global surgeries.

4 For Medicare, a new global period begins with modifier 79.

5 If more than two procedures are performed during the postoperative period and are unrelated, modifier 79 is appended to all unrelated procedures, not just the first procedure.

6 If a procedure is related to the first procedure and performed during the postoperative period, modifier 78 is used instead of modifier 79.

7 For Medicare and many other payers, when procedures are performed on the right and left sides of the body (same procedure) at different operative sessions during the postoperative period, modifier RT or LT is used with modifier 79.

Modifiers 80 to 82: Assistant Surgeons

Introduction

When billing is done for an assistant-at-surgery, the service should be indicated with one of the following modifiers:
- **80** Assistant surgeon
- **81** Minimum assistant surgeon
- **82** Assistant surgeon (when qualified resident surgeon not available)
- **AS** Physician assistant, nurse practitioner, or clinical nurse specialist services for assistant at surgery

Co-surgeon vs Assistant Surgeon

An assistant-at-surgery serves as an additional pair of hands for the operating surgeon. Assistants-at-surgery do not carry primary responsibility for or "perform distinct parts" of the surgical procedure.

Co-surgeons share responsibility for a surgical procedure, each serving as a primary surgeon during some portion of the surgery. Both must be surgeons, and they are frequently of different specialties. Co-surgeons may also have preoperative responsibility, are always responsible for dictating the operative report for the portion of the surgery that is their primary responsibility, and always have the responsibility for some of the postoperative care.

Which personnel qualify for reimbursement when performing as an assistant-at-surgery? Medicare will reimburse for the services of a physician, clinical nurse specialist (CNS), physician assistant (PA), and nurse practitioner (NP) when the primary surgeon requires an assistant and the surgical procedure meets Medicare's requirements. Medicare will not reimburse for surgical assistants such as registered nurse first assists (RNFAs), orthopedic physician assistants (OPAs), licensed practical nurses (LPNs), certified surgical technologists (CSTs), or other licensed or nonlicensed personnel employed by the physician practice.

Modifier 80: Assistant Surgeon

Definition

Surgical assistant services may be identified by adding the modifier 80 to the usual procedure number(s).

AMA Guidelines

One physician assists another physician in performing a procedure. If an assistant surgeon assists a primary surgeon and is present for the entire operation, or a substantial portion of the operation, then the assisting physician reports the same surgical procedure as the operating surgeon. The operating surgeon does not append a modifier to the procedure that he or she reports. The assistant surgeon reports the same CPT code as the operating physician, with modifier 80 appended.

For example, to report closure of an intestinal cutaneous fistula, the primary operating surgeon reports code 44640 and the assistant surgeon reports 44640 80. The individual operative report submitted by each surgeon should indicate the distinct service provided by each surgeon.

CMS Guidelines

To qualify as an assistant surgeon, the surgeon must actively assist when a physician performs a Medicare-covered surgical procedure. The assistant must be involved in the actual performance of the procedure, not simply provide ancillary services. The assistant would not be available to perform another surgical procedure during the same time period.

Fewer than 5% of cases nationwide utilize assistant surgeons. Physicians may not report assistant surgeons for procedure codes that are not approved for assistant surgery.

Current law requires the approved amount for assistant surgeons to be set at the lower of the actual charge or 16% of the global surgical approved amount. In addition, the law requires that payment for services of assistant surgeons be made only when the most recent national Medicare claims data indicate that a procedure has used assistants in at least 5% of cases based on a national average percentage. Full payment for the assistant surgeon's services may be made for some procedures if documentation is provided establishing medical necessity.

First, as the words denote, an assistant-at-surgery must actively assist when a physician performs a Medicare-covered surgical procedure. This necessarily entails that the assistant be involved in the actual performance of the procedure, not simply in other ancillary services. Since an assistant would be occupied during the surgical procedure, the assistant would not be available to perform and could not bill for another surgical procedure during the same time period.

To determine whether a surgical procedure is approved and subject to the assistant-at-surgery restriction, the Medicare Physician Fee Schedule Data Base (MPFSDB) should be consulted. This information can be found on the CMS Web site at www.cms.hhs.gov or by ordering *Medicare RBRVS: The Physician's Guide* from the American Medical Association. Section 15044 of the MCM gives specific instructions about CMS policy for assistant surgeons.

If a physician is not participating in the Medicare program, the limiting charge is 115% of 16% of the nonparticipating fee schedule amount. If it is within the state licensure of a limited-license practitioner to be an assistant-at-surgery, the payment is 10.4% of the fee schedule amount for the particular surgery. A PA or other nonphysician provider who assists at surgery, for example, would not use modifier 80. The modifier a nonphysician provider would use is the HCPCS modifier AS.

To qualify for the CMS definition of an assistant surgeon (modifier 80), the assistant surgeon needs to be able to take over the surgery should the primary surgeon become incapacitated. The surgical note should clearly document what the assistant surgeon did during the operative session. Medicare Part B does not pay for stand-by services.

CMS uses four indicators in the database to indicate whether modifier 80 (assistant surgery) is approved for payment:

1   An indicator of 0 indicates that the procedure would require medical necessity documentation for Medicare to pay for an assistant-at-surgery.

2   An assistant surgery indicator of 1 identifies procedures that are restricted and not payable under the Medicare Fee Schedule.

3   An indicator of 2 indicates a procedure that will allow payment for an assistant-at-surgery for this procedure with modifier 80.

4   An indicator of 9 indicates that the assistant surgery concept does not apply.

Table 6-2 gives the MPFSDB indicators for assistant surgery.

TABLE 6-2 **Assistant Surgery Rules (Modifier 80)**	
Indicator	**Definition**
0	Assistant surgeon may be paid with documentation. Use modifier 80.
1	Assistant surgeon cannot be paid.
2	Assistant surgeon can be paid. Use modifier 80.
9	Assistant surgeon concept does not apply.

Medicare will not cover an assistant surgeon's claim for services that do not require the presence of an assistant surgeon more than 5% of the time. Physicians are prohibited from billing a Medicare beneficiary for assistant-at-surgery services for procedure codes subject to the limit. Physicians who knowingly and willfully violate this prohibition and bill a beneficiary for an assistant-at-surgery for these procedures may be subject to the penalties contained under section 1842(j)(2) of the Social Security Act.

Assistant surgeon coverage is limited to fully qualified physicians and nonphysician practitioners (ie, PAs, NPs) if it is within the scope of their license. The services of an assistant are necessary in a number of operative procedures. Some simple procedures do not require the services of an assistant surgeon, and an assistant surgeon's services would not be covered.

Coverage is provided only when the use of an assistant is medically necessary. Some surgical procedure codes may be covered for two assistant surgeons. The

CMS CODING TIP

To determine whether a surgical procedure is approved for use of an assistant-at-surgery by CMS, refer to the MPFSDB.

AMA CODING TIP

Other modifiers may be used if applicable when modifier 80 is used.

THIRD-PARTY PAYER CODING TIP

Survey your commercial payers to determine the reimbursement rules when billing is done for nonphysician providers and get the information in writing.

allowance for the assistant surgeon, when covered, is 16% of the Medicare Physician Fee Schedule. A nonphysician practitioner's allowance for assisting at surgery is 85% of the 16% that physicians are allowed. The appropriate assistant surgeon modifier (80 or AS) must be submitted with surgical code(s) when billing is done for an assistant-at-surgery.

- Medicare will reimburse only if medical necessity of the assistant is documented.
- Medicare will not pay for an assistant when there is an assistant-at-surgery restriction.
- Medicare will reimburse for an assistant surgeon (MD, PA, NP, or CNS).

A primary surgeon may request that another provider assist with a surgical case. Depending on the procedure(s) performed, and the qualifications and training of the assisting provider, these services may be separately billable to Medicare. Medicare will reimburse only licensed personnel as assistants-at-surgery.

Claims from an assistant-at-surgery are subject to the same edits that are applied to the claims from a primary surgeon or other physician providing care during the global period of a procedure. All claims for a second assistant must have an operative report attached. Lack of documentation to support the medical necessity for an assistant-at-surgery will cause the service to be denied with the following remittance advice message: "Medicare does not usually pay for this service for the reported condition or surgical assistant for this kind of surgery is not covered."

When the indicator is "0" or "1," which indicates an assistant at surgery may not be paid for this procedure in the MFSDB, CMS had determined the procedure generally is not medically necessary. The carrier uses group code CO on the remittance advice. This signifies that the physician may not bill the beneficiary (patient) and may be subject to penalties if he or she bills the patient for the assistant surgeon.

Third-Party Payer Guidelines

Many third-party payers have varying payment rates for assistant-at-surgery with the use of modifiers 80 to 82. Multiple-procedure fee reduction applies to an assistant-at-surgery the same as it would apply to the primary surgeon. Individual consideration may be made when there are extenuating circumstances.

Modifiers 80 and 82 will be reimbursed at between 15% and 20% of the allowance for the primary surgeon in most cases. Many insurance carriers surveyed follow CMS policy for assistant surgeon allowance. Most insurance carriers require submission of documentation to determine what role the assistant surgeon played in the procedure. Non-Medicare payers may reimburse for the RNFA, OPA, or CST assisting in surgery. Commercial payers should be surveyed to determine their reimbursement rules and appropriate modifier use when nonphysician provider services are billed for. It is wise to obtain this information in writing.

Examples

The following chart illustrates the reimbursement of an assistant at surgery for CMS with modifier 80 used for the assistant surgeon in Los Angeles, California.

Assistant Surgeon Reduction

Code	Definition	Physician Fee Amount	Assistant-at-Surgery Reduction	Final Allowance
33300	Repair of heart wound	$1152.46	$1152.46 × 16% = $184.39	$184.39

> **CMS CODING TIP**
>
> Payment for an assistant-at-surgery is set at 16% of the actual charge of the global procedure amount.

The next chart illustrates the reimbursement of an assistant-at-surgery for CMS with modifier AS used for an NP, PA, or CNS in Los Angeles, California.

Assistant-at-Surgery Reduction

Code	Definition	Physician Fee Amount	Assistant-at-Surgery Reduction (85%)	Nonphysician Practitioner	Final Allowance
33300	Repair of heart wound	$1154.46	$1154.46 × 16% = $184.39	$184.39 × 85% =$156.73	$156.73

Example 1

A 50-year-old man underwent an anterior arthrodesis of the lumbar spine for degenerative disease. Through a retroperitoneal approach, the disc was excised and the end plates were prepared for fusion. In addition, an anterior fusion of L5-S1 was performed. A retroperitoneal incision was made and an arthrodesis was performed by means of an interbody lumbar fusion cage (BAK Cage). A distractor was placed in the interspace, a hole was drilled in the interspace, and the cage was placed in the hole. The spacer was removed and replaced with another cage. Both cages were filled with bone graft harvested from the iliac crest through a separate incision in the fascia. Two surgeons were necessary for the anterior fusion (22558 62). The general surgeon assisted the spinal surgeon with anterior instrumentation (22851) and harvesting an autograft (20937).

CPT Code(s) Billed by Spine Surgeon: 22558 62, 22851, and 20937

CPT Code(s) Billed by General Surgeon: 22558 62, 22851 80, and 20937 80

22558	Arthrodesis, anterior interbody technique, including minimal diskectomy to prepare interspace (other than for decompression); lumbar
22851	Application of intervertebral biomechanical device(s) (eg, synthetic cage[s], threaded bone dowel[s], methylmethacrylate) to vertebral defect or interspace
20937	Autograft for spine surgery only (includes harvesting the graft); morselized (through separate skin or fascial incision)

Spine Surgeon:

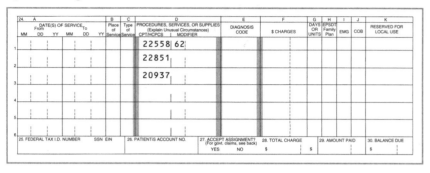

General Surgeon:

Rationale for Using Modifiers 62 and 80

Because the general surgeon acted as a co-surgeon and assistant surgeon during the same operative session, modifiers to explain the assistant surgeon's participation are required, as shown in Table 6-3.

TABLE 6-3 Co-surgeon and Assistant Surgeon Table

Procedure	Spinal Surgeon	General Surgeon
Anterior fusion	22558 62	22558 62
Anterior instrumentation	22851	22851 80
Iliac crest graft	20937	20937 80

Example 2

A 70-year-old male Medicare patient with coronary artery disease and chronic obstructive pulmonary disease arrived by ambulance with a 1-hour history of excruciating abdominal and back pain. His blood pressure was 70/40 mm Hg, heart rate was 140/min, and he had a distended abdomen with a tender pulsatile mass. Emergent repair of a ruptured infrarenal abdominal aortic aneurysm was performed by placement of a tube graft. An assistant surgeon was needed to assist in placing the tube graft while the cardiac surgeon repaired the ruptured abdominal aortic aneurysm through an open abdominal incision.

CPT Code(s) Billed by Cardiac Surgeon: 35082

CPT Code(s) Billed by Assistant Surgeon: 35082 80

35082   Direct repair of aneurysm, pseudoaneurysm, or excision (partial or total) and graft insertion, with or without patch graft; for ruptured aneurysm, abdominal aorta

Rationale for Using Modifier 80

Since the primary surgeon requested an assistant surgeon, the assistant surgeon would bill the same procedure code with modifier 80. Since this procedure is on the MPFSDB as an approved procedure, using an assistant surgeon would be allowed.

Example 3

A 40-year-old right-handed patient with hypertension and insulin-dependent diabetes had chronic renal failure. He had never had a previous hemoaccess procedure. Neither cephalic vein was an acceptable conduit for arteriovenous fistula access. As an outpatient, he had an arteriovenous graft with polytetrafluoroethylene inserted in the left arm with local anesthesia and intravenous sedation (by an anesthesiologist). The primary surgeon inserted a thermoplastic graft while the assistant surgeon assisted in creating the arteriovenous fistula.

CPT Code(s) Billed by Primary Surgeon: 36830
CPT Code(s) Billed by Assistant Surgeon: 36830 80

36830   Creation of arteriovenous fistula by other than direct arteriovenous anastomosis (separate procedure); nonautogenous graft (eg, biological collagen, thermoplastic graft)

Rationale for Using Modifier 80

Since the primary surgeon requested an assistant surgeon, the assistant surgeon would bill the same procedure code with modifier 80. Documentation may be required to support medical necessity for the use of an assistant surgeon with many insurance carriers.

Example 4

A 4-year-old boy presented with cardiomegaly and a prominent thrill over the precordium. Echocardiogram and catheterization demonstrate severe left ventricular outflow tract obstruction at both the subvalvar and valvar levels. The outflow gradient is 90 mm Hg. Dr Jones, assisted by Dr Moore, performed an aortic valve replacement with allograft in the hospital surgery department.

CPT Code(s) Billed by Dr Smith: 33413
CPT Code(s) Billed by Dr Moore: 33413 80

33413   Replacement, aortic valve; by translocation of autologous pulmonary valve with allograft replacement of pulmonary valve (Ross procedure)

Rationale for using Modifier 80

The second surgeon provided the extra pair of hands by assisting for the entire procedure. The primary surgeon will report the procedure without a modifier, while the assistant reports the same procedure with modifier 80. It is not necessary for the assistant surgeon to dictate an operative report, but the operative report must clearly define the role and extent of the assistant's involvement.

Review of Modifier 80

1 Modifier 80 is used when a surgical assistant is used for the entire procedure to assist the primary surgeon.

2 Medicare and many other insurance carriers do not allow payment for an assistant when the assistant is a nonlicensed physician or a nonphysician in the operating room (surgical technician).

3 CMS pays for the assistant surgeon only if the procedure is approved for assistant-at-surgery coverage (MPSFDB) and if the procedure is medically necessary.

4 If the procedure requires the use of co-surgeons or a team of surgeons, modifier 62 or 66 is used.

5 The MPFSDB indicates whether a surgical procedure is approved for use of an assistant-at-surgery for CMS.

6 Physicians are prohibited from charging a Medicare beneficiary for an assistant-at-surgery when a procedure is not covered. If they willfully violate this rule, physicians could be subject to penalties and/or sanctions through the Medicare program under the Social Security Act and to fraud and abuse penalties under the Health Insurance Portability and Accountability Act of 1996, as well as the Balanced Budget Act of 1997.

7 The operative note should clearly document what the assistant surgeon did during the operative session.

8 Commercial payers should be surveyed to determine their reimbursement rules and appropriate modifier use when billing is done for nonphysician provider services. These instructions should be obtained in writing.

9 Other modifiers may be used if applicable when modifier 80 is appended.

Modifier 81: Minimum Assistant Surgeon

Definition

Minimum surgical assistant services are identified by adding the modifier 81 to the usual procedure number.

AMA Guidelines

At times, although a primary operating physician may plan to perform a surgical procedure alone, during the operation circumstances may arise that require the services of an assistant surgeon for a relatively short time. In this instance, the second surgeon provides minimal assistance, for which he or she reports the surgical procedure code with modifier 81 appended.

CMS Guidelines

CMS rarely recognizes modifier 81 except in extreme cases. Modifier 81 does not appear in the MPFSDB. When modifier 81 is used with a procedure code that has a maximum allowable payment, the maximum allowable payment for the procedure will be no more than 13% of the maximum allowable payment listed in the CMS rules or the billed charge, whichever is less. When modifier 81 is with a "by report" procedure, the maximum allowable payment for the procedure is no more than 13% of the reasonable amount paid for the primary procedure.

Third-Party Payer Guidelines

Many third-party payers have varying payment rates for a minimal assistant-at-surgery billed with modifier 81. Multiple-procedure fee reduction applies to an assistant-at-surgery the same as it would apply to the primary surgeon. Individual consideration may be made when there are extenuating circumstances. Carriers that allow a minimal assistant surgeon in many cases require documentation to support the medical necessity of using an assistant surgeon for a portion of the procedure.

AMA CODING TIP

The services provided by the surgeon who provides "minimal assistance" during the surgery would be reported with modifier 81 appended to the surgical procedure code.

Example 1

At 6 weeks of age, after neonatal colostomy, a neonate underwent a sacroperineal repair that included repair of the urethral fistula, reconstruction of the muscular components, and repair of an imperforate anus. An assistant surgeon assisted with the reconstruction only.

CPT Code(s) Billed by Primary Surgeon: 46716
CPT Code(s) Billed by Minimal Assistant Surgeon: 46716 81

46716   Repair of low imperforate anus; with transposition of anoperineal or anovestibular fistula

Rationale for Using Modifier 81

Since the primary surgeon requested a minimal assistant surgeon, the assistant surgeon would bill the same procedure code with modifier 81. An assistant surgeon provided assistance with the reconstruction only, which may be considered minimal assistance by most insurance carriers, since he or she participated with only a portion of the surgical procedure. Documentation (operative note) is normally required to support the medical necessity as well as to determine what participation the assistant surgeon provided.

Example 2

A 35-year-old woman was evaluated because of a lesion approximately 2 cm in largest diameter that was confined to the cervix. A biopsy specimen showed a well-differentiated squamous cell cancer. The patient then underwent a radical abdominal hysterectomy, with bilateral total pelvic lymphadenectomy and selected periaortic lymph node sampling. An assistant surgeon assisted with lymph node sampling.

CPT Code(s) Billed by Primary Surgeon: 58210
CPT Code(s) Billed by Minimal Assistant Surgeon: 58210 81

58210   Radical abdominal hysterectomy, with bilateral total pelvic lymphadenectomy and para-aortic lymph node sampling (biopsy), with or without removal of tube(s), with or without removal of ovary(s)

Rationale for Using Modifier 81

In this example, the assistant is assisting the surgeon for only a part of the procedure and would report the CPT code 58210 with modifier 81. The primary surgeon would report 58210 without a modifier. The individual operative report submitted by each of these surgeons should indicate the distinct service provided by each of them.

Example 3

A 28-year-old male presented with an expansile lesion of the left maxilla with extension into the infraorbital region. He had biopsy-proven ameloblastoma of the maxilla with infiltration of the maxillary sinus and adjacent soft tissues. Medical imaging revealed an 8 x 6 cm radiopaque/radiolucent lesion that originated from the left third molar region and extended into the maxillary sinus with disruption and distortion of the anterior maxillary wall extending above the infraorbital nerve foramen. The ENT surgeon, Dr Smythe, enlisted the assistance of another surgeon, Dr Johnston, to minimally assist with the procedure.

At operation, surgical excision required an extra-oral Weber-Ferguson approach to access the superior extent of the maxillary tumor. The lesion is resected with a left posterior maxillectomy and an anterior osteotomy, with clear margins. The large antral opening is packed, and the patient is fitted with a custom-made surgical obturator to close the dead space. A split thickness skin graft is taken from the lateral thigh, cut, and placed in the defect by Dr Johnston. The pre-made temporary obturator is loaded with a thermo plastic compound and seated in the defect against the skin graft to customize the superior aspect of the obturator. The appliance is removed and the excess compound is removed. It is heated again and replaced for final contour and to support the skin graft against the surgical defect.

CPT Code(s) Billed by Dr Smythe: *21049*
CPT Code(s) Billed by Dr Johnston: *21049 81*

21049   Excision of benign tumor or cyst of maxilla; requiring extra-oral osteotomy and partial maxillectomy (eg, locally aggressive or destructive lesion(s))

Rationale for Using Modifier 81

Because the physician only assisted minimally with obtaining and placing the graft, modifier 81 would be appended to the procedure for the portion of the procedure that he or she assisted with (grafting).

Review of Modifier 81

1   CMS rarely reimburses when a minimal assistant surgeon is used except under extenuating circumstances.

2   Documentation is required by most insurance carriers to support medical necessity for the assistant surgeon.

3   Modifier 81 is used when an assistant surgeon does not participate in the entire procedure, but is needed only for a short time.

4   Modifier 81 is not used for nonphysicians or nonphysician assistants who do not meet the criteria for payment, which includes surgical technicians. Payment for nonphysician assistants who do not qualify are bundled into the payment for the hospital or ASC and should not be billed to the insurance carrier or to the beneficiary.

Modifier 82: Assistant Surgeon (When Qualified Resident Surgeon Not Available)

Definition

The unavailability of a qualified resident surgeon is a prerequisite for use of modifier 82 appended to the usual procedure code number(s).

AMA Guidelines

The prerequisite for using modifier 82 is the unavailability of a qualified resident surgeon. In certain programs (eg, teaching hospitals), the physician acting as the assistant surgeon is usually a qualified resident surgeon.

CMS CODING TIP

Medicare rarely recognizes modifier 81 except in extreme cases.

CMS CODING TIP

Documentation is required by most insurance carriers to support the medical necessity of using a minimal assistant surgeon.

However, there may be times (eg, during rotational changes) when a qualified resident surgeon is not available and another surgeon assists in the operation. In these instances, the services of the nonresident assistant surgeon are reported with modifier 82 appended to the appropriate code. This indicates that another surgeon is assisting the operating surgeon instead of a qualified resident surgeon.

Although the intent of the assistant surgeon modifiers is to report physician services, many physicians and/or coders report the modifiers incorrectly for a variety of nonphysician surgical assistant services. The most common misinterpretation of the assistant surgeon modifiers is to report PA or NP assistant surgical services.

Although from a CPT perspective this is not the intended use of the assistant surgeon modifiers, some third-party payers consider this an acceptable means of reporting nonphysician assistants during surgery. Many have established their own guidelines for reporting assistant surgeon services. Since each third-party payer may establish reporting guidelines that vary from coding guidelines, a clear understanding of CPT coding guidelines, as well as third-party payer reporting guidelines, is essential.

CMS Guidelines

Some surgical procedures require an assistant surgeon. The CMS has identified those surgical procedures for which an assistant surgeon may be reimbursed. Payment will not be made for services of assistants-at-surgery furnished in a teaching hospital that has a training program related to the surgical specialty required for the surgical procedure and has a qualified resident available to perform the service, unless exceptional medical circumstances exist. If the procedure is deemed ineligible, the cost cannot be passed on to the patient.

> **NOTE:** CMS defines a teaching hospital as one that has a graduate education program in the field of medicine, osteopathy, dentistry, or podiatry, approved by the appropriate accrediting body for graduate education in each of these fields. This definition does not include hospitals that only participate in the approved programs of other hospitals or have only nonapproved programs. In some cases in a teaching hospital, there may not be a qualified resident available. This might be because of other involvement in activities, the complexity of the surgery, numbers of residents in the program, or other reasons that may be validated.

Exceptional Medical Circumstances

Payment is made for the services of assistants-at-surgery in teaching hospitals despite the availability of a qualified resident to furnish the services in the following circumstances:

- In emergency or life-threatening situations where multiple traumatic injuries require immediate treatment

- If the primary surgeon has an across-the-board policy of never involving residents in the preoperative, operative, or postoperative care of his or her patients

Claims for assistants-at-surgery furnished in teaching hospitals based on the unavailability of qualified residents are payable only on the basis of the following certification:

I understand that Section 1842(b)(6)(D) of the Social Security Act generally prohibits Medicare Part B reasonable charge payment for the services of assistants at surgery in teaching hospitals when qualified residents are available to furnish such service. I certify that the services for which payment is claimed were medically necessary and that no qualified resident was available to perform the service. I further understand that these services are subject to post-payment review by the Medicare carrier.

For surgical procedures that require a primary surgeon and an assistant surgeon, the primary surgeon reports the procedure code for the surgery without a modifier, and the assistant surgeon reports the procedure code for the surgical procedure with a modifier to indicate that he or she was an assistant surgeon.

Assistant-at-Surgery Modifiers

The following modifiers are to be used when billing for assistance-at-surgery services:

- **Modifier 80:** This modifier is used in a nonteaching setting or in a teaching setting when a resident was available but the surgeon opted not to use the resident. In the latter case, the service is generally not covered by Medicare.
- **Modifier 82:** The unavailability of a qualified resident surgeon is a prerequisite for use of this modifier. This modifier is used in teaching hospitals if there is no approved training program related to the medical specialty required for the surgical procedure or no qualified resident is available.
- **Modifier AS:** This is used for assistant-at-surgery services performed by a PA or NP.

When modifier 82 is used and the assistant surgeon is a licensed doctor of medicine, doctor of osteopathic medicine and surgery, doctor of podiatric medicine, or doctor of dental surgery, the maximum level of reimbursement is the same as for modifier 80. If the assistant surgeon is a PA, the maximum level of reimbursement is the same as for modifier 81. If a person other than a physician or a certified PA bills with modifier 82, the charge and payment for the service are reflected in the facility fee.

CMS CODING TIP

CMS will deny payment for services of assistants-at-surgery furnished in a teaching hospital that has a training program related to the surgical specialty required for the surgical procedure and has a qualified resident available to perform the service.

THIRD-PARTY PAYER CODING TIP

A teaching hospital is one that has a graduate education program in the field of medicine, osteopathy, dentistry, or podiatry, approved by the appropriate accrediting body for graduate education in each of these fields.

If the physician (MD, NP, PA, or CNS) is not paid when CMS is billed for the assistant surgeon, it is likely that the surgical procedure is not on Medicare's approved list. In that event, the physician should take the following steps:

1 Check the resource book Medicare RBRVS: The Physician's Guide to see if the surgical procedure is on the approved list of codes.

2 Ask the Medicare intermediary to provide a list of approved surgical procedures.

3 Ask the primary surgeon to clearly dictate the reason for the assistant's presence and role during the surgical case.

4 If the procedure performed is on the approved list, contact the payer, first by phone and, if unsuccessful, through an appeal.

5 For non-Medicare payers, obtain a list of approved modifiers to denote the assistant-at-surgery. If a non-Medicare provider was billed and the payer does not pay for the assistant, review your contracts and determine whether the contract allows for nonphysician providers as assistants. Ideally, the payers were surveyed before the practice made this investment.

Example 1

One year after a frontal skull fracture with bone loss, an adolescent was admitted to the hospital for reconstruction of most of the forehead and superior orbital rims with the use of methylmethacrylate cranioplasty or bone allograft. The procedure was performed in a teaching hospital. All qualified residents were unavailable, and the neurosurgeon requested the assistance of a colleague to assist with the procedure.

CPT Code(s) Billed by Primary Neurosurgeon: 21179
CPT Code(s) Billed by Assistant Surgeon: 21179 82

21179   Reconstruction, entire or majority of forehead and/or supraorbital rims; with grafts (allograft or prosthetic material)

Rationale for Using Modifier 82

Since the primary surgeon requested an assistant surgeon, the assistant surgeon would bill the same procedure code with modifier 82. Since a qualified resident was not available, it would be appropriate for the physician to submit the claim with modifier 82 appended to the procedure. A certification statement should be submitted with the claim to validate the procedure.

Example 2

A neurosurgeon in a teaching hospital performed surgery on a 63-year-old man who had a spontaneous intracerebral hemorrhage into the basal ganglia in the minor hemisphere. The patient was hypertensive, with normal clotting factors and no arrhythmia. A computed tomographic scan at admission showed a large hematoma with shift and displacement of the medial temporal lobe into the incisura. The patient had a large sluggish pupil on the same side, suggesting early uncal herniation. A craniotomy was done with exposure and evacuation of the hematoma. The neurosurgeon enlisted the help of another surgeon for the entire procedure because no qualified resident surgeon was available.

CPT Code(s) Billed by Primary Surgeon: 61313
CPT Code(s) Billed by Assistant Surgeon: 61313 82

61313   Craniectomy or craniotomy for evacuation of hematoma, supratentorial; intracerebral

Rationale for Using Modifier 82

Since the primary surgeon requested an assistant surgeon, the assistant surgeon would bill the same procedure code with modifier 82. Since a qualified resident was not available, it would be appropriate for the physician to submit the claim with modifier 82 appended to the procedure. A certification statement should be submitted with the claim to validate the procedure.

Example 3

A male patient presented to a teaching hospital with bilateral upper extremity amputation at the wrist, requiring tendon transfers and interosseous releases to allow abduction and adduction of the radius from the ulna. There was not an orthopedic resident available to assist with the procedures, so the primary surgeon called in another teaching orthopedic surgeon to assist.

At operation, tendons were transferred and the interosseous membrane was released. The skin flaps were rotated as needed, and the arm was placed in a bulky dressing. During subsequent hospital and office visits, through the 90-day global period, sutures were removed, dressings were changed, and rehabilitation progress was monitored.

CPT Code(s) Billed by Primary Orthopedic Surgeon: 25915
CPT Code(s) Billed by Assistant Orthopedic Surgeon: 25915 82

25915   Krukenberg procedure

Rationale for Using Modifier 82

Since a resident is not available in the teaching setting in this example, the physician must call another teaching physician to assist. Use of modifier 82 identifies that the resident is not available at the time of the procedure or service.

Review of Modifier 82

1 Modifier 82 is used for an assistant-at-surgery only if a qualified resident is not available or the surgeon never uses residents in surgery in a teaching facility.

2 Modifier 82 is used to indicate that an assistant-at-surgery was used when a qualified resident was not available in a teaching facility.

3 For most payers, overuse of modifier 82 consistently by physicians in a teaching facility would flag potential abuse.

4 Modifier 82 should not be used when a resident is available and assists with the procedure.

5 CMS fee allowance is the same as with modifier 80.

6 Certification for using modifier 82 must be on file for each claim. Many carriers require the certification to be submitted with the claim and the operative report.

Test Your Knowledge

Multiple Choice

1 Modifiers 76 and/or 77 are used to:
   a. Explain why the patient returned to the operating room during the postoperative period
   b. Comply with CMS compliance guidelines
   c. Only supply information; reimbursement will not be affected
   d. Explain why a procedure was duplicated, usually with a report, so the physician will be reimbursed appropriately

2 When using modifier 80, assistant surgeon, the primary surgeon must use:
   a. Modifier 81
   b. Modifier 66
   c. Modifier 62
   d. No modifier is necessary for the primary surgeon.

3 The main difference between modifier 80 and modifier 81 is:
   a. The board certification of the assistant surgeon
   b. The amount of time the assistant surgeon spends in the surgery suite
   c. Modifier 81 is used to indicate the primary surgeon and modifier 80 is for the assistant surgeon
   d. Modifier 80 is used for the primary surgeon, 81 for the assistant

4 If a procedure must be performed because of a complication of a previous surgery and is performed during the global surgical period, the correct modifier to append to the procedure code is:
   a. Modifier 58
   b. Modifier 79
   c. Modifier 78
   d. Modifier 76

5 Modifier 62 is used for:
   a. Two surgeons, both are primary
   b. Surgical team, one primary and one assistant surgeon
   c. Repeat procedure by same physician, same procedure billed
   d. Assistant surgeon, assistant is available for the entire operation

True or False

6 _____ When reporting a procedure using modifier 82 in a teaching facility, the teaching hospital must use a resident in all cases when reporting the services.

7 _____ The definition of modifier 79 is return to the operating room for a related procedure.

8 _____ Modifier 66 is reported for team surgery.

9 _____ When reporting services for unrelated procedures during the post-operative procedure, the correct modifier to use is modifier 76.

10 _____ Surgical assistants are reported with modifier 80.

Fill in the Blanks

11 _____ _____ must be supported when a claim is submitted with modifiers 76 and 77.

12 Each surgeon reports modifier _____ when performing team surgery.

13 Modifier 76 is used when a procedure is repeated by _____ _____.

14 The difference between modifiers 76 and 77 is _____.

15 Physician A performs a procedure in the morning, and the procedure needs to be repeated in the afternoon. Physician A is not available, so Physician B performs the same procedure on the same day as the original surgery. Physician B reports the procedure with _____.

CHAPTER 7

Modifiers 90 to 99

Modifier 90: Reference (Outside) Laboratory

Definition

When laboratory procedures are performed by a party other than the treating or reporting physician, the procedure may be identified by adding modifier 90 to the usual procedure number.

AMA Guidelines

cpt This modifier is used by a physician or clinic when laboratory tests for a patient are performed by an outside or reference laboratory. This modifier is used to indicate that, although the physician is reporting the performance of a laboratory test, the actual testing component was a service from a laboratory.

When the physician bills the patient for lab work that was performed by an outside or (reference) lab, modifier 90 is added to the lab procedure codes. Physicians use this modifier when laboratory procedures are performed by a party other than the treating or reporting physician.

CMS Guidelines

CMS Physicians should never bill Medicare or Medicaid patients for lab work done outside their office. The laboratory performing the service will bill for the laboratory procedures. CMS does not recognize the use of modifier 90. The physician may bill the insurance carrier only for the actual laboratory testing performed in the office.

Third-Party Payer Guidelines

With managed care and commercial insurance carriers that have contracts with specific laboratories, modifier 90 would not be recognized. When the beneficiary has a "carve out," which means a specific laboratory at which the specimen must be examined or the lab work performed, the physician may not act as the "agent" and bill the patient's insurance company for the specimen collection and the lab work performed if the specimen is sent to an independent lab.

While this was the standard practice in the 1970s and early 1980s, very few insurance carriers will allow the physician to bill for the lab work if the services are not performed in the office. It is important that the clinic or medical practice check with the individual insurance carrier to determine whether this practice is allowed.

Example 1

Dr Jones, an internist, examined a non-Medicare patient and, as part of the exam, ordered a complete blood cell count. He did not perform in-office lab testing. He had an arrangement with a laboratory to bill him for the testing procedure, and, in turn, he would bill the patient. The physician's staff performed the venipuncture. The physician reported the appropriate evaluation and management code, the venipuncture (36415), and 85025 90 for the complete blood cell count performed by the outside lab.

CPT Code(s) Billed by Physician: 36415—Collection of venous blood by venipuncture

> *85025 90—Blood count; complete (CBC), automated (Hgb, Hct, RBC, WBC and platelet count) and automated differential WBC count*

24.	A DATE(S) OF SERVICE		B Place of Service	C Type of Service	D PROCEDURES, SERVICES, OR SUPPLIES (Explain Unusual Circumstances) CPT/HCPCS MODIFIER	E DIAGNOSIS CODE	F $ CHARGES	G DAYS OR UNITS	H EPSDT Family Plan	I EMG	J COB	K RESERVED FOR LOCAL USE
	From MM DD YY	To MM DD YY										
1					36415							
2					85025 90							
3												
4												
5												
6												

25. FEDERAL TAX I.D. NUMBER SSN EIN	26. PATIENTIS ACCOUNT NO.	27. ACCEPT ASSIGNMENT? (For govt. claims, see back) YES NO	28. TOTAL CHARGE $	29. AMOUNT PAID $	30. BALANCE DUE $

Rationale for Using Modifier 90

The physician may bill 36415 without a modifier for the venipuncture since the work is performed in the office. The specimen is sent to a laboratory with which the physician has an agreement to handle the billing. The laboratory will bill the physician and the physician will bill the patient and/or insurance company.

> **NOTE:** The Clinical Laboratory Improvement Amendments allow an uncertified lab to perform a limited number of laboratory procedures in the office. For patient ease, most physicians draw the blood for the lab work in the office and send it to an outside facility for performance of the test. Some physicians have contracts with the outside labs and bill the patient. Other physicians provide the blood drawn and the outside lab bills directly.

Example 2

A physician's office drew blood for a lipid panel. The physician's office coded the chemistry panel, but indicated that an outside lab performed the procedure by using the modifier 90. The primary care physician did not have a Clinical Laboratory Improvement Act-approved lab on site and indicated by use of modifier 90 that the lab procedure was performed off site to maintain compliance.

> *CPT Code(s) Billed:* *36415—Collection of venous blood by venipuncture*
>
>   *80061 90—Lipid panel. This panel must include the following: Cholesterol, serum, total (82465); Lipoprotein, direct measurement, high density cholesterol (HDL cholesterol) (83718); Triglycerides (84478)*

Rationale for Using Modifier 90

The venipuncture is performed in the physician's office and the specimen is sent to the laboratory for analysis. The laboratory bills the physician for the service and the physician bills for the venipuncture and the laboratory analysis. The venipuncture (36415) would not need a modifier because the service was performed in the physician's office.

Example 3

A 56-year-old patient visited her internist for her annual physical examination. The physician documented a preventive medicine E/M service for the patient, and a Pap and pelvic were performed with specimen collection by endocervical scraping. The specimen was placed in a preservative suspension and sent to the laboratory. The laboratory performed the Pap evaluation under a physician's supervision. The laboratory billed the patient's insurance company for the analysis of the specimen.

> *CPT Code(s) Reported by the Internist:* *99396—Periodic comprehensive preventive medicine reevaluation and management of an individual including an age and gender appropriate history, examination, counseling/anticipatory guidance/risk factor reduction interventions, and the ordering of appropriate immunization(s), laboratory/ diagnostic procedures, established patient; 40–64 years*
>
>   *99000—Handling and/or conveyance of specimen for transfer from the physician's office to a laboratory*

24.	A					B	C	D	E	F	G	H	I	J	K
	DATE(S) OF SERVICE From — To					Place of Service	Type of Service	PROCEDURES, SERVICES, OR SUPPLIES (Explain Unusual Circumstances) CPT/HCPCS | MODIFIER	DIAGNOSIS CODE	$ CHARGES	DAYS OR UNITS	EPSDT Family Plan	EMG	COB	RESERVED FOR LOCAL USE
	MM	DD	YY	MM	DD	YY										
1									99396							
2									99000							
3																
4																
5																
6																

25. FEDERAL TAX I.D. NUMBER	SSN EIN	26. PATIENTIS ACCOUNT NO.	27. ACCEPT ASSIGNMENT? (For govt. claims, see back) YES NO	28. TOTAL CHARGE $	29. AMOUNT PAID $	30. BALANCE DUE $

CPT Code(s) Reported by the Laboratory: 88142—Cytopathology, cervical or vaginal (any reporting system), collected in preservative fluid, automated thin layer preparation; manual screening under physician supervision

24.	A DATE(S) OF SERVICE						B Place of Service	C Type of Service	D PROCEDURES, SERVICES, OR SUPPLIES (Explain Unusual Circumstances) CPT/HCPCS | MODIFIER		E DIAGNOSIS CODE	F $ CHARGES	G DAYS OR UNITS	H EPSDT Family Plan	I EMG	J COB	K RESERVED FOR LOCAL USE
	From MM	DD	YY	To MM	DD	YY											
1									88142 |								
2																	
3																	
4																	
5																	
6	25. FEDERAL TAX I.D. NUMBER SSN EIN						26. PATIENTIS ACCOUNT NO.		27. ACCEPT ASSIGNMENT? (For govt. claims, see back) YES NO		28. TOTAL CHARGE $		29. AMOUNT PAID $		30. BALANCE DUE $		

Rationale for Not Using Modifier 90

Because the physician is not billing the laboratory for the laboratory/pathology services, an outside reference lab would not apply. The physician reports the E/M service and may report specimen handling for transfer from the physician's office to the laboratory. Keep in mind, however, that not every insurance carrier will reimburse for specimen handling.

The laboratory will report code 88142 for the cytopathology and will submit the claim for the service provided.

Review of Modifier 90

1 A claim with modifier 90 should not be submitted for a Medicare patient. Medicare does not recognize the use of modifier 90.

2 The insurance carrier should be consulted to determine whether it recognizes an "outside reference laboratory," since many managed care plans and commercial carriers do not recognize the outside reference laboratory concept.

Modifier 91: Repeat Clinical Diagnostic Test

Definition

In the course of treatment of the patient, it may be necessary to repeat the same laboratory test on the same day to obtain subsequent (multiple) test results. Under these circumstances, the laboratory test performed can be identified by its usual procedure number and the addition of the modifier 91. **Note:** This modifier may not be used when tests are rerun to confirm initial results; due to testing problems with specimens or equipment; or for any other reason when a normal, one-time, reportable result is all that is required. This modifier may not be used when other code(s) describe a series of test results (eg, glucose tolerance tests, evocative/

suppression testing). This modifier may only be used for laboratory test(s) performed more than once on the same day on the same patient.

AMA Guidelines

Modifier 91 was created to replace the CMS national level II modifier QR, which was deleted from the Health Care Common Procedure Coding System (HCPCS) 2000 manual. Modifier 91 may be appended to a laboratory code to indicate that a laboratory test was performed multiple times on the same day, for the same patient, and that it was necessary to obtain multiple results in the course of treatment. The note included in the text of the modifier indicates that modifier 91 is not intended to be used when laboratory tests are rerun:

- To confirm initial test results
- Due to testing problems encountered with specimens or equipment
- For any other reason when a normal, one-time, reportable result is all that is required

Modifier 91 may not be used when there are other code(s) to describe a series of test results (eg, glucose tolerance tests, evocative/suppression testing). Modifier 91 would be reported only when laboratory tests are performed more than once during the same day for the same patient.

Examples may include:

- Follow-up with potassium level after treatment of hyperkalemia
- Repeat arterial blood gas to monitor a patient's condition

Specific laboratory tests that may include multiple samples being drawn, such as a glucose tolerance test, should be reported with the appropriate CPT® code for the entire test and should not be reported as multiple individual tests. An examples of a procedure for which modifier 91 should not be reported is a glucose tolerance test. This test is used to monitor disorders of carbohydrate metabolism. This test usually is performed using an oral dose of glucose but may also be performed using intravenous glucose. A blood specimen is obtained prior to glucose administration and at intervals following glucose administration. The test is repeated at specific time intervals. Since the description of the code includes three specimens, modifier 91 would not be reported.

82951   Glucose; tolerance test (GTT), three specimens (includes glucose)

Modifier 59 vs Modifier 91

Since the introduction of modifier 91, many questions have been raised regarding its use vs modifier 59. Some third-party payers have suggested that modifier 91 can be appended to every laboratory code that is reported more than one time on the same date of service. However, per the CPT coding guidelines, this is not the appropriate method of reporting modifier 91.

The descriptor of modifier 59 is as follows:

Under certain circumstances, the physician may need to indicate that a procedure or service was distinct or independent from other services performed on the same day. Modifier 59 is used to identify procedures/services that are not normally reported together, but are appropriate under the circumstances. This may represent a different session or patient encounter, different procedure or surgery, different site or organ system, separate incision/excision, separate lesion, or separate injury (or area of injury in extensive injuries) not ordinarily encountered or performed on the same day by the same physician. However, when another already established modifier is appropriate it should be used rather than modifier 59. Only if no more descriptive modifier is available, and the use of modifier 59 best explains the circumstances, should modifier 59 be used.

Modifier 59 was added to report instances when distinct and separate multiple services are provided to a patient on a single date of service. As the description indicates, some examples of common uses of this modifier may include separate sessions or patient encounters, different procedures or surgeries, surgery directed to different sites or organ systems, surgery directed to separate incision/excision or separate lesions, or treatment to separate injuries. When laboratory services are performed, modifier 59 should be used to report procedures that are distinct or independent, such as performing the same procedure (which uses the same procedure code) for a different specimen. As indicated in the guidelines, this modifier should not be used when a more descriptive modifier is available.

For example, if four bacterial blood cultures are tested, including isolation and presumptive identification of isolates, then code 87040, *Culture, bacterial; blood, aerobic, with isolation and presumptive identification of isolates (includes anaerobic culture, if appropriate),* should be used to identify each culture procedure performed. Modifier 59 should be appended to the additional procedures to identify each additional culture performed as a distinct service.

Modifier 91, on the other hand, is intended to identify a laboratory test that is performed more than once on the same day for the same patient, when it is necessary to obtain subsequent (multiple) results in the course of the treatment. In addition, modifier 91 is not intended for use when there are CPT codes available to describe the series of results (eg, glucose tolerance tests, evocative/suppression testing).

For example, if three subsequent blood tests for determination of potassium level are ordered and performed on the same date as the initial test to obtain multiple results in the course of potassium replacement therapy, then code 84132 (Potassium; serum) should be reported once for each blood test performed, and modifier 91 should be appended to the subsequent test codes to identify the repeat clinical diagnostic laboratory tests performed.

To assist with the appropriate use of this series of codes, additional instructions for use of modifiers 59 and 91 are given in the Microbiology subsection of the CPT book. The Microbiology guidelines state:

> Presumptive identification of microorganisms is defined as identification by colony morphology, growth on selective media, Gram stains, or up to three tests (eg, catalase, oxidase, indole, urease). Definitive identification of microorganisms is defined as identification to the genus or species level that requires additional tests (eg, biochemical panels, slide cultures). If additional studies involve molecular probes, chromatography, or immunologic techniques, these should be separately coded in addition to definitive identification codes (87140-87158). For multiple specimens/sites, use modifier 59. For repeat laboratory tests performed on the same day, use modifier 91.

CMS Guidelines

CMS understands that "In the course of patient treatment, it may be necessary to repeat the same laboratory test on the same day to obtain subsequent (multiple) test results." To be covered by Medicare, the repeat diagnostic laboratory test must be rendered the same day, the same test as originally rendered, and for the same patient (beneficiary).

If the above criteria are fulfilled, the repeat test may be billed with modifier 91 appended to it.

Third-Party Payer Guidelines

Modifier 91 must be appended to laboratory tests that are repeated and are medically necessary. Recent data trends indicate that providers are unsure when to use this modifier, resulting in denials for duplicate bills. The rationale behind modifier 91 is to ensure that a same-day, same-clinical laboratory test is recognized as a separate procedure. When requested, documentation to support subsequent testing procedures may be required to support the medical necessity of the second procedure.

Example 1

A 14-year-old boy presented as an outpatient to the laboratory for aerobic and anaerobic culture of two sites of a single vertical wound to the anterior left foreleg, which was a result of a scooter mishap. The laboratory technologist obtained independent specimens, one from the proximal wound site and one from the distal wound site, for aerobic culture of the drainage material for testing, using the appropriate type of aerobic culturettes. The laboratory technologist also obtained independent specimens by means of anaerobic culturettes, one from the proximal wound site and one from the distal wound site, for anaerobic culture of the drainage material for testing.

AMA CODING TIP

Review the guidelines in the Microbiology subsection of the Pathology and Laboratory section of the CPT book for additional instructions on the use of modifiers 59 and 91.

CPT Code(s) Billed: 87071, 87071 59, 87073, 87073 59

87071   Culture, bacterial; quantitative, aerobic with isolation and presumptive identification of isolates, any source except urine, blood or stool

87073   Culture, bacterial; quantitative, anaerobic with isolation and presumptive identification of isolates, any source except urine, blood or stool

Rationale for Using Modifier 59 vs Modifier 91

The cultures were from two separate wound sites, and two separate types of cultures (aerobic and anaerobic) were performed. Since there was no indication that the lab tests were repeated on the same day, modifier 91 would not be appropriate. However, since two separate cultures were identified at two separate sites, modifier 59 would be appropriate (distinct and separate).

Example 2

A 65-year-old male patient with diabetic ketoacidosis had multiple blood tests performed to check the potassium level after potassium replacement and low-dose insulin therapy. After the initial potassium value was measured, three subsequent blood tests were ordered and performed on the same date after the administration of potassium to correct the patient's hypokalemic state.

CPT Code(s) Billed: 84132, 84132 91, 84132 91, 84132 91

84132   Potassium; serum

Rationale for Using Modifier 91

Since multiple blood tests were performed to check the potassium level after potassium replacement and low-dose insulin therapy, it would be appropriate to bill the initial blood test and all three subsequent blood tests on the same date with modifier 91 used for each subsequent blood test.

Example 3

An 18-year-old non-pregnant woman with previous symptoms of weakness, light-headedness, shortness of breath, and a sweating/clammy feeling after exertion presented as an outpatient to the laboratory for a fasting blood glucose test and a repeat random blood glucose test after ingestion of a full breakfast. Both blood specimens were ordered and testing was performed on the same date.

CPT Code(s) Billed: 82947—Glucose; quantitative, blood (except reagent strip)

82950 59—Glucose; post glucose dose (includes glucose)

Rationale for Not Using Modifier 91

It is not necessary to use modifier 91 in this circumstance, since there are codes available to describe the series of glucose tests and they are not identical tests repeated. Modifier 59 may be used to indicate the procedures are distinct and separate.

Example 4

A 2-year-old child was taken to the emergency department after ingesting lead paint. A lead toxicity test was performed, and IV infusion consisting of normal saline and D5W was started to detoxify the effects of the lead. Two hours later a lead test was run to determine the level of lead in the patient's blood. The lead test indicated the level had been reduced dramatically, and the IV was removed. The patient was released and advised to follow up with the pediatrician the next day.

CPT Code(s) Billed: 90760—Intravenous infusion, hydration; initial, up to 1 hour

90761—Intravenous infusion, hydration; each additional hour, up to 8 hours (List separately in addition to code for primary procedure)

83655—Lead

83655 91—Lead

Rationale for Using Modifier 91

The initial lead toxicity test was to measure the current lead level in the patient's bloodstream, and the repeat lead toxicity test (83655 91) was performed to make sure the toxicity level was decreased and the IV infusion was effective. The IV infusion is reported with 90760 for the first hour and 90761 for each additional hour. Because the patient was on the IV for 2 hours, 90761 is reported with 90760.

Review of Modifier 91

1   Modifier 91 is not used when the second test or culture is from a different site; modifier 59 is used on the same date of service unless a second culture (same CPT code) is performed on the same day for the same site.

2   To be covered by CMS, the repeat diagnostic laboratory test must be rendered the same day, must be the same test as originally rendered (same procedure code), and must be for the same patient (beneficiary).

3   Modifier 91 may not be used when there is a HCPCS/CPT code that describes a series of results (glucose tolerance tests, evocative/suppression testing).

4   The Microbiology subsection of the CPT book provides additional coding instructions.

Modifier 99: Multiple Modifiers

Definition

Under certain circumstances two or more modifiers may be necessary to completely delineate a service. In such situations modifier 99 should be added to the basic procedure, and other applicable modifiers may be listed as part of the description of the service.

AMA Guidelines

 This modifier is used to alert third-party payers that several modifiers are being used to report the service.

For example, a physician who assisted on a bilateral subcutaneous mastectomy (19182) would code *19182 99 80 50,* since there are two modifiers appended to the procedure.

24.	A DATE(S) OF SERVICE		B Place of Service	C Type of Service	D PROCEDURES, SERVICES, OR SUPPLIES (Explain Unusual Circumstances) CPT/HCPCS | MODIFIER	E DIAGNOSIS CODE	F $ CHARGES	G DAYS OR UNITS	H EPSDT Family Plan	I EMG	J COB	K RESERVED FOR LOCAL USE
	From MM DD YY	To MM DD YY										
1					19182 99 80 50							
2												
3												
4												
5												
6												
25. FEDERAL TAX I.D. NUMBER SSN EIN				26. PATIENT'S ACCOUNT NO.		27. ACCEPT ASSIGNMENT? (For govt. claims, see back) YES NO	28. TOTAL CHARGE $		29. AMOUNT PAID $		30. BALANCE DUE $	

CMS Guidelines

CMS recognizes the use of modifier 99. Modifier 99 is informational only and does not affect reimbursement. It alerts the carrier that additional modifiers are to follow.

Third-Party Payer Guidelines

Many carriers require that there be a charge for each line used on the claim form. Thus, it may be necessary to string the modifiers together on the same line on the claim form. This can be done by putting the 99 modifier next to the code in the procedure column and listing the other modifiers in the procedure description column.

Example 1

An orthopedic surgeon assisted with multiple procedures performed on a patient with multiple trauma resulting from a motorcycle crash. The patient underwent a craniotomy with debridement for an extradural hematoma, cranial decompression of the posterior fossa, and treatment of a rib fracture with external fixation. The patient tolerated the procedures well.

CPT Code(s) Billed: *61312 80—Craniectomy or craniotomy for evacuation of hematoma, supratentorial; extradural or subdural*

61345 99 80 51—Other cranial decompression, posterior fossa

21810 99 80 59—Treatment of rib fracture requiring external fixation (flail chest)

24. A DATE(S) OF SERVICE						B Place of Service	C Type of Service	D PROCEDURES, SERVICES, OR SUPPLIES (Explain Unusual Circumstances) CPT/HCPCS | MODIFIER	E DIAGNOSIS CODE	F $ CHARGES	G DAYS OR UNITS	H EPSDT Family Plan	I EMG	J COB	K RESERVED FOR LOCAL USE
From MM	DD	YY	To MM	DD	YY										
1								61312 | 80							
2								61345 | 99 | 80 51							
3								21810 | 99 | 80 59							
4															
5															
6															

25. FEDERAL TAX I.D. NUMBER	SSN EIN	26. PATIENTIS ACCOUNT NO.	27. ACCEPT ASSIGNMENT? (For govt. claims, see back) YES NO	28. TOTAL CHARGE $	29. AMOUNT PAID $	30. BALANCE DUE $

Example 2

A 68-year-old retired salesman with a 50-pack-year smoking history presented with gastric outlet obstruction. He had had a 9 kg weight loss in the past 3 months, had known peptic ulcer disease, and had been treated with histamine$_2$ blockers. Despite medical advice, he continued to smoke and drink socially until the week of the examination, when he was unable to keep anything down. A decision was made to operate, and the surgeon reviewed laboratory and X ray/imaging studies to plan the operative approach; discussed the procedure with the patient; and obtained informed consent. Initial lab studies showed the following values: potassium, 3.0 mEq/L; total protein, 5.0 g/dL; albumin, 2.5 g/dL; and hemoglobin, 10.8 g/dL. Arterial blood gas values indicated metabolic alkalosis. Pulmonary function tests showed mild chronic obstructive pulmonary disease. The surgeon decided to use an assistant surgeon to help dissect the area around the ulcer. At operation, a large prepyloric anterior/superior benign ulcer was found. A careful dissection of the chronically scarred and inflamed area around the ulcer was performed, including the duodenum and common bile duct. Before the procedure could be completed, the patient went into cardiac arrest and the procedure was discontinued. The patient was stabilized in the operating room. Drains were placed in the operative area as needed. The patient was extubated, and ventilation returned to an acceptable level.

CPT Code(s) Billed by the Primary Surgeon: 43631 53

CPT Code(s) Billed by the Assistant Surgeon: 43631 99 80 53

43631   Gastrectomy, partial, distal; with gastroduodenostomy

Review of Modifier 99

1 Modifier 99 is used when more than two modifiers are appended to the procedure code.

2 Modifier 99 is informational only and does not affect reimbursement.

3 Most carriers recognize the use of modifier 99.

Test Your Knowledge

Indicate the Appropriate Modifier

1 _____ This modifier indicates that an outside reference laboratory was used.

2 _____ This modifier was created to replace the HCPCS level II QR modifier.

3 _____ This modifier is not recognized by CMS.

4 _____ This modifier identifies that additional modifiers are to follow.

5 _____ This modifier is not to be used when laboratory tests are rerun to confirm the initial results.

Fill in the Blanks

6 Modifier _____ is used when more than two modifiers are appended to the procedure code.

7 Physicians use modifier _____ when laboratory procedures are performed by a party other than the treating or reporting physician.

8 Modifier _____ is often confused with modifier 91.

9 According to CMS, to cover modifier _____, the service must be rendered the same day, must be the same test as originally rendered, and must be for the same patient.

10 Modifier _____ might be used to report a situation when multiple modifiers are used.

11 _____ A patient with a history of seizure disorder returned to the neurologist for follow up. The patient's blood test indicated the patient's level of Phenobarbital was not effective in treating the seizures. The physician ordered a Phenobarbital level drawn the next morning before meals, followed by the Phenobarbital level redrawn in the late afternoon after the patient had taken his medication. What modifier would the lab report in addition to the procedure code?

12 _____ A family physician in a rural town in Alabama sent a patient's blood to the laboratory for a TSH and Chem 7. The laboratory and the physician had a written agreement that the physician would bill the insurance carriers and/or patient for the interpretation and the physician would pay the laboratory monthly for their services. What modifier should be reported for each laboratory procedure?

13 _____ When a managed care or commercial insurance carrier has a specific contract with the laboratory and the beneficiary has a "carve-out," which modifier may not be used?

14 This Amendment allows an uncertified laboratory to perform a limited number of laboratory procedures in the office. What is this amendment called? _____ _____ _____ _____.

15 _____ CMS recognizes this modifier, which is informational only. This modifier does not affect reimbursement, but alerts the carrier that additional modifiers are to follow. What modifier is this?

CHAPTER 8

HCPCS Level II Modifiers

HCPCS is the acronym for the Health Care Common Procedure Coding System developed by the Centers for Medicare and Medicaid Services (CMS), formerly the Health Care Financing Administration (HCFA). HCPCS level II codes are alphanumeric codes developed by the CMS as an adjunct coding system to the American Medical Association (AMA) Current Procedural Terminology (CPT®) code sets. HCPCS level II codes describe procedures, services, and supplies not found in the CPT manual, such as ambulance services and durable medical equipment. HCPCS was implemented in 1983 to provide a uniform system for coding a procedure, service, or supply for reimbursement for government programs. HCPCS level II was developed to accomplish the following:

- Report services, procedures, and supplies to meet the operational needs of Medicare and Medicaid
- Allow providers and suppliers to communicate their services in a consistent manner
- Provide a manner of reporting and coordinating programs uniformly with CMS policies
- Ensure the validity of fee schedules and profiles through standardized coding
- Provide a vehicle for local, regional, and national comparison of code utilization to enhance medical research

The level II national codes are alphanumeric, beginning with a letter (A-V) followed by four digits. HCPCS level II codes are updated annually by CMS. CMS receives input from commercial insurance companies when updating HCPCS level II. The codes are grouped by type of service or supplies provided to Medicare, Medicaid, and most private and commercial insurance carriers.

HCPCS level II also contains alphabetic modifiers consisting of two characters (AA-VP) and can be used with all levels of HCPCS codes (CPT and HCPCS). The HCPCS level II codes are maintained by the HCPCS National Panel, consisting of representatives of CMS, the Health Insurance Association of America, and the Blue Cross/Blue Shield Association.

As with CPT nomenclature, HCPCS level II modifiers (extenders) further define services, procedures, and supplies without changing the definition of the code. HCPCS level II modifiers are different from CPT modifiers in that they are alphanumeric or alphabetic characters.

HCPCS level II is published and updated yearly and may be purchased from various publishers and bookstores across the country. Because HCPCS code(s) and modifiers may change and some may be added throughout the year, the CMS Web site at www.cms.gov/providers should be checked periodically for HCPCS modifier updates.

The secretary of Health and Human Services (HHS) delegated authority in October 2003, under HIPAA legislation to CMS, to maintain and distribute HCPCS Level II codes. CMS has a HCPCS internal workgroup that is comprised of representatives of the major components of CMS and consultants from other federal agencies.

On August 17, 2000, the regulation 45 CFR 162.10002 to implement the HIPAA requirement for standardized coding systems was enacted, establishing

HCPCS Level II codes as the standardized coding system. The system was created to describe and identify health care equipment and supplies in health care transactions that are not identified in HCPCS Level I, CPT codes. The HCPCS coding system is widely recognized and accepted by both private and public insurers. Public and private insurers were required to be in compliance with the August 2000 regulation by October 1, 2002.

Reporting HCPCS Modifiers According to HIPAA Rules

In accordance with the Transaction Rule of the Health Insurance Portability and Accountability Act (HIPAA), CMS requires all providers to report HCPCS modifiers that are valid at the time a service is performed. Providers should take the appropriate steps to ensure that the reported HCPCS modifiers are valid for the time the service was performed.

If the modifiers are determined to be invalid, the provider will receive a rejection notice. The rejection notice will indicate that the modifier was not valid for the date of service reported. The provider will then need to resubmit the service with a correct modifier. This reporting requirement applies to both paper claims and electronic claims.

HCPCS Modifiers and the National Correct Coding Initiative

Modifiers E1 through E4, FA, F1 through F9, LC, LD, LT, RC, RT, TA, and T1 through T9, created by CMS, and CPT modifiers 25, 58, 59, 78, 79, and 91 have been designated specifically for use with the National Correct Coding Initiative. When one of these modifiers is used, it identifies the circumstances for which both services rendered to the same beneficiary, on the same date of service, by the same provider should be allowed separately because one service was performed at a different site, in a different session, or as a distinct service.

For purpose of clarification and ease of reading, the HCPCS modifiers have been categorized in this book by specific category of use.

Modifiers Used for Ambulance Services

The following modifiers are typically used for ambulance services.

GY	Item or service statutorily excluded or does not meet the definition of any Medicare benefit
GM	Multiple patients on one ambulance trip
QL	Patient pronounced dead after ambulance called

QM	Ambulance service provided under arrangement by a provider of services
QN	Ambulance furnished directly by provider of services
TP	Medical transport, unloaded vehicle
TQ	Basic life support transport by a volunteer ambulance provider

> **MEDICAID CODING TIP**
>
> Each individual state defines its own Medicaid coverage and does not impose Medicare requirements for the Medicaid program(s).

Reporting Ambulance HCPCS Modifiers

Effective January 1, 1997, providers are required to report HCPCS modifiers to distinguish between ambulance services provided under arrangement with a provider of services and ambulance service furnished directly to the provider (modifiers QM and QN). In addition, providers are required to report HCPCS modifiers along with additional modifiers to describe the type of ambulance service provided, including pickup origin and destination.

The first character indicates the transport's place of origin, and the second character describes the destination. The pickup origin and destination modifier is placed after the modifier QM or QN. Also, the name of the hospital or facility should be included on the claim form. If a pickup at the scene of an accident or acute event (eg, collapse of a building) is reported, the scene or event must be indicated on the claim form with a written report describing the actual location of the scene or event.

The origin and destination modifiers most commonly used are as follows:

D	Diagnostic or therapeutic other than the physician's office or hospital when these codes are used as origin codes
E	Residential, domiciliary, custodial facility (other than an 1819 facility)
G	Hospital-based dialysis facility (hospital or hospital-related)
H	Hospital
I	Site of transfer (eg, airport or helicopter pad) between types of ambulances
J	Non-hospital-based dialysis facility
N	Skilled nursing facility (1819)
P	Physician's office (includes health maintenance organization ASC hospital facility, clinic, etc)
R	Residence
S	Scene of accident or acute event
X	(Destination code only) Intermediate stop at physician's office on the way to the hospital (includes health maintenance organization ASC hospital facility, clinic, etc)

Example 1

ABC Ambulance Service was called to pick up a 68-year-old woman at her residence. The caller stated that the patient was experiencing severe numbness of the right arm with chest pain. The ambulance service arrived at the patient's home, provided basic life support, and transported her to St Mary's Hospital.

HCPCS Code(s) Billed: A0429—Ambulance service, basic life support, emergency transport (BLS-emergency)

This patient encounter will need two modifiers. Before the modifier is appended, the question that must be asked is whether the ambulance was provided under arrangement to a provider of services. This means that the ambulance service is contracted or has an arrangement with the hospital or facility to provide these services. If the hospital or facility has its own ambulance or emergency transport, modifier QN would be appended to the code.

If the ambulance belongs to St Mary's Hospital, the claim would be coded A0429 QN. Once it is determined that St Mary's owns the ambulance, the next step is to determine the origin and destination. The origin in this example is the patient's home, which is modifier R, and the destination is the hospital, which is modifier H. The encounter should be coded *A0429 QN RH*.

Rationale for Using Modifiers QN and RH

The patient was transported on basic life support in an emergency from her home (R) to the hospital (H) in an ambulance that is provided by St Mary's Hospital (QN).

Anesthesia HCPCS Level II Modifiers

CPT codes used for anesthesia service are 00100 to 01999 and are approved for use with modifier AA. Modifier AA is used when a physician assists the surgeon with anesthesia service in the care of a patient and the anesthesia is considered personally performed by the physician. Modifier AA affects Medicare and other third-party payer reimbursement. Guidance for billing anesthesia for CMS claims can be found in the Medicare Carriers' Manual sections 15018 and 4830 and on the CMS Web site (www.cms.hhs.gov).

Medically Directed Anesthesia Services and CMS

The guidelines for CMS indicate that the provider is to adjust the base unit for physician anesthesia services in accordance with section 8313B, where the physician medically directs the services of two or more nurse anesthetists on or after April 1, 1988, and before January 1, 1996. Section 8313C explains the application of base unit adjustments for cataract and iridectomy anesthesia furnished on or after January 1, 1989. The procedures in 8312E indicate how to determine the base units and modifier units assigned to medically directed anesthesia services furnished on or after January 1, 1989.

Qualified Anesthetists

Qualified anesthetists are certified registered nurse anesthetists (CRNAs) and anesthesiologist assistants (AAs). A qualified AA is a person who (1) is permitted by state law to administer anesthesia, and (2) has successfully completed a 6-year program for AAs of which 2 years consist of specialized academic and clinical training in anesthesia. A CRNA is a registered nurse who is licensed by the state in which the nurse practices and who (1) is currently certified by the Council on Certification of Nurse Anesthetists or the Council on Recertification of Nurse Anesthetists, or (2) has graduated within the past 18 months from a nurse anesthesia program that meets the standards of the Council on Accreditation of Nurse Anesthesia educational programs and is awaiting initial certification.

HCPCS Modifiers Used for Anesthesia Services

The following HCPCS modifiers are typically used for anesthesia services.

AA	Anesthesia services performed personally by anesthesiologist
AD	Medical supervision by a physician; more than four concurrent anesthesia procedures
GY	Item or service statutorily excluded or does not meet the definition of any Medicare benefit
G8	Monitored anesthesia care (MAC) for deep complex, complicated, or markedly invasive surgical procedure
G9	Monitored anesthesia care for patient who has history of severe cardio-pulmonary condition
QK	Medical direction of two, three, or four concurrent anesthesia procedures involving qualified individuals
QS	Monitored anesthesia care service
QX	CRNA service: with medical direction by a physician

QY   Medical direction of one CRNA by an anesthesiologist

QZ   CRNA service: without medical direction by a physician

Modifier AD is used when the anesthesiologist/physician is supervising more than four anesthesia procedures at one time. The physician may not need to stay in one surgical suite during the entire procedure, but may monitor several rooms at one time. Medicare has a set fee schedule for this type of procedure(s). If the physician medically directs two or more nurse anesthetists concurrently, the number of base units recognized by CMS with respect to medical direction for each concurrent procedure is reduced as follows:

- Concurrent medical direction of two nurse anesthetists—10%
- Concurrent medical direction of three nurse anesthetists—25%
- Concurrent medical direction of four nurse anesthetists—40%

If the physician medically directs two, three, or four nurse anesthetists concurrently and any of the medically directed procedures are cataract or iridectomy anesthesia, the number of base units for each cataract or iridectomy anesthesia procedure would be reduced by 10% effective for cataract or iridectomy anesthesia furnished on or after January 1, 1989.

Modifier G8 is applicable to CPT codes 00100, 00400, 00160, 00300, 00532, and 00920. The G8 modifier should not be reported in conjunction with the QS modifier, but it must be reported with the pertinent anesthesia payment modifier for personally performed anesthesia (AA) or medical supervision (AD).

Modifier G9 is used for MAC for a patient who has a history of a severe cardiopulmonary condition (CMS transmittal No. B-99-38, November 1999).

Modifier QK is used when a physician uses qualified individuals such as CRNAs to perform anesthesia services. The physician supervises two to four qualified individuals during the surgical procedures.

The QS modifier is reported in addition to other anesthesia modifiers to indicate that MAC was provided. The QS modifier should always be reported in the second position. MAC involves the intraoperative monitoring of the patient's vital physiological signs in anticipation of the need for administration of general anesthesia or of the development of an adverse physiological reaction to the surgical procedure. The QS modifier is closely monitored by most carriers to ensure that medical necessity is documented. The diagnosis code should be specific to support the rationale for using monitored anesthesia. CMS monitors MAC procedures even though reimbursement is the same as with general anesthesia. The QS modifier should always be reported in addition to the other anesthesia modifiers in the second position (second modifier) to indicate that MAC was provided.

Example 1

A patient was taken to the operating room for removal of a deep hemangioma of the cheek in an ambulatory surgery center. The MAC was administered personally by the anesthesiologist. The patient was a normal healthy adult.

CPT Code(s) Billed: 00300 AA QS—Anesthesia for all procedures on the integumentary system, muscles and nerves of head, neck, and posterior trunk, not otherwise specified

24.	A					B	C	D		E	F	G	H	I	J	K	
	DATE(S) OF SERVICE					Place of Service	Type of Service	PROCEDURES, SERVICES, OR SUPPLIES (Explain Unusual Circumstances)		DIAGNOSIS CODE	$ CHARGES	DAYS OR UNITS	EPSDT Family Plan	EMG	COB	RESERVED FOR LOCAL USE	
	From			To				CPT/HCPCS	MODIFIER								
	MM	DD	YY	MM	DD	YY											
1									00300	AA QS							
2																	
3																	
4																	
5																	
6																	
25. FEDERAL TAX I.D. NUMBER SSN EIN						26. PATIENT'S ACCOUNT NO.		27. ACCEPT ASSIGNMENT? (For govt. claims, see back) YES NO		28. TOTAL CHARGE $		29. AMOUNT PAID $				30. BALANCE DUE $	

Rationale for Using Multiple Modifiers

The anesthesiologist is providing MAC (QS), along with personally participating in the procedure (AA). Both modifiers are necessary to explain to the carrier that the procedure was monitored by the physician personally.

Modifier QX is used when a CRNA provides anesthesia services under medical direction of a physician. Medicare limits payment to 55% of the amount allowed if performed personally by the physician or CRNA without medical direction.

HCPCS modifier QY was implemented after January 1, 1998, for medical direction of one certified registered nurse anesthetist (CRNA) by an anesthesiologist.

Billing for CRNA services without physician direction (QZ) should have no effect on payment. Payment should be equal to the amount received if it was performed personally by the physician.

Example 2

A 79-year-old female with mild hypertension underwent a bronchoscopy. The anesthesiologist supervised the CRNA during the procedure. The surgeon completed the procedure and the patient was wheeled into the recovery room in good condition.

CPT Code(s) Billed: 00520 P2 QX, 99100

24.	A					B	C	D		E	F	G	H	I	J	K	
	DATE(S) OF SERVICE					Place of Service	Type of Service	PROCEDURES, SERVICES, OR SUPPLIES (Explain Unusual Circumstances)		DIAGNOSIS CODE	$ CHARGES	DAYS OR UNITS	EPSDT Family Plan	EMG	COB	RESERVED FOR LOCAL USE	
	From			To				CPT/HCPCS	MODIFIER								
	MM	DD	YY	MM	DD	YY											
1									00520	P2 QX							
2									99100								
3																	
4																	
5																	
6																	
25. FEDERAL TAX I.D. NUMBER SSN EIN						26. PATIENT'S ACCOUNT NO.		27. ACCEPT ASSIGNMENT? (For govt. claims, see back) YES NO		28. TOTAL CHARGE $		29. AMOUNT PAID $				30. BALANCE DUE $	

Rationale for Using HCPCS QX and P2

Because the patient has mild hypertension, the patient is at more risk. Modifier P2 indicates the patient has a mild systemic disease. Modifier QX identifies the CRNA services under medical direction. In addition, 99100 is reported because there is an additional risk since the patient is of extreme age (over 70).

Dressings, Wounds, and Supplies

Wound dressings are listed with modifiers A1 to A9. Selection of the modifier is determined by the number of wounds treated. The following HCPCS modifiers might be used for treating wounds:

A1	Dressing for 1 wound
A2	Dressing for 2 wounds
A3	Dressing for 3 wounds
A4	Dressing for 4 wounds
A5	Dressing for 5 wounds
A6	Dressing for 6 wounds
A7	Dressing for 7 wounds
A8	Dressing for 8 wounds
A9	Dressing for 9 or more wounds
EY	No physician or other licensed health care provider order for this item or service
GY	Item or service statutorily excluded or does not meet the definition of any Medicare benefit
KX	Specific required documentation on file
AW	Item furnished in conjunction with a surgical dressing

Modifiers A1 to A9 were added to HCPCS 2003. However, initially CMS did not recognize these modifiers for payment, but determined that modifiers A1 to A9 would be carrier priced, which means that the individual carriers would determine coverage. The category of HCPCS codes used with these modifiers are A4550 to A4649 (supplies), A6010 to A6512 (dressings), and A9270 (non-covered item or service). If a physician applies surgical dressings as part of a professional service, the surgical dressings are considered incident to the professional services of the health care practitioner and should not be separately billed to the insurance carrier. For CMS, if dressing changes are sent home with the patient, claims for the dressings may be submitted by using the place-of-service code corresponding to the patient's residence. The CMS Coverage Issues Manual 45-12 addresses documentation guidelines as well as medical necessity for coding dressings and wound care with modifiers A1 to A9.

Modifiers A1 to A9 have been established to indicate that a particular item is being used as a primary or secondary dressing on a surgical or debrided wound and also to indicate the number of wounds on which that dressing is being used. When modifier A9 is appended, information must be submitted with the claim indicating the number of wounds. Modifiers A1 to A9 are informational for CMS and convey information to facilitate correct claim processing and medical review; they should be used whenever appropriate.

If GY is used, a brief description of the reason for noncoverage must be indicated, which would be included with the hard copy of the claim or in the narrative field of the electronic claim form.

For example,

A6216 GY   Gauze, non-impregnated, nonsterile, pad size 16 sq. in. or less, without adhesive border, each dressing, noncovered

indicates to the carrier the service is a noncovered service.

Clinical information to support medical necessity of the type and quantity of surgical dressings provided should be present in the patient's medical record. The patient's wound(s) must be evaluated on a monthly basis unless documentation in the medical record justifies why an evaluation could not be performed within this time frame and what other monitoring methods were used to evaluate the patient's need for dressing. The evaluation could be performed by the physician, nurse, or other health care professional. The evaluation should include the following:

- Type of wound (surgical, pressure ulcer, burn, etc)
- Location
- Size (length multiplied by width, in centimeters)
- Depth
- Amount of drainage
- Other relevant information

The information does not necessarily need to be submitted with each claim, unless the carrier specifically mandates it be submitted, but a brief statement documenting the medical necessity of any quantity billed that exceeds the quantity needed for the usual dressing change frequency should be submitted with the claim whether the claim is submitted as a hard copy or electronically.

Modifier AW is for use with any items furnished with surgical dressings, and modifier AX is used for items furnished along with dialysis services. Claims for tape (A4450 and A4452) should be billed with modifier AW appended.

Drugs and Enteral/Parenteral Therapy, Supplies, and Infusion

The following are codes used for drug formulation, monitoring, and/or administration of infusion therapy. These modifiers may be used in conjunction with CPT codes or the HCPCS level II codes as appropriate.

BA	Item furnished in conjunction with parenteral-enteral nutrition services
BO	Orally administered nutrition, not by feeding tube
EJ	Subsequent claims for a defined course of therapy, eg, EPO, sodium hyaluronate, infliximab
EY	No physician or other licensed health care provider order for this item or service
GY	Item or service statutorily excluded or does not meet the definition of any Medicare benefit
JW	Drug amount discarded/not administered to any patient
KO	Single drug unit dose formulation
KP	First drug of a multiple drug unit dose formulation
KQ	Second or subsequent drug of a multiple drug unit dose formulation
KS	Glucose monitor supply for diabetic beneficiary not treated with insulin
KX	Specific required documentation on file
SJ	Third or more concurrently administered infusion therapy
SH	Second concurrently administered infusion therapy
SK	Member of high risk population (use only with codes for immunization)
SL	State supplied vaccine
SV	Pharmaceuticals delivered to patient's home but not utilized

Modifier BO alters the allowance for the procedure code and is used when nutritional supplements are administered without a feeding tube, orally. Enteral nutrition is the provision of nutritional supplements through a tube into the stomach or small intestine.

For CMS, enteral nutrition products administered orally and related supplies are currently considered not covered. Modifier BO is appended to HCPCS codes B4150-B4156 when enteral nutrients are administered by mouth. For example:

B4155 BO   Enteral formulae; category V: modular components, administered through an enteral feeding tube, 100 calories = 1 unit

Third-Party Payer Guidelines

Each third-party payer or commercial insurance carrier determines coverage for enteral nutrition by oral administration individually; it normally is based on the member's health care benefits plan and should be verified before administration.

Medicaid Guidelines

Some state Medicaid carriers are accepting the use of modifier BO for special orally administered formulas under the Early Periodic Screening Diagnosis and Treatment Program (EPSDT), which is available to individuals under the age of 21 years in whom an EPSDT screening has identified specific nutrition problems that require special treatment. Regular baby formula, which is typically sold in grocery or drug stores, is not covered. State guidelines will indicate whether this modifier is accepted for the Medicaid carrier.

Modifier BA may be used, for example, when an intravenous pole (E0776) is used for enteral nutrition administered by gravity or pump. For CMS, E0776 is the only code with which a BA modifier may be used.

Example 1

A patient was given enteral formula, one unit through a feeding tube in a nursing home. An intravenous pole was used to administer the feeding.

HCPCS Code(s) Billed: B4153, E0776 BA

B4153   Enteral formulae; category III: hydrolyzed protein/amino acids, administered through an enteral feeding tube, 100 calories = 1 unit

E0776   IV pole, item furnished in conjunction with parental enteral nutrition (PEN) services

Glucose Monitoring and Supplies

Modifiers KS and KX are used for glucose monitoring and supplies. To support their medical necessity, the patient must have diabetes (International Classification of Diseases, Ninth Revision, Clinical Modification [ICD-9-CM] codes 250.00-250.93) and be treated by a physician. The glucose monitor and related accessories and supplies have been ordered by a physician who is treating the patient's diabetes and the treating physician maintains records reflecting the care provided, including evidence of medical necessity for the prescribed frequency of testing.

CMS mandates the following for coverage:

- The patient or caregiver has successfully completed training or is scheduled to begin training in the use of the monitor, test strips, and lancing devices and is capable of using the test results to ensure the patient's appropriate glycemic control. The device must be designed for home use.
- The HCPCS codes used for home blood glucose monitors are E2100 (Blood glucose monitor with integrated voice synthesizer) and E2101 (Blood glucose monitor with integrated lancing/blood sample).
- Typically lancets, blood glucose test reagent strips, glucose control solutions, spring-powered devices for lances, and replacement lens shield cartridges are covered. When a patient is not taking insulin, HCPCS modifier KS must be appended to the HCPCS code.

Example 1

An endocrinologist was treating a non-insulin-dependent diabetic patient (a Medicare recipient) whose blood glucose levels had risen during the past 3 months and wanted the patient to monitor glucose levels at home. The physician performed and documented an expanded problem-focused history and examination with a moderate level of decision making (99213). The patient was given instruction on how to use the monitor along with information regarding supplies. The physician documented the order in the medical record. The physician had a supply of monitors in the office along with supplies to dispense to his diabetic patients. The patient was instructed to monitor her glucose levels three times a day for the next 3 months and return for reevaluation at that time. The patient was also instructed to keep a daily log and to report the finding to the office weekly.

CPT and HCPCS Code(s) Billed: 99213—Office or other outpatient visit for the evaluation and management of an established patient, which requires at least two of these three components: an expanded problem focused history; an expanded problem focused examination; medical decision making of low complexity.

E2101 KS—Blood glucose monitor with integrated lancing/blood sample

A4253 KS—Blood glucose test or reagent strips for home blood glucose monitor, per 50 strips

A4259 KS—Lancets, per box of 100

Rationale for Using Modifier KS

Since the patient is not insulin-dependent, the KS modifier would be appropriate. Many carriers now cover glucose monitoring at home and will reimburse physicians and/or suppliers for these items. However, there is more information the provider must supply.

Documentation Requirements for CMS

An order must be signed and dated by the physician who is treating the patient's diabetes. It must be kept on file and made available to a Durable Medical Equipment Regional Carrier (DMERC) on request. Items billed to the DMERC before a signed and dated order has been received by the supplier must be submitted with an EY modifier added to each HCPCS code. The order for home blood glucose monitors and/or diabetes testing supplies must include the following elements:

- The items to be dispensed
- The quantity of the item(s) to be dispensed
- The specific frequency of testing
- Whether the patient has insulin-treated or non-insulin-treated diabetes

- The treating physician's signature
- The date of the treating physician's signature
- A start date of the order if different from the signature date

Documentation showing "as needed" is not sufficient and is not considered to demonstrate medical necessity. The supplier is required to have a renewal order from the treating physician every 12 months.

HCPCS CODING TIP

Modifier KX is used with any CPT or HCPCS code when the carrier mandates that a written order must be on file with the appropriate documentation.

Example 2

An endocrinologist was treating a non-insulin-dependent diabetic patient (a Medicare recipient) whose blood glucose levels had risen during the past 3 months and wanted the patient to monitor glucose levels at home. The physician performed and documented an expanded problem-focused history and examination with a moderate level of decision making (99213). The patient was given instruction on how to use the monitor along with information regarding supplies. The patient was instructed to monitor her glucose levels three times a day for the next 3 months and return for reevaluation at that time. The patient was also instructed to keep a daily log and to report the findings to the office weekly. A written order was given to the patient, who took it to the pharmacy to fill.

CPT and HCPCS Code(s) Billed: 99213, E2101 KS KX, A4253 KS KX, A4259 KS KX

> *E2101 KS KX—Blood glucose monitor with integrated lancing/blood sample*
>
> *A4253 KS KX—Blood glucose test or reagent strips for home blood glucose monitor, per 50 strips*
>
> *A4259 KS KX—Lancets, per box of 100*

24.	A				B	C	D	E	F	G	H	I	J	K
	DATE(S) OF SERVICE From To				Place of Service	Type of Service	PROCEDURES, SERVICES, OR SUPPLIES (Explain Unusual Circumstances) CPT/HCPCS MODIFIER	DIAGNOSIS CODE	$ CHARGES	DAYS OR UNITS	EPSDT Family Plan	EMG	COB	RESERVED FOR LOCAL USE
	MM	DD	YY	MM	DD	YY									
1								99213						
2								E2101 KS KX						
3								A4253 KS KX						
4								A4259 KS KX						
5														
6														

25. FEDERAL TAX I.D. NUMBER SSN EIN	26. PATIENTıS ACCOUNT NO.	27. ACCEPT ASSIGNMENT? (For govt. claims, see back) YES NO	28. TOTAL CHARGE $	29. AMOUNT PAID $	30. BALANCE DUE $

Rationale for Using Modifiers KS and KX

Since the patient is not insulin-dependent, the KS modifier would be appropriate. Many carriers now cover glucose monitoring at home and will reimburse physicians and/or suppliers for these items. Modifier KX is also needed to report that an order is on file with the appropriate documentation.

When drugs are coded, an order for each item billed must be signed and dated by the treating physician, kept on file by the supplier, and made available to the carrier on request. Modifier KX indicates that the required documentation is on file. Also, if the drug administered is a single drug unit dose, modifier KO is appended to the procedure code. Documentation must clearly specify the type of drug dispensed, administration method and/or instruction, name of drug and concentration, and unit dosage. If the drug is a multiple drug unit dose, modifier KP is appended when the drug is administered the first time. The second or subsequent administration of the drug should be appended with the modifier KQ along with modifier KX if the required documentation is on file. If there is no order on file, modifier EY (no physician or other licensed health care provider order for this item or service) is appended as the second modifier.

Example 3

A physician ordered a nebulizer with compressor (E0570) and albuterol (J7619), 1-mg single unit dose, for a patient with obstructive pulmonary disease. The order was documented appropriately in the medical record.

HCPCS Code(s) Billed: E0570 KO KK—Nebulizer, with compressor

J7613 KO KK—Albuterol, all formulations including separated isomers, inhalation solution administered through DME, unit dose, per 1 mg (Albuterol) or per 0.5 mg (Levalbuterol)

Durable Medical Equipment and Orthotic/Prosthetic Devices

Durable medical equipment (DME) is equipment that can withstand repeated use, such as prosthetic devices or braces. DME is generally not useful to a person in the absence of an illness or injury but is used to serve a medical purpose generally for use in the home. Supplies and accessories that are required for effective use of medically necessary DME are covered by most insurance carriers, including Medicare. Supplies that include biologicals and drugs that must be put directly into DME, such as infusion pumps and nebulizers, to achieve therapeutic benefit of equipment are normally covered by the carrier as well. Also normally included are medically necessary repairs, skilled maintenance, and replacement of medically necessary DME.

The following codes are typically used with orthotics, prosthetics, or DME.

AU	Item furnished in conjunction with a urological, ostomy, or tracheostomy supply
AV	Item furnished in conjunction with a prosthetic device, prosthetic, or orthotic
BP	The beneficiary has been informed of the purchase and rental options and has elected to purchase the item
BR	The beneficiary has been informed of the purchase and rental options and has elected to rent the item

BU   The beneficiary has been informed of the purchase and rental options and after 30 days has not informed the supplier of his/her decision

EY   No physician or other licensed health care provider order for this item or service

GY   Item or service statutorily excluded or does not meet the definition of any Medicare benefit

K0   Lower extremity prosthesis functional level 0—does not have the ability or potential to ambulate or transfer safely with or without assistance and a prosthesis does not enhance the quality of life or mobility

K1   Lower extremity prosthesis functional level 1—has the ability or potential to use a prosthesis for transfers or ambulation on level surfaces at fixed cadence. Typical of the limited and unlimited household ambulator

K2   Lower extremity prosthesis functional level 2—has the ability or potential for ambulation with the ability to transverse low level environmental barriers such as curbs, stairs, or uneven surfaces. Typical of the limited community ambulator

K3   Lower extremity prosthesis functional level 3—has the ability or potential for ambulation with variable cadence. Typical of the community ambulator who has the ability to traverse most environmental barriers and may have vocational, therapeutic, or exercise activity that demands prosthetic utilization beyond simple locomotion

K4   Lower extremity prosthesis functional level 4—has the ability or potential for prosthetic ambulation that exceeds the basic ambulation skills, exhibiting high impact, stress, or energy levels, typical of the prosthetic demands of the child, active adult, or athlete

KA   Add-on option/accessory for wheelchair

KH   DMEPOS item, initial claim, purchase or first month rental

KI   DMEPOS item, second or third month rental

KJ   DMEPOS item, parenteral-enteral nutrition (PEN) pump or capped rental, months four to fifteen

NOTE: DMEPOS is the acronym for durable medical equipment, prosthetics, orthotics, and supplies.

KM   Replacement of facial prosthesis including new impression/moulage

KN   Replacement of facial prosthesis using previous master model

KR	Rental item, billing for partial month
KX	Specific required documentation on file
LL	Lease/rental (use the 'LL' modifier when DME equipment rental is to be applied against the purchase price)
LT	Left side (used to identify procedures performed on the left side of the body)
MS	Six-month maintenance and servicing fee for reasonable and necessary parts and labor that are not covered under any manufacturer or supplier warranty
NR	New when rented (use the 'NR' modifier when DME which was new at the time of rental is subsequently purchased)
NU	New equipment
QA	FDA investigational device exemption
RP	Replacement and repair (RP may be used to indicate replacement of DME, orthotic, and prosthetic devices which have been in use for some time. The claim shows the code for the part, followed by the 'RP' modifier and the charge for the part.)
RR	Rental (use the 'RR' modifier when DME is to be rented)
RT	Right side (used to identify procedures performed on the right side of the body)
TW	Back-up equipment
UE	Used DME

Modifiers **KH, KI,** and **KJ** indicate that the item is considered a capped rental, which means that payment will be made only on a rental basis. A rent-purchase option must be offered in the 10th rental month, as with all capped rental items.

Modifier **KH** is used in conjunction with modifier NU or UE to identify the purchase of new or used equipment. Modifier **KH** is reported in conjunction with modifier LL or RR to identify the first month equipment was rented.

Modifier **KI** is used in conjunction with modifier RR or LL for equipment rented for the second or third month.

Modifier **KJ** is reported in conjunction with modifier RR or LL for equipment rentals for the 4th to 15th month.

The **LL** modifier is used when DME rental is to be applied against the purchase price. **LL** is reported in conjunction with modifier KH, KI, or KJ to identify the item as a lease or rental.

LT and **RT** are used to report procedures performed on the left and right sides of the body, respectively.

Modifier **NR** is used when DME that was new at the time of rental is subsequently purchased. Modifier **NU** is used when new DME is purchased.

RP may be used to indicate replacement of DME, orthotics, and prosthetic devices that have been in use for some time. The claim shows the code for the part, followed by the RP modifier and the charge for the part.

Modifier **RR** is used when DME is to be rented. **RR** is reported in conjunction with modifier KH, KI, or KJ to identify the item as a rental.

Modifier **UE** is reported when used DME is purchased.

When urological supplies such as indwelling catheters (A4311-A4316, A4338-A4346) are coded, modifier **KX** must be appended and an order must be on file when billing is done for a Medicare patient. In the physician's office, urological supplies may be covered under the prosthetic device benefit for Medicare only if the patient's condition meets the definition of permanence. Documentation of medical necessity must be evident in the patient's medical record. Some carriers will also cover catheter insertion trays (A4310-A4316, A4353, A4354). Medicare will cover one insertion tray per episode of an indwelling catheter insertion.

Documentation Guidelines

An order for each item billed must be signed and dated by the treating physician, kept on file by the supplier, and made available to the insurance carrier on request. A copy must be kept in the patient's medical record. The order must include the type of supplies ordered and the approximate quantity to be used per unit of time. If the supplier is billing for items that are not covered, modifier GY must be added to the procedure code.

Ostomy Supplies

Ostomy supplies are appropriately used for colostomies, ileostomies, and urinary ostomies. Ostomy supplies may be found in the Medical and Surgical sections of HCPCS. For example, tape (A4450) would require modifier AU to indicate that the item was furnished in conjunction with the ostomy supply. Without modifier AU, the claim might be denied as not medically necessary. When A4450 and A4452 are coded, they must be billed with modifier AU. Medicare will allow modifier AU only with these two codes:

A4450 AU   Tape, non-waterproof, per 18 square inches

A4452 AU   Tape, waterproof, per 18 square inches

Coders should contact the individual carriers about what ostomy supplies may be billed with modifier AU or contact the Statistical Analysis Durable Medical Equipment Regional Carrier for further guidance.

Example 1

An indwelling catheter was inserted for a patient with permanent urinary incontinence. Tape was used to secure the catheter to the patient's body.

HCPCS Code(s) Billed: A4346 KX, A4452 AU KX, A4316 AU KX, A4355 AU KX

A4346   Indwelling catheter; Foley type, three-way for continuous irrrigation, each

A4452   Tape, waterproof, per 18 square inches

A4316   Insertion tray with drainage bag with indwelling catheter, Foley type, three-way, for continuous irrigation

A4355   Irrigation tubing set for continuous bladder irrigation through a three-way indwelling Foley catheter, each

Rationale for Using Modifiers AU and KX

Modifier AU is used to support that the item was furnished in conjunction with the ostomy supply. Modifier KX indicates that the specific required documentation is on file. Since A4346 is for the indwelling catheter, modifier AU would not be necessary since it is the ostomy supply.

Lower-Limb Prostheses

HCPCS modifiers applicable to lower limb prostheses are EY, K0, K1, K2, K3, K4, LT, RP, and RT. Replacement of components is billed by means of the code for the component with the addition of the RP modifier. The only exception is for the replacement of sockets (L5700-L5702). Since the codes are defined as replacement in the code descriptor, the modifier RP is not used.

Example 1

A socket was replaced below the knee of the right leg for a patient.

HCPCS Code(s) Billed: L5700 RT—Replacement, socket, below knee, molded to patient model

Rationale for Using Modifier RT

Modifier RP is not required because replacement is part of the code descriptor. However, modifier RT (right side) is necessary to identify on which side of the body the socket is replaced.

Example 2

A patient's prosthetic sheath was replaced below the right knee.

HCPCS Code(s) Billed: L8400 RP RT—Prosthetic sheath, below knee, each

Rationale for Using Modifiers RP and RT

In this example, modifier RT is necessary to identify that the sheath was replaced on the right side of the body. RP is used because the code L8400 does not specify replacement.

For Medicare patients, an order for each item billed must be signed and dated by the treating physician and kept on file for prosthetic devices ordered. Documentation must be supported in the medical record. When a replacement or repair is indicated, reimbursement may be made without a new physician's order if it is determined that the prosthesis as originally ordered, considering the time it was furnished, still fills the patient's medical need. The prosthetist must retain documentation of the prosthesis or prosthetic component replaced, the reason for replacement or repair, and a description of the labor involved regardless of the time since the prosthesis was provided to the patient. If replacement for the entire prosthesis or socket is billed, the claim should be accompanied by an explanation of the medical necessity of the replacement. A few examples to support medical necessity are changes in the residual limb, functional need changes, and irreparable damage or wear and tear due to excessive patient weight. The examples are not all-inclusive.

The HCPCS codes for prosthetics that require modifiers K0 to K4 are L5610 to L5616, L5780, L5810 to L5840, L5981, and L5982 to L5986. Modifiers K0 to K4 indicate the expected patient functional level. The expectation of the patient's functional ability should be clearly documented and retained in the prosthetist's records as well as in the ordering physician's medical record. The entry of a K modifier in the record is not sufficient. There must be information about the patient's history and current condition that supports the designation of the functional level by the prosthetist.

Example 3

A patient was fitted for a lower-extremity prosthesis of the left leg. The expected functioning level was level 2, which gave the patient the ability of limited ambulation. The order for the prosthesis was written by the physician who treated the patient.

HCPCS Code(s) Billed: L5981 K2 LT KX—All lower extremity prostheses, flex-walk system or equal

24. A DATE(S) OF SERVICE						B Place of Service	C Type of Service	D PROCEDURES, SERVICES, OR SUPPLIES (Explain Unusual Circumstances) CPT/HCPCS | MODIFIER	E DIAGNOSIS CODE	F $ CHARGES	G DAYS OR UNITS	H EPSDT Family Plan	I EMG	J COB	K RESERVED FOR LOCAL USE
From MM	DD	YY	To MM	DD	YY										
1								L5981 K2 LT KX							
2															
3															
4															
5															
6															
25. FEDERAL TAX I.D. NUMBER SSN EIN						26. PATIENT'S ACCOUNT NO.		27. ACCEPT ASSIGNMENT? (For govt. claims, see back) YES NO	28. TOTAL CHARGE $		29. AMOUNT PAID $		30. BALANCE DUE $		

Rationale for Using Multiple Modifiers

Modifier K2 indicates that the patient will have a functional level 2, which will allow limited ambulation and will enable the patient to manage curbs, stairs, and uneven surfaces. In addition, modifier LT indicates that the prosthesis was provided for the left extremity. The use of modifier KX indicates that there is an order for the item or service on file.

Pathology and Laboratory Services

Regardless of whether a diagnostic laboratory test is performed in a physician's office, by an independent laboratory, or by a hospital laboratory for its outpatients or nonpatients, it is considered a laboratory service. When a hospital laboratory performs diagnostic laboratory tests for nonhospital patients, the laboratory is functioning as an independent laboratory. Also, when physicians and laboratories perform the same test, whether manually or with automated equipment, the services are deemed similar.

Modifiers typically used for laboratory services include the following:

LR	Laboratory round trip
QP	Documentation is on file showing that the laboratory test(s) was ordered individually or ordered as a CPT-recognized panel other than automated profile codes 80002-80019, G0058, G0059, G0060
QW	CLIA waived test

Modifier LR

In addition to a specimen collection fee allowed under section 5114.1.D of the Medicare Carriers' Manual, a travel allowance can be made to cover the costs of travel to collect a specimen from a nursing home or homebound patient. The additional allowance can be made only where a specimen collection fee is also payable, ie, no travel allowance is made where the technician merely performs a messenger service to pick up a specimen drawn by a physician or nursing home personnel. The travel allowance may not be paid to a physician unless the trip to the home or nursing home was solely for the purpose of drawing a specimen. Otherwise, travel costs are considered to be associated with the other purposes of the trip. The allowance is intended to cover the estimated travel costs of collecting a specimen and is an allowance reflecting the technician's salary and travel costs. The following HCPCS codes are used for travel allowances:

P9603	Travel allowance one way in connection with medically necessary laboratory specimen collection drawn from homebound or nursing home bound patient; prorated miles actually traveled

P9604   Travel allowance one way in connection with medically necessary laboratory specimen collection drawn from homebound or nursing home bound patient; prorated trip charge

Identify round-trip travel by use of modifier LR.

Modifier QP

Modifier QP is appended to a laboratory procedure code to allow laboratories to attest that documentation exists to show that the ordering physician or authorized health professional ordered the test(s) individually or as a CPT-recognized panel. This modifier cannot be used for automated profile tests. The use of this modifier is optional and does not ensure payment. While this modifier is helpful to use, its use will not preclude a request from the insurance carrier for additional documentation to support the medical necessity of the ordered laboratory test(s).

Modifier QW

Modifier QW, CLIA waived test, is used for all codes (CPT and HCPCS) that are designated waived tests after 1996 under the Clinical Laboratory Improvement Amendments (CLIA). The CPT codes for these new tests must have the modifier QW to be recognized as a waived test. A complete list of the waived tests can be found on the Medicare Web site at www.medicarenhic.com.

CMS regulates all laboratory testing (except research) performed on humans in the United States through the CLIA. In total, CLIA covers approximately 175,000 laboratory entities. The Division of Laboratory Services, within the Survey and Certification Group, under the Center for Medicaid and State Operations has the responsibility for implementing the CLIA program.

The objective of the CLIA program is to ensure quality laboratory testing. Although all clinical laboratories must be properly certified to receive Medicare or Medicaid payments, CLIA has no direct Medicare or Medicaid program responsibilities.

Congress passed the CLIA in 1988, establishing quality standards for all laboratory testing to ensure the accuracy, reliability, and timeliness of patient test results regardless of where the test was performed. A laboratory is defined by CLIA as any facility that performs laboratory testing on specimens derived from humans for the purpose of providing information for the diagnosis, prevention, or treatment of disease, or impairment of, or assessment of health. CLIA is funded by user fees; therefore, all costs of administering the program must be covered by the regulated facilities, including certificate and survey costs.

The final CLIA regulations were published on February 28, 1992, and are based on the complexity of the test method; thus, the more complicated the test, the more stringent the requirements. Three categories of tests have been established: waived complexity, moderate complexity, including the subcategory of provider-performed microscopy (PPM), and high complexity. CLIA specifies quality standards for proficiency testing, patient test management, quality control, personnel qualifications, and quality assurance for laboratories performing moderate- and/or high-complexity tests. Waived laboratories must enroll in CLIA, pay the applicable fee, and follow manufacturers' instructions. Because problems in cytology laboratories were the impetus for CLIA, there are also specific cytology requirements.

The CMS is charged with the implementation of CLIA, including laboratory registration, fee collection, surveys, surveyor guidelines and training, enforcement, approvals of proficiency-tested providers, accrediting organizations, and exempt states. The Centers for Disease Control and Prevention is responsible for the CLIA studies, convening the Clinical Laboratory Improvement Amendments Committee and providing scientific and technical support/consultation to Department of Health and Human Services/CMS. The Food and Drug Administration (FDA) is responsible for test categorization.

To enroll in the CLIA program, laboratories must first register by completing an application, pay fees, be surveyed, if applicable, and become certified. Waived and PPM laboratories may apply directly for their certificate, as they are not subject to routine inspections. Laboratories that must be surveyed routinely, ie, those performing moderate- and/or high-complexity testing, can choose whether they wish to be surveyed by CMS or by a private accrediting organization. The CMS survey process is outcome oriented and utilizes a quality assurance focus and an educational approach to assess compliance.

Waived and Provider-Performed Microscopy (PPM) Tests

By the CLIA law, waived laboratories perform only tests that are determined by FDA or Centers for Disease Control and Prevention to be so simple that there is little risk of error. Laboratories with a PPM certificate perform tests, using a microscope, during the course of a patient visit on specimens that are not easily transportable.

Waived laboratories must meet only the following requirements under CLIA:
- Enroll in the CLIA program
- Pay applicable certificate fees biannually
- Follow manufacturers' test instructions

The number and types of tests waived under CLIA have increased from eight tests to approximately 40 since the inception of the program in 1992; thereby, the number of waived laboratories has grown exponentially from 20% to 56% of the total 174,500 laboratories enrolled.

PPM laboratories must meet only the following requirements under CLIA:
- Enroll in the CLIA program
- Pay applicable certificate fees biannually
- Fulfill certain quality and administrative requirements

Example 1

An established Medicare patient visited her family physician for follow-up for hypertension and diabetes mellitus. During the encounter, the patient mentioned having experienced burning on urination. The physician performed a urinalysis without microscopy. It was determined after the performance of the urinalysis that the patient had a urinary tract infection. The physician performed a detailed history and examination and determined that the patient's hypertension and diabetes mellitus were stable, made no adjustments in medications, and wrote a prescription for treating the urinary tract infection. The patient was asked to return in 10 days for follow-up of the infection.

CPT Code(s) Billed: 99214—Office or other outpatient visit for the evaluation and management of an established patient, which requires at least two of these three key components: a detailed history; a detailed examination; medical decision making of moderate complexity

81003 QW—Urinalysis, by dip stick or tablet reagent for bilirubin, glucose, hemoglobin, ketones, leukocytes, nitrite, pH, protein, specific gravity, urobilinogen, any number of these constituents; automated, without microscopy

Rationale for Using Modifier QW

Since procedure 81003 is a CLIA-waived lab test, the QW indicates that the service was performed by a physician who has a certificate to perform the service in the office.

Radiology

HCPCS level II modifiers for radiology include the following.

GG	Performance and payment of a screening mammogram and diagnostic mammogram on the same patient, same day
GH	Diagnostic mammogram converted from screening mammogram on same day
TC	Technical component. Under certain circumstances, a charge may be made for the technical component alone. Under those circumstances the technical component charge is identified by adding modifier 'TC' to the usual procedure number. Technical component charges are institutional charges and not billed separately by physicians. However, portable X ray suppliers only bill for technical components and should utilize modifier TC. The charge data from portable X ray suppliers will then be used to build customary and prevailing profiles.

Modifiers GG and GH

Modifier GG is used when a screening mammogram and a diagnostic mammogram are performed on the same patient on the same day. Modifier GH is used when a diagnostic mammogram is converted from a screening mammogram on the same day. These modifiers may be used with the following CPT and HCPCS screening codes:

76092   Screening mammography, bilateral (two view film study of each breast)

G0202   Screening mammography, producing direct digital image, bilateral, all views

G0204   Diagnostic mammography, producing direct digital image, bilateral, all views

G0206   Diagnostic mammography, producing direct digital image, unilateral, all views

The diagnostic CPT codes are as follows:

76090   Mammography; unilateral

76091   Mammography; bilateral

Modifier GG is appended to both the CPT code and the HCPCS code when a screening mammogram and a diagnostic mammogram are performed on the same day for the same patient. Carriers will pay for both the screening and diagnostic mammograms. The physician may order a screening mammogram, which indicates a problem, and then have the patient come back for a diagnostic mammogram on the same day. This modifier is for tracking purposes only.

When a screening mammogram (CPT code 76092) indicates a potential problem, the interpreting radiologist can order additional films during the same visit on the same day, without an additional order from the treating physician. The radiologist must report to the treating physician the condition of the patient. These additional films, with the report to the treating physician, convert a screening mammogram to a diagnostic mammogram. The procedure code is reported with modifier GH to indicate that the radiologist converted the screening mammogram to a diagnostic mammogram.

The difference between GG and GH is that with modifier GG, the screening mammogram is reported and the diagnostic mammogram is reported (different encounters on the same day). Modifier GH is reported when, because of a potential problem detected by the interpreting radiologist, the radiologist will also perform a diagnostic mammogram at the same visit.

When additional mammography views are ordered because of potential problems during the same visit on the same day when a screening mammogram is ordered, CPT code 76092 for the original screening test should not be submitted. Instead, CPT code 76090 (unilateral) or 76091 (bilateral) should be submitted, with modifier GH (diagnostic mammogram converted from screening mammogram on the same day). The ICD-9 code V76.12 is required on the claim for it to be processed, or it will be returned. Moreover, the unique physician identification number of the treating physician should be on the claim.

Example 1

A 67-year-old female visited the hospital radiology department for a screening mammogram. The screening mammogram was performed bilaterally with direct digital imaging, and the physician interpreting the test noticed a small lump in the left breast and wanted further investigation. The patient was contacted and asked to return immediately for the diagnostic mammogram. The diagnostic mammogram indicated the lump was suspicious, and the patient was referred to a surgeon for a biopsy.

CPT Code(s) Billed: G0202—Screening mammography, producing direct digital image, bilateral, all views

76090 GG—Mammography; unilateral

Rationale for Using Modifier GG

Modifier GG identifies that the procedure or service was performed on the same day for a specified reason. In this example, if modifier GG were not appended, the mammography might be denied.

Medicare Guidelines

Medicare provides coverage for screening mammographies for women. Screening mammographies are radiologic procedures for early detection of breast cancer and include a physician's interpretation of the results. A physician's prescription or referral is not necessary for the procedure to be covered. The woman's age and statutory frequency parameter determine whether payment can be made.

Screening and diagnostic mammography services have been updated on the basis of section 104 of the Benefits Improvement and Protection Act of 2000, which amends section 1848(j)(3) of the act to include screening mammography as a physician's service for which payment is made under the Medicare Physician Fee Schedule Data Base. The payment limitation for screening mammography no longer applies for claims with dates of service on or after January 1, 2002. Medicare payment for the service is 80% of the allowed charge. The Part B deductible is waived and does not apply to screening mammography.

Diagnostic mammography and screening mammography can both be paid when performed on the same day when provided to the same beneficiary. Medicare provides for annual screening mammographies for women older than 39 years and waives the deductible.

Coverage applies as follows: age 35 to 39 years: baseline (only one screening allowed for women in this age group); age greater than 39 years: annual (11 full months must have elapsed since the month of last screening). For example, if a patient received a screening mammography examination in January 2004, counting begins the next month (February 2004) until 11 months have elapsed. Payment can be made for another screening mammography in January 2005.

Specific codes used with mammography claims on or after January 1, 2002, are listed below. The CPT codes and G codes will be paid under the Medicare Physician Fee Schedule Database.

76090	Mammography; unilateral
76091	Mammography; bilateral
76092	Screening mammography, bilateral (two view film study of each breast)
G0202	Screening mammography, producing direct digital image, bilateral, all views
G0204	Diagnostic mammography, producing direct digital image, bilateral, all views
G0206	Diagnostic mammography, producing direct digital image, unilateral, all views
G0236	Digitization of film radiographic images with computer analysis for lesion detection, or computer analysis of digital mammogram for lesion detection, and further physician review for interpretation, diagnostic mammography (list separately in addition to code for primary procedure)

CMS Documentation Requirements

The clinical medical record must contain documentation that justifies a diagnostic mammogram, including the results of an abnormal screening mammogram, if applicable. If a radiologist who interprets the screening mammogram justifiably orders additional films during the same visit on the same day, the radiologist must document that the condition of the patient has been reported to the treating physician.

Computer-Aided Detection Codes

The following CPT codes were added in 2004 for computer-aided detection for mammography:

- The CPT code 76082, Computer aided detection (computer algorithm analysis of digital image data for lesion detection) with further physician review for interpretation, with or without digitization of film radiographic images; diagnostic mammography (list separately in addition to code for primary procedure)
- The CPT code 76083, screening mammography (list separately in addition to code for primary procedure)

These add-on codes are intended to be reported with mammography procedure codes 76090, 76091, and 76092.

Modifier TC

Under certain circumstances, a charge may be made for the technical component alone. Under those circumstances, the technical component charge is identified by adding modifier TC to the usual procedure number. Technical component charges are institutional charges and not billed separately by physicians. However, portable X ray suppliers only bill for the technical component and should use modifier TC. The charge data from portable X ray suppliers will then be used to build customary and prevailing profiles.

Modifier TC is not limited to radiology procedures but may be used for any procedure that has a professional and a technical component, and the technical component is performed by one provider and the professional component by another (modifier 26).

Modifier TC is reported with the procedure code. The payment includes the practice and malpractice expense. There are CPT codes and HCPCS codes that describe the technical component only and do not include the professional component. The TC modifier should not be used with any of these codes. Technical components are the facilities services and should not be billed separately by the physician or clinical provider.

A "complete" procedure (ie, professional plus technical component), billed with no modifier attached to the procedure code, is eligible for reporting and reimbursement only when that provider owns the equipment and is also providing the professional component.

CMS Guidelines for Modifier TC

A complete service, as defined by CMS, is one in which the physician provides the entire service, including equipment, supplies, technical personnel, and the physician's professional services. The complete service can then be divided into a technical and a professional component. The HCPCS level II modifier TC was developed by CMS to identify the technical component vs the professional component. CMS recognizes the use of modifier 26 when the professional component is billed on the claim.

When a technical service is rendered in a hospital inpatient or outpatient setting, nursing facility, or comprehensive outpatient rehabilitation facility (CORF), Medicare Part B does not pay for it. The cost is submitted to Medicare Part A by the facility.

Technical services rendered in an ambulatory surgery center (ASC) are not covered as a charge separate from the facility fee. They are included in the reimbursement of the facility fee charge.

CMS published, in the National Physician Fee Schedule, CPT and HCPCS procedures eligible for the modifier TC. Typically, when the procedure is submitted with modifier TC, reimbursement is based on the technical component associated with the procedure.

The technical component includes providing the equipment, supplies, technical personnel, and costs attendant to the performance of the procedure other than the professional services.

Third-Party Payer Guidelines

Many third-party payers have established modifier and/or specific reporting policies for reporting the technical component. Many carriers recognize the TC modifier for reporting the technical component. Some carriers have developed their own guidelines for reporting the professional and technical component(s) separately. When reporting the technical component, providers should be familiar with reporting requirements of the individual insurance carrier policies in their area, because reimbursement policies vary among insurance companies.

Example 2

A stand-alone radiology center performed a complete cervical spine series on a 25-year-old patient. The films were sent to the radiologist to be read. The radiologist was located in another office.

CPT Code(s) Billed by Radiology Center: 72052 TC

CPT Code(s) Billed by Radiologist: 72052 26

72052   Radiologic examination, spine, cervical; complete, including oblique and flexion and/or extension studies

Rationale for Using Modifier TC

Since the radiology center performed only the technical portion, which covers the technical staff, films, equipment, and facility, modifier TC indicates that only the technical portion was performed.

Example 3

A physician ordered a fetal nonstress test for a patient in her second trimester of pregnancy. The patient was sent to the outpatient radiology department of the hospital. The patient arrived at the radiology department; the test was performed and the nonstress test was read by the radiologist (not employed by the hospital). A written report was sent back to the requesting physician.

CPT Code(s) Billed by Facility: 59025 TC

CPT Code(s) Billed by Radiologist: 59025 26

59025   Fetal non-stress test

Rationale for Using 59025 TC

Since the outpatient radiology department does not employ the physician who read the stress test, the global component could not be billed. Modifier TC indicates to the insurance carrier that only the technical component was performed by the facility.

Dialysis/Hemodialysis

The following modifiers are typically billed for dialysis, hemodialysis, and/or end-stage renal disease (ESRD).

AX	Item furnished in conjunction with dialysis services
EM	Emergency reserve supply (for ESRD benefit only)
G1	Most recent URR reading of less than 60
G2	Most recent URR reading of 60 to 64.9
G3	Most recent URR reading of 65 to 69.9
G4	Most recent URR reading of 70 to 74.9
G5	Most recent URR reading of 75 or greater
G6	ESRD patient for whom less than 6 dialysis sessions have been provided in a month

Medicare Guidelines

When reporting dialysis, the treatment must include the adequacy of hemodialysis data measured by the urea reduction ratio (URR). Dialysis facilities must monitor the adequacy of dialysis treatments monthly for facility patents. Home dialysis patients are monitored less frequently but no less than quarterly, based on CMS criteria. When a home hemodialysis patient is not monitored during the month, the most recent URR for the dialysis patient is reported.

All hemodialysis claims must indicate the most recent URR for the dialysis patient with a G modifier. If the modifier is missing, the claim will be denied. CPT code 90999 (unlisted dialysis procedure, inpatient or outpatient) must be reported along with the appropriate G modifier for patients who received seven or more dialysis treatments in a month. For patients who have received six or fewer sessions of dialysis in a month, the modifier G6 is used.

Documentation Guidelines

Claims for dialysis treatments must include the adequacy of dialysis data as measured by URR. Dialysis facilities must monitor the adequacy of dialysis treatments monthly for facility patients. Patients receiving home hemodialysis and peritoneal dialysis may be monitored less frequently, but not less than quarterly.

The techniques to be used to draw the predialysis and postdialysis serum urea nitrogen samples are listed in the National Kidney Foundation Dialysis Outcomes Quality Initiative Clinical Practice Guidelines for Hemodialysis Adequacy: Guideline 8, Acceptable Methods for BUN Sampling (New York, National Kidney Foundation, 1997, pp 53–60).

Other

GW   Service not related to the hospice patient's terminal condition

Q3   Live kidney donor surgery and related services

Report postoperative medical complications directly related to the donation. Replace local modifier definition ("no financial hardship-Medicare only") with the national definition.

ST   Related to trauma or injury

TH   Obstetrical treatment/services, prenatal or postpartum

TJ   Program group, child and/or adolescent

TK   Extra patient or passenger, nonambulance

TL   Early intervention/individualized family service plan (IFSP)

TM   Individualized education program (IEP)

TR   School-based individualized education program (IEP) services provided outside the public school district responsible for the student

Example 1

A 65-year-old Medicare ESRD patient received hemodialysis at the Dialysis Center from February 1 to March 1. The patient's physician evaluated the patient on February 10, and the patient received seven dialysis treatments in a 30-day period. The patient's most recent URR was 74.5.

HCPCS Code(s) Billed: G0319 G4

G0319   End Stage Renal Disease (ESRD) related services during the course of treatment, for patients 20 years of age and over; with 1 face-to-face physician visit per month.

Rationale for Using Modifier G4

Because the patient is a Medicare patient, HCPCS code G0319 is reported for the dialysis service for the month. Also, as required by CMS, a modifier must be appended to the claim to report the most recent urea reduction ratio (URR).

38					39 CODE	VALUE CODES AMOUNT	40 CODE	VALUE CODES AMOUNT	41 CODE	VALUE CODES AMOUNT	
					a						a
					b						b
					c						c
					d						d

	42 REV. CD.	43 DESCRIPTION	44 HCPCS / RATES	45 SERV. DATE	46 SERV. UNITS	47 TOTAL CHARGES	48 NON-COVERED CHARGES	49	
1			G0319 G4						1
2									2
3									3
4									4
5									5
6									6
7									7
8									8
9									9
10									10

Oxygen and Monitoring

These modifiers are used to identify home oxygen therapy when the treating physician has determined that the patient has a severe lung disease or hypoxia-related symptoms that might be expected to be improved with oxygen therapy. CMS has specific guidelines in the DMERC medical policy manual when oxygen services are covered.

CMS will cover only rented oxygen systems and not purchased oxygen systems. The appropriate modifier must be used if the prescribed flow rate is less than 1 L/min (QE) or greater than 4 L/min (QG). These modifiers are used only with stationary compressed gaseous oxygen systems (E0424) or stationary liquid oxygen systems (E0439), or with an oxygen concentrator (E1390-E1391). They should not be used with codes for portable systems or oxygen contents.

Documentation Requirements

An order for each item billed must be signed and dated by the treating physician, kept on file by the supplier, and made available to the carrier upon request. A certificate of medical necessity that is completed, dated, and signed may act as a written order if sufficiently detailed. The certificate of medical necessity for home oxygen is CMS form 484 for Medicare and Medicaid.

The following modifiers are applicable to oxygen services:

EY	No physician or other licensed health care provider order for this item or service
QE	Prescribed amount of oxygen is less than 1 liter per minute (LPM)
QF	Prescribed amount of oxygen exceeds 4 liters per minute (LPM) and portable oxygen is prescribed
QG	Prescribed amount of oxygen is greater than 4 liters per minute (LPM)
QH	Oxygen conserving device is being used with an oxygen delivery system

THIRD-PARTY PAYER CODING TIP

Many carriers, including Medicare and Medicaid, do not cover refractions.

Vision Services

Modifiers typically used for vision services are the following:

AP	Determination of refractive state was not performed in the course of diagnostic ophthalmological examination
LS	FDA-monitored intraocular lens implant
LT	Left side (used to identify procedures performed on the left side of the body)
PL	Progressive addition lenses
RT	Right side (used to identify procedures performed on the right side of the body)
VP	Aphakic patient

In determining the refractive state, the provider examines the patient's eyes for refractive errors. The keratometer and retinoscope may be used by the provider when performing the refraction. Some common examples of refractive errors are hyperopia (farsightedness), astigmatism, and myopia (nearsightedness). The refraction determines the patient's eyeglass prescription.

Interpretation and report by the physician are an integral part of special ophthalmological services where indicated. Technical procedures (which might be performed by the physician personally) are often part of the service, but should not be mistaken to constitute the service itself. The physician may prescribe corrective lens to help relieve the symptoms caused by refractive error. As the prescription of the lens is included in the determination of the refractive state, it would not be reported separately. However, the fitting of the eyeglasses themselves is a separately reportable service when performed by the physician and would be reported by using codes. Prescription of lenses, when required, is included in 92015. Determination of refractive state includes specification of lens type (monofocal, bifocal, other), lens power, axis, prism, absorptive factor, impact resistance, and other factors. Fitting of eyeglasses is a separate service. When the determination of the refractive state is not performed, modifier AP is appended.

Medicare does not cover 92015 (refractive state) and considers the determination as part of the general ophthalmoscopic examination.

Example 1

A 65-year-old established patient with a recent onset of decreased vision and a history of cataracts visited the ophthalmologist for a 6-month examination. A comprehensive ophthalmological examination was performed. Since the diagnosis was cataracts and the recommendation was cataract extraction, the ophthalmologist did not perform a refraction.

CPT Code(s) Billed: 92014 AP

92014 Ophthalmological services: medical examination and evaluation, with initiation or continuation of diagnostic and treatment program; comprehensive, established patient, one or more visits

Rationale for Using Modifier AP

Because the ophthalmologist did not perform a refraction during the diagnostic examination, modifier AP identifies the fact that the service was not performed.

Modifier LS

Special coverage rules apply to situations in which an ophthalmologist is involved in an FDA-monitored study of the safety and efficacy of an investigational intraocular lens (IOL). The investigation process for IOLs is unique in that there is a core period and an adjunct period. The core study is a traditional, well-controlled clinical investigation with full record keeping and reporting requirements. The adjunct study is essentially an extended distribution phase for lenses in which only limited safety data are compiled. Depending on the lens being evaluated, the adjunct study may be an extension of the core study or may be the only type of investigation to which the lens is subject.

The FDA has taken the position that, during the entire investigation period, including the core and adjunct periods, all eye care services related to the investigation of the IOL must be provided by the investigator (ie, the implanting ophthalmologist) or another practitioner (including a doctor of optometry) who provides services at the direction or under the supervision of the investigator and who has an agreement with the investigator that information on the patient is given to the investigator so that he or she may report on the patient to the IOL manufacturer.

Eye care services furnished by anyone other than the investigator (or a practitioner who assists the investigator) are not covered by CMS during the period the IOL is being investigated, unless the services are not related to the investigation. To ensure that this policy is properly applied, all ophthalmologists in a service area must be informed that, when they are involved in an FDA-monitored study of an IOL, the modifier LS must be added to the procedure code for initial and subsequent claims for each beneficiary who is implanted with the investigational lens. This is the HCPCS two-digit modifier for an FDA-monitored IOL implant. The ophthalmologist should provide the names of any other practitioners who will be assisting in the study and inform the other practitioners to use the LS modifier on their claims. The FDA is currently phasing out the adjunct period of the IOL investigation process. However, until an IOL is approved for general marketing, it is considered investigational.

Modifier VP

Refractive lenses are covered when they are medically necessary to restore the vision normally provided by the natural lens of the eye of an individual lacking the organic lens because of surgical removal or congenital absence. Covered diagnoses are limited to pseudophakia (ICD-9 V43.1), aphakia (ICD-9 379.31), and congenital aphakia (ICD-9 743.35). Lenses provided for other diagnoses may be denied by the insurance carriers.

If a Medicare beneficiary has a cataract extraction with IOL insertion in one eye, subsequently has a cataract extraction with IOL insertion in the other eye, and does not receive eyeglasses or cataract lenses between the two surgical procedures, Medicare covers only one pair of eyeglasses or contact lenses after the second surgery. If a beneficiary has a pair of eyeglasses, has a cataract extraction with IOL insertion, and receives only new lenses but not new frames after the surgery, the benefit would not cover new frames at a later date (unless it follows subsequent cataract extraction in the other eye).

For patients who are aphakic who do not have an IOL (ICD-9 379.31, 743.35), the following lenses or combinations of lenses are covered by CMS when determined to be medically necessary:

- Bifocal lenses in frames
- Lenses in frames for far vision and lenses in frames for near vision
- When a contact lens(es) for far vision is prescribed (including cases of binocular and monocular aphakia), payment will be made for the contact lens(es), and lens(es) in frames for near vision to be worn at the same time as the contact lens(es), and lenses in frames to be worn when the contacts have been removed.

Documentation and Coding Guidelines for CMS

Appropriate modifiers (RT and LT) must be used with the procedure code(s) on the claim. When lenses are provided bilaterally and the same code is used for both lenses, both are billed on the same claim line with the LT/RT modifier and two units of service on the claim form.

An order for the lens(es) that is signed and dated by the treating physician must be kept on file by the supplier. The order must include the ICD-9 diagnosis code for the condition necessitating the lens(es). If the ordering physician is also the supplier, the prescription is an integral part of the patient's record.

If aphakia is the result of the removal of a previously implanted lens, the date of the surgical removal of the lens must accompany the claim.

Example 2

A 67-year-old Medicare patient, who had a cataract extraction of the left eye with intraocular lens implant 120 days ago, went to the ophthalmologist for a follow-up visit. The patient underwent the same procedure on the right eye 6 months prior. The ophthalmologist examined the patient, performing a problem-focused history and examination with low complexity decision making, and determined the patient was ready for contact lenses to improve vision in both eyes. The physician's technician determined the patient's corneal curvature, fitting the patient for power, size, flexibility and lens type. The technician determined a gas-permeable, toric lens would work well for the patient. The technician performed the fitting and instruction, and advised the patient to return in 1 week to make sure the lens fit well and vision was improved.

CPT Code(s) Billed: 99212 25—Office or other outpatient visit for the evaluation and management of an established patient, which requires at least two of these three key components: a problem focused history; a problem focused examination; straightforward medical decision making

92312 VP—Prescription of optical and physical characteristics of and fitting of contact lens, with medical supervision of adaptation; corneal lens for aphakia, both eyes

V2511 VP—Contact lens, gas permeable, toric, prism ballast, per lens

24. A DATE(S) OF SERVICE						B Place of Service	C Type of Service	D PROCEDURES, SERVICES, OR SUPPLIES (Explain Unusual Circumstances) CPT/HCPCS | MODIFIER		E DIAGNOSIS CODE	F $ CHARGES	G DAYS OR UNITS	H EPSDT Family Plan	I EMG	J COB	K RESERVED FOR LOCAL USE
	From			To												
MM	DD	YY	MM	DD	YY											
1								99212	25							
2								92312	VP							
3								V2511	VP							
4																
5																
6																

25. FEDERAL TAX I.D. NUMBER	SSN EIN	26. PATIENT'S ACCOUNT NO.	27. ACCEPT ASSIGNMENT? (For govt. claims, see back) YES NO	28. TOTAL CHARGE $	29. AMOUNT PAID $	30. BALANCE DUE $

Rationale for Using Modifier VP

Modifier VP would not be necessary for reporting the E/M service, but many carriers require VP for the contact and/or lens fitting and for the prescription identifying the aphakia, which in this instance is the absence of human lens removed via cataract extraction. For CMS, the VP identifies coverage of the contact lens material, fitting, and training, which is covered only under certain circumstances.

Medicaid-Only Modifiers

Each state identifies the level of care with modifiers U1-UD. Most state Medicaid carriers identify the levels of service as type of service (ie, dental, medical). HCPCS T codes have been added to the HCPCS book to identify Medicaid patient encounters. For example, if a Medicaid patient visited a clinic, code T1015 (Clinic visit/encounter) would be used with modifier U1 (All-inclusive, medical service) as a medical service modifier. Modifier U1 is defined individually by each state. In this example, the Medicaid carrier defined a clinic visit with modifier U1.

The Medicaid modifiers are as follows:

U1	Medicaid level of care 1, as defined by each state
U2	Medicaid level of care 2, as defined by each state
U3	Medicaid level of care 3, as defined by each state
U4	Medicaid level of care 4, as defined by each state
U5	Medicaid level of care 5, as defined by each state
U6	Medicaid level of care 6, as defined by each state
U7	Medicaid level of care 7, as defined by each state
U8	Medicaid level of care 8, as defined by each state
U9	Medicaid level of care 9, as defined by each state
UA	Medicaid level of care 10, as defined by each state
UB	Medicaid level of care 11, as defined by each state
UC	Medicaid level of care 12, as defined by each state
UD	Medicaid level of care 13, as defined by each state
EP	Service provided as part of Medicaid early periodic screening diagnosis and treatment program
FP	Service provided as part of Medicaid Family Planning Program

Providers and coders must check with their state Medicaid carrier to determine proper usage of these modifiers. Modifier EP is appended to the procedure code to identify that the service is part of the Early Periodic Screening Diagnosis and Treatment Program. For example, if a well visit was performed for a 5-year-old established patient as part of the program, the code selected would be 99393 with modifier EP appended. Coverage is based on the patient's eligibility for the program.

99393 EP	Periodic comprehensive preventive medicine reevaluation and management of an individual including an age and gender appropriate history, examination, counseling/anticipatory guidance/risk factor reduction interventions, and the ordering of appropriate immunization(s), laboratory/diagnostic procedures, established patient; late childhood (age 5 through 11 years)

The following example shows a claim submitted to Medicaid with modifier U2.

Example 3

21. DIAGNOSIS OR NATURE OF ILLNESS OR INJURY. (RELATE ITEMS 1,2,3 OR 4 TO ITEM 24E BY LINE)					22. MEDICAID RESUBMISSION CODE		ORIGINAL REF. NO.
1. V23 9		3.			23. PRIOR AUTHORIZATION NUMBER		
2.		4.					

	A. DATE(S) OF SERVICE		B. Place of Service	C. Type of Service	D. PROCEDURES, SERVICES, OR SUPPLIES (Explain Unusual Circumstances) CPT/HCPCS | MODIFIER	E. DIAGNOSIS CODE	F. $ CHARGES		G. DAYS OR UNITS	H. EPSDT Family Plan	I. EMG	J. COB	K. RESERVED FOR LOCAL USE
	From MM DD YY	To MM DD YY											
1	11 15 03		11		H1000	1	XXX	XX	1.0				
2	11 15 03		11		H1002 U2	1	XX	XX	4.0				
3	11 20 03		11		H1003	1	XX	XX	2.7				
4	11 20 03		11		H1003 TT	1	XX	XX	6.7				
5	12 28 03		11		H1002	1	XX	XX	2.7				
6	12 28 03		11		H1004	1	XX	XX	4.0				

25. FEDERAL TAX I.D. NUMBER SSN EIN	26. PATIENT'S ACCOUNT NO. 1234JED	27. ACCEPT ASSIGNMENT? (For govt. claims, see back) YES NO	28. TOTAL CHARGE $ XXX XX	29. AMOUNT PAID	30. BALANCE DUE $ XXX XX

Professional Service Modifiers

Modifiers in this category identify what type of provider and/or practitioner is providing care. Many insurance carriers require the use of these modifiers.

AM   Physician, team member service

AE   Registered dietician

AF   Specialty physician

AG   Primary physician

AK   Non-participating physician

AQ   Physician providing services in a HPSA [Health Professional Shortage Area]

AR   Physician scarcity area

AS   Physician assistant, nurse practitioner, or clinical nurse specialist services for assistant at surgery

EY   No physician or other licensed health care provider order for this item or service

GF   Non-physician service Critical Access Hospital

HM   Less than bachelors degree level

HN   Bachelors degree level

HO   Masters degree level

HP   Doctoral level

HT   Multidisciplinary team

HL   Intern

Q5   Service furnished by a substitute physician under a reciprocal billing arrangement

Q6	Service furnished by a locum tenens physician
SA	Nurse practitioner rendering service in collaboration with a physician
SB	Nurse midwife
SD	Services provided by registered nurse with specialized, highly technical home infusion training
SW	Service by certified diabetes educator
TD	RN [registered nurse]
TE	LPN/LVN [licensed practical nurse/licensed visiting nurse]

CMS does not recognize HCPCS modifiers HN, HO, and HP since coverage for services is not available on the basis of these modifiers. However, Medicaid in many states does recognize the use of these modifiers for services such as training and education services and skilled nursing services provided in a day care center, to name a few.

Modifiers Used in Mental Health

These modifiers typically represent providers of service, such as a clinical social worker, and types of programs (eg, substance abuse program, group setting). Even though CMS does not recognize all of these types of services, many carriers cover these services or programs if the patient's coverage includes mental health and/or counseling services. These modifiers should be used when mental health services are provided to patients.

AH	Clinical psychologist
AJ	Clinical social worker
HE	Mental health program
HF	Substance abuse program
HG	Opioid addiction treatment program
HH	Integrated mental health/substance abuse program
HI	Integrated mental health and mental retardation/developmental disabilities program
HK	Specialized mental health programs for high-risk populations
HQ	Group setting
HR	Family/couple with client present
HS	Family/couple without client present

Where appropriate, modifiers must be used to denote the services that are rendered by a clinical psychologist and a licensed clinical social worker.

The modifiers are as follows:

AH   Clinical psychologist

AJ   Clinical social worker

Billing/Coding for Clinical Psychologists (CP)

The following identifies the billing requirements for CP services:
- CPs must submit assigned claims for all of their services.
- CPs must bill appropriate codes with modifier AH immediately after the procedure/service code (eg, 90826 AH).

Example 1

A woman sought counseling because she claimed she "let things get to her," obsessing over painful thoughts and feeling depressed. She decided to seek therapeutic services after a friend encouraged her to do so. The client stated that she broke up with her boyfriend 5 months previously and indicated that the relationship had been very intense; although they had not been living together, they had planned to get married. She stated that it was her idea to break up and that she was feeling paranoid and could not trust her behavior any longer. The client stated that she was jealous of her boyfriend's former wife and could not tolerate his responsibility to his children. The client was a single parent with two children who were 9 months and 4 years of age. She worked full time as a bank manager. She indicated that her symptoms of depression were lack of ambition, lack of interest in her job and children, difficulty concentrating, difficulty falling asleep, and weight loss of 4 kg during the past 3 weeks. The client did indicate, however, that her appetite had improved in the past 2 days. She denied suicidal ideas or plans but was having panic attacks, although not often. Symptoms of panic included heart palpitations, heart flutters, shortness of breath, shakiness, and a feeling of impending disaster.

Previous Psychiatric History: None

Family History: Development and current problem.

The client reported that she was born and raised in Anderson, Indiana. Her father was also a banker who suffered from diabetes and eventually lost his sight. He died at age 50 when she was 11 years old. Her mother was emotionally and financially dependent on her parents and never worked outside the home. The client stated that her mother had developed Alzheimer disease and had died 2 years ago after a lengthy illness. The patient had been responsible for her mother's care for 4 years until she died, and felt a great deal of loss because of it. She reported that she had five siblings; the oldest sister was 45 years old, and youngest brother was 30. The client was the second child. She indicated that one brother and one sister lived in

California, and the other three siblings lived in Illinois. The client was a college graduate and had been married for 5 years before her divorce. She was not on good terms with her former husband. She denied the use of alcohol or street drugs, but she smoked two to three packs of cigarettes a day and had been smoking for approximately 10 years. She consumed five cups of coffee per day.

Mental Status Examination: The patient was appropriately well dressed and displayed good hygiene. She displayed mild tension. Her mannerisms and posture were associated with her tension. She displayed a moderate level of motor retardation. The patient was moderately withdrawn emotionally and somewhat sensitive. No conceptual disorganization or altered association was observed. She displayed midlevel guilt feelings and a moderate level of suspiciousness. There was no hallucinatory or delusional behavior; the patient was moderately anxious and depressed with a restrictive range of affective expression. Her insight and judgment appeared mildly impaired.

Impression: The patient was a mature single parent 40 years of age, who was experiencing a severe level of anxiety and panic. In addition, she was experiencing some depressive feelings and symptomology and was genuinely motivated to ameliorate these difficulties.

Axis I: Panic disorder w/o agoraphobia, R/O adjustment disorder with mixed emotional features (300.01)

Axis II: Diagnosis deferred (799.90)

Axis III: None

Axis IV: Mild breakup with boyfriend and difficulties at work and concerns about single parenthood

Axis V: Current Global Assessment Functioning (GAF) 70; Highest GAF over the past year 75

Plan: Begin individual cognitive insight-oriented therapy from 12 to 24 sessions. Patient will return in 1 week.

CPT Code(s) Billed: 90801 AH—Psychiatric diagnostic interview examination-provided by a clinical psychologist

Rationale for Using Modifier AH

The service was provided by a CP (clinical psychologist), and the AH modifier indicates that that type of provider performed the service(s).

Covered services rendered by CPs are extended to all appropriate places of service. The following is a list of the CPT procedure codes and modifier, where appropriate, that may be reported for services rendered by CPs. Further, the single asterisk indicates the services that are subject to the outpatient psychiatric services limitation for Medicare. The double asterisk indicates that the service is subject to the outpatient psychiatric services limitation in certain settings.

90801AH	90847AH**
90802AH	90849AH**
90804AH*	90853AH**
90806AH*	90857AH**
90808AH*	96101
90810AH*	96102
90812AH*	96103
90814AH*	96105
90816AH**	96110
90818AH**	96111
90821AH**	96116
90823AH**	96118
90826AH**	96119
90828AH**	96120
90845AH	

Clinical Social Worker (Modifier AJ)

A clinical social worker is defined by CMS as an individual who:
- Possesses a masters or doctoral degree in social work
- Has performed at least 2 years of supervised clinical social work, and either:
  - ~ Is licensed or certified as a clinical social worker by the state in which the services are performed, or
  - ~ In the case of an individual in a state that does not provide for licensure or certification, has completed at least 2 years or 3000 hours of post masters degree supervised clinical social work practice under the supervision of a masters-level social worker in an appropriate setting such as a hospital, skilled nursing facility, or clinic

Clinical social worker services are defined by CMS as those services that the licensed clinical social worker (LCSW) is legally authorized to perform under state law (or the state regulatory mechanism provided by state law) of the state in which such services are performed for the diagnosis and treatment of mental illnesses.

Billing and/or Coding Issues for CMS

The following list identifies the billing requirements for LCSW services.
- LCSWs must submit assigned claims for all of their services.
- LCSWs must bill all appropriate codes with modifier AJ immediately after the procedure/service code.

- LCSWs must bill appropriate codes under their identification number or, if the patient is a Medicare patient, the unique physician identification number.

Example 2

Patient: Mary Jones

Date: 06/30/20XX

Time Spent With Patient: 45 minutes

Session Focus: To cope with lifestyle changes, which are a cause of depression.

The patient stated, "I have had a bad week. I am still having crying spells and tension." The patient stated that crying spells had decreased in frequency but depression had worsened. The patient discussed her anger, need for distraction, and anger at loss of a travel opportunity. She reported a solid block of sleep at night, and added that she had been spending a lot of time in bed.

Assessment and Plan: The patient presented in a depressed state after 4 of 12 planned counseling sessions. She will continue therapy as planned, with the next session in 2 weeks, and continue current medications.

CPT Code(s) Billed: 90806 AJ—Individual psychotherapy, insight oriented, behavior modifying and/or supportive, in an office or outpatient facility, approximately 45 to 50 minutes face-to-face with the patient; performed by a licensed clinical social worker

Rationale for Using Modifier AJ

Since the service was provided by a licensed social worker, modifier AJ would indicate what type of provider performed the service(s).

Covered Procedure Codes

Covered services rendered by LCSWs are extended to all appropriate places of service. The following is a list of the CPT procedure codes (with modifier) that may be reported for services rendered by LCSWs. The asterisk indicates services that are subject to the outpatient psychiatric services limitation.

90801 AJ	90845 AJ
90802 AJ*	90847 AJ*
90847 AJ*	90849 AJ*
90806 AJ*	90853 AJ*
90808 AJ*	90857 AJ*

90810 AJ*   97532 AJ

90812 AJ*   97533 AJ

90814 AJ*

Federal, State, and County Agencies

These modifiers are not covered by CMS, but may be covered by other third-party payers and some state Medicaid providers. They are used when, for example, a patient is ordered into a drug treatment program by the courts. If the patient must seek treatment for the addition, a procedure code such as a physician office visit (99213 *Expanded problem-focused history and examination with low-complexity decision making*) with modifier H9 appended will indicate that the court has ordered that the patient participate in the treatment program.

H9	Court-ordered
HU	Funded by child welfare agency
HV	Funded by state addictions agency
HW	Funded by state mental health agency
HX	Funded by county/local agency
HY	Funded by juvenile justice agency
HZ	Funded by criminal justice agency
QJ	Services/items provided to a prisoner or patient in state or local custody; however, the state or local government, as applicable, meets the requirements in 42 CFR 411.4 (b)
SE	State and/or federally funded programs/services
TR	School-based individualized education program (IEP) services provided

Miscellaneous Modifiers

AT	Acute treatment (used when reporting chiropractic manipulative treatment [98940, 98941, 98942])
ET	Emergency services
G7	Pregnancy resulted from rape or incest or pregnancy certified by physician as life threatening
GQ	Via asynchronous telecommunications system
GT	Via interactive audio and video telecommunication systems
HA	Child/adolescent program
HB	Adult program, nongeriatric

HC	Adult program, geriatric
HD	Pregnant/parenting women's program
HJ	Employee assistance program
ST	Related to trauma or injury
TF	Intermediate level of care
TG	Complex/high-tech level of care
UF	Services provided, morning
UG	Services provided, afternoon
UH	Services provided, evening
UJ	Services provided, night
UK	Service on behalf of the client to someone other than the client (collateral relationship)

Regulatory and Informational Modifiers

CA	Procedure payable inpatient
CB	ESRD Beneficiary Part A (SNF) separate payment
CC	Procedure code change (use CC when the procedure code submitted was changed either for administrative reasons or because an incorrect code was filed). Modifier CC indicates the procedure code was incorrect. The carrier will determine reimbursement based on the new procedure code.
CD	AMCC Test for ESRD or MCP MD
CF	AMCC Test not composite rate
CG	Innovator drug dispensed
GA	Waiver of liability statement on file
GB	Claim being resubmitted for payment because it is no longer covered under a global payment demonstration
GC	This service has been performed in part by a resident under the direction of a teaching physician
GE	This service has been performed by a resident without the presence of a teaching physician under the primary care exception
GJ	"Opt out" physician or practitioner emergency or urgent care

GK	Actual item/service ordered by physician, item associated with GA or GZ modifier
GL	Medically unnecessary upgrade provided instead of standard item, no charge, no advance beneficiary notice (ABN)
GY	Item or service statutorily excluded or does not meet the definition of any Medicare benefit
GZ	Item or service expected to be denied as not reasonable and necessary
KB	Beneficiary requested upgrade for ABN, more than four modifiers identified on claim
KC	Replace special power WC interface
KD	Drug/biological/DME infused
KF	FDA Class III device
KX	Specific required documentation on file
KZ	New coverage not implemented by M+C
Q2	HCFA/ORD demonstration project procedure/service
Q4	Service for ordering/referring physician qualifies as a service exemption
QC	Single-channel monitoring
QD	Recording and storage in solid-state memory by digital recorder
QT	Recording and storage on tape by an analog tape recorder
QV	Item or service provided as routine care in a Medicare qualifying clinical trial
QW	CLIA waived test
RD	Drug provided to beneficiary, but not administered incident-to
SC	Medically necessary service or supply
SF	Second opinion ordered by a professional review organization per section 9401, pp 199–272 (100% reimbursement-no Medicare deductible or coinsurance)
SG	Ambulatory surgical center (ASC) facility service. ASC services should be coded with modifier appended to all procedure codes. When other CPT modifiers are used, the CPT modifiers should be listed first, followed by the SG modifier.

SU	Procedure performed in physician's office (to denote use of facility and equipment)
SY	Contact with high-risk population
TC	Technical component
TN	Rural/outside service providers' customary service area
TR	School-based individualized education program (IEP) services provided outside the public school district responsible for the student
TS	Follow-up service
TT	Individualized service provided to more than one patient in the same setting
TU	Special payment rate, overtime
TV	Special payment rates, holidays/weekends

Modifiers GA, GY, and GZ

Effective January 1, 2002, new modifiers were developed to allow physicians, practitioners, and suppliers to report services that are statutorily noncovered or that may be determined by Medicare not to be medically necessary or reasonable and necessary by Medicare. Modifier GX was deleted from the HCPCS book in 2002 and replaced by GA, GY, and GZ.

The GY modifier is used when a physician, practitioner, and/or supplier needs to report that an item or service is statutorily noncovered or is not a Medicare benefit. Modifier GY is appended to the code for the procedure or service when the patient indicates that he or she wants the claim submitted to Medicare.

The GA modifier is reported when the physician, practitioner, or supplier expects that Medicare will deny an item or service as not reasonable and necessary and the practitioner has a waiver of liability statement on file (ABN). The ABN is completed before the service is provided to the patient. The claim may be submitted to CMS with the GA modifier, which advises CMS that an ABN is on file for the patient and the patient has been advised that the claim for services will most likely be denied. If the practitioner or supplier does not obtain a signed ABN before rendering service, and the claim is denied, the practitioner or supplier must not bill the patient for the denied service(s). CMS guidelines for these modifiers may be found in the Medicare Carriers' Manual, sections 4508 and 4509. In the past, practitioners were allowed to modify the ABN to meet the office's needs. However, effective January 1, 2001, this is no longer allowed. CMS developed a standard ABN with instructions on proper use. The ABN is available in an English version and a Spanish version and can be located on the CMS Web site.

The CMS ABN form is shown on the next page.

PATIENT'S NAME: MEDICARE # (HICN): _____

ADVANCE BENEFICIARY NOTICE (ABN)

NOTE: You need to make a choice about receiving these health care items or services.

We expect that Medicare will not pay for the item(s) or service(s) that are described below. Medicare does not pay for all of your health care costs. Medicare only pays for covered items and services when Medicare rules are met. The fact that Medicare may not pay for a particular item or service does not mean that you should not receive it. There may be a good reason your doctor recommended it. Right now, in your case, **Medicare probably will not pay for:**

Items or Services:

Because:

The purpose of this form is to help you make an informed choice about whether or not you want to receive these items or services, knowing that you might have to pay for them yourself. Before you make a decision about your options, you should **read this entire notice carefully.**

- Ask us to explain, if you don't understand why Medicare probably won't pay.
- Ask us how much these items or services will cost you
  (**Estimated Cost:** $_____), in case you have to pay for them yourself or through other insurance.

PLEASE CHOOSE **ONE** OPTION. CHECK **ONE** BOX. **SIGN & DATE** YOUR CHOICE.

☐ **Option 1.   YES. I want to receive these items or services.**
I understand that Medicare will not decide whether to pay unless I receive these items or services. Please submit my claim to Medicare. I understand that you may bill me for items or services and that I may have to pay the bill while Medicare is making its decision. If Medicare does pay, you will refund to me any payments I made to you that are due to me. If Medicare denies payment, I agree to be personally and fully responsible for payment. That is, I will pay personally, either out of pocket or through any other insurance that I have. I understand I can appeal Medicare's decision.

☐ **Option 2.   NO. I have decided not to receive these items or services.**
I will not receive these items or services. I understand that you will not be able to submit a claim to Medicare and that I will not be able to appeal your opinion that Medicare won't pay.

_____   _____
Date   **Signature of patient or person acting on patient's behalf**

NOTE: Your health information will be kept confidential. Any information that we collect about you on this form will be kept confidential in our offices. If a claim is submitted to Medicare, your health information on this form may be shared with Medicare. The health information Medicare sees will be kept confidential by Medicare.

OMB Approval No. 0938-0566 Form No. CMS-R-131-G (June 2001)

Modifier GZ must be used when a physician, practitioner, and/or supplier wants to indicate that it expects Medicare will deny the service submitted as not medically necessary, but it failed to obtain an ABN signed by the patient. This lets the Medicare carrier understand that the provider of services failed to obtain the ABN, is aware that the service may be denied, and will not bill the patient for the service if denied by CMS.

The GY, GA, and GZ modifiers may be used with CPT codes or with HCPCS codes.

HCPCS code A9270 is only to be used in cases where there is no specific procedure code (CPT or HCPCS) for an item or supply and no appropriate unlisted or "not otherwise classified" HCPCS code available. HCPCS code A9270 (Noncovered item or service) is for suppliers who bill for DMERCS for statutorily noncovered items and items that do not meet the definition of a Medicare benefit.

The information below for modifiers GA, GY and GZ can be a helpful tool in determining which of the three modifiers to use. This information can be found in table format on the CMS Web site.[1]

GA modifier "Waiver of liability on file."

Description
Item or service expected to be denied as not reasonable and necessary and an advance beneficiary notice was given to the beneficiary. These are so-called "medical necessity" denials. The GA modifier also may be used with assigned and unassigned claims for DMEPOS where one of the following Part B "technical denials" may apply:
- prohibited telephone solicitation
- no supplier number
- failure to obtain an advance determination of coverage

When to use the GA modifier
When you think a service will be denied because it does not meet the Medicare program standards for medically necessary care and you gave the beneficiary an advance beneficiary notice. You are required to include the GA modifier on your claim anytime you obtain a signed ABN, or have a patient's refusal to sign an ABN witnessed properly in an assigned claim situation (except an assigned claim for one of the specified DMEPOS technical denials). Use a GA modifier on an assigned claim if you gave an ABN to a patient but the patient refused to sign the ABN and you did furnish the services. (In these circumstances, on all unassigned claims, as well as an assigned claim for a specified DMEPOS technical denial, use the GZ modifier.)

Examples of its use
All instances in which you deliver an ABN to a Medicare patient and services are furnished, eg, after having a patient sign an ABN, you fur-

---

1. Beneficiary Notices Initiative, available at www.cms.hhs.gov/medicare/bni/.

nish a service covered by Medicare but likely to be denied as "too fre-quent" by Medicare.

What happens if you use the GA modifier?

The claim will be reviewed by Medicare like any other claim and may or may not be denied. The carrier will NOT use the presence of the GA modifier to influence its determination of Medicare coverage and pay-ment of the service. If Medicare pays the claim, the GA modifier is irrelevant. If the claim is denied, the beneficiary will be fully and per-sonally liable to pay you for the service, personally or through other insurance. Medicare will not pay you for the service since your giving an ABN to the patient is evidence that you knew Medicare probably would not pay for the service.

What happens if you don't use the GA modifier?

The claim will be reviewed by Medicare like any other claim and may or may not be denied. If the claim is denied, the beneficiary will be held not liable and you will be held liable. Medicare will not pay you nor allow you to collect from the beneficiary. In order to remedy this situation, you will need to appeal Medicare's action limiting the beneficiary's liability. The question of an abusive billing pattern could arise. It is possible that fraud and abuse implications may arise out of your omission of the fact of hav-ing had an ABN signed by the patient under these circumstances, espe-cially if there is a consistent pattern of such omissions (viz., a pattern of failure to include the GA modifier when it is applicable).

GY modifier "Item or service statutorily excluded or does not meet the definition of any Medicare benefit."

Description

These are the so-called "statutory exclusions" or "categorical exclu-sions" and the "technical denials." ABNs are not an issue for these ser-vices. There are no advance beneficiary notice (ABN) requirements for statutory exclusions. There are no ABN requirements for technical denials (except three types of DMEPOS denials, and they are listed under modifiers GZ and GA).

When to use the GY modifier

1) When you think a claim will be denied because it is not a Medicare benefit or because Medicare law specifically excludes it.
2) When you think a claim will be denied because the service does not meet all the requirements of the definition of a benefit in Medicare law.
3) When you submit a claim to obtain a Medicare denial for secondary payer purposes.

Examples of its use

1) Routine physicals, laboratory tests in absence of signs or symptoms, hearing aids, air conditioners, services in a foreign country, services to a family member.

2) Surgery performed by a physician not legally authorized to perform surgery in the State.

What happens if you use the GY modifier?

The claim will be denied by Medicare. The carrier may "auto-deny" claims with the GY modifier. This action may be quicker than if you do not use a GY modifier. The beneficiary will be liable for all charges, whether personally or through other insurance. If Medicare pays the claim, the GY modifier is irrelevant.

What happens if you don't use the GY modifier?

The claim will be reviewed by Medicare and probably will be denied. This action may be slower than if you had used a GY modifier. If the claim is denied as an excluded service or for failure to meet the definition of a benefit, the beneficiary will be liable for all charges, whether personally or through other insurance.

GZ modifier "Item or service expected to be denied as not reasonable and necessary." (No signed ABN on file.)

Description

Item or service expected to be denied as not reasonable and necessary and an advance beneficiary notice (ABN) was not signed by the beneficiary. These are the so-called "medical necessity" denials. The GZ modifier also may be used with assigned and unassigned claims for DMEPOS where one of the following Part B "technical denials" may apply:

- Prohibited telephone solicitation

- No supplier number

- Failure to obtain an advance determination of coverage

When to use the GZ modifier

When you think a service will be denied because it does not meet Medicare program standards for medically necessary care and you did not obtain a signed ABN from the beneficiary. When you gave an ABN to a patient who refused to sign the ABN and you, nevertheless, did furnish the services, use a GZ modifier on unassigned claims for all physicians' services and DMEPOS; and also on assigned claims for which one of the DMEPOS technical denials is expected. If you wish to indicate to the carrier that one of the above situations exists, in your opinion, then you may elect to include the GZ modifier on your claim.

Examples of its use

When you would have given an ABN to a patient but could not because of an emergency care situation, eg, in an EMTALA covered situation in an emergency room, or in an ambulance transport. When a patient was not personally present at your premises and could not be reached to timely sign an ABN, eg, before a specimen is tested. When you realize too late, only after furnishing a service, that you should have given the patient an ABN.

What happens if you use the GZ modifier?

The claim will be reviewed by Medicare like any other claim and may or may not be denied. The carrier will NOT use the presence of the GZ modifier to influence its determination of Medicare coverage and payment of the service. If Medicare pays the claim, the GZ modifier is irrelevant. If the claim is denied, the beneficiary generally will not be liable to pay you for the service. However, even though the beneficiary is found not liable, if you are also found not liable with respect to an unassigned claim, or an assigned claim denied for one of the DMEPOS technical denial reasons specified, you may be allowed to collect from the beneficiary. Medicare may or may not hold you liable depending whether you knew that payment would be denied when you furnished the service. In cases where you gave an ABN to the patient, or attempted to, but could not obtain a beneficiary signature, most likely Medicare will hold you liable.

What happens if you don't use the GZ modifier?

You never need to use the GZ modifier when you expect Medicare to pay. You are always free to elect not to use a GZ modifier. The claim will be reviewed by Medicare like any other claim and may or may not be denied. NOTE: The GZ modifier is provided for physicians and suppliers that wish to submit a claim to Medicare, that know that an ABN should have been signed but was not, and that do not want any risk of allegation of fraud or abuse for claiming services that are not medically necessary. By notifying Medicare, by the GZ modifier, that you expect Medicare will not cover the service, you can greatly reduce the risk of a mistaken allegation of fraud or abuse.

Example 1

A 68-year-old Medicare patient visited her internist for her annual visit. The physician performed and documented a comprehensive history and examination, and counseled the patient on diet, exercise, and maintaining a healthy lifestyle. In addition, labs were ordered. The patient indicated it was time for her Pap, pelvic, and breast exams, which had last been performed 1 year ago. The physician failed to get the ABN signed and realized after the patient left that both services were unlikely to be covered.

The physician advised the patient the service is only covered by Medicare every 2 years. The patient also was advised that the preventive visit was not covered by Medicare unless it was her first exam after obtaining Medicare insurance, which was not the case. The patient insisted the physician file the claim because she had supplemental coverage that would pay for the preventive visit along with the other preventive services.

CPT Code(s) Billed: 99397 GZ, G0101 GZ, Q0091 GZ

99397 Periodic comprehensive preventive medicine reevaluation and management of an individual including an age and gender appropriate history, examination, counseling/anticipatory guidance/risk factor reduction interventions, and the ordering of appropriate immunization(s), laboratory/diagnostic procedures, established patient; 65 years and over

G0101 Cervical or vaginal cancer screening; pelvic and clinical breast examination

Q0091 Screening papanicolaou smear; obtaining, preparing and conveyance of cervical or vaginal smear to laboratory

24. A DATE(S) OF SERVICE From / To	B Place of Service	C Type of Service	D PROCEDURES, SERVICES, OR SUPPLIES (Explain Unusual Circumstances) CPT/HCPCS | MODIFIER	E DIAGNOSIS CODE	F $ CHARGES	G DAYS OR UNITS	H EPSDT Family Plan	I EMG	J COB	K RESERVED FOR LOCAL USE
1			99397 | GZ							
2			G0101 | GZ							
3			Q0091 | GZ							
4										
5										
6										

25. FEDERAL TAX I.D. NUMBER SSN EIN	26. PATIENT'S ACCOUNT NO.	27. ACCEPT ASSIGNMENT? (For govt. claims, see back) YES NO	28. TOTAL CHARGE $	29. AMOUNT PAID $	30. BALANCE DUE $

Rationale for Using Modifier GZ

The preventive medicine visit and the Pap, pelvic, and breast examinations would not likely be covered since the services had been provided the previous year. The preventive medicine exam was only covered at the patient's initial visit after obtaining Medicare. The physician failed to obtain the ABN and cannot hold the patient financially liable for the services unless the ABN was signed prior to receiving the services. Modifier GZ tells CMS that the provider failed to provide the proper notice to the patient.

Modifiers Used in Outpatient Rehabilitation

GN Services delivered under an outpatient speech language pathology plan of care

GO Services delivered under an outpatient occupational therapy plan of care

GP   Services delivered under an outpatient physical therapy plan of care

These modifiers are used for outpatient rehabilitation services for speech/language, occupational therapy, and physical therapy modalities. They are for informational purposes only and have no effect on reimbursement. Providers report procedures with modifiers to distinguish the type of therapist who performed the outpatient rehabilitation service; if the service was not delivered by a therapist, the discipline of the plan of treatment under which the service is delivered should be reported.

If an audiology procedure is performed by an audiologist, these modifiers are not required to be reported.

Example 2

A patient underwent knee replacement surgery. Six weeks later, the patient began physical therapy for 60 minutes three times a week.

CPT Code(s) Billed: *97116 GP—Therapeutic procedure, one or more areas,*
each 15 minutes; gait training (includes stair climbing)

24.	A DATE(S) OF SERVICE From To MM DD YY MM DD YY	B Place of Service	C Type of Service	D PROCEDURES, SERVICES, OR SUPPLIES (Explain Unusual Circumstances) CPT/HCPCS | MODIFIER	E DIAGNOSIS CODE	F $ CHARGES	G DAYS OR UNITS	H EPSDT Family Plan	I EMG	J COB	K RESERVED FOR LOCAL USE
1				97116|GP			4				
2											
3											
4											
5											
6											
	25. FEDERAL TAX I.D. NUMBER SSN EIN		26. PATIENTíS ACCOUNT NO.		27. ACCEPT ASSIGNMENT? (For govt. claims, see back) YES NO	28. TOTAL CHARGE $		29. AMOUNT PAID $		30. BALANCE DUE $	

Rationale for Using Modifier GP

The GP modifier is appended to the physical therapy code to indicate it was delivered under an outpatient physical therapy plan of care. Since the patient underwent 60 minutes per session, and the procedure code is based on each 15 minutes, the units billed would be 4 in the units column on the claim form.

Anatomic Modifiers

The anatomic-specific modifiers, such as RT, LT, E1, and LC, designate the area or part of the body on which the procedure is performed. Generally, these modifiers have been added to streamline the claims processing system by allowing for automated payment without having to request additional documentation to rule out duplicate or other inappropriate billing.

In addition to the modifiers that have been approved by the National Uniform Billing Committee for hospital outpatient reporting, the use of other HCPCS level II modifiers may be required by various third-party payers.

When eyelid procedures are coded, instead of modifier RT or LT, the procedure code should be appended with modifiers E1 to E4 to indicate upper and lower eyelid. For example, if the physician performed an ectropion repair on the lower right eyelid of each eye, the procedure would be coded as follows:

67916   Repair of ectropion; blepharoplasty, excision tarsal wedge

Without the appropriate modifier to identify upper or lower and which eye (right or left) was affected, the carrier would suspend the claim for more information or may request documentation. By appending HCPCS modifier E4 to the procedure code, the carrier can identify which eye and what side of the body the surgery was performed on.

Correct coding: 67916 E4

Modifiers to identify digits for hands and feet are also helpful when surgeons perform hand surgery; the modifiers inform the insurance carrier which hand and what digit the procedure was performed on.

The following anatomic modifiers may be used:

E1	Upper left, eyelid
E2	Lower left, eyelid
E3	Upper right, eyelid
E4	Lower right, eyelid
F1	Left hand, second digit
F2	Left hand, third digit
F3	Left hand, fourth digit
F4	Left hand, fifth digit
F5	Right hand, thumb
F6	Right hand, second digit
F7	Right hand, third digit
F8	Right hand, fourth digit
F9	Right hand, fifth digit
FA	Left hand, thumb
LC	Left circumflex coronary artery
LD	Left anterior descending coronary artery
LT	Left side (used to identify procedures performed on the left side of the body)
RC	Right coronary artery

RT	Right side (used to identify procedures performed on the right side of the body)
T1	Left foot, second digit
T2	Left foot, third digit
T3	Left foot, fourth digit
T4	Left foot, fifth digit
T5	Right foot, great toe
T6	Right foot, second digit
T7	Right foot, third digit
T8	Right foot, fourth digit
T9	Right foot, fifth digit
TA	Left foot, great toe

Modifiers LT and RT

Modifiers LT (left side) and RT (right side) are used to identify procedures performed on either the left or right side of the body. Modifiers LT and RT do not, however, indicate bilateral procedures (modifier 50). For example, lesions removed from the left leg and the right leg should be coded with RT and LT, since it may not be the same exact site on each leg.

Modifiers LC, LD, and RC

These modifiers are used to identify stents, balloon angioplasty, and atherectomy. Each procedure has two codes, for a single vessel and each additional vessel if applicable. The National Correct Coding Initiative edits state that modifier 59 does not need to be included with these procedures.

Example 1

The decision was made to place a stent in a patient, and this decision was discussed fully with the patient and his family. The patient was prepared for the procedure, which includes sterilization of the access site and cannulation with an indwelling sheath (typically the femoral artery is used). A guide catheter was positioned in the appropriate coronary ostium and baseline arteriograms were obtained. A guidewire was passed down the target vessel across the target stenosis. The stent was loaded on a carrying catheter (which had an expandable balloon), which was inserted into the guiding catheter and advanced under fluoroscopic guidance in the right coronary artery. The physician positioned the stent in the target vessel and confirmed the location by fluoroscopy and comparison with previous contrast injections; the balloon was inflated to expand and secure the stent. The carrying catheter balloon was deflated and the catheter removed over the guidewire. Then a larger or less compliant balloon was passed over the guidewire into the stent, expanded until the stent was fully dilated, and then removed. An additional stent (loaded on a separate carrying catheter) was inserted through the guiding catheter and advanced into the left descending coronary artery under fluoroscopic guidance. The physician positioned the stent in the target vessel and confirmed the location by fluoroscopy and comparison with previous contrast injections. The carrying catheter balloon was deflated and the catheter was removed over the guidewire. A balloon was passed over the guidewire into the stent, expanded until the stent was fully dilated, and then removed.

NOTE: At the time of initial stent placement, it was determined that an additional stent was required. This additional service represents only the intraservice work of placing the additional stent. It does not include any prework or postwork, as these portions of the service are captured in the initial stent placement code. The patient returned to the recovery room in good condition.

CPT Code(s) Billed: 92980 RC, 92981 LD

92980   Transcatheter placement of an intracoronary stent(s), percutaneous, with or without other therapeutic intervention, any method; single vessel

92981   Transcatheter placement of an intracoronary stent(s), percutaneous, with or without other therapeutic intervention, any method; each additional vessel (List separately in addition to code for primary procedure)

Rationale for Using Modifiers RC and LD
The documentation indicates a stent was placed in the right coronary artery and the left anterior descending coronary artery.

Example 2

A 45-year-old female patient with some compressive symptoms and a right thyroid goiter underwent a right thyroid lobectomy in the hospital surgery department. The physician removed the lobe with isthmusectomy, exposing the thyroid with a transverse incision in the skin line. The platysma was divided, and the strap muscles were separated in the midline. The thyroid lobe was isolated, and the superior and inferior thyroid vessels were ligated. The thyroid gland was divided in the midline of the isthmus over the anterior trachea and was resected. The platysmas and skin were closed, and the patient tolerated the procedure well.

CPT Code(s) Billed: 60220 RT

60220   Total thyroid lobectomy, unilateral; with or without
              isthmusectomy

Rationale for Using Modifier RT

The thyroid lobectomy was performed on the right thyroid, and the modifier identifies that the lobectomy was performed on that side of the body. If the modifier was not appended, the carrier might query the physician as to the side of the body. The modifier attempts to eliminate a denial or suspension of the claim for more information.

Foot Care Modifiers

National modifiers were established by CMS to allow class findings to be reported without writing a narrative description. The following modifiers should be used in conjunction with "covered routine" foot care procedures (eg, 11719, 11720, 11721) to indicate the severity of the patient's systemic condition.

Q7   One class A finding

Q8   Two class B findings

Q9   One class B and two class C findings

Class A Findings

- Nontraumatic amputation of foot or integral skeletal portion thereof

Class B Findings

- Absent posterior tibial pulse
- Absent dorsalis pedis pulse
- Advanced trophic changes such as (3 of the following are required to equal 1 class B finding):
  - ~ Hair growth (decrease or absence)
  - ~ Nail changes (thickening)
  - ~ Pigmentary changes (discloration)
  - ~ Skin texture (thin, shiny)
  - ~ Skin color (elevation pallor or dependence rubor)

Class C Findings

- Claudication
- Temperature changes (eg, cold feet)
- Edema
- Paresthesias (abnormal spontaneous sensations in feet)
- Burning

- Markedly diminished or absent sensation in the foot, secondary to systemic disease or injury resulting in damage to the sensory nerves to the lower extremity
- Vascular grafts (aortic, lower extremity)
- Joint implants
- Heart valve replacement
- Active chemotherapy

National Modifiers Not Payable by Medicare

The following HCPCS modifiers are considered national HCPCS modifiers and are not recognized by Medicare; they should not be used when claims are submitted to Medicare.

H9	Court-ordered
HA	Child adolescent program
HB	Adult program, nongeriatric
HC	Adult program, geriatric
HD	Pregnant/parenting women's program
HE	Mental health program
HF	Substance abuse program
HG	Opioid addiction treatment program
HH	Integrated mental health/substance abuse program
HI	Integrated mental health and mental retardation/developmental disabilities program
HJ	Employee assistance program
HK	Specialized mental health programs for high-risk populations
HL	Intern
HM	Less than bachelor degree level
HN	Bachelors degree level
HO	Masters degree level
HP	Doctoral level
HQ	Group setting
HR	Family/couple with client present
HS	Family/couple without client present
HT	Multidisciplinary team
HU	Funded by child welfare agency

HV   Funded by state addictions agency

HW   Funded by state mental health agency

HX   Funded by county/local agency

HY   Funded by juvenile justice agency

HZ   Funded by criminal justice agency

SE   State and/or federally funded programs/services

SK   Member of high-risk population (use only with codes for immunization)

SL   State-supplied vaccine

ST   Related to trauma or injury

SU   Procedure performed in physician's office (to denote use of facility and equipment)

SV   Pharmaceuticals delivered to patient's home but not utilized

TK   Extra patient or passenger, nonambulance

TL   Early intervention/individualized family planning service plan (IFSP)

TM   Individualized education program (IEP)

TN   Rural/outside service providers' customary service area

TP   Medical transport, unloaded vehicle

TQ   Basic life support transport by a volunteer ambulance provider

TR   School-based individualized education program (IEP) services provided outside the public school district responsible for the student

TS   Follow-up service

TT   Individualized service provided to more than one patient in the same setting

TU   Special payment rate, overtime

TV   Special payment rates, holidays/weekends

TW   Back-up equipment

U1   Medicaid level of care 1, as defined by each state

U2   Medicaid level of care 2, as defined by each state

U3   Medicaid level of care 3, as defined by each state

U4   Medicaid level of care 4, as defined by each state

U5   Medicaid level of care 5, as defined by each state

U6	Medicaid level of care 6, as defined by each state
U7	Medicaid level of care 7, as defined by each state
U8	Medicaid level of care 8, as defined by each state
U9	Medicaid level of care 9, as defined by each state
UA	Medicaid level of care 10, as defined by each state
UB	Medicaid level of care 11, as defined by each state
UC	Medicaid level of care 12, as defined by each state
UD	Medicaid level of care 13, as defined by each state
UF	Services provided, morning
UG	Services provided, afternoon
UH	Services provided, evening
UJ	Services provided, night
UK	Service on behalf of client someone other than the client (collateral relationship)

Test Your Knowledge

Multiple Choice

1   Modifiers RT and LT are:
   a. Right and left
   b. Sometimes used with modifier 50
   c. Never used with multiple procedures
   d. All of the above

2   HCPCS modifiers are only used with Medicare and Medicaid claims.
   a. True
   b. False

3   Modifier CC indicates:
   a. An ABN is on file
   b. Acute treatment
   c. The code submitted had to be changed
   d. A subsequent claim

4   Modifier RC
   a. Can be used with any procedure code
   b. Is used to indicate a right coronary artery
   c. Can only be used by a locum tenens physician
   d. None of the above

5   A licensed social worker performed an initial psychiatric diagnostic inter-view on a 15-year-old female who was having problems coping with peer pressure at school. What procedure code(s) would be reported for this service?
   a. 90806 AJ
   b. 90801 AJ
   c. 90806 AH
   d. 90801 AM

6   Modifier U3 can be submitted to a third-party payer.
   a. True
   b. False

7   A 30-year-old man with complex congenital heart disease that had been surgically repaired in childhood presented with progressive shortness of breath. Chest X ray showed cardiomegaly. Cardiac magnetic resonance imaging was indicated to assess the morphology of cardiac chambers and great vessels. The imaging protocol was prepared and the procedure was monitored by the physician, who requested additional sequences on the basis of initial observations. What modifier is used to identify the facility portion of the service?
   a. 75552 26
   b. 75552 LD

    c. 75552 TC

    d. None of the above

8 Some reasons that the HCPCS coding system was developed were to:

    a. Report services, procedures, and supplies to meet the operational needs of Medicare and Medicaid

    b. Provide a coding system for the Outpatient Prospective System

    c. Provide a method to report hospital services

    d. All of the above

9 Providers are required to report HCPCS modifiers for ambulance services by using two modifiers, one to report the type of ambulance service provided, and the other for the origin and destination.

    a. True

    b. False

10 If the supplier is billing for an item or service that is noncovered, which modifier should be used?

    a. GA

    b. QW

    c. GY

    d. TN

11 Which modifier is used to report when a CRNA provides anesthesia service under the medical direction of a physician?

    a. QX

    b. QS

    c. QY

    d. QZ

12 A 68-year-old patient was transported by ambulance to a hospital facility in an urban area. The patient had suffered an acute myocardial infarction. Which origin and destination modifier would be reported?

    a. R

    b. E

    c. H

    d. X

13 A physician performed an enucleation of patient's right eye with placement of an implant. The muscles were attached to the implant during the same operative session. During the same operative session, the physician performed a surgical repair of the conjunctiva with conjunctival graft. Select the procedure code(s) for this patient encounter.

    a. 65103 RT, 68320 51 RT

    b. 65105 LT

    c. 68320 LT

    d. 65105 RT, 68320 51 RT

14   A physician performed a urinalysis in the office, automated with microscopy. How should these services be reported?
   a. 81000 QP
   b. 81001 QW
   c. 81002 QP
   d. 81003 LR

15   What HCPCS modifier is used to report a screening mammogram and a diagnostic mammogram performed on the same day?
   a. GH
   b. TC
   c. GG
   d. A HCPCS modifier is not reported under this circumstance

CHAPTER 9

Ambulatory Surgery Center and Hospital Outpatient Modifiers

When the Medicare statute was originally enacted, Medicare payment for hospital outpatient services was based on hospital-specific costs. In an effort to ensure that Medicare and its beneficiaries pay appropriately for services and to encourage more efficient delivery of care, Congress mandated replacement of the cost-based payment methodology with a prospective payment system (PPS).

Section 4523 of the Balanced Budget Act of 1997 provides authority for the Centers for Medicare and Medicaid Services (CMS) to implement PPS under Medicare for hospital outpatient services, certain Part B services furnished to hospital inpatients who have no Part A coverage, and partial hospitalization services. (Partial hospitalization is an intensive outpatient program of psychiatric services provided to patients in place of inpatient psychiatric care. A partial hospitalization program may be provided by a hospital to its outpatients or by a Medicare-certified community mental health center).

The primary objective of the Hospital Outpatient Prospective Payment System (OPPS) is to simplify the payment system, encourage efficient delivery of care, and encourage hospital efficiency in providing outpatient services, while ensuring adequate compensation, and reducing the Medicare beneficiary share of outpatient hospital payment(s). Section 4523 of the Balanced Budget Act also changed the way beneficiary coinsurance is determined for the services included under the PPS. The Balanced Budget Refinement Act of 1999 provides that no coinsurance amount can be greater than the hospital inpatient deductible in a given year.

Ambulatory Payment Classifications

CMS's Final Rule for the new payment system was published in the Federal Register on April 7, 2000 (65 FR 18434). All services paid under the PPS are classified into groups called "ambulatory payment classifications" (APCs), which contain all outpatient services included in the payment schedule. The services within each group are clinically similar and require comparable resources. APCs group together services, supplies, drugs, and devices used in a particular procedure. A payment rate is established for each APC. Depending on the services provided, hospitals may be paid for more than one APC for an encounter. Each year, the Secretary of the Department of Health and Human Services (HHS) must review and adjust as necessary the APC groupings, relative payment weights, and adjustments to ensure that they are consistent with current clinical practice.

APC Development and Structure

To better correlate the use of Current Procedural Terminology (CPT®) and Health Care Current Procedure Coding System (HCPCS) level II modifiers for Medicare reporting under OPPS, it is helpful to understand how a particular CPT or HCPCS code appears in a given APC. The initial design and development of OPPS began in the early 1990s with the development of ambulatory patient groups (APGs). In 1994, Iowa Medicaid became the first major payer to implement an APG-based OPPS. In September 1998, the CMS published the proposed regulations for the Medicare OPPS.

In the proposed regulations, the basis of payment was APCs, which are a modification of APGs resulting from the evaluation of newer and more comprehensive outpatient data. The proposed regulation generated approximately 10,500 comments, the majority of which were on issues relating to the APCs.

In November 1999, the Balanced Budget Refinement Act of 1999 made major changes to the proposed OPPS. With respect to APCs, the act limited the variation in resource use among procedures or services within an APC such that the highest-cost procedure or service within an APC could not be more than twice the cost of the lowest-cost procedure or service within the same APC. The one exception to this "2-times" rule was for low-volume procedures or services.

As a result of the comments and the 2-times rule, the APCs in the proposed regulation were modified to have fewer codes and a narrower range of costs. In particular, because of the 2-times rule, some otherwise clinically homogeneous APCs were split into smaller groups.

In the evolution from APGs to proposed APCs to final APCs, several basic concepts have been consistent:

- **Significant procedure, therapy, or service:** Procedures, therapies, or services that are normally scheduled, constitute the reason for the visit, and dominate the time and resources expended during the visit (eg, skin excision)
- **Medical visit:** Diagnostic, therapeutic, or consultative services provided to a patient by a health care professional that do not include a significant procedure, therapy, or service (eg, emergency department visit for chest pain)
- **Ancillary tests and procedures:** Tests and procedures ordered to assist in patient diagnosis and treatment but not dominating the time and resources expended during the visit (eg, chest X ray)
- **Incidental services:** Services that are an integral part of or incidental to a medical visit or significant procedure, therapy, or service (eg, range of motion measurement)
- **Packaging:** The inclusion of certain costs into the payment amount for an APC (eg, room charges)
- **Multiple significant procedure discounting:** The reduction of the standard payment amount for an APC to recognize that the marginal cost of providing a second procedure to a patient during a single visit is less than the cost of providing the procedure by itself.

CPT/HCPCS Level II Modifiers Approved for Use in the Ambulatory Surgery Center

The Medicare OPPS represents the most significant change in the method of hospital payment since the inception of the inpatient PPS. Appropriate payment is primarily determined by the accuracy and completeness of the CPT and HCPCS codes and modifiers on the claim. The adjudication process for an outpatient claim includes extensive edits and payment rules, which can result in loss of revenue and cash flow delays should a claim not be appropriately coded.

To facilitate the use of the OPPS, modifier usage has had reporting relevance since the implementation of the new CMS payment methodology for procedures performed in freestanding ambulatory surgery centers (ASC), hospital outpatient departments, and hospital-based ASCs. Before October 1, 1997, CPT modifiers were not used for hospital outpatient reporting to the Medicare program. On the basis of approval by the National Uniform Billing Committee, CMS instructed its Medicare fiscal intermediaries to accept those approved level 1 (CPT) and level II (HCPCS) modifiers applicable to outpatient reporting. CMS required Medicare fiscal intermediaries to accept certain CPT modifiers beginning April 1, 1998, and providers were required to use them for Medicare reporting purposes by July 1, 1998.

The OPPS was first implemented for services furnished on or after August 1, 2000. Additional information about the Outpatient Prospective Payment System may be found on the CMS Web site at www.cms.hhs.gov/hospitals.

Purpose of Modifiers

A modifier provides the means by which the reporting facility can indicate that the service or procedure has been altered by some specific circumstance(s) while not changing the definition of the code. The judicious application of modifiers obviates the necessity for separate procedure listings that may describe the modifying circumstance. Modifiers may be used in the ASC to indicate that:

- A service or procedure has been increased or reduced
- Only part of the intended service or procedure could be performed
- An evaluation and management (E/M) service was performed on the same date as a procedure
- A patient received multiple E/M services performed by the same or different physician(s) in multiple hospital outpatient settings
- An adjunctive service was performed
- A bilateral procedure was performed
- A service or procedure was provided more than once
- A service or procedure was planned prospectively at the time of the original procedure
- Unusual events occurred (ie, procedure terminated because of alteration in patient's status).

Occasionally semantic differences have led to difficulties in the use of certain CPT code sets and modifiers for hospital outpatient reporting. The language in modifiers 58, 78, and 79 might be confusing since hospital outpatient reporting represents a 24-hour period or a range of dates. To alleviate the confusion, the reference to the "postoperative period" does not alter the use of these modifiers, as the individual circumstance depicted by each modifier continues to have reimbursement or tracking relevance to the carrier. The use of modifiers enables the insurance carriers to appropriately pay for the procedure and any associated postoperative services performed within or subsequent to the global period (eg, 0 days, 10 days, 90 days). In addition, modifier usage allows the carrier to electronically differentiate instances where duplicate billing or duplicate services may have been reported.

Table 9-1 is a listing of CPT modifiers approved for use in the hospital outpatient department. Table A-3 in Appendix A lists the complete code descriptors for CPT (HCPCS Level 1) modifiers that are approved for ambulatory surgery centers (ASC).

TABLE 9-1	CPT (HCPCS Level I) Modifiers Approved for Ambulatory Surgery Centers
CPT Modifier	**Description**
25	Significant, Separately Identifiable Evaluation and Management Service by the Same Physician on the Same Day of the Procedure or Other Service
27	Multiple Outpatient Hospital E/M Encounters on the Same Date
50	Bilateral Procedures
52	Reduced Services
58	Staged or Related Procedure or Service by the Same Physician During the Postoperative Period
59	Distinct Procedural Service
73	Discontinued Outpatient Hospital/Ambulatory Surgery Center (ASC) Procedure Prior to the Administration of Anesthesia
74	Discontinued Outpatient Hospital Ambulatory Surgery After Administration of Anesthesia
76	Repeat Procedure by Same Physician
77	Repeat Procedure by Another Physician
78	Return to the Operating Room for a Related Procedure During the Postoperative Period
79	Unrelated Procedure or Service by the Same Physician During the Postoperative Period
91	Repeat Clinical Diagnostic Laboratory Test

National (HCPCS Level II) Modifiers

The following are some key modifiers used in the hospital outpatient department or ASC. Appendix B lists all the national (HCPCS Level II) modifiers.

CA	Procedure payable only in the inpatient setting when performed emergently on an outpatient who expires prior to admission
E1-E4	*Modifiers identify anatomical sites on the eyelids*
FA-F9	*Modifiers identify different fingers on each hand*

GA   Waiver of liability statement on file

GG   Performance and payment of a screening mammogram and diagnostic mammogram on the same patient, same day

Modifier GG is appended to the diagnostic code, and Medicare will separately reimburse both services

GH   Diagnostic mammogram converted from screening mammogram on same day

GM   Multiple patients on one ambulance trip

GN   Services delivered under an outpatient speech language pathology plan of care

GO   Services delivered under an outpatient occupational therapy plan of care

GP   Services delivered under an outpatient physical therapy plan of care

LC   Left circumflex coronary artery

Hospitals use with codes 92980-92982, 92995, 92996.

LD   Left anterior descending coronary artery

Hospitals use with codes 92980-92982, 92995, 92996.

LT   Left side (used to identify procedures performed on the left side of the body)

QA   FDA investigational device exemption

QL   Patient pronounced dead after ambulance called

QM   Ambulance service provided under arrangement by a provider of services

QN   Ambulance service furnished directly by a provider of services

QP   Documentation is on file showing that the laboratory test(s) was ordered individually or ordered as a CPT-recognized panel other than automated profile codes 80002-80019, G0058, G0059, and G0060

QV   Item or service provided as routine care in a Medicare qualifying clinical trial

RC   Right coronary artery

Hospitals use with codes 92980-92982, 92995, 92996.

RT   Right side (used to identify procedures performed on the right side of the body)

TA-T9   *Modifiers identify different toes on each foot*

TK	Extra patient or passenger, nonambulance
TP	Medical transport, unloaded vehicle
TQ	Basic life support transport by a volunteer ambulance provider

Miscellaneous Modifiers

The **CA modifier** is used for those services billed on bill type 13x for a procedure that is on the inpatient list and assigned the payment status indicator (SI) "C." Conditions to be met for hospital payment for a claim reporting a service billed with modifier CA include a patient with an emergent, life-threatening condition on whom a procedure on the inpatient list is performed on an emergency basis to resuscitate or stabilize the patient.

The **GA modifier** must be used when practitioners want to indicate that they expect Medicare will deny a service as not reasonable and necessary, and they do have on file an Advanced Beneficiary Notice (ABN) signed by the beneficiary.

The **GY modifier** must be used when practitioners want to indicate that the item or service is statutorily noncovered (as defined in the Program Integrity Manual [PIM] Chapter 1, S2.3.3.B), or is not a Medicare benefit (as defined in the PIM Chapter 1, S2.3.3.a).

The **GZ modifier** is used for an item or service expected to be denied as not reasonable and necessary. The GZ modifier must be used when practitioners want to indicate that they expect Medicare will deny an item or service as not reasonable and necessary, and they have not had an ABN signed by the beneficiary.

The GY and GZ modifiers should be used with the specific, appropriate HCPCS code when one is available. In cases where there is no specific procedure code to describe services, a "not otherwise classified code" (NOC) must be used with either the GY or GZ modifier.

For more information on the GA, GY, and GZ modifiers, refer to Chapter 8.

CMS Policy for General Use of Modifiers

The October 5, 2000, Program Memorandum (transmittal No. A-00-73) provided clarification of modifier usage in the reporting of outpatient hospital services. The memorandum stated that the use of modifiers is an integral part of the OPPS, and the following guidelines have been provided for modifier use:

1   A modifier should not be used if the narrative definition of a code indicates multiple occurrences.

   20553   Injection(s); single or multiple trigger point(s), three or more muscle(s)

2   A modifier should not be used if the narrative definition of a code indicates that the procedure applies to different body parts.

   11305   Shaving of epidermal or dermal lesion, single lesion, scalp, neck, hands, feet, genitalia; lesion diameter 0.5 cm or less

When the use of a modifier is considered, it may be applicable if adding the modifier will add more information regarding the anatomic site of the procedure. If the modifier will help eliminate the appearance of duplicate billing, it may be appropriate to append a modifier to the CPT code.

When to Use HCPCS Level II Modifiers Approved for Outpatient Hospital Reporting

The HCPCS level II (national) modifiers are generally required to add specificity to the reporting of procedures performed on eyelids, fingers, toes, and arteries.

Accurate, comprehensive code assignment has become even more important with the implementation of the OPPS. It is important that all outpatient care areas (ambulatory surgery, endoscopy suites, emergency department, urgent care center, hospital-based clinics, and ancillary services) supply quality information for coding, which has been a challenge for hospitals.

After determining the appropriateness of International Classification of Diseases, Ninth Revision, Clinical Modification diagnosis and procedure code assignments, hospital coders may forget to assign or incorrectly assign unlisted procedure codes. Many questions also arise for coders regarding the assignment of modifiers when faced with the need to code "bilateral procedures" or "separate procedures."

The facility should apply the CMS-endorsed coding policy/instruction when outpatient services are billed, and these should be applied for all payers, unless other specific directives have been received.

The key to any quality monitoring program for coding is complete and timely documentation. Keeping apprised of all the changes that have occurred (and continue to occur) with the OPPS has also proven to be a challenge to outpatient coding staff. Coders need to make time to read the transmittals, because this is the method by which CMS releases information to providers on how to report codes for services provided in the outpatient setting. CMS program memoranda and transmittals may be obtained by accessing the CMS Web site at www.cms.gov.

HCPCS level II modifiers must be used to identify the therapist performing speech language therapy, occupational therapy, and physical therapy.

- **GN** Service delivered personally by a speech language pathologist or under an outpatient speech-language pathology plan of care
- **GO** Service delivered personally by an occupational therapist or under an outpatient occupational therapy plan of care
- **GP** Service delivered personally by a physical therapist or under an outpatient physical therapy plan of care.

The modifiers may be appended to CPT codes. If more than one level II HCPCS modifier applies, indicating two surgical procedures, the CPT code should be repeated on another line with the appropriate level II modifier. For example, if a patient underwent a simple drainage of the finger for an abscess on

CODING TIP

When appending a modifier under OPPS, do not list the code as a one-line item with both modifiers appended. List the procedure code twice with the modifier appended to each line item.

THIRD-PARTY PAYER CODING TIP

Not all third-party payers will accept the use of the APC system of reimbursement for ASC and outpatient hospital facility services. Many major payers are satisfied with the APG method of reimbursement for facility services.

the left-hand thumb and second finger, each would be listed as a two-line item with the appropriate HCPCS level II modifier appended.

CPT Code(s) Billed: 26010 FA, 26010 F1

26010   Drainage of finger abscess, simple

Guidelines for UB-92 Reporting With Modifiers

Modifiers are reported on the hard-copy UB-92 (CMS-1450) in FL 44 next to the HCPCS code. There is a space for two modifiers on the hard-copy form (four of the nine positions). On the UB-92 flat file, providers use record type 61, field numbers 6 and 7. There is a space for two modifiers, one in field 6 and one in field 7.

The dash often seen preceding a modifier should *never* be reported on the claim form. When it is appropriate to use a modifier, the most specific modifier should be listed first. For example, LT, RT, and 59 should never be used before modifiers E1 to E4, FA to F9, LC, RC, and TA to T9. For example, a separately distinct procedure performed on the left thumb would be listed as 26010 59 FA.

As a part of the Health Insurance Portability and Accountability Act, the inclusion of a hyphen, when referring to a modifier, is extraneous to the submission of health care data (for both UB-92 and HCFA-1500 reporting). Reference to the modifier appears with the number (ie, 59 or '59'). The hyphen was removed completely commencing with *CPT® 2005*.

The HCPCS level II modifiers apply whether Medicare is the primary or secondary insurance payer.

Modifier 25: Significant, Separately Identifiable Evaluation and Management Service by the Same Physician on the Same Day of the Procedure or Other Service

Definition

The physician may need to indicate that on the day a procedure or service identified by a CPT code was performed, the patient's condition required a significant, separately identifiable E/M service above and beyond the other service provided or beyond the usual preoperative and postoperative care associated with the procedure that was performed. The E/M service may be prompted by the symptom or condition for which the procedure and/or service was provided. As such, different diagnoses are not required for reporting of the E/M services on the same date. This circumstance may be reported by adding the modifier 25 to the appropriate level of E/M service. **Note:** This modifier is not used to report an E/M service that resulted in a decision to perform surgery. See modifier 57.

The OPPS distinguishes three levels of service for payment purposes which are referred to as "low-level," "mid-level," and "high-level" emergency or clinic visits. Again, for 2003 OPPS reporting purposes, low-level clinic and emergency visits include CPT codes for level one and two services (for example, CPT codes 92012, 99201, 99202, 99211, 99212, 99241, 99242, 99281, 99282, 99431, and HCPCS codes G0101, G0245, and G0246); mid-level visits include level three services (for example, CPT codes 92002, 99203, 99213, 99243, and 99283), and high-level visits include level four and five services (for example, CPT codes 92004, 92014, 99204, 99205, 99214, 99215, 99244, 99245, 99275, 99284, 99285, and HCPCS code G0175). There is a single APC for critical care services (99291), as hospitals are required to use CPT code 99291 to report outpatient encounters in which critical care services are furnished. The hospital is required to use CPT code 99291 in place of, but not in addition to, a code for a medical visit or for an emergency department service.

To address the need for facilities to comply with the requirements of the Health Insurance Portability and Accountability Act (HIPAA) and audit and compliance program issues, CMS has proposed development of new Level II HCPCS codes for facility visits in the emergency department and clinic setting to ensure accurate payment. CMS proposes to implement new evaluation and management codes only when it is also ready to implement guidelines for their use, after allowing ample opportunity for public comment, systems change, and provider education. CMS will continue to work with hospitals to develop documentation guidelines for the use of the new facility emergency and clinic visit Level II HCPCS codes. CMS plans to make any proposed guidelines available to the public for comment on the OPPS Web site as soon as they are complete. CMS anticipates providing at least 6 to 12 months notice prior to implementation of the new evaluation and management codes and guidelines. CMS will continue working to develop and test the new codes even though it has not yet made plans for their implementation. CMS will notify the public through listserv when these proposed guidelines become available. To subscribe to this listserv, please go to the following Web site: www.cms.hhs.gov/medlearn/listserv.asp and follow the directions to the OPPS listserv. The OPPS is updated and further clarified each year in the Federal Register, which also is available on the CMS Web site.

AMA Guidelines

To append modifier 25 appropriately to an E/M code, the service provided must meet the definition of "significant, separately identifiable E/M service" as defined by the CPT code set.

Modifier 25 should be appended only to the following E/M service(s) as defined by the AMA in the CPT codebook:

- E/M codes 92002–92014
- E/M codes 99201–99499
- E/M codes 99281–99285

CMS Guidelines

Modifier 25 was approved for hospital outpatient use on June 5, 2000. Although CMS transmittal No. A-00-40 states that Medicare requires that modifier 25 always be appended to the emergency department E/M codes when provided, the outpatient code editor only requires the use of modifier 25 on an E/M code when it is reported with a procedure code that has a status indicator of S or T. Nevertheless, such an edit does not preclude the reporting of modifier 25 on E/M services that are reported with procedure codes that have a status indicator of S or T. (See CMS transmittal No. A-01-90.) Table 9-2 provides more information on status indicators.

Status Indicators

Payment for hospital services are made using a status indicator methodology. The status indicator determines under what payment system the services are paid. A payment status indicator is assigned to every HCPCS code to identify how the service or procedure described by the code would be paid under the OPPS. Services paid by other methodology include:

- Pulmonary rehabilitation clinical trial
- DME and prosthetics
- Physical, occupational, and speech therapy
- Ambulance
- EPO and ESRD patients
- Physician services for ESRD patients
- Clinical diagnostic laboratory services
- Screening mammography
- Physician professional services

Historically, CMS has used status indicator E to identify certain codes that are recognized by Medicare but that are not payable under the OPPS when they are submitted on an outpatient hospital Part B bill type (12x, 13x, or 14x). Beginning with implementation of the 2004 final rule, CMS has assigned status indicator B to codes that are not payable under OPPS when submitted on an outpatient hospital Part B bill type (12x, 13x, and 14x), but that may be payable by intermediaries to other provider types when submitted on an appropriate bill type, such as bill type 75x submitted by a CORF. In some cases, another code may be submitted by hospitals on an outpatient hospital Part B bill type to receive payment for a service or code that is assigned status indicator B.

Not every service delivered by a hospital outpatient department is paid under OPPS. Every HCPCS code is assigned 1 of the 19 APC status indicators (see Table 9-2). HCPCS codes with status indicators G, H, K, N, P, Q, S, T, V, and

	TABLE 9-2 **Payment Status Indicators for the Hospital Outpatient Prospective Payment System[1]**

Indicator	Item/Code/Service	OPPS Payment Status
A	Services furnished to a hospital outpatient that are paid under a fee schedule or payment system other than OPPS, for example: • Ambulance Services • Clinical Diagnostic Laboratory Services • Non-Implantable Prosthetic and Orthotic Devices • EPO for ESRD Patients • Physical, Occupational, and Speech Therapy • Routine Dialysis Services for ESRD Patients Provided in a Certified Dialysis Unit of a Hospital • Diagnostic Mammography • Screening Mammography	Not paid under OPPS. Paid by fiscal intermediaries under a fee schedule or payment system other than OPPS.
B	Codes that are not recognized by OPPS when submitted on an outpatient hospital Part B bill type (12x,13x, and 14x)	Not paid under OPPS. • May be paid by intermediaries when submitted on a different bill type, for example, 75x (CORF), but not paid under OPPS. • An alternate code that is recognized by OPPS when submitted on an outpatient hospital Part B bill type (12x, 13x, and 14x) may be available.
C	Inpatient Procedures	Not paid under OPPS. Admit patient. Bill as inpatient.
D	Discontinued Codes	Not paid under OPPS.
E	Items, Codes, and Services: • That are not covered by Medicare based on statutory exclusion. • That are not covered by Medicare for reasons other than statutory exclusion.	Not paid under OPPS.

---

1. Source: Payment Status Indicators for the Hospital Outpatient Prospective Payment System, available at www.cms.hhs.gov/providers/hopps/2006p/1501p.asp.

Indicator	Item/Code/Service	OPPS Payment Status
	• That are not recognized by Medicare but for which an alternate code for the same item or service may be available. • For which separate payment is not provided by Medicare.	
F	Corneal Tissue Acquisition; Certain CRNA Services and Hepatitis B Vaccines	Not paid under OPPS. Paid at reasonable cost.
G	Pass-Through Drugs and Biologicals	Paid under OPPS; Separate APC payment includes pass-through amount.
H	(1) Pass-Through Device Categories (2) Brachytherapy Sources (3) Radiopharmaceutical Agents	Paid under OPPS; (1) Separate cost-based pass-through payment. (2) Separate cost-based non-pass-through payment. (3) Separate cost-based non-pass-through payment.
K	Non-Pass-Through Drugs, Biologicals, and Radiopharmaceuticals Agents	Paid under OPPS; Separate APC payment.
L	Influenza Vaccine; Pneumococcal Pneumonia Vaccine	Not paid under OPPS. Paid at reasonable cost; Not subject to deductible or coinsurance.
M	Items and Services Not Billable to the Fiscal Intermediary	Not paid under OPPS.
N	Items and Services Packaged into APC Rates	Paid under OPPS; Payment is packaged into payment for other services, including outliers. Therefore, there is no separate APC payment.
P	Partial Hospitalization	Paid under OPPS; Per diem APC payment.
Q	Packaged Services Subject to Separate Payment Under the OPPS Payment Criteria	Paid under OPPS; (1) Separate APC payment based on OPPS payment criteria. (2) If criteria are not met, payment is packaged into payment for other services, including outliers. Therefore, there is no separate APC payment.

Indicator	Item/Code/Service	OPPS Payment Status
S	Significant Service, Separately Payable	Paid under OPPS; Separate APC payment.
T	Significant Procedure, Multiple Reduction Applies	Paid under OPPS; Separate APC payment.
V	Clinic or Emergency Department Visit	Paid under OPPS; Separate APC payment.
Y	Non-Implantable Durable Medical Equipment	Not paid under OPPS. All institutional providers other than home health agencies bill to DMERC.
X	Ancillary Services	Paid under OPPS; Separate APC payment.

X are assigned to an APC and are paid under OPPS. The subset of drugs, biologicals, and devices that are eligible for pass-through payments under OPPS are assigned to status indicators G and H.

For 2006, CMS created two new status indicators: M to indicate services that are only billable to carriers and not to fiscal intermediaries, and that are not payable under the OPPS; and Q to indicate packaged services subject to separate payment under OPPS payment criteria.

The remaining drugs, biologicals, and devices are assigned a status indicator of N along with other incidental services, which means their cost is packaged into an APC with a status indicator of S, T, or V. Packaged incidental services include the use of operating and recovery rooms, anesthesia, medical/surgical supplies, observation, and various services such as venipuncture.

Although incidental services are packaged and not paid separately, a hospital still is compensated for these services because the cost of the incidental services is incorporated into the payment amount of the type S, T, or V service with which the incidental service is associated. Services with status indicators of A and F are not paid under OPPS, but rather are paid by other methods such as a fee schedule. Status indicator C is assigned to inpatient procedures that are not payable under the OPPS. Services with a status indicator of D, L, and Y are either deleted codes, discontinued services, or items or services not covered by CMS statutes. Services with a status indicator E are not covered by Medicare for reasons other than statutory exclusion or for which an alternate code for the same item or service may be available.

These status indicators are important in determining payment for services under the OPPS because they determine whether a CPT or HCPCS code is payable under OPPS or another payment system such as PPS or fee schedule.

Only one status indicator is assigned to an APC and to each CPT or HCPCS code, and each code has the same status indicator as the APC to which it is assigned.

Confusion sometimes occurs with physician billing for multiple E/M services on the same day. The examples that follow will help to clarify this situation.

Example 1

An established patient saw his family physician in the morning in follow-up for hypertension and diabetes mellitus. The patient's blood pressure was mildly elevated. After the physician performed an E/M visit, which included a detailed history and examination, he adjusted the patient's medication for hypertension. Later in the day, the patient's blood pressure became elevated to an alarming level, and he visited the family physician again.

CPT Code(s) Billed: *99214—Office or other outpatient visit for the evaluation and management of an established patient, which requires at least two of these three key components: a detailed history; a detailed examination; medical decision making of moderate complexity*

Rationale for Not Using Modifier 25
The modifiers approved for the ASC or a hospitalized outpatient department were not intended to be used by the physician in the office, where multiple visits are occasionally necessary. The patient is visiting the physician for the same or a similar problem, but the E/M services should be included in one E/M code on the same day.

Example 2

After sustaining a facial laceration in a car accident, a man went to the emergency department for treatment. The emergency department physician took a detailed history and examination with moderate decision making. After the evaluation, the physician repaired one wound, an intermediate repair on the forehead measuring 1.5 cm. The patient was released from the emergency department in good condition.

CPT Code(s) Billed: *99284 25—Emergency department visit for the evaluation and management of a patient, which requires these three key components: a detailed history; a detailed examination; and medical decision making of moderate complexity*

12051—Layer closure of wounds of face, ears, eyelids, nose, lips and/or mucous membranes; 2.5 cm or less

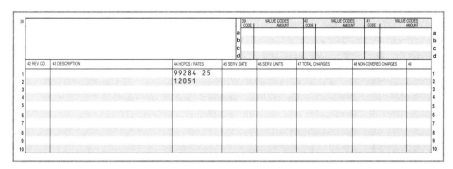

The CMS Program Memorandum TR A-02-082 (August 21, 2002) for the October 2003 Outpatient Code Editor Specifications updates the "Rules for Medical Procedures and Visits on the Same Day." According to CMS,

> Under some circumstances, medical visits on the same date as a procedure will result in additional payments. A modifier 25 with the Evaluation and Management (E/M) (service indicator V) code is used to indicate that the medical visit was unrelated to any procedure performed with a type T or S status indicator.

E/M codes on the same day and same claim as a procedure or type T or S will have the medical APC assigned to all lines with E/M codes. However, if any E/M code occurs on a claim with a type T or S procedure and does not have a modifier 25, it will incur a line item rejection for the procedure.

Example 3

A tourist was mugged by two men in a subway and suffered a laceration on the scalp. The patient went to the emergency room of a local hospital. The ER physician performed and documented a mid-level E/M service and determined that the scalp wound was in need of repair. The laceration measured 1.6 cm. A complex repair was performed in the ER.

CPT Code(s) Billed: 99283 25—Emergency department mid-level visit
13120 Repair, complex, scalp, arms, and/or legs;
1.1 cm to 2.5 cm

Review of Modifier 25

1　Modifier 25 is appended only to the E/M service.

2　The modifier that will affect reimbursement is listed first.

3　Modifier 25 is always appended to the emergency department E/M service when a separately identifiable, significant service and/or procedure is performed during the patient encounter.

4　Use of modifier 25 does not require different or separate diagnosis codes based on CPT guidelines.

5　Modifier 25 should be used cautiously, as it is scrutinized by CMS and many third-party payers.

Modifier 27: Multiple Outpatient Hospital E/M Encounters on the Same Date

Definition

For hospital outpatient reporting purposes, utilization of hospital resources related to separate and distinct E/M encounters performed in multiple outpatient hospital settings on the same date may be reported by adding the modifier 27 to each appropriate level outpatient and/or emergency department E/M code(s). This modifier provides a means of reporting circumstances involving evaluation and management services provided by physician(s) in more than one (multiple) outpatient hospital setting(s) (eg, hospital emergency department, clinic).

NOTE: This modifier is not to be used for physician reporting of multiple E/M services performed by the same physician on the same date. For physician reporting of all outpatient evaluation and management services provided by the same physician on the same date and performed in multiple outpatient setting(s) (eg, hospital emergency department, clinic), see Evaluation and Management, Emergency Department, or Preventive Medicine Service codes.

AMA Guidelines

Modifier 27 is intended to facilitate hospital outpatient reporting to delineate a circumstance wherein a patient receives multiple E/M services performed by different physician(s) in multiple hospital outpatient settings (eg, hospital emergency department, clinic) on the same date.

Modifier 27 should be appended only to the following E/M codes:

- 92002–92014
- 99201–99499
- HCPCS level II G0175

CMS Guidelines

CMS indicates that October 1, 2001, is the implementation date for the use of modifier 27, intended to facilitate hospital outpatient reporting to delineate a circumstance wherein a patient receives multiple E/M encounters performed by the same or different physician(s) in multiple hospital outpatient settings. Hospitals may append modifier 27 to the second and subsequent E/M code when more than one E/M service is provided to indicate that the E/M service is a "separate and distinct E/M encounter" from the service previously provided that same day in the same or different hospital outpatient setting. When modifier 27 is reported, the condition code G0 should be reported. G0 specifies that multiple medical visits occurred on the same day with the same revenue center and these visits were distinct and independent visits (eg, two visits in the emergency department). The patient's medical record documentation should support the use of modifier 27.

The difference between the CPT modifier definition and the CMS interpretation is that CMS allows the use of modifier 27 when E/M services are reported for the same physician, whereas CPT guidelines state that the service(s) must be reported by different physicians, although it may be in the same department.

Hospitals may append modifier 27 to the second and subsequent E/M code(s) when reporting more than one E/M service, to indicate that the E/M service is a "separate and distinct E/M encounter" provided that same day in the same or different hospital outpatient setting. In addition to the E/M code with modifier 27, the condition code GO is assigned when the service provided is the same revenue center. The medical APC is also assigned to each line item with the E/M code.

CMS CODING TIP

Make sure the patient's medical record documentation supports the use of modifier 27.

Example 1

A 70-year-old man presented in the emergency department after a fall from his porch, which was slippery with ice. He complained of pain in the right hip and foot. The emergency department physician performed a comprehensive history and examination and ordered X rays. According to the radiology report, there were no broken bones or substantial injuries other than a sprained right foot. The patient's foot was wrapped in an elastic bandage and the patient was given instructions for care of the sprain. Medication was prescribed for pain, and the patient was instructed to see his family physician the next week. Later in the day, the patient arrived back in the emergency department and a different physician was on duty. The patient had been fixing lunch and had burned his right arm on the gas stove. The emergency department physician performed an expanded problem-focused history and examination, determined that the burn was minor and of the first degree, dressed the area, and gave the patient instructions on care of the wound. During the encounter, the physician noted that the patient's blood pressure was abnormally high, and on finding out that the patient was hypertensive, he adjusted the patient's medication. The patient was released and sent home in good condition.

CPT Code(s) Billed: 99284—Emergency department visit for the evaluation and management of a patient, which requires these three key components: a detailed history; a detailed examination; and medical decision making of moderate complexity

99283 27 G0—Emergency department visit for the evaluation and management of a patient, which requires these three key components: an expanded problem-focused history; an expanded problem-focused examination; and medical decision making of moderate complexity

38					39 CODE	VALUE CODES AMOUNT	40 CODE	VALUE CODES AMOUNT	41 CODE	VALUE CODES AMOUNT		
				a								a
				b								b
				c								c
				d								d
42 REV. CD.	43 DESCRIPTION		44 HCPCS / RATES	45 SERV. DATE	46 SERV. UNITS	47 TOTAL CHARGES		48 NON-COVERED CHARGES	49			
1			99284									1
2			99283 27									2
3												3
4												4
5												5
6												6
7												7
8												8
9												9
10												10

Example 2

A 67-year-old woman presented in the emergency department after being involved in a minor car accident at 7am while driving to her daughter's home. She complained of a headache from hitting her head against the steering wheel. The emergency department physician performed a comprehensive history and examination and determined that, other than minor bruises on her arms and legs, the patient was not hurt. Medication was prescribed for the headache and the patient was advised to rest for a few days. At 1pm, the patient arrived back in the emergency department complaining of chest pain and shortness of breath. A different emergency department physician decided to admit the patient for observation and ordered an electrocardiogram. Later that evening, after the patient had been observed for 9 hours and no physical problems were found, the patient was released with a diagnosis of anxiety disorder.

CPT Code(s) Billed: *99284—Emergency department visit for the evaluation and management of a patient, which requires these three key components: a detailed history; a detailed examination; and medical decision making of moderate complexity*

99234 27 GO—Observation or inpatient hospital care, for the evaluation and management of a patient including admission and discharge on the same date which requires these three key components: a detailed or comprehensive history; a detailed or comprehensive examination; and medical decision making that is straightforward or of low complexity

Example 3

A patient presented for a clinic visit in a teaching hospital. The level billed for the procedure was 99214. The physician sent the patient to the cardiology clinic for a consultation on the same date of service. The service performed and documented in the cardiology clinic was 99243. Both visits were coded and billed; however, the cardiology service included modifier 27 to indicate a significant, separate service.

CPT Code(s) Billed by Internal Medicine Clinic: 99214—Detailed E/M service

CPT Code(s) Billed by Cardiology Clinic: 99243 27 G0—Detailed Consultation

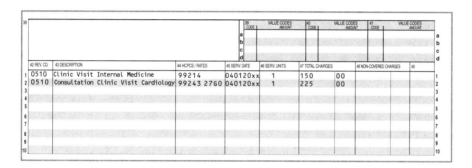

Review of Modifier 27

1   As of January 2001, modifier 27 is not used to report the technical component of a procedure, since modifier 27 is now defined as "multiple outpatient hospital E/M encounters on the same date." The correct modifier to use to report the technical component is TC.

2   It is not appropriate to add clinic or hospital outpatient E/M visits together without the condition code G0 when two physicians are billed for the same date in the same revenue center.

3   When multiple E/M encounters are coded in the same revenue center, both E/M services are coded with modifiers 27 and G0.

Modifier 50: Bilateral Procedure

Definition

Unless otherwise identified in the listings, bilateral procedures that are performed at the same operative session should be identified by adding the modifier 50 to the appropriate five-digit code. Modifier 50 in the ASC has several reporting uses:

- Modifier 50 is used to report bilateral procedures that are performed at the same operative session as a single line item.

- When modifier 50 is used, HCPCS level II modifiers RT and LT are not used.
- A code for an inherently bilateral procedure should not be submitted with modifier 50 appended.
- Modifier 50 applies to any bilateral procedure performed on both sides of the body at the same operative session.
- Modifier 50 is not restricted to surgical codes.

Modifier 50 may not be used in the following instances:
- To report surgical procedures that are identified in the code terminology as "bilateral"
- To report surgical procedures identified in the terminology as "unilateral or bilateral"

CMS Guidelines

When modifier 50 is used, the reimbursement is for two procedures. If the procedure is an approved ASC service, the multiple procedure rules apply. Since the procedures are in the same payment group, the ASC Pricer program calculates the payment at the full rate for one procedure and 50% of the rate for the other procedure.

According to CMS, the bilateral indicators were updated in the January 1, 2001, Medicare Physician Fee Schedule (MPFS) with bilateral indicators 1, 2, and 3, which are used to indicate "conditional, inherent and independent" bilateral use in the outpatient code editor. These bilateral codes were designed exclusively by CMS as a subset of those with indicator "1" on the Medicare Fee Schedule List. The list was updated in the July 2002 release. The CMS Program Memorandum (transmittal No. A-02-082), August 21, 2002, states that bilateral procedures having the following values in the "bilateral" field of the October 2002 Outpatient Code Editor (OCE):

1   Conditional bilateral (procedure considered bilateral if modifier 50 is present)

2   Inherent bilateral (procedure in and of itself is bilateral in definition)

3   Independent bilateral (procedure is considered bilateral when modifier 50 is present, but full payment should be made for each procedure)

The Outpatient Prospective Payment System (OPPS) discounting process utilized an APC payment amount file. The discounting factor for bilateral procedure is the same as the discounting factor for multiple type "T" procedures. Inherent bilateral procedures are treated as nonbilateral procedures because the bilaterality of the procedure is encompassed in the code. For bilateral procedures the type "T" procedure discounting rules take precedence over the discounting specified in the physician's fee schedule.

Example 1

A 35-year-old recreational skier injured both right and left knees, with peripheral longitudinal tears of both medial and lateral menisci, and underwent arthroscopic meniscus repair of both knees by a suture technique.

CPT Code(s) Billed: 29883 50—Arthroscopy, knee, surgical; with meniscus repair (medial AND lateral)

Conditional Bilateral

This represents procedures/services for which it is appropriate to append modifier 50, for example, 67916 Repair of ectropion; excision tarsal wedge (with the modifier 50 appended).

Inherent Bilateral

It is not appropriate to append modifier 50 to procedures/services that are designated inherent bilateral, which means that the code descriptor indicates bilateral in the description. These procedures/services involve physiology or anatomy on both the left and right sides of the body. The CPT code descriptors for these procedures may be worded in one of the following ways:

1 Specifically state the procedure may be performed either "unilaterally or bilaterally"
    Example: 31231—Nasal endoscopy, diagnostic, unilateral or bilateral
    Example: 52290—Cystourethroscopy; with ureteral meatotomy, unilateral or bilateral

2 Specify that the procedure is bilateral
    Example: 75803—Lymphangiography, extremity only, bilateral, radiological supervision and interpretation
    Example: 55041—Excision of hydrocele; bilateral

3 Reflect multiple anatomy
    Example: 46600—Anoscopy; diagnostic, with or without collection of specimen(s) by brushing or washing (separate procedure)
    Example: 67805—Excision of chalazion; multiple, different lids

Independent Bilateral

CPT codes having an "independent bilateral" designation represent procedures/services that may be performed independently of one another as the anatomic structures exist bilaterally. It is appropriate to append modifier 50 when the identical procedure is performed independent of the other, on both sides of the body.
    Example: 92135—Scanning computerized ophthalmic diagnostic imaging (eg, scanning laser) with interpretation and report, unilateral
    Example: 73100—Radiologic examination, wrist; two views

The OPPS discounting process used an APC payment amount file. The discounting factor for bilateral procedure is the same as the discounting factor for multiple type T procedures. Inherent bilateral procedures are treated in the same way as a nonbilateral procedure because the bilaterality of the procedure is encompassed in the code. For bilateral procedures, the type T procedure discounting rules take precedence over the discounting specified in the physician fee schedule.

HCPCS Level II Modifiers LT and RT

Modifiers LT and RT apply to codes that identify procedures that can be performed on paired organs such as ears, eyes, nostrils, kidneys, lungs, and ovaries. Modifiers LT and RT should be used whenever a procedure is performed on only one side. Hospitals use the appropriate RT and LT modifiers to identify which one of the paired organs was operated on. CMS requires these modifiers whenever appropriate.

Example 2

A patient with a history of fibrocystic breast disease and a family history of breast cancer underwent a percutaneous needle core biopsy in the ASC of a hospital. A mammogram and ultrasound indicated two suspicious masses; one in the right upper quadrant of the left breast and one in the lower quadrant of the right breast. A needle core biopsy was performed bilaterally using CT guidance.

CPT Code(s) Billed: 19102 50, 76360 RT, 76360 LT

19102   Biopsy of breast; percutaneous, needle core, using imaging guidance

76360   Computed tomography guidance for needle placement (eg, biopsy, aspiration, injection, localization device), radiological supervision and interpretation

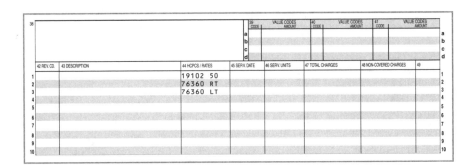

Rationale for Using Modifier 50

Since the procedure was the exact same procedure performed on both breasts, modifier 50 would be appropriate in reporting the patient encounter.

CT guidance was used for imaging and should be reported in addition to the needle core biopsies. The radiology procedures are reported using RT (right side of the body), and LT (left side of the body). Modifier 50 is not universally accepted by insurance carriers for reporting, and it is appropriate to report with HCPCS modifiers versus modifier 50.

Review of Modifier 50

1 Bilateral procedures that are performed at the same operative session are reported with modifier 50.

2 Modifier 50 is not used when the description of the procedure/service code is bilateral in its definition.

3 Modifier 50 is not used if the description of the procedures/service indicates "unilateral or bilateral" in its definition.

4 Modifier 50 is not used for CPT codes having independent designations (services that can be reported independently of one another).

5 Modifier 50 is reported for procedures/services that are performed on both sides of the body at the same operative session.

6 Modifier 50 is used with the procedure/service code with a 1-line item.

7 RT and LT are not used when modifier 50 is applicable.

Modifier 52: Reduced Services

Definition

Under certain circumstances a service or procedure is partially reduced or eliminated at the physician's discretion. Under these circumstances the service provided can be identified by its usual procedure number and the addition of the modifier 52, signifying that the service is reduced. This provides a means of reporting reduced services without disturbing the identification of the basic service. **Note:** For hospital outpatient reporting of a previously scheduled procedure/service that is partially reduced or canceled as a result of extenuating circumstances or those that threaten the well being of the patient prior to or after administration of anesthesia, see modifiers 73 and 74.

AMA Guidelines

cpt Because of the varying nature of procedures described by the CPT codes, the modifier 52 has several uses. The modifier 52 may be used to represent any of the following:

- A service or procedure that is partially reduced or eliminated at the provider's discretion

> **CODING TIP**
>
> Modifier 50 should not be appended when the code descriptor indicates that the service or procedure is bilateral by definition, or includes the HCPCS level II modifiers LT and RT.

- A service that is not performed for the entire time specified in the code descriptor
- A situation in which an inherently bilateral procedure cannot be performed as such

Modifier 52 Use Indicating a "Reduced Service"

Modifier 52 may be used to indicate that a service or procedure is partially reduced or eliminated at the provider's discretion. To code for this, the service provided can be identified by its usual procedure number and the addition of modifier 52, signifying that the service is reduced. As reflected in the following clinical example, this provides a means of reporting reduced services without disturbing the identification of the basic service. The next clinical example reflects the CMS reporting requirement that is a departure from the CPT intent.

Example 1

A patient was to undergo a flexible fiber-optic upper gastrointestinal endoscopy. Although the procedure was attempted, the physician could not complete the entire procedure because of obstruction at the distal esophagus.

CPT Code(s) Billed: *43235 52—Upper gastrointestinal endoscopy including esophagus, stomach, and either the duodenum and/or jejunum as appropriate; diagnostic, with or without collection of specimen(s) by brushing or washing (separate procedure); reduced service*

Rationale for Using Modifier 52

In this instance, for non-Medicare reporting, CPT code 43235 with the modifier 52 appended indicates that the intended procedure was reduced.

CMS Guidelines

CMS does not allow the use of modifier 52 when the endoscopic procedure is incomplete and there is a CPT or HCPCS level II code to describe the actual service performed.

In this instance, CMS requires the reporting of a code describing only the anatomy examined at that endoscopic procedure. Therefore, if a code is available that fully describes the hospital outpatient procedure performed, this code choice supersedes the reporting of a code describing the intended (albeit not performed) procedure.

Example 2

A patient was to undergo a flexible fiber-optic upper gastrointestinal endoscopy. Although the procedure was attempted, the physician could not complete the entire procedure because of obstruction at the distal esophagus.

CPT Code(s) Billed: 43200—Esophagoscopy, rigid or flexible; diagnostic, with or without collection of specimen(s) by brushing or washing (separate procedure)

Rationale for Not Using Modifier 52

In this instance, for Medicare reporting, CPT code 43200 describes only the procedure performed. The previous examples illustrate the importance of recognizing the difference between CPT instructional usage and CMS OPPS policy requirements. Specifically, the CPT introductory notes to the Endoscopy subsection of the Digestive System section instruct users to use a colonoscopy code with the modifier 52 appended.

According to an August 1, 2003, Program Memorandum (TR-AB-03-114) regarding payment and claims processing for incomplete colonoscopies, Medicare covers colorectal cancer screening test/procedures for the early detection of colorectal cancer when coverage conditions are met. Among the screening procedures covered are screening colonoscopies: G0105 Colorectal cancer screening; colonoscopy on individual at high risk; and G0121 Colorectal screening; colonoscopy on individual not meeting criteria for high risk. Coverage of these services is subject to certain frequency limitations.

In some instances, a provider may begin a screening colonoscopy but, because of extenuating circumstances, be unable to complete the procedure. At another time, the provider may attempt and complete the intended screening colonoscopy on the patient. This situation parallels those of diagnostic colonoscopies in which the provider is unable to complete the colonoscopy because of extenuating circumstances and must attempt a complete colonoscopy at a later time. If coverage conditions are met, Medicare pays for both the uncompleted colonoscopy and the completed colonoscopy whether the colonoscopy is screening or diagnostic. Because screening colonoscopies G0105 and G0121 are subject to frequency limitations, the common working file must be able to distinguish between those services that are subject to the frequency limitation and those that are not. It is not appropriate to count the incomplete colonoscopy toward the beneficiary's frequency limit for a screening colonoscopy because that would preclude the beneficiary's being able to obtain a covered completed colonoscopy. The common working file must be changed so that it ignores incomplete screening colonoscopies when it calculates frequency limitations for this benefit.

Policy for Carriers

When a covered colonoscopy is attempted but cannot be completed because of extenuating circumstances (refer to Medicare Carriers' Manual section 15100B), Medicare will pay for the interrupted colonoscopy at a rate consistent with that of a flexible sigmoidoscopy as long as coverage conditions are met for the

---

CMS CODING TIP

Make certain the appropriate CPT or HCPCS code is reported. CMS OPPS policy created two HCPCS level II screening colonoscopy codes, which might be required for CMS reporting: G0104 Colorectal cancer screening; flexible sigmoidoscopy, to be used for flexible screening sigmoidoscopy; and G0105 Colorectal cancer screening; colonoscopy for an individual at risk, to be used for screening colonoscopy.

THIRD-PARTY PAYER CODING TIP

Medicare would expect the provider to maintain adequate information in the patient's medical record in case it is needed by the contractor to document the incomplete procedure.

incomplete procedure. When a covered colonoscopy is next attempted and completed, Medicare will pay for that colonoscopy according to its payment methodology for this procedure as long as coverage conditions are met. This policy is applied to both screening and diagnostic colonoscopies. When submitting a claim for the interrupted colonoscopy, professional providers are to suffix the colonoscopy code with a modifier 53 to indicate that the procedure was interrupted. When submitting a claim for the facility fee associated with this procedure, ASCs are to suffix the colonoscopy code with 73 or 74 as appropriate. Payment for covered screening colonoscopies, including that for the associated ASC facility fee when applicable, will be consistent with payment for diagnostic colonoscopies, whether the procedure is complete or incomplete. The medical record must have sufficient documentation to support the incomplete colonoscopy.

Modifier 52 Use for Decreased Time of Service

Modifier 52 may also be used to indicate when a service is not performed for the entire time specified in the code descriptor. Therefore, another use for modifier 52 includes instances associated with time-based CPT codes.

Example 3

A 72-year-old woman with dysthymic disorder and dependent personality disorder was seen in the office for individual psychotherapy. She also had chronic obstructive pulmonary disease and congestive heart failure. She was taking antidepressant medication and had attempted an overdose 4 months earlier but had been stable since that time. Comorbid medical diagnoses, interaction of medications, and laboratory screening and interpretation were considered. The session lasted 40 minutes.

CPT Code(s) Billed: 90806 52—*Individual psychotherapy, insight oriented, behavior modifying and/or supportive, in an office or outpatient facility, approximately 45 to 50 minutes face-to-face with the patient*

Rationale for Using Modifier 52

In this instance, modifier 52 is used to identify the reduced service performed. Since the code descriptor for 90806 is 45 to 50 minutes and is time based, modifier 52 should be appended indicating the reduced service.

Modifier 52 Use for Inherently Bilateral Procedures

Modifier 52 may also be used to indicate that an inherently bilateral procedure cannot be performed as bilateral. Some CPT codes indicate that associated services described by that code are inherently bilateral. However, sometimes a procedure cannot be performed as described in the CPT book.

Example 4

A 65-year-old man who had previously undergone left femoral angioplasty complained of increasing recurrent claudication. There was a diminished posterior tibial pulse. Ankle-brachial indices were obtained to compare with the immediate post-procedure ankle-brachial indices. The patient had a previous above-the-knee amputation on the right leg.

CPT Code(s) Billed: 93922 52—*Noninvasive physiologic studies of upper or lower extremity arteries, single level, bilateral (eg, ankle/brachial indices, Doppler waveform analysis, volume plethysmography, transcutaneous oxygen tension measurement)*

Rationale for Using Modifier 52

In this example, modifier 52 would be appended to code 93922 to indicate that this test was not performed in its entirety because of the previous amputation.

Review of Modifier 52

1 This modifier is not used to reduce a fee for a patient.

2 Modifier 52 is used to indicate that under certain circumstances a service or procedure is partially reduced or eliminated at the physician's discretion.

3 Modifier 52 is not used for CMS for incomplete endoscopic procedures.

4 Modifier 52 is used when a service is not performed in its entirety (time specified) with time-based codes.

5 Modifier 52 is used when an inherently bilateral procedure cannot be performed as such.

Checkpoint Exercises 1

Fill in the blanks.

1 The modifier that indicates that multiple E/M encounters occurred on the same day at different times is modifier _____.

2 This modifier indicates that a procedure was partially reduced or eliminated at the physician's discretion: _____.

3   This modifier is not to be used to report an E/M service that resulted in the decision to perform surgery: _____.

4   These modifiers identify the left and right sides of the body: _____ and _____.

5   ASC stands for _____.

6   Conditional bilateral means _____
    _____.

7   Section 4523 of the _____ of 1997 provides authority for CMS to implement the PPS under Medicare for hospital outpatient services, certain Part B services furnished to hospital inpatients who have no Part A coverage, and partial hospitalization services furnished by community mental health centers.

Modifier 58: Staged or Related Procedure or Service by the Same Physician During the Postoperative Period

Definition

The physician may need to indicate that the performance of a procedure or service during the postoperative period was: (a) planned prospectively at the time of the original procedure (staged); (b) more extensive than the original procedure; or (c) for therapy following a diagnostic surgical procedure. This circumstance may be reported by adding the modifier 58 to the staged or related procedure. **Note:** This modifier is not used to report the treatment of a problem that requires a return to the operating room. See modifier 78.

AMA Guidelines

At times it is necessary for a surgeon to perform one surgical procedure and then, during the postoperative period associated with the original procedure, perform a "staged" or related procedure. Modifier 58 should be appended for surgeries planned prospectively, at the time of the original procedure, for follow-up surgeries that are more extensive than the original procedure, or for therapy after a diagnostic surgical procedure.

Commonly asked is why and how modifier 58 is used for hospital outpatient reporting. It is recognized that the reference to the "postoperative period" in the language of modifier 58 does not have strict relevance in hospital outpatient reporting. However, the individual circumstance depicted by modifier 58 continues to have reimbursement or tracking relevance to the CMS fiscal intermediary (FI).

Because hospital outpatient reporting represents services performed within a given 24-hour period or a range of dates, the original intent and use of modifier 58 is not altered for hospital outpatient reporting. Modifier 58 delineates the following circumstances for the reported procedure:

- It is related to the original procedure, intended to be performed sometime in the future as a "staged" procedure, and may represent:
  - ~ a procedure performed by the original surgeon or provider
  - ~ a follow-up surgery more extensive than the original procedure
  - ~ a therapy after a diagnostic surgical procedure.
- The performance of the "staged" procedure may occur during the postoperative period (ie, global period) associated with the original surgery.

CMS Guidelines

The use of the modifier 58 enables the CMS FI or other payers/carriers to appropriately pay for the procedure per se and other associated postoperative services performed within or subsequent to its assigned global period (eg, 0 days, 10 days, 90 days). In addition, the modifier usage allows the instance where duplicate billing or duplicate services may have been reported to be differentiated electronically.

Example 1

A 65-year-old man presented with essential tremor that had become quite severe and was disabling. He had had the disease for 8 years and had failed to obtain tremor relief with the use of various oral medications and physical therapy. The physician decided to perform a deep brain stimulation in two separate stages. The physician performed the craniotomy for implantation of a neurostimulator on April 13 and the neurostimulator pulse generator was implanted on April 25. The services were performed in the outpatient surgery department of the hospital.

CPT Code(s) Billed: (April 13) 61863; (April 25) 61885 58

61863   Twist drill, burr hole, craniotomy, or craniectomy for stereotactic implantation of neurostimulator electrode array in subcortical site (eg, thalamus, globus pallidus, subthalamic nucleus, periventricular, periaqueductal gray), without use of intraoperative microelectrode recording; first array

61885   Incision and subcutaneous placement of cranial neurostimulator pulse generator or receiver, direct or inductive coupling; with connection to a single electrode array

Rationale for Using Modifier 58

In the above-described patient, a two-stage operation is planned for deep brain stimulation (ie, the neurostimulator electrode array is placed and connected to an external generator, then, if successful in allaying symptoms, the stimulator generator is subcutaneously placed at a later date). Deep brain stimulation is used to treat movement disorders (eg, rigidity, tremors, balance control). For example, with the electrode array placed in the thalamus, stimulation is used for treatment of essential tremor or tremor resulting from Parkinson disease.

The trial implantation of one stereotactically guided deep brain stimulator electrode array is performed, CPT code 61862 (status indicator T) is reported for the stereotactic implantation of neurostimulator array(s) into the thalamus for treatment of tremor (implantation of electrodes into the globus pallidus or subthalamic nucleus for stimulation to treat/monitor rigidity, dyskinesia, or tremor). Should the trial implantation be successful, at a future date, the subcutaneous placement of the neurostimulator pulse generator would be performed and is reported with CPT code 61885 (status indicator T) with modifier 58 appended. Code 61886 (status indicator T) would be reported with the modifier 58 appended for subcutaneous placement of a cranial neurostimulator pulse generator or receiver when the connection is to two or more electrode arrays.

Example 2

A diabetic patient with advanced circulatory problems had three gangrenous toes removed from the left foot in the hospital surgery center on June 1. On June 15 the patient returned to the ambulatory surgery center for amputation of the left foot.

CPT Code(s) Billed on June 1: 28820, 28820 51, 28820 51

CPT Code(s) Billed on June 15: 28805 58

28820   Amputation, toe; metatarsophalangeal joint
28805   Amputation, foot; transmetatarsal

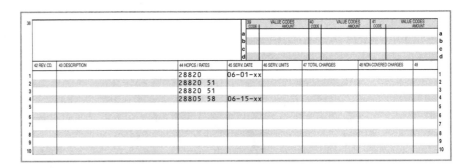

Rationale for Using Modifier 58

Since the amputation is related to the reason for the previous amputation of the toes (diabetic gangrene), modifier 58 is used. The amputation of the foot was not due to a complication of the first surgery, but to the underlying disease.

The intent of modifier 58 precludes its use to report the treatment of a problem that requires a return to the operating room. For that circumstance, modifier 78 is used. Modifier 58 is also not used to report a related or unrelated procedure performed on the same date as the original procedure. For that circumstance, modifier 59 is used.

Example 3

On July 25, a 32-year-old female patient with a breast lump on the left breast was taken to the operating room in a regional hospital for a biopsy. The patient previously underwent a mastectomy of the right breast due to a malignancy. The physician discussed with the patient that if he found another malignancy, the recommendation would be to immediately perform a mastectomy on the left breast. The patient signed the consent for surgery including a possible mastectomy. An open incisional biopsy was performed. The physician sent the mass along with surrounding tissue to pathology for a "stat" report. The pathology report came back positive for cancer, and a complete mastectomy was immediately performed along with reconstruction consisting of a breast prosthesis.

CPT Code(s) Billed: 19100—Biopsy of breast; open, incisional

19180 58—Mastectomy, simple, complete

19340 58—Immediate insertion of breast prosthesis following mastopexy, mastectomy or in reconstruction

Rationale for Using Modifier 58

The biopsy performed was diagnostic in nature, which confirmed the suspected malignancy. Since the outcome of the biopsy determined the second procedure (mastectomy, 19180), modifier 58 should be appended to indicate it was a staged procedure. The third procedure, the reconstruction, also is reported with modifier 58 because it immediately followed the mastectomy. If the pathology had indicated the lump was benign, both the mastectomy and breast prosthesis would not be necessary and the only service reported would be 19100.

CMS Interpretation of Modifier 58 and Breast Procedures[2]

According to CMS,

Because of the unique nature of procedures developed to address breast disease, a section of CPT (19000-19499) is set aside for such services.

> **CMS CODING TIP**
>
> Check with your FI regarding local policy associated with the use of the modifier 58 for staged procedures on the same date.

---

2. Source: NCCI Policy Manual, available at http://www.cms.hhs.gov/physicians/cciedits/nccmanual.asp.

Fine needle aspiration biopsies, core biopsies, open incisional or excisional biopsies, and related procedures performed to procure tissue from a lesion for which an established diagnosis exists are not to be reported separately at the time of a lesion excision unless performed on a different lesion or on the contralateral breast. However, if a diagnosis is not established and the decision to perform the excision or mastectomy is dependent on the results of the biopsy, then the biopsy is separately reported. Modifier 58 may be used appropriately to indicate that the biopsy and the excision or mastectomy are staged or planned procedures.

Modifier 59: Distinct Procedural Service

Definition

Under certain circumstances, the physician may need to indicate that a procedure or service was distinct or independent from other services performed on the same day. Modifier 59 is used to identify procedures/services that are not normally reported together, but are appropriate under the circumstances. This may represent a different session or patient encounter, different procedure or surgery, different site or organ system, separate incision/excision, separate lesion, or separate injury (or area of injury in extensive injuries) not ordinarily encountered or performed on the same day by the same physician. However, when another already established modifier is appropriate it should be used rather than modifier 59. Only if no more descriptive modifier is available, and the use of modifier 59 best explains the circumstances, should modifier 59 be used.

AMA Guidelines

cpt By identifying procedures/services that are not normally reported together, but are appropriate under the circumstances, the distinct procedural service modifier 59 is used to clearly designate instances when distinct and separate multiple services are provided to a patient on a single date of service. Although the modifier 59 has several reporting uses, it is only to be used if no more descriptive modifier is available and its use best explains the circumstances. As the description of this modifier indicates, some examples of common uses of the 59 modifier include separate sessions or patient encounters, different procedures or surgeries, surgery directed to different sites or organ systems, surgery directed to separate incision/excision or separate lesions, or treatment to separate injuries.

Modifier 59 is also intended to assist in reporting those procedures/services that may be considered a component of another procedure, but have been carried out independently or considered unrelated or distinct from other procedures/services provided at that time. In this instance, the procedure/service may be reported by itself, or in addition to other procedures/services, by appending modifier 59 to the specific procedure code reported.

CMS Guidelines

The CMS National Correct Coding Initiative (NCCI) edits provide many specific instructions on the use of modifier 59, which is the most commonly used CPT modifier to report distinct services performed on the same date. Modifier 59 replaced the HCPCS level II modifier GB to indicate that multiple but distinct services were provided by the same provider on the same date of service to the same patient. If this modifier is not used appropriately, the insurance claim may be denied, with the explanation for denial on the remittance advice reading, "Medicare does not pay for this service because it is part of another service that was performed at the same time."

When certain services are reported together on a patient by the same physician on the same date of service, there may be a perception of "unbundling" when, in fact, the services were performed under circumstances that did not involve this practice at all. Because carriers cannot identify this simply on the basis of CPT coding on either electronic or paper claims, modifier 59 was established to permit services of such a nature to bypass correct coding edits if the modifier is present.

Modifier 59 indicates that the procedure represents a distinct service from others reported on the same date of service. This may represent a different session, different surgery, different site, different lesion, or different injury or area of injury (in extensive injuries). Frequently, another already established modifier has been defined that describes this situation more specifically. In the event that a more descriptive modifier is available, it should be used in preference to modifier 59.

> **NOTE:** According to CMS, modifier 59 should be the modifier of "last resort."

Example 1

A patient required placement of a flow-directed pulmonary artery catheter for hemodynamic monitoring. The procedure was performed via the subclavian vein. Later in the day, the catheter had to be removed and a central venous catheter was inserted through the femoral vein.

CPT Code(s) Billed: 93503—Insertion and placement of flow-directed catheter (eg, Swan-Ganz) for monitoring purposes

36010 59—Introduction of catheter, superior or inferior vena cava

Rationale for Using Modifier 59

Because the pulmonary artery catheter requires passage through the vena cava, it may appear that the service for the pulmonary artery catheter was being "unbundled" if both services were reported on the same day. Accordingly, the central venous catheter code should be reported with modifier 59 (CPT code 36010 59) indicating that this catheter was placed in a different site as a different service on the same day. The carrier may request documentation to support submission of both services on the same day even with modifier 59 appended.

Modifier 59 is often misused. The two codes in a code pair edit often by definition represent different procedures. The provider cannot use the 59 modifier for such an edit because the two codes are for different procedures. However, if the two procedures are performed at separate sites or at separate patient encounters on the same date of service, modifier 59 may be appended. In addition, modifier 59 cannot be used with E/M services (CPT codes 99201-99499) or radiation treatment management (CPT code 77427).

Example 2

An orthopedic surgeon performed surgery on a 45-year-old patient with a foreign body in his left heel after stepping on some glass at the beach. He also was complaining about knee pain, and X rays indicated he had right knee degenerative joint disease. The physician decided to proceed with surgery for both problems. Once prepped and draped, an Esmarch was used as a tourniquet for about 10 minutes. An elliptical incision was made over the foreign body, and it appeared to be an embedded piece of glass within the dermis. It was excised without difficulty. The underlying sub-Q was exposed. An approximate 1-cm incision was made, and hemostasis had been achieved. The right knee was sterilely prepped and injected with 40 mg of Kenalog and 2 cc of Marcaine.

CPT code(s) billed: *28190—Removal of foreign body, foot; subcutaneous*

20610 59—Arthrocentesis, aspiration and/or injection; major joint or bursa (eg, shoulder, hip, knee joint, subacromial bursa)

Rationale for Using Modifier 59

Since both procedures were not related and were distinct and separate, it would be appropriate to append modifier 59 to the second procedure for the facility.

Reporting Radiology Procedures

Multiple radiology procedures often are performed on the same day.

Example 3

A construction worker presented to the emergency department after falling three floors from a high-rise building. He received a single-view cervical spine X ray prior to the removal of a cervical collar. Several hours after his release, he returned complaining of headache and neck pain, and received a complete cervical X ray series.

CPT Code(s) Billed for the First Visit: *72020—Radiologic examination, spine, single view, specify level*
CPT Code(s) Billed for the Second Visit: *72052 59—Radiologic examination, spine, cervical; complete, including oblique and flexion and/or extension studies*

38			39 CODE	VALUE CODES AMOUNT	40 CODE	VALUE CODES AMOUNT	41 CODE	VALUE CODES AMOUNT		
			a							a
			b							b
			c							c
			d							d

42 REV. CD.	43 DESCRIPTION	44 HCPCS / RATES	45 SERV. DATE	46 SERV. UNITS	47 TOTAL CHARGES	48 NON-COVERED CHARGES	49	
1		72020						1
2		72052 59						2
3								3
4								4
5								5
6								6
7								7
8								8
9								9
10								10

NOTE: Keep in mind that with situations like the one in the radiology example, the carrier may request documentation to support the reason for the two procedures.

Reporting Laboratory Procedures

Both modifier 59 and modifier 91 are used to report repeat clinical diagnostic laboratory tests performed on the same patient on the same day. According to CMS, modifier 59 is appropriate for reporting multiple claims submissions by a clinical laboratory for the same CPT code for the same patient on the same day. To clarify, according to the NCCI guidelines, it would not be appropriate to append the modifier 59 in the following instances: "If after a test is ordered and performed, additional related procedures are necessary to provide or confirm the result, these would be considered part of the ordered test. As another example, if a patient has an abnormal test result and repeat performance of the test is done to verify the result, the test is reported as one unit of service rather than two." NCCI also directs, "Multiple tests to identify the same analyte marker, or infectious agent should not be reported separately. For example, it would not be appropriate to report both direct probe and amplified probe technique tests for the same infectious agent."

Modifier 59 is used, for example, to report procedures that are distinct or independent, such as performing the same procedure (which uses the same procedure code) for testing of a different specimen (eg, aerobic culture of two independent wound site specimens).

Example 4

A 67-year-old woman presented as an outpatient to the laboratory for aerobic and anaerobic culture of two sites of a single vertical wound to the anterior left foreleg incurred as a result of a fall over a metal lawn chair. The laboratory technologist obtained independent specimens, one from the proximal wound site and one from the distal wound site, for aerobic culture of the drainage material for testing, using the appropriate type of aerobic culturettes. The laboratory technologist also obtained independent specimens with anaerobic culturettes, one from the proximal wound site and one from the distal wound site, for anaerobic culture of the drainage material for testing.

CPT Code(s) Billed: 87071, 87071 59, 87073, 87073 59

87071   Culture, bacterial; quantitative, aerobic with isolation and pre-sumptive identification of isolates, any source except urine, blood or stool

87073   Culture, bacterial; quantitative, anaerobic with isolation and presumptive identification of isolates, any source except urine, blood or stool

Review of Modifier 59

1   Modifier 59 is reported when two procedures are reported on the same day that are "distinct and separate."

2   Modifier 59 is used to report the following:
   a. Separate sessions or patient encounters
   b. Different procedures or surgeries
   c. Different sites or organ systems
   d. Separate injuries
   e. Separate lesions
   f. Separate incision/excision(s)

3   Caution should be used with modifier 59.

4   The NCCI provides instructions on the use of modifier 59. The NCCI edits should be checked before modifier 59 is appended.

5   Modifier 59 is not used when the procedures are considered multiple procedures.

6   Modifier 59 is not used with E/M services 99201-99499 or radiation treatment management CPT code 77427.

7   Modifier 59 replaced the HCPCS level II modifier GB to indicate that multiple, but distinct, services were provided by the same provider on the same date of service to the same patient.

Modifier 73: Discontinued Outpatient Hospital/ Ambulatory Surgery Center (ASC) Procedure Prior to the Administration of Anesthesia

Definition

Due to extenuating circumstances or those that threaten the well being of the patient, the physician may cancel a surgical or diagnostic procedure subsequent to the patient's surgical preparation (including sedation when provided, and being taken to the room where the procedure is to be performed), but prior to the administration of anesthesia (local, regional block[s], or general). Under these circumstances, the intended service that is prepared for but canceled can be reported by its usual procedure number and the addition of the modifier 73. **Note:** The elective cancellation of a service prior to the administration of anesthesia and/or surgical preparation of the patient should not be reported. For physician reporting of a discontinued procedure, see modifier 53.

AMA Guidelines

Effective January 1, 1999, a new CPT modifier 73 replaced modifier 52 for identifying discontinued services occurring under the stated circumstances. Before the establishment of modifier 73, CPT modifier 53 was used to specify when a procedure was terminated after the induction of anesthesia (eg, local, regional block[s], or general anesthesia), or after the procedure was started (incision made, intubation started, scope inserted).

Modifier 73 was established specifically to assist hospital outpatient reporting associated with the utilization of resources in the event a surgical or diagnostic procedure is canceled due to extenuating circumstance or those that threaten the well-being of the patient. In this instance, the cancellation occurs subsequent to the patient's surgical preparation (including sedation when provided), while the patient is in the room where the procedure is to be performed, and before the administration of anesthesia.

CMS Guidelines

With the OPPS, modifiers for discontinued procedures/services were implemented so that hospitals would have a way under the system to be reimbursed for expenses incurred in preparing a patient for surgery and scheduling a room for performing the procedure. Modifier 52 was implemented for use when a procedure is terminated after the patient has been prepared for surgery (including sedation when provided) and taken to the room where the procedure is performed but before the induction of local, regional, or general anesthesia. However, in 1999, modifier 73 replaced modifier 52 for reporting discontinued procedures.

If modifier 73 is reported and the procedure is an approved ASC service, payment will be 50% of the facility rate, subject to the ASC payment calculation. If modifier 74 is reported, there is no payment reduction. This is because the resources of the facility are consumed in essentially the same manner and the same extent as they would have been had the procedure been completed. The Medicare carriers apply these same guidelines to discontinued services performed in ASCs. In this instance, the cancellation occurs:

- Prior to the administration of anesthesia (local, regional block(s), or general) including conscious sedation
- Subsequent to the patient's surgical preparation (including sedation when provided)

- Subsequent to the patient being taken to the room where the procedure is to be performed

Appending this modifier helps to reimburse the facility for the costs incurred to prepare the patient for the procedure, as well as for the resources expended in the procedure room and recovery room (if required), even though the procedure has been discontinued.

When one or more of the planned procedures is completed, the completed procedures are reported as usual. The other(s) that were planned but not started are not reported. When none of the planned procedures is completed, the first planned procedure is reported with modifier 73 as appropriate. The others are not reported.

If a procedure is terminated before the induction of anesthesia and before the patient is wheeled into the procedure room, the procedure should not be reported. The patient has to be taken to the room where the procedure is to be performed for modifier 73 to be reported. A diagnosis code from the V64.X series should be included to indicate the reason for cancellation.

Example 1

A 70-year-old man was brought to the operating room for elective repair of a recurrent inguinal hernia. The usual surgical preparation and positioning was carried out. Before the administration of general anesthesia, the patient complained of radiating chest pain, with the cardiac monitor reflecting ST-segment changes. Because of the possibility of an evolving cardiac event, the procedure was canceled.

CPT Code(s) Billed: 49520 73—Repair recurrent inguinal hernia, any age; reducible

Rationale for Using Modifier 73

Under these circumstances, the intended service that is prepared for but canceled can be reported by its usual procedure code with modifier 73 appended. This modifier is not intended for reporting by a physician or other qualified health care provider. Modifier 73 is also not used to depict the elective cancellation of a service before the administration of anesthesia and/or surgical preparation of the patient.

Example 2

A 65-year-old man presented to the emergency department with lower abdominal pain and voiding small amounts of grossly bloody urine with clots. On physical examination, his bladder was tender and distended. Several urethral catheters were placed, but they rapidly obstructed because of clots. Because of inadequate bladder drainage, the patient was taken to the operating room. Before the induction of general anesthesia, the patient's blood pressure dropped and the surgeon elected to cancel the procedure.

CPT Code(s) Billed: 52001 73—Cystourethroscopy with irrigation and evacuation of multiple obstructing clots

Rationale for Using Modifier 73

Since the patient's surgery was discontinued prior to the administration of anesthesia because of the patient's blood pressure dropping, it would be appropriate for the facility to report modifier 73.

Example 3

In the ASC, a patient underwent drainage of a right nasal abscess via an internal approach. Prior to the administration of anesthesia, the patient (who has a seizure disorder) suffered a Grand Mal seizure, and the physician elected to discontinue the procedure. The physician contacted the patient's neurologist, who admitted the patient to the hospital.

CPT Code(s) Billed: 30000 73—Drainage abscess or hematoma, nasal, internal approach

Rationale for Using Modifier 73

Because the patient suffered a seizure before administration of anesthesia and the physician elected to cancel the procedure and address the patient's medical condition, it would be appropriate to append modifier 73 to the surgical procedure for ASC reimbursement.

Review of Modifier 73

1 Modifier 73 is used when the facility reports the service was canceled before the induction of anesthesia at the physician's discretion.

2 Modifier 73 is used when the patient has been prepared, but anesthesia has not been induced (local, regional block, or general anesthesia).

3 For physician reporting of a discontinued procedure, modifier 53 is used.

4 Modifier 73 is used only with outpatient hospital or ASC reporting.

5 Modifier 73 is not used for reporting outpatient hospital or ASC procedures that were discontinued before administration of anesthesia.

6 Modifier 73 is not to be used for elective cancellation of a procedure before the administration of anesthesia.

7 When procedure is terminated before the induction of anesthesia and before the patient is wheeled into the procedure room, the procedure should not be reported.

Modifier 74: Discontinued Outpatient Hospital/Ambulatory Surgery Center (ASC) Procedure After Administration of Anesthesia

Definition

Due to extenuating circumstances or those that threaten the well-being of the patient, the physician may terminate a surgical or diagnostic procedure after the administration of anesthesia (local, regional block[s], general) or after the procedure was started (incision made, intubation started, scope inserted, etc). Under these circumstances, the procedure started but terminated can be reported by its usual procedure number and the addition of the modifier 74. **Note:** The elective cancellation of a service prior to the administration of anesthesia and/or surgical preparation of the patient should not be reported. For physician reporting of a discontinued procedure, see modifier 53.

AMA Guidelines

Before the establishment of modifier 74, the CPT modifier 53 was used to report when a procedure was terminated after the induction of anesthesia (eg, local, regional block[s], or general anesthesia), or after the procedure was started (incision made, intubation started, scope inserted).

Modifier 74 was established specifically to assist hospital outpatient reporting associated with the utilization of resources in the event a surgical or diagnostic procedure is terminated because of extenuating circumstances or those that threaten the well-being of the patient after the procedure was started (incision made, intubation started, scope inserted, etc), and after the administration of anesthesia. In this instance, the cancellation occurs subsequent to:

- the administration of anesthesia (local, regional block(s) or general)
- the patient's surgical preparation (including sedation when provided)
- the patient being taken into the room where the procedure is to be performed

If modifier 74 is reported, there is no payment reduction. This is because the resources of the facility are consumed in essentially the same manner and to the same extent as they would have been had the procedure been completed. The Medicare carriers apply these same guidelines to discontinued services performed in ambulatory surgical centers.

CMS Guidelines

Effective January 1, 1999, modifier 74 replaced modifier 53 for reporting these discontinued services, with modifier 53 no longer being an acceptable modifier for hospital reporting.

Coinciding with the establishment of modifiers 73 and 74, the language of modifier 53 was revised to reflect its sole usage for physician reporting. The language of modifier 74 instructs that the elective cancellation of a procedure should not be reported. When used to indicate discontinued procedures, modifiers 52 and 53 (and the replacement modifiers 73 and 74) are applicable only to surgical and certain diagnostic procedures.

When a procedure is reported with modifier 74, there is no payment reduction. This is because the resources of the facility are consumed in essentially the same manner and to the same extent as they would have been had the procedure been completed. The Medicare carriers apply these same guidelines to discontinued services performed in ASCs. Use of modifiers 73 and 74 is approved by CMS in the hospital outpatient department as well as the Ambulatory Surgery Center.

Termination When Multiple Procedure Are Planned

When one or more of the planned procedures is completed, the completed procedures are reported as usual. The other(s) that were planned but not started are not reported. When none of the procedures that were planned is completed, and the patient had been prepared for the procedure and taken into the procedure room, the first procedure is reported with modifier 73. However, if the first procedure had begun (ie, incision made, scope inserted), and/or the patient had received anesthesia, then modifier 74 is reported with the first procedure only. The additional planned procedures are not reported.

Example 1

A 66-year-old woman was taken to the operating room for a laparoscopic cholecystectomy. After making the incisional port entry, the anesthesiologist detected ventricular fibrillation on the cardiac monitor. Ventilation continued while defibrillator pads and paddles were brought into the surgical field. On the second defibrillation effort, the arrhythmia abated, but ventricular irritability was present. The procedure was canceled pending further cardiac consultation/stabilization.

CPT Code(s) Billed: 47562 74—Laparoscopy, surgical; cholecystectomy

38				39 CODE	VALUE CODES AMOUNT	40 CODE	VALUE CODES AMOUNT	41 CODE	VALUE CODES AMOUNT	
				a						a
				b						b
				c						c
				d						d
42 REV. CD.	43 DESCRIPTION		44 HCPCS / RATES	45 SERV. DATE	46 SERV. UNITS	47 TOTAL CHARGES		48 NON-COVERED CHARGES	49	
1			47562 74							1
2										2
3										3
4										4
5										5
6										6
7										7
8										8
9										9
10										10

Rationale for Using Modifier 74

Under these circumstances, the procedure started but terminated can be reported by its usual procedure code with modifier 74 appended. This modifier is not intended for reporting physicians or other qualified health care providers.

Modifier 74 is also not used to report the elective cancellation of a service before the administration of anesthesia and/or surgical preparation of the patient.

Example 2

A 54-year-old woman had a 3-cm renal cell carcinoma in the lower pole of the left kidney, discovered on CT scan for suspected gallbladder disease. The gallbladder was found to be normal. The patient's surgery was scheduled in the outpatient department of the hospital. The patient was placed under sedation and the laparoscope was inserted. The patient went into cardiac arrest, and the physician stopped the procedure and treated the patient. The patient suffered an acute myocardial infarction, and once stabilized was transferred to the critical care unit.

CPT Code(s) Billed: 50545 74—Laparoscopy, surgical; radical nephrectomy (includes removal of Gerota's fascia and surrounding fatty tissue, removal of regional lymph nodes, and adrenalectomy)

Rationale for Using Modifier 74

Because the patient had received anesthesia before going into cardiac arrest, the surgical procedure is reported with modifier 74. There should be no reduction in reimbursement for the facility since resources were utilized for the surgery.

Review of Modifier 74

1   Modifier 74 is not used for physician services; modifier 53 is used.

2   Modifier 74 is for use in outpatient hospital or ASC procedures when the service/procedure is discontinued after administration of anesthesia (local, regional, general).

3   Modifier 53 is not used for outpatient hospital or ASC procedures.

4   When one or more of the procedures planned is completed, the completed procedure is reported as usual. The others planned that were not started after induction of anesthesia are not reported.

5   For CMS, there is no payment reduction for use of modifier 74 because the resources of the facility are consumed in essentially the same manner and to the same extent as they would have been had the procedure been completed.

Checkpoint Exercises 2

1   Which modifier replaced modifier 53 when a surgical procedure is reported that is canceled before administration of anesthesia?

2   This modifier is used when a procedure is planned prospectively that is more extensive than the original procedure or that follows a diagnostic surgical procedure.

3   The modifier used specifically to assist hospital outpatient reporting associated with the cancellation after administration of anesthesia is _____ .

4   CMS reimburses payment by _____ of the facility rate, subject to the ASC payment calculation with modifier 73.

5   When two procedures are performed through separate incisions, the modifier used to report the second procedure is _____ .

Modifiers 76, 77, 78, and 79

CMS Guidelines

The individual circumstances described by modifiers 76, 77, 78, and 79 continue to have reimbursement or tracking relevance to the CMS FI, which enables the FI or other payers/carriers to appropriately pay for the procedure per se and other associated postoperative services performed within or subsequent to its assigned global period (eg, 0 days, 10 days, 90 days). In addition, use of these modifiers allows instances where duplicate billing or duplicate services may have been reported to be differentiated electronically.

Modifier 76: Repeat Procedure by Same Physician

Definition

The physician may need to indicate that a procedure or service was repeated subsequent to the original procedure or service. This circumstance may be reported by adding the modifier 76 to the repeated procedure/service.

AMA Guidelines

Modifier 76 is used to indicate that a procedure or service was repeated in a separate operative session on the same day by the same physician.

Similar to modifier 58, the reference to the "postoperative period" in the language of the "repeat" procedure modifiers does not have strict relevance in hospital outpatient reporting.

CMS Guidelines

As outlined in the October 5, 2000, Program Memorandum, CMS implemented the two repeat procedure modifiers for hospital use. CMS directs that, should there be a question regarding who the ordering physician was and whether the same physician ordered the second procedure, code choice is based on whether the physician performing the procedure is the same. The procedure must be the same procedure. It is listed once and then listed again with the appropriate modifier. This modifier is appended to a procedure or service that was repeated subsequent to the original procedure or service. **For OPPS purposes, the postoperative period is the same day.**

Example 1

A 68-year-old woman had an unfortunate landing while bicycling, sustaining a mildly displaced closed fracture of the right distal ulna. Because of the patient's condition and the nature of the injury, closed manipulation was performed under anesthesia in the operating room, with placement of a long-arm plaster splint. After postanesthesia recovery, the patient was discharged. The patient presented to the emergency department later that evening, after having tripped over her dog. Radiographs were taken, indicating mild slippage at the fracture site. The patient underwent outpatient closed manipulation, performed by the same physician who performed the original procedure, with placement of a long-arm fiberglass cast.

CPT Code(s) Billed: 25535, 25535 76 (same date)

25535   Closed treatment of ulnar shaft fracture; with manipulation

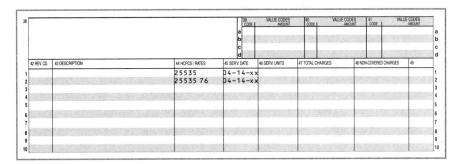

Rationale for Using Modifier 76

In this instance, the same closed reduction code is reported with the modifier 76 appended, as this is the same procedure (ie, "repeat procedure") performed by the same physician.

Example 2

A 38-year-old male developed medial elbow instability after a waterskiing accident. Surgical repair of the medial collateral ligament was performed using local tissues in the outpatient surgery department of the hospital. The patient was released in good condition later that afternoon. In the evening, the patient fell going down a staircase and re-injured the elbow. The patient was taken to the emergency department of the same hospital, and the surgeon who performed the initial procedure took the patient back into the operating room to redo the procedure.

CPT Code(s) Billed: 24345, 24345 76 (same date)

24345   Repair medial collateral ligament, elbow, with local tissue

38			39 CODE	VALUE CODES AMOUNT	40 CODE	VALUE CODES AMOUNT	41 CODE	VALUE CODES AMOUNT	
			a						a
			b						b
			c						c
			d						d

	42 REV. CD.	43 DESCRIPTION	44 HCPCS / RATES	45 SERV. DATE	46 SERV. UNITS	47 TOTAL CHARGES	48 NON-COVERED CHARGES	49	
1			24345	08-11-xx					1
2			24345 76	08-11-xx					2
3									3
4									4
5									5
6									6
7									7
8									8
9									9
10									10

Rationale for Using Modifier 76

Both procedures were performed during the postoperative period, which for the hospital facility reporting, is the initial date of service. Since the same exact procedure was repeated by the same physician, modifier 76 would be appended to the second procedure for reporting to receive reimbursement for the claim.

> **NOTE:** If a procedure is performed twice, add a modifier to the code on the subsequent claim line. If a procedure is performed more than two times, either report with the number of services in the units field of the subsequent claim line or report each procedure as a separate line item with the correct modifier. Some Medicare fiscal intermediaries recognize the use of modifier 76 to procedures such as radiological, laboratory, and some Medicare section codes, and not surgical procedures. Modifier 91 is used to identify repeat performance of the same laboratory test on the same day to obtain subsequent (multiple) test results.

Modifier 77: Repeat Procedure by Another Physician

Definition

The physician may need to indicate that a basic procedure or service performed by another physician had to be repeated. This situation may be reported by adding modifier 77 to the repeated procedure/service.

AMA Guidelines

Modifier 77 is used to indicate that a procedure or service was repeated in a separate operative session on the same day by another physician. The original intent and use of modifier 77 is not altered for hospital outpatient reporting.

This modifier is similar to modifier 76, but it differs slightly in that it indicates that a basic procedure or service performed by another physician had to be repeated. The clinical example given for modifier 76 may also be used to illustrate modifier 77, but Physician A was not available to perform the procedure, so Physician B performed a second closed manipulation. Physician B reports the closed reduction procedure with the modifier 77 appended.

CMS Guidelines

As outlined in the October 5, 2000, Program Memorandum, CMS implemented the two repeat procedure modifiers for hospital use. CMS directs that, should there be a question regarding who the ordering physician was and whether the same physician ordered the second procedure, code choice is based on whether the physician performing the procedure is the same. The procedure must be the same procedure. It is listed once and then listed again with the appropriate modifier. When the second procedure is performed by a different physician, modifier 77 is the appropriate modifier to append to the procedure code.

Example 1

Thoracentesis with insertion of a chest tube was performed on a 45-year-old patient who suffered a gunshot wound during an armed robbery of his convenience store. Dr Smythe performed the procedure in the morning of September 2 and removed the chest tube in the late afternoon. At 11pm the chest tube had to be reinserted, and Dr Luther, the surgeon on call, performed thoracentesis with a chest tube insertion.

CPT Code(s) Billed by Dr Smythe: 32002

CPT Code(s) Billed by Dr Luther: 32002 77

32002   Thoracentesis with insertion of tube with or without water seal (eg, for pneumothorax) (separate procedure)

Rationale for Using Modifier 77

Modifier 77 is used only when reporting the second surgical procedure. Without modifier 77, the insurance carrier would assume the claim submitted was a duplicate and thus would deny the claim. Since a different physician performed the second procedure, which was the exact same procedure as Dr Smythe performed, modifiers 76, 78, or 79 would not be appropriate.

Modifier 78: Return to the Operating Room for a Related Procedure During the Postoperative Period

Definition

The physician may need to indicate that another procedure was performed during the postoperative period of the initial procedure. When this subsequent procedure is related to the first, and requires the use of the operating room, it may be reported by adding the modifier 78 to the related procedure. (For repeat procedures on the same day, see 76.)

Little explanation is required for this modifier, as the title clearly describes its use. However, the issues surrounding its use occur when providers and carriers disagree as to whether the procedure is actually "unrelated" to the original procedure.

An example of this includes a postoperative complication and hemorrhage at the operative site that requires the patient to return to the operating room for treatment. It is important to note that the postoperative period for the facility is the date of the initial surgery, and the global surgical package does not apply.

CMS Guidelines

As with modifiers 76 and 77, for OPPS purposes, the postoperative period is the same day. Modifier 78 is appended to procedures that are performed during the postoperative period that require a patient to return to the operating room and are directly associated with the performance of the initial operation. For example, if a patient's operative site bleeds after an initial surgery and requires a return to the operating room to stop the bleeding, the same procedure is not repeated.

Example 1

On July 15, a 69-year-old man underwent endoscopic nasal polypectomy with an anterior and posterior ethmoidectomy. Later that day, the patient experienced increased bleeding with clots and presented to the emergency department for treatment.

After unsuccessful manual pressure, packing insertion, and local administration of vasoconstrictors performed in the emergency department, the patient was returned to the operating room, where bleeding was controlled by repair of a posterior arterial hemorrhage.

CPT Code(s) Billed: 31255, 30905 78 (same date)

31255   Nasal/sinus endoscopy, surgical; with ethmoidectomy, total (anterior and posterior)

30905   Control nasal hemorrhage, posterior, with posterior nasal packs and/or cautery, any method; initial

Rationale for Using Modifier 78

In this instance, the medical documentation reflected that the postprocedure bleeding was attributable to the initial operation. Therefore, a different code describing the procedure would be reported with modifier 78 appended. Since the same procedure is not repeated, modifier 76 would not be appropriate.

Modifier 79: Unrelated Procedure or Service by the Same Physician During the Postoperative Period

Definition

The physician may need to indicate that the performance of a procedure or service during the postoperative period was unrelated to the original procedure. This circumstance may be reported by using the modifier 79. (For repeat procedures on the same day, see modifier 76.)

Example 1

A 68-year-old woman had an unfortunate landing while bicycling, sustaining a mildly displaced closed fracture of the right distal ulna. Because of the patient's condition and the nature of the injury, closed manipulation was performed in the operating room, with placement of a long-arm plaster splint. The patient was discharged. Later in the day, the patient presented to the emergency department after experiencing nasal bleeding with clots. After unsuccessful pressure packing insertion and use of local vasoconstrictors, the patient was returned to the operating room, where bleeding was controlled by repair of a posterior arterial hemorrhage.

CPT Code(s) Billed: 25535, 30905 79 (same date)

25535   Closed treatment of ulnar shaft fracture; with manipulation

30905   Control nasal hemorrhage, posterior, with posterior nasal packs and/or cautery, any method; initial

Rationale for Using Modifier 79

In this instance, the medical documentation reflected that the postprocedure bleeding was not attributable to the initial operation. Therefore, a different code describing the procedure would be reported with modifier 79 appended. Since the same procedure is not repeated and is unrelated, modifier 76 would not be appropriate. The unrelated procedure is reported with modifier 79 appended (30905 79).

Example 2

A patient underwent a rotator cuff repair 4 weeks after an ACL repair of the right knee. The patient had been involved in a motor accident 1 year ago that resulted in the necessity of multiple surgeries. A longitudinal incision was made along the anterior portion of the shoulder, and the skin was reflected back. The deltoid fibers and the underlying tissues were divided. The coracoacromial ligament was divided, and the supraspinatus tendon was detached by a transverse incision along the greater tuberosity. The distal frayed edges of the tendon were removed. A trench was chiseled into the humeral bone along the level of the anatomical neck of the humerus. The supraspinatus tendon flap was buried in it. The flap was fixed with sutures tied to the tendon and passed through holes drilled in the bone. The repair was completed with side-to-side sutures of the supraspinatus to the adjacent subscapularis and infraspinatus tendons. The incision was closed, and a soft dressing was applied.

CPT Code(s) Billed: 23412—Repair of ruptured musculotendinous cuff (eg, rotator cuff) open; chronic

Rationale for Not Using Modifier 79

The procedure for the rotator cuff repair is unrelated to the ACL repair of the knee. However, in the outpatient facility hospital or ASC, the global period is considered only the day of the procedure. In this example, the patient's ACL repair was 4 weeks prior to the rotator cuff repair, so modifier 79 would not be required for the outpatient hospital facility. However, the surgeon who reports the professional services would report the procedure with modifier 79.

Review of Modifiers 76, 77, 78, and 79

1 Modifier 76 is used for reporting a repeat procedure (same procedure code) on the same day for outpatient hospital or ASC procedures by the same physician.

2 Modifier 77 is used when repeat procedures (same procedure code) are reported on the same day by a different physician for outpatient hospital or ASC procedures.

3 Modifiers 76 and 77 may be used to report services performed by a technician when ordered by a physician.

4 Modifiers 76 and 77 may be used for radiology procedures.

5 Modifier 78 is used for a related procedure performed during the postoperative period. The procedure is not the same but may be necessitated by a complication of the original procedure (same day for outpatient hospital and/or ASC reporting).

6 Modifier 79 is used when the surgical procedure is unrelated to the initial procedure during the postoperative period (same day for outpatient hospital and/or ASC reporting).

Modifier 91: Repeat Clinical Diagnostic Laboratory Test

Definition

In the course of treatment of the patient, it may be necessary to repeat the same laboratory test on the same day to obtain subsequent (multiple) test results. Under these circumstances, the laboratory test performed can be identified by its usual procedure number and the addition of the modifier 91. **Note:** This modifier may not be used when tests are rerun to confirm initial results; due to testing problems with specimens or equipment; or for any other reason when a normal, one-time, reportable result is all that is required. This modifier may not be used when other code(s) describe a series of test results (eg, glucose tolerance tests, evocative/suppression testing). This modifier may only be used for laboratory test(s) performed more than once on the same day on the same patient.

AMA Guidelines

Modifier 91 is used to report repeat clinical diagnostic laboratory tests performed on the same patient on the same day. As indicated in the descriptor language for use of modifier 91, it is used to identify repeat performance of the same laboratory test on the same day to obtain subsequent (multiple) test results.

For example, if a second culture was performed of the same wound site on the same day, then modifier 91 would be appended.

Modifier 91 is not intended to be used when tests are rerun to confirm initial results because of testing problems with the specimen(s) or equipment, or for any other reason when a normal, one-time reportable result is all that is required. In addition, modifier 91 is not intended for use when there are CPT codes available to describe the series of results (eg, glucose tolerance tests, evocative/suppression testing).

CMS Guidelines

Modifier 91 is appropriate when, in the course of treatment of the patient, it is necessary to repeat the same laboratory test on the same day to obtain subsequent test results. For example, modifier 91 would be used to report repeated blood testing for the same patient, using the same CPT code, performed at different intervals during the same day (eg, initial and three subsequent blood potassium levels).

Example 1

On July 14, a 65-year-old man with diabetic ketoacidosis had multiple blood tests performed to check the potassium level after potassium replacement and low-dose insulin therapy. After the initial potassium value was determined, three subsequent blood tests were ordered and performed on the same date at different times after the administration of potassium to correct the patient's hypokalemic state.

CPT Code(s) Billed: 84132, 84132 91 x 3 (units) (same day)
84132   Potassium; serum

38			39 CODE	VALUE CODES AMOUNT	40 CODE	VALUE CODES AMOUNT	41 CODE	VALUE CODES AMOUNT	
			a						a
			b						b
			c						c
			d						d
42 REV. CD.	43 DESCRIPTION	44 HCPCS / RATES	45 SERV. DATE	46 SERV. UNITS	47 TOTAL CHARGES		48 NON-COVERED CHARGES	49	
1		84132	07 14 XX						1
2		84132 91	07 14 XX	3					2
3									3
4									4
5									5
6									6
7									7
8									8
9									9
10									10

Rationale for Using Modifier 91

Code 84132 should be reported for the initial evaluation and 84132 with the modifier 91 appended should be reported three times for the three subsequently repeated blood potassium levels described in the preceding example.

To further clarify, the CPT Microbiology guidelines in the Pathology and Laboratory section state:

> Presumptive identification of microorganisms is defined as identification by colony morphology, growth on selective media, Gram stains, or up to three tests (eg, catalase, oxidase, indole, urease). Definitive identification of microorganisms is defined as an identification to the genus or species level that requires additional tests (eg, biochemical panels, slide cultures). If additional studies involve molecular probes, chromatography, or immunologic techniques, these should be separately coded in addition to definitive identification codes (87140-87158). For multiple specimens/sites, use modifier 59. For repeat laboratory tests performed on the same day, use modifier 91.

Review of Modifier 91

1   Modifier 91 should not be used when the second test or culture is from a different site; modifier 59 is used on the same date of service unless a second culture (same CPT code) is performed on the same day for the same site.

2   It must be medically necessary to perform the repeat procedure on the same day.

3   To be covered by CMS, the repeat diagnostic laboratory test must be rendered the same day, the same test as originally rendered (same procedure code), and for the same patient (beneficiary).

4   Modifier 91 may not be used when there is a HCPCS/CPT code that describes a series of results (glucose tolerance tests, evocative/ suppression testing).

5   If several of the same services (same CPT code) are performed for the same beneficiary on the same day by the physician, modifier 91 should be used to indicate that multiple clinical diagnostic laboratory tests were done on the same day. For example, a comprehensive metabolic panel (80053) is ordered. Later that day the physician orders a glucose test (82947) to follow up on an abnormal laboratory result.

6   Coding instructions are given in the Microbiology subsection of the CPT book.

Checkpoint Exercises 3

1   Modifier _____ is used to report a procedure by a different physician on the same day in the ASC.

2   What two modifiers were implemented to report discontinued procedures for hospital use? _____ _____ What modifiers did they replace? _____ _____

3   This modifier is used to report the same laboratory procedure on the same day. _____

4   Indicate the ways in which modifier 78 may be used. _____ _____ _____

5   Modifier _____ is used when the surgical procedure is unrelated to the original procedure and is performed on the same day in the ASC.

HCPCS Level II (National) Modifiers Approved for the ASC

Generally, HCPCS modifier codes are required to add specificity to the reporting of procedures performed on eyelids, fingers, toes, and arteries. They may be appended to CPT codes. If more than one level II modifier applies, the HCPCS code is repeated on another line with the appropriate level II modifier.

For example, code 26010 (Drainage of finger abscess; simple) done on the left hand thumb and second finger would be reported with the following codes:
   · 26010 FA (left hand, thumb)
   · 26010 F1 (left hand, second digit)

The level II modifiers apply whether Medicare is the primary or secondary payer. Previous modifier information and instruction were published by CMS in the Medicare Intermediary Manual (CMS publication 13-3), transmittal 1729, and the Medicare Hospital Manual (CMS publication 10), transmittal 726. These transmittals were dated January 1998 and were effective July 1, 1998.

Transmittal A-00-07 gives further clarification of the HCPCS outpatient hospital and ASC modifiers. These are available in Medicare manuals or at www.cms.hhs.gov. The hospital manual (CMS publication 10) as well as an index is also available at www.cms.hhs.gov.

Modifiers LT and RT

Modifiers LT and RT apply to codes for procedures that can be performed on paired organs, eg, ears, eyes, nostrils, kidneys, lungs, and ovaries. Modifiers LT and RT should be used whenever a procedure is performed on only one side. Hospitals use the appropriate RT or LT modifier to identify which of the paired organs was operated on.

NOTE: Modifiers LT and RT should not be used to report bilateral surgical procedures. (Modifier 50 is used for reporting bilateral procedures.)

Example 1

On November 14, a patient visited the ophthalmologist for an eye examination. The patient lost the left eye in an industrial accident 10 years prior. The ophthalmologist performed and documented an intermediate examination in the hospital clinic. The focus of the visit was related only to the right eye.

CPT Code(s) Billed: 92002 52 RT

92002   Ophthalmological services: medical examination and evaluation with initiation of diagnostic and treatment program; intermediate, new patient

Rationale for Using Modifier RT

Because the focus of the service was confined to the right eye, RT identifies that the service was performed only on the right side of the body. The service is reported for the outpatient facility, which includes a hospital clinic. The professional services will be reported on a CMS 1500, and the ophthalmologist will report 92002 with modifier 52 as well as the reduced services.

Modifiers E1 to E4 (Eyelids), F1 to F9 (Fingers), and TA to T9 (Toes)

- The most specific modifier available should be used.
- If more than one HCPCS level II modifier applies, the code should be repeated with each of the appropriate modifiers.
- These modifiers should not be used if the procedure/service code indicates multiple occurrences.
- The modifiers should not be used if the code indicates that the procedure applies to different body parts.

Example 2

A patient was admitted to the ASC on July 21 for a tenotomy of the left foot, second digit. A small incision was made at the crease of the toes on the bottom of the foot, the skin was reflected back, and the tendon was exposed. The tendon was released from its attachment. The incision was repaired with a layered closure, and a dressing was applied.

CPT Code(s) Billed: 28234 T1—Tenotomy, open, extensor, foot or toe, each tendon

Rationale for Using Modifier T1

Modifier T1 identifies the specific foot and digit on which the physician performed the procedure. This sometimes helps process the claim more smoothly and avoids suspended claims for documentation when the carrier needs to clarify the anatomy involved.

Modifiers LC, LD, and RC

- These modifiers are used to identify the vessel on which the procedure was performed.
- If more than one level II HCPCS modifier applies, the HCPCS code should be repeated on another line with the level II modifier on the CMS-1450 claim form or the UB-92 form.

Review of HCPCS Level II Approved Outpatient Hospital and ASC Modifiers

1   Only valid modifiers should be reported.

2   HCPCS modifiers may be applied to surgical, radiology, and other diagnostic procedures.

3   As with CPT modifiers, the hyphen (-) preceding the modifier has been eliminated.

4   The most specific modifiers available should always be used.

5   HCPCS level II modifiers should not be used if the code indicates multiple occurrences.

6   HCPCS level II modifiers should not be used if the code indicates that the procedure applies to different body parts.

7   HCPCS level II modifiers may be used with the CPT code set as well as the HCPCS level II codes.

Test Your Knowledge

Multiple Choice

1 _____ The modifiers RT and LT are:
   a. Right and left
   b. Sometimes used with the 50 modifier
   c. HCPCS modifiers
   d. All of the above

2 _____ A hammer-toe correction was performed on both big toes. Which of the following would be the appropriate code(s) to report?
   a. 28285 50
   b. 28285 LT and 28285 RT
   c. 28285 TA and 28285 T5
   d. None of the above

3 _____ A colonoscopy was scheduled for a Medicare patient. The scope was inserted but could not be passed beyond the splenic flexure. The procedure was discontinued. Select the appropriate procedure code(s).
   a. 45378
   b. 45378 52
   c. 45330 52
   d. 45330

4 _____ How is a bilateral tubal ligation reported?
   a. 58600
   b. 58600 50
   c. 58600 RT, LT
   d. 58600 76

5 _____ Two different lesions of the left breast were excised through two separate incisions. Select the appropriate procedure code(s).
   a. 19120, units of 2
   b. 19120 LT and 19120 RT
   c. 19120 LT and 19120 59 RT
   d. 19120, 19120 59

6 _____ A patient presented to radiology for an upper gastrointestinal series with a kidney-ureter-bladder study, but because of equipment failure, the procedure was canceled and rescheduled. Which of the following should be coded?
   a. No code is assigned
   b. 74241 52
   c. 74240
   d. 74240 52

7 _____ A Medicare patient was seen in the emergency department after a fall. On examination, he was found to have a 2-cm laceration

of the thigh and a 0.5-cm laceration of the wrist. The thigh was repaired as a layered closure, and the wrist was a simple repair. Select the correct procedure code(s).

a. 99281 25, 12031, and 12001 59
b. 99281 25, 12031, and 12001
c. 12031 and 12001
d. 12001 and 12031 58

8 _____ Excision of a chalazion of the left upper eyelid and a biopsy of the left lower eyelid were performed during the same operative session. Select the appropriate procedure code(s).

a. 67800 and 67810
b. 67800 and 67810 59
c. 67800 E1 and 67810 E2
d. 67800 E1 and 67810 59 E2

9 _____ A surgeon placed a temporary self-retaining indwelling ureteral stent after a cystourethroscopic procedure. Later in the evening the patient returned to the operating room for removal of the stent by the same surgeon. Select the appropriate modifier.

a. 78
b. 58
c. 79
d. 76

10 _____ The reason for using modifiers 76 and 77 is to:

a. Explain why the patient returned to the operating room during the postoperative period (same day in the ASC).
b. Comply with CMS compliance guidelines.
c. Only supply information; reimbursement will not be affected.
d. Explain why a procedure was duplicated, usually with a report, so the provider will be reimbursed appropriately.

11 _____ A 5-year-old male was taken to the emergency department at the local hospital. The child had swallowed lead paint that had peeled from a bedroom in his babysitter's house. A lead toxicity test was performed immediately, and the patient was started on IV infusion of a detoxification agent. Three hours later, a lead test was repeated to determine if the IV infusion was reducing the level of lead in the patient's blood. How should these lab services be reported?

a. 83655 × 2
b. 83655 91
c. 83655
d. 83655, 83655 91

12 _____ A 4-year-old with acute and chronic serous otitis media and hypertrophy of the adenoids presented to the ASC and under-

went an initial adenoidectomy and insertion of ventilation tubes under general anesthesia. Select the correct code(s).

a. 42830, 64936 51, 00120

b. 42830, 64936 59

c. 42820, 69433, 00120

d. 42835, 69421 59

13 _____ In the outpatient hospital surgery department, a patient with hypercalcemia of both hips underwent arthroscopy. After being prepped and draped, a needle was carefully inserted under fluoroscopic guidance into the joint of the right hip. Using the Seldinger technique, a wire was introduced through the needle. A small skin incision was made, and a trocar was placed over the wire and advanced to the hip capsule, where the sharpened end broke through the hip capsule into the joint. A fiberoptic arthroscope was placed over the trocar into the joint. A second port was created at the anterolateral position to assist in examination and passing of instruments. The hip was examined, and hypercalcemia was identified and removed. The same procedure was performed on the left hip. Select the correct code(s).

a. 29861 RT, LT

b. 29860, 29861

c. 29862 50, RT, LT

d. 29861 50

14 _____ A patient presented to the ASC for an excision of a 4.8 cm malignant melanoma of the left inner thigh. A 6-cm × 6-cm rotation flap was created for closure. What is the correct procedural code(s) for this encounter?

a. 15100 LT

b. 11606 LT, 15130 LT

c. 14300 LT

d. 11606 LT, 14300 LT

15 _____ A patient presented with a crush injury of the right middle finger distal phalanx with open fracture of the right middle finger and underwent surgery in the outpatient department at the local hospital. After adequate prepping and draping of the right upper extremity, it was extended on the hand table. There was noted to be a stellate laceration of the nailbed of the right middle finger; this was explored and debrided. The fracture site then was identified, was cleared of fracture hematoma, and was debrided. Fracture fragments were adequately realigned manually utilizing forceps, and the fracture site was copiously irrigated with normal sterile saline. Nailbed repair was carried out with oversided laceration repair using interrupted sutures. Sterile nonadherent dressings and a dorsal AlumaFoam splint was applied. The patient

was sent to recovery in stable condition. Provide the procedure code and diagnosis code for this encounter.

a. 26765 F7, 11760 59, F7
b. 26775, 11760 59, F7
c. 26746 F7, 11762 51
d. 26735 F7, 11760 59

CHAPTER 10

Genetic Testing Modifiers and Category II Modifiers

Genetic Modifiers

CPT® 2005 featured a new appendix that lists numeric-alpha genetic modifiers. These modifiers are appended to the molecular diagnostics codes 83890-83912 when molecular diagnostic procedures are performed to test for infectious disease, oncology, hematology, neurology, or inherited disorders, to specify the probe type or condition tested. The genetic modifiers also may be appended to the cytogenetic studies codes 88245-88291 when molecular diagnostic procedures are performed to test for oncologic or inherited disorders to specify the probe type or condition tested.

Why These Modifiers Were Established

New CPT codes typically are established to describe a specific laboratory test procedure. However, the CPT nomenclature uses modifiers as an integral part of its structure. The CPT code set instructs the use of a modifier in an instance where the reporting of a procedure or service could potentially require the addition of a large number of new codes and/or use of a large number of code combinations.

The molecular diagnostic and cytogenetic studies depict this circumstance as these CPT codes (see Table 10-1) are reported multiple times and/or in multiple combinations to describe a broad range of complex testing.

For example, a deoxyribonucleic acid (DNA) sample can be obtained from any tissue or body fluid, including blood. For some types of gene tests, laboratories design short pieces of DNA called probes, whose sequences are complementary to the mutated sequences. These probes will seek their complement among the 3 billion base pairs of an individual's genome. If the mutated sequence is present in the patient's genome, the probe will bind to it and flag the mutation. Another type of DNA testing involves comparing the sequence of DNA bases in a patient's gene to a normal version of the gene.

The information in DNA is stored as a "code" made up of four chemical bases: adenine (A), guanine (G), cytosine (C), and thymine (T). Human DNA consists of about 3 billion bases, and more than 99% of those bases are the same in all people. The order, or sequence, of these bases determines the information available for building and maintaining an organism, similar to the way in which letters of the alphabet appear in a certain order to form words and sentences. The number and types of testing depend on the sizes of the genes and the number of mutations tested.

When molecular diagnostic testing has been performed, for example, to determine whether a person carries a genetic mutation associated with cystic fibrosis, multiple nucleic acid probes are used to detect both the normal and mutant variants within the gene. Code 83896, Molecular diagnostics; nucleic acid probe, each, should be used to report the use of nucleic acid probes in molecular diagnostic testing. Code 83896 should be reported for each nucleic acid probe used in traditional assays. If 25 nucleic acid probes are used to detect 25 gene mutations when testing for cystic fibrosis, then code 83896 is reported 25 times.

One can only imagine how many CPT codes would be required to report the number, types, and possible molecular diagnostic test combinations related to all types of infectious disease, oncology, hematology, neurology, or inherited disorders and cytogenetic studies for all types of oncologic and inherited disorders.

Reporting Solution: Genetic Modifiers

To capture the gene- and disease-specific data necessary for utilization tracking, the numeric-alpha modifier option addresses concerns expressed by laboratories and payers regarding significant problems of granularity in the molecular diagnostic CPT codes.

The genetic modifiers denote gene type and mutation to allow providers to submit complete and specific information and for payers to adjudicate claims. While CPT genetic modifiers will not likely provide a permanent solution to the expected growth of molecular genetics in clinical practice, they do supply a method of standard modifier usage to offer a more stable environment for claims submission and processing.

How to Use CPT Genetic Modifiers

The CPT numeric-alpha genetic modifier model logic will yield 260 potential combinations and is intended for use with certain CPT molecular diagnostic and cytogenetic codes (see Table 10-2). Specifically, implementation is intended to:

- Provide an accurate method of reporting and identifying different molecular genetic diagnostic analyses
- Provide disease- or gene-specific identifiers to allow the ability to track utilization of genetic tests
- Maintain the CPT code set as the most appropriate procedural coding system for the medical laboratory

While CPT modifiers are two-digit numeric indicators (except for the physical status modifiers), the CPT genetic numeric-alpha modifiers are arranged in a hierarchical system with the first numeric character indicating the disease category and the second alpha character denoting the disease or gene. This new level of granularity enables providers to communicate complete and specific information to assist payers to adjudicate claims for such analyses without written explanation or chart review. While this number will not allow complete capture of the human genome, it will provide a short-term, viable solution to the expected growth of molecular genetics in clinical practice over the next decade as technology and nomenclature systems mature. It should be noted that each disease category list ends with a "not otherwise specified" code, usually denoted by the Z placement that can be used when specific genes are being tested that do not have a specific modifier assigned (eg, 2Z, lymphoid/hematopoetic neoplasia, not otherwise specified).

When using the CPT genetic modifiers, codes 83890-83912 are intended for use with molecular diagnostic techniques for analysis of nucleic acids. Codes 83890-83912 are reported by procedure rather than analyte. Each procedure used in an analysis should be coded separately. For example, a procedure requiring isolation of DNA, restriction endonuclease digestion, electrophoresis, and nucleic acid probe amplification would be coded as 83890, 83892, 83894, and 83898.

Example 1

A 32-year-old woman in otherwise good health presented with deep vein thrombosis. During the evaluation, her physician learned of a family history of thrombotic disorders and ordered a DNA evaluation for Factor V Leiden, prothrombin, and MTHFR. The laboratory performs an evaluation for R506Q (Leiden) mutation in the Factor V gene, the G20210A mutation in the Factor II (prothrombin) gene, and the C677T and A1298C mutations in the MTHFR gene.

CPT Code(s) and Genetic Modifiers Reported:

83890—Molecular diagnostics; molecular isolation or extraction

83892 3A—Molecular diagnostics; enzymatic digestion

83892 3F—Molecular diagnostics; enzymatic digestion

83892 3G—Molecular diagnostics; enzymatic digestion

83894 3A—Molecular diagnostics; separation by gel electrophoresis (eg, agarose, polyacrylamide)

83894 3F—Molecular diagnostics; separation by gel electrophoresis (eg, agarose, polyacrylamide)

83894 3G—Molecular diagnostics; separation by gel electrophoresis (eg, agarose, polyacrylamide)

83898 3A (x2)—Molecular diagnostics; amplification of patient nucleic acid (eg, PCR, LCR), single primer pair, each primer pair

83898 3F (x2)—Molecular diagnostics; amplification of patient nucleic acid (eg, PCR, LCR), single primer pair, each primer pair

83898 3G—Molecular diagnostics; amplification of patient nucleic acid (eg, PCR, LCR), single primer pair, each primer pair

83912 3A—Molecular diagnostics; interpretation and report

83912 3F—Molecular diagnostics; interpretation and report

83912 3G—Molecular diagnostics; interpretation and report

Rationale for Using the Genetic Modifiers

The use of the genetic modifiers is only applicable when the procedure described by the CPT code is used exclusively for the genetic analysis encoded by the modifier. In this example, the extraction step is being used for all three gene analyses, hence negating the applicability of the modifiers. As each mutation analysis requires a digestion, electrophoresis, amplification, and interpretation step, the

CODING TIP

Although this reporting method reflects the intent and use of the CPT codes and genetic modifiers, third-party payers may request that these services be reported differently.

modifier for Factor V Leiden (3A) would be applied to one set of the 83892/83894/83898/83912 codes, and the modifiers for the MTHFR gene (3F) and Factor II (3G) would be used on the second and third sets, respectively. It should be noted that as two DNA primer segments are amplified for Factor V Leiden (one for normal germline and one for the mutated forms) and for MTHFR (one for C677T and another for A1298C), each of these modified is used twice.

Example 2

A 25-year-old female patient, presenting with a strong family history of ovarian and breast carcinomas, recently learned that her mother tested positive for the BRCA1 gene. Following genetic counseling, she expected to be tested for the same gene. The clinician requested analysis for BRCA1. The laboratory performs known mutation, single-site DNA analysis for BRCA1.

CPT Code(s) and Genetic Modifiers Reported:

83891 0A—Molecular diagnostics; isolation or extraction of highly purified nucleic acid

83898 0A—Molecular diagnostics; amplification of patient nucleic acid (eg, PCR, LCR), single primer pair, each primer pair

83894 0A—Molecular diagnostics; separation by gel electrophoresis (eg, agarose, polyacrylamide)

83904 0A—Molecular diagnostics; mutation identification by sequencing, single segment, each segment

83912 0A—Molecular diagnostics; interpretation and report

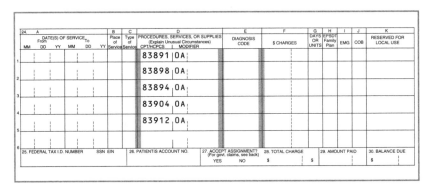

Rationale for Using the Genetic Modifiers

As was true in the first example, the use of the genetic modifiers is only applicable when the procedure described by the CPT code is exclusively used for the genetic analysis encoded by the modifier. In this example, the extraction, amplification, and interpretation steps are being used exclusively for the BRCA1 mutation analysis. It would be appropriate to use the modifier 0A for these services in addition to its use in the other procedural codes encompassing this analysis.

TABLE 10-1	**CPT Codes Currently Used with CPT Genetic Modifiers**
83890	Molecular diagnostics; molecular isolation or extraction
83891	Molecular diagnostics; isolation or extraction of highly purified nucleic acid
83892	Molecular diagnostics; enzymatic digestion
83893	Molecular diagnostics; dot/slot blot production
83894	Molecular diagnostics; separation by gel electrophoresis (eg, agarose, polyacrylamide)
83896	Molecular diagnostics; nucleic acid probe, each
83897	Molecular diagnostics; nucleic acid transfer (eg, Southern, Northern)
83898	Molecular diagnostics; amplification of patient nucleic acid, each nucleic acid sequence
83900	Molecular diagnostics; amplification of patient nucleic acid, multiplex, first two nucleic acid sequences
83901	Molecular diagnostics; amplification of patient nucleic acid, multiplex, each additional nucleic acid sequence (List separately in addition to code for primary procedure)
83902	Molecular diagnostics; reverse transcription
83903	Molecular diagnostics; mutation scanning, by physical properties (eg, single strand conformational polymorphisms (SSCP), heteroduplex, denaturing gradient gel electrophoresis (DGGE), RNA'ase A), single segment, each
83904	Molecular diagnostics; mutation identification by sequencing, single segment, each segment
83905	Molecular diagnostics; mutation identification by allele specific transcription, single segment, each segment
83906	Molecular diagnostics; mutation identification by allele specific translation, single segment, each segment
83907	Molecular diagnostics; lysis of cells prior to nucleic acid extraction (eg, stool specimens, paraffin embedded tissue)
83908	Molecular diagnostics; signal amplification of patient nucleic acid, each nucleic acid sequence
83909	Molecular diagnostics; separation and identification by high resolution technique (eg, capillary electrophoresis)
83912	Molecular diagnostics; interpretation and report

TABLE 10-1 CPT Codes Currently Used with CPT Genetic Modifiers, *continued*

83914	Mutation identification by enzymatic ligation or primer extension, single segment, each segment (eg, oligonucleotide ligation assay (OLA), single base chain extension (SBCE), or allele-specific primer extension (ASPE))
88245	Chromosome analysis for breakage syndromes; baseline Sister Chromatid Exchange (SCE), 20-25 cells
88248	Chromosome analysis for breakage syndromes; baseline breakage, score 50-100 cells, count 20 cells, 2 karyotypes (eg, for ataxia telangiectasia, Fanconi anemia, fragile X)
88249	Chromosome analysis for breakage syndromes; score 100 cells, clastogen stress (eg, diepoxybutane, mitomycin C, ionizing radiation, UV radiation)
88261	Chromosome analysis; count 5 cells, 1 karyotype, with banding
88262	Chromosome analysis; count 15-20 cells, 2 karyotypes, with banding
88263	Chromosome analysis; count 45 cells for mosaicism, 2 karyotypes, with banding
88264	Chromosome analysis; analyze 20-25 cells
88267	Chromosome analysis; amniotic fluid or chorionic villus, count 15 cells, 1 karyotype, with banding
88269	Chromosome analysis, in situ for amniotic fluid cells, count cells from 6-12 colonies, 1 karyotype, with banding
88271	Molecular cytogenetics; DNA probe, each (eg, FISH)
88272	Molecular cytogenetics; chromosomal in situ hybridization, analyze 3-5 cells (eg, for derivatives and markers)
88273	Molecular cytogenetics; chromosomal in situ hybridization, analyze 10-30 cells (eg, for microdeletions)
88274	Molecular cytogenetics; interphase in situ hybridization, analyze 25-99 cells
88275	Molecular cytogenetics; interphase in situ hybridization, analyze 100-300 cells
88280	Chromosome analysis; additional karyotypes, each study
88283	Chromosome analysis; additional specialized banding technique (eg, NOR, C-banding)
88285	Chromosome analysis and additional cells counted, each study

| 88289 | Chromosome analysis; additional high resolution study |
| 88291 | Cytogenetics and molecular cytogenetics, interpretation and report |

Table 10-2 includes all genetic testing code modifiers in the CPT® codebook.

TABLE 10-2 Genetic Testing Code Modifiers[1]

This listing of modifiers is intended for reporting with molecular laboratory procedures related to genetic testing. Genetic test modifiers should be used in conjunction with CPT and HCPCS codes to provide diagnostic granularity of service to enable providers to submit complete and precise genetic testing information without altering test descriptors. These modifiers are categorized by mutation. The first (numeric) character indicates the disease category and the second (alpha) character denotes gene type. Introductory guidelines in the molecular diagnostic and molecular cytogenetic code sections of CPT provide further guidance in interpretation and application of genetic test modifiers.

Neoplasia (solid tumor, excluding sarcoma and lymphoma)

0A	BRCA1 (Hereditary breast/Ovarian cancer)
0B	BRCA2 (Hereditary breast cancer)
0C	Neurofibromin (Neurofibromatosis, type 1)
0D	Merlin (Neurofibromatosis, type 2)
0E	c-RET (Multiple endocrine neoplasia, types 2A/B, familial medullary thyroid carcinoma)
0F	VHL (Von Hippel Lindau disease, renal carcinoma)
0G	SDHD (Hereditary paraganglioma)
0H	SDHB (Hereditary paraganglioma)
0I	ERRB2, commonly called Her-2/neu
0J	MLH1 (HNPCC, mismatch repair genes)
0K	MSH2, MSH6, or PMS2 (HNPCC, mismatch repair genes)
0L	APC (Hereditary polyposis coli)
0M	Rb (Retinoblastoma)
0N	TP53, commonly called p53
0O	PTEN (Cowden's syndrome)
0P	KIT, also called CD117 (gastrointestinal stromal tumor)
0Z	Solid tumor gene, not otherwise specified

1. Source: Appendix I—Genetic Testing Code Modifiers, *CPT® 2006.*

TABLE 10-2 Genetic Testing Code Modifiers, *continued*

Neoplasia (Sarcoma)

1A   WT1 or WT2 (Wilm's tumor)

1B   PAX3, PAX7, or FOXO1A (Alveolar rhabdomyosarcoma)

1C   FLI1, ERG, ETV1, or EWSR1 (Ewing's sarcoma, desmoplastic round cell)

1D   DDIT3 or FUS (Myxoid liposarcoma)

1E   NR4A3, RBF56, or TCF12 (Myxoid chondrosarcoma)

1F   SSX1, SSX2, or SYT (Synovial sarcoma)

1G   MYCN (Neuroblastoma)

1H   COL1A1 or PDGFB (Dermatofibrosarcoma protruberans)

1I   TFE3 or ASPSCR1 (Alveolar soft parts sarcoma)

1J   JAZF1 or JJAZ1 (Endometrial stromal sarcoma)

1Z   Sarcoma gene, not otherwise specified

Neoplasia (lymphoid/hematopoetic)

2A   RUNX1 or CBFA2T1, commonly called AML1 or ETO, genes associated with t(8;21) AML1-also ETO (Acute myelogenous leukemia)

2B   BCR or ABL1, genes associated with t(9;22) (Chronic myelogenous or acute leukemia) BCR-also ABL (Chronic myeloid, acute lymphoid leukemia)

2C   PBX1 or TCF3, genes associated with t(1;19) (Acute lymphoblastic leukemia) CGF1

2D   CBFB or MYH11, genes associated with inv 16 (Acute myelogenous leukemia) CBF beta (Leukemia)

2E   MLL (acute leukemia)

2F   PML or RARA, genes associated with t(15;17) (Acute promyelocytic leukemia) PML/RAR alpha (Promyelocytic leukemia)

2G   ETV6, commonly called TEL, gene associated with t(12;21) (acute leukemia) TEL (Leukemia)

2H   BCL-2 (B cell lymphoma, follicle center cell origin) bcl-2 (Lymphoma)

2I   CCND1, commonly called BCL1, cyclin D1 (Mantle cell lymphoma, myeloma) bcl-1 (Lymphoma)

2J	MYC (Burkitt lymphoma) c-myc (Lymphoma)
2K	IgH (Lymphoma/leukemia)
2L	IGK (Lymphoma/leukemia)
2M	TRB, T cell receptor beta (Lymphoma/leukemia)
2N	TRG, T cell receptor gamma (Lymphoma/leukemia)
2O	SIL or TAL1 (T cell leukemia)
2T	BCL6 (B cell lymphoma)
2Q	API1 or MALT1 (MALT lymphoma)
2R	NPM or ALK, genes associated with t(2;5) (Anaplastic large cell lymphoma)
2S	FLT3 (acute myelogenous leukemia)
2Z	Lymphoid/hematopoetic neoplasia, not otherwise specified

Non-neoplastic hematology/coagulation

3A	F5, commonly called Factor V (Leiden, others) (Hypercoagulable state)
3B	FACC (Fanconi anemia)
3C	FACD (Fanconi anemia)
3D	HBB, beta globin (Thalassemia, Sickle cell anemia, other hemoglobinopathies)
3E	HBA, commonly called alpha globin (Thalassemia)
3F	MTHFR (Elevated homocystinemia)
3G	F2, commonly called prothrombin (20210, others) Hypercoagulable state) Prothrombin (Factor II, 20210A) (Hypercoagulable state)
3H	F8, commonly called Factor VIII (Hemophilia A/VWF)
3I	F9, commonly called Factor IX (Hemophilia B)
3K	F13, commonly called Factor XIII (bleeding or hypercoagulable state) Beta globin
3Z	Non-neoplastic hematology/coagulation, not otherwise specified

Histocompatability/blood typing/identity/microsatellite

4A	HLA-A
4B	HLA-B
4C	HLA-C

TABLE 10-2 **Genetic Testing Code Modifiers,** *continued*

4D	HLA-D
4E	HLA-DR
4F	HLA-DQ
4G	HLA-DP
4H	Kell
4I	Fingerprint for engraftment (post-allogeneic progenitor cell transplant)
4J	Fingerprint for donor allelotype (allogeneic transplant)
4K	Fingerprint for recipient allelotype (allogeneic transplant)
4L	Fingerprint for leukocyte chimerism (allogeneic solid organ transplant)
4M	Fingerprint for maternal versus fetal origin
4N	Microsatellite instability
4O	Microsatellite loss (loss of hererozygosity)
4Z	Histocompatability/blood typing, not otherwise specified
Neurologic, non-neoplastic	
5A	ASPA, commonly called Aspartoacylase A (Canavan disease)
5B	FMR-1 (Fragile X, FRAXA, syndrome)
5C	FRDA, commonly called Frataxin (Freidreich's ataxia)
5D	HD, commonly called Huntington (Huntington's disease)
5E	GABRA5, NIPA1, UBE3A, or ANCR GABRA (Prader Willi-Angelman syndrome)
5F	GJB2, commonly called Connexin-26 (Hereditary hearing loss) Connexin-32 (GJB2) (Hereditary deafness)
5G	GJB1, commonly called Connexin-32 (X-linked Charcot-Marie-Tooth disease)
5H	SNRPN (Prader Willi-Angelman syndrome)
5I	SCA1, commonly called Ataxin-1 (Spinocerebellar ataxia, type 1)
5J	SCA2, commonly called Ataxin-2 (Spinocerebellar ataxia, type 2)
5K	MJD, commonly called Ataxin-3 (Spinocerebellar ataxia, type 3, Machado-Joseph disease)

5L	CACNA1A (Spinocerebellar ataxia, type 6)
5M	ATXN7 Ataxin-7 (Spinocerebellar ataxia, type 7)
5N	PMP-22 (Charcot-Marie-Tooth disease, type 1A)
5O	MECP2 (Rett syndrome)
5Z	Neurologic, non-neoplastic, not otherwise specified

Muscular, non-neoplastic

6A	DMD, commonly called dystrophin (Duchenne/Becker muscular dystrophy)
6B	DMPK (Myotonic dystrophy, type 1)
6C	ZNF-9 (Myotonic dystrophy, type 2)
6D	SMN1/SMN2 (Autosomal recessive spinal muscular atrophy)
6E	MTTK, commonly called tRNAlys (myotonic epilepsy, MERRF)
6F	MTTL1, commonly called tRNAleu (mitochondrial encephalomyopathy, MELAS)
6Z	Muscular, not otherwise specified

Metabolic, other

7A	APOE, commonly called apolipoprotein E (Cardiovascular disease or Alzheimer's disease)
7B	NPC1 or NPC2, commonly called sphingomyelin phosphodiesterase (Nieman-Pick disease)
7C	GBA, commonly called acid beta glucosidase (Gaucher disease)
7D	HFE (Hemochromatosis)
7E	HEXA, commonly called hexosaminidase A (Tay-Sachs disease)
7F	ACADM (medium chain acyl CoA dehydrogenase deficiency)
7Z	Metabolic, other, not otherwise specified

Metabolic, transport

8A	CFTR (Cystic fibrosis)
8B	PRSS1 (Hereditary pancreatitis)
8Z	Metabolic, transport, not otherwise specified

Metabolic-pharmacogenetics

9A	TPMT commonly called (thiopurine methyltransferase) (patients on antimetabolite therapy)

TABLE 10-2 **Genetic Testing Code Modifiers,** *continued*	
9B	CYP2 genes, commonly called cytochrome p450 (drug metabolism)
9C	ABCB1, commonly called MDR1 or p-glycoprotein (drug transport)
9D	NAT2 (drug metabolism)
9L	Metabolic-pharmacogenetics, not otherwise specified
Dysmorphology	
9M	FGFR1 (Pfeiffer and Kallmann syndromes)
9N	FGFR2 (Crouzon, Jackson-Weiss, Apert, Saethre-Chotzen syndromes)
9O	FGFR3 (Achondroplasia, Hypochondroplasia, Thanatophoric dysplasia, types I and II, Crouzon syndrome with acanthosis nigricans, Muencke syndromes)
9P	TWIST (Saethre-Chotzen syndrome)
9Q	DCGR, commonly called CATCH-22 (DiGeorge and 22q11 deletion syndromes)
9Z	Dysmorphology, not otherwise specified

Terminology

Deoxyribonucleic acid (DNA): DNA is the hereditary material in humans and almost all other organisms. Nearly every cell in a person's body has the same DNA. Inside each human cell lies a nucleus, a membrane-bounded region that provides a sanctuary for genetic information. The nucleus contains long strands of DNA that encode this genetic information. Most DNA is located in the cell nucleus (where it is called nuclear DNA), but a small amount of DNA can also be found in the mitochondria (where it is called mitochondrial DNA or mtDNA).

Gene: The gene is the basic physical and functional unit of heredity. Genes, which are made up of DNA, act as instructions to make molecules called proteins. In humans, genes vary in size from a few hundred DNA bases to more than 2 million bases. The Human Genome Project has estimated that humans have between 30,000 and 40,000 genes. Every person has two copies of each gene, one inherited from each parent. Most genes are the same in all people, but a small number of genes (less than 1% of the total) are slightly different between people. Alleles are forms of the same gene with small differences in their sequence of DNA bases. These small differences contribute to each person's unique physical features.

Genetics: Genetics is the science of heredity (the genetic properties and phenomena of an organism), dealing with resemblances and differences of related organisms resulting from the interaction of their genes and the environment.

Genome: The biological information contained in a genome is encoded in its DNA and divided into discrete units called genes. Genes code for proteins that attach to the genome at the appropriate positions and switch on a series of reactions called gene expression.

Molecular marker: A gene or DNA sequence that can be used to identify an organism, species, or strain or phenotypic trait(s) associated with it.

Category II Modifiers

Category II Modifiers were added to CPT in 2006. There are two modifiers that have been included for exclusionary circumstances.

Definition of Category II Modifiers

Performance Measurement Inclusion/Exclusion Modifiers indicate that a service specified by a performance measure was considered, but due to certain circumstances documented in the medical record, the service was not provided.

These modifiers are used to identify services specified by a performance measure that was considered but not provided due to the following rationale:
- medical reasons
- patient circumstances

They are intended to be appended only to Category II codes. Category II codes are intended to facilitate data collection about the quality of care rendered by coding certain services and test results that support nationally established performance measures, and that have an evidence base as contributing to quality patient care. Use of Category II codes and modifiers is optional.

Category II modifiers should not be used with Category I or Category III codes. The Category II modifiers are reported according to whether the cause for exclusion is due to medical reasons or patient reasons.

Medical reasons (modifier 1P) include:
- Patient allergic history,
- Potential adverse drug interactions,
- Acquired or congenital absence of an organ/limb,
- Other documented clinical contraindications.

Patient reasons (modifier 2P) include:
- Patient refusal of treatment
- Economic
- Social
- Religious

Example 1

A patient with persistent arthritis returned to her physician for follow-up care. The physician performed and documented a detailed history and examination, and attempted to prescribe an anti-inflammatory drug. The patient indicated she had adverse reactions to various anti-inflammatory drugs in the past and refused the prescription. The physician reported the E/M service with code 99214. In addition, the physician documented the patient's refusal for the anti-inflammatory medication.

CPT Code(s) Billed: *99214—Office or other outpatient visit for the evaluation and management of an established patient, which requires at least two of these three key components: a detailed history; a detailed examination; medical decision making of moderate complexity.*

4016F 1P—Anti-inflammatory/analgesic agent prescribed

24.	A DATE(S) OF SERVICE						B Place of Service	C Type of Service	D PROCEDURES, SERVICES, OR SUPPLIES (Explain Unusual Circumstances) CPT/HCPCS | MODIFIER		E DIAGNOSIS CODE	F $ CHARGES	G DAYS OR UNITS	H EPSDT Family Plan	I EMG	J COB	K RESERVED FOR LOCAL USE
	From MM	DD	YY	To MM	DD	YY											
1									99214								
2									4016F	1P							
3																	
4																	
5																	
6																	
25. FEDERAL TAX I.D. NUMBER				SSN EIN			26. PATIENT/S ACCOUNT NO.		27. ACCEPT ASSIGNMENT? (For govt. claims, see back) YES NO		28. TOTAL CHARGE $		29. AMOUNT PAID $		30. BALANCE DUE $		

Rationale for Using Modifier 1P

Because the patient was prescribed the anti-inflammatory and refused the drug due to adverse reactions in the past, Category II code 4016F would be reported. Modifier 1P indicates that even though therapy was prescribed, the exclusion is due to a medical circumstance.

Example 2

A 45-year-old patient visiting a new family practitioner underwent a preventive medicine examination. The patient was a 25-year, two-pack-a-day smoker with a family history of heart disease. After completing the physical examination the physician provided counseling and offered pharmacologic intervention to help the patient quit smoking. The patient indicated he was not interested because he enjoyed smoking, and he would not further discuss the issue with the physician.

CPT Code(s) Billed: *99386—Initial comprehensive preventive medicine evaluation and management of an individual including an age and gender appropriate history, examination, counseling/anticipatory guidance/risk factor reduction interventions, and the ordering of appropriate immunization(s), laboratory/diagnostic procedures, new patient; 40–64 years*

4000F 2P—Tobacco use cessation intervention, counseling

Rationale for Using Modifier 2P

Because the physician attempted smoking cessation intervention but the patient refused, modifier 2P is appended to 4000F for smoking cessation intervention. Make sure the Category II codes are not reported as the primary procedure on the claim form.

As is true with other CPT modifiers, these modifiers should be appended to the specific Category II code(s) for which they apply.

NOTE: Only append the Category II modifiers to Category II codes. Do not append these modifiers to Category I or Category III codes.

Test Your Knowledge

Select the appropriate Modifier

1. _____ F13, commonly called Factor XIII (bleeding or hypercoagulable state) Beta globin

2. _____ VHL (Von Hippel Lindau disease, renal carcinoma)

3. _____ MTTK, commonly called tRNAlys (myotonic epilepsy, MERRF)

4. _____ HLA-C

5. _____ Exclusion due to economic reasons

6. _____ HEXA, commonly called Hexosaminidase A (Tay-Sachs disease)

7. _____ Microsatellite loss (loss of hererozygosity)

8. _____ NAT2 (drug metabolism)

9. _____ COL1A1 or PDGFB (Dermatofibrosarcoma protruberans)

10. _____ TWIST (Saethre-Chotzen syndrome)

11. _____ CBFB or MHY11, genes associated with inv 16 (Acute myelogenous leukemia) CBF beta (Leukemia)

12. _____ Dysmorphology, not otherwise specified

13. _____ Exclusion due to an acquired absence of a limb

14. _____ GJB1, commonly called Connexin-32 (X-linked Charcot-Marie-Tooth disease)

15. _____ PRSS1 (Hereditary pancreatitis)

APPENDIX A

HCPCS (Level I) CPT Modifiers

CPT Modifiers

The following list includes all of the modifiers applicable to the CPT® code set.

NOTE: All CPT modifiers in references to the five-digit modifier codes have been deleted.

TABLE A-1 CPT Modifiers

CPT Modifier	Description
21	**Prolonged Evaluation and Management Services** When the face-to-face or floor/unit service(s) provided is prolonged or otherwise greater than that usually required for the highest level of evaluation and management service within a given category, it may be identified by adding modifier 21 to the evaluation and management code number. A report may also be appropriate.
22	**Unusual Procedural Services** When the service(s) provided is greater than that usually required for the listed procedure, it may be identified by adding modifier 22 to the usual procedure number. A report may also be appropriate.
23	**Unusual Anesthesia** Occasionally, a procedure, which usually requires either no anesthesia or local anesthesia, because of unusual circumstances must be done under general anesthesia. This circumstance may be reported by adding the modifier 23 to the procedure code of the basic service.
24	**Unrelated Evaluation and Management Service by the Same Physician During a Postoperative Period** The physician may need to indicate that an evaluation and management service was performed during a postoperative period for a reason(s) unrelated to the original procedure. This circumstance may be reported by adding the modifier 24 to the appropriate level of E/M service.
25	**Significant, Separately Identifiable Evaluation and Management Service by the Same Physician on the Same Day of the Procedure or Other Service** The physician may need to indicate that on the day a procedure or service identified by a CPT code was performed, the patient's condition required a significant, separately identifiable E/M service above and beyond the other service provided or beyond the usual preoperative and postoperative care associated with the procedure that was performed. A significant, separately identifiable E/M service is defined or substantiated by documentation that satisfies the relevant criteria for the respective E/M service to be reported

TABLE A-1	**CPT Modifiers,** *continued*

CPT Modifier	Description
	(see **Evaluation and Management Services Guidelines** for instructions on determining level of E/M service). The E/M service may be prompted by the symptom or condition for which the procedure and/or service was provided. As such, different diagnoses are not required for reporting of the E/M service. **Note:** This modifier is not used to report an E/M service that resulted in a decision to perform surgery (see modifier 57).
26	**Professional Component** Certain procedures are a combination of a physician component and a technical component. When the physician component is reported separately, the service may be identified by adding the modifier 26 to the usual procedure number.
27	**Multiple Outpatient Hospital E/M Encounters on the Same Date** For hospital outpatient reporting purposes, utilization of hospital resources related to separate and distinct hospital E/M encounters performed in multiple outpatient hospital settings on the same date may be reported by adding the modifier 27 to each appropriate level outpatient and/or emergency department E/M code(s). This modifier provides a means of reporting circumstances involving evaluation and management services provided by physician(s) in more than one (multiple) outpatient hospital setting(s) (eg, hospital emergency department, clinic). **Note:** This modifier is not to be used for physician reporting of multiple E/M services performed by the same physician on the same date. For physician reporting of all outpatient evaluation and management services provided by the same physician on the same date and performed in multiple outpatient setting(s) (eg, hospital emergency department, clinic), see **Evaluation and Management, Emergency Department,** or **Preventive Medicine Services** codes.
32	**Mandated Services** Services related to mandated consultation and/or related services (eg, PRO, third-party payer, governmental, legislative, or regulatory requirement) may be identified by adding the modifier 32 to the basic procedure.
47	**Anesthesia by Surgeon** Regional or general anesthesia provided by the surgeon may be reported by adding the modifier 47 to the basic service. (This does not include local anesthesia.) **Note:** Modifier 47 would not be used as a modifier for the anesthesia procedures.

CPT Modifier	Description

50   **Bilateral Procedure**

Unless otherwise identified in the listings, bilateral procedures that are performed at the same operative session should be identified by adding the modifier 50 to the appropriate five-digit code.

51   **Multiple Procedures**

When multiple procedures, other than E/M services, are performed at the same session by the same provider, the primary procedure or service may be reported as listed. The additional procedure(s) or service(s) may be identified by appending the modifier 51 to the additional procedure or service code(s). **Note:** This modifier should not be appended to designated "add-on" codes (see Appendix D).

52   **Reduced Services**

Under certain circumstances, a service or procedure is partially reduced or eliminated at the physician's discretion. Under these circumstances, the service provided can be identified by its usual procedure number and the addition of the modifier 52, signifying that the service is reduced. This provides a means of reporting reduced services without disturbing the identification of the basic service. **Note:** For hospital outpatient reporting of a previously scheduled procedure/service that is partially reduced or canceled as a result of extenuating circumstances or those that threaten the well-being of the patient prior to or after administration of anesthesia, see modifiers 73 and 74 (see modifiers approved for ASC hospital outpatient use).

53   **Discontinued Procedure**

Under certain circumstances, the physician may elect to terminate a surgical or diagnostic procedure. Due to extenuating circumstances or those that threaten the well-being of the patient, it may be necessary to indicate that a surgical or diagnostic procedure was started but discontinued. This circumstance may be reported by adding the modifier 53 to the code reported by the physician for the discontinued procedure. **Note:** This modifier is not used to report the elective cancellation of a procedure prior to the patient's anesthesia induction and/or surgical preparation in the operating suite. For outpatient hospital/ambulatory surgery center (ASC) reporting of a previously scheduled procedure/service that is partially reduced or canceled as a result of extenuating circumstances or those that threaten the well-being of the patient prior to or after administration of anesthesia, see modifiers 73 and 74 (see modifiers approved for ASC hospital outpatient use).

54   **Surgical Care Only**

When one physician performs a surgical procedure and another provides preoperative and/or postoperative management, surgical

TABLE A-1 CPT Modifiers, *continued*

CPT Modifier	Description
	services may be identified by adding the modifier 54 to the usual procedure number.
55	**Postoperative Management Only** When one physician performed the postoperative management and another physician performed the surgical procedure, the postoperative component may be identified by adding the modifier 55 to the usual procedure number.
56	**Preoperative Management Only** When one physician performed the preoperative care and evaluation and another physician performed the surgical procedure, the preoperative component may be identified by adding the modifier 56 to the usual procedure number.
57	**Decision for Surgery** An evaluation and management service that resulted in the initial decision to perform the surgery may be identified by adding the modifier 57 to the appropriate level of E/M service.
58	**Staged or Related Procedure or Service by the Same Physician During the Postoperative Period** The physician may need to indicate that the performance of a procedure or service during the postoperative period was: (a) planned prospectively at the time of the original procedure (staged); (b) more extensive than the original procedure; or (c) for therapy following a diagnostic surgical procedure. This circumstance may be reported by adding the modifier 58 to the staged or related procedure. **Note:** This modifier is not used to report the treatment of a problem that requires a return to the operating room. See modifier 78.
59	**Distinct Procedural Service** Under certain circumstances, the physician may need to indicate that a procedure or service was distinct or independent from other services performed on the same day. Modifier 59 is used to identify procedures/services that are not normally reported together, but are appropriate under the circumstances. This may represent a different session or patient encounter, different procedure or surgery, different site or organ system, separate incision/excision, separate lesion, or separate injury (or area of injury in extensive injuries) not ordinarily encountered or performed on the same day by the same physician. However, when another already established modifier is appropriate, it should be used rather than modifier 59. Only if no more descriptive modifier is available, and the use of modifier 59 best explains the circumstances, should modifier 59 be used.

CPT Modifier	Description

62

Two Surgeons

When two surgeons work together as primary surgeons performing distinct part(s) of a procedure, each surgeon should report his/her distinct operative work by adding the modifier 62 to the procedure code and any associated add-on code(s) for that procedure as long as both surgeons continue to work together as primary surgeons. Each surgeon should report the cosurgery once using the same procedure code. If additional procedure(s) (including add-on procedure[s]) are performed during the same surgical session, separate code(s) may also be reported with the modifier 62 added. **Note:** If a co-surgeon acts as an assistant in the performance of additional procedure(s) during the same surgical session, those services may be reported using separate procedure code(s) with the modifier 80 or modifier 82 added as appropriate.

63

Procedure Performed on Infants Less than 4 kg

Procedures performed on neonates and infants up to a present body weight of 4 kg may involve significantly increased complexity and physician work commonly associated with these patients. This circumstance may be reported by adding the modifier 63 to the procedure number. **Note:** Unless otherwise designated, this modifier may only be appended to procedures/services listed in the 20000-69990 code series. Modifier 63 should not be appended to any CPT code listed in the Evaluation and Management Services, Anesthesia, Radiology, Pathology/Laboratory, or Medicine sections of the CPT book.

66

Surgical Team

Under some circumstances, highly complex procedures (requiring the concomitant services of several physicians, often of different specialties, plus other highly skilled, specially trained personnel, various types of complex equipment) are carried out under the "surgical team" concept. Such circumstances may be identified by each participating physician with the addition of the modifier 66 to the basic procedure number used for reporting services.

76

Repeat Procedure by Same Physician

The physician may need to indicate that a procedure or service was repeated subsequent to the original procedure or service. This circumstance may be reported by adding the modifier 76 to the repeated procedure/service.

77

Repeat Procedure by Another Physician

The physician may need to indicate that a basic procedure or service performed by another physician had to be repeated. This situation may be reported by adding the modifier 77 to the repeated procedure/service.

TABLE A-1	**CPT Modifiers,** *continued*
CPT Modifier	**Description**
78	**Return to the Operating Room for a Related Procedure During the Postoperative Period** The physician may need to indicate that another procedure was performed during the postoperative period of the initial procedure. When this subsequent procedure is related to the first, and requires the use of the operating room, it may be reported by adding the modifier 78 to the related procedure. (For repeat procedures on the same day, see 76.)
79	**Unrelated Procedure or Service by the Same Physician During the Postoperative Period** The physician may need to indicate that the performance of a procedure or service during the postoperative period was unrelated to the original procedure. This circumstance may be reported by using the modifier 79. (For repeat procedures on the same day, see 76.)
80	**Assistant Surgeon** Surgical assistant services may be identified by adding the modifier 80 to the usual procedure number(s).
81	**Minimum Assistant Surgeon** Minimum surgical assistant services are identified by adding the modifier 81 to the usual procedure number.
82	**Assistant Surgeon (when qualified resident surgeon not available)** The unavailability of a qualified resident surgeon is a prerequisite for use of modifier 82 appended to the usual procedure code number(s).
90	**Reference (Outside) Laboratory** When laboratory procedures are performed by a party other than the treating or reporting physician, the procedure may be identified by adding the modifier 90 to the usual procedure number.
91	**Repeat Clinical Diagnostic Laboratory Test** In the course of treatment of the patient, it may be necessary to repeat the same laboratory test on the same day to obtain subsequent (multiple) test results. Under these circumstances, the laboratory test performed can be identified by its usual procedure number and the addition of the modifier 91. **Note:** This modifier may not be used when tests are rerun to confirm initial results; due to testing problems with specimens or equipment; or for any other reason when a normal, one-time, reportable result is all that is required. This modifier may not be used when other code(s)

CPT Modifier	Description
	describe a series of test results (eg, glucose tolerance tests, evocative/suppression testing). This modifier may only be used for laboratory test(s) performed more than once on the same day on the same patient.
99	**Multiple Modifiers** Under certain circumstances two or more modifiers may be necessary to completely delineate a service. In such situations modifier 99 should be added to the basic procedure, and other applicable modifiers may be listed as part of the description of the service.

Anesthesia Physical Status Modifiers

The Physical Status modifiers are consistent with the American Society of Anesthesiologists ranking of patient physical status and distinguish various levels of complexity of the anesthesia service provided. All anesthesia services are reported by use of the anesthesia five-digit procedure code (00100-03108) with the appropriate physical status modifier appended.

Example: 00100 P4 33

TABLE A-2 **Physical Status Modifiers**	
Physical Status Modifier	**Description**
P1	A normal healthy patient
P2	A patient with mild systemic disease
P3	A patient with severe systemic disease
P4	A patient with severe systemic disease that is a constant threat to life
P5	A moribund patient who is not expected to survive without the operation
P6	A declared brain-dead patient whose organs are being removed for donor purposes

Modifiers Approved for Ambulatory Surgery Center (ASC) Hospital Outpatient Use

The following includes all of the CPT level I modifiers approved for ASC hospital outpatient use.

TABLE A-3	**CPT (HCPCS Level 1) Modifiers Approved for the ASC**
CPT Level I Modifier	**Description**
25	**Significant, Separately Identifiable Evaluation and Management Service by the Same Physician on the Same Day of the Procedure or Other Service** The physician may need to indicate that on the day a procedure or service identified by a CPT code was performed, the patient's condition required a significant, separately identifiable E/M service above and beyond the other service provided or beyond the usual preoperative and postoperative care associated with the procedure that was performed. A significant, separately identifiable E/M service is defined or substantiated by documentation that satisfies the relevant criteria for the respective E/M service to be reported (see **Evaluation and Management Services Guidelines** for instructions on determining level of E/M service). The E/M service may be prompted by the symptom or condition for which the procedure and/or service was provided. As such, different diagnoses are not required for reporting of the E/M service. **Note:** This modifier is not used to report an E/M service that resulted in a decision to perform surgery (see modifier 57).
27	**Multiple Outpatient Hospital E/M Encounters on the Same Date** For hospital outpatient reporting purposes, utilization of hospital resources related to separate and distinct E/M encounters performed in multiple outpatient hospital settings on the same date may be reported by adding the modifier 27 to each appropriate level outpatient and/or emergency department E/M code(s). This modifier provides a means of reporting circumstances involving evaluation and management services provided by physician(s) in more than one (multiple) outpatient hospital setting(s) (eg, hospital emergency department, clinic). **Note:** This modifier is not to be used for physician reporting of multiple E/M services performed by the same physician on the same date. For physician reporting of all outpatient evaluation and management services provided by the same physician on the same date and performed in multiple outpatient setting(s) (eg, hospital emergency department, clinic), see **Evaluation and Management, Emergency Department,** or **Preventive Medicine Services** codes.

CPT Level I Modifier	Description

50

Bilateral Procedure

Unless otherwise identified in the listings, bilateral procedures that are performed at the same operative session should be identified by adding the modifier 50 to the appropriate five-digit code.

52

Reduced Services

Under certain circumstances a service or procedure is partially reduced or eliminated at the physician's discretion. Under these circumstances the service provided can be identified by its usual procedure number and the addition of the modifier 52, signifying that the service is reduced. This provides a means of reporting reduced services without disturbing the identification of the basic service. **Note:** For CPT Level I Modifiers, hospital outpatient reporting of a previously scheduled procedure/service that is partially reduced or canceled as a result of extenuating circumstances or those that threaten the well-being of the patient prior to or after administration of anesthesia, see modifiers 73 and 74.

58

Staged or Related Procedure or Service by the Same Physician During the Postoperative Period

The physician may need to indicate that the performance of a procedure or service during the postoperative period was: (a) planned prospectively at the time of the original procedure (staged); (b) more extensive than the original procedure; or (c) for therapy following a diagnostic surgical procedure. This circumstance may be reported by adding the modifier 58 to the staged or related procedure. **Note:** This modifier is not used to report the treatment of a problem that requires a return to the operating room. See modifier 78.

59

Distinct Procedural Service

Under certain circumstances, the physician may need to indicate that a procedure or service was distinct or independent from other services performed on the same day. Modifier 59 is used to identify procedures/services that are not normally reported together, but are appropriate under the circumstances. This may represent a different session or patient encounter, different procedure or surgery, different site or organ system, separate incision/excision, separate lesion, or separate injury (or area of injury in extensive injuries) not ordinarily encountered or performed on the same day by the same physician. However, when another already established modifier is appropriate it should

TABLE A-3 **CPT (HCPCS Level 1) Modifiers Approved for the ASC,** *continued*	
CPT Level I Modifier	**Description**
	be used rather than modifier 59. Only if no more descriptive modifier is available, and the use of modifier 59 best explains the circumstances, should modifier 59 be used.
73	**Discontinued Outpatient Hospital/Ambulatory Surgery Center (ASC) Procedure Prior to the Administration of Anesthesia** Due to extenuating circumstances or those that threaten the well-being of the patient, the physician may cancel a surgical or diagnostic procedure subsequent to the patient's surgical preparation (including sedation when provided, and being taken to the room where the procedure is to be performed), but prior to the administration of anesthesia (local, regional block(s), or general). Under these circumstances, the intended service that is prepared for but canceled can be reported by its usual procedure number and the addition of the modifier 73. **Note:** The elective cancellation of a service prior to the administration of anesthesia and/or surgical preparation of the patient should not be reported. For physician reporting of a discontinued procedure, see modifier 53.
74	**Discontinued Outpatient Hospital/Ambulatory Surgery Center (ASC) Procedure After Administration of Anesthesia** Considering the well-being of the patient, the physician may terminate a surgical or diagnostic procedure after the administration of anesthesia (local, regional block[s], general), or after the procedure was started (incision made, intubation started, scope inserted, etc). Under these circumstances, the procedure started but terminated can be reported by its usual procedure number and the addition of the modifier 74. **Note:** The elective cancellation of a service prior to the administration of anesthesia and/or surgical preparation of the patient should not be reported. For physician reporting of a discontinued procedure, see modifier 53.
76	**Repeat Procedure by Same Physician** The physician may need to indicate that a procedure or service was repeated subsequent to the original procedure or service. This circumstance may be reported by adding the modifier 76 to the repeated procedure/service.

CPT Level I Modifier	Description

77

Repeat Procedure by Another Physician

The physician may need to indicate that a basic procedure or service performed by another physician had to be repeated. This situation may be reported by adding modifier 77 to the repeated procedure/service.

78

Return to the Operating Room for a Related Procedure During the Postoperative Period

The physician may need to indicate that another procedure was performed during the postoperative period of the initial procedure. When this subsequent procedure is related to the first and requires the use of the operating room, it may be reported by adding the modifier 78 to the related procedure. (For repeat procedures on the same day, see 76.)

79

Unrelated Procedure or Service by the Same Physician During the Postoperative Period

The physician may need to indicate that the performance of a procedure or service during the postoperative period was unrelated to the original procedure. This circumstance may be reported by using the modifier 79. (For repeat procedures on the same day, see 76.)

91

Repeat Clinical Diagnostic Laboratory Test

In the course of treatment of the patient, it may be necessary to repeat the same laboratory test on the same day to obtain subsequent (multiple) test results. Under these circumstances, the laboratory test performed can be identified by its usual procedure number and the addition of the modifier 91. **Note:** This modifier may not be used when tests are rerun to confirm initial results; due to testing problems with specimens or equipment; or for any other reason when a normal, one-time, reportable result is all that is required. This modifier may not be used when other code(s) describe a series of test results (eg, glucose tolerance tests, evocative/suppression testing). This modifier may only be used for laboratory tests(s) performed more than once on the same day on the same patient.

APPENDIX B

HCPCS (Level II) Modifiers

HCPCS Modifiers

The following is a list of the HCPCS (Level II) modifiers.

TABLE B-1 **Level II HCPCS Modifiers**	
HCPCS Modifier	**Description**
A1	Dressing for one wound
A2	Dressing for two wounds
A3	Dressing for three wounds
A4	Dressing for four wounds
A5	Dressing for five wounds
A6	Dressing for six wounds
A7	Dressing for seven wounds
A8	Dressing for eight wounds
A9	Dressing for nine or more wounds
AA	Anesthesia services performed personally by anesthesiologist
AD	Medical supervision by a physician; more than four concurrent anesthesia procedures
AE	Registered dietician
AF	Specialty physician
AG	Primary physician
AH	Clinical psychologist
AJ	Clinical social worker
AK	Non-participating physician
AM	Physician, team member service
AP	Determination of refractive state was not performed in the course of diagnostic ophthalmological examination
AQ	Physician providing a service in an unlisted health professional shortage area (HPSA)
AR	Physician provider services in a physician scarcity area
AS	Physician assistant, nurse practitioner, or clinical nurse specialist services for assistant at surgery
AT	Acute treatment (This modifier should be used when reporting service 98940, 98941, 98942)

TABLE B-1 **Level II HCPCS Modifiers,** *continued*	
HCPCS Modifier	**Description**
AU	Item furnished in conjunction with a urological, ostomy, or tracheostomy supply
AV	Item furnished in conjunction with a prosthetic device, prosthetic, or orthotic
AW	Item furnished in conjunction with a surgical dressing
AX	Item furnished in conjunction with dialysis services
BA	Item furnished in conjunction with parenteral enteral nutrition (PEN) services
BL	Special acquisition of blood and blood products
BO	Orally administered nutrition, not by feeding tube
BP	The beneficiary has been informed of the purchase and rental options and has elected to purchase the item
BR	The beneficiary has been informed of the purchase and rental options and had elected to rent the item
BU	The beneficiary has been informed of the purchase and rental options and after 30 days has not informed the supplier of his/her decision
CA	Procedure payable only in the inpatient setting when performed emergently on an outpatient who expires prior to admission
CB	Service ordered by a renal dialysis facility (RDF) physician as part of the ESRD Beneficiary's dialysis benefit, is not part of the composite rate, and is separately reimbursable
CC	Procedure code change (use CC when the procedure code submitted was changed either for administrative reasons or because an incorrect code was filed)
CD	AMCC test that has been ordered by an ERSD facility or MCP physician that is part of the composite rate and is not separately billable
CE	AMCC test has been ordered by an ESRD facility or MCP physician that is a composite rate test but is beyond the normal frequency covered under the rate and is separately reimbursable based on medical necessity
CF	AMCC test has been ordered by an ESRD facility or MCP physician that is not part of the composite rate and is separately billable

HCPCS Modifier	Description
CR	Catastrophe/disaster related
E1	Upper, left eyelid
E2	Lower, left eyelid
E3	Upper, right eyelid
E4	Lower, right eyelid
EJ	Subsequent claims for a defined course of therapy, (eg, EPO, Sodium Hyaluronate, Infliximab)
EM	Emergency reserve supply (for ESRD benefit only)
EP	Service provided as part of Medicaid early periodic screening diagnosis and treatment (EPSDT) program
ET	Emergency services
EY	No physician or other licensed health care provider order for this item or service
F1	Left hand, second digit
F2	Left hand, third digit
F3	Left hand, fourth digit
F4	Left hand, fifth digit
F5	Right hand, thumb
F6	Right hand, second digit
F7	Right hand, third digit
F8	Right hand, fourth digit
F9	Right hand, fifth digit
FA	Left hand, thumb
FB	Item provided without cost to provider, supplier, or practitioner (examples, but not limited to: covered under warranty, replaced due to defect, free samples)
FP	Service provided as part of Family Planning Program
G1	Most recent URR reading of less than 60
G2	Most recent URR reading of 60 to 64.9
G3	Most recent URR reading of 65 to 69.9
G4	Most recent URR reading of 70 to 74.9
G5	Most recent URR reading of 75 or greater

TABLE B-1 **Level II HCPCS Modifiers,** *continued*

HCPCS Modifier	Description
G6	ESRD patient for whom less than six dialysis sessions have been provided in a month
G7	Pregnancy resulted from rape or incest or pregnancy certified by physician as life threatening
G8	Monitored anesthesia care (MAC) for deep complex, complicated, or markedly invasive surgical procedure
G9	Monitored anesthesia care for patient who has history of severe cardiopulmonary condition
GA	Waiver of liability statement on file
GB	Claim being re-submitted for payment because it is no longer covered under a global payment demonstration
GC	This service has been performed in part by a resident under the direction of a teaching physician
GE	This service has been performed by a resident without the presence of a teaching physician under the primary care exception
GF	Non-physician (eg, nurse practitioner (NP), certified registered nurse anesthetist (CRNA), certified registered nurse (CRN), clinical nurse specialist (CNS), physician assistant (PA)) services in a Critical Access Hospital
GG	Performance and payment of a screening mammogram and diagnostic mammogram on the same patient, same day
GH	Diagnostic mammogram converted from screening mammogram on same day
GJ	"Opt Out" physician or practitioner emergency or urgent care
GK	Actual item/service ordered by physician, item associated with GA or GZ modifier
GL	Medically unnecessary upgrade provided instead of standard item, no charge, no advance beneficiary notice (ABN)
GM	Multiple patients on one ambulance trip
GN	Services delivered under an outpatient speech language pathology plan of care
GO	Services delivered under an outpatient occupational therapy plan of care
GP	Services delivered under an outpatient physical therapy plan of care

HCPCS Modifier	Description
GQ	Via asynchronous telecommunication system
GR	This service was performed in whole or in part by a resident in a department of veterans affairs medical center or clinic, supervised in accordance with VA policy
GS	Dosage of EPO or Darbepoietin Alfa has been reduced 25% of preceding month's dosage
GT	Via interactive audio and video telecommunication systems
GV	Attending physician not employed or paid under arrangement by the patient's hospice provider
GW	Service not related to the hospice patient's terminal condition
GY	Item or service statutorily excluded or does not meet the definition of any Medicare benefit
GZ	Item or service expected to be denied as not reasonable and necessary
H9	Court-ordered
HA	Child/adolescent program
HB	Adult program, non geriatric
HC	Adult program, geriatric
HD	Pregnant/parenting women's program
HE	Mental health program
HF	Substance abuse program
HG	Opioid addiction treatment program
HH	Integrated mental health/substance abuse program
HI	Integrated mental health and mental retardation/developmental disabilities program
HJ	Employee assistance program
HK	Specialized mental health programs for high-risk populations
HL	Intern
HM	Less than bachelor degree level
HN	Bachelors degree level
HO	Masters degree level
HP	Doctoral level
HQ	Group setting

TABLE B-1 **Level II HCPCS Modifiers,** *continued*

HCPCS Modifier	Description
HR	Family/couple with client present
HS	Family/couple without client present
HT	Multi-disciplinary team
HU	Funded by child welfare agency
HV	Funded by state addictions agency
HW	Funded by state mental health agency
HX	Funded by county/local agency
HY	Funded by juvenile justice agency
HZ	Funded by criminal justice agency
J1	Competitive Acquisition Program no-pay submission for a prescription number
J2	Competitive Acquisition Program, restocking of emergency drugs after emergency administration
J3	Competitive Acquisition Program (CAP), drug not available through CAP as written, reimbursed under Average Sales Price Methodology
JW	Drug amount discarded/not administered to any patient
K0	Lower extremity prosthesis functional level 0—does not have the ability or potential to ambulate or transfer safely with or without assistance and a prosthesis does not enhance their quality of life or mobility
K1	Lower extremity prosthesis functional level 1—has the ability or potential to use a prosthesis for transfers or ambulation on level surfaces at fixed cadence. Typical of the limited and unlimited household ambulator.
K2	Lower extremity prosthesis functional level 2—has the ability or potential for ambulation with the ability to traverse low level environmental barriers such as curbs, stairs, or uneven surfaces. Typical of the limited community ambulator.
K3	Lower extremity prosthesis functional level 3—has the ability or potential for ambulation with variable cadence. Typical of the community ambulator who has the ability to traverse most environmental barriers and may have vocational, therapeutic or exercise activity that demands prosthetic utilization beyond simple locomotion.

HCPCS Modifier	Description
K4	Lower extremity prosthesis functional level 4-has the ability or potential for prosthetic ambulation that exceeds the basic ambulation skills, exhibiting high impact, stress, or energy levels, typical of the prosthetic demands of the child, active adult, or athlete.
KA	Add-on option/accessory for wheelchair
KB	Beneficiary requested upgrade for ABN, more than 4 modifiers identified on claim
KC	Replacement of special power wheelchair interface
KD	Drug or biological infused through DME
KF	Item designated by FDA as Class III device
KH	DMEPOS item, initial claim, purchase or first month rental
KI	DMEPOS item, second or third month rental
KJ	DMEPOS item, parenteral enteral nutrition (PEN) pump or capped rental, months four to fifteen
KM	Replacement of facial prosthesis including new impression/moulage
KN	Replacement of facial prosthesis using previous master model
KO	Single drug unit dose formulation
KP	First drug of a multiple drug unit dose formulation
KQ	Second or subsequent drug of a multiple drug unit dose formulation
KR	Rental item, billing for partial month
KS	Glucose monitor supply for diabetic beneficiary not treated with insulin
KX	Specific required documentation on file
KZ	New coverage not implemented by Managed Care
LC	Left circumflex coronary artery
LD	Left anterior descending coronary artery
LL	Lease/rental (use the "LL" modifier when DME equipment rental is to be applied against the purchase price)
LR	Laboratory round trip
LS	FDA-monitored intraocular lens implant
LT	Left side (used to identify procedures performed on the left side of the body)

TABLE B-1 Level II HCPCS Modifiers, *continued*

HCPCS Modifier	Description
MS	Six month maintenance and servicing fee for reasonable and necessary parts and labor which are not covered under any manufacturer or supplier warranty
NR	New when rented (use "NR" modifier when DME which was new at the time of the rental is subsequently purchased)
NU	New equipment
PL	Progressive addition lenses
Q2	HCFA/ORD demonstration project procedure/service
Q3	Live kidney donor surgery and related services
Q4	Service for ordering/referring physician qualifies as a service exemption
Q5	Service furnished by a substitute physician under a reciprocal billing arrangement
Q6	Service furnished by a locum tenens physician
Q7	One class A finding
Q8	Two class B findings
Q9	One class B and two class C findings
QA	FDA investigational device exemption
QB	Physician providing service in a rural HPSA
QC	Single channel monitoring
QD	Recording and storage in solid state memory by a digital recorder
QE	Prescribed amount of oxygen is less than 1 liter per minute (LPM)
QF	Prescribed amount of oxygen exceeds 4 liters per minute (LPM) and portable oxygen is prescribed
QG	Prescribed amount of oxygen is greater than 4 liters per minute (LPM)
QH	Oxygen conserving device is being used with an oxygen delivery system
QJ	Services/items provided to a prisoner or patient in state or local custody, however the state or local government, as applicable, meets the requirements in 42 CFR 411.4 (b)

HCPCS Modifier	Description
QK	Medical direction of two, three, or four concurrent anesthesia procedures involving qualified individuals
QL	Patient pronounced dead after ambulance called
QM	Ambulance service provided under arrangement by a provider of services
QN	Ambulance service furnished directly by a provider of services
QP	Documentation is on file showing that the laboratory test(s) was ordered individually or ordered as a CPT-recognized panel other than automated profile codes 80002-80019, G0058, G0059, and G0060
QR	Item or service provided in a Medicare specified study
QS	Monitored anesthesia care service
QT	Recording and storage on tape by an analog tape recorder
QV	Item or service provided as routine care in a Medicare qualifying clinical trial
QW	CLIA waived test
QX	CRNA service: with medical direction by a physician
QY	Medical direction of one certified registered nurse anesthetist (CRNA) by an anesthesiologist
QZ	CRNA service: without medical direction by a physician
RC	Right coronary artery
RD	Drug provided to beneficiary, but not administered "Incident-To"
RP	Replacement and repair; RP may be used to indicate replacement of DME, orthotic and prosthetic devices which have been in use for some time. The claim shows the code for the part, followed by the "RP" modifier and the charge for the part.
RR	Rental (use of "RR" modifier when DME is to be rented)
RT	Right side (used to identify procedures performed on the right side of the body)
SA	Nurse practitioner rendering service in collaboration with a physician
SB	Nurse midwife
SC	Medically necessary service or supply

TABLE B-1 Level II HCPCS Modifiers, *continued*

HCPCS Modifier	Description
SD	Services provided by registered nurse with specialized, highly technical home infusion training
SE	State and/or federally funded programs/services
SF	Second opinion ordered by a professional review organization (PRO) per section 9401, P.L. 99-272 (100% reimbursement-no Medicare deductible or coinsurance)
SG	Ambulatory surgical center (ASC) facility service
SH	Second concurrently administered infusion therapy
SJ	Third or more concurrently administered infusion therapy
SK	Member of high risk population (use only with codes for immunization)
SL	State supplied vaccine
SM	Second surgical opinion
SN	Third surgical opinion
SQ	Item ordered by Home Health
SS	Home infusion services provided in the infusion suite of the IV therapy provider
ST	Related to trauma or injury
SU	Procedure performed in physician's office (to denote use of facility and equipment)
SV	Pharmaceuticals delivered to patient's home but not utilized
SW	Services provided by a certified diabetic educator
SY	Persons who are in close contact with member of high-risk population (use only with codes for immunization)
T1	Left foot, second digit
T2	Left foot, third digit
T3	Left foot, fourth digit
T4	Left foot, fifth digit
T5	Right foot, great toe
T6	Right foot, second digit
T7	Right foot, third digit

HCPCS Modifier	Description
T8	Right foot, fourth digit
T9	Right foot, fifth digit
TA	Left foot, great toe
TC	Technical component. Under certain circumstances, a charge may be made for the technical component alone. Under those circumstances the technical component charge is identified by adding modifier "TC" to the usual procedure number. Technical component charges are institutional charges and not billed separately by physicians. However, portable x-ray suppliers only bill for technical component and should utilize modifier TC. The charge data from portable x-ray suppliers will then be used to build customary and prevailing profiles.
TD	RN
TE	LPN/LVN
TF	Intermediate level of care
TG	Complex/high tech level of care
TH	Obstetrical treatment/services, prenatal or postpartum
TJ	Program group, child and/or adolescent
TK	Extra patient or passenger, non-ambulance
TL	Early intervention/individualized family service plan (IFSP)
TM	Individualized education program (IEP)
TN	Rural/outside service providers' customary service area
TP	Medical transport, unloaded vehicle
TQ	Basic life support transport by a volunteer ambulance provider
TR	School-based individualized education program (IEP) services provided outside the public school district responsible for the student
TS	Follow-up service
TT	Individualized service provided to more than one patient in the same setting
TU	Special payment rate, overtime
TV	Special payment rates, holidays/weekends
TW	Back-up equipment
U1	Medicaid level of care 1, as defined by each state

TABLE B-1 **Level II HCPCS Modifiers,** *continued*

HCPCS Modifier	Description
U2	Medicaid level of care 2, as defined by each state
U3	Medicaid level of care 3, as defined by each state
U4	Medicaid level of care 4, as defined by each state
U5	Medicaid level of care 5, as defined by each state
U6	Medicaid level of care 6, as defined by each state
U7	Medicaid level of care 7, as defined by each state
U8	Medicaid level of care 8, as defined by each state
U9	Medicaid level of care 9, as defined by each state
UA	Medicaid level of care 10, as defined by each state
UB	Medicaid level of care 11, as defined by each state
UC	Medicaid level of care 12, as defined by each state
UD	Medicaid level of care 13, as defined by each state
UE	Used durable medical equipment
UF	Services provided in the morning
UG	Services provided in the afternoon
UH	Services provided in the evening
UJ	Services provided at night
UK	Service on behalf of the client to someone other than the client (collateral relationship)
UN	Two patients served
UP	Three patients served
UQ	Four patients served
UR	Five patients served
US	Six or more patients served
VP	Aphakic patient

APPENDIX C

Genetic Testing Modifiers

See Chapter 10 for a list of CPT® codes currently used with CPT genetic modifiers.

TABLE C-1	**Genetic Testing Modifiers**
Modifier	**Description**
Neoplasia (solid tumor, excluding sarcoma and lymphoma)	
0A	BRCA1 (Hereditary breast/Ovarian cancer)
0B	BRCA2 (Hereditary breast cancer)
0C	Neurofibromin (Neurofibromatosis, type 1)
0D	Merlin (Neurofibromatosis, type 2)
0E	c-RET (Multiple endocrine neoplasia, types 2A/B, familial medullary thyroid carcinoma)
0F	VHL (Von Hippel Lindau disease, renal carcinoma)
0G	SDHD (Hereditary paraganglioma)
0H	SDHB (Hereditary paraganglioma)
0I	ERRB2, commonly called Her-2/neu
0J	MLH1 (HNPCC, mismatch repair genes)
0K	MSH2, MSH6, or PMS2 (HNPCC, mismatch repair genes)
0L	APC (Hereditary polyposis coli)
0M	Rb (Retinoblastoma)
0N	TP53, commonly called p53
0O	PTEN (Cowden's syndrome)
0P	KIT, also called CD117 (gastrointestinal stromal tumor)
0Z	Solid tumor gene, not otherwise specified
Neoplasia (Sarcoma)	
1A	WT1 or WT2 (Wilm's tumor)
1B	PAX3, PAX7, or FOXO1A (Alveolar rhabdomyosarcoma)
1C	FLI1, ERG, ETV1, or EWSR1 (Ewing's sarcoma, desmoplastic round cell)
1D	DDIT3 or FUS (Myxoid liposarcoma)
1E	NR4A3, RBF56 or TCF12 (Myxoid chondrosarcoma)
1F	SSX1, SSX2, or SYT (Synovial sarcoma)
1G	MYCN (Neuroblastoma)

TABLE C-1	**Genetic Testing Modifiers,** *continued*

Modifier	Description
1H	COL1A1 or PDGFB (Dermatofibrosarcoma protruberans)
1I	TFE3 or ASPSCR1 (Alveolar soft parts sarcoma)
1J	JAZF1 or JJAZ1 (Endometrial stromal sarcoma)
1Z	Sarcoma gene, not otherwise specified
Neoplasia (lymphoid/hematopoetic)	
2A	RUNX1 or CBFA2T1, commonly called AML1 or ETO, genes associated with t(8;21) AML1-also ETO (Acute myelogenous leukemia)
2B	BCR or ABL1, genes associated with t(9;22) (Chronic myelogenous or acute leukemia) BCR-also ABL (Chronic myeloid, acute lymphoid leukemia)
2C	PBX1 or TCF3, genes associated with t(1;19) (Acute lymphoblastic leukemia) CGF1
2D	CBFB or MYH11, genes associated with inv 16 (Acute myelogenous leukemia) CBF beta (Leukemia)
2E	MLL (acute leukemia)
2F	PML or RARA, genes associated with t(15;17) (Acute promyelocytic leukemia) PML/RAR alpha (Promyelocytic leukemia)
2G	ETV6, commonly called TEL, gene associated with t(12;21) (acute leukemia) TEL (Leukemia)
2H	BCL-2 (B cell lymphoma, follicle center cell origin) bcl-2 (Lymphoma)
2I	CCND1, commonly called BCL1, cyclin D1 (Mantle cell lymphoma, myeloma) bcl-1 (Lymphoma)
2J	MYC (Burkitt lymphoma) c-myc (Lymphoma)
2K	IgH (Lymphoma/leukemia)
2L	IGK (Lymphoma/leukemia)
2M	TRB, T cell receptor beta (Lymphoma/leukemia)
2N	TRG, T cell receptor gamma (Lymphoma/leukemia)
2O	SIL or TAL1 (T cell leukemia)
2T	BCL6 (B cell lymphoma)
2Q	API1 or MALT1 (MALT lymphoma)
2R	NPM or ALK, genes associated with t (2;5) (Anaplastic large cell lymphoma)

Modifier	Description
2S	FLT3 (Acute myelogenous leukemia)
2Z	Lymphoid/hematopoetic neoplasia, not otherwise specified

Non-neoplastic hematology/coagulation

Modifier	Description
3A	F5, commonly called Factor V (Leiden, others) (Hypercoagulable state)
3B	FACC (Fanconi anemia)
3C	FACD (Fanconi anemia)
3D	HBB, beta globin (Thalassemia, Sickle cell anemia, other hemoglobinopathies)
3E	HBA, commonly called alpha globin (Thalassemia)
3F	MTHFR (Elevated homocystinemia)
3G	F2, commonly called prothrombin (20210, others) Hypercoagulable state) Prothrombin (Factor II, 20210A) (Hypercoagulable state)
3H	F8, commonly called Factor VIII (Hemophilia A/VWF)
3I	F9, commonly called Factor IX (Hemophilia B)
3K	F13, commonly called Factor XIII (bleeding or hypercoagulable state) Beta globin
3Z	Non-neoplastic hematology/coagulation, not otherwise specified

Histocompatability/blood typing/identity/microsatellite

Modifier	Description
4A	HLA-A
4B	HLA-B
4C	HLA-C
4D	HLA-D
4E	HLA-DR
4F	HLA-DQ
4G	HLA-DP
4H	Kell
4I	Fingerprint for engraftment (post-allogeneic progenitor cell transplant)
4J	Fingerprint for donor allelotype (allogeneic transplant)
4K	Fingerprint for recipient allelotype (allogeneic transplant)
4L	Fingerprint for leukocyte chimerism (allogeneic solid organ transplant)

TABLE C-1 **Genetic Testing Modifiers,** *continued*

Modifier	Description
4M	Fingerprint for maternal versus fetal origin
4N	Microsatellite instability
4O	Microsatellite loss (loss of hererozygosity)
4Z	Histocompatability/blood typing, not otherwise specified

Neurologic, non-neoplastic

Modifier	Description
5A	ASPA, commonly called Aspartoacylase A (Canavan disease)
5B	FMR-1 (Fragile X, FRAXA, syndrome)
5C	FRDA, commonly called Frataxin (Freidreich's ataxia)
5D	HD, commonly called Huntington (Huntington's disease)
5E	GABRA5, NIPA1, UBE3A, or ANCR GABRA (Prader Willi-Angelman syndrome)
5F	GJB2, commonly called Connexin-26 (Hereditary hearing loss) Connexin-32 (GJB2) (Hereditary deafness)
5G	GJB1, commonly called Connexin-32 (X-linked Charcot-Marie-Tooth disease)
5H	SNRPN (Prader Willi-Angelman syndrome)
5I	SCA1, commonly called Ataxin-1 (Spinocerebellar ataxia, type 1)
5J	SCA2, commonly called Ataxin-2 (Spinocerebellar ataxia, type 2)
5K	MJD, commonly called Ataxin-3 (Spinocerebellar ataxia, type 3, Machado-Joseph disease)
5L	CACNA1A (Spinocerebellar ataxia, type 6)
5M	ATXN7 Ataxin-7 (Spinocerebellar ataxia, type 7)
5N	PMP-22 (Charcot-Marie-Tooth disease, type 1A)
5O	MECP2 (Rett syndrome)
5Z	Neurologic, non-neoplastic, not otherwise specified

Muscular, non-neoplastic

Modifier	Description
6A	DMD, commonly called dystrophin (Duchenne/Becker muscular dystrophy)
6B	DMPK (Myotonic dystrophy, type 1)
6C	ZNF-9 (Myotonic dystrophy, type 2)

Modifier	Description
6 D	SMN1/SMN2 (Autosomal recessive spinal muscular atrophy)
6 E	MTTK, commonly called tRNAlys (myotonic epilepsy, MERRF)
6 F	MTTL1, commonly called tRNAleu (mitochondrial encephalomyopathy, MELAS)
6 Z	Muscular, not otherwise specified

Metabolic, other

Modifier	Description
7 A	APOE, commonly called apolipoprotein E (Cardiovascular disease or Alzheimer's disease)
7 B	NPC1 or NPC2, commonly called sphingomyelin phosphodiesterase (Nieman-Pick disease)
7 C	GBA, commonly called acid beta glucosidase (Gaucher disease)
7 D	HFE (Hemochromatosis)
7 E	HEXA, commonly called hexosaminidase A (Tay-Sachs disease)
7 F	ACADM (medium chain acyl CoA dehydrogenase deficiency)
7 Z	Metabolic, other, not otherwise specified

Metabolic, transport

Modifier	Description
8 A	CFTR (Cystic fibrosis)
8 B	PRSS1 (Hereditary pancreatitis)
8 Z	Metabolic, transport, not otherwise specified

Metabolic-pharmacogenetics

Modifier	Description
9 A	TPMT commonly called (thiopurine methyltransferase) (patients on antimetabolite therapy)
9 B	CYP2 genes, commonly called cytochorme cytochrome p450 (drug metabolism)
9 C	ABCB1, commonly called MDR1 or p-glycoprotein (drug transport)
9 D	NAT2 (drug metabolism)
9 L	Metabolic-pharmacogenetics, not otherwise specified

Dysmorphology

Modifier	Description
9 M	FGFR1 (Pfeiffer and Kallmann syndromes)
9 N	FGFR2 (Crouzon, Jackson-Weiss, Apert, Saethre-Chotzen syndromes)

TABLE C-1	**Genetic Testing Modifiers,** *continued*

Modifier	Description
9 O	FGFR3 (Achondroplasia, Hypochondroplasia, Thanatophoric dysplasia, types I and II, Crouzon syndrome with acanthosis nigricans, Muencke syndromes)
9 P	TWIST (Saethre-Chotzen syndrome)
9 Q	DCGR, commonly called CATCH-22 (DiGeorge and 22q11 deletion syndromes)
9 Z	Dysmorphology, not otherwise specified

APPENDIX D

Logic Trees

MODIFIER 21

Prolonged Services

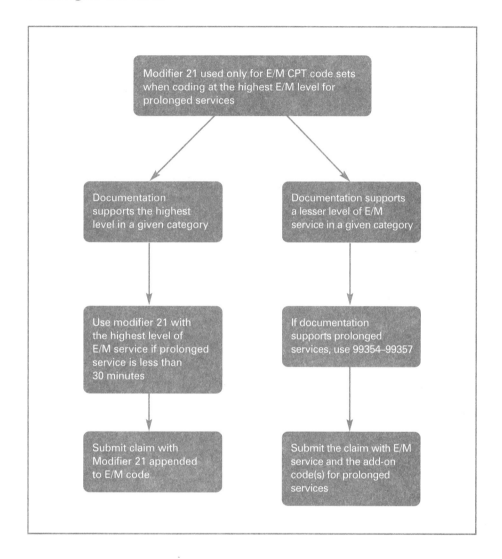

Modifier 21 used only for E/M CPT code sets when coding at the highest E/M level for prolonged services

Documentation supports the highest level in a given category

Documentation supports a lesser level of E/M service in a given category

Use modifier 21 with the highest level of E/M service if prolonged service is less than 30 minutes

If documentation supports prolonged services, use 99354–99357

Submit claim with Modifier 21 appended to E/M code

Submit the claim with E/M service and the add-on code(s) for prolonged services

MODIFIER 22

Unusual Procedure or Service

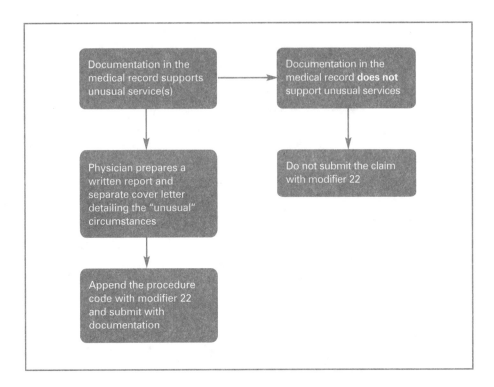

MODIFIER 23

Unusual Anesthesia

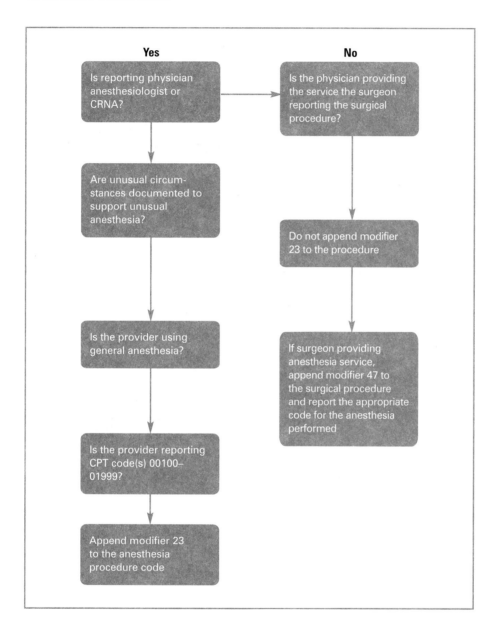

MODIFIER 24

Unrelated E/M Service by the Same
Physician During a Postoperative Period

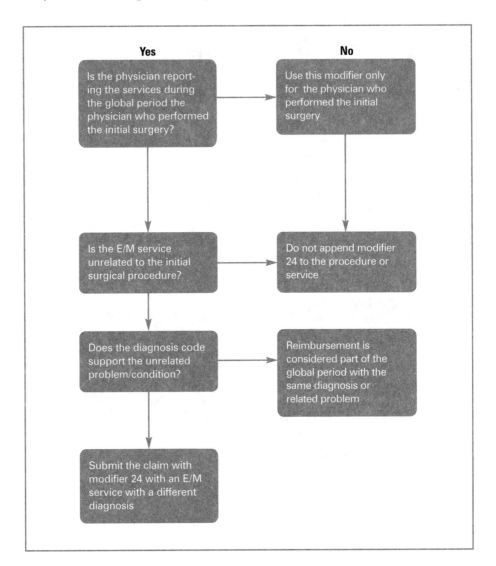

MODIFIER 25

Significant, Separately Identifiable E/M Service by the Same
Physician on the Same Day of the Procedure or Other Service

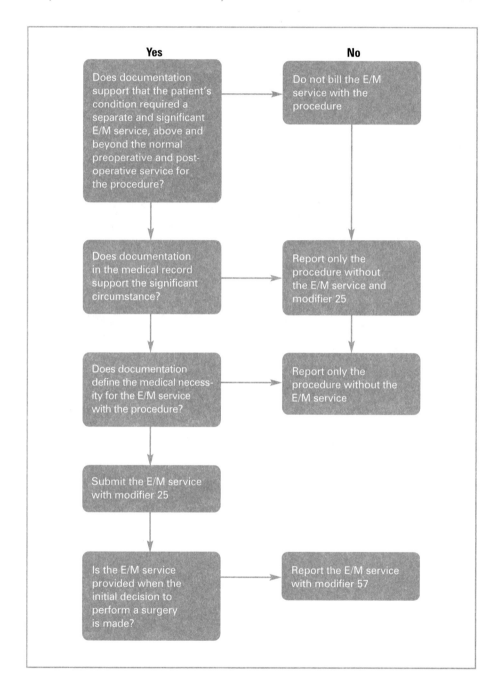

MODIFIER 26

Professional Component

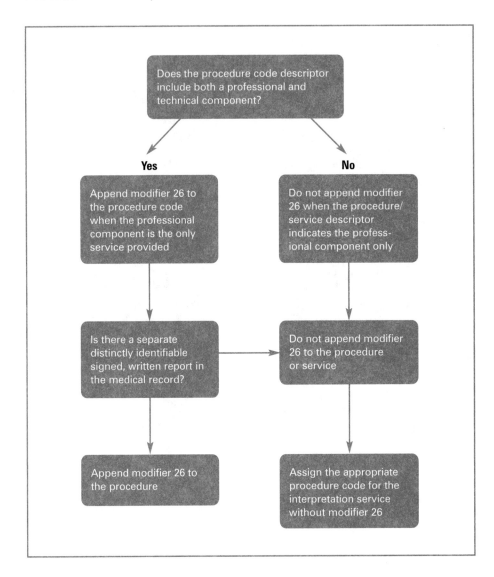

MODIFIER 27

Multiple Outpatient Hospital E/M Encounters
on the Same Date

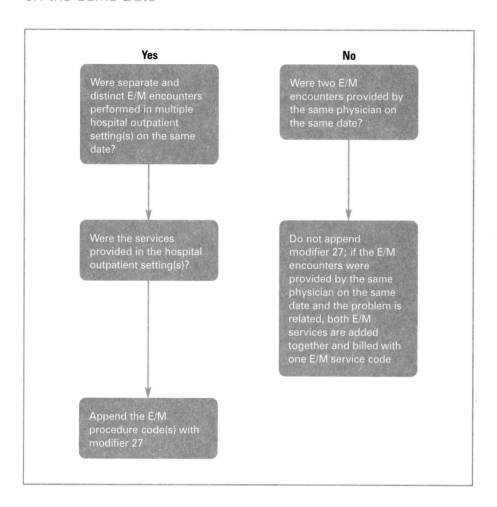

Yes

Were separate and distinct E/M encounters performed in multiple hospital outpatient setting(s) on the same date?

Were the services provided in the hospital outpatient setting(s)?

Append the E/M procedure code(s) with modifier 27

No

Were two E/M encounters provided by the same physician on the same date?

Do not append modifier 27; if the E/M encounters were provided by the same physician on the same date and the problem is related, both E/M services are added together and billed with one E/M service code

MODIFIER 32

Mandated Services

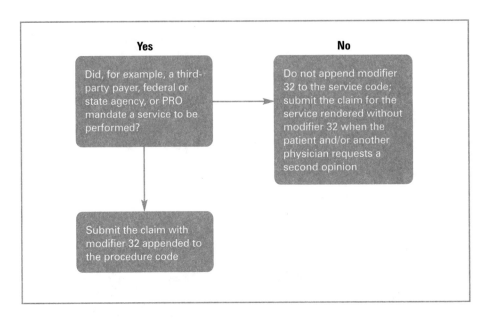

MODIFIER 47

Anesthesia by Surgeon

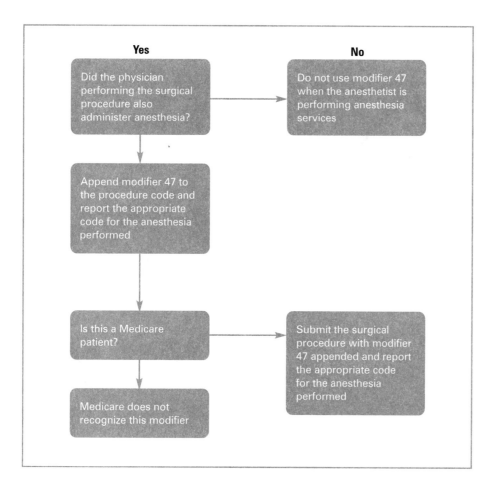

MODIFIER 50

Bilateral Procedures

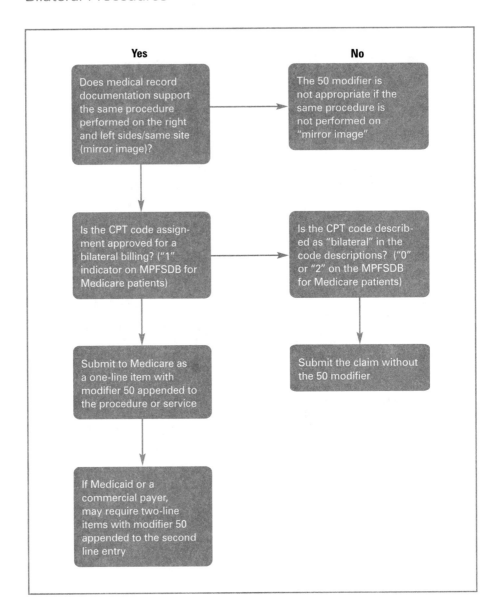

Yes

Does medical record documentation support the same procedure performed on the right and left sides/same site (mirror image)?

No

The 50 modifier is not appropriate if the same procedure is not performed on "mirror image"

Is the CPT code assignment approved for a bilateral billing? ("1" indicator on MPFSDB for Medicare patients)

Is the CPT code described as "bilateral" in the code descriptions? ("0" or "2" on the MPFSDB for Medicare patients)

Submit to Medicare as a one-line item with modifier 50 appended to the procedure or service

Submit the claim without the 50 modifier

If Medicaid or a commercial payer, may require two-line items with modifier 50 appended to the second line entry

MODIFIER 51

Multiple Procedures

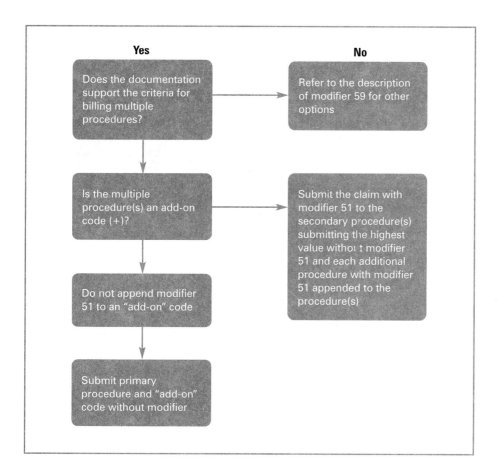

Yes / **No**

Does the documentation support the criteria for billing multiple procedures?

Refer to the description of modifier 59 for other options

Is the multiple procedure(s) an add-on code (+)?

Submit the claim with modifier 51 to the secondary procedure(s) submitting the highest value without modifier 51 and each additional procedure with modifier 51 appended to the procedure(s)

Do not append modifier 51 to an "add-on" code

Submit primary procedure and "add-on" code without modifier

MODIFIER 52

Reduced Services

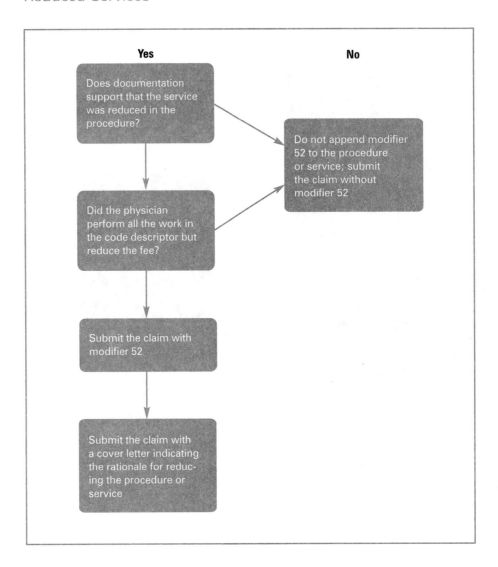

MODIFIER 53

Discontinued Procedure

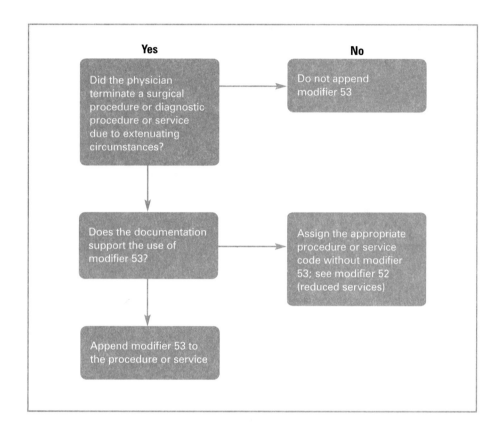

MODIFIER 54

Surgical Care Only

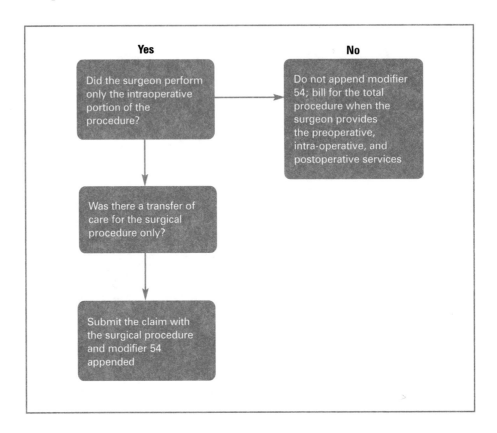

MODIFIER 55

Postoperative Management Only

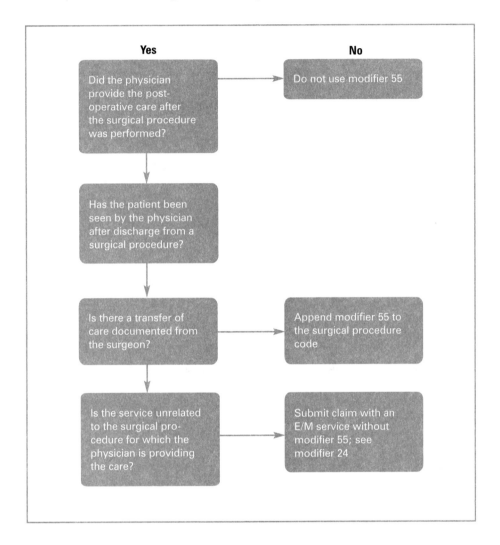

MODIFIER 56

Preoperative Management Only

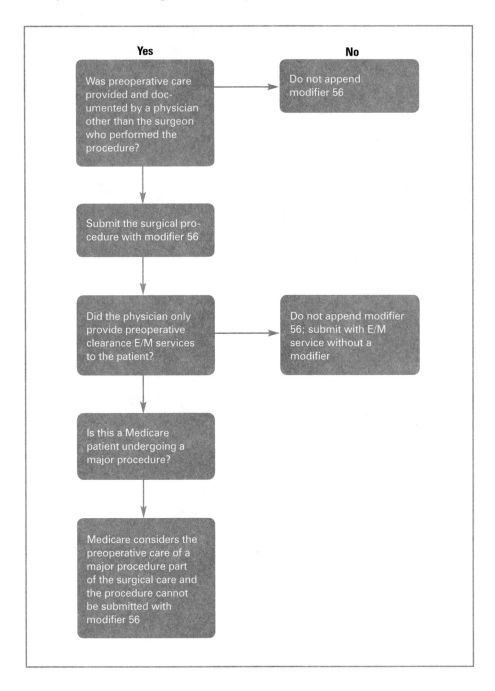

MODIFIER 57

Decision for Surgery

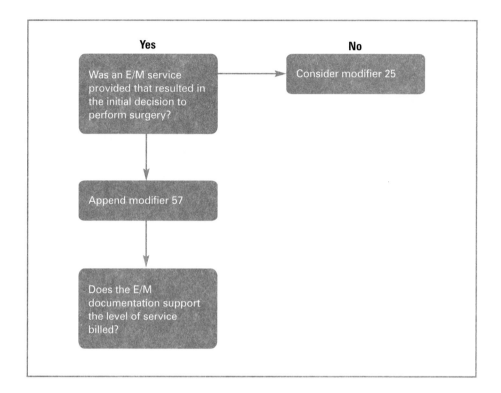

MODIFIER 58

Staged or Related Procedure or Service by the
Same Physician During the Postoperative Period

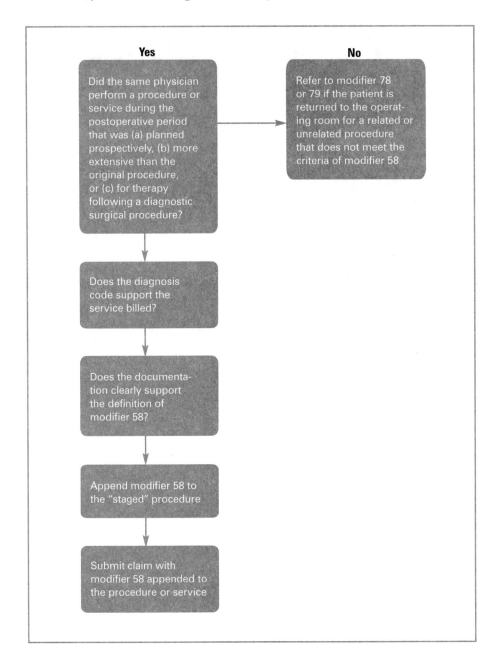

MODIFIER 59

Distinct Procedural Service

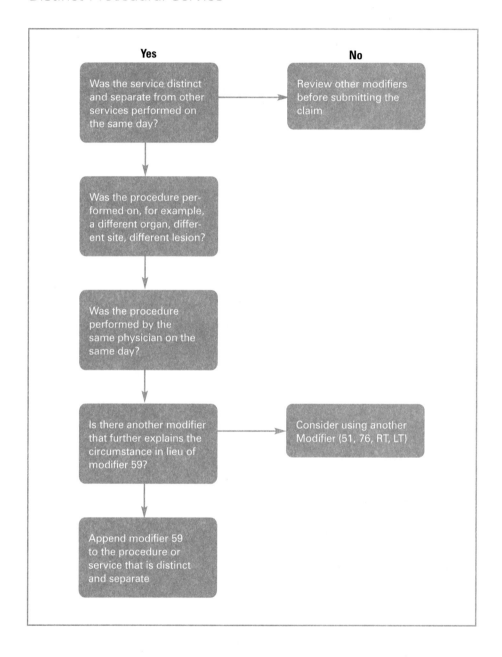

Yes

No

Was the service distinct and separate from other services performed on the same day?

Review other modifiers before submitting the claim

Was the procedure performed on, for example, a different organ, different site, different lesion?

Was the procedure performed by the same physician on the same day?

Is there another modifier that further explains the circumstance in lieu of modifier 59?

Consider using another Modifier (51, 76, RT, LT)

Append modifier 59 to the procedure or service that is distinct and separate

MODIFIER 62

Two Surgeons

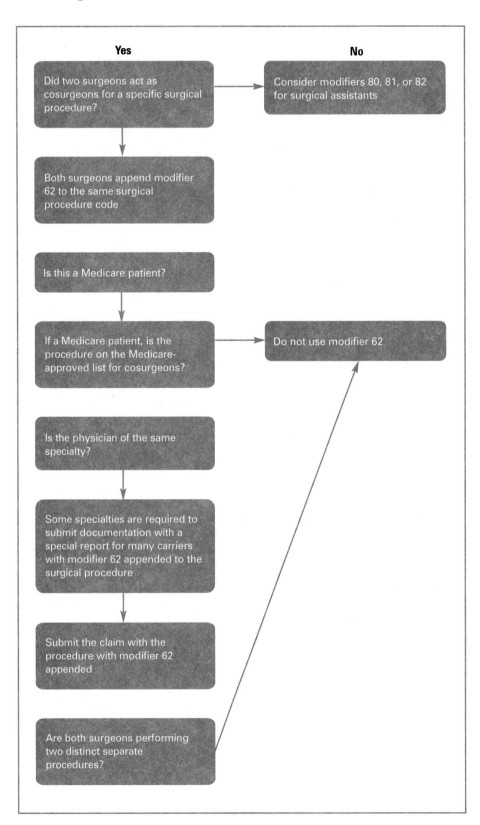

MODIFIER 63

Procedure Performed on Infants Less than 4 kg

Unless otherwise designated, this modifier may only be appended to procedures/services listed in the 20000–69990 code series.

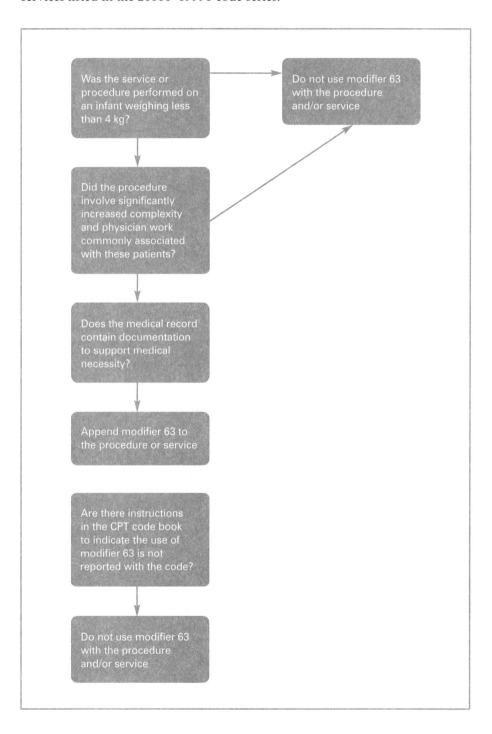

MODIFIER 66

Team Surgery

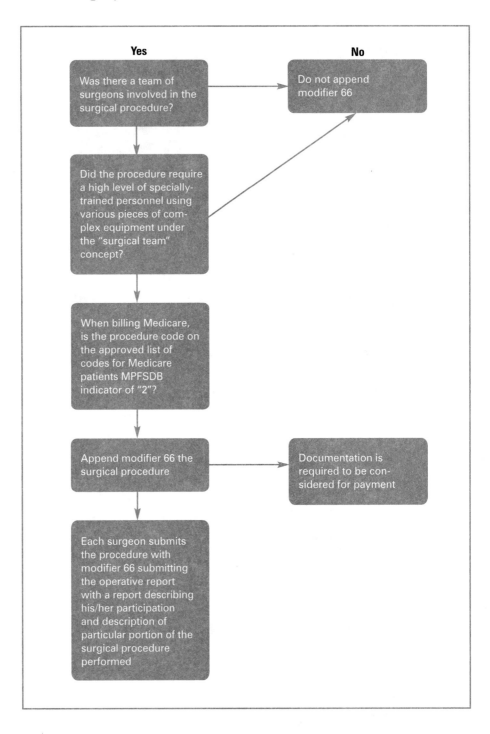

MODIFIER 73

Discontinued Outpatient Hospital/Ambulatory Surgery Center (ASC) Procedure Prior to the Administration of Anesthesia

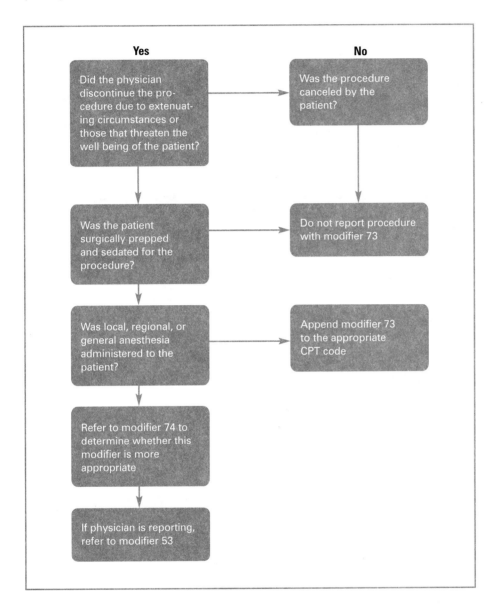

MODIFIER 74

Discontinued Outpatient Hospital/Ambulatory Surgery Center (ASC) Procedure After Administration of Anesthesia

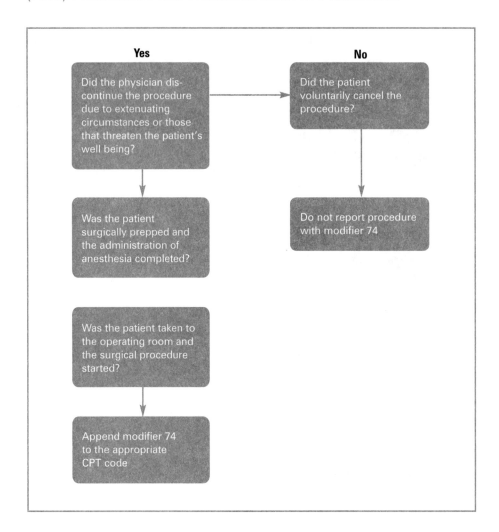

MODIFIER 76

Repeat Procedure by Same Physician

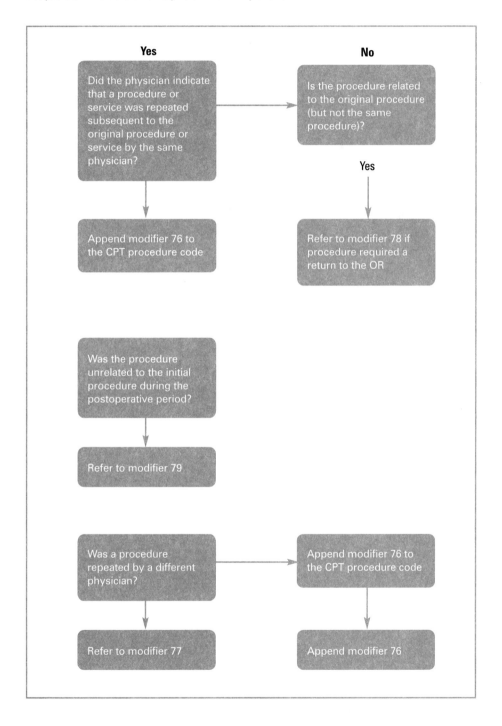

Yes

Did the physician indicate that a procedure or service was repeated subsequent to the original procedure or service by the same physician?

No

Is the procedure related to the original procedure (but not the same procedure)?

Append modifier 76 to the CPT procedure code

Yes

Refer to modifier 78 if procedure required a return to the OR

Was the procedure unrelated to the initial procedure during the postoperative period?

Refer to modifier 79

Was a procedure repeated by a different physician?

Append modifier 76 to the CPT procedure code

Refer to modifier 77

Append modifier 76

MODIFIER 77

Repeat Procedure by Another Physician

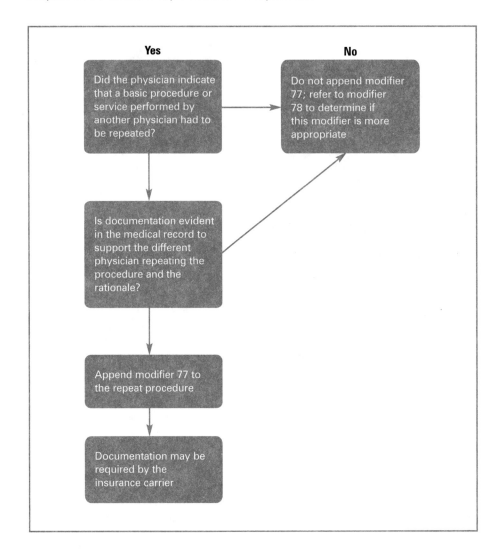

MODIFIER 78

Return to the Operating Room for a Related Procedure
During the Postoperative Period

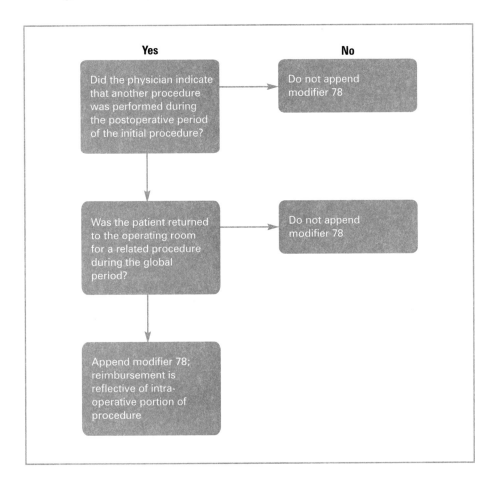

MODIFIER 79

Unrelated Procedure or Service by the Same Physician During the Postoperative Period

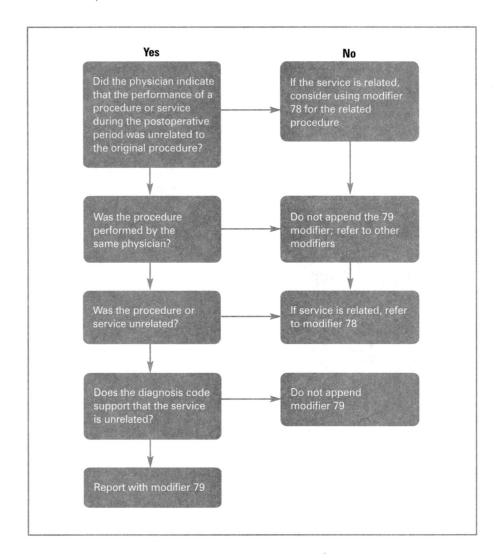

MODIFIER 80

Assistant Surgeon

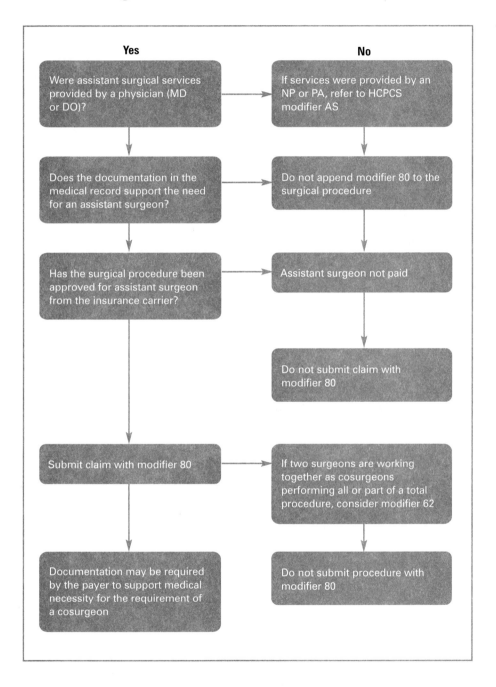

Yes

No

Were assistant surgical services provided by a physician (MD or DO)?

If services were provided by an NP or PA, refer to HCPCS modifier AS

Does the documentation in the medical record support the need for an assistant surgeon?

Do not append modifier 80 to the surgical procedure

Has the surgical procedure been approved for assistant surgeon from the insurance carrier?

Assistant surgeon not paid

Do not submit claim with modifier 80

Submit claim with modifier 80

If two surgeons are working together as cosurgeons performing all or part of a total procedure, consider modifier 62

Documentation may be required by the payer to support medical necessity for the requirement of a cosurgeon

Do not submit procedure with modifier 80

MODIFIER 81

Minimum Assistant Surgeon

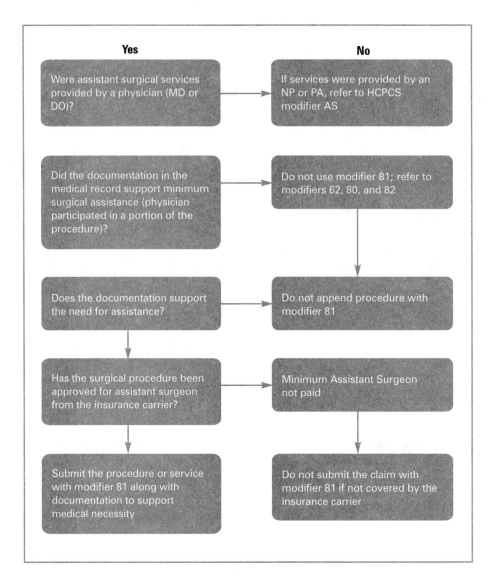

MODIFIER 82

Assistant Surgeon When Qualified Resident Surgeon
Not Available

The unavailability of a qualified resident surgeon is a prerequisite for use of a modifier.

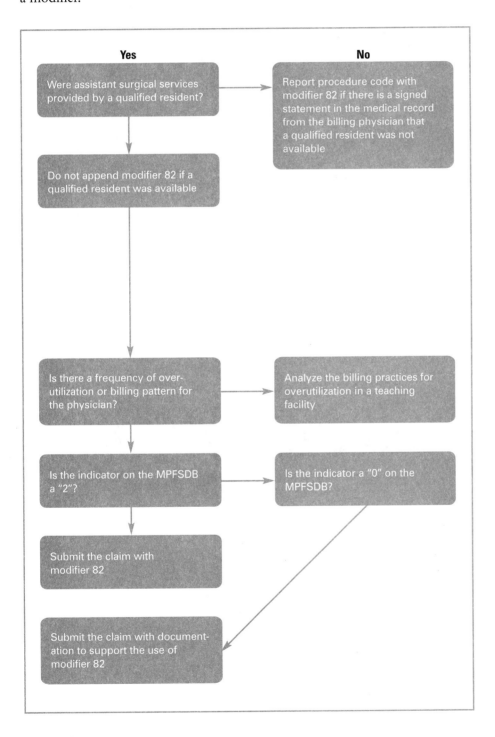

Yes

Were assistant surgical services provided by a qualified resident?

Do not append modifier 82 if a qualified resident was available

No

Report procedure code with modifier 82 if there is a signed statement in the medical record from the billing physician that a qualified resident was not available

Is there a frequency of over-utilization or billing pattern for the physician?

Analyze the billing practices for overutilization in a teaching facility

Is the indicator on the MPFSDB a "2"?

Is the indicator a "0" on the MPFSDB?

Submit the claim with modifier 82

Submit the claim with document-ation to support the use of modifier 82

MODIFIER 90

Reference (Outside) Laboratory

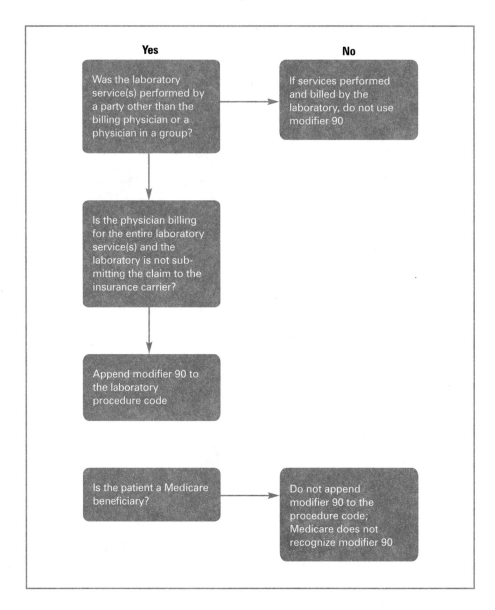

MODIFIER 91

Repeat Clinical Diagnostic Laboratory Test

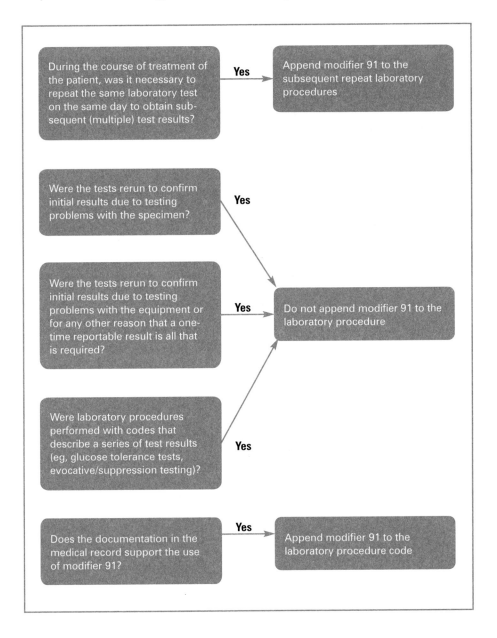

MODIFIER 99

Multiple Modifiers

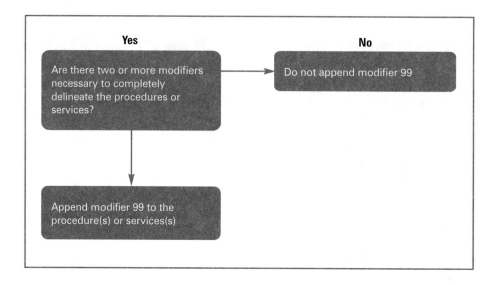

APPENDIX E

Exams

Midterm Exam

Match the modifier definition to the correct modifier.

1 _____ Modifier 21   a. Mandated Services

2 _____ Modifier 22   b. Multiple Procedures

3 _____ Modifier 23   c. Unusual Procedural Services

4 _____ Modifier 24   d. Bilateral Procedures

5 _____ Modifier 25   e. Surgical Care Only

6 _____ Modifier 26   f. Postoperative Management Only

7 _____ Modifier 32   g. Anesthesia by Surgeon

8 _____ Modifier 47   h. Discontinued Procedure

9 _____ Modifier 50   i. Unrelated E/M Service by the Same Physician During the Postoperative Period

10 _____ Modifier 51   j. Professional Component

11 _____ Modifier 52   k. Prolonged E/M Services

12 _____ Modifier 53   l. Unusual Anesthesia

13 _____ Modifier 54   m. Preoperative Management Only

14 _____ Modifier 55   n. Reduced Services

15 _____ Modifier 56   o. Significant Separately Identifiable E/M Service by the Same Physician on the Same Day of the Procedure or Other Service

Select the correct answer.

16 _____ The modifier that identifies the physician component.
   a. Modifier 22
   b. Modifier 26
   c. Modifier 24
   d. Modifier 32

17 _____ Using anesthesia procedure codes 00100-01999, code general anesthesia for repair of ruptured aortic aneurysm with graft. The patient was noted to have severe systemic disease at the time of the anesthesia, and a pump oxygenator was used during the procedure.
   a. 00566 P3
   b. 00563 P3
   c. 00562 P3
   d. 00563 P2

18 _____ A patient underwent a percutaneous needle core biopsy of the left breast with imaging guidance. The specimen was sent to pathology and the findings indicated a malignancy. The next morning the patient was taken to surgery and a partial mastectomy with removal of lymph nodes was performed on the left breast. Select the appropriate code for the second procedure.
   a. No code is necessary because the second procedure falls within the 90-day global period.
   b. 19162 58
   c. 19102, 76095 51 58
   d. 19102, 76095, 19162 58

19 _____ A second opinion regarding surgery was required by the insurance company to assure maximum reimbursement for the performing physician. The patient was seen in the physician's office. The following key components were performed: comprehensive history and examination with moderate complexity medical decision making.
   a. 99241 22
   b. 99254 22
   c. 99253 32
   d. 99244 32

20 _____ Code for the following: arthroscopy, knee, surgical, with synovectomy, limited, in the medial compartment, and with lateral meniscectomy.
   a. 29880 50, 29875 51
   b. 29870, 29880 51, 29875 59
   c. 29881 22
   d. 29881, 29875 59

21 _____ What modifier indicates that a bilateral procedure was performed?
   a. Modifier 50
   b. Modifier 32
   c. Modifier 51
   d. Modifier 99

22 _____ Modifiers 54 and 55 are often used:
   a. In primary care
   b. To indicate the procedure is on the right or left side of the body
   c. Together on the same claim
   d. Submitted with the same surgical procedure code by each physician who provided the service

23 _____ Modifier 24 should always be used with:
   a. Surgical procedures
   b. Evaluation and management services
   c. Radiology procedures
   d. Laboratory and pathology procedures

24 _____ Modifier 25 is:
   a. Used to report unusual services
   b. Used for the initial evaluation of a problem for which a procedure is performed
   c. Never appended to E/M services
   d. Used only for the decision for surgery

25 _____ Payment using modifier 51 may be impacted by:
   a. Multiple procedures during the same operative session; same incision
   b. Discontinued procedure; amount of time spent before discontinuing a procedure
   c. Multiple procedures performed in different body areas
   d. Procedures performed bilaterally

26 _____ The portion of a test or procedure that the physician performs (reading an X ray, EKG, and so on) is known as the:
   a. Professional component
   b. Technical component
   c. Limiting component
   d. Complete procedural component

27 _____ A national uniform coding structure developed by the Centers for Medicare and Medicaid for reporting physician/supplier services for government programs is known as:
   a. HIMA
   b. HCFA
   c. HCPCS
   d. None of the above

28 _____ A patient returning within the global surgical time frame for a mole excision presents to the physician's office for treatment of acne. Which modifier should be attached?
   a. Modifier 24
   b. Modifier 25
   c. Modifier 78
   d. Modifier 79
   e. None of the above

29 _____ After a consultation for a new patient, the surgeon decided to operate on the patient the same day. The procedure is a major procedure with a 90-day global surgical time frame and the patient's insurance company is a third-party payer. What modifier is appended to the consultation code?
   a. Modifier 78
   b. Modifier 51
   c. Modifier 25
   d. Modifier 57

30 _____ How many physical status modifiers are there?
a. None
b. 3
c. 5
d. 6

True or false.

31 _____ The modifier used to indicate that a procedure is less extensive than the description given in CPT is 53.

32 _____ The modifier that indicates that surgical care only was provided for a procedure is modifier 55.

33 _____ An insurance carrier requires a patient to obtain a second opinion before approving a surgical procedure. Modifier 22 would be used to indicate that this was a mandated service.

34 _____ If a patient had multiple procedures during the same operative session, modifier 51 is added to the lesser of the two codes.

35 _____ It is always incorrect to use modifier 21 and a code from the code series 99354-99359 in conjunction with each other.

36 _____ Modifier 23 is the modifier used to report anesthesia services performed by the surgeon.

37 _____ Modifier 55 is used to indicate only the preoperative management of the patient.

38 _____ Modifiers 51 and 59 may be appended to an add-on code.

39 _____ Modifier 47 is used by the physician—not the anesthesiologist—who provides regional or general anesthesia during a surgical procedure; the modifier is attached to the appropriate anesthesia code.

40 _____ Modifier 25 may be used with an E/M service when a surgical procedure is the only service provided to a patient on the same day.

Code the following scenarios including modifiers.

41 _____ A patient required arthroplasty of the tibial plateaus of both knees. Code this procedure for the surgeon.

42 _____ A patient presented to the operating room for a diagnostic arthroscopy of the knee. The physician inserted the arthroscope and the patient suddenly went into respiratory distress. The arthroscope was withdrawn and the procedure was terminated.

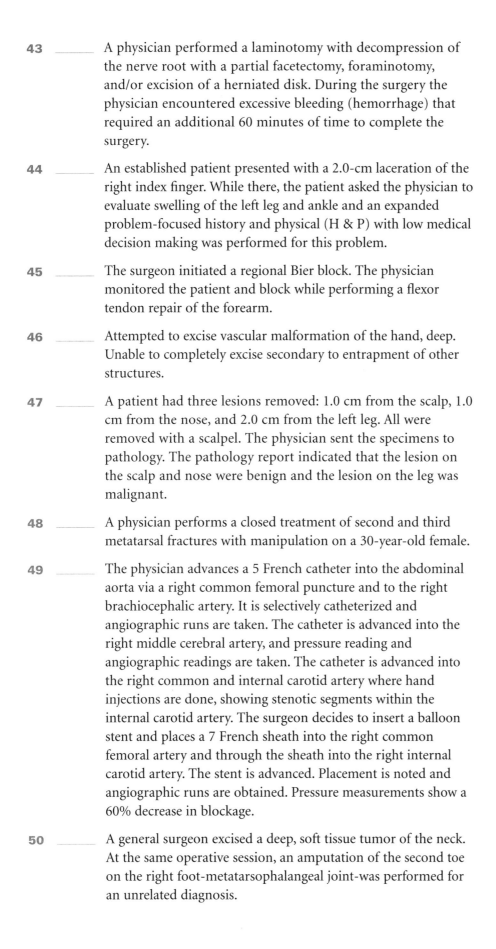

43 _____ A physician performed a laminotomy with decompression of the nerve root with a partial facetectomy, foraminotomy, and/or excision of a herniated disk. During the surgery the physician encountered excessive bleeding (hemorrhage) that required an additional 60 minutes of time to complete the surgery.

44 _____ An established patient presented with a 2.0-cm laceration of the right index finger. While there, the patient asked the physician to evaluate swelling of the left leg and ankle and an expanded problem-focused history and physical (H & P) with low medical decision making was performed for this problem.

45 _____ The surgeon initiated a regional Bier block. The physician monitored the patient and block while performing a flexor tendon repair of the forearm.

46 _____ Attempted to excise vascular malformation of the hand, deep. Unable to completely excise secondary to entrapment of other structures.

47 _____ A patient had three lesions removed: 1.0 cm from the scalp, 1.0 cm from the nose, and 2.0 cm from the left leg. All were removed with a scalpel. The physician sent the specimens to pathology. The pathology report indicated that the lesion on the scalp and nose were benign and the lesion on the leg was malignant.

48 _____ A physician performs a closed treatment of second and third metatarsal fractures with manipulation on a 30-year-old female.

49 _____ The physician advances a 5 French catheter into the abdominal aorta via a right common femoral puncture and to the right brachiocephalic artery. It is selectively catheterized and angiographic runs are taken. The catheter is advanced into the right middle cerebral artery, and pressure reading and angiographic readings are taken. The catheter is advanced into the right common and internal carotid artery where hand injections are done, showing stenotic segments within the internal carotid artery. The surgeon decides to insert a balloon stent and places a 7 French sheath into the right common femoral artery and through the sheath into the right internal carotid artery. The stent is advanced. Placement is noted and angiographic runs are obtained. Pressure measurements show a 60% decrease in blockage.

50 _____ A general surgeon excised a deep, soft tissue tumor of the neck. At the same operative session, an amputation of the second toe on the right foot-metatarsophalangeal joint-was performed for an unrelated diagnosis.

Final Exam

Match the modifier definition to the correct modifier.

1 _____ Modifier 27

2 _____ Modifier 57

3 _____ Modifier 58

4 _____ Modifier 59

5 _____ Modifier 62

6 _____ Modifier 63

7 _____ Modifier 66

8 _____ Modifier 73

9 _____ Modifier 74

10 _____ Modifier 76

11 _____ Modifier 77

12 _____ Modifier 78

13 _____ Modifier 79

14 _____ Modifier 80

15 _____ Modifier 81

16 _____ Modifier 82

17 _____ Modifier 90

18 _____ Modifier 91

19 _____ Modifier 99

a. Repeat Clinical Diagnostic Laboratory Tests

b. Surgical Team

c. Minimum Assistant Surgeon

d. Repeat Procedure by Same Physician

e. Multiple Modifiers

f. Staged or Related Procedure or Service by the Same Physician During the Postoperative Period

g. Repeat Procedure by Another Physician

h. Multiple Outpatient Hospital E/M Encounters on the Same Date

i. Unrelated Procedure or Service by the Same Physician During the Postoperative Period

j. Reference (Outside) Laboratory

k. Assistant Surgeon

l. Procedures Performed on Infants Less than 4 kg

m. Distinct Procedural Service

n. Discontinued Outpatient Hospital/Ambulatory Surgery Center (ASC) Procedure After Administration of Anesthesia

o. Return to the Operating Room for a Related Procedure or Service During the Postoperative Period

p. Two Surgeons

q. Assistant Surgeon (When Qualified Resident Surgeon Not Available)

r. Discontinued Outpatient Hospital/Ambulatory Surgery Center (ASC) Procedure Prior to Administration of Anesthesia

s. Decision for Surgery

Select the correct answer.

20 _____ The two-digit modifier 57 means:
a. Prolonged E/M services
b. Reduced services
c. Decision for surgery
d. Mandated services

21 _____ When coding for X ray films taken of both knees:
a. List the proper X ray code twice and use modifier 76 (repeat procedure by same physician) with the second code
b. List the proper X ray code twice and use modifier 51 (multiple procedure) with the second code
c. List the proper X ray code once and modify it with modifier 51 (multiple procedure)
d. List the proper X ray code twice and use modifier RT (right) with the first code and modifier LT (left) with the second code

22 _____ Modifiers 73 and 74 are most appropriate in:
a. Emergency room services
b. Physician services
c. Inpatient hospital services
d. Outpatient hospital and ambulatory surgery centers (ASC)

23 _____ Modifier 62 is used:
a. Two surgeons, two are primary
b. Surgical team, one primary and one assistant surgeon
c. When a qualified resident is not available
d. Assistant surgeon, assistant is available for the entire operation

24 _____ The main difference between modifier 80 and modifier 81 is:
a. Modifier 81 is used to indicate the primary surgeon and modifier 80 for the assistant
b. Modifier 80 is used for the primary surgeon and modifier 81 is for the assistant
c. Modifier 80 is used for the assistant surgeon and modifier 81 is a minimum assistant surgeon
d. The amount of time the surgeon spends in the operating room determines the use of modifiers 80 and 81

25 _____ Modifier 91 is used:
a. When there are testing problems with either the specimen or equipment
b. To obtain subsequent (multiple) readings of a test on the same day and it is medically necessary
c. When specimens are lost or not sent to the laboratory appropriately
d. To obtain subsequent (multiple) readings of a test on the same day for the patient's peace of mind

26 _____ Modifiers 76 and 77 are used:
  a. To explain why the patient returned to the operating room during the postoperative period
  b. To supply information only and does not affect reimbursement
  c. To explain why a procedure was duplicated, usually by submitting an operative report which supports medical necessity for repeating the procedure
  d. Only when the procedures are unrelated or related

27 _____ Modifier 59 is used:
  a. Only with radiology procedures
  b. Only to specify separate incision on an existing site
  c. To report distinct procedural services
  d. None of the above

28 _____ Modifier 27 is used:
  a. For multiple outpatient E/M encounters by the physician
  b. To report outpatient hospital services
  c. To report the second and subsequent E/M code(s) when reporting more than one evaluation and management service to indicate that each of the E/M services is a "separate and distinct E/M encounter" (provided that same day in the same or different hospital outpatient setting)
  d. B and C

29 _____ Modifier 74 was established specifically to assist hospital outpatient reporting associated with the utilization of resources in the event a surgical or diagnostic procedure is canceled due to extenuating circumstance or those that threaten the well-being of the patient. In this instance, modifier 74 can be used:
  a. Subsequent to the patient's surgical preparation (including sedation when provided) before administration of anesthesia
  b. Subsequent to the patient's surgical preparation (including sedation when provided) after administration of anesthesia
  c. By the physician to report discontinued procedures
  d. Only for inpatient procedures

30 _____ Modifier 58 is used:
  a. When the description of the code indicates one or more visits or one or more sessions
  b. When the procedure was planned prospectively because it was more extensive than the original procedure or represents a therapeutic or diagnostic procedure or service
  c. For a return to the operating room for an unrelated procedure during the postoperative period
  d. None of the above

True or false.

31 _____ Modifier 77 is used to indicate a repeat procedure by the same physician.

32 _____ Modifier 66 is used for team surgery.

33 _____ Modifiers 73 and 74 are not used to indicate discontinued radiology procedures.

34 _____ Modifier 90 is used to indicate that although the physician is reporting the performance of a laboratory test, the actual testing component was a service from a laboratory.

35 _____ If surgeons of different specialties are each performing a different procedure (with specific CPT codes), neither co-surgery nor multiple surgery rules apply even if the procedure(s) are performed through the same incision.

36 _____ Modifier 91 (Repeat Clinical Diagnostic Laboratory Test) was created to replace the Centers for Medicare and Medicaid (CMS) National Level II modifier QR.

37 _____ Modifier LD may be used with procedure codes 92975-92984, 92995, and 92996 for hospital use.

38 _____ Modifier 59 is not designed to provide reimbursement for separate procedures that are performed as an integral part of another procedure and is watched closely by carriers.

39 _____ Modifier TC is a HCPCS modifier indicating the technical component was provided only.

40 _____ Modifier GA is reported when the physician, practitioner, or supplier expects that Medicare will not deny an item or service as reasonable and necessary.

Code the following scenarios including modifiers.

41 _____ A physician performed an internal and external destruction of hemorrhoids on a patient during a 90-day follow-up period for a second (staged) destruction procedure in regard to infrared coagulation of hemorrhoids.

42 _____ A primary care physician performed a chest X ray and observes a suspicious mass. He sent the patient to a pulmonologist who, on the same day, repeated the chest X ray.

43 _____ A full-thickness graft was performed 10 days following an allograft application of pigskin to allow the underlying tissues time to heal. The surgeon knew at the time of the allograft that grafting would be performed at a later date. Provide the procedure and modifier for the graft.

44 _____ A 46-year-old patient with a history of seizure disorder, and who was taking Phenobarbital for seizure control, went to the lab to have her blood drawn to measure the Phenobarbital level to determine if the dosage was providing proper therapeutic value. She had her blood drawn prior to taking the drug in the morning. In the afternoon, the patient had the labs redrawn to determine if the level in the afternoon was providing appropriate seizure control.

45 _____ An orthopedic surgeon performed an arthroscopy on the right knee for loose body removal. One week later (during the postoperative period), the patient tripped and fell, and fractured the right radial shaft. The orthopedic surgeon who performed the arthroscopy was contacted and performed a closed manipulation of the radial shaft and applied a short arm cast.

46 _____ A 66-year-old male patient suffered a right ankle injury while attempting to clear a sidewalk of snow. The patient presented to the emergency department where the emergency room physician ordered ankle films, three views. After reviewing the X rays, the physician applied a short leg splint (calf to foot) and advised the patient to see his family physician in 10 days.

47 _____ A 60-year-old male with an enlarged spleen and past history of Hodgkin disease presented to the emergency room. After the ER physician examined the patient, the ER physician contacted the patient's physician (surgeon) who came down to the emergency room to see the patient. The surgeon evaluated the patient and performed a comprehensive history and examination with high complexity decision making, and determined the patient needed an immediate spleenectomy. Once the decision was made to operate, the surgeon reviewed laboratory and X ray/imaging studies to plan the operative approach, discussed the procedure with the patient, and obtained informed consent. Medical and anesthesiology consults are requested. At operation, a subcostal incision was performed, the spleen mobilized, and the vessels doubly ligated. Postoperatively, the wound was monitored for infection and injectable pain medications were tapered as tolerated. The patient was discharged from the hospital when stable and comfortable on oral pain medications.

48 _____ A 21-year-old college tennis player sprained her ankle during a game. She could hardly walk and needs to be helped off the court. The next day she saw her orthopedist who noted considerable swelling, bruising, and pain about her ankle and foot. She was on crutches. The physician sent the patient to the outpatient radiology department for X rays. Two views were taken of the ankle. The order indicated that the orthopedist would read the films. The patient brought the films back to the orthopedist's office and the physician read the films. Ankle and subtalar range of motion were reduced due to pain and guarding. She was neurovascularly intact. Clinically, there was a suggestion of anterior translation of the talus on the tibia when pulling her foot forward. She was treated in a cast for several weeks. Code for the hospital outpatient radiology services only.

49 _____ A 20-year-old patient, who was having trouble hearing out of her left ear, underwent a screening test (pure tone, air only) in her left ear.

50 _____ Anesthesia for procedures on a major blood vessel in the abdomen for a patient with severe systemic disease that is hypotensive and an emergency situation.

APPENDIX F

Answer Key

CHAPTER 1

Test Your Knowledge

1 C

2 D

3 A

4 B

5 C

6 B

7 D

8 B

9 B

10 A

CHAPTER 2

Test Your Knowledge

1 False—only with E/M

2 True—many carriers require documentation to support additional time worked before paying additional reimbursement.

3 False—unusual anesthesia

4 False—unrelated

5 False

6 False

7 False

8 False

9 True

10 True

11 24

12 P3

13 22

14 24

15 21

CHAPTER 3

Checkpoint Exercises 1

1 D

2 A

3 C

4 A

5 D

Checkpoint Exercises 2

1 True

2 False

3 False

4 True

5 True

Test Your Knowledge

1 B

2 B

3 C

4 A

5 C

6 26

7 25

8 26

9 47

10 32

11 26

12 25

13 47

14 32

15 26

CHAPTER 4

Checkpoint Exercises 1

1 52

2 50

3 51

4 No modifier is reported for physician services.

5 53

Checkpoint Exercises 2

1 surgical package

2 54

3 medical record

4 56

5 preoperative, intraoperative, and postoperative

Test Your Knowledge

1 True

2 False

3 False

4 True

5 False

6 False

7 False

8 55

9 52

10 51

11 50

12 51

13 51

14 53

15 52

CHAPTER 5

Checkpoint Exercises 1

1 58

2 57

3 58

4 57

5 57

Checkpoint Exercises 2

1 59

2 62

3 63

4 62

5 58

Test Your Knowledge

1 False

2 True

3 True

4 False (no modifier is required)

5 False

6 63

7 57

8 59

9 57

10 58

11 51

12 57

13 59

14 63

15 58

CHAPTER 6

Checkpoint Exercises 1

1 False

2 False

3 True

4 False

5 True

Test Your Knowledge

1 A

2 D

3 B

4 C

5 A

6 False

7 False

8 True

9 False

10 True

11 Medical Necessity

12 66

13 The same physician

14 Both are repeat procedures, but modifier 76 is used when the same physician performed the initial surgery, and modifier 77 is when it's performed by another physician during the postoperative period.

15 Modifier 77

CHAPTER 7

Test Your Knowledge

1 91

2 91

3 90

4 99

5 91

6 99

7 90

8 59

9 91

10 99

11 91

12 90

13 90

14 Clinical Laboratory Improvement Amendment (CLIA)

15 99

CHAPTER 8

Test Your Knowledge

1 A

2 B

3 C

4 B

5 B

6 B

7 C

8 A

9 A

10 A

11 A

12 C

13 D

14 B

15 C

CHAPTER 9

Checkpoint Exercises 1

1 27

2 52

3 25

4 RT (right side), LT (left side)

5 Ambulatory Surgery Center

6 Bilateral indicators from CMS in the Medicare Physician Fee Schedule (MPFS) in the Outpatient Code Editor (means modifier 50 is present).

7 Balanced Budget Act

Checkpoint Exercises 2

1 73

2 58

3 74

4 50%

5 59

Checkpoint Exercises 3

1 77

2 73 and 74; replaced 52 and 53

3 91

4 To perform a procedure that was related to the first procedure, but not the same procedure. Examples include postsurgical hemorrhage, postoperative bleeding, postoperative complication requiring a related procedure, and so on.

5 79

Test Your Knowledge

1 A

2 C

3 B

4 A

5 D

6 A

7 A (In the outpatient hospital or ASC, modifier 51 is not recognized)

8 D

9 B

10 A

11 D

12 B

13 D

14 C

15 A

CHAPTER 10

Test Your Knowledge

1 3K

2 0F

3 6E

4 4C

5 2P

6 7E

7 4O

8 9D

9 1H

10 9P

11 2D

12 9Z

13 1P

14 5G

15 8B

MIDTERM EXAM

1 K

2 C

3 L

4 I

5 O

6 J

7 A

8 G

9 D

10 B

11 N

12 H

13 E

14 F

15 M

16 B

17 C

18 B

19 D

20 D

21 A

22 D

23 B

24 B

25 A

26 A

27 C

28 E

29 D

30 D

31 False (Modifier 52)

32 False (Modifier 54)

33 False (Modifier 32)

34 True

35 True

36 False (Modifier 47)

37 False (Modifier 56)

38 False (An add-on code does not require the use of modifier 51 or 59.)

39 False (The modifier is appended to the surgical procedure code.)

40 False (When the only service provided is the surgical procedure, only the procedure is reported unless there is a significant separately identifiable service or procedure on the same day.)

41 27440 50

42 29870 53

43 63020 22

44 99213 25, 12001

45 25260 47

46 26116 52

47 11421, 11441 51, 11602 59

48 28475, 28475 51

49 36217, 37205, 75660 26, 75665 26, 75960 26

50 28820 T6, 21556 59

FINAL EXAM

1 H

2 S

3 F

4 M

5 P

6 L

7 B

8 R

9 N

10 D

11 G

12 O

13 I

14 K

15 C

16 Q

17 J

18 A

19 E

20 C

21 D

22 D

23 A

24 C

25 B

26 C

27 C

28 D

29 B

30 B

31 False (Modifier 77 is used to report a repeat procedure by another physician.)

32 True

33 True

34 True

35 True

36 True

37 False (Modifier LD may be used with codes 92980-92984, 92995, and 92996 for hospital use.)

38 True

39 True

40 False (The GA modifier is reported when the physician, practitioner, or supplier expects that Medicare will deny an item or service as reasonable and necessary.)

41 46936 58

42 71020 77

43 15760 58

44 80184 (initial laboratory procedure), 80184 91 (repeat laboratory procedure)

45 25505 79

46 29515 RT, 73610 RT

47 99215 57, 38100

48 73600 TC

49 92551 52

50 00770 P4, 99140, 99135

Index

References to table or figure items are in *italic*.

**Engineering Thermodynamics
Work and Heat Transfer**

Contents

v

xii

Preface to the Fourth Edition

Over the years the publisher has kindly allowed the authors to make improvements at many of the reprintings but, as this was always subject to no change in pagination, the revised material was not always in the best location or expressed as clearly as it could have been. The authors were pleased that Longman offered to reset completely this new edition, enabling them to make a thorough revision and to enjoy seeing their work in a more aesthetically pleasing form.

Presented with this opportunity, the authors asked themselves whether their methodology, based on Keenan's *Thermodynamics* published in 1941, was still appropriate for the 1990s. Having looked again at the chief contenders, namely the Born–Carathéodory and Keenan–Hatsopolous approaches, the authors remain convinced that the well-established route still provides the best way of introducing thermodynamics to engineering students. One fundamental change was required, however: it seemed wise to adopt the sign convention for work transfer which is now widely used by physicists and chemists and by an increasing number of engineers abroad. Although the change may appear to be trivial it has repercussions throughout much of the book. So too do some of the minor changes of notation and methods of handling units necessitated by international agreements.

Some important topics were in need of a revised presentation, and others, having grown in importance, required a more extensive coverage. The way in which the perfect gas was introduced was less than perfect; it has been given a more rigorous treatment. Most books including our own had worked with an unsound definition of the equilibrium constant; this has been rectified as part of a general updating of the presentation of thermochemical concepts. We have revised the treatment of axial-flow turbines, adopting the modern convention of measuring blade angles from the axial instead of the tangential direction. This change arose from experimental work on flow through cascades of blades, stimulated by the advent of the gas turbine and its axial-flow compressor. Growing concern with energy conservation and the environment has led us to make more space available for discussion of combined cycle plant, cogeneration schemes, low-temperature power cycles, and pollution problems.

Numerous books devoted solely to heat transfer have appeared since this book was first published in 1957. We still feel, however, that the coverage provided in Part IV is worth retaining; for many students it is all they are likely to need on the subject, while for others it is a succinct introduction. We have been able to deal with some new topics, if only briefly, and improve the treatment of others. We made some changes in the previous edition in recognition of the growth in computational techniques; we have not carried this further because we believe that what is important at undergraduate level is a firm grasp of physical principles.

The worked examples and problems have been revised and increased in number. At the suggestion of teachers we have added a section in the Prologue with what we hope are helpful hints on how the book might be used in conjunction with a course of lectures.

In conclusion, we particularly wish to thank Carrie Pharaoh for retracing the figures so good humouredly, and Jennifer Scherr of Queen's Building Library for checking references. Our wives deserve special thanks for putting up with less attention than they had a right to expect from two semi-retired academics.

Bristol 1992

G.F.C.R.
Y.R.M.

Preface to the Third Edition

Although minor additions and improvements have been made to the text and references to take account of recent work and current applications of thermodynamics, no substantial changes have been made in this third edition. Its prime purpose is to convey to students the outcome of much international effort to standardise nomenclature, units and methods of presenting technical data. The importance of this should not be underestimated. If the ever-increasing output of technical literature is to be assimilated, unremitting attention must be paid to ways of making it easily digestible. Readers can no longer afford the time to battle with ambiguities and idiosyncrasies. It is vital that students — the authors of tomorrow — should acquire good habits during their undergraduate studies.

When preparing the second edition in 1966 it was necessary to anticipate certain decisions relating to the introduction of SI (Système International d'Unités). The authors failed to anticipate the choice of K instead of °K as a symbol for the kelvin unit of temperature, and failed to foresee the new definition of the mole. (The formal decisions were taken in 1968 and 1971 respectively.) This third edition has afforded the authors the opportunity to bring the book up to date in these respects, and in others associated with a more rigorous attitude to the concept of a physical quantity and its units which has repercussions in the way equations should be written and data presented in graphs and tables. The reader is referred particularly to the rewritten Appendix A on dimensions and units.

G.F.C.R.

Bristol 1980

Y.R.M.

Preface to the Second Edition

This edition of the book in SI units has been produced in the hope that it will play its part in furthering the change from British to metric units which is to take place during the next few years. Examples and problems have been worked out using data contained in the second edition of *Thermodynamic and Transport Properties of Fluids (SI Units)* (Basil Blackwell, 1967). The first edition of the book, and the tables in British units, will continue to be available as long as required.

While preparing this edition, the opportunity has been taken to bring the material up to date in some major and many minor respects. A large part of Chapter 8 has been rewritten to accommodate changes in the approach to the definition of temperature units and the adoption of the triple point as the datum state for steam tables. The treatment of regenerative cycles has been revised. Material has been added to Chapters 7 and 15 to include an introduction to the concept of availability and the closely associated use of the Gibbs function and other chemical thermodynamic data; the section on calorific values has been brought into line with the new British Standard. A chapter has been added on direct conversion; although inevitably little more than descriptive, it is hoped that it will encourage some students to pursue the subject further as a postgraduate study. Owing to the widespread use of computers, numerical methods of dealing with non-steady heat flow problems have been substituted for the less flexible graphical methods described in the previous edition. Additional material is included on liquid metals as heat transfer media, and on boiling. Various other topics which have assumed importance since the book was first written, such as cycles for nuclear power plant and the Wankel engine, have also been included, and the references have been revised to bring greater benefit from further reading.

The general plan of the book is unchanged. The authors still believe that classical macroscopic thermodynamics provides the best introduction to the subject for mechanical engineers, and that any real attempt to deal with statistical thermodynamics and irreversible thermodynamics is best left to postgraduate courses.

We wish to acknowledge the invaluable help given by Dr M. Hollingsworth, who reworked the problems of Appendix B in SI units to provide the reader with answers. And once again we thank Mr C. J. Spittal, our librarian, for his work in checking the references.

Bristol 1967

G.F.C.R.

Y.R.M.

Preface to the First Edition

This book is intended for engineering students and covers the fundamentals of applied thermodynamics courses up to honours degree standard. The following presentation has been adopted.

An exposition of the principles of thermodynamics is given in Part I without reference to the behaviour of any particular substance. Part II opens with a discussion of the properties of fluids, and the principles of Part I are then applied to closed and open systems assuming that the properties are best related (a) in tables and (b) by simple equations. This is followed by an analysis of power and refrigeration cycles. Part II ends with a study of gas and vapour mixtures and combustion processes.

Parts I and II are chiefly concerned with relations between fluid properties and the quantities of work and heat which accompany changes of state. The way in which the work and heat transfers are effected in practice is described in Parts III and IV respectively. Part III is divided broadly into work transfers associated with (a) positive-displacement machines and (b) nonpositive-displacement machines. For the latter, a more detailed analysis of flow processes is required than is given in Parts I and II, and therefore a chapter on one-dimensional flow is included. This chapter is designed as a bridge between the sciences of thermodynamics and fluid dynamics and, to avoid obscuring the fundamental links, concepts such as total temperature and Mach number have not been used. The usual classification of modes of heat transfer is adopted in Part IV, with the emphasis placed on methods of approach rather than on the presentation of established empirical data.

We do not suggest that our order of presentation is suitable as a direct introduction to the subject, and the book is not designed as a substitute for a course of lectures. Most students are best introduced to a subject by a careful juxtaposition of principle and application, and the book leaves it open to the lecturer to choose any preferred order of presentation. But, although a mixture of principle and application is necessary in a lecture course, it can leave the student with serious misconceptions, and it by no means follows that he will gain a sufficient grasp of the principles to be able to tackle unfamiliar problems. Our object has been to produce a book which will enable the student to distinguish principle from application; a reading of the first six chapters, as revision late in his first year, should enable him to make this distinction. It should also help him to appreciate the elegance and power, as well as the limitations, of the science he is using.

Our second concern has been to provide a book of reference to which the student can turn for the elucidation of difficult points. A rigorous approach cannot often be used in a lecture course, partly for lack of time and partly because it would be inappropriate when introducing the student to a new idea. In this book, however, a rigorous proof or explanation is given wherever practicable for the benefit of the better student who is not satisfied with simplifications.

A few words are necessary about two of the appendixes. Many of the problems provided in Appendix B are intended to amplify points only touched on in the text. To this extent they should be regarded as an integral part of the book. The answers to the problems, and to the worked examples in the text, have been obtained using the abridged tables of properties arranged by us and published separately as *Thermodynamic Properties of Fluids and Other Data* (Basil Blackwell, 1957). Most of the references, given in Appendix C, are to be regarded as suggestions for further reading and also as acknowledgement of sources. A few classical papers of academic interest are also included.

Finally we wish to acknowledge our particular indebtedness to two books which we have found a source of inspiration: J. H. Keenan's *Thermodynamics* (Wiley, 1941), and E. R. G. Eckert's *Introduction to the Transfer of Heat and Mass* (McGraw-Hill, 1950). We also wish to thank our colleagues at Bristol — Dr B. Crossland, Mr T. V. Lawson and Dr P. Woodward — for their useful suggestions after reading parts of the manuscript. Mr C. J. Spittal, of the University Library, has been most helpful in obtaining papers and checking the references.

Bristol 1957

G.F.C.R.

Y.R.M.

Prologue

Why study thermodynamics?

Since the Industrial Revolution there has been an exponential growth of population and of material wealth. This growth has been associated with the ever-increasing use of energy in machines. The revolution began with coal, and has progressed through the use of petroleum, natural gas and uranium. Hydroelectric and geothermal power have made, and can make, only a small contribution on a world scale, although they are highly significant to certain countries with no indigenous resources of fossil fuel. Easily exploited reserves of both fossil fuel and uranium are limited, and many will approach exhaustion in the lifetime of present students. There are two obvious consequences: first, ways have to be found of using our energy resources more efficiently; and secondly, in the long term, other sources of power must be developed.

It is the science of thermodynamics which enables us to deal quantitatively with the analysis of machines which are used to convert chemical or nuclear energy into useful work. It is therefore an essential study for those hoping to improve the effectiveness with which we use our existing energy resources. The optimisation of total energy schemes involving combined electricity production and process or district heating, or the assessment of combined gas and steam turbine plant (Cogas plant), to take but two examples, inevitably involve thermodynamic analysis. One of the important consequences of the Second Law of Thermodynamics is that unnecessarily large temperature differences used for the transfer of heat incur a waste of energy. A knowledge of the associated subject of heat transfer, dealt with in Part IV of this book, is also essential in an energy-conscious world.

Thermodynamics is likely to play a vital role in the solution of the long-term problem also. It may not help in itself to throw up suggestions for new sources of power, but it is an essential tool for evaluating correctly the potential of new ideas. For example, it will be used to assess proposals for more effective ways of using solar energy, whether in devices which convert it into electricity, or less directly by photosynthesis in plant life from which alcohol or methane fuels can be obtained. It will also be used if ways can be found of harnessing the fusion process. Like fission, fusion will provide heat which can be converted to electricity in more or less conventional power plant. Such solutions would provide mankind with safe and non-polluting sources of power for an indefinitely long period.

Are these massive sources of power really needed? Certainly it is possible for a few small groups to live in self-supporting communes. However, if we care for the bulk of mankind (approximately 5.3×10^9 and probably doubling in under 40 years), continued expansion of power production is essential if only to produce the energy required for modern methods of food production. But it is needed not merely for this: experience in the developed nations suggests that the world population will be stabilised only when the standard of living has been raised substantially in the developing countries. Failure to stabilise it will lead inevitably to famine and conflict over living space. Finally, some of the other reasons why more energy is likely to be needed in the future are:

(a) To enable lower-grade metallic ores to be used, and to operate waste reclamation plant to recover scarce materials

(b) To produce secondary fuels for land, sea and air transport, and the necessary hydrocarbon feedstock for the chemical industry, when natural oil and gas become scarce

(c) To reduce environmental pollution from power plant and industrial processes, which will become increasingly important as the population increases.

The increase in demand will be offset to some extent by energy conservation measures, and by new inventions which will enable society's needs to be met with a smaller expenditure of scarce resources. The development of micro-electronics, and of optical fibres as a substitute for copper wire, are two recent examples of such inventiveness. There is little doubt, however, that there will be a large net increase in demand from the world as a whole because, at present, two-thirds of the world uses energy at about one-tenth of the rate used in the developed countries. In studying engineering in general, and thermodynamics in particular, the student is laying a foundation which will enable him to make a substantial contribution to the welfare of mankind.

To whet the appetite, the accompanying diagram shows the range of energy resources at man's disposal and the ways in which they might be used. Not all of the devices mentioned have been developed to date, and some may never be economic, but most of them receive some attention in this book. Other devices dealt with, which do not appear in this schematic diagram because they do not involve the production of power, are refrigerators, heat pumps, air-conditioning plant and heat exchangers.

How to use this book

Some suggestions as to how the book might be used were given in the Preface to the First Edition, but few new readers feel inclined to read an old preface. In response to requests for guidance, we will repeat here some of what was said there and enlarge upon it.

The first point we made was as follows: 'We do not suggest that our order of presentation is suitable as a direct introduction to the subject, and the book is not designed as a substitute for a course of lectures. Most students are best introduced to a subject by a careful juxtaposition of principle and application, and the book leaves it open to the lecturer to choose any preferred order of

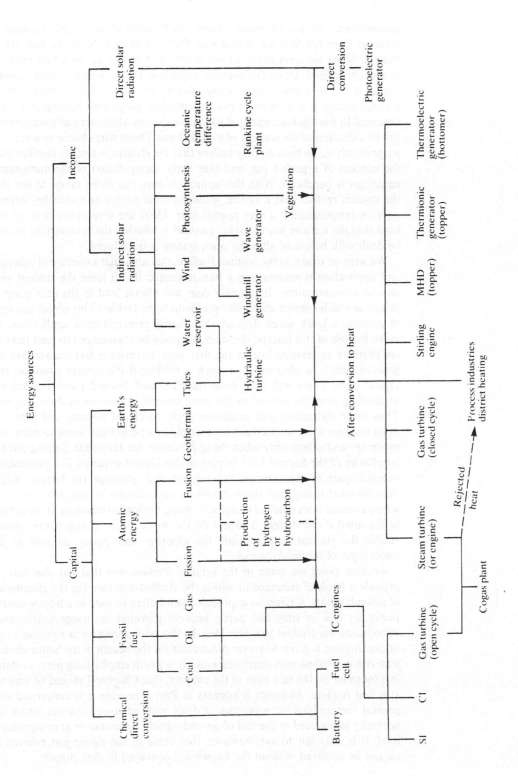

presentation.' Thus a first-year course can be built from an interweaving of material from the first six chapters of Part I with that from the first six of Part II. Some lecturers prefer to use steam, and others air, as a first example of a working fluid. Using the authors' superheat tables, which include internal energy data, the former can give the student an early feel for systems whose internal energy is a function of two independent properties. Principles are not obscured by the algebraic manipulation of equations which normally accompany the introduction of the concept of a perfect gas. Those who choose to start with air probably do so because they believe that the student is already familiar with the concept of a perfect gas, and that early manipulation of thermodynamic equations is beneficial. With this approach, care has to be taken to see that the student realises that a system whose internal energy and enthalpy depend only on temperature is a very special case. There are several decisions of this kind that the lecturer has to make; another is whether the Second Law should be dealt with before or after the open system is introduced.

We went on to say, in the original Preface, that although a mixture of principle and application is necessary in a lecture course, it can leave the student with serious misconceptions. It certainly does not always lead to the firm grasp of principle which enables unfamiliar problems to be tackled. Our object has been to produce a book which distinguishes clearly principle from application. To make full use of this feature, the student should be encouraged to read the first six chapters as revision late in the first year. Experience has shown that the greatest benefit is obtained from such a reading if the student produces two logical trees. These will start from the First and Second Laws respectively, proceeding from the general to the more specific as one moves down the tree. Thus some statements and equations apply to closed systems and others to open systems; some to any fluid, others only to a perfect gas; some to particular processes and others only when those processes are reversible. Setting out the corollaries of the Second Law as part of this logical sequence is a particularly valuable part of the exercise. We suggest that although the lecturer might indicate what is required, there should be no handouts of complete trees. The whole exercise loses much of its value in fixing the logical structure of the subject in the mind if the student does not do the work. Effort of this nature should enable the student to appreciate the elegance and power, as well as the limitations, of thermodynamics.

Another point we made in the original Preface was that our aim was 'to provide a book of reference to which the student can turn for the elucidation of difficult points. A rigorous approach cannot often be used in a lecture course, partly for lack of time and partly because it would be inappropriate when introducing the student to a new idea. In this book, however, a rigorous proof or explanation is given wherever practicable for the benefit of the better student who is not satisfied with simplifications.' It is worth emphasising here, as stated in a footnote on the first page of the chapter, that Chapter 7 should be omitted at a first reading. Although it appears in Part I, because it is concerned with general thermodynamic principles, it deals with advanced matters which are normally introduced at the end of an undergraduate course or at postgraduate level. It is only fair to say, however, that some of the rigour just referred to cannot be achieved without the knowledge conveyed in that chapter.

The widespread adoption of SI has made life for students both easier and more difficult. When using properly constructed physical equations in conjunction with coherent SI units, everything drops out easily and correctly but without requiring much thought. As a consequence, students can lose an awareness of the pitfalls which may be encountered when using non-SI units or even legitimate SI multiples; the latter, though legitimate, are not part of the *coherent* set of units. The student is well advised to digest Appendix A, on dimensions and units, early in the first year.

One final word of warning. A manual of solutions to the problems in Appendix B has been produced for the benefit of teachers and students who do not have easy access to helpful discussions with others. Students who look at any solutions manual before attempting the problems are wasting their time; not only will they learn little, but worse still they will be deceiving themselves into thinking they know something when they do not.

Part I

Principles of Thermodynamics

Introduction

In this book the student will be introduced to a wide range of engineering plant: steam turbines, reciprocating engines, turbo-jets and rockets, combustion systems, refrigerators and heat pumps, direct conversion devices such as fuel cells, compressors, boilers, condensers, cooling towers and heat exchangers. What determines their place in the book is that they are concerned with the transfer of heat and work, in many cases with the ultimate object of converting one form of energy into another. In every case they make use of the way a fluid behaves as it is compressed or expanded, heated or cooled. These features imply that the design of the equipment must involve the science of *thermodynamics*, because this is the science dealing with the relations between the properties of a substance and the quantities of 'work' and 'heat' which cause a change of state. Before a satisfactory analysis of such changes can be made, it is necessary to introduce some carefully defined concepts.

The idea of a *system* plays an important part in thermodynamics; it may be defined as a region in space containing a quantity of matter whose behaviour is being investigated. This quantity of matter is separated from its surroundings by a *boundary*, which may be a physical boundary, such as the walls of a vessel, or some imaginary surface enveloping the region. Before any thermodynamic analysis is attempted it is essential to define the boundary of the system, because it is across the boundary that work and heat are said to be transferred. The term *surroundings* is restricted to those portions of matter external to the system which are affected by changes occurring within the system. When the same matter remains within the region throughout the process under investigation it is called a *closed system*, and only work and heat cross the boundary. An *open system*, on the other hand, is a region in space defined by a boundary across which matter may flow in addition to work and heat.

Part I is primarily concerned with the behaviour of a particular form of matter — a *simple fluid*. A simple fluid may be a gas (e.g. oxygen), a vapour (e.g. steam), a liquid, or a mixture of such substances provided they do not react chemically with one another (e.g. dry or humid air). Closed and open systems containing such fluids are the main concern of engineering thermodynamics. Chemical and physical thermodynamics deal with a wider variety of systems and phenomena, e.g. solids, surface films, electric cells, mixtures undergoing chemical reactions, thermoelectric effects, and magnetic substances (see Refs 5 and 8). These are not the main concern of this book, although some consideration is given in Part II to the chemical reactions involved in the combustion of fuel, and in Part III there is a brief introduction to thermoelectric and other phenomena which make possible the direct conversion of an energy source into electricity.

It follows that in Part I, and indeed for most of the book, a system may be defined less generally as a region in space containing a quantity of fluid. If the fluid is flowing into, out of, or through the region, it is an open system. Some examples are (a) a gas expanding from a container through a nozzle, (b) steam flowing through a turbine, and (c) water entering a boiler and leaving as steam. Examples of a closed system are (a) a mixture of water and steam in a closed vessel, and (b) a gas expanding in a cylinder by displacing a piston. From the last example it will be seen that the boundary separating a closed system from its surroundings need not be fixed; it may expand or contract to accommodate any change of volume undergone by the fixed quantity of fluid. The processes undergone by the fluid in a closed system are described as *non-flow processes*, whereas those undergone by the fluid in an open system are referred to as *flow processes*.

When chemical, surface tension, electrical and magnetic effects are absent, any closed system can only change its condition or state for one or both of the following reasons: (a) there will be a change of state if a part of the boundary is displaced by a force so that some mechanical work is done, e.g. when a force is applied to a piston to compress a gas; (b) there will be a change of state if the system is brought into contact with a portion of the surroundings which is at a different temperature, i.e. if heat is allowed to flow across the boundary. Thus the engineer is concerned to know the way in which the state of a system changes when work and heat cross the boundary.

The *state** of a system at any given instant is determined by the values of its *properties* at that instant. The sort of characteristic which can be used to describe the condition of any object under investigation must always be found by experience, and will depend upon the nature of the investigation. From the standpoint of thermodynamics, many observable characteristics will be irrelevant; for example, shape and colour are irrelevant characteristics of the systems considered in this book. On the other hand, shape would be an important characteristic of any thermodynamic system involving surface tension effects. Those characteristics of a system which can be used to describe its condition or state, and which are relevant to the investigation, are termed the properties of the system. These properties are not all independent of one another; for example, for a perfect gas it is known that the temperature must have a definite value if the pressure and volume are fixed, in accordance with the well-known equation of state $pv = RT$. Classical thermodynamics has been built up from a

---

* The term 'state' is sometimes used in textbooks on heat to refer to the solid, liquid or vapour form of a substance, but these forms are referred to as 'phases' in thermodynamics.

study of closed systems, and it has been found by experiment* that *only two properties are necessary and sufficient to determine the state of a closed system containing a simple fluid.* This state may be termed the *thermodynamic state* of the fluid, and the properties of the fluid from which these two may be chosen are called the *thermodynamic properties.* When the thermodynamic state has been determined by a knowledge of two thermodynamic properties, any third thermodynamic property can be found from a relation expressing it as a function of the two known properties. It will be assumed in Part I that these relations have been determined by experiment for all the fluids likely to be used in engineering systems; the equation of state of a perfect gas is merely one such relation.

The study of open systems is complicated by the fact that the fluid is in motion. If attention is concentrated on a portion of the fluid entering the system, it will be realised that it posseses a relevant *mechanical state* in addition to a thermodynamic state. The *mechanical properties* necessary to determine its mechanical state are (a) velocity relative to the fixed boundary of the system and (b) position in the gravitational field, i.e. height above some datum level. Both these characteristics may change during the passage of the fluid through the system, and they may affect events which occur within the system and the work and heat which cross the boundary; they cannot therefore be omitted from an analysis of open systems. The two mechanical properties are independent of one another and, moreover, are independent of the thermodynamic properties. For example, the fact that a perfect gas is flowing through a pipe with a certain velocity in no way changes the fact that at any point the pressure, volume and temperature of an element of the gas are related by $pv = RT$. All the relations between the thermodynamic properties which will be developed in the following pages are similarly independent of whether the fluid is in motion or changing its position in the gravitational field. Thus the mechanical state is something which can be superimposed upon the thermodynamic state without disturbing the relations between the thermodynamic properties. It will appear later that this makes it possible for the body of knowledge built up from a study of closed systems to be applied to the analysis of open systems.

We are now in a position to summarise the contents of Part I, which present the fundamentals of thermodynamics *without reference to any particular fluid.* First, we note that experiment has shown that the state of a closed system is determined when two thermodynamic properties are known, and that all the other thermodynamic properties are then determined. We shall assume that sufficient experimental information is available to enable any third thermodynamic property to be found if two are known. Secondly, the state of a system changes when work or heat cross the boundary. Thermodynamics provides a means of relating the quantities of heat and work with the change of state, i.e. with the variation of the properties of the fluid. The structure of thermodynamics

---

* Advanced students will find an interesting logical analysis of this procedure in Ref. 2, Chapter 1.

rests upon two important principles called the *First and Second Laws of Thermodynamics*. These cannot be proved and are treated as axioms; their validity rests upon the fact that neither they, nor any deductions made from them, have ever been disproved by experience.

The First Law is initially stated with reference to closed systems, and it is applied to various processes which such systems may undergo. It is then applied to open systems. The First Law is an expression of the principle of the conservation of energy. With the aid of this law it is possible to calculate the quantities of heat and work which cross the boundary of a system when given changes in properties occur, e.g. the work done by steam expanding through a given range of pressure in a turbine, the work required to produce a given pressure rise in an air compressor, or the heat required to generate steam at a given pressure in a boiler.

A second class of problems is concerned with how much of the heat, normally supplied by burning fuel, can be converted into work by a heat engine; or, again, how much work is required to extract a given amount of heat from a body in a refrigerator. These are problems concerning the efficiency of power plant, and they can be solved with the aid of the Second Law of Thermodynamics. The Second Law is an expression of the fact that it is impossible to convert all the heat supplied to an engine into work; some heat must always be rejected, representing a waste of energy. As with the First Law, the second is enunciated with reference to closed systems, and then its consequences for open systems are deduced.

In the final chapter, *which may be omitted on a first reading*, some important general relations between the thermodynamic properties are deduced from the First and Second Laws.

This introduction opened with a list of engineering plant, in the design of which thermodynamics plays a vital role. It may not be out of place to end it with a reminder that the complete design of any of the plant mentioned must involve other engineering sciences, such as mechanics of machines and properties of materials. The engineer will be concerned not only with the behaviour of the working fluid, but also with the stresses and strains and vibration problems that are inevitable consequences of trying to meet the thermodynamic require-ments as economically as possible. No student of engineering — however science based his courses may be — should forget that his ultimate aim is the design of new equipment which is both more efficient in operation, and cheaper to produce and maintain, than its predecessor. The natural resources of our planet are not unlimited.

1

Fundamental Concepts

Before the basic structure of thermodynamics can be outlined, it is necessary to define some of the concepts more thoroughly than has been attempted in the Introduction to Part I, paying particular attention to temperature, work and heat. Accordingly, this chapter is devoted to a discussion of such fundamental concepts. We shall have in mind here only closed systems, consisting of a simple fluid in the absence of chemical, surface tension, electrical and magnetic effects.

1.1 Thermodynamic properties

The idea of a system has been presented in the Introduction to Part I. A closed system is fully defined when the following details are known:

(a) The fluid, e.g. air, hydrogen or water
(b) The boundary between the fluid under consideration and its surroundings
(c) The mass of fluid with the boundary.

The state of the system has yet to be determined; for this a knowledge of its properties is required.

To define the state of a closed system, only the thermodynamic properties of the fluid are relevant. Any such property must be some characteristic that can be measured, and it must have a unique numerical value when the fluid is in any particular state. Pressure, volume and temperature are obvious examples. The value of a property must be independent of the process through which the fluid has passed in reaching that state. It follows that a *change in the value of a property depends only on the initial and final states of the systems, and is independent of the process undergone by the system during the change of state.*

Using pressure as an example, a gas at state 1 may have a pressure of 5 atm, and after a compression process to state 2 a pressure of 8 atm. The change in pressure is an increase of 3 atm however the compression is carried out. If dP is any infinitesimal change in a property during a process, the total change between states 1 and 2 can be written as

$$\int_1^2 dP = P_2 - P_1$$

Mathematically speaking, dP is an *exact differential.**

Consider the following mechanical analogy. A cyclist travels from point 1 at a height z_1 above sea level, to point 2 on a hill z_2 above sea level. Treating the cyclist as the system, his height above sea level can be regarded as a property of the system because the change in height $(z_2 - z_1)$ is independent of the path, i.e. the process, by which the cyclist travels from 1 to 2. The work done by the cyclist, however, is not independent of the process; it clearly depends upon whether he has chosen a short or long route between 1 and 2 and whether he has a following or head wind. Consequently the work done, although a measurable quantity, is not a property. If, during any infinitesimal part of a process, a measurable quantity which depends upon the process is denoted by dX, dX is not an exact differential and

$$\int_1^2 dX \neq X_2 - X_1$$

When the quantity is not a property, the integration between state 1 and state 2 must be written as

$$\int_1^2 dX = X_{12} \quad \text{(or simply as } X\text{)}$$

Further discussion of quantities which are not properties will be deferred to section 1.3, which deals with the concepts of work and heat.

We have already noted the experimental fact that when the values of two properties are known, the state of a closed system is completely determined. An important assumption is implicit in this statement, i.e. that the system is in *thermodynamic equilibrium*. A system is said to be in thermodynamic equilibrium if no further changes occur within it when it is isolated from the surroundings in such a way that no heat and work can cross the boundary. The properties, such as pressure and temperature, must be uniform throughout the system when it is in equilibrium. If the pressure is not uniform, owing to turbulence for example, spontaneous internal changes occur in the isolated system until the turbulence has died down and the pressure has become uniform. Similarly, if there are temperature gradients in the isolated system, a spontaneous redistribution of temperature occurs until all parts of the system are at the same temperature. Only under conditions of equilibrium can single values of pressure and temperature be ascribed to the system, and thus be used to determine its state. *It will always be assumed in this book that the system is in equilibrium at the beginning and end of any process, and therefore that the end states are determined when the values of two properties are fixed.*

It follows that the initial and final states of any closed system can be located

---

* The concept of an exact differential is defined in Chapter 7.

as points on a diagram using two properties as coordinates. If the system is imagined to pass through a continuous series of equilibrium states during the process, the intermediate states could also be located on the diagram, and a line representing the *path* of the process could be drawn through all the points. Such a process is called a *reversible process*; it will be found to be an ideal process analogous to the frictionless process so often referred to in mechanics. In all real processes, however, the system is not in equilibrium in any of the intermediate states. These states cannot be located on the coordinate diagram because the properties do not have single unique values throughout the system. Such processes are called *irreversible processes*. They are best represented on a diagram by a dotted line joining the initial and final state points, to indicate that the intermediate points are indeterminate. Such a line indicates mean values of the properties during the process. The full significance of the ideas of reversibility and irreversibility will appear later.

Pressure, specific volume and temperature are three properties observable by the senses. Pressure p is defined as the force exerted by the fluid on unit area of the boundary, and the unit* we normally employ is the *bar* (1 bar = 10^5 N/m^2 = 1/1.013 25 atm). The specific volume v is the volume of unit mass of fluid, usually quoted in m^3/kg. It is the reciprocal of the density ρ, defined as mass per unit volume, but it is conventional to use specific volume rather than density as one of the properties in thermodynamics. Temperature is a property deserving special attention and it will be introduced in section 1.2. Three more thermodynamic properties — internal energy, enthalpy and entropy — will emerge as consequences of the First and Second Laws of Thermodynamics. Although they are not directly observable by the senses, they are essential to the structure of thermodynamics.

From these six properties, two may be selected to determine the state of a closed system in thermodynamic equilibrium, and the values of the remaining four are then fixed. Care must be taken to see that the two chosen properties are *independent* of one another, i.e. it must be possible to vary one of these properties without changing the other. Obviously ρ and v are not independent properties because one is simply the reciprocal of the other; this fact is recognized in that density is not included in the six properties to which reference was made. But, less obviously, pressure and temperature are not always independent properties: when a liquid is in contact with its vapour in a closed vessel, it is found that the temperature at which the liquid and vapour are in equilibrium is always associated with a particular pressure and one cannot be changed without the other. Pressure and temperature cannot be used to determine the state of such systems, although other pairs, such as pressure and specific volume, may be so used.

As stated in the Introduction, it will be assumed throughout Part I that if any two independent properties are known, the others can be found from experimental data relating to the particular fluid under consideration. If, for example, p and v are known, any third property x must be a function of these

---

* The N/m^2 is called the pascal (Pa), so 1 bar = 10^5 Pa. Dimensions and units are discussed in Appendix A.

Fig. 1.1
Table of properties

	v_a	v_b	— — — — — — —	v_y	v_z
p_a	•	•		•	•
p_b	•	•		•	•
⋮			Values of temperature (or internal energy or enthalpy or entropy)		
p_y	•	•		•	•
p_z	•	•		•	•

two, i.e. $x = \phi(p, v)$. For some fluids the functions are simple, and algebraic equations are used to relate the properties; for others the function is complicated and the experimental data are most conveniently presented in tabular form. Fig. 1.1 shows such a table, the dots denoting values of temperature corresponding to the various combinations of p and v. Similar tables can be prepared with internal energy, enthalpy or entropy as the third property. It is assumed in Part I that either a set of equations or a set of tables is available for each fluid likely to be encountered in engineering systems.

1.2 Temperature

Two systems are said to have *equal temperatures* if there is no change in any of their observable characteristics when they are brought into contact with one another. Consider a system A consisting of a gas enclosed in a vessel of fixed volume fitted with a pressure gauge. If there is no change of pressure when this system is brought into contact with a second system B, say a block of metal, then the two systems are said to have the same temperature. Experiment shows that if the system A is brought into contact with a third system C, again with no change of pressure, then B and C when brought into contact will also show no change in their characteristics. That is, if two bodies are each equal in temperature to a third body they are equal in temperature to each other. This principle of *thermal equilibrium* is often called the *zeroth law of thermodynamics*; the possibility of devising a means of measuring temperature rests upon this principle.

The temperatures of any group of systems may be compared by bringing a particular system, known as the thermometer, into contact with each in turn. System A performs this function in the foregoing example. Such a system must possess an easily observable characteristic termed a *thermometric property*, e.g. the pressure of a gas in a closed vessel, the length of a column of mercury in a capillary tube, or the resistance of a platinum wire. A scale of temperature could be defined by assigning numbers to divisions on the pressure gauge, to points spaced at intervals on the capillary tube, or to divisions on the meter registering the resistance of the wire; units so formed are called degrees of temperature. These temperatures scales would be quite arbitrary, and each instrument would have its own scale. The necessary conditions for a temperature scale to be reproducible when any given thermometric property is used will be discussed in Chapter 8, as well as the means adopted for comparing scales resulting from the use of different thermometric properties.

The reason for postponing the definition of temperature scales is that the practical procedure of constructing an empirical scale of temperature is irrelevant to the structure of thermodynamics. It will be shown that a temperature scale can be defined as a consequence of the Second Law of Thermodynamics without reference to any particular thermometric property, and consequently this has been adopted as the ultimate standard. In Part I, where the analysis is carried out only in symbolic form, no numerical scale need be assigned to the property temperature. The qualitative terms 'high' and 'low' will be used, however, thereby adopting the conventional terminology which originates from our sense of hotness and coldness.

1.3   Work and heat

The limitations placed upon the closed systems considered here* imply that only the application of work or heat can cause a change of state, or conversely that a change of state must be accompanied by the appearance of work or heat at the boundary.

As in mechanics, work is said to be done when a force moves through a distance. If part of the boundary of a system undergoes a displacement under the action of a pressure, the work done W is the product of the force (pressure × area) and the distance it moves in the direction of the force. Fig. 1.2a illustrates this with the conventional piston and cylinder arrangement, the heavy line defining the boundary of the system. The base unit of work in the SI system is the newton metre (N m), also called the joule (J); we shall use the more convenient kilojoule (kJ) which is 10^3 N m. Fig. 1.2b illustrates another way in which work might be applied to a system. Here the boundary really consists of the inner surface of the vessel and the surfaces of the paddle. A force is exerted by the paddle as it changes the momentum of the fluid, and since this force moves during the rotation of the paddle some work is done. To calculate the paddle work it would be necessary to know all the forces acting on the paddle

Fig. 1.2
Work due to movement of
part of a boundary

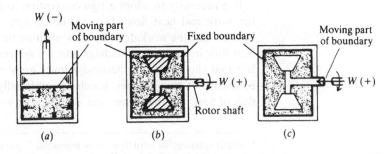

* See Chapter 20 for a brief discussion of a broader concept of work.

11

or rotor surfaces and their displacements; this information would be difficult to obtain in practice. For this reason, when work is transmitted via a shaft it is more convenient to include within the system boundary the paddle (or rotor) and the shaft up to the section at the boundary, as shown in Fig. 1.2c. The work transmitted across the boundary so defined is then calculated from the product of the torque and the angular displacement of the shaft.

The analogy of the cyclist was used in section 1.1 to indicate that work is a quantity which is *not* a property of a system. Work is a transient quantity which only appears at the boundary while a change of state is taking place within a system. *Work is 'something' which appears at the boundary when a system changes its state due to the movement of a part of the boundary under the action of a force.* Although there cannot be said to be any work in a system either before or after the change has taken place, work may be said to 'flow' or 'be transferred' across the boundary. This is a somewhat loose way of speaking; it will be shown in the next chapter that it is 'energy' which is transferred, and that work is the particular form of energy transfer associated with the movement of a force at the boundary.

Heat, denoted by the symbol Q, may be defined in an analogous way to work as follows. *Heat is 'something' which appears at the boundary when a system changes its state due to a difference in temperature between the system and its surroundings.* Again anticipating the next chapter, the 'something' is a form of energy transfer, this time the form associated with a temperature difference. Heat, like work, is a transient quantity which only appears at the boundary while a change is taking place within the system. It is apparent that neither dW nor dQ is an exact differential (section 1.1), and therefore any integration of the elemental quantities of work or heat which appear during a change from state 1 to state 2 must be written as

$$\int_1^2 dW = W_{12} \ \text{(or } W) \quad \text{and} \quad \int_1^2 dQ = Q_{12} \ \text{(or } Q)$$

Although in thermodynamics there cannot be said to be any heat *in* a system either before or after a change of state, loosely speaking heat may be said to 'flow' or 'be transferred' across the boundary. Strictly speaking it is energy which is transferred, but to say 'the heat transferred' is a shorthand way of saying 'the energy transferred by virtue of a temperature difference'.*

It is necessary to adopt a sign convention to indicate the direction in which the work and heat flow. The traditional sign convention in engineering has been to take the work done by the system on the surroundings as positive, and heat flow from the surroundings into the system as positive. It arose from the fact that the science of thermodynamics grew out of the need to explain the behaviour of heat engines, which are essentially devices where there is a net flow of heat into the system and a net flow of work out of it. It seemed natural

---

* Strictly speaking, the word 'heat' alone means this — just as the word 'pedestrian' means 'a man transporting himself on foot'. However, our language requires an explicit verb in a sentence; so we say 'heat is transferred from A to B' and 'there is a pedestrian walking in the road'.

to choose these as the positive quantities. Thermodynamics now has much wider application, and physicists, chemical engineers and most European engineers have found it more logical to take all flows *into* a system as positive — whether of heat, work, or fluid mass and momentum which play a prominent part in open systems. We propose to adopt the newer convention for this and subsequent editions of the book. Thus:

> *Work done by the surroundings on the system and heat flowing from the surroundings into the system are taken as positive.*

Conversely:

> *Work done by the system on the surroundings and heat flowing from the system into the surroundings are taken as negative.*

The exact definition of the *unit of heat* must be deferred until the concept of energy has been introduced formally. The old calorimetric definition may be mentioned, however; it is so called because it originates from the early experiments on heat carried out with calorimeters. The unit of heat was defined as that quantity which would raise the temperature of unit mass of water, at standard atmospheric pressure, through one degree on some temperature scale. Not only does the unit depend upon the temperature scale used, but careful experiments showed that a slightly different quantity of heat was necessary at different points on the chosen temperature scale, i.e. the unit depended on the temperature of the water at the beginning of the one-degree rise. Thus a unit called the *kilocalorie* (kcal) was defined originally as the heat required to raise one kilogram of water one degree on the Celsius scale of temperature. (Similarly, the *British thermal unit* (Btu) and *Celsius heat unit* (Chu) were defined as the quantities of heat required to raise one pound of water one degree Fahrenheit and one degree Celsius respectively.) Later, more carefully defined units were used, such as the 15 °C kcal for which the temperature rise must be from 14.5 to 15.5 °C. So-called calorimetric heat units are still in use; for most practical purposes these are identical with calorimetric units defined in terms of the properties of water, but these calorimetric units are now defined in terms of work units. This is discussed further in section 2.3.

Summarising: neither heat nor work is a property of a system, but both are transient quantities, only appearing at the boundary while a change of state occurs within the system. Although they cannot, therefore, be used to describe the state of a system, heat and work can be used to describe the process undergone by the system during a change of state. For example, using the cyclist analogy, the work done by the cyclist might indicate whether he had chosen a short or long route. Or again, consider a vessel of constant volume containing a gas. Let the gas undergo a change of state in such a way that the pressure and temperature are increased. This change could be obtained by placing the vessel in contact with a body at a higher temperature, or as in Fig. 1.2b by churning the gas with a rotating paddle. Thus the same final state could be

13

reached by the provision of either heat or work. Moreover, both heat and work could be added simultaneously in an infinite number of different proportions to produce the same final state. From this example it is clear that *quantities of heat and work are functions not only of the initial and final states of the system, but also of the process undergone by the system.*

2

The First Law of Thermodynamics

The structure of thermodynamics rests upon two fundamental laws. The First Law, introduced in this chapter, is concerned with the principle of conservation of energy as applied to closed systems which undergo changes of state due to transfers of work and heat across the boundary. The First Law cannot be proved; its validity rests upon the fact that neither it, nor any of its consequences, have ever been contradicted by experience.

2.1 The cycle

A closed system is said to undergo a cyclic process, or *cycle*, when it passes through a series of states in such a way that its final state is equal in all respects to its initial state. This implies that all its properties have regained their initial values. The system is then in a position to be put through the same cycle of events again, and the procedure may be repeated indefinitely. Work can be transferred continuously by devising machines which undergo cyclic processes.

Consider the simple, idealised, mechanical system consisting of a frictionless pulley and a weightless rope shown in Fig. 2.1a. Let a force be applied to raise the weight through a certain distance, a force only infinitesimally greater than the weight. Work is done on the system, and hence the quantity is positive. Now let the weight descend slowly to its original position by reducing the force until it is infinitesimally smaller than the weight (Fig. 2.1b). Since the pulley is frictionless, an infinitesimal difference between the weight and the applied force is sufficient to set the system in motion. The system does work on the surroundings in overcoming the applied force (it could, in fact, be used to raise another weight), so that this time the quantity is negative. The system has now returned to its original state and, in the limit, both quantities of work are equal in magnitude. For the whole cyclic process, therefore,

$$\sum \delta W = 0$$

A circle on the summation sign is used to signify that the algebraic summation of all the increments of work δW is carried out over a complete cycle.

Now consider what happens if, for the second part of the cycle, the force is removed from the rope and a brake shoe is applied to the pulley to restrain the downward acceleration of the weight (Fig. 2.1c). When the weight has been

Fig. 2.1
A cyclic process

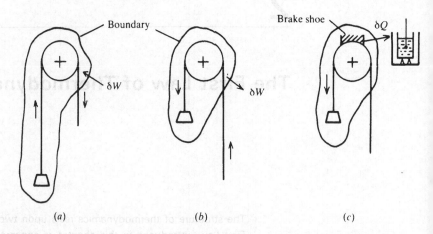

restored to its original position, it will be noticed that the system has not reached
its initial state in *all respects*, for the temperature of the pulley and brake shoe
is higher than it was originally. To restore the system to its original state and
so complete the cycle, heat may be permitted to flow across the boundary of
the system. If desired, the quantity of heat may be measured by allowing it to
raise the temperature of water in a calorimeter. This process is illustrated
diagrammatically in Fig. 2.1c.

As no force moves in the surroundings of the system during the last part of
the cycle, no work is done, and

$$\sum \delta W \neq 0$$

The net work done during this cycle is a positive quantity equal to the work
required to raise the weight initially. On the other hand, a quantity of heat has
crossed the boundary into the surroundings (i.e. the calorimeter). Since no heat
crosses the boundary in the first part of the cycle and a negative quantity
appears in the second,

$$\sum \delta Q \neq 0$$

and is negative.

From this experiment it appears that when a system is taken through a
complete cycle, the algebraic summation of the quantities of either work or
heat which cross the boundary may have some value other than zero. Since the
change in the value of any property over a complete cycle must be zero, because
the initial and final states are identical, this is a further illustration of the fact
that work and heat are *not* properties of a system.

2.2   The First Law of Thermodynamics

Experiments similar to those described in section 2.1 were first carried out by
Joule (1843). He found that the net quantity of heat delivered by the system
was directly proportional to the net quantity of work done on the system during
the cycle. The First Law of Thermodynamics may be expressed as a generalisation

of this result covering all cyclic processes, irrespective of whether net amounts of heat and work are supplied to the system or to the surroundings; the only constraint is that if one is net *into* the system, the other must be net *out* of the system. Because of the historical association of the first law with heat engine cycles, namely cycles producing a net amount of work on the surroundings, the law is usually stated in the following form:

> *When any closed system is taken through a cycle, the net work delivered to the surroundings is proportional to the net heat taken from the surroundings.*

However, the converse is also true, namely:

> *When a closed system is taken through a cycle, the net work done on the system is proportional to the net heat delivered to the surroundings.*

In this latter form, the statement relates to heat pump and refrigerator cycles. These statements may be expressed in mathematical form by

$$\underset{\text{net in}}{\sum \delta Q} \propto \underset{\text{net out}}{\sum \delta W} \quad \text{and} \quad \underset{\text{net out}}{\sum \delta Q} \propto \underset{\text{net in}}{\sum \delta W} \tag{2.1}$$

In section 2.3 we shall reconcile these mathematical statements with our sign convention, thereby merging the two statements into one.

A simple type of cyclic process is indicated in Fig. 2.2. The system is a gas enclosed by a cylinder and piston. If a source of heat is applied to the system the gas expands, pushing the piston before it and doing work on the surroundings; the gas may then be returned to its original state by applying a sink of heat, i.e. a body at a lower temperature than the gas. In the second part of the cycle, the gas contracts and some work is done by the surrounding as the piston moves inwards. This is a straightforward closed system undergoing a series of non-flow processes during which the fluid does not move bodily but merely expands and contracts.

The First Law is adopted as an axiom and provides one of the two foundation stones upon which the structure of classical thermodynamics rests. Joule's experiments, and others of the same nature, are not *proofs* of the First Law; they merely lend support for its adoption as an axiom by providing instances which do not contradict the law. A proof could only be formulated if the First Law could be shown to be a consequence of some even broader and more general

Fig. 2.2
A simple cycle undergone
by a gas

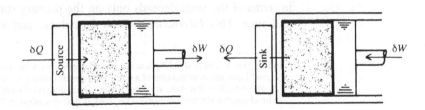

proposition about nature.* Certain propositions about the behaviour of thermodynamic systems can be deduced from the laws of thermodynamics; they may be termed corollaries. These corollaries are often most conveniently proved by *reductio ad absurdum*, i.e. the contrary of a proposition is assumed to be true, and the consequences are then shown to lead to a contradiction of the fundamental axiom.

Before deducing the corollaries of the First Law, which help to bring out all its implications, the constant of proportionality implicit in the expression (2.1) will be discussed.

2.3 Mechanical equivalent of heat

If the constant of proportionality is denoted by $\mathscr{J}$, and taking due account of the sign convention, expression (2.1) can be rewritten as

$$\mathscr{J}\sum \delta Q + \sum \delta W = 0 \qquad (2.2)$$

$\mathscr{J}$ is called the *mechanical equivalent of heat* or *Joule's equivalent*; it expresses the number of work units which are equivalent to one heat unit. Once a work unit and a heat unit have been adopted, experiments such as those carried out by Joule can be used to find the value of $\mathscr{J}$. For such experiments it has been customary to use a calorimetric definition of the unit of heat. If the kJ and the kcal are chosen as the units of work and heat respectively, the value of $\mathscr{J}$ is found to be approximately 4.19 kJ/kcal. Similarly in the older, but now obsolete, systems of units,

$$\mathscr{J} \approx 427\,\frac{\text{kgf m}}{\text{kcal}} \approx 778\,\frac{\text{ft lbf}}{\text{Btu}} \approx 1400\,\frac{\text{ft lbf}}{\text{Chu}}$$

These values are sufficiently accurate for most engineering calculations when both calorimetric and mechanical units are employed.

Strictly speaking, once the First Law has been established and heat and work are interpreted as forms of energy transfer, the need for separate units vanishes. Certainly there is no justification for two sets of absolute standards, e.g. the primary standards of mass, length and time to which the unit of work may be referred, and a standard thermometer and mass of water of a certain purity to which the unit of heat may be referred. This was recognised in 1929 when the First International Steam Table Conference decided to *define* a heat unit in terms of a work unit. The definition accepted today was laid down at the Fifth International Conference on the Properties of Steam (1956) in terms of the joule (J) as the standard unit of work (see Appendix A). A heat unit defined in terms of the joule depends only on the primary standards of mass, length and time. This *International Table kilocalorie*, unit symbol kcal_{IT} although

---

* Indeed this has been done by Keenan and Hatsopoulos, who showed that both the First and Second Laws are consequences of a more basic generalisation about the existence of stable states (i.e. about the fact that there are states which cannot undergo a finite change without a permanent finite change in the environment). This work is best described in Ref. 11.

often written without the subscripts, is defined as

$$1 \text{ kcal}_{IT} = 4.1868 \text{ kJ}$$

The number was chosen so that calorimetric methods of measuring quantities of heat can still be used for ordinary purposes.* Another kilocalorie defined in terms of the joule, and still used in physical chemistry, is the *thermochemical kilocalorie* defined as

$$1 \text{ kcal}_{th} = 4.184 \text{ kJ}$$

Since no fundamental distinction can now be made between the unit of heat and the unit of work, and the 'mechanical equivalent of heat' $\mathscr{J}$ is recognised merely to be a conversion factor between different units, $\mathscr{J}$ can be dropped from equation (2.2), which can now be written as

$$\sum \delta Q + \sum \delta W = 0 \tag{2.3}$$

It is understood that the same unit, for us the kJ, is used consistently for both heat and work. *Equation (2.3), in conjunction with our sign convention, can now be taken to express the First Law.*

Some of the corollaries of the First Law may now be considered.

2.4   Corollaries of the First Law

> *Corollary 1*   There exists a property of a closed system such that a change in its value is equal to the sum of the net heat and work transfers during any change of state.

Proof   Assume that the converse of the proposition is true; i.e. that $\sum_1^2 (\delta Q + \delta W)$ depends upon the process, as well as upon the end states 1 and 2, and so cannot be equal to the change in a property. The procedure is to show that this contradicts the First Law.

Consider any two processes A and B by which a system can change from state 1 to state 2 (Fig. 2.3). The assumption is that in general

$$\sum (\delta Q + \delta W)_A \neq \sum (\delta Q + \delta W)_B \tag{2.4}$$

The subscripts A and B are used to indicate the process for which the summation is carried out. In each case let the system return to its original state by a third

---

* Bearing in mind that 1 kgf = 9.806 65 N, the kcal is related to the metric technical unit of work by

$$1 \text{ kcal} = \frac{4.1868 \times 10^3}{9.806\,65} \text{ kgf m} = 426.935 \text{ kgf m}$$

The old British units are related to the kJ by the definitions

$$1.8 \frac{\text{Btu}}{\text{lb}} = 1 \frac{\text{Chu}}{\text{lb}} = 4.1868 \frac{\text{kJ}}{\text{kg}} \quad \text{which lead to} \quad 1 \text{ ft lbf} = \frac{1}{778.169} \text{ Btu} = \frac{1}{1400.70} \text{ Chu}$$

These definitions ensure that specific heat capacities in calorimetric units are numerically identical in all systems of units — see section 8.2.2.

19

Fig. 2.3
Proof of existence of a
property 'internal energy'

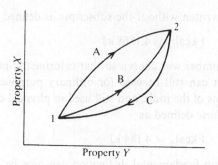

process C. For each of the complete cycles AC and BC so formed, we have

$$\sum (\delta Q + \delta W)_{AC} = \sum_{1}^{2} (\delta Q + \delta W)_{A} + \sum_{2}^{1} (\delta Q + \delta W)_{C}$$

$$\sum (\delta Q + \delta W)_{BC} = \sum_{1}^{2} (\delta Q + \delta W)_{B} + \sum_{2}^{1} (\delta Q + \delta W)_{C}$$

If the assumption described by the inequality (2.4) is true, it follows that

$$\sum (\delta Q + \delta W)_{AC} \neq \sum (\delta Q + \delta W)_{BC}$$

But this contradicts the First Law expressed by equation (2.3), which implies that these quantities must be equal since they are both zero. Therefore the original proposition, that $\sum_{1}^{2} (\delta Q + dW)$ is independent of the process, must be true.

If the property so discovered is denoted by U, the corollary can be expressed mathematically as

$$\sum_{1}^{2} (\delta Q + \delta W) = U_2 - U_1$$

Or, writing Q_{12} and W_{12} for the net quantities of heat and work crossing the boundary during the change of state,

$$Q_{12} + W_{12} = (U_2 - U_1) \tag{2.5}$$

Q and W carry the subscript 12 to indicate that the process follows some path between states 1 and 2 at which the internal energies are U_1 and U_2. Normally we shall omit the subscript on Q and W when the end states are self-evident. When considering a succession of processes, however, it will often be helpful to indicate the steps by retaining the subscripts and writing $(Q_{12} + W_{12})$, $(Q_{23} + W_{23})$ and so on.

The property U is called the *internal energy* of the system, and equation (2.5) is called the *non-flow energy equation*. Expressed verbally: the increase in internal energy of a closed system is equal to the heat supplied *to* the system plus the work done *on* the system. The adjective 'internal' has been adopted to distinguish this form of energy from mechanical forms which might be superimposed on the system. Thus if the system is moving as a whole and changing its position

Fig. 2.4
The importance of defining
the boundary of a system

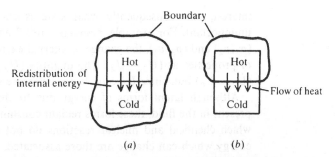

in the gravitational field, we know from mechanics that the system will possess kinetic and potential energy in addition to internal energy.

It should be noted that the First Law is more than a mere definition of the internal energy by a statement to the effect that $\delta U = \delta Q + \delta W$. It states that the internal energy is a quantity *different in kind* from the quantities of work and heat. Internal energy, being a property, can be said to reside in the system and it can be increased or decreased by a change of state. It is only energy which can truly be said to flow across the boundary, and the terms 'work' and 'heat' simply refer to two different causes of the flow of energy. As already stated, if the flow occurs as the result of the movement of a force at the boundary it is termed work, and if it occurs because of a temperature difference between the system and surroundings it is called heat.

Suppose a system consists of two bodies at different temperatures, the boundary being imagined to be an insulating wall isolating the two bodies from their surroundings (Fig. 2.4a). This would represent a system in a non-equilibrium state, since at least one property, temperature, is not uniform throughout the system. Energy will flow from one body to another until the temperatures are identical, when the system will be in equilibrium and any property will have the same value in all parts of the system. The term 'heat' has no meaning in this situation as no energy crosses the boundary. On the other hand, if one body is considered to be the system and the other to be part of its surroundings as in Fig. 2.4b, and energy flows from one to the other owing to the temperature difference, then heat is said to cross the boundary. It follows that the first step in the enunciation of any thermodynamic problem must be to define the system.

The terms in any physical equation must have the same dimensions and be expressed in the same units. Since Q and W are to be expressed in kJ, U must be in kJ; but if Q and W were in kcal then U would also be in kcal. It is important to notice that the energy equation is concerned with *changes* in internal energy. The First Law suggests no means for assigning an absolute value to the internal energy of a system at any given state. For practical purposes, however, it is possible to adopt some state, say state 0, at which the energy is arbitrarily taken to be zero, and then find the changes of energy when the system proceeds from this reference state to a series of states 1, 2, 3 etc. In this way values of U_1, U_2, U_3 etc. can be found and tabulated as in Fig. 1.1, although they are strictly values of $(U_1 - U_0), (U_2 - U_0), (U_3 - U_0)$ etc. In all engineering applications of thermodynamics only changes in energy are of interest, and consequently what state is chosen as the reference state is unimportant. For example, between states 2 and 3, defined say by the values (p_2, v_2) and (p_3, v_3), the change of internal energy can be found from the table of properties as $(U_3 - U_2)$. The quantity $(U_3 - U_2)$ is strictly $(U_3 - U_0) - (U_2 - U_0)$ but, since U_0 cancels, the reference state is irrelevant.

Although latent forms of energy due to chemical and nuclear bonds are present in the fluid, these forms remain constant in any change of state during which chemical and nuclear reactions do not take place. The only forms of energy which can change are those associated, on the kinetic theory of fluids, with the kinetic energy of the molecules and the potential energy due to intermolecular forces; 'random molecular energy' might be used as a collective term when thinking of the mechanical model. It is this random molecular energy which is envisaged when the term 'internal energy' is applied to a closed system in equilibrium. When the system is not in equilibrium, the internal energy can include macroscopic mechanical forms, both kinetic and potential, associated with the movement of relatively large-scale elements of fluid; under these circumstances the symbol E will be used in place of U. The internal energy quoted in tables of properties always refers to the fluid when in a state of equilibrium.

Corollary 2 The internal energy of a closed system remains unchanged if the system is isolated from its surroundings.

No formal proof of this proposition is required once the first corollary has been established; it follows directly from equation (2.5). If the system is isolated from its surroundings, Q and W are both zero and hence ΔU must be zero. The system represented by Fig. 2.4a is an example of an isolated system. All that happens in this case is a spontaneous redistribution of energy between parts of the system which continues until a state of equilibrium is reached; there is no change in the total quantity of energy within the system during the process.

Corollary 2 is often called the *Law of Conservation of Energy*. It is sometimes loosely applied to the whole universe to suggest that the energy of the universe is constant. Such an extrapolation may be admissible only if the universe can be regarded as finite, because the proposition has been inferred from our experience of finite systems.

Corollary 3 A perpetual motion machine of the first kind is impossible.

The perpetual motion machine was originally conceived as a purely mechanical contrivance which, when once set in motion, would continue to run for ever. Such a machine would be merely a curiosity of no practical value, and we know that the presence of friction makes it impossible. What would be of immense value is a machine producing a continuous supply of work without absorbing energy from the surroundings; such a machine is called a *perpetual motion machine of the first kind.*

It is always possible to devise a machine to deliver a limited quantity of work without requiring a source of energy in the surroundings. For example, a gas compressed behind a piston will expand and do work at the expense of the internal energy of the gas. Such a device cannot produce work continuously, however; for this to be achieved the machine must be capable of undergoing a succession of cyclic processes. But equation (2.3) states that if a net amount of heat is not supplied by the surroundings during a cycle, no net amount of work can be delivered by the system. Thus the First Law implies that a perpetual motion machine of the first kind is impossible.

3

Non-Flow Processes

In this chapter the non-flow energy equation expressing the First Law will be given particular forms relating to various special processes which occur in closed systems. It will be shown that these processes may be classified further into reversible and irreversible processes. For the former class the energy equation may be expressed in a particularly useful form because the quantities of heat and work can each be stated in terms of changes in the properties of the system. The equations so derived are quite general in that they apply to any fluid.

3.1 The energy equation and reversibility

In section 2.4 the non-flow energy equation was presented in the form

$$Q + W = (U_2 - U_1)$$

It has already been stated that we shall only consider systems which are in equilibrium in their initial and final states. When the system is in equilibrium, all the properties are uniform throughout the system and, in particular, each unit mass of the system will have the same internal energy.* Thus, if u represents the internal energy of unit mass, and m is the mass of the system, it is possible to write $U = mu$. In the same circumstances the volume V is equal to mv. u is termed the *specific internal energy* just as v is the specific volume, although the adjective 'specific' is often omitted when referring to internal energy. It is often convenient to work with specific quantities throughout an analysis and then multiply the final result by the mass of the system. Thus the non-flow energy equation is usually written as

$$Q + W = (u_2 - u_1) \tag{3.1}$$

implying that Q and W are the quantities of heat and work per unit mass of fluid.

For the particular class of processes known as reversible processes, the system is imagined to pass through a continuous series of equilibrium states. In such cases the equation may be applied to any infinitesimal part of the process between the end states, and the energy equation may be written in the differential

---

* This statement only applies to systems consisting of a fluid in a single phase or, when more than one phase is present, if the phases are homogeneously mixed.

form

$$dQ + dW = du \qquad (3.2)$$

The analysis of a reversible process may therefore be carried out by considering an infinitesimal part of the process undergone by unit mass, and overall changes which occur between the end states can be found by an integration performed at the conclusion of the analysis followed by multiplication by the mass of the system.

During irreversible processes, on the other hand, the system does not pass through a series of equilibrium states. It is not possible to write mu for the internal energy of the system in any intermediate state because (a) a single value of u cannot be used to define the random molecular energy of the fluid, and (b) this energy is not the only relevant form if the fluid is turbulent. Each elemental mass δm may have a different specific internal energy e which must include the kinetic and potential energy of the mass δm. It is possible to consider an infinitesimal part of an irreversible process, but only by writing

$$dQ + dW = dE$$

where $E = \Sigma(e\,\delta m)$. Consequently, to evaluate dE it would be necessary to find the change in the specific internal energy of each of the elemental masses of which the system is composed — an impossible task. When considering irreversible processes, therefore, the energy equation can be used only in the integrated form of equation (3.1), and it is then sufficient to be able to assign values of u to the end states. This can be done because these are always assumed to be states of equilibrium.

For the system to pass through a series of equilibrium states, and therefore to undergo a reversible process, it may be shown that the work and heat must cross the boundary under certain particular conditions. These conditions will be discussed for work and heat in turn.

3.1.1   Work and reversibility

Let us consider a closed system where a part of the boundary is allowed to move under such conditions that the external restraining force is only infinitesimally smaller than that produced by the pressure of the system. Fig. 3.1 illustrates such a system. The area of the piston is A, the pressure of the fluid at any instant is p, and the restraining force exerted by the surroundings is infinitesimally smaller than pA. If p is assumed constant during an infinitesimal movement of the piston over a distance dl, the work done in moving the external force pA through this distance must be $pA\,dl$. But $A\,dl = dV$, the infinitesimal change of volume, and therefore

$$dW = -p\,dV$$

The negative sign is required because in an expansion dV is positive, whereas dW is negative because work is being done on the surroundings. If the expansion occurs from a pressure p_1 to a pressure p_2, in such a way that the restraining

25

Fig. 3.1
A reversible process

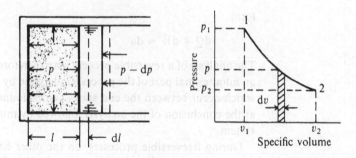

force is changed continuously so that it is never materially different from pA, the total work done can be found by summing all the increments of work:

$$W = -\int_1^2 p\,dV \qquad (3.3)$$

The conditions under which this expansion has been imagined to proceed are just those necessary for the expansion to be reversible. No pressure gradients or eddies are set up in the fluid, and the properties are uniform throughout the system at all times. The system passes through a series of equilibrium states, and the process may be represented by a full line on the p–v diagram (Fig. 3.1). The area under this curve is given by $\int_1^2 p\,dv$. Comparison with equation (3.3) shows that the area represents the *magnitude* of the work done per unit mass of fluid.

The reason for the use of the term 'reversible' is now apparent; the expansion may be stopped at any point and reversed by only an infinitesimal change in the external force. The system will then return through the same series of states, and exactly the same quantity of work will be done by the surroundings on the system as has been done by the system on the surroundings in the original process. dV would be negative for the compression, and hence $-p\,dV$ would appear as a positive quantity in agreement with the sign convention adopted for work.

It is easy to show that $-\int p\,dv$ is not always equal to the work done per unit mass, and that the equality only holds when the system passes through a series of equilibrium states. Fig. 3.2a shows a container divided into two compartments by a sliding partition. One part contains a mass of gas at a pressure p_1 and specific volume v_1, and the other is evacuated. When the partition is withdrawn, the gas undergoes an expansion which is not restrained in any way by an opposing force at the moving boundary; the process is called a *free expansion*. When the system has settled down to a new state of equilibrium it may have a pressure p_2 and specific volume v_2. The end states could be located on the p–v diagram, but the fact that a process had occurred could only be indicated by a dashed line. Each intermediate state is indeterminate because no single values of p and v can be ascribed to the system as a whole. Some intermediate points could be found, however, if the process were carried out in a number of steps as in Fig. 3.2b. After each partition is withdrawn, and the gas has settled down to an equilibrium state, the pressure and volume could be measured and

Fig. 3.2
The free expansion and
irreversibility

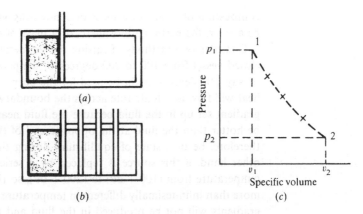

(a)

(b)

(c)

the corresponding state point plotted on the p–v diagram. If a dashed curve is drawn through all such points, as in Fig. 3.2c, the area under the curve could be found and this would be equal to $\int_1^2 p\,dv$. Yet no work has been done by the system on the surroundings at all, because no external force has been moved through a distance.

This is an extreme case; in general there is some restraining force at a moving boundary, and some work will be done by the fluid during the expansion. But, unless the process is reversible, the magnitude of the work done per unit mass will always be less than $\int p\,dv$. This point will be elaborated in section 5.4, where it is also noted that for a compression the magnitude of the work done on the system is always greater than $\int p\,dv$ unless the process is reversible. When it is helpful to emphasise that equation (3.3) is valid only for reversible processes, the equation may be written as

$$W_{\mathrm{rev}} = -\int_1^2 (p\,dv) \quad \text{or} \quad W = -\int_1^2 (p\,dv)_{\mathrm{rev}}$$

The condition for reversibility, that the external force in the surroundings should differ only infinitesimally from the internal force due to the pressure of the fluid, means that there is no excess force available for accelerating the fluid or boundary. Thus it implies that the reversible expansion or compression is an infinitely slow process. Since any real process must occur within a finite time, it is clear that the reversible process is an ideal process, i.e. one which may be approached but is never actually achieved in practice.

3.1.2   Heat and reversibility

The part of the surroundings which exchanges energy with a system by virtue of the fact that it is at a different temperature is called a *heat reservoir*; it may be a source or sink of heat. Usually the term 'reservoir' is restricted to mean a source or sink of such capacity that any quantity of heat which crosses the boundary during a process is insufficient to change its temperature. A practical source of large capacity might be the gases produced by the continuous combustion of a fuel, or a mass of condensing vapour; a practical sink might be a river, the earth's atmosphere, or a mass of melting solid.

Consider two methods of raising the temperature of a fluid contained in a closed vessel from 100 to 200 degrees of temperature. An infinite heat source of, say, 300 degrees might be used for the purpose. Under these circumstances heat will flow at a finite rate across the boundary. There will be a temperature gradient set up in the fluid because the fluid nearest to the source will always be hotter than the fluid at the opposite end of the vessel. The system cannot, therefore, be in a state of equilibrium during the transfer of energy. On the other hand, if this source is replaced by a series of heat sources ranging in temperature from $(100 + d\theta)$ to $(200 + d\theta)$, so that the active source is never more than infinitesimally different in temperature from the system, temperature gradients will not be produced in the fluid and the system may be presumed to pass through a series of equilibrium states. Moreover, at any point in the process only an infinitesimal change in the temperature of the source is necessary for it to become a sink and for the direction of the process to be reversed.

Thus a transfer of energy by virtue of a temperature difference can be carried out reversibly only if the temperature difference is infinitesimally small. This implies that the rate at which the transfer can proceed is infinitely slow, and once again it appears that the reversible process cannot be completely achieved in practice. Practical methods by which a reversible heat transfer process can be approached are available, and one is described in section 12.9.

A number of particular non-flow processes may now be considered, each of which may or may not be performed reversibly. When they are performed irreversibly, the non-flow energy equation may be applied in the integrated form

$$Q + W = (u_2 - u_1)$$

because the end states are always assumed to be states of equilibrium. When they are performed reversibly, the energy equation may also be applied in the differential form

$$dQ + dW = du$$

And, in addition, the work transfer can be expressed in terms of the properties of the system, i.e. $dW = -p\,dv$, so that

$$dQ - p\,dv = du$$

It might be supposed, by analogy, that when heat is transferred during a reversible process it too can be expressed in terms of properties. As temperature is clearly associated with heat, it might be one of the properties. For example, we might be able to write $dQ = \theta\,dx$, where θ is the temperature and x some other property. This is in fact the case. As a consequence of the Second Law of Thermodynamics it will be shown that two suitable properties can be defined, and that $dQ = T\,ds$, where T is the *absolute thermodynamic temperature* and s is the property *entropy*. We shall not, at this stage, presuppose the relation $dQ = T\,ds$, but will point out the type of problem in which it might prove useful.

3.2   Constant volume process

The discussion in section 1.3 has already shown that there are an infinite number of processes which can produce a given change of state and during which the volume remains constant. Any combination of quantities of heat and work can be used which will satisfy the equation

$$Q + W = (u_2 - u_1)$$

remembering that u_1 and u_2 are fixed when the initial and final states are given. The only restriction is that W must be zero or positive, because during a constant volume process work can only be done in practice by some method of churning the fluid.

The process of increasing the internal energy of a system by using the viscous or frictional effects inherent in any movement of a fluid is one to be avoided. Such a process involves a degradation of energy because, as will be shown later, no practical method exists of making all the internal energy available again as work. Consequently, whenever reference is made to a constant volume process, it will always be to one in which the work is zero unless otherwise stated. Thus the energy equation for a constant volume process is usually written as

$$Q = (u_2 - u_1) \tag{3.4}$$

That is, the quantity of heat is equal to the change of internal energy.

If, in addition to the work being zero, it is stipulated that the heat is transferred by virtue of an infinitesimally small temperature difference, then the process is reversible and the energy equation can be written in differential form as

$$dQ = du \tag{3.5}$$

There is one, and only one, constant volume process which can join two given end states when the process is reversible.

It is worth noting that the integrated form of equation (3.5) is (3.4), so that the overall quantity of heat transferred during a constant volume process from state 1 to state 2 does not depend upon the provision of a reversible method of transferring the heat, but merely on the assumption that the work is zero.

3.3   Constant pressure process

A closed system undergoing a process at constant pressure is illustrated in Fig. 3.3. The fluid is enclosed in a cylinder by a piston on which rests a constant weight. If heat is supplied, the fluid expands and work is done by the system in overcoming the constant force; if heat is extracted, the fluid contracts and work is done on the system by the constant force. In the general case,

$$Q + W = (u_2 - u_1)$$

Work might also be done on the system simultaneously by churning the fluid with a paddle, and this positive quantity of work must then be included in the

Fig. 3.3

A process at constant pressure

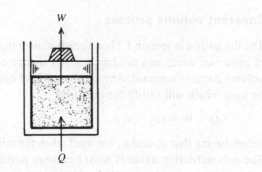

term W. If no paddle work is done on the system, and the process is reversible,

$$dQ - p\,dv = du \qquad (3.6)$$

Since p is constant, this can be integrated to give

$$Q - p(v_2 - v_1) = (u_2 - u_1) \qquad (3.7)$$

If the initial and final states are known, e.g. if p, v_1 and v_2 are given, a definite quantity of heat Q is transferred during the process which can be calculated from (3.7). There is therefore only one reversible constant pressure process which can join the two given states.

A further simplification of the energy equation is possible if a new property is introduced. Since p is constant, $p\,dv$ is identical with $d(pv)$. Thus the energy equation can be written as

$$dQ - d(pv) = du$$

or

$$dQ = d(u + pv)$$

The quantity $(u + pv)$ occurs so frequently in thermodynamics, particularly in equations relating to open systems, that it has been given a special name and symbol, the *specific enthalpy h*. Because enthalpy is defined merely as a combination of the properties u, p and v, it is itself a property. That is, a change in enthalpy between two states depends only upon the end states, and is independent of the process. Values of the enthalpy are included in tables of properties of fluids and, as with internal energy, the values given are always differences between the enthalpy at various states and the enthalpy at some reference state where it is arbitrarily assumed to be zero. Since only changes of enthalpy are of interest, this information is adequate. In terms of specific quantities,

$$h = u + pv \qquad (3.8)$$

and for any mass of fluid m, in a state of equilibrium,

$$H = U + pV \qquad (3.9)$$

where $H = mh$, $U = mu$ and $V = mv$. The units of enthalpy must be those of energy; therefore we shall express enthalpy in kJ and the specific enthalpy in kJ/kg.

Using this derived property, the energy equation corresponding to (3.6) becomes

$$dQ = dh \qquad (3.10)$$

or, in the integrated form,

$$Q = (h_2 - h_1) \qquad (3.11)$$

Thus the heat added in a reversible constant pressure process is equal to the increase of enthalpy,* whereas it was equal to the increase of internal energy in the reversible constant volume process. Equation (3.11) does not apply if the process is irreversible; it is an integrated form of the special equation (3.6), and has not been deduced directly from the general equation.

3.4 Polytropic process

The constant volume and constant pressure processes can be regarded as limiting cases of a more general type of process in which both the volume and the pressure change, but in a certain specified manner. In many real processes it is found that the states during an expansion or compression can be described approximately by a relation of the form $pv^n = $ constant, where n is a constant called the *index of expansion or compression*, and p and v are average values of pressure and specific volume for the system. Compressions and expansions of the form $pv^n = $ constant are called *polytropic* processes. When $n = 0$ the relation reduces to $p = $ constant, and when $n = \infty$ it can be seen to reduce to $v = $ constant by writing it in the form $p^{1/n}v = $ constant.

For the *reversible* polytropic process, single values of p and v can truly define the state of a system, and $dW = -p\,dv$. The work done per unit mass during a change from state 1 to state 2 may then be found by integration as follows. For the initial, final and any intermediate state,

$$p_1 v_1^n = p_2 v_2^n = pv^n$$

Therefore

$$W = -\int_1^2 p\,dv = -p_1 v_1^n \int_1^2 \frac{dv}{v^n} = \frac{p_1 v_1^n (v_2^{1-n} - v_1^{1-n})}{n-1}$$

$$= \frac{p_2 v_2^n v_2^{1-n} - p_1 v_1^n v_1^{1-n}}{n-1} = \frac{p_2 v_2 - p_1 v_1}{n-1} \qquad (3.12)$$

The integrated form of the energy equation for a reversible polytropic process

---

* It is this particular relation which led to the adoption of the term 'total heat' as an alternative to enthalpy. Such a name is misleading because the enthalpy is related to the heat supplied only in the special case of a reversible constant pressure process, whereas the property is used in the analysis of many other processes where it bears no direct relation to a quantity of heat.

31

Fig. 3.4
Polytropic processes

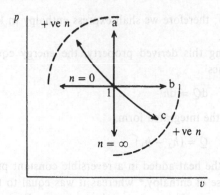

may therefore be written as

$$Q + \frac{(p_2 v_2 - p_1 v_1)}{n - 1} = (u_2 - u_1) \tag{3.13}$$

For any given reversible polytropic process, i.e. one joining two given end states, definite quantities of heat and work cross the boundary. For example, if the end states are defined by (p_1, v_1) and (p_2, v_2), the index n can be found, and W and Q calculated from (3.12) and (3.13).

Some reversible polytropic processes are represented in Fig. 3.4 on the p–v diagram. The lower right-hand quadrant contains expansion processes starting from an initial state represented by point 1, and the upper left-hand quadrant contains compression processes starting from the same initial state. The area under the curve or line represents the *magnitude* of the work done in each case, i.e. under a it is zero, under b it is $p(v_2 - v_1)$, and under c it is $(p_2 v_2 - p_1 v_1)/(1 - n)$. The larger the value of n, the more nearly does the polytropic curve approach the vertical line representing the constant volume process. This fact could also be found by differentiating $pv^n = $ constant to give

$$v^n \, dp + pnv^{n-1} \, dv = 0$$

or

$$\frac{dp}{dv} = -\frac{np}{v} \tag{3.14}$$

Thus the slope of the curve increases in the negative direction with increase of n.

Although it is physically possible for processes to fall into the other two quadrants, they do not often arise in practical systems. These would be processes during which the pressure and volume increase or decrease simultaneously, and would imply a negative value of n if they were polytropic processes. An example of a system in which p and v increase simultaneously is illustrated in Fig. 3.5, wherein a piston is controlled by a spring. When heat is supplied to the fluid the restraining force increases as the expansion of fluid compresses the spring. The pressure of the fluid is always equal to the spring force divided by the piston area, and consequently the pressure must increase linearly with volume as shown on the p–v diagram. The process would be represented by a straight line in the upper right-hand quadrant of Fig. 3.4; it would of course only be a

Fig. 3.5
Simultaneous increase of
pressure and volume

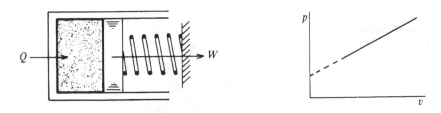

polytropic process if the projected line passed through the origin (i.e. when
$n = -1$).

3.5 Adiabatic process

The term *adiabatic* is used to describe any process during which heat is prevented
from crossing the boundary of the system. That is, an adiabatic process is one
undergone by a system which is thermally insulated from its surroundings. For
adiabatic non-flow processes, therefore, the energy equation reduces to

$$W = (u_2 - u_1) \tag{3.15}$$

In an adiabatic expansion, work is done by the system at the expense of its
internal energy; in an adiabatic compression, the internal energy is increased
by an amount equal to the work done on the system. If the initial and final
states are known, the values u_1 and u_2 are determined and the work done can
be calculated. We shall proceed to show that in the case of a *reversible* adiabatic
process there is only one process which can join the end states, i.e. that there
is a definite relation between p and v. In this case, therefore, the work done can
be predicted when the initial state and only one property of the system in its
final state are known.

We shall suppose that p_1 and v_1 are known, and that it is required to find
the work done by the system during a reversible adiabatic expansion to p_2. For
this process the energy equation may be written in differential form as

$$p \, dv = -du \tag{3.16}$$

If a known algebraic equation $u = \phi(p, v)$ relates p, v and u, (3.16) may be
rewritten as

$$p \, dv = -d\phi(p, v)$$

and integrated. The result will be a definite relation between p and v, e.g. $v = f(p)$.
v_2 can be found by putting $p = p_2$ in $f(p)$. Consequently u_2 and u_1 can be found
from $\phi(p, v)$, and the work can be calculated using equation (3.15).

If no simple algebraic equation relates p, v and u, the following graphical
method could, in principle, be used:

(a) First, a series of constant pressure lines are drawn on a diagram using u
and v as coordinates, from the information contained in the table of
properties (Fig. 1.1). For each pressure in the table a series of values of
u and v are given, and these pairs of values can be represented by points
on the diagram. All points relating to one pressure, p_a, say, are joined up

33

Fig. 3.6
The reversible adiabatic
process

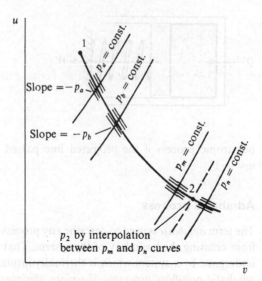

to form a constant pressure line. This is repeated for a series of pressures $p_b, \ldots, p_m, p_n$ covering the range p_1 to p_2 as shown in Fig. 3.6.

(b) Secondly, the path of the reversible process is traced out on the diagram starting from the initial state 1. Recasting equation (3.16) in the form $du/dv = -p$, it is seen that at any point in the process the slope of the curve is negative and equal in magnitude to the pressure at that point. Through each constant pressure line a series of short parallel lines can be drawn with a slope equal to $-p$. The path of the process will be represented by a curve drawn from point 1 so that its slope is always the same as that of the short parallel line where it intersects each constant pressure line.

(c) Lastly, since the final pressure p_2 is known, the final state can be located on the curve, and the value of u_2 can be read off the diagram. The work done can then be calculated from (3.15).

The foregoing graphical procedure is very lengthy. Looking ahead, it is easy to show that the calculation can be considerably simplified if we can write $dQ = T\,ds$ for a reversible process, where T is the absolute thermodynamic temperature (section 6.2) and s is the property entropy (section 6.4). Then, since $dQ = 0$ for an adiabatic process, $ds = 0$ when it is reversible and the entropy must remain constant. The foregoing problem may be solved by finding s_1 corresponding to p_1 and v_1 from the tables of properties, and then, since $s_2 = s_1$, finding v_2 corresponding to p_2 and s_2. Corresponding values of u_1 and u_2 can also be found from the tables, and the problem is solved. This illustrates one possible use of the property entropy.

3.6 Isothermal process

When the quantities of heat and work are so proportioned during an expansion or compression that the temperature of the fluid remains constant, the process is said to be *isothermal*. Since temperature gradients are excluded by the definition, the reversibility of an isothermal process is implied. If it were not reversible a single value of the temperature could not be allotted to the system as a whole in all the intermediate states. It should be noted, however, that the term 'isothermal' is often ascribed to processes which are not reversible but during which the average temperature of the bulk of the fluid remains constant.

It is possible to show that for a reversible isothermal process a certain definite relation must exist between p and v, and consequently the work done has a definite value which can be predicted. For any reversible process the energy equation is

$$dQ - p\,dv = du$$

or

$$Q - \int_1^2 p\,dv = (u_2 - u_1)$$

A relation between p, v and temperature θ must exist, either as some equation of state $\theta = \phi(p, v)$, or in the form of a table of properties. Consequently, if the temperature remains constant, a definite relation exists between p and v which may be determined analytically or graphically. If p_1, v_1 and p_2 are given, v_2 can be found from this particular p–v relation. The work done may be found either by integrating $p\,dv$ between these limits, or by finding the area under the curve on a p–v diagram. Since the end states are known, u_1 and u_2 can be found, and consequently Q can be calculated from the energy equation if it is required.

There is no need to outline the graphical procedure required if no simple function relates p, v and the temperature θ, because once again, looking ahead, the problem is much more easily solved by the use of the entropy s and the absolute thermodynamic temperature T. For a reversible process $dQ = T\,ds$, and since T is constant in the case of an isothermal process it is possible to integrate this expression directly. Thus for a reversible isothermal process, $Q = T(s_2 - s_1)$, where $T = T_1 = T_2$. If p_1 and v_1 are known, s_1, T_1 and u_1 can be found from tables of properties. Since p_2 and T_2 ($= T_1$) are known, s_2 and u_2 can also be found from the tables. Thus Q can be calculated from $T(s_2 - s_1)$, and the work transfer can then be found from

$$W = (u_2 - u_1) - Q$$

4

Flow Processes

This chapter is devoted to a discussion of various flow processes which occur in open systems. Since the energy equation expressing the First Law has been deduced with reference to closed systems, the first step is to deduce an equivalent equation for open systems. Flow processes may be classified into steady-flow and nonsteady-flow processes, and since the former are of greater interest they are considered first. Finally, the idea of a cycle consisting of steady-flow processes is presented. The application of the concept of reversibility to flow processes will be deferred until Chapters 5 and 6.

4.1 The steady-flow energy equation

A diagrammatic sketch of a typical open system is shown in Fig. 4.1. Fluid flows through the system at a uniform rate, while heat and work are transferred between the fluid and surroundings also at a uniform rate. The work is done in this instance by allowing the fluid to impinge on a row of turbine blades. Useful work done by the turbine is transferred to the surroundings via a shaft and is called *shaft work*. Note that the boundary has been drawn outside the container for clarity, although it should be imagined to encompass only the fluid.* If the rotor is included also, with the boundary cutting the shaft, then the work done can be deduced from the torque in the shaft and the angular displacement; detailed knowledge of the forces exerted by the fluid on the turbine blading is then unnecessary. The idea behind this procedure was introduced in section 1.3 when dealing with paddle work in closed systems. With any *open* system, the boundary is assumed to cut the entrance and exit ducts where the properties of the fluid are known, i.e. at cross-sections 1 and 2 in Fig. 4.1.

At any given point in the flow, an element of the fluid has a relevant mechanical state in addition to a thermodynamic state. Any of the mechanical and thermodynamic properties may change as the element passes through the system, so that both types of property are relevant to the analysis. For the flow to be regarded as *steady*, the rate of mass flow (kg/s say) must be constant and the

---

* In fluid mechanics the boundary is often referred to as a *control surface* and the system as a *control volume*.

36

Fig. 4.1
Open system with heating
chamber and turbine

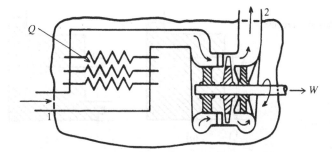

same at inlet and outlet, and the properties of the fluid at any point in the open system must not vary with time. The latter condition means that all elements of fluid flowing past a given point will always have the same mechanical and thermodynamic states. The properties will, in general, be different at different points in the system, and therefore any given element of fluid passes through a series of states on its way through the system.

It is possible to regard the continuous-flow process as a series of non-flow processes undergone by an imaginary closed system, and Fig. 4.2 illustrates this.* The boundary of the closed system includes the fluid contained in the open system at any instant, plus a portion of the fluid about to enter the system. The imaginary closed system must then be supposed to undergo a deformation as indicated by the succession of Figs 4.2a, b and c. Continuous flow may be regarded as a succession of these non-flow processes, carried out for every element of fluid entering the open system. It now becomes possible to apply the energy equation which has been developed from a study of closed systems.

First consider the state of the imaginary closed system in the configuration shown in Fig. 4.2a. Fig. 4.3 shows an enlarged view of the part of the system containing the element of fluid which is about to enter the open system. The thermodynamic and mechanical states of the element of mass δm may be assumed to be known. The random molecular energy of the element is U_1 say, and if the element is moving with a velocity C_1 at a height z_1 above some reference level, it also possesses kinetic energy $\frac{1}{2}\delta m\, C_1^2$ and potential energy $\delta m\, gz_1$. The total energy of the mass δm is therefore

$$U_1 + \tfrac{1}{2}\delta m\, C_1^2 + \delta m\, gz_1$$

If we assume that the element is small enough for the thermodynamic properties to be uniform throughout its extent, this becomes

$$\delta m(u_1 + \tfrac{1}{2}C_1^2 + gz_1)$$

At the instant when mass δm reaches the boundary of the open system, let the fluid within the open system possess a total quantity of internal energy E'. E' includes the kinetic and potential energies of the fluid elements within the boundary of the open system; the possibility of using the term 'internal energy'

---

* This approach was suggested in a paper by Gillespie and Coe (Ref. 9), and used by Keenan in his *Thermodynamics* (Ref. 6).

Fig. 4.2
Imaginary non-flow process

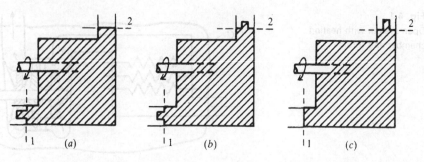

(a)   (b)   (c)

in this way has already been noted in section 2.4. For reasons which will appear later, however, there is no need to specify the different forms of energy of which E' consists; nor does it matter that this quantity of fluid is not in a state of equilibrium and that the mass of fluid is unknown. The total internal energy of the imaginary closed system in its initial state (Fig. 4.2a) is

$$E' + \delta m(u_1 + \tfrac{1}{2}C_1^2 + gz_1)$$

Now consider the state of the closed system in the configuration shown in Fig. 4.2c. Since, for steady flow, the properties of the fluid at any point in the open system do not change with time, the quantity of energy contained within the original boundary must still be E'. Therefore, if a mass δm leaves the open system at some part of the boundary where the properties are denoted by subscript 2, the final internal energy of the imaginary closed system (Fig. 4.2c) will be

$$E' + \delta m(u_2 + \tfrac{1}{2}C_2^2 + gz_2)$$

Lastly, we must consider how the imaginary closed system changes its state from that in Fig. 4.2a to that in Fig. 4.2c. In this period of time we may assume that δQ units of energy are transferred to the system as heat, and that δW units of energy are transferred to the system as work via a shaft. The shaft work δW is not the only work transferred as far as the imaginary closed system is concerned

Fig. 4.3
Elemental mass crossing inlet
plane 1

Internal energy	$\delta m\, u_1$
Kinetic energy	$\tfrac{1}{2}\delta m\, C_1^2$
Potential energy	$\delta m\, g z_1$

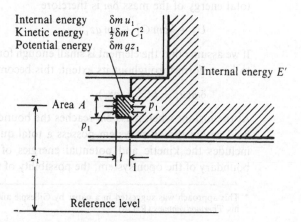

Internal energy E'

Area A

p_1

p_1

z_1

l

Reference level

because parts of its boundary move at sections 1 and 2. For the element δm to enter the open system, the imaginary closed system must be compressed, its volume decreasing by $\delta m\, v_1$. This is accompanied by a force $p_1 A$ moving a distance $l = \delta m\, v_1/A$, where A is the cross-sectional area of the element, as illustrated in Fig. 4.3. The work done by the surroundings on the system is therefore $\delta m\, p_1 v_1$. Similarly, it can be shown that the work done by the closed system on the surroundings, as δm is expelled from the open system, is $\delta m\, p_2 v_2$.* The net work done on the system during the change represented in Fig. 4.2 is therefore

$$\delta W - \delta m(p_2 v_2 - p_1 v_1)$$

We may now apply the energy equation to the imaginary closed system and write

$$\delta Q + \{\delta W - \delta m(p_2 v_2 - p_1 v_1)\}$$
$$= \{E' + \delta m(u_2 + \tfrac{1}{2}C_2^2 + gz_2)\} - \{E' + \delta m(u_1 + \tfrac{1}{2}C_1^2 + gz_1)\} \qquad (4.1)$$

The quantity E' cancels, and by writing the enthalpy h for $(u + pv)$, the equation reduces to

$$\delta Q + \delta W = \delta m(h_2 + \tfrac{1}{2}C_2^2 + gz_2) - \delta m(h_1 + \tfrac{1}{2}C_1^2 + gz_1)$$

The continuous steady-flow process consists of the sum total of all the elemental mass transfers across sections 1 and 2; it may therefore be represented by the equation

$$\Sigma \delta Q + \Sigma \delta W = \Sigma \delta m(h_2 + \tfrac{1}{2}C_2^2 + gz_2) - \Sigma \delta m(h_1 + \tfrac{1}{2}C_1^2 + gz_1)$$

This equation can be simplified considerably if the properties are uniform over the cross-section of flow at inlet and outlet. Thus if every δm enters the system with the properties h_1, C_1, z_1 and leaves with the properties h_2, C_2, z_2, the equation can be written as

$$\Sigma \delta Q + \Sigma \delta W = (h_2 + \tfrac{1}{2}C_2^2 + gz_2)\Sigma \delta m - (h_1 + \tfrac{1}{2}C_1^2 + gz_1)\Sigma \delta m$$

We may now write m, Q and W for $\Sigma \delta m$, $\Sigma \delta Q$ and $\Sigma \delta W$, where these quantities are associated with any *arbitrary time interval*. The equation then becomes

$$Q + W = m\{(h_2 - h_1) + \tfrac{1}{2}(C_2^2 - C_1^2) + g(z_2 - z_1)\}$$

If we divide throughout by m, we can write the equation as

$$Q + W = \{(h_2 - h_1) + \tfrac{1}{2}(C_2^2 - C_1^2) + g(z_2 - z_1)\}$$

where Q and W are the heat and work transfers *per unit mass* flowing through the system. Here care must be taken in checking units: if Q and W are expressed

---

* The product pv has been called flow work, flow energy and pressure energy by various authors. Such names may be misleading, and there is no need to give this quantity any special name at all. The term arises out of the need to view the flow process as a series of non-flow processes, and so far as the open system is concerned it is merely the product of two properties, pressure and specific volume; it is not a part of the energy of the system, nor does it represent any work done on or by the *open* system.

in terms of energy, then there is implied a factor of unit mass before the brace; while if Q and W are expressed in terms of energy per unit mass, no dimensional factor is implied before the brace.

The most useful form of these equations is obtained when we consider *unit time interval* during which the mass flowing through the system is the mass flow rate $\dot{m}$, and Q and W become the rates $\dot{Q}$ and $\dot{W}$. The equation then assumes the form

$$\dot{Q} + \dot{W} = \dot{m}\{(h_2 - h_1) + \tfrac{1}{2}(C_2^2 - C_1^2) + g(z_2 - z_1)\} \qquad (4.2)$$

Equation (4.2) expresses the relation between rates of heat and work transfer and the properties of the fluid at inlet and outlet of an open system. It is called the *steady-flow energy equation*, and provides the basic means for studying most open systems of importance in engineering.

The assumptions upon which equation (4.2) is based may be summarised as follows:

(a) The mass flow at inlet is constant with respect to time, and equal to the mass flow at outlet.

(b) The properties at any point within the open system do not vary with time.

(c) The properties are constant over the cross-section of the flow at inlet and outlet.

(d) Any heat or work crossing the boundary does so at a uniform rate.

Note that no assumption has been made about the nature or configuration of the steady flow *within* the open system, and the steady-flow energy equation applies whether there is viscous friction or not. It corresponds to the general non-flow energy equation (3.1).

It is not possible for all these conditions to be satisfied in any practical process. For example, when a fluid flows through a pipe, it is known that viscous friction causes the velocity to fall rapidly to zero in the layer adjacent to the wall. Friction between the layers of fluid will also slightly affect the distribution of the thermodynamic properties across the pipe. Thus assumption (c) is not completely justified. Nevertheless, experiments have shown that equation (4.2) can be applied in these circumstances with sufficient accuracy for practical purposes if mean values of the properties are used. To take another example, it is not necessary for assumption (b) to be satisfied rigorously. The properties at any point within the open system may be allowed to fluctuate. Provided that they return to the same values periodically, the equation can still be applied. Under these circumstances, the quantities Q and W represent the average heat transferred and work done per unit mass, over a period of time appreciably longer than that required for one cyclic variation of the internal energy E'.

Finally we must note an important equation which follows directly from assumptions (a) and (c). It is known as the *continuity equation*, and expresses the principle of conservation of mass in steady flow. If $\dot{m}$ is the rate of mass flow, we have

$$\dot{m} = \frac{A_1 C_1}{v_1} = \frac{A_2 C_2}{v_2} \qquad (4.3)$$

The steady-flow energy equation will now be applied to various open systems of particular importance. In all these examples the potential energy term $g(z_2 - z_1)$ is either zero or negligible compared with the other terms. It has been included in equation (4.2) for the sake of completeness, but will henceforth be omitted. It may appear, for example, in the analysis of hydraulic machinery where the fluid is a liquid and the enthalpy and heat terms are negligible; but such systems are not considered in this book.

4.2   Open systems with steady flow

4.2.1   Boiler and condenser

Fig. 4.4 illustrates a boiler, the fluid entering as a liquid and leaving as a vapour at a constant rate. In this case no work is done on or by the fluid as it passes through the system, and hence $\dot{W} = 0$. The velocities of flow are usually quite low, so that the difference between the kinetic energies at inlet and outlet is negligible compared with the other terms of the equation. This is verified by a numerical example in section 10.1. The steady-flow energy equation for this open system reduces to

$$\dot{Q} = \dot{m}(h_2 - h_1) \tag{4.4}$$

where $\dot{Q}$ is the rate of heat transferred to the boiler. All that is necessary to calculate $\dot{Q}$ is a knowledge of the thermodynamic state of the fluid as it enters and leaves the boiler, and the mass flow.

Fig. 4.5 illustrates a simple surface condenser. The vapour passes over a bank of tubes, and is condensed as it comes into contact with the surface of the tubes. The tubes are maintained at a lower temperature than the vapour by a flow of cooling water. The cooling water is not part of the fluid of this open system, but acts as a sink of heat in the surroundings. Equation (4.4) also applies to this system, although in this case h_1 is greater than h_2 and $\dot{Q}$ is negative.

Fig. 4.4
Simple water-tube boiler

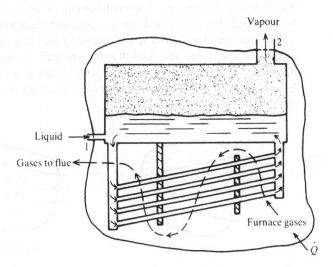

Fig. 4.5
Simple shell-and-tube
condenser

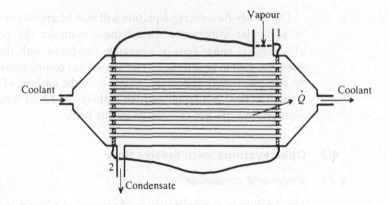

Coolant

Coolant

$\dot{Q}$

Vapour

1

2

Condensate

4.2.2 Nozzle and diffuser

A nozzle is a duct of varying cross-sectional area so designed that a drop in pressure from inlet to outlet accelerates the flow. A simple convergent nozzle is shown in Fig. 4.6a. The flow through a nozzle usually occurs at very high speed, and there is little time for the fluid to gain or lose energy by a flow of heat through the walls of the nozzle as the fluid passes through it. The process is therefore always assumed to be adiabatic. Also, no work crosses the boundary during the process. The steady-flow energy equation becomes

$$\tfrac{1}{2}(C_2^2 - C_1^2) = (h_1 - h_2) \qquad (4.5)$$

i.e. the gain in kinetic energy is equal to the decrease of enthalpy.

If the thermodynamic state at inlet and outlet and the inlet velocity are known, the final velocity can be calculated. Normally only one property in the final thermodynamic state is known, namely the pressure, and some additional assumption must be made about the flow before h_2, and hence the final velocity, can be predicted. This additional assumption is that the flow is reversible. The way in which the concept of reversibility can be applied to flow processes will be described after the second law has been introduced (sections 5.4 and 6.6).

The function of a diffuser is the reverse of that of a nozzle; the diffuser is a duct so shaped that the fluid flowing through it decelerates, the pressure increasing from inlet to outlet. Fig. 4.6b shows a simple divergent diffuser. Equation (4.5) applies to this system also, although in this case both sides of the equation will be negative.

Fig. 4.6
Simple forms of open system
with no work or heat
transfer

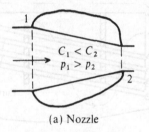

1

$C_1 < C_2$
$p_1 > p_2$

2

(a) Nozzle

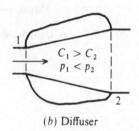

1

$C_1 > C_2$
$p_1 < p_2$

2

(b) Diffuser

Fig. 4.7
An axial-flow turbine

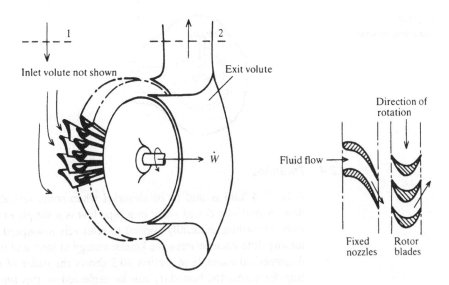

4.2.3   Turbine and compressor

A turbine is a means of extracting work from a flow of fluid expanding from a high pressure to a low pressure. Fig. 4.7 is a diagrammatic sketch of one type of turbine. Briefly, the fluid is accelerated in a set of fixed nozzles, and the resulting high-speed jets of fluid then change their direction as they pass over a row of curved blades attached to a rotor. A force is exerted on the blades equal to the rate of change of momentum of the fluid, and this produces a torque at the rotor shaft. At the same time the velocity of the fluid is reduced to somewhere near the value it possessed before entering the nozzles. As a first approximation the velocity of flow at the inlet and outlet of the turbine can be assumed equal. Also, because the average velocity of flow through a turbine is very high, the process can be assumed to be adiabatic. Hence the energy equation becomes

$$\dot{W} = \dot{m}(h_2 - h_1) \tag{4.6}$$

A turbine does work on the surroundings, so $\dot{W}$ is negative according to our sign convention, and $h_2 < h_1$.

The rotary compressor can be regarded as a reversed turbine, work being done to the fluid to raise its pressure. In this case work is done on the fluid by a bladed rotor driven from an external source. This increases the velocity of the fluid. The velocity is then reduced in a set of fixed diffusers to some value approximating to that at the inlet to the compressor, and the pressure is increased. Equation (4.6) is applicable, but in this case $\dot{W}$ is positive because work is done on the system, and $h_2 > h_1$.

Again, normally the final thermodynamic state is not known. The outlet pressure p_2 may be known, but a second property must be determined by making some additional assumption about the flow before h_2 can be found and the work of expansion or compression can be predicted.

43

Fig. 4.8
Throttling process

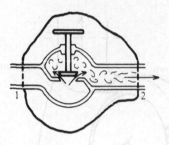

4.2.4 Throttling

A flow of fluid is said to be *throttled* when some restriction is placed in the flow. A partially closed valve in a pipe line is a simple example (Fig. 4.8). The term 'throttling' is usually applied to relatively low-speed flow, i.e. low enough for any difference between the kinetic energy at inlet and outlet to be negligible. A numerical example in section 10.3 shows the order of magnitude. Any heat transfer across the boundary can be neglected — this time for the reason that throttling takes place in such a short length of pipe that the surface area across which heat can flow is very small. Also, no work crosses the boundary. Thus the energy equation reduces to

$$h_2 = h_1 \qquad\qquad (4.7)$$

i.e. the throttling process is an adiabatic steady-flow process such that the enthalpy is the same at inlet and outlet.

4.2.5 Reciprocating compressor

Fig. 4.9 illustrates a reciprocating compressor. The remarks made about assumption (b) at the end of section 4.1 apply to this system. If a receiver is inserted in the pipe line at the outlet of the compressor, of sufficient capacity to damp out the pulsations, the properties of the fluid at the outlet can be

Fig. 4.9
Reciprocating compressor

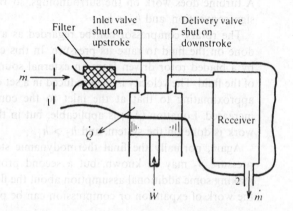

assumed to be constant. Ambient conditions usually determine the properties at the inlet. The steady-flow energy equation can then be applied to relate the average rates of heat and work transfers to the properties of the fluid at inlet and outlet. Some heat transfer does occur in a reciprocating compressor because the flow occurs at a relatively low speed, and the surface area of the cylinder is appreciable in relation to the volume. Moreover, the cylinder is normally finned and air-cooled, or jacketed and water-cooled, so that $\dot{Q}$ is negative and significant in practice; this is in contrast with rotary compressors which can be assumed to be adiabatic. The difference between the kinetic energies at inlet and outlet, however, can be neglected. Thus the equation becomes

$$\dot{Q} + \dot{W} = \dot{m}(h_2 - h_1) \qquad (4.8)$$

$\dot{Q}$ is the rate of heat transfer for the whole plant between the inlet and exit planes where the properties are measured, and will include any heat loss from the receiver.

4.3 Nonsteady-flow processes

A fluid expanding through an orifice in the side of a vessel provides a simple example of an open system undergoing a nonsteady-flow process. Neither the mass of fluid within the open system, nor the quantity of internal energy possessed by this mass, remains constant with respect to time. That is, the quantity denoted by E' varies, and it cannot be eliminated from the energy equation. Moreover, in the general case, the properties of the fluid at inlet and outlet of the open system also vary during the process. If E' is to be capable of being specified at any instant, the mechanical and thermodynamic state of each element of fluid within the system must be known. The total change $\Sigma \delta E = (E'' - E')$ between the initial and final states of the system, denoted by single and double primes respectively, can be calculated from

$$(E'' - E') = \sum_{V''} \delta m \left(u'' + \frac{C''^2}{2} + gz'' \right) - \sum_{V'} \delta m \left(u' + \frac{C'^2}{2} + gz' \right)$$

where V', V'' denote that the summations are carried out over the initial and final volumes of the system.

We shall now simplify the problem by assuming that the initial and final states of the system are (a) states of thermodynamic equilibrium, implying that u is uniform throughout the volume of the system initially and finally, and (b) states of rest, implying that the kinetic energy terms are zero. For most practical nonsteady-flow processes it is possible to choose a boundary and some boundary conditions which fulfil these assumptions. This is fortunate because otherwise the determination of E' and E'' would be very difficult. The above expression then reduces to

$$(E'' - E') = m''(u'' + gz'') - m'(u' + gz')$$

where z' and z'' must be interpreted as the heights of the centre of gravity of the initial and final masses m' and m''. Even if the position of the centre of gravity does not change, the potential energy would change if the mass of the system changes.

We shall consider the general case depicted in Fig. 4.1, starting as before with the elemental process undergone by an imaginary closed system as illustrated in Fig. 4.2. The difference in this case is that as the imaginary closed boundary is deformed, a mass δm_1 enters the system and a different mass δm_2 leaves it. During this elemental process, increments of heat δQ and work δW cross the boundary of the open system, and the total internal energy of the fluid within the original open boundary changes by an amount $\delta E'$. The primed quantities refer to the whole mass contained in the open system — a single prime for the initial equilibrium state and a double prime for the final equilibrium state. Subscripts 1 and 2 are used to denote the properties of the fluid as it enters and leaves the system at any instant. The energy equation for the non-flow process becomes

$$\delta Q + \{\delta W - (\delta m_2 p_2 v_2 - \delta m_1 p_1 v_1)\}$$
$$= \delta E' + \delta m_2(u_2 + \tfrac{1}{2}C_2^2 + gz_2) - \delta m_1(u_1 + \tfrac{1}{2}C_1^2 + gz_1)$$

Although the properties at inlet and outlet may again be assumed constant during this elemental process, they may have different values for each successive elemental process, i.e. the properties vary with time. The quantities δQ, δW and $\delta E'$ may also vary. We may write down similar equations for each elemental process between the initial and final states of the open system. Adding these equations, we have

$$\Sigma \, \delta Q + \{\Sigma \, \delta W - (\Sigma \, \delta m_2 p_2 v_2 - \Sigma \, \delta m_1 p_1 v_1)\}$$
$$= \Sigma \, \delta E' + \Sigma \, \delta m_2(u_2 + \tfrac{1}{2}C_2^2 + gz_2) - \Sigma \, \delta m_1(u_1 + \tfrac{1}{2}C_1^2 + gz_1)$$

If we write Q and W for the total quantities of heat and work crossing the boundary during the whole non-steady-flow process, substitute $m''(u'' + gz'') - m'(u' + gz')$ for $\Sigma \, \delta E'$, and introduce the property enthalpy, this reduces to

$$Q + W = \{m''(u'' + gz'') - m'(u' + gz')\} + \Sigma \, \delta m_2(h_2 + \tfrac{1}{2}C_2^2 + gz_2)$$
$$- \Sigma \, \delta m_1(h_1 + \tfrac{1}{2}C_1^2 + gz_1) \qquad (4.9)$$

Although this equation is still very cumbersome in its general form, it can be simplified further when it is applied to particular systems. One example will be considered in general terms, and other numerical examples are given in section 10.7.

Consider the system shown in Fig. 4.10. A fluid under pressure in a container is allowed to expand through a turbine to atmospheric pressure. We require an expression for the work done by the turbine as the fluid in the container changes from one state of equilibrium to another, i.e. during the time the valve is allowed to remain open. The state of the fluid in the container is assumed to be known before the valve is opened and after it is closed. For this system the potential energy terms can be neglected.

A major simplification in equation (4.9) is achieved because no mass enters the system. Also, since the process will be rapid, it may be assumed adiabatic.

Fig. 4.10
A nonsteady-flow process

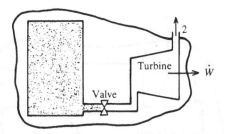

Finally, as a first approximation the kinetic energy of the fluid leaving the turbine will be ignored; a turbine is usually designed for this to be small as it represents a waste of energy. Thus equation (4.9) reduces to

$$-W = (m'u' - m''u'') - \Sigma \, \delta m_2 h_2 \qquad (4.10)$$

In other words, the *magnitude* of the work done *by* the turbine is equal to the decrease of internal energy in the system minus the enthalpy of the fluid that has left the system. A description of the way in which this equation can be applied in a practical case must be left to Part II.

4.4   Cycles consisting of steady-flow processes

During a steady-flow process the open system itself does not, strictly speaking, undergo any process, because the properties remain constant at every point within it; nevertheless, individual elements of fluid undergo a process as they flow through the system. It is therefore possible to imagine a series of open systems through which the fluid circulates continuously, each element of fluid passing through a cycle of mechanical and thermodynamic states.

Fig. 4.11 illustrates a simple steam power plant in which the fluid undergoes a continuous series of cyclic processes. Water at a certain pressure and temperature enters the boiler and is converted to steam; the steam expands to a low pressure in the turbine and is condensed at that low pressure; finally, the water is returned to the boiler by the feed pump at its original pressure and temperature. The individual components — boiler, turbine, condenser and feed

Fig. 4.11
Closed-cycle plant

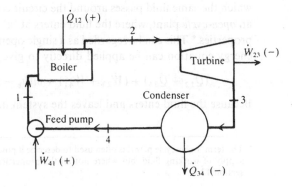

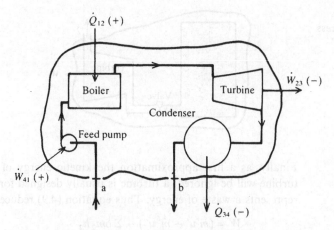

Fig. 4.12
Open-cycle plant

pump—are open systems, and the energy equation for each may be written as:

Boiler: $\dot{Q}_{12} = \dot{m}(h_2 - h_1)$
Turbine: $\dot{W}_{23} = \dot{m}(h_3 - h_2)$
Condenser: $\dot{Q}_{34} = \dot{m}(h_4 - h_3)$
Feed pump: $\dot{W}_{41} = \dot{m}(h_1 - h_4)$

Adding these equations, we have

$$(\dot{Q}_{12} + \dot{Q}_{34}) + (\dot{W}_{23} + \dot{W}_{41}) = 0$$

or

$$\sum \delta\dot{Q} + \sum \delta\dot{W} = 0$$

Thus the sum of the net rates of heat and work transferred to the whole plant is zero.

This equation is analogous to the original expression of the First Law made for a closed system undergoing a cycle of non-flow processes. It could have been deduced by regarding the whole plant as a closed system. The total internal energy of this system does not vary because the properties are constant with respect to time at every point within it. Consequently if heat and work cross the boundary at various points at uniform rates, the algebraic sum must be zero. If this were not so, the total internal energy would increase or decrease.

Fig. 4.11 is an example of a plant operating on a *closed cycle*, i.e. one in which the same fluid passes around the circuit continuously. Fig. 4.12 illustrates an *open-cycle* plant, where the fluid enters at 'a' and leaves at 'b' with the same properties.* This can be regarded as a single open system, so that the steady-flow energy equation can be applied directly to give

$$(\dot{Q}_{12} + \dot{Q}_{34}) + (\dot{W}_{23} + \dot{W}_{41}) = \dot{m}(h_b - h_a) + \tfrac{1}{2}(C_b^2 - C_a^2)$$

Because the fluid enters and leaves the system in the same state, the right-hand

---

* The term 'open-cycle plant' is often used to describe a power plant which uses a continuous fresh supply of working fluid, but where not all the properties are identical at inlet and outlet: see section 12.1.

side of the equation is zero, and again

$$\sum \delta \dot{Q} + \sum \delta \dot{W} = 0$$

All the properties revert to their initial values, and the fact that fresh quantities of fluid act as a vehicle for these properties is irrelevant.

5

The Second Law of Thermodynamics and Reversibility

In this chapter the idea of a cycle efficiency is introduced, and the Second Law is then stated and distinguished from the First. One of the corollaries of the Second Law is deduced, but the development of the other corollaries requires a fuller treatment of the concept of reversibility than has so far been given. These corollaries are therefore dealt with in the next chapter, while the remainder of this chapter is devoted to the formal definition of a reversible process and to a discussion of its implications both for non-flow and steady-flow processes.

5.1 Cycle efficiency

When a closed system undergoes a series of non-flow processes, during which the fluid passes through a cycle of thermodynamic states, it has been seen that the First Law is expressed by equation (2.3), i.e.

$$\sum \delta Q + \sum \delta W = 0$$

Up to now the symbol Q has been used for both positive and negative quantities of heat. The important arguments which follow in this chapter, and through part of the next, will be easier to understand if *we use separate symbols for positive and negative quantities.* Thus, when considering engine cycles, we shall collect the positive quantities of heat under the symbol Q_1 and the negative quantities under the symbol Q_2. Furthermore, the symbols will stand for the *magnitudes* of the quantities of heat (i.e. their absolute values or moduli). The symbol W will also represent a magnitude, irrespective of sign, but in this case of the *net work transferred in the cycle.* Where it may be helpful to emphasise that these symbols stand for magnitudes, we will enclose them in the mathematical modulus sign $|\quad|$. The First Law applied to a heat engine cycle can then be written

$$|Q_1| - |Q_2| = |W| \tag{5.1}$$

where $|Q_1| > |Q_2|$, and $|W|$ is the net work delivered *to* the surroundings.

The concept of the efficiency of a heat engine cycle will play a prominent part in what follows, and it can be defined quite unambiguously. The greater the fraction of the heat supplied $|Q_1|$ that is converted into net work output

$|W|$, the better the engine, and consequently the *cycle efficiency* η is defined as

$$\eta = \frac{\text{net work done}}{\text{heat supplied}} = \frac{|W|}{|Q_1|} \tag{5.2}$$

Hence, from equations (5.1) and (5.2), we have

$$\eta = \frac{|Q_1| - |Q_2|}{|Q_1|} \tag{5.3}$$

The quantities $|Q_1|$ and $|Q_2|$ may be expressed per unit mass of the system, or they may be regarded as the rate of heat supplied and rejected. The latter alternative is possible because the numerator and denominator of equation (5.2) can be multiplied by the number of cycles per unit time without affecting their ratio.

The efficiency of any heat engine cycle consisting of a sequence of steady-flow processes, whether the cycle is open or closed (see section 4.4), can also be expressed by equation (5.3). In this case $|Q_1|$ and $|Q_2|$ must be interpreted either as the heat supplied and rejected per unit mass flowing round the circuit, or as the rates of heat supplied and rejected, namely $|\dot{Q}_1|$ and $|\dot{Q}_2|$.

5.2 The Second Law of Thermodynamics

There is nothing implicit in the First Law of Thermodynamics to say that some proportion of the heat supplied to an engine must be rejected, and therefore that the cycle efficiency cannot be unity. All that the First Law states is that net work cannot be produced during a cycle without *some* supply of heat, i.e. that a perpetual motion machine of the first kind is impossible. The Second Law is an expression of the fact that some heat must always be rejected during the cycle, and therefore that the cycle efficiency is always less than unity. The law may be stated in the following form:*

> *It is impossible to construct a system which will operate in a cycle, extract heat from a reservoir, and do an equivalent amount of work on the surroundings.*

Thus the First Law says that the net work can never be greater than the heat supplied, while the Second Law goes further and states that it must always be less. If $|W| < |Q_1|$, then it follows from equation (5.1) that $|Q_2|$ must have some finite value.

If energy is to be supplied to a system in the form of heat, the system must be in contact with a reservoir at a temperature higher than that of the fluid at some point in the cycle. Similarly, if heat is to be rejected, the system must at some time be in contact with a reservoir of lower temperature than the fluid. Thus the Second Law implies that if a system is to undergo a cycle and produce work, it must operate between at least two reservoirs of different temperature, however small this difference may be. Fig. 5.1a will be used to represent a heat

---

* This is essentially the statement given by Planck in Ref. 7.

Fig. 5.1
Schematic representation of
(a) heat engine and (b) heat
pump or refrigerator

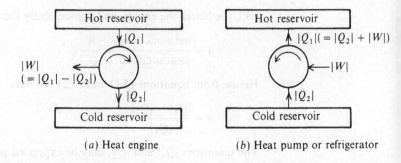

(a) Heat engine   (b) Heat pump or refrigerator

engine. A machine which will produce work continuously, while exchanging heat with only a single reservoir, is known as a perpetual motion machine of the second kind; such a machine would contradict the Second Law.

It is now possible to see why a ship could not be driven by an engine using the ocean as a source of heat, or why a power station could not be run using the atmosphere as a source of heat. There is nothing in the First Law to say that these desirable projects are not feasible. Neither project would contravene the principle of conservation of energy; their impossibility is a consequence of the Second Law. They are impossible because there is no natural infinite sink of heat at a lower temperature than the atmosphere or ocean, and they would therefore be perpetual motion machines of the second kind. These remarks require some qualification because in practice there is temperature stratification, and the atmosphere and ocean are not strictly single heat reservoirs. It is possible, both in principle and in practice, to make use of the temperature difference between the surface and a deeper layer of the ocean. Schemes of this kind are considered briefly in section 11.9.

The cycles described so far have all been those of heat engines. However, we can devise cycles during which the net work is done *on* the system while a net amount of heat is *rejected*. In this case the quantities in equation (5.1) are of opposite sign, i.e. Q_1 is the heat rejected, Q_2 is the heat supplied, and W is the net work done on the system. This would be the cycle of a *heat pump* or *refrigerator*, and it can be regarded as a reversed heat engine cycle. The heat pump or refrigerator is represented symbolically by Fig. 5.1b. It should be noted that the Second Law does not imply that work cannot be continuously and completely converted into heat. Indeed, any process involving friction achieves this without the need for the system to operate in a cycle. For example, a fluid in a closed vessel may have work done on it by a paddle at the same time as heat is allowed to cross the boundary into the surroundings. The rates of flow of work and heat may be made equal, the internal energy of the system remaining constant. But this is an extremely wasteful method of producing heat because, by using the work to drive a heat pump, a larger quantity of heat may be delivered to the surroundings for the same expenditure of work. The quantity of heat delivered is then greater than the net work done on the system by an amount equal to the heat drawn from the colder reservoir. An important consequence of the Second Law is, therefore, that *work is a more valuable form of energy transfer than heat*; heat can never be transformed continuously and completely into work, whereas work can always be transformed continuously and completely into heat and, if properly used, can even result in a supply of heat which is greater than the quantity of work expended.

This section has been devoted primarily to distinguishing between the First and Second Laws. It should be clear that the Second Law cannot be deduced from the First; it is a separate axiom. Like the First Law, its validity rests upon the fact that neither the law, nor any of its consequences, has ever been disproved by experience. The following statements summarise the more obvious consequences of the Second Law:

(a)   If a system is taken through a cycle and does a net amount of work on the surroundings, it must be exchanging heat with at least two reservoirs at different temperatures.
(b)   If a system is taken through a cycle while exchanging heat with only one reservoir, the work transfer must be either zero or positive.
(c)   Since heat can never be converted continuously and completely into work, whereas work can always be converted continuously and completely into heat, work is a more valuable form of energy transfer than heat.

Other consequences of the Second Law will be developed in the form of corollaries, and the first is deduced in the next section.

5.3   The Clausius statement of the Second Law

The first corollary of the Second Law has often been used as a statement of the law; it was first used in this way by Clausius. When so used, the statement of the law already given can easily be shown to be a corollary of this.

Corollary 1   It is impossible to construct a system which will operate in a cycle and transfer heat from a cooler to a hotter body without work being done on the system by the surroundings.

Proof   Suppose that the converse of the proposition be true. The system could be represented by a heat pump for which $|W| = 0$, as in Fig. 5.2. If it takes $|Q|$ units of heat from the cold reservoir, it must deliver $|Q|$ units to the hot reservoir to satisfy the First Law. A heat engine could also be operated between the two reservoirs; let it be of such a size that it delivers $|Q|$ units of

Fig. 5.2
Can a heat pump operate without a work input?

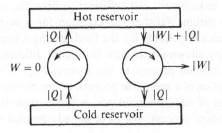

heat to the cold reservoir while performing $|W|$ units of work. Then the First Law states that the engine must be supplied with $(|W| + |Q|)$ units of heat from the hot reservoir. In the combined plant the cold reservoir becomes superfluous because the heat engine could reject its heat directly into the heat pump. The combined plant represents a heat engine extracting $(|W| + |Q|) - |Q| = W$ units of heat from a reservoir, and delivering an equivalent amount of work. This is impossible according to the Second Law. Consequently the converse of the proposition cannot be true and the original proposition must be true.

5.4 Reversibility and irreversibility

The idea of a reversible process has so far only been developed with respect to non-flow processes. It was presented as a process between two states during which the system passes through a series of equilibrium states. For this to happen, it was shown that the heat and work must be transferred across the boundary in a particular way, that is:

(a) Heat must flow by virtue of an infinitesimally small temperature difference.
(b) Work must be done only when the force exerted by the surroundings on the moving boundary is infinitesimally different from the force due to the pressure of the fluid in the system.

When these conditions are fulfilled, only an infinitesimal change is necessary in the temperature of the reservoir, or in the force applied to the boundary by the surroundings, to reverse the process and make the system return through the same series of equilibrium states to the initial state. If this is done, any work previously delivered to the surroundings is returned to the system, and any heat supplied to the system is returned to the reservoir. No effects of either the original process or the reversed process are left in the system or the surroundings, because any changes required to reverse the process are infinitesimal.

So that the idea of reversibility can be applied to non-flow and steady-flow processes, the following criterion of reversibility will be adopted:

> *When a fluid undergoes a reversible process, both the fluid and its surroundings can always be restored to their original states.*

Steady-flow processes undergone by a fluid in an open system can easily be imagined to be reversible according to this criterion. For example, imagine that a fluid, after expanding adiabatically in a turbine, is compressed adiabatically in a rotary compressor. If this can be carried out so that the fluid is returned to its initial thermodynamic and mechanical states, and so that the work obtained from the turbine is just sufficient to drive the compressor, then the expansion in the turbine satisfies the criterion for a reversible process. Similarly, it is theoretically possible for the fluid leaving a nozzle to be returned to its initial state, by allowing it to flow through a diffuser, without leaving any effects of the combined process in the surroundings. On the other hand the original conception of a reversible process, as one during which a system passes through a series of equilibrium states, is too narrow to enable it to be applied to a steady-flow process. We have already pointed out that a steady-flow system, as such, cannot be said to undergo a process at all, because the properties of the fluid within it are everywhere constant with respect to time; moreover, it is clearly never in a state of equilibrium.

We shall proceed to show that if either of the following phenomena is present during a process it cannot be reversible:

(a)   Friction
(b)   Heat transfer across a finite temperature difference.

Since at least one of these is always present in some degree, no real process can be reversible. The reversible process must be regarded as a limiting case – an ideal which can never quite be achieved. Any particular process involving (a) or (b) can be shown to be irreversible, although no general proof can be given. The procedure will be to find processes by which the fluid can be returned to its initial state, and then show that the surroundings cannot also be returned to their state without contradicting the Second Law.

5.4.1   Friction

Friction is always present when one part of a fluid moves relatively to another, or to a solid boundary, with finite velocity. This is inherent in the viscous nature of fluids. The effect of viscous friction is always to produce a conversion of some of the kinetic energy of the fluid into random molecular energy. Non-flow and steady-flow processes will be considered in turn.

Friction in non-flow processes
Consider the simple case of a fixed volume of fluid being stirred by a paddle. Work is done on the system, and the First Law states that

$$W = (u_2 - u_1)$$

If the process is reversible it must be possible to return the quantity W to the surroundings, and restore the internal energy of the system to u_1 without change of volume. The internal energy can be restored to its original value by allowing heat to flow across the boundary into the surroundings equal in amount to the former increase in internal energy. We then have to think of a device which will convert all this heat into work without itself introducing further changes of state in the surroundings. Only a cyclic device, i.e. a heat engine, could do this, but such an engine is impossible according to the Second Law. Therefore the stirring process does not satisfy the criterion of reversibility.

In practical processes, any deliberate stirring of the fluid is avoided whenever possible. Nevertheless it might be supposed that friction would make its presence felt during the ordinary non-flow expansion or compression of a fluid in the cylinder of a reciprocating machine operating at a reasonable speed. With any such process there will always be a finite difference between the force displaced in the surroundings, and the opposing force due to the pressure of the fluid in the system. Thus the process must be accompanied by an acceleration of the moving boundary and working fluid, and there will be some conversion of kinetic energy into random molecular energy due to friction. As an example,

Fig. 5.3
Irreversibility due to friction
in non-flow processes

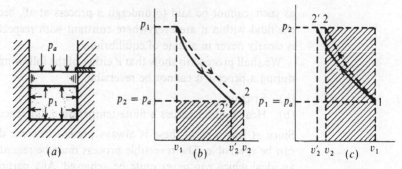

consider the behaviour of the adiabatic system containing unit mass of fluid
shown in Fig. 5.3a. For simplicity the piston may be assumed weightless and
frictionless, so that the surroundings exert a constant force on the fluid due to
the atmospheric pressure p_a. Let the initial pressure of the fluid p_1 be greater
than this, a stop holding the piston in position. When the stop is removed, the
fluid expands and the piston accelerates under the action of the unbalanced
force $(p_1 - p_a)A$, where A is the area of the piston.

Before the system can settle down to a new state of equilibrium, where the
pressure of the fluid has fallen to p_a, the kinetic energy of the fluid must be
dissipated. This is accomplished by an oscillation which is damped out by the
viscous forces in the fluid. Since the system is thermally insulated from the
surroundings, the whole of the kinetic energy is reconverted to random molecular
energy u by fluid friction.* The decrease of internal energy from one equilibrium
state to the other is therefore smaller than it would have been had the expansion
from p_1 to p_a proceeded infinitely slowly, i.e. less internal energy has left the
system.

The expansion process can be represented approximately on the p–v diagram
as the dashed curve in Fig. 5.3b. The end states are defined by (p_1, v_1) and
(p_a, v_2). Although the pressure is not uniform throughout the system during the
process, average pressures might be measured to give the intermediate points
some meaning. From the First Law for an adiabatic non-flow process, the work
is done at the expense of the internal energy, and

$$|W| = (u_1 - u_2)$$

When carried out infinitely slowly, this might be written

$$|W'| = (u_1 - u_2')$$

where $u_2' < u_2$ and $|W'| > |W|$. When the pressure is constant, a decrease of
internal energy of a fluid is normally accompanied by a decrease of volume
(water between 0°C and 4°C being an exception). Thus v_2' is less than v_2, and
the perfectly restrained process might be shown by the full line 1–2'.

The magnitude of the work done during the actual process, in moving the
constant force $p_a A$ a distance $(v_2 - v_1)/A$, is equal to $p_a(v_2 - v_1)$. This is

---

* A column of air in the surroundings will also have been accelerated and viscous forces in the
surroundings will contribute to the damping; for simplicity we may neglect this effect, e.g. by
assuming the surroundings to have negligible viscosity.

represented by the area of the shaded rectangle. It is clearly less than the area under the dotted curve, which is given by $\int_1^2 p\, dv$, where p is interpreted as the average pressure at any point in the expansion.

By a similar argument it can be shown that a compression, carried out under similar conditions, would require an amount of work equal to $p_2(v_1 - v_2)$ to be done on the system by a constant force $p_2 A$ in the surroundings. This work is equal to the area of the shaded rectangle in Fig. 5.3c. In this case the work done is greater than the magnitude of $\int_1^2 p\, dv$.

The magnitude of the work of expansion can be increased, and that of compression reduced, by applying the external force in a series of steps decreasing successively from $p_1 A$ to $p_a A$ in the former case, and increasing successively from $p_a A$ to $p_2 A$ in the latter. The difference between the magnitudes is then reduced. In the limit, when the external force never departs by more than an infinitesimal amount from that due to the pressure of the fluid, the work done will be numerically equal to $\int_1^2 p\, dv$ in each case and the processes become reversible.

In an actual reciprocating engine the mass of the piston and other moving parts is considerable, but most of the kinetic energy acquired by these is stored in the flywheel and recovered. The piston is prevented from undergoing the oscillation which would occur if the piston were free, and the kinetic energy acquired by the fluid exists in the form of eddies which are damped out by viscous friction. The creation and dissipation of kinetic energy is therefore a continuous process throughout the expansion or compression. With normal piston speeds the quantity of energy dissipated in this way is very small, and the effect of fluid friction can usually be ignored. Thus, when a calculation of the work done during a practical non-flow expansion or compression is made on the assumption that it is a reversible process, it provides not only a criterion of perfection but also a close approximation to the actual value.* It will not be such a good approximation when special devices are used to introduce turbulence, as in some compression-ignition engines.

Friction in steady-flow processes
When considering the effect of friction during flow processes, it is usually found to be by no means negligible. In nozzles, turbines and rotary compressors, the speed of flow is high and fluid friction is considerable.

Consider first the effect of friction in a nozzle. Let the thermodynamic state of the fluid at the inlet be defined by (p_1, h_1), and let the inlet velocity be C_1. Assume that the outlet pressure is fixed at some value p_2, this being chosen as the independent property of the final state. The appropriate steady-flow energy equation (4.5) states that

$$\tfrac{1}{2}(C_2^2 - C_1^2) = (h_1 - h_2)$$

---

* We are here referring to the work done on or by the fluid. Some of this work will be dissipated externally by piston friction, but this is expressed separately by the mechanical efficiency of the machine — see section 16.2.

Fig. 5.4
Irreversibility due to friction
in flow processes

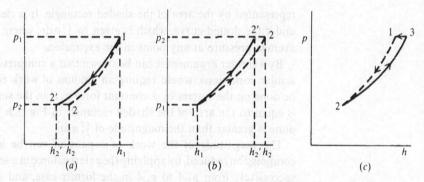

$$(a) \qquad\qquad\qquad (b) \qquad\qquad\qquad (c)$$

Friction always produces a force opposing the motion, and after the expansion to pressure p_2 the stream of fluid moves more slowly than it would have done had there been no friction. If the values which the dependent properties would have after frictionless flow are denoted by primes, this means that $C_2 < C'_2$. Consequently it follows that $h_2 > h'_2$, since the First Law must be satisfied, i.e.

$$\tfrac{1}{2}(C_2'^2 - C_1^2) = (h_1 - h_2')$$

During the process with friction, some of the directional kinetic energy $(\tfrac{1}{2}C^2)$ is being continually transformed into random molecular energy (u). But at any given pressure an increase of u must involve an increase in the specific volume v, and consequently an increase in enthalpy $(u + pv)$. In effect, some of the initial enthalpy which could have produced an increase in kinetic energy has been prevented from doing so by friction.

It is often helpful to represent a steady-flow process on a coordinate diagram, although it cannot be completely defined in this way. The thermodynamic state of the fluid at the inlet and outlet may be represented by points on a diagram using two thermodynamic properties as coordinates, and a line joining the points can be used to represent the process.* A full line will always be used to denote a frictionless process, and a dashed line to denote a process where friction is present. Such diagrams only partially represent the process because the changes in mechanical properties are not shown. Fig. 5.4a shows the expansion process in a nozzle on a p–h diagram.

Fig. 5.4a can equally well represent the expansion in a turbine between pressures p_1 and p_2. With the usual assumptions, i.e. adiabatic flow and equal inlet and outlet velocities, the energy equation is

$$|\dot{W}| = \dot{m}(h_1 - h_2)$$

If the flow is frictionless it may be written

$$|\dot{W}'| = \dot{m}(h_1 - h_2')$$

where $|\dot{W}'| > |\dot{W}|$ and $h'_2 < h_2$. Similarly, Fig. 5.4b can represent the processes

---

* Strictly speaking, the intermediate points only have meaning if every element of fluid flowing through the system passes through the same series of thermodynamic states. This implies that the properties are uniform at right angles to the flow throughout the system — not merely at the inlet and outlet, which was all we had to assume when deriving the steady-flow energy equation. When this additional assumption can be made, the flow is called 'one-dimensional' (see Chapter 18).

in either a diffuser or a rotary compressor. As always, friction results in the final enthalpy being greater than it would have been after a frictionless process to the same final pressure. Considering the case of a rotary compressor, this means that the actual work of compression $\dot{m}(h_2 - h_1)$ is greater than the frictionless work $\dot{m}(h'_2 - h_1)$.

As an example, we may show that friction makes an expansion in a turbine irreversible. The dashed curve 1–2 in Fig. 5.4c illustrates this process. As before, we shall find processes by which the fluid can be returned to its initial state, and then show that the surroundings cannot be returned to their initial state without contradicting the Second Law. Let the fluid flow through a rotary compressor on leaving the turbine, so that it is compressed without friction to the original pressure (curve 2–3). The enthalpy drop in the turbine must have been less than the enthalpy rise in the compressor, because friction was present in the expansion. Therefore some net work, given by

$$\dot{m}\{(h_3 - h_2) - (h_1 - h_2)\} = \dot{m}(h_3 - h_1)$$

must be supplied by the surroundings. The fluid can be returned to its final state by cooling it at constant pressure without change of velocity, the quantity of heat entering the surroundings being equal to $\dot{m}(h_3 - h_1)$ from equation (4.4). To return the surroundings to their initial state, a heat engine would be required to convert $\dot{m}(h_3 - h_1)$ units of heat into $\dot{m}(h_3 - h_1)$ units of work. This is impossible according to the Second Law, and therefore the process in the turbine cannot have been reversible.

5.4.2 Transfer of heat across a finite temperature difference

Consider the process of allowing heat to flow from a source to a fluid at a lower temperature, when the difference between the temperature of the source and the fluid is finite. If the fluid is a closed system having fixed boundaries, the quantity of heat supplied is equal to the increase of internal energy. Alternatively, if the heat is supplied to a fluid flowing in a duct under conditions such that the velocity remains unchanged, the quantity of heat is equal to the increase of enthalpy, equation (4.4). In either case the fluid may be restored to its initial state by allowing the same quantity of heat to flow across the boundary into a sink. Even if this second process is carried out so that the temperature of the sink is never more than infinitesimally lower than that of the fluid, the difference in temperature between the source and the sink will be finite. If the original process is to be reversible, it must be possible to transfer the quantity of heat from the sink to the source without incurring any further changes in the surroundings. This is impossible because, according to corollary 1 of the Second Law (section 5.3), some work would have to be supplied by the surroundings. Thus the process of heat transfer across a finite temperature difference is irreversible. We have already noted that a temperature difference is essential if any heat transfer is to take place in a finite time, so that all real transfers of heat must be irreversible.

5.5 Reversible and irreversible cycles

A cycle is reversible if it consists only of reversible processes. When such a cycle is reversed, all the quantities of work and heat crossing the boundary are reversed in direction without their magnitude being affected. The cycle may consist of reversible non-flow processes, or it may be an open or closed cycle consisting of reversible steady-flow processes.

The original conception of a reversible cycle was due to Sadi Carnot (Ref. 4). He conceived of a particular cycle, called the *Carnot cycle*, which will be examined in detail in Part II. It is sufficient to note here that it is one of a special class of reversible cycles during which all the heat enters the system from a source at constant temperature, and all the heat leaving it is rejected to a sink at constant temperature. It follows that the processes during which heat is exchanged with the surroundings must be isothermal, the temperature of the fluid never differing by more than an infinitesimal amount from the fixed temperature of the source or sink.

A cycle may be thought of as reversible without this limitation. If the temperature of the fluid changes during any heat transfer process, all that is necessary is that the source or sink be a series of reservoirs covering the required range of temperature. At any instant during the process, heat must be exchanged between the system and the particular source or sink which differs only infinitesimally in temperature from the fluid in the system. This idea has already been introduced in section 3.1.2. Engines operating on this type of reversible cycle will be shown symbolically by Fig. 5.5. The quantity Q_1, for example, can be regarded as the sum of the infinitesimal quantities of heat received from the hot reservoirs.

It is the limited class of reversible cycles, of which the Carnot cycle is a member, that plays an important part in the deduction of the corollaries of the Second Law. If the term 'reservoir' is restricted, in the manner suggested in section 3.1.2, to a source or sink of invariable temperature, then this class of reversible cycles will comprise those of engines or heat pumps operating between only two reservoirs.

If any of the processes in a cycle are irreversible, the whole cycle is irreversible. The efficiency of an engine in which irreversible processes occur must always be less than that of the hypothetical reversible engine. For example, if friction

Fig. 5.5

Representation of reversible engine operating between more than two reservoirs

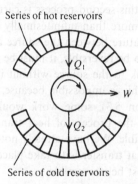

Series of hot reservoirs

Q_1

W

Q_2

Series of cold reservoirs

occurs during the expansion in the turbine of the steam power plant shown in Fig. 4.11, the work output of the turbine is reduced. The enthalpy at exit from the turbine is thereby increased, and more heat must be rejected in the condenser to bring the fluid back to the same state before it passes through the feed pump. The First Law is still satisfied, i.e. $|Q_1| = |W| + |Q_2|$, but the cycle efficiency $|W|/|Q_1|$ is reduced. If the efficiency of a cycle is calculated on the assumption that all the processes are reversible, this provides a figure for the maximum possible efficiency of power plant operating on that cycle.

6

Corollaries of the Second Law

The Clausius statement of the Second Law has been presented in section 5.3 as the first corollary. Other corollaries are concerned with: (a) the characteristics of reversible engines operating between only two reservoirs, (b) the thermo-dynamic scale of temperature, (c) the characteristics of engines operating between a series of reservoirs, and (d) the property entropy.

The way in which entropy can be used to simplify calculations concerning non-flow processes has already been indicated in Chapter 3. This chapter ends with a description of the way entropy may be used in the analysis of steady-flow processes, followed by a few remarks on the limitations of the laws of thermodynamics and a summary of Chapters 1 to 6.

The reader is reminded that for much of this chapter the symbols Q_1 and Q_2 refer to the *magnitudes* of the heat transfers.

6.1 Reversible engines operating between only two reservoirs

> *Corollary 2* It is impossible to construct an engine operating between only two heat reservoirs which will have a higher efficiency than a reversible engine operating between the same two reservoirs.

Proof Assume the converse of this proposition to be true; let X be such an engine, having an efficiency η_X. Let it receive heat Q_1 from the source, do work W_X, and reject heat $(Q_1 - W_X)$ to the sink. Then it is assumed that $\eta_X > \eta_R$, where η_R is the efficiency of a reversible engine R operating between the same two reservoirs (Fig. 6.1a). If the reversible engine also receives heat Q_1 from the source, it will do work W_R such that $W_R < W_X$, and the heat rejected will be $(Q_1 - W_R)$ which is greater than $(Q_1 - W_X)$.

Let the reversible engine be reversed and act as a heat pump (Fig. 6.1b). It now receives heat $(Q_1 - W_R)$ from the low-temperature reservoir, receives work W_R from the surroundings, and rejects heat Q_1 to the high-temperature reservoir. If the engine X is coupled to the heat pump, and the latter feeds heat Q_1 directly

Fig. 6.1
Can an engine have a higher
efficiency than its reversible
equivalent?

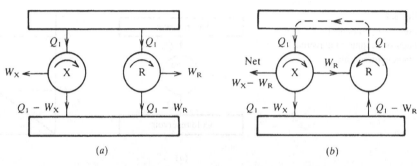

(a)   (b)

into the former, the combined plant represents a heat engine receiving heat
$(Q_1 - W_R) - (Q_1 - W_X) = (W_X - W_R)$ from the surroundings, and delivering an
equivalent amount of work. According to the Second Law this is impossible, and
the assumption that $\eta_X > \eta_R$ cannot be true. Consequently the original proposition
must be true.

> *Corollary 3* All reversible engines operating between the same
> two reservoirs have the same efficiency.

Once the second corollary has been proved, no special proof is required for the
third. If two reversible engines differ in efficiency when operating between the
same two reservoirs, then one must have a higher efficiency than the other. This
is impossible if corollary 2 is true. Since all reversible engines operating between
the same two reservoirs have the same efficiency, this efficiency must depend
upon the only feature which is common to them all, namely the temperatures
of the reservoirs: it is called the *Carnot efficiency*.

6.2 Thermodynamic temperature scale

> *Corollary 4* A scale of temperature can be defined which is
> independent of any particular thermometric substance, and which
> provides an absolute zero of temperature.

Proof Let us consider the reversible engine operating between only
two reservoirs represented symbolically in Fig. 6.2a. Corollary 3 implies that its
efficiency depends only on the temperature of the reservoirs, and therefore that
it is independent of the particular properties of the working fluid and of the
quantity of heat Q_0 supplied to the engine. But

$$\eta = \frac{Q_0 - Q}{Q_0} = 1 - \frac{Q}{Q_0}$$

and hence it follows that Q/Q_0 is a function only of the temperatures of the
reservoirs.

Fig. 6.2
Use of a hypothetical
reversible engine to construct
a temperature scale

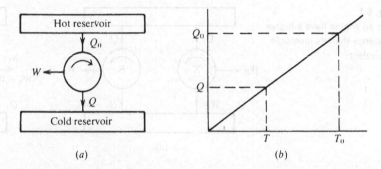

(a) (b)

Let us now allot a positive number T_0 to some reservoir in a convenient reference state which is easily reproducible (e.g. a pure substance melting at a definite pressure); further, let us define the temperature T of any other reservoir by the equation

$$T = T_0 \frac{Q}{Q_0} \tag{6.1}$$

The value T is then fully and uniquely determined by (a) the arbitrary choice of T_0 and (b) the ratio Q/Q_0 which, as a consequence of the Second Law, is a fixed and definite quantity for the two given reservoirs. If Q is measured for several sinks at different temperatures and plotted against T obtained from (6.1), we obtain by definition a scale of temperature which is linear in Q. The slope of the line in Fig. 6.2b is Q_0/T_0. The *unit of temperature* now follows as the fraction $1/T_0$ of the interval from $T = 0$ to T_0. The temperature scale defined in this way is called the *thermodynamic scale*, because it is dependent solely on the laws of thermodynamics and not upon the properties of any particular substance. It is an *absolute* scale because it presents us with the idea of an absolute zero, i.e. $T = 0$ when $Q = 0$. The Second Law implies that Q can in fact never be zero, and we may therefore deduce that absolute zero is a conceptual limit and not a temperature which can ever be reached in practice.*

It may be helpful if we visualise the scale as being constructed by a series of reversible engines (Fig. 6.3a), each operating between only two reservoirs and *each producing the same quantity of work*. Each sink is a source for the following engine, the heat entering a reservoir being equal to the heat leaving it. If the temperatures of the reservoirs are defined in the way suggested by equation (6.1), then

$$\frac{Q_0}{Q_1} = \frac{T_0}{T_1}, \quad \frac{Q_1}{Q_2} = \frac{T_1}{T_2}, \quad \frac{Q_2}{Q_3} = \frac{T_2}{T_3}, \quad \dots \tag{6.2}$$

And the efficiencies of the engines therefore become

$$\eta_0 = \frac{T_0 - T_1}{T_0}, \quad \eta_1 = \frac{T_1 - T_2}{T_1}, \quad \eta_2 = \frac{T_2 - T_3}{T_2}, \quad \dots \tag{6.3}$$

---

* Strictly speaking, it is necessary to invoke the Third Law (see end of section 7.9.1) to deduce the unattainability of absolute zero: this is discussed in Ref. 8.

Fig. 6.3
An absolute thermodynamic
temperature scale

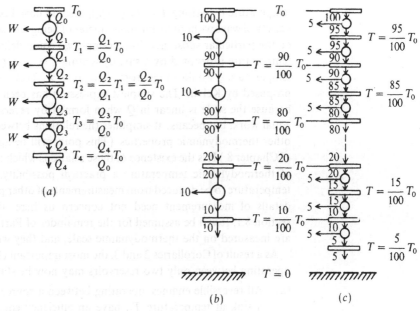

$$W = \eta_0 Q_0 = \eta_1 Q_1 = \eta_2 Q_2 = \dots$$

it follows that

$$\frac{Q_0}{T_0}(T_0 - T_1) = \frac{Q_1}{T_1}(T_1 - T_2) = \frac{Q_2}{T_2}(T_2 - T_3) = \dots$$

Using equations (6.2), this reduces to

$$(T_0 - T_1) = (T_1 - T_2) = (T_2 - T_3) = \dots \tag{6.4}$$

Thus the differences between the temperatures of successive reservoirs are the same and can provide intervals or units of temperature. T_0 may be as high as we wish to make it, and the intervals may be made as small as desired by increasing the number of engines in the series. The series of reservoirs could theoretically be used as a standard set of temperatures with which to calibrate any practical thermometer.

Figs 6.3b and c illustrate the effect of increasing the number of engines. The last possible engine in the series is one which rejects an amount of heat equal to the work W; according to the Second Law the next engine in the series is an impossibility. It is evident that the temperature of the sink of the last possible engine is reduced as the number of engines is increased, but as long as W is finite the scale must stop short of absolute zero. Note that the choice of 100 units for Q_0 in the scales of Figs 6.3b and c is quite arbitrary; a discussion of the accepted way in which numbers are assigned to the thermodynamic scale is left to section 8.1.

Although it has been internationally agreed to define the thermodynamic

65

temperature by writing $T = T_0(Q/Q_0)$, it could have been defined in an infinite variety of ways without losing its character of being independent of the properties of any particular substance. For example we could define a scale, on which the temperature is denoted by ξ say, by writing $\xi = \xi_0 \ln(Q/Q_0)$; on this scale the temperature ξ would range from $-\infty$ to $+\infty$. This was in fact the first scale proposed by Kelvin. The simplest expression has been adopted, however, not because the scale is linear in Q when formed by reversible engines producing equal work, but because it simplifies the relations between temperature and the other thermodynamic properties. (This point will be appreciated after a study of Chapter 8.) It is the existence of these relations which makes the measurement of thermodynamic temperature a practical possibility, since they enable the temperature to be deduced from measurements of other properties. The practical details of measurement need not concern us here; they are referred to in section 8.1. It will be assumed for the remainder of Part I that all temperatures are measured on the thermodynamic scale, and they will be denoted by T.

As a result of Corollaries 2 and 3, the most important characteristics of engines operating between only two reservoirs may now be stated as follows:

(a)   All reversible engines, operating between a source at temperature T_1 and a sink at temperature T_2, have an efficiency equal to $(T_1 - T_2)/T_1$; see equation (6.3).

(b)   For a given value of T_2, the efficiency increases with increase of T_1. Since the lowest possible temperature of a practical infinite sink is fixed within close limits, i.e. the temperature of the atmosphere or ocean, it may be said that a given quantity of heat is more useful for producing work the higher the temperature of the source from which it is received.

(c)   For all reversible engines operating between only two reservoirs, $Q_1/T_1 = Q_2/T_2$. If an engine is irreversible, its efficiency is less than $(T_1 - T_2)/T_1$. For the same heat received Q_1, the heat rejected Q_2 must be greater than that rejected by a reversible engine operating between the same two reservoirs. Therefore, for irreversible engines operating between only two reservoirs, $Q_1/T_1 < Q_2/T_2$.

It is important to note that when applying statements (a), (b) and (c) to reversible engines, the temperature T refers both to the temperature of the reservoir and to the temperature of the fluid exchanging heat with it. On the other hand, when considering irreversible engines, T refers to the temperature of the reservoir only; the temperature of the fluid may then not be the same as that of the reservoir and different parts of the fluid may have different temperatures.

The three results (a), (b) and (c) will now be used in the deduction of the characteristics of reversible engines operating between more than two reservoirs.

6.3   Engines operating between more than two reservoirs

In many practical cycles the heat is received and rejected during processes which involve a continuous change in the temperature of the fluid. It has been explained that these cycles can still be considered reversible if the source and sink are each assumed to consist of an infinite number of reservoirs differing infinitesimally from one another in temperature. At any instant during a heating and cooling process, heat must be exchanged between the system and a source or sink which differs only infinitesimally in temperature from the fluid in the system.

We have seen that the efficiency with which a given quantity of heat can be converted into work by a reversible engine operating between reservoirs at T_1 and T_2 is given by $(T_1 - T_2)/T_1$ or $(1 - T_2/T_1)$. Now let T'_1 and T'_2 be the maximum and minimum temperatures of the working fluid in a reversible engine operating between more than two reservoirs. Only a fraction of the heat supplied can be received at T'_1 and only a fraction of the heat rejected can be rejected at T'_2. The remaining part of the heat supplied must be converted into work with an efficiency less than $(1 - T'_2/T'_1)$, because the temperatures of the remaining sources are less than T'_1 and the temperatures of the remaining sinks are greater than T'_2. Thus the efficiency with which the total heat received is converted into work must be less than $(T'_1 - T'_2)/T'_1$. This result may be summarised as the following corollary.

> *Corollary 5* The efficiency of any reversible engine operating between more than two reservoirs must be less than that of a reversible engine operating between two reservoirs which have temperatures equal to the highest and lowest temperatures of the fluid in the original engine.

The most important characteristic of engines operating between more than two reservoirs is presented as the sixth corollary of the Second Law; it is known as the *Clausius Inequality*.

> *Corollary 6* Whenever a system undergoes a cycle, $\oint(dQ/T)$ is zero if the cycle is reversible and negative if irreversible, i.e. in general $\oint(dQ/T) \leqslant 0$.

Proof First consider an engine operating between a finite number of reservoirs. The engine is represented in Fig. 6.4a; it may be reversible *or* irreversible. Let quantities of heat $Q_{1a}, Q_{1b}, \ldots, Q_{1n}$ be supplied from sources at temperatures $T_{1a}, T_{1b}, \ldots, T_{1n}$, and quantities of heat $Q_{2p}, Q_{2q}, \ldots, Q_{2z}$ be rejected to sinks at $T_{2p}, T_{2q}, \ldots, T_{2z}$. Now let the sources be supplied with their quantities of heat by a series of *reversible* heat pumps receiving quantities of heat $Q_{0a}, Q_{0b}, \ldots, Q_{0n}$ from a single reservoir at T_0. Similarly, let the sinks reject their quantities of heat to a series of *reversible* heat engines which in turn reject quantities of heat $Q_{0p}, Q_{0q}, \ldots, Q_{0z}$ to the single reservoir at T_0. T_0 may be any temperature, providing it is less than the temperature of any of the reservoirs of the original engine. The whole plant is represented in Fig. 6.4b.

The work delivered by the original engine is given by

$$\sum_a^n Q_1 - \sum_p^z Q_2$$

Fig. 6.4
Proof of the Clausius
inequality

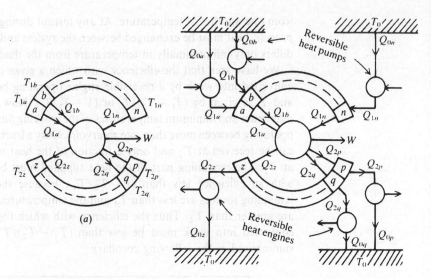

(a)

The work delivered by the auxiliary engines is

$$\sum_{p}^{z}(Q_2 - Q_0)$$

and the work supplied to the heat pumps must be

$$\sum_{a}^{n}(Q_1 - Q_0)$$

The series of sources and sinks plays no effective part in the transformations of energy, and the complete plant is a system undergoing a cyclic process while exchanging heat with a single reservoir (of temperature T_0). It follows from the Second Law that the net work *overall* cannot be into the surroundings, but must be either zero or into the plant. Thus we can write, for the composite cyclic system,

(net work *from* main engine) + (net work *from* set of reversible engines)

$$- \text{(net work } to \text{ set of reversible heat pumps)} \leqslant 0$$

This statement can be rewritten, from the First Law, as

$$\sum_{a}^{n}Q_1 - \sum_{p}^{z}Q_2 + \sum_{p}^{z}(Q_2 - Q_0) - \sum_{a}^{n}(Q_1 - Q_0) \leqslant 0$$

which reduces to

$$\sum_{a}^{n}Q_0 - \sum_{p}^{z}Q_0 \leqslant 0$$

But for each of the reversible heat engines and heat pumps which operate between only two reservoirs, we can write equations of the form

$$\frac{Q_1}{T_1} = \frac{Q_0}{T_0} \quad \text{between } a \text{ and } n$$

$$\frac{Q_2}{T_2} = \frac{Q_0}{T_0} \quad \text{between } p \text{ and } z$$

Therefore, substituting for the Q_0 terms in the previous inequality, we have

$$\sum_a^n \frac{Q_1}{T_1} T_0 - \sum_p^z \frac{Q_2}{T_2} T_0 \leqslant 0$$

Dividing throughout by the constant temperature T_0, we get finally

$$\sum_a^n \frac{Q_1}{T_1} - \sum_p^z \frac{Q_2}{T_2} \leqslant 0 \tag{6.5}$$

We may now revert to the *original convention of writing Q for any quantity of heat whether positive or negative* (see beginning of section 5.1), so that the algebraic summation of all such quantities as $(\delta Q/T)$ for the original cycle becomes

$$\sum \frac{\delta Q}{T} \leqslant 0$$

In the limiting case, where the temperature changes continuously during the heat exchanges, the number of reservoirs becomes infinite and the individual quantities of heat become infinitesimal. The equation can then be written as

$$\oint \frac{dQ}{T} \leqslant 0 \tag{6.6}$$

which is the *Clausius Inequality*.

We have now to show that the equality holds in the special case of a reversible engine. The foregoing argument can be repeated for a heat pump, all the quantities of heat and work flowing in directions opposite to those shown in Fig. 6.4b. If the quantities of heat are denoted by symbols with primes, we should find that equations (6.5) and (6.6) are unchanged in other respects, e.g. equation (6.6) is simply

$$\oint \frac{dQ'}{T} \leqslant 0 \tag{6.7}$$

Now if an engine is reversible, and it is reversed to form a heat pump, all the quantities of heat will be unchanged in magnitude although reversed in sign. It follows that $dQ' = -dQ$. Equation (6.7) can therefore be written as

$$-\oint \frac{dQ}{T} \leqslant 0 \quad \text{or} \quad \oint \frac{dQ}{T} \geqslant 0$$

The only way in which this result can be satisfied simultaneously with equation (6.6) is for the equality to hold. Therefore, if the engine is reversible,

$$\oint \frac{dQ}{T} = 0$$

Fig. 6.5
A cycle regarded as
equivalent to an infinite
number of elementary Carnot
cycles

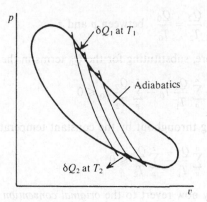

The engine operating between only two reservoirs is easily seen to provide a special example of the Clausius Inequality. In this case

$$\oint \frac{dQ}{T} = \frac{|Q_1|}{T_1} - \frac{|Q_2|}{T_2}$$

and we have already noted that the right-hand side is zero if the engine is reversible and negative if irreversible (section 6.2, result (c)).

From this specific case, a simpler though less rigorous proof of the Clausius Inequality can be derived. As indicated in Fig. 6.5, any cycle in which the temperature of the fluid changes during the processes in which heat is transferred can be replaced in principle by an infinite number of elementary cycles each of which operates between only two reservoirs. Summing $dQ/T \leqslant 0$ for all elementary cycles yields $\sum dQ/T \leqslant 0$, and therefore the Clausius Inequality applies also to cycles operating between more than two reservoirs.

It must be emphasised that the Clausius Inequality is a relation between the quantities of heat received or rejected by a series of reservoirs and the temperatures of those reservoirs, when a system is taken through a cycle. Only in the special case of a reversible cycle can the temperature be associated with the temperature of the fluid undergoing the cycle. This is a most important case, however, and the following section will show how it may be used to deduce a new property of a system.

So far, the Second Law has been stated with reference to cycles, and various characteristics of these cycles have been deduced. All the conclusions refer equally to cycles composed of either non-flow or steady-flow processes. The implication of the Second Law for the individual processes of which the cycles may be composed must now be considered. It will be necessary to deal with non-flow and steady-flow processes separately, and the former class will be considered first.

6.4 Consequences of the Second Law for non-flow processes

> *Corollary 7*   There exists a property of a closed system such that a
> change in its value is equal to $\int_1^2 dQ/T$ for any reversible process
> undergone by the system between state 1 and state 2.

Proof   Assume that the converse is true, i.e. that $\int_1^2 dQ/T$ depends
upon the reversible process as well as upon the end states. The procedure is to
show that this contradicts Corollary 6. Here the temperature T under consideration
is the temperature of the fluid undergoing the process. However, since the
process is to be reversible, T must also be equal to the temperature of the
reservoir with which the system is exchanging the quantity of heat dQ. This is
why we can base the proof upon Corollary 6.

Consider any two *reversible* processes A and B by which a system can change
from state 1 to state 2 (Fig. 6.6). The assumption is that

$$\int_1^2 \left(\frac{dQ}{T}\right)_A \neq \int_1^2 \left(\frac{dQ}{T}\right)_B$$

In each case let the system return to its original state by a third reversible
process C. For each of the complete reversible cycles AC and BC we have

$$\oint \left(\frac{dQ}{T}\right)_{AC} = \int_1^2 \left(\frac{dQ}{T}\right)_A + \int_2^1 \left(\frac{dQ}{T}\right)_C$$

$$\oint \left(\frac{dQ}{T}\right)_{BC} = \int_1^2 \left(\frac{dQ}{T}\right)_B + \int_2^1 \left(\frac{dQ}{T}\right)_C$$

If the assumption described by the inequality is true, it follows that

$$\oint \left(\frac{dQ}{T}\right)_{AC} \neq \oint \left(\frac{dQ}{T}\right)_{BC}$$

But these cyclic integrals must be equal because, according to Corollary 6, they
are zero for any reversible cycle. Therefore the original proposition, that $\int_1^2 dQ/T$
is independent of the path of the reversible process and represents the change
in a property of the system, must be true.

Fig. 6.6
Proof of existence of a
property 'entropy'

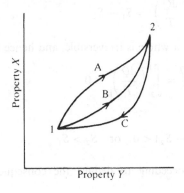

71

If the property is denoted by S, this corollary can be expressed mathematically as

$$\int_1^2 \left(\frac{dQ}{T}\right)_{rev} = S_2 - S_1 \tag{6.8}$$

or in differential form as

$$dS = \left(\frac{dQ}{T}\right)_{rev} \tag{6.9}$$

The subscript 'rev' is added as a reminder of the fact that the relation only holds for a reversible process. The property S is called the *entropy* of the system. Before describing the property entropy in more detail, one final corollary will be deduced.

Corollary 8   The entropy of any closed system which is thermally isolated from the surroundings either increases or, if the process undergone by the system is reversible, remains constant.

Proof   There are two cases to be considered; that of a closed system undergoing a reversible process presents no difficulty. For any thermally insulated system $dQ = 0$. But for any reversible process $dS = (dQ/T)$. Therefore for any reversible adiabatic process the change of entropy must be zero. For this reason the reversible adiabatic process is called an *isentropic process*. That the entropy of a system undergoing an irreversible adiabatic process must increase may be proved as follows.

Let any closed system change from state 1 to state 2 by an irreversible adiabatic process A. There may be a change of entropy of the fluid in this case because equation (6.9) is not applicable. But since the process is adiabatic, $dQ = 0$ and therefore

$$\int_1^2 \left(\frac{dQ}{T}\right)_A = 0$$

Now let the system be returned to its original state by some reversible process B, in this case not necessarily adiabatically. For this process it is possible to write

$$\int_2^1 \left(\frac{dQ}{T}\right)_B = S_1 - S_2$$

The cycle as a whole is irreversible, and hence from corollary 6

$$\oint \frac{dQ}{T} = \int_2^1 \left(\frac{dQ}{T}\right)_B < 0$$

Therefore

$$(S_1 - S_2) < 0 \quad \text{or} \quad S_2 > S_1$$

Before proceeding to deduce the consequences of the Second Law for steady-flow processes, we shall discuss some of the more important characteristics of the property entropy.

6.5 Characteristics of entropy

6.5.1 Determination of values of entropy

The property entropy arises as a consequence of the Second Law, in much the same way as the property internal energy arises from the First Law. There is, however, an important difference. The change in internal energy can be found directly from a knowledge of the heat and work crossing the boundary during *any* non-flow process undergone by a closed system. The change in entropy, on the other hand, can be found from a knowledge of the quantity of heat transferred only during a *reversible* non-flow process.

Since equations (6.8) and (6.9) apply to reversible processes, during which the system passes through a series of equilibrium states, they may be applied to any unit mass of the system. The entropy per unit mass, or *specific entropy*, will be denoted by s, and $S = ms$ when the system is in equilibrium. It is possible, therefore, to write the equations as

$$\int_1^2 \left(\frac{dQ}{T} \right)_{rev} = s_2 - s_1 \tag{6.10}$$

$$ds = \left(\frac{dQ}{T} \right)_{rev} \tag{6.11}$$

implying that dQ is the increment of heat transferred per unit mass of fluid in the system.

As with internal energy, only changes of entropy are normally of interest. The entropy at any arbitrary reference state can be made zero, and the entropy at any other state can then be found by evaluating (dQ/T) for any reversible process by which the system can change from the reference state to this other state. Since no real process is reversible, values of entropy cannot be found from measurements of Q and T in a direct experiment. The entropy is a thermodynamic property, however, and it can be expressed as a function of other thermodynamic properties which can be measured in experiments involving real processes. Two important relations of this kind can be obtained by combining the equations expressing the First and Second Laws. Thus the First Law yields the equation

$$(dQ)_{rev} = du + p\,dv$$

and combining this with equation (6.11) we have

$$T\,ds = du + p\,dv \tag{6.12}$$

Alternatively, substituting $du = dh - d(pv)$, we get

$$T\,ds = dh - v\,dp \tag{6.13}$$

Fig. 6.7
Graphical determination of
entropy

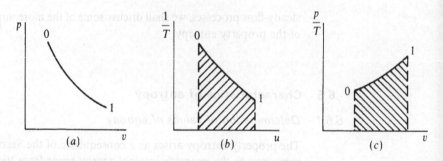

(a)   (b)   (c)

Equations (6.12) and (6.13) are general relations between properties which apply to any fluid. Moreover, when integrated they give the difference in entropy between any two equilibrium states, regardless of whether any particular process joining them is carried out reversibly or not.* We may show how equation (6.12) can be used for compiling tables of values of entropy as follows.

The entropy at state 1, defined by (p_1, v_1) say, relative to the entropy at some reference state 0, defined by (p_0, v_0), is given by

$$s_1 - s_0 = \int_0^1 \frac{1}{T}\,du + \int_0^1 \frac{p}{T}\,dv \tag{6.14}$$

The integrals can be evaluated graphically by the following procedure. The end states can be plotted on a p–v diagram and joined by any arbitrary curve as in Fig. 6.7a. (The curve can be chosen arbitrarily because the change of entropy depends only on the end states.) For several pairs of values of p and v along the curve, equilibrium values of u and T can be found from tables of properties. Finally, curves of $1/T$ versus u, and p/T versus v, can be plotted as in Figs 6.7b and c. The shaded areas under these curves will be equal to the integrals on the right-hand side of equation (6.14), and hence s_1 can be found assuming s_0 is arbitrarily chosen to be zero. Values of s for any other state, defined by different values of p and v, may be obtained in a similar way, and the results can be presented in a table of the form shown in Fig. 1.1.

When the properties of a fluid can be related by simple algebraic equations, the integrals of equation (6.14) can be evaluated analytically, and a simple equation for s in terms of p and v, or any other two independent properties, can be determined. Once the functions relating the entropy and other properties have been established, whether expressed algebraically or in the form of a table, there is no need to find the change of entropy by evaluating $\int(dQ/T)_{\text{rev}}$. It can be found directly from a knowledge of other properties in the initial and final states.

---

* The only proviso is that the states must be capable of being joined *in principle* by a reversible process, because this is assumed in deriving (6.12) and (6.13). Normally this is so. An example to the contrary is when a vapour in a metastable state (supersaturated) changes to a wet vapour in a stable state (see sections 8.2.1 and 18.2). Tables of entropy do not refer to metastable states and this special case can be ignored here.

6.5.2 *Entropy as a criterion of reversibility*

One use of the property entropy has already been indicated in sections 3.5 and 3.6, where it was shown to simplify calculations concerned with reversible adiabatic and isothermal non-flow processes. Another use is suggested by Corollary 8, namely that the change of entropy can be used as a criterion of reversibility. If a non-flow process is adiabatic, this corollary can be applied directly; it states that the entropy will remain unchanged if the process is reversible. When the process is not adiabatic the criterion may be applied in the following way. Any system together with its surroundings can be regarded as one single system. If the term 'surroundings' is used in a special sense to mean only that portion of matter outside a system which is affected by the changes under consideration, the system plus surroundings may be called the 'universe'. The quotation marks will be retained as a reminder that the word is used in this restricted sense. The 'universe' is an isolated system, and its entropy must either increase or remain constant in accordance with Corollary 8. If its entropy is determined before and after a change, an increase indicates that the process must have been irreversible. The way in which the entropy changes can therefore still be used as a criterion of reversibility, although when the process is not adiabatic it is necessary to refer to the entropy of the 'universe' and not merely to that of the system.

Before presenting an example of this use of the property entropy, we must see how the change in the entropy of a reservoir may be evaluated. It will be remembered that a reservoir is assumed to be a source or sink of such capacity that the quantity of heat leaving or entering it does not cause its temperature to change by more than an infinitesimal amount. Any change in the specific entropy (or any other specific property) is similarly infinitesimal, but since the mass of the reservoir is large, the total entropy change is finite. Because the elements of the reservoir undergo only infinitesimal changes, the process undergone by the reservoir as a whole when the quantity of heat Q enters or leaves it must be considered reversible. If the constant temperature of the reservoir is T, it follows that the entropy change of a reservoir is simply Q/T.

Let us now consider the process of transferring a quantity of heat Q from a reservoir at T_1 to a system at a constant lower temperature T_2, via an intervening medium which is a poor conductor (Fig. 6.8a). The source and conductor are the surroundings of the system. There is a temperature gradient along the conductor during the passage of energy through it. The heat Q enters the system

Fig. 6.8
External irreversibilities

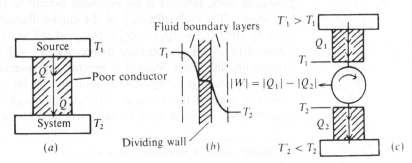

75

by virtue of an infinitesimal temperature difference at the boundary. The system therefore passes through a series of equilibrium states and, *as far as the system is concerned*, it undergoes a reversible change. Since its temperature remains constant at T_2, there is an increase in the entropy of the system equal to Q/T_2. The entropy change in the surroundings must now be considered. The change in the entropy of the reservoir is a decrease of Q/T_1. No change of entropy occurs in the conductor because it is in exactly the same state after the quantity of energy has passed through it as it was initially. Thus the entropy of the 'universe' has increased because $Q/T_2 > Q/T_1$. The complete process must therefore be irreversible.

The form of irreversibility just discussed is usually described as *external* because no dissipation of energy takes place within the system; the irreversibility occurs in the surroundings. Energy can be said to be 'wasted' or 'degraded' because the quantity Q has been transferred to a lower temperature level without producing any of the work of which it is capable. If T_0 is the lowest temperature of any natural infinite sink, such as the atmosphere or ocean, the maximum efficiency with which a quantity of heat at temperature T can be transformed into work is $(T - T_0)/T$. Therefore the maximum quantity of work which Q at T_1 could theoretically have produced is $Q(T_1 - T_0)/T_1$, while after its conduction to T_2 it is capable of producing only $Q(T_2 - T_0)/T_2$ units of work. No means exist for returning this quantity of heat to the original temperature level without some expenditure of work (Corollary 1), and so some energy has been irretrievably degraded in the sense that its capacity for producing work has been permanently decreased.

An external irreversibility is inevitably present when heat is conducted from one fluid to another through a dividing wall.* For example, when heat is transferred from the furnace gases to the water in a boiler, there is always a considerable temperature difference between the main body of hot gas and the main body of water. Briefly, this is because there are relatively stationary boundary layers of fluid on both sides of the boiler tube which are poor conductors of heat (Fig. 6.8b). The temperature drop across them is therefore considerable. The quantity of heat transferred to the working fluid in an engine can be calculated from the change in the average values of the properties of the fluid during the heat transfer process, and this quantity is the same whether the source is at a much higher, or only an infinitesimally higher, temperature. Thus although an external irreversibility results in the loss of some capacity for producing work, this loss is *not* expressed directly in the cycle efficiency of a heat engine. The cycle efficiency of the engine illustrated in Fig. 6.8c is still given by $|W|/|Q_1| = (|Q_1| - |Q_2|)/|Q_1|$, and the values of $|Q_1|$ and $|Q_2|$ are independent of the temperature differences $(T'_1 - T_1)$ and $(T_2 - T'_2)$. The temperature differences adopted in practice are governed by the area of heat transfer surface that is regarded as economic. If the cycle were modified to operate over nearly the full range of temperature available, T'_1 to T'_2, a higher cycle efficiency would be achieved but a very large heat exchange surface would

---

* A detailed analysis of this process is given in Part IV.

be required, so putting up the capital cost. The importance of balancing capital and running costs when designing power plant is discussed in section 11.11.

The other source of irreversibility, fluid friction, does cause a dissipation of energy within the system, and it is said to produce an *internal* irreversibility. The changes in the fluid properties are affected by friction, as explained in section 5.4.1, and the cycle efficiency is always reduced by this form of irreversibility.

6.6   Consequences of the Second Law for steady-flow processes

It must be emphasised that entropy is a thermodynamic property. The entropy of any element of fluid is a function only of the thermodynamic state and, as already pointed out, such functions are independent of whether the fluid is flowing or not. Each element of fluid of mass δm in an open system may have a different value of the specific entropy s'. The total entropy S' of the fluid in the system at any given moment is given by $S' = \Sigma(\delta m\, s')$. During any steady-flow process, S' remains constant because the properties at all points within the system do not change with time. We may imagine the steady-flow process to consist of a succession of elementary non-flow processes as in section 4.1.

First, let us consider a steady-flow process during which no heat is allowed to cross the boundary, although work may do so. The entropy of the imaginary closed system in its initial configuration (Fig. 4.2a) is given by

$$\delta m\, s_1 + S'$$

where s_1 denotes the specific entropy of the element of fluid which is about to enter the open system. Similarly, the entropy of the closed system in its final configuration is

$$\delta m\, s_2 + S'$$

Since the imaginary non-flow process is adiabatic, the final entropy of the closed system must be either greater than or equal to the initial entropy (Corollary 8). Therefore

$$\delta m\, s_2 + S' \geqslant \delta m\, s_1 + S' \quad \text{or} \quad \delta m\, s_2 \geqslant \delta m\, s_1$$

For the steady-flow process we therefore have

$$\Sigma(\delta m\, s_2) \geqslant \Sigma(\delta m\, s_1)$$

Since each element of fluid enters the open system with the same properties, denoted by subscript 1, and leaves with the same properties, denoted by subscript 2, this expression reduces to

$$s_2 \geqslant s_1 \tag{6.15}$$

Thus for an adiabatic steady-flow process, the specific entropy of the fluid leaving the system must be greater than or equal to the specific entropy at entry. If the process is reversible, i.e. frictionless, $s_2 = s_1$; otherwise $s_2 > s_1$. The reversible adiabatic steady-flow process may therefore be called an isentropic steady-flow process.

Since a large number of practical steady-flow processes may be assumed adiabatic, relation (6.15) is most useful. First, the principle of increasing entropy informs us of the direction of any real adiabatic flow process; it must occur so that the fluid changes from a state of lower entropy to a state of higher entropy. Sometimes this principle can be used effectively to show that certain flow processes are impossible. For example, in the study of gas dynamics it is used to show that a flow of gas through a shock wave can only be accompanied by a rise in pressure because a fall in pressure implies a decrease of entropy of the gas. Secondly, the equality of entropy at the inlet and outlet of an open system, when the adiabatic process is reversible, can simplify the analysis of many steady-flow processes.

Consider for example an adiabatic expansion in a turbine, where the fluid enters with an initial thermodynamic state defined by (p_1, v_1), and leaves with a pressure p_2. The values of h_1 and s_1 can be found from tables of properties. If the expansion is assumed to be reversible, s_2 will be known because it is equal to s_1. The final state is now completely determined by the properties p_2 and s_2, and the value of h_2 can also be found from the appropriate tables. The work done can then be found from the steady-flow energy equation

$$\dot{W} = \dot{m}(h_2 - h_1)$$

If the adiabatic process is irreversible, the final state cannot be predicted; all that is known is that $s_2 > s_1$. For the same value of p_2 this can be found from the tables of properties to imply that h_2 is greater than it would have been after a reversible expansion. This result is in agreement with the earlier discussion of the effect of irreversibility on the expansion in a turbine (section 5.4). But, as already pointed out, the effect of friction cannot be neglected in most steady-flow processes. In practice it is usual to calculate the required quantity on the assumption that the process is reversible, and then multiply the result by a *process efficiency* to give a more realistic estimate. The process efficiency in the case of a turbine is defined by

$$\text{turbine efficiency} = \frac{\text{work done during the real expansion}}{\text{work done during an isentropic expansion}}$$

Process efficiencies must be found empirically, i.e. by carrying out tests on actual components. Their definition is somewhat arbitrary, and no fixed form can be adopted which will apply to all processes.

So far we have only considered adiabatic steady-flow processes. The analysis leading up to relation (6.15) must now be repeated for the case of an open system which is exchanging heat with the surroundings. Consider the case of the reversible steady-flow process. When it is reversible, the individual non-flow processes of which it is assumed to consist must also be reversible. In general the heat crosses the boundary along a finite length of the system as the temperature of the fluid changes in the direction of flow. Let increments of heat $\delta Q_a, \delta Q_b, \ldots, \delta Q_n$ cross the boundary at points where the fluid temperature is

$T_a, T_b, \ldots, T_n$, during the change of configuration of the imaginary closed system (Fig. 4.2). Then equation (6.8) applied to this process becomes

$$(\delta m\, s_2 + S') - (\delta m\, s_1 + S') = \sum_a^n \frac{\delta Q}{T}$$

and hence

$$\delta m\, s_2 - \delta m\, s_1 = \sum_a^n \frac{\delta Q}{T}$$

Similar equations can be written for every elemental mass passing through the open system. Adding these equations we have, for the whole steady-flow process,

$$\sum(\delta m\, s_2) - \sum(\delta m\, s_1) = \sum\left(\sum_a^n \frac{\delta Q}{T}\right)$$

To simplify this equation we must assume not only that each elemental mass δm enters with the specific entropy s_1 and leaves with s_2, but also that each element exchanges $\delta Q_a, \delta Q_b, \ldots$ with the surroundings when the temperature is $T_a, T_b, \ldots$. If we make this additional assumption the equation reduces to

$$s_2 - s_1 = \sum_a^n \frac{\delta Q}{T}$$

where δQ is the quantity of heat *per unit mass* transferred across the boundary at the point where the fluid temperature is T. Also, if the temperature increases continuously from T_1 to T_2 during the process, the equation may be written in the form

$$s_2 - s_1 = \int_1^2 \frac{dQ}{T} \tag{6.16}$$

In the special case where T is constant during the process, e.g. when the fluid is a liquid which is being vaporised at constant pressure, equation (6.16) becomes

$$s_1 - s_2 = \frac{1}{T} \int_1^2 dQ$$

and therefore

$$Q = T(s_2 - s_1)$$

where Q is the heat transfer per unit mass between inlet and outlet. Or, if $\dot{m}$ is the rate of mass flow and $\dot{Q}$ the rate of heat transfer per unit time,

$$\dot{Q} = \dot{m}T(s_1 - s_1) \tag{6.17}$$

It must be emphasised that equations (6.16) and (6.17) apply only to an internally reversible process, i.e. a frictionless process,* because they are derived

---

* Since friction results in an increase of entropy, it is possible to imagine an irreversible steady-flow process in which the amount of heat rejected results in a decrease of entropy which is just equal to the increase caused by friction. In such circumstances s_2 will equal s_1. Although strictly speaking this would be an isentropic process, it is an unimportant kind. Less ambiguity arises if the term 'isentropic' is restricted to mean a reversible adiabatic process, as will be done throughout this book.

from equation (6.8). Nevertheless, in many practical cases where heat is received or rejected during a steady-flow process these equations can be applied with sufficient accuracy. For example, the velocity of flow in a boiler or condenser is low, and the effect of friction is negligible.

6.7 Validity and limitations of the laws of thermodynamics

With its emphasis on logical structure, and its reference to axioms and corollaries, this account of thermodynamics may have obscured the important fact that thermodynamics is essentially an experimental science. It is not a branch of mathematics, like Euclidean geometry, although it makes use of mathematical tools as do all the physical sciences. The two 'axioms' of thermodynamics are hypotheses put forward to explain a wide variety of phenomena and a vast range of experimental data. Every experiment which confirms a deduction from a hypothesis confirms and strengthens the validity of the hypothesis itself. The mathematical tools are merely used to draw every possible observable and verifiable consequence from the hypothesis.

When a hypothesis is sufficiently well established, it achieves the status of a law. The First and Second Laws of thermodynamics are so well established that we may confidently assume they will remain unchanged in the face of new developments. They may, of course, be shown to be of more limited application than was first supposed, and to be special cases of a more general hypothesis — in much the same way that Newtonian mechanics has been subsumed in the theory of relativity. Indeed this has already happened to some extent with the discovery that mass can be transformed into energy. But this has in no way invalidated the application of classical thermodynamic theory to systems in which mass is effectively conserved.

It is worth noting some possible restrictions upon the generality of the laws of thermodynamics.* We have already observed that it may not be permissible to apply the First Law to the whole universe to suggest that its total energy is constant. A similar extrapolation of the Second Law is sometimes made which is equally questionable. Since all real processes are irreversible, the entropy of all 'universes' must increase whenever a change occurs within them. This has led to the broad generalisation that the entropy of the universe as a whole is increasing. But the Second Law, like the first, is an expression of the observed behaviour of finite systems and it is not certain that the universe can be regarded as finite. Moreover, the significance of the Second Law for systems consisting of living organisms is not yet clear.

There is a definite limit to the applicability of the laws of thermodynamics at the other end of the scale of magnitude; the laws cannot be applied to microscopic systems which contain only a small number of molecules. The reasons for making this statement are as follows.

The thermodynamic state of any system can be completely described by 'macroscopic' properties, i.e. properties which are directly observable by the

---

* Advanced students will find a stimulating discussion of this in Ref. 2.

senses, such as pressure, volume and temperature. Other properties defined in terms of these or deduced as consequences of the laws of thermodynamics are also used but, though more abstract, they are none the less macroscopic in the sense that they are quite independent of any theory as to the molecular or atomic structure of matter. By constructing hypotheses about the 'microscopic' nature of matter, it is possible to regard these macroscopic properties as averages of microscopic quantities. Thus pressure can be regarded, on the kinetic theory of fluids, as the average value of all the rates of change of momentum due to molecular impacts on a unit area of the boundary. These hypotheses must yield results in agreement with the observed macroscopic behaviour of matter, and changes in such hypotheses do not require any modification to be made to the structure of classical thermodynamics. An assumption as to the nature of matter can, however, place a restriction on the field of application of thermodynamics. The kinetic theory indicates that a thermodynamic system must be large enough to contain a great number of molecules. If a system consists of only a few molecules the concept of pressure, for example, is meaningless. The force exerted by the system on its boundaries would be finite at the points of impact of the molecules and zero at all other points: thus the 'pressure' would not be uniform over the surface nor constant with respect to time, and it would be useless as a characteristic for describing the state of the system. Since, for example, one cubic centimetre of air at atmospheric pressure and temperature contains about 25×10^{18} molecules, this restriction is of little practical importance to engineers.

The way in which the laws of thermodynamics lose their meaning when applied to microscopic systems is illustrated by the following discussion of a microscopic engine which appears to contradict the Second Law. On the kinetic theory, the molecules of a gas are rushing about at random with various velocities. If a plate is suspended in the gas it will be bombarded on both faces by the molecules and, on the average, the number and force of the impacts on each face will be equal. If the plate is made so small that only a few molecules are bombarding each face at any given instant, then sometimes the force exerted on one side will be larger than that on the other. The plate could be made to operate a ratchet mechanism, the ratchet wheel only moving when the force on one particular side of the plate predominates. The wheel might turn a winch and raise a weight, so doing work on the surroundings. This microscopic engine does work continuously by merely extracting energy from the gas, e.g. the atmosphere, and no second reservoir is necessary. Such an engine contradicts the Second Law of Thermodynamics. This argument is open to refutation, on the grounds that the microscopic engine is impossible in principle because it would itself be subject to the random motion of the molecules.

We have shown how the Second Law loses its meaning when applied to microscopic systems or to an infinite universe. When applied to macroscopic finite systems it has been found to be valid, but it is worth emphasising that its usefulness is limited. The limitation can be seen more clearly from some of the corollaries, such as the Clausius Inequality, rather than from the statement of the law itself. The limitation results from the fact that the corollaries of the Second Law only provide definite quantitative statements about *reversible* processes. Only for such processes is it possible to predict the work and heat transfers crossing the boundary of a system. For irreversible processes the law merely provides statements of trend, e.g. that the entropy of an isolated system must increase, and quantitive predictions of energy transfers cannot be made.

In engineering calculations empirical 'correction factors' (e.g. process efficiencies) are often used to supplement the Second Law. In effect they express the degree of reversibility of real processes, and they will be introduced formally in Part II. Sometimes a process efficiency is insufficiently illuminating and recourse is made to additional empirical relations which are found to be applicable to a limited range of phenomena. Relations of this kind are used in Part IV, i.e. Fourier's law of heat conduction and Newton's law of viscosity. They all take the form of proportionalities between a quantity transferred in an irreversible process and a property gradient. The constants of proportionality in the examples mentioned are the 'thermal conductivity' and 'viscosity' respectively. These 'laws' are approximate empirical relations, whose accuracy can be determined by direct experiment; their inaccuracy is manifested by the fact that the 'constants of proportionality' are not in fact constant but vary with the conditions of the experiment (temperature, pressure, or their gradients etc.). The laws of thermodynamics, like Newton's laws of motion, are quite different in kind, being fundamental hypotheses upon which the respective sciences as a whole are based, and which can only be true, false, or shown to be part of an even broader generalisation about nature.

We began this section by trying to dispel a misconception that might have resulted from the systematic presentation of the theory, and we may end on the same note. It should not be supposed from this exposition that the science of thermodynamics developed historically in neat logical steps. In common with every science, the concepts which led to a systematic ordering and satisfactory understanding of experience, and which now seem so obvious, required for their birth centuries of experiment and the flashes of insight of some remarkable men. Although a definitive history of thermodynamics has yet to be written, some brief but stimulating accounts can be found. The student will be well advised to supplement his systematic study with a reading of the short historical survey given in Ref. 10.

6.8   Summary of Chapters 1 to 6

With the thoughts of section 6.7 in mind, we may now return to our logical account, and survey briefly the ground we have covered. We opened by defining terms such as 'system', 'property', 'temperature', 'work' and 'heat', although they did not all permit of simple definition with equal rigour. For example, we were able to note a few of the characteristics of the concepts of work and heat, such as the fact that they are not properties, but we were unable to define them completely until the First Law was enunciated. This is always the case with any really fruitful concept in an experimental science. Such concepts cannot be described completely in everyday language, and are only definable in terms of the way in which they play their part in the logical framework of the theory.

The more fruitful they are in enabling observable consequences to be deduced from the general law, the more they must rely on the logical structure for their definition;* energy and entropy are excellent examples of such concepts.

The notion of energy arose when we applied the First Law to a non-cyclic process. We saw that when heat and work cross the boundary of a closed system, there is a property of the system which increases by an amount equal to the net quantity of heat and work entering the system. We called this property the 'internal energy', and we explained the phenomenon by suggesting that heat and work are merely different ways in which 'energy' can be transferred between a system and its surroundings. Energy is the first outstandingly fruitful concept in thermodynamics, and it should be noted that it cannot be defined in terms we have already used without circularity. For example, it is pointless to say that energy is the capacity for doing work, and then define work as a form of transfer of energy. It is nearer the truth to say that energy is a concept which is necessary for the deduction of a variety of observable consequences from the First Law.

The First Law refers to any cycle, whether that of a heat engine or a heat pump — and there is nothing in it to say that heat and work are not equivalent in all respects. We might have a cycle (a) in which all the heat supplied is converted into work, or (b) in which all the work supplied is converted into heat. The necessity for the Second Law arises from the fact that heat and work are *not* equivalent in all respects. The Second Law is not reciprocal like the first, in the sense that it states (a) to be impossible without denying the possibility of (b). It is this lack of reciprocity in the behaviour of cycles which is the fundamental reason why the concept of reversibility has to be introduced. When the consequences of the Second Law for a non-cyclic process were deduced, we found that only in the absence of friction and heat transfer across a temperature difference can a change take place without a degradation of energy. When either of these causes of irreversibility is present during a process, some inherent capacity for producing work, in the system or its surroundings, is permanently lost. When the process is reversible, on the other hand, any changes brought about in the system and its surroundings can be undone; nothing irretrievable has occurred.

The implications of the Second Law can only be properly expressed in terms of measurable consequences, by using our mathematical tools to deduce a new property of a system — namely entropy. This property could not be deduced in quite such a direct way as internal energy. We had first to show that all reversible engines operating between the same two reservoirs must have the same efficiency. This, in turn, led us to infer that the efficiency must be a function only of the temperature of the reservoirs — since in every other respect the engines may differ from one another. When the temperatures of the two reservoirs are defined in such a way that their ratio is equal to the ratio of the quantities of heat leaving and entering the reservoirs, we found that we could devise a

---

* For the advanced student who is philosophically inclined, an interesting discussion of why this is so can be found in Ref. 1.

temperature scale which was independent of the behaviour of any particular substance and which was an absolute scale in the sense that a meaning could be given to the idea of zero temperature.

Once we had decided to use temperatures measured on this thermodynamic scale, we were able to widen the scope of our enquiry and investigate the behaviour of engines operating between more than two reservoirs. We found that when the cycle is reversible, the integration of all such quantities as (dQ/T) round the complete cycle must be equal to zero. If the cycle is reversible, there can be no more than an infinitesimal difference in temperature between the reservoirs and the system undergoing the cycle at the points where each quantity of heat dQ is transferred across the boundary. Therefore T can refer to the system as well as the reservoir. It becomes probable that (dQ/T) represents a change in a property of the system, since the total change for the complete reversible cycle is zero. We proved that this is in fact the case, by showing that the integral of (dQ/T) between the end states of any reversible process is independent of the process. The property whose change is given by $\int(dQ/T)_{rev}$ is called the entropy of the system. It differs from the internal energy, whose change is given by $\int(dQ + dW)$, because the change in entropy can be evaluated from $\int(dQ/T)$ only when the process is reversible. This is no great drawback since we can usually find a reversible process which can be imagined to connect any two given end states and for which we can evaluate $\int(dQ/T)$ in terms of other properties.

The lack of reciprocity in the Second Law can now be expressed in terms of the property entropy. We showed that for any isolated system the entropy must either remain constant or increase; it increases if any process occurring in the isolated system is irreversible. The degradation of energy consequent upon an irreversibility is thereby manifested as an increase in the entropy of the system plus surroundings, or 'universe'. All real processes must occur in such a direction that the state of the 'universe' changes from one of lower to one of higher entropy.

Although the reasoning required to deduce the existence of entropy from the Second Law is more complex than that required to deduce the internal energy from the First, the two concepts are of the same type. They are both consequences of empirical laws and are to this extent grounded in experience. If entropy appears the more mysterious, it is only because it is less familiar; the student meets the concept of energy in his early study of mechanics. It is because each is the consequence of an empirical law of great generality that these properties have such significance — much greater significance, for example, than the property enthalpy which was arbitrarily defined as a combination of other properties purely for convenience.

The utility of the concepts of internal energy and entropy only becomes apparent when the principles of thermodynamics are applied to particular systems. For the closed systems we are considering, it is an experimental fact that any property can be expressed as a function of two other independent properties when the system is in equilibrium. This fact, together with the laws of thermodynamics, enables a great many useful relations between the properties to be deduced which are universally valid for all such systems. These general relations are deduced in the next chapter, although they need concern only the advanced student. They are necessary because values of the internal energy and entropy are most conveniently obtained indirectly from measurements of other properties; indeed the latter can be obtained in no other way since no system can be put through a reversible process in practice. The next chapter indicates how these general relations may be used when tables of properties are to be compiled. So far we have assumed, and we shall do so again in Part II, that tables of properties are available for any substance we need consider, e.g. that given the values of p and v at any state we shall know the corresponding values of the other properties. We have already shown that this information enables the behaviour of both closed and open systems to be analysed and predicted when the processes are reversible, and also that some of the calculations would be extremely tedious, or even impossible, without the use of the concept of entropy. All this part of the exposition in these first six chapters will be further illustrated in Part II by numerical calculations relating to systems consisting of particular fluids.

7

General Thermodynamic Relations*

With the aid of the two laws of thermodynamics and the differential calculus, it is possible to deduce general relations between the thermodynamic properties which hold for any of the limited class of systems considered in this book. Since relations between thermodynamic properties are independent of whether the substance is in motion or not, we need refer only to closed systems.

The distinguishing characteristics of the systems considered here are that, when in equilibrium, (a) they only change their state when heat and mechanical work cross the boundary, and (b) only two independent properties are necessary to determine their thermodynamic state. These conditions are satisfied, in the absence of surface, gravitational, electric and magnetic effects, by any system consisting of a single substance, even if more than one phase is present. They are also satisfied by systems consisting of a mixture of substances, provided that no chemical reaction is taking place; for example, air is normally treated as a single substance. When mixtures which react chemically are considered, it must be emphasised that only for *stable* states of chemical equilibrium are two properties sufficient to define the system completely. A mixture of H_2 and O_2 at atmospheric temperature is in an *apparently* stable state only because the reaction $H_2 + \frac{1}{2}O_2 \rightarrow H_2O$ leading to the most stable state is very slow at that temperature. When such quasi-stable states of chemically reacting systems are to be considered, more than two properties are required to define the state: in our foregoing example, the proportions of H_2, O_2 and H_2O in the mixture must be specified as a third property. For a treatment of systems whose composition is variable, the reader is referred to texts on chemical thermodynamics.

Some of the more important thermodynamic relations are deduced in this chapter — principally those which are useful when tables of properties are to be compiled from limited experimental data, and those which may be used when calculating the work and heat transfers associated with processes undergone by a liquid or solid. It should be noted that the relations only apply to a substance in the solid phase when the stress, i.e. the pressure, is uniform

---

* This chapter should be omitted on the first reading.

in all directions; if it is not, a single value for the pressure cannot be allotted to the system as a whole. The chapter ends with an introduction to the concept of exergy and its relation to the Gibbs function.

7.1 Properties to be related

We are already acquainted with six properties which may be used to describe the thermodynamic state of a system: pressure, volume, temperature, internal energy, enthalpy and entropy. The first three are directly measurable characteristics. The absolute measurement of pressure and volume presents no difficulty, and we have seen that the introduction of the thermodynamic scale as a consequence of the Second Law makes an absolute measurement of temperature possible. The internal energy u was shown to be a property as a consequence of the First Law and, since the enthalpy h is defined as a function of u, p and v, h is itself a property. Lastly, the entropy s was shown to be a property as a consequence of the Second Law.

Two other properties will be added to the list, although they are of less significance to engineers. These are the *Helmholtz function f* and the *Gibbs function g*, arbitrarily defined in a similar way to enthalpy by the expressions:

$$f = u - Ts$$

$$g = h - Ts$$

h, f and g are sometimes referred to as *thermodynamic potentials*, and g is often referred as the *free energy* for reasons which will be apparent after a reading of section 7.9. Both f and g are useful when considering chemical reactions, and the former is of fundamental importance in statistical thermodynamics. The Gibbs function is also useful when considering processes involving a change of phase.

Of the eight properties p, v, T, u, h, s, f and g, only the first three are directly measurable. We shall find it convenient to introduce other combinations of properties which are relatively easy to measure and which, together with measurements of p, v and T, enable the values of the remaining properties to be determined. These combinations of properties might be called 'thermodynamic gradients'; they are all defined as the rate of change of one property with another while a third is kept constant. Before proceeding to define them, and to deduce general relations between the properties, it is necessary to review certain theorems concerning the mathematical properties of differentials

7.2 Exact differentials

When the state of a system can be defined by two independent properties, it follows that any third property must be a function of these two. In general terms, any property z can be expressed as $z = z(x, y)$, where x and y are two independent properties. This implies that if x and y change to new values x'

Fig. 7.1
Geometric interpretation of
partial differentials

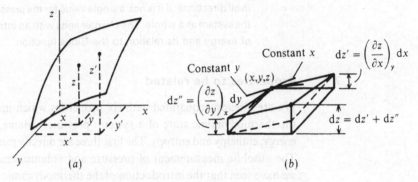

and y', z will have a new definite value z' irrespective of the process. The function can therefore be represented by a three-dimensional surface, as in Fig. 7.1a. Now consider an infinitesimal change from a state defined by the point x, y to that defined by $(x + dx)$, $(y + dy)$. It should be clear from Fig. 7.1b that the change in z is given by

$$dz = \left(\frac{\partial z}{\partial x}\right)_y dx + \left(\frac{\partial z}{\partial y}\right)_x dy \qquad (7.1)$$

In mathematics it is common to omit the subscripts on the partial differential coefficients because it is obvious which variable is being maintained constant. However, in thermodynamics it is often necessary to refer to these coefficients out of context of such equations as (7.1). Since any one of the many thermodynamic properties might be kept constant during the change, it is essential to retain the subscript so that we know which third property is being considered.

Equation (7.1) is quite general and applies to any infinitesimal change of state. Suppose an infinitesimal change occurs in such a way that z is a constant. Then dz is zero, and

$$\left(\frac{\partial z}{\partial x}\right)_y dx = -\left(\frac{\partial z}{\partial y}\right)_x dy$$

But since z is constant,

$$dx = \left(\frac{\partial x}{\partial y}\right)_z dy$$

and substituting for dx in the previous equation we have

$$\left(\frac{\partial z}{\partial x}\right)_y \left(\frac{\partial y}{\partial z}\right)_x \left(\frac{\partial x}{\partial y}\right)_z = -1 \qquad (7.2)$$

This is a relation between the three gradients at any point on the three-dimensional surface of Fig. 7.1a, i.e. it is a general relation between the three properties x, y and z at any state and does not refer to a process.

Equations frequently arise in thermodynamics in the form

$$dz = M\,dx + N\,dy \tag{7.3}$$

where, although x and y are known to be properties, z is not necessarily a property. The coefficients M and N may be constants or functions of x and y. An example is provided by the energy equation for a reversible non-flow process: $dQ = du + p\,dv$. If an equation such as (7.3) can be expressed in the form of (7.1), it may be inferred that z is a property and that $z = z(x, y)$. If this cannot be done, the equation cannot be directly integrated to give $z = z(x, y)$; z is not a property, and the change in z depends upon the path of the process as well as on the values of x and y at the end states.

A simple test by which equations (7.1) and (7.3) can be compared for identity may be devised as follows. Equations (7.1) and (7.3) are identical if

$$M = \left(\frac{\partial z}{\partial x}\right)_y \quad \text{and} \quad N = \left(\frac{\partial z}{\partial y}\right)_x$$

Differentiating these equations, we have

$$\left(\frac{\partial M}{\partial y}\right)_x = \left\{\frac{\partial}{\partial y}\left(\frac{\partial z}{\partial x}\right)_y\right\}_x = \frac{\partial^2 z}{\partial x \partial y}$$

$$\left(\frac{\partial N}{\partial x}\right)_y = \left\{\frac{\partial}{\partial x}\left(\frac{\partial z}{\partial y}\right)_x\right\}_y = \frac{\partial^2 z}{\partial y \partial x}$$

But if $z = z(x, y)$, the magnitude of the second derivative of z with respect to x and y is independent of the order of differentiation, and hence

$$\left(\frac{\partial M}{\partial y}\right)_x = \left(\frac{\partial N}{\partial x}\right)_y \tag{7.4}$$

It follows that if (7.4) is satisfied, equations (7.1) and (7.3) are identical, and the quantity z in (7.3) must be capable of being expressed as a function of x and y. dz is then referred to as an *exact* or *perfect differential*. Conversely, if the quantity z in (7.3) is known to be a property, (7.4) must be satisfied.

Reverting to the example provided by the energy equation for a closed system, $M = 1$ and $N = p$ in this case. Therefore

$$\left(\frac{\partial M}{\partial y}\right)_x = \left(\frac{\partial 1}{\partial v}\right)_u = 0 \quad \text{and} \quad \left(\frac{\partial N}{\partial x}\right)_y = \left(\frac{\partial p}{\partial u}\right)_v$$

Reflection on the process of heating a gas at constant volume indicates that in general the rate of change of pressure with internal energy at constant volume cannot be zero. Thus the two partial differential coefficients are not equal, so that dQ cannot be an exact differential and Q is not a property. In order to integrate such an equation the path of the process must be specified in addition to the end states. In this case the path is fixed when the variation of p with v is known.

When $(M\,dx + N\,dy)$ is not an exact differential, it can always be made exact by multiplying throughout by an *integrating factor*. For our example the integrating factor is $1/T$, because the expression then becomes equal to (dQ/T), the differential of the property entropy. ds can be substituted for (dQ/T) in this case because the equation $dQ = du + p\,dv$ applies to a reversible process. It is important to realise that we have not introduced entropy in the same way as h, f or g — as an arbitrary combination of other properties. The fact that $(du + p\,dv)/T$ is an exact differential is a consequence of the Second Law; it is neither self-evident nor a purely mathematical deduction.* This accounts for the considerable significance which attaches to entropy. As the following sections will show, it is possible to deduce a large number of useful relations between the properties of a substance which do not contain entropy at all, but which could not have been deduced without its help.

7.3 Some general thermodynamic relations

The First Law applied to a closed system undergoing a reversible process states that

$$dQ = du + p\,dv$$

From the Second Law,

$$ds = \left(\frac{dQ}{T}\right)_{rev}$$

Combining these equations we have

$$T\,ds = du + p\,dv$$

or

$$du = T\,ds - p\,dv \tag{7.5}$$

The properties h, f and g may also be put in terms of T, s, p and v as follows:

$$dh = du + p\,dv + v\,dp$$

$$= T\,ds + v\,dp \tag{7.6}$$

$$df = du - T\,ds - s\,dT$$

$$= -p\,dv - s\,dT \tag{7.7}$$

$$dg = dh - T\,ds - s\,dT$$

$$= v\,dp - s\,dT \tag{7.8}$$

Each of these equations is a result of the two laws of thermodynamics.

---

* In this book we are dealing mainly with systems whose state is determined by two independent properties. The Second Law is not required to show that an integrating factor *exists* for a total differential which is a function of two variables; this is an established fact in the theory of functions. But the same does not necessarily apply to functions of more than two variables, and the Second Law tells us that even for such cases (e.g. systems involving electric, magnetic or surface tension effects) there always exists an integrating factor for dQ, *and* that this factor is $1/T$.

Since du, dh, df and dg are exact differentials, we can express them as

$$du = \left(\frac{\partial u}{\partial s}\right)_v ds + \left(\frac{\partial u}{\partial v}\right)_s dv$$

$$dh = \left(\frac{\partial h}{\partial s}\right)_p ds + \left(\frac{\partial h}{\partial p}\right)_s dp$$

$$df = \left(\frac{\partial f}{\partial v}\right)_T dv + \left(\frac{\partial f}{\partial T}\right)_v dT$$

$$dg = \left(\frac{\partial g}{\partial p}\right)_T dp + \left(\frac{\partial g}{\partial T}\right)_p dT$$

Comparing these equations with (7.5) to (7.8), we may equate the corresponding coefficients. For example, from the two equations for du we have

$$\left(\frac{\partial u}{\partial s}\right)_v = T \quad \text{and} \quad \left(\frac{\partial u}{\partial v}\right)_s = -p$$

The complete group of such relations may be summarised as follows:*

$$\left(\frac{\partial u}{\partial s}\right)_v = T = \left(\frac{\partial h}{\partial s}\right)_p \qquad (7.9)$$

$$\left(\frac{\partial u}{\partial v}\right)_s = -p = \left(\frac{\partial f}{\partial v}\right)_T \qquad (7.10)$$

$$\left(\frac{\partial h}{\partial p}\right)_s = v = \left(\frac{\partial g}{\partial p}\right)_T \qquad (7.11)$$

$$\left(\frac{\partial f}{\partial T}\right)_v = -s = \left(\frac{\partial g}{\partial T}\right)_p \qquad (7.12)$$

Finally, making use of the fact that equation (7.4) must hold for equations (7.5) to (7.8), we have

$$\left(\frac{\partial T}{\partial v}\right)_s = -\left(\frac{\partial p}{\partial s}\right)_v \qquad (7.13)$$

$$\left(\frac{\partial T}{\partial p}\right)_s = \left(\frac{\partial v}{\partial s}\right)_p \qquad (7.14)$$

$$\left(\frac{\partial p}{\partial T}\right)_v = \left(\frac{\partial s}{\partial v}\right)_T \qquad (7.15)$$

---

* These relations may be obtained by an alternative argument. Consider equation (7.5), for example; it is quite general and applies to any infinitesimal process. Applying it first to an infinitesimal process at constant volume, we have $(du)_v = T(ds)_v$ or $(\partial u/\partial s)_v = T$. Applying it to an infinitesimal process at constant entropy, we have $(du)_s = -p(dv)_s$ or $(\partial u/\partial v)_s = -p$.

$$\left(\frac{\partial v}{\partial T}\right)_p = -\left(\frac{\partial s}{\partial p}\right)_T \qquad (7.16)$$

These last four equations are known as the *Maxwell relations*.

It must be emphasised that equations (7.9) to (7.16) do not refer to a process, but simply express relations between properties which must be satisfied when any system is in a state of equilibrium. Each partial differential coefficient can itself be regarded as a property of state. The state may be defined by a point on a three-dimensional surface, the surface representing all possible states of stable equilibrium. Suppose, for example, that the coordinates of Fig. 7.1a are u, v and s. If u and v are specified, s is determined, and any gradient of the surface at the point (u, v, s) is also determined. The gradient of a curve formed by the intersection of a horizontal plane with the surface is $(\partial u/\partial v)_s$, and equation (7.10) informs us that the gradient at any point on this curve is always negative and numerically equal to the pressure at that point. All the relations (7.9) to (7.16) can be interpreted graphically in this way.

To deduce equations (7.9) to (7.12) we took four forms of the equation expressing the laws of thermodynamics, and compared each with an equation expressing one property in terms of two others. The two independent properties were so chosen that a direct comparison could be made of the differential coefficients, e.g. we took $u = u(s, v)$ for comparison with equation (7.5). However, we need not limit the analysis in this way. For example, writing $u = u(T, v)$ we have

$$du = \left(\frac{\partial u}{\partial T}\right)_v dT + \left(\frac{\partial u}{\partial v}\right)_T dv$$

Equating this to (7.5) we get

$$\left(\frac{\partial u}{\partial T}\right)_v dT + \left(\frac{\partial u}{\partial v}\right)_T dv = T\,ds - p\,dv$$

or

$$T\,ds = \left(\frac{\partial u}{\partial T}\right)_v dT + \left\{p + \left(\frac{\partial u}{\partial v}\right)_T\right\} dv$$

In this case we may take $s = s(T, v)$ to provide an equation for direct comparison of coefficients, i.e.

$$ds = \left(\frac{\partial s}{\partial T}\right)_v dT + \left(\frac{\partial s}{\partial v}\right)_T dv$$

Then

$$\left(\frac{\partial s}{\partial T}\right)_v = \frac{1}{T}\left(\frac{\partial u}{\partial T}\right)_v \qquad (7.17)$$

$$\left(\frac{\partial s}{\partial v}\right)_T = \frac{1}{T}\left\{p + \left(\frac{\partial u}{\partial v}\right)_T\right\} \qquad (7.18)$$

Since there are eight properties, and in general each can be written as a function of any other two, it is clear that a very large number of relations can be derived. No attempt will be made here to expand the number of relations systematically,* although a few others will be deduced in the course of illustrating the use of these general relations.

It must be remembered that relations obtained by using expressions of the form $z = z(x, y)$ are only valid if x and y are independent. Thus relations based on the assumption that p and T are independent cannot be applied to a mixture of phases. For example, the right-hand equations of (7.11) and (7.12) were obtained by writing $g = g(p, T)$. It is shown in section 7.7 that when the temperature or pressure of a mixture of phases is maintained constant, g is constant also. If equations (7.11) and (7.12) were valid they would imply that v and s are zero under these conditions, which is obviously untrue.

7.4 Measurable quantities

Of the eight thermodynamic properties listed in section 7.1, only p, v and T are directly measurable. We must now examine the information that can be obtained from measurements of these primary properties, and then see what other easily measurable quantities can be introduced.

7.4.1 Equation of state

Imagine a series of experiments in which the volume of a substance is measured over a range of temperature while the pressure is maintained constant, this being repeated for various pressures. The results might be represented graphically by a three-dimensional surface, or by a family of constant pressure lines on a v–T diagram. It is useful if an equation can be found to express the relation between p, v and T, and this can always be done over a limited range of states. No single equation will hold for all phases of a substance, and usually more than one equation is required even in one phase if the accuracy of the equation is to match that of the experimental results. Equations relating p, v and T are called *equations of state* or *characteristic equations*. Accurate equations of state are usually complicated, a typical form being

$$pv = A + \frac{B}{v} + \frac{C}{v^2} + \dots$$

where $A, B, C, \dots$ are functions of temperature which differ for different substances.

An equation of state of a particular substance is an empirical result, *and it cannot be deduced from the laws of thermodynamics*. Nevertheless the general form of the equation may be predicted from hypotheses about the microscopic structure of matter. This type of prediction has been developed to a high degree of precision for gases, and to a lesser extent for liquids and solids. The simplest postulates about the molecular structure of gases lead to the concept of the

---

* A comprehensive collection can be found in Ref. 3.

perfect gas, which has the equation of state $pv = RT$. Experiments have shown that the behaviour of real gases at low pressure and high temperature agrees well with this equation. Additional refinements to the assumptions lead to the more complicated equations of state. A brief statement of the main assumptions is given in Chapter 8, but for a description of the theory itself the reader is referred to books on the kinetic theory of gases and statistical mechanics.

7.4.2 Coefficient of expansion and compressibility

An equation of state is not the only useful information that can be obtained from $p-v-T$ measurements. When the experimental results are plotted as a series of constant pressure lines on a $v-T$ diagram, as in Fig. 7.2a, the slope of a constant pressure line at any given state is $(\partial v/\partial T)_p$. If the gradient is divided by the volume at that state, we have the value of a property of the substance called its *coefficient of cubical expansion β*. That is,

$$\beta = \frac{1}{v}\left(\frac{\partial v}{\partial T}\right)_p \qquad (7.19)$$

Values of β can be tabulated for a range of pressures and temperatures, or plotted graphically as in Fig. 7.2b. For solids and liquids over the normal working range of pressure and temperature, the variation of β is small and can often be neglected. In tables of physical properties β is usually quoted as an average value over a small range of temperature, the pressure being atmospheric. This average coefficient may be symbolised by $\bar{\beta}$, and it is defined by

$$\bar{\beta} = \frac{v_2 - v_1}{v_1(T_2 - T_1)}$$

Fig. 7.2a can be replotted to show the variation of volume with pressure for various constant values of temperature, as in Fig. 7.3a. In this case the gradient of a curve at any state is $(\partial v/\partial p)_T$. When this gradient is divided by the volume at that state, we have a property known as the *compressibility κ* of the substance. Since this gradient is always negative, i.e. the volume of a substance always decreases with increase of pressure when the temperature is constant, the

Fig. 7.2

Determination of coefficient of expansion from $p-v-T$ data

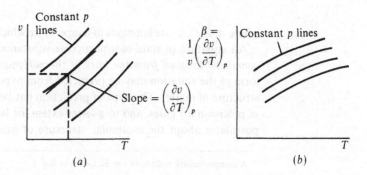

Constant p lines

Slope $= \left(\dfrac{\partial v}{\partial T}\right)_p$

$\beta = \dfrac{1}{v}\left(\dfrac{\partial v}{\partial T}\right)_p$

Constant p lines

(a)

(b)

Fig. 7.3
Determination of
compressibility from p–v–T
data

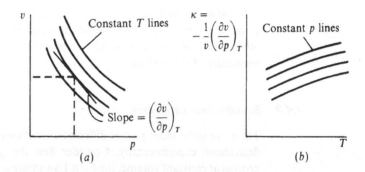

(a)   (b)

compressibility is usually made a positive quantity by defining it as

$$\kappa = -\frac{1}{v}\left(\frac{\partial v}{\partial p}\right)_T \tag{7.20}$$

Again, for solids and liquids κ can be regarded as a constant for many purposes. In tables of properties it is often quoted as an average value over a small range of pressure at atmospheric temperature, i.e.

$$\bar{\kappa} = -\frac{v_2 - v_1}{v_1(p_2 - p_1)}$$

When β and κ are known, equation (7.2) may be used to find the third partial differential coefficient involving p, v and T. Thus (7.2) becomes

$$\left(\frac{\partial p}{\partial T}\right)_v \left(\frac{\partial T}{\partial v}\right)_p \left(\frac{\partial v}{\partial p}\right)_T = -1$$

Since

$$\left(\frac{\partial v}{\partial T}\right)_p = \beta v \quad \text{and} \quad \left(\frac{\partial v}{\partial p}\right)_T = -\kappa v$$

we have

$$\left(\frac{\partial p}{\partial T}\right)_v = \frac{\beta}{\kappa} \tag{7.21}$$

When the equation of state is known, the coefficients of cubical expansion and compressibility can be found by differentiation. For a perfect gas, for example, we have

$$\left(\frac{\partial v}{\partial T}\right)_p = \frac{R}{p} \quad \text{and} \quad \left(\frac{\partial v}{\partial p}\right)_T = -\frac{RT}{p^2}$$

Hence

$$\beta = \frac{1}{v}\left(\frac{\partial v}{\partial T}\right)_p = \frac{R}{pv} = \frac{1}{T}$$

$$\kappa = -\frac{1}{v}\left(\frac{\partial v}{\partial p}\right)_T = \frac{RT}{p^2 v} = \frac{1}{p}$$

It will be found in section 7.5 that information about the relation between p, v and T is not sufficient to enable the other properties to be determined, and other measurable quantities must be introduced. These will be discussed in the remainder of this section.

7.4.3 Specific heat capacities

There are three more partial differential coefficients which are relatively easily determined experimentally. Consider first the quantity $(\partial u/\partial T)_v$. During a process at constant volume, the First Law informs us that an increase of internal energy is equal to the heat supplied. If a calorimetric experiment is conducted with a known mass of substance at constant volume, the quantity of heat Q required to raise the temperature of unit mass by ΔT may be measured. We can then write

$$\left(\frac{\Delta u}{\Delta T}\right)_v = \left(\frac{Q}{\Delta T}\right)_v$$

The quantity obtained in this way is known as the mean specific heat capacity at constant volume over the temperature range ΔT. It is found to vary with the conditions of the experiment, i.e. with the temperature range and the specific volume of the substance. As the temperature range is reduced the value approaches that of $(\partial u/\partial T)_v$, and the true *specific heat capacity at constant volume* is defined by

$$c_v = \left(\frac{\partial u}{\partial T}\right)_v$$

This is a *property* of the substance, and in general its value varies with the state of the substance, e.g. with temperature and pressure.

The First Law also implies that the heat supplied is equal to the increase of enthalpy during a reversible constant pressure process. Therefore a calorimetric experiment carried out with a substance at constant pressure gives us

$$\left(\frac{\Delta h}{\Delta T}\right)_p = \left(\frac{Q}{\Delta T}\right)_p$$

which is the mean specific heat capacity at constant pressure. As the range of temperature is made infinitesimally small, this becomes the rate of change of enthalpy with temperature at a particular state defined by T and p, and the true *specific heat capacity at constant pressure* is defined by

$$c_p = \left(\frac{\partial h}{\partial T}\right)_p$$

c_p also varies with the state, e.g. with pressure and temperature.

Descriptions of experimental methods of determining c_p and c_v can be found in texts on physics. When solids and liquids are considered, it is not easy to measure c_v owing to the stresses set up when such a substance is prevented from expanding. Fortunately a relation between c_p, c_v, β and κ can be found as follows, from which c_v may be obtained if the remaining three properties have been measured.

From equations (7.5) and (7.6) we can write

$$T\,ds = du + p\,dv = dh - v\,dp$$

Putting $u = u(T, v)$ and $h = h(T, p)$, we can also write respectively

$$du = \left(\frac{\partial u}{\partial T}\right)_v dT + \left(\frac{\partial u}{\partial v}\right)_T dv = c_v\,dT + \left(\frac{\partial u}{\partial v}\right)_T dv$$

$$dh = \left(\frac{\partial h}{\partial T}\right)_p dT + \left(\frac{\partial h}{\partial p}\right)_T dp = c_p\,dT + \left(\frac{\partial h}{\partial p}\right)_T dp$$

Substituting for du and dh in the above equation for $T\,ds$, we arrive at

$$c_v\,dT + \left\{p + \left(\frac{\partial u}{\partial v}\right)_T\right\}dv = c_p\,dT - \left\{v - \left(\frac{\partial h}{\partial p}\right)_T\right\}dp$$

As this equation is true for any process, it will also be true for the case when $dp = 0$, and hence

$$(c_p - c_v)(dT)_p = \left\{p + \left(\frac{\partial u}{\partial v}\right)_T\right\}(dv)_p$$

or

$$c_p - c_v = \left\{p + \left(\frac{\partial u}{\partial v}\right)_T\right\}\left(\frac{\partial v}{\partial T}\right)_p$$

Now from equations (7.15) and (7.18) we have

$$\left(\frac{\partial p}{\partial T}\right)_v = \left(\frac{\partial s}{\partial v}\right)_T = \frac{1}{T}\left\{p + \left(\frac{\partial u}{\partial v}\right)_T\right\}$$

and therefore

$$c_p - c_v = T\left(\frac{\partial p}{\partial T}\right)_v\left(\frac{\partial v}{\partial T}\right)_p$$

Finally, from equations (7.19) and (7.21),

$$c_p - c_v = \frac{\beta^2 Tv}{\kappa} \tag{7.22}$$

Thus at any state defined by T and v, c_v can be found if c_p, β and κ are known for the substance at that state.

The values of T, v and κ are always positive and, although β may sometimes be negative (e.g. between 0 and 4 °C water contracts on heating at constant pressure), β^2 is always positive. It follows that c_p is always greater than c_v.

By making use of equation (7.9), other expressions for c_p and c_v can be obtained. Thus since

$$c_v = \left(\frac{\partial u}{\partial T}\right)_v = \left(\frac{\partial u}{\partial s}\right)_v \left(\frac{\partial s}{\partial T}\right)_v$$

we have

$$c_v = T\left(\frac{\partial s}{\partial T}\right)_v \tag{7.23}$$

Similarly,

$$c_p = \left(\frac{\partial h}{\partial T}\right)_p = \left(\frac{\partial h}{\partial s}\right)_p \left(\frac{\partial s}{\partial T}\right)_p$$

and consequently

$$c_p = T\left(\frac{\partial s}{\partial T}\right)_p \tag{7.24}$$

These two relations will be found useful when expressing entropy in terms of measurable quantities (section 7.5).

7.4.4 Joule-Thomson coefficient

Consider the partial differential coefficient $(\partial T/\partial p)_h$. We have already noted in section 4.2 that if a fluid is flowing through a pipe, and the pressure is reduced by a throttling process, the enthalpies on either side of the restriction may be equal. Fig. 7.4a illustrates the process: the velocity increases at the restriction, with a consequent decrease of enthalpy, but this increase of kinetic energy is dissipated by friction as the eddies die down after the restriction. The steady-flow energy equation implies that the enthalpy of the fluid is restored to its initial value if the flow is adiabatic and if the velocity before the restriction is equal to that downstream of it. These conditions are very nearly satisfied in the following experiment; it was first carried out by Joule and Thomson (Lord Kelvin), and is usually referred to as the Joule-Thomson experiment.

Fig. 7.4
Determination of
Joule–Thomson coefficient

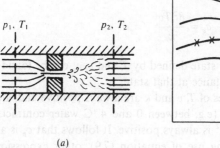

p_1, T_1 p_2, T_2

(a)

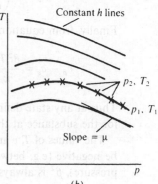

(b)

A fluid is allowed to flow steadily from a high pressure to a low pressure through a porous plug inserted in a pipe. The pipe is well lagged so that any heat flow to or from the fluid is negligible when steady conditions have been reached. Furthermore, the velocity of flow is kept low, and any difference between the kinetic energy upstream and downstream of the plug is negligible. A porous plug is used because the local increase of directional kinetic energy, caused by the restriction, is rapidly reconverted to random molecular energy by viscous friction in the fine passages of the plug. Irregularities in the flow die out a very short distance downstream of the plug, and temperature and pressure measurements taken there will be values for the fluid in a state of thermodynamic equilibrium.

With the upstream pressure and temperature maintained constant at p_1 and T_1, the downstream pressure p_2 is reduced in steps and the corresponding temperature T_2 is measured. The fluid in the successive states defined by the values of p_2 and T_2 must always have the same value of the enthalpy, namely the value of the enthalpy corresponding to the state defined by p_1 and T_1. From these results, points representing equilibrium states of the same enthalpy can be plotted on a T–p diagram, and joined up to form a curve of constant enthalpy. The curve does *not* represent the throttling process itself, which is irreversible. During the actual process the fluid undergoes first a decrease and then an increase of enthalpy, and no single value of the specific enthalpy can be ascribed to all elements of the fluid. If the experiment is repeated with different values of p_1 and T_1, a family of curves may be obtained covering a range of values of enthalpy (Fig. 7.4b). The slope of a curve at any point in the field is a function only of the state of the fluid; it is the *Joule-Thomson coefficient* μ, defined by

$$\mu = \left(\frac{\partial T}{\partial p} \right)_h$$

The change of temperature due to a throttling process is small and, if the fluid is a gas, it may be an increase or a decrease. At any particular pressure there is a temperature, the *temperature of inversion*, above which a gas can never be cooled by a throttling process. If a gas is to be liquefied by the Linde process, it must first be cooled below the temperature of inversion.

It may be seen that both c_p and μ are defined in terms of p, T and h. The third partial differential coefficient based on these three properties can therefore be found from equation (7.2), i.e.

$$\left(\frac{\partial h}{\partial p} \right)_T \left(\frac{\partial p}{\partial T} \right)_h \left(\frac{\partial T}{\partial h} \right)_p = -1$$

Hence

$$\left(\frac{\partial h}{\partial p} \right)_T = -\mu c_p \qquad (7.25)$$

Summarising: experimental methods are available for determining the p–v–T relation (and hence β and κ), and also values of c_p, c_v and μ at any state. We must now see how the values of the remaining properties (s, h, u, f and g) can be determined from these experimental data.

7.5 Graphical determination of entropy and enthalpy

Let us assume that v is expressed as a function of p and T in the form of a family of curves (Fig. 7.5). For practical purposes, and in particular for compiling tables of properties, it is sufficient if we can determine the change in entropy and enthalpy between any state (p, T) and an arbitrary reference state (p_0, T_0). The values of these properties at the reference state may be denoted by s_0 and h_0; they are usually put equal to zero. Since the change in a property is independent of the process, any convenient path may be considered. We shall proceed from the reference state to any other state by means of a reversible constant pressure process at p_0 followed by a reversible isothermal process at T (Fig. 7.5).

The change in entropy along any constant pressure line can be found by integrating $(\partial s/\partial T)_p$ with respect to T. It is not possible to derive an expression for $(\partial s/\partial T)_p$ in terms of p, v and T, but we may make use of equation (7.24) in the form

$$\left(\frac{\partial s}{\partial T}\right)_p = \frac{c_p}{T}$$

The change of entropy between state (p_0, T_0) and state (p_0, T) is then given by

$$s_{0T} - s_0 = \left\{ \int_{T_0}^{T} \frac{c_p}{T} \, dT \right\}_{p_0}$$

where s_{0T} is used to denote the entropy at a state defined by p_0 and any temperature T. Experimental data for c_p at pressure p_0 may be expressed by a single curve of c_p versus T, from which Fig. 7.6a can easily be constructed. The integral is then given by the area under the curve between T_0 and any required temperature T.

The change of entropy along any isothermal can be found by integrating $(\partial s/\partial p)_T$ with respect to p. This coefficient can be expressed in terms of primary

Fig. 7.5
A possible path between the reference state and any other state

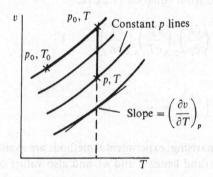

Fig. 7.6
Graphical determination of
entropy

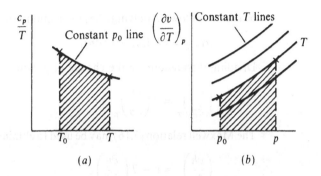

properties, since the Maxwell relation (7.16) states that

$$\left(\frac{\partial s}{\partial p}\right)_T = -\left(\frac{\partial v}{\partial T}\right)_p$$

Hence, on integration between the state (p_0, T) and the state (p, T), we have

$$s - s_{0T} = -\left\{\int_{p_0}^{p}\left(\frac{\partial v}{\partial T}\right)_p dp\right\}_T$$

The integration may be performed graphically if values of $(\partial v/\partial T)_p$ are plotted against pressure as in Fig. 7.6b. This can be done by measuring the slopes of the constant pressure lines in Fig. 7.5 at the required temperature T. The integral is then given by the area under the curve between p_0 and p.

The complete expression for the entropy at any state defined by (p, T), in terms of the entropy at the reference state and the measurable properties p, v, T and c_p, becomes

$$s = s_0 + \left\{\int_{T_0}^{T}\frac{c_p}{T}dT\right\}_{p_0} - \left\{\int_{p_0}^{p}\left(\frac{\partial v}{\partial T}\right)_p dp\right\}_T \tag{7.26}$$

An expression for the enthalpy of a substance can be found in a similar way. The change in enthalpy along a constant pressure line can be found by integrating $(\partial h/\partial T)_p$. Since this partial differential coefficient is equal to c_p, the change of enthalpy between the reference state (p_0, T_0), and any other state where the pressure is also p_0, is given by

$$h_{0T} - h_0 = \left\{\int_{T_0}^{T}c_p dT\right\}_{p_0}$$

In this case the integral can be evaluated directly from the curve of c_p versus T. Again, only values of c_p at the pressure p_0 need be known.

To find the change of enthalpy along the isothermal path, we must integrate the partial differential coefficient $(\partial h/\partial p)_T$. This quantity may be expressed in terms of p, v and T, although the expression is not given directly by a Maxwell relation as in the case of $(\partial s/\partial p)_T$. The required expression can be obtained by repeating the analysis used to determine equation (7.18), but in this case starting with the equations expressing h as a function of p and T. Alternatively, the argument contained in the footnote indicated just before equation (7.9) may

101

be used as follows. Applying (7.6) to an infinitesimal isothermal process, we have

$$(dh)_T = (T\,ds)_T + (v\,dp)_T$$

Dividing throughout by the change of pressure, this becomes

$$\left(\frac{\partial h}{\partial p}\right)_T = T\left(\frac{\partial s}{\partial p}\right)_T + v$$

The Maxwell relation (7.16) may be used to eliminate the entropy term to give

$$\left(\frac{\partial h}{\partial p}\right)_T = v - T\left(\frac{\partial v}{\partial T}\right)_p. \tag{7.27}$$

Equation (7.27) could now be integrated as it stands, although it would involve the evaluation of two integrals. By substituting τ for $1/T$, one of the integrals is eliminated. Thus (7.27) can be written as

$$\left(\frac{\partial h}{\partial p}\right)_T = v - \frac{1}{\tau}\left(\frac{\partial v}{\partial \tau}\right)_p\left(\frac{\partial \tau}{\partial 1/\tau}\right)_p = v + \tau\left(\frac{\partial v}{\partial \tau}\right)_p$$

and hence

$$\left(\frac{\partial h}{\partial p}\right)_T = \left(\frac{\partial v\tau}{\partial \tau}\right)_p \tag{7.28}$$

Integrating between state (p_0, T) and state (p, T), we have

$$h - h_{0T} = \left\{\int_{p_0}^{p}\left(\frac{\partial v\tau}{\partial \tau}\right)_p dp\right\}_T$$

The integration can be performed graphically if Figs 7.7a and b are constructed. Fig. 7.7a can be deduced directly from the p–v–T data in Fig. 7.5. Then, by measuring the slopes of the constant pressure lines at the required temperature T (and therefore a particular value of τ), the appropriate curve of Fig. 7.7b is obtained. The integral is equal to the area under this curve between the limits p_0 and p.

The complete expression for the enthalpy may be written as

$$h = h_0 + \left\{\int_{T_0}^{T} c_p\,dT\right\}_{p_0} + \left\{\int_{p_0}^{p}\left(\frac{\partial v\tau}{\partial \tau}\right)_p dp\right\}_T \tag{7.29}$$

Fig. 7.7
Graphical determination of enthalpy

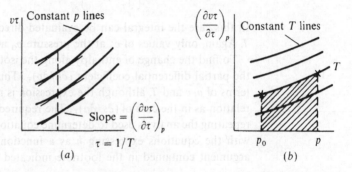

(a)　(b)

As already stated, s_0 and h_0 are usually assigned the arbitrary value of zero.

It is worth emphasising that the p–v–T data alone are insufficient for the determination of the entropy and enthalpy. Some additional information about the substance along a line of reference states is evidently necessary. It is not essential for the additional data to consist of experimental values of c_p; values of the Joule-Thomson coefficient can be used instead. Thus from equation (7.25) we have

$$c_p = -\frac{1}{\mu}\left(\frac{\partial h}{\partial p}\right)_T$$

and hence from (7.28),

$$c_p = -\frac{1}{\mu}\left(\frac{\partial v\tau}{\partial \tau}\right)_p$$

The partial differential coefficient $(\partial v\tau/\partial\tau)_p$ is already used in equation (7.29), and values of this quantity at the reference pressure p_0 and any temperature T can be read from Fig. 7.7b. The required values of c_p can then be determined if μ is known for various temperatures at pressure p_0.

Once the entropy and enthalpy have been obtained, the remaining properties u, f and g are easily found. For example, $u = (h - pv)$ and both h and v are known for any pair of values of p and T. Similarly, f is found from $(u - Ts)$ and g from $(h - Ts)$. Note that the value of u at the reference state cannot be zero if h_0 is put equal to zero. At the reference state (p_0, T_0), the internal energy is

$$u_0 = h_0 - p_0 v_0 = -p_0 v_0$$

It should also be noted that it has been assumed that no discontinuity occurs in the experimental curves during the change from the reference state to the state (p, T). This assumption is invalid if a change of phase occurs, and in such cases it is necessary to determine the changes of entropy and enthalpy in more than two steps. This matter will be referred to again in section 7.7.

The following section shows how expressions for the entropy and enthalpy may be deduced when the p–v–T data are given in the form of an equation of state. After a general example, we shall consider two important hypothetical substances which are characterised by two particular equations of state. When the equation of state is known, it is usually easier to work from first principles rather than use equations (7.26) and (7.29).

7.6   Analytical determination of entropy and enthalpy

A typical equation of state giving v as an explicit function of p and T is provided by

$$v = \frac{RT}{p} + A - \frac{B}{T^2}$$

where R, A and B are constants. We have seen that in addition to this information we require a knowledge of c_p or μ along a line of reference states. Let us assume that, over the required range of temperature, experiment shows c_p to vary linearly with T at zero pressure. That is, when $p = 0$,

$$c_p = C + DT$$

where C and D are constants. The problem is to find expressions for s and h at any state defined by pressure p and temperature T, and we may assume that the values of s and h are put equal to zero at an arbitrary reference state (p_0, T_0). We shall work from first principles, and check the result by applying (7.26) and (7.29).

Considering s as a function of p and T,

$$ds = \left(\frac{\partial s}{\partial T}\right)_p dT + \left(\frac{\partial s}{\partial p}\right)_T dp,$$

Using equation (7.24) and the Maxwell relation (7.16), this becomes

$$ds = \frac{c_p}{T} dT - \left(\frac{\partial v}{\partial T}\right)_p dp \qquad (7.30)$$

The next step is to find an expression for c_p in terms of p and T. This can be done because the variation of c_p along a line of reference states is given. Using (7.24) again and differentiating,

$$c_p = T\left(\frac{\partial s}{\partial T}\right)_p \quad \text{and} \quad \left(\frac{\partial c_p}{\partial p}\right)_T = T\left(\frac{\partial^2 s}{\partial T \partial p}\right)$$

On substitution of the Maxwell relation (7.16), this becomes

$$\left(\frac{\partial c_p}{\partial p}\right)_T = -T\left(\frac{\partial^2 v}{\partial T^2}\right)_p$$

Differentiating the characteristic equation, treating p as constant,

$$\left(\frac{\partial v}{\partial T}\right)_p = \frac{R}{p} + \frac{2B}{T^3} \quad \text{and} \quad \left(\frac{\partial^2 v}{\partial T^2}\right)_p = -\frac{6B}{T^4}$$

Hence

$$\left(\frac{\partial c_p}{\partial p}\right)_T = \frac{6B}{T^3}$$

Integrating, and remembering that when $p = 0$, $c_p = C + DT$, we have

$$c_p = \left(\int \frac{6B}{T^3} dp\right)_T = C + DT + \frac{6Bp}{T^3}$$

Substituting for $(\partial v/\partial T)_p$ and c_p in equation (7.30),

$$ds = \left(C + DT + \frac{6Bp}{T^3}\right)\frac{dT}{T} - \left(\frac{R}{p} + \frac{2B}{T^3}\right) dp$$

$$= \left(\frac{C}{T} + D\right)dT - \frac{R}{p}dp + 2B\left(\frac{3p}{T^4}dT - \frac{1}{T^3}dp\right)$$

$$= \left(\frac{C}{T} + D\right)dT - \frac{R}{p}dp - 2B\,d\left(\frac{p}{T^3}\right) \qquad (7.31)$$

By integration between the reference state (p_0, T_0) and any other state (p, T), we obtain

$$s = C\ln\left(\frac{T}{T_0}\right) + D(T - T_0) - R\ln\left(\frac{p}{p_0}\right) - 2B\left(\frac{p}{T^3} - \frac{p_0}{T_0^3}\right)$$

The enthalpy can be obtained from equation (7.6),

$$dh = T\,ds + v\,dp$$

Substituting for $T\,ds$ from (7.31), and for v from the equation of state, we have

$$dh = \left(C + DT + \frac{6Bp}{T^3}\right)dT - \left(\frac{RT}{p} + \frac{2B}{T^2}\right)dp + \left(\frac{RT}{p} + A - \frac{B}{T^2}\right)dp$$

$$= (C + DT)\,dT + A\,dp + 3B\left(\frac{2p}{T^3}dT - \frac{1}{T^2}dp\right)$$

$$= (C + DT)\,dT + A\,dp - 3B\,d\left(\frac{p}{T^2}\right)$$

Therefore

$$h = C(T - T_0) + \frac{D}{2}(T^2 - T_0^2) + A(p - p_0) - 3B\left(\frac{p}{T^2} - \frac{p_0}{T_0^2}\right)$$

As a check, we may deduce these expressions for s and h from equations (7.26) and (7.29). We have already obtained expressions for c_p and $(\partial v/\partial T)_p$, so equation (7.26) becomes

$$s = s_0 + \left\{\int_{T_0}^{T}\left(\frac{C}{T} + D + \frac{6Bp}{T^4}\right)dT\right\}_{p_0} - \left\{\int_{p_0}^{p}\left(\frac{R}{p} + \frac{2B}{T^3}\right)dp\right\}_{T}$$

$$= s_0 + C\ln\frac{T}{T_0} + D(T - T_0) - 2Bp_0\left(\frac{1}{T^3} - \frac{1}{T_0^3}\right) - R\ln\frac{p}{p_0} - \frac{2B}{T^3}(p - p_0)$$

$$= s_0 + C\ln\frac{T}{T_0} + D(T - T_0) - R\ln\frac{p}{p_0} - 2B\left(\frac{p}{T^3} - \frac{p_0}{T_0^3}\right)$$

Since $s = 0$ when $p = p_0$ and $T = T_0$, $s_0 = 0$, and this becomes identical with the previous result.

In order to use (7.29) we must first find $(\partial v\tau/\partial \tau)_p$. From the equation of state,

$$v\tau = \frac{R}{p} + A\tau - B\tau^3 \quad \text{and} \quad \left(\frac{\partial v\tau}{\partial \tau}\right)_p = A - 3B\tau^2$$

Hence (7.29) becomes

$$h = h_0 + \left\{ \int_{T_0}^{T} \left(C + DT + \frac{6Bp}{T^3} \right) dT \right\}_{p_0} + \left\{ \int_{p_0}^{p} (A - 3B\tau^2)\, dp \right\}_T$$

$$= h_0 + C(T - T_0) + \frac{D}{2}(T^2 - T_0^2) - 3Bp_0 \left(\frac{1}{T^2} - \frac{1}{T_0^2} \right)$$

$$+ A(p - p_0) - \frac{3B}{T^2}(p - p_0)$$

$$= h_0 + C(T - T_0) + \frac{D}{2}(T^2 - T_0^2) + A(p - p_0) - 3B \left(\frac{p}{T^2} - \frac{p_0}{T_0^2} \right)$$

This again equals the former result when h_0 is put equal to zero.

We may now consider two simple characteristic equations which are of particular significance. All gases at low pressures and high temperatures have an equation of state approximating to the perfect gas equation

$$pv = RT$$

A better approximation is provided by the van der Waals equation

$$\left(p + \frac{a}{v^2} \right)(v - b) = RT$$

R, a and b are constants for any particular gas. The significance of these equations is discussed more fully in Chapter 8, but a few of their consequences will appear here in the course of deducing the relevant expressions for entropy and enthalpy.

7.6.1 Perfect gas

Certain information about the internal energy, enthalpy and specific heat capacities of a perfect gas is implicit in the equation of state. Transforming equation (7.18), we have

$$\left(\frac{\partial u}{\partial v} \right)_T = T \left(\frac{\partial s}{\partial v} \right)_T - p$$

which, on substituting the Maxwell relation (7.15), can be written

$$\left(\frac{\partial u}{\partial v} \right)_T = T \left(\frac{\partial p}{\partial T} \right)_v - p \tag{7.32}$$

But from the equation of state $pv = RT$,

$$\left(\frac{\partial p}{\partial T} \right)_v = \frac{R}{v} = \frac{p}{T}$$

Therefore

$$\left(\frac{\partial u}{\partial v} \right)_T = 0$$

This means that when T is constant, u does not vary with v. But the existence of an equation of state of any kind implies that when T is constant, p and v are not independent properties. Consequently it also follows that u does not vary with p when T is constant. The final conclusion must be that *for a perfect gas u is a function only of T.*

Since the enthalpy is defined as $(u + pv)$, and $pv = RT$, it follows immediately that h also is a function only of T. It is of interest to note that this implies that the temperatures before and after a throttling process must be equal, and therefore that the Joule-Thomson coefficient μ of a perfect gas is zero.

The specific heat capacities are defined by

$$c_v = \left(\frac{\partial u}{\partial T} \right)_v \quad \text{and} \quad c_p = \left(\frac{\partial h}{\partial T} \right)_p$$

But for a perfect gas u and h are not functions of v and p, and the partial notation may be dropped. Thus

$$c_v = \frac{du}{dT} \quad \text{and} \quad c_p = \frac{dh}{dT}$$

and c_v and c_p are either constants or functions of temperatures only. A relation between c_p, c_v and R follows immediately. Since $dh = du + d(pv)$, we have in this case

$$dh = du + R \, dT$$

and hence

$$c_p - c_v = R \tag{7.33}$$

Thus, although c_p and c_v may vary with temperature, their difference is constant. This important result can also be obtained in another way. From (7.22) we have the general relation

$$c_p - c_v = \frac{\beta^2 \, Tv}{\kappa}$$

When $pv = RT$ it has already been shown in section 7.4.2 that β and κ are equal to $1/T$ and $1/p$ respectively. Therefore

$$c_p - c_v = \frac{pv}{T} = R$$

Expressions for enthalpy and internal energy can now be written as

$$h = h_0 + \int_{T_0}^{T} c_p \, dT \quad \text{and} \quad u = u_0 + \int_{T_0}^{T} c_v \, dT$$

In this case h and u may be put equal to zero along a line of reference states at T_0, since they are independent of pressure.

We have seen that the perfect gas equation implies that c_p and c_v are independent of p and v; they must therefore be either constant or some function of temperature. A perfect gas is sometimes defined as one which both satisfies the equation $pv = RT$, and has constant specific heat capacities. The enthalpy and internal energy of a perfect gas defined in this way are therefore given by the expressions

$$h = c_p(T - T_0) \quad \text{and} \quad u = c_v(T - T_0)$$

when u_0 and h_0 are put equal to zero. And the changes in these properties between any two states at T_1 and T_2 are

$$h_2 - h_1 = c_p(T_2 - T_1) \tag{7.34}$$

$$u_2 - u_1 = c_v(T_2 - T_1) \tag{7.35}$$

It now remains to find an expression for the entropy. The simplicity of the equation of state enables equation (7.6) to be used. Writing $c_p \, dT$ for dh, and R/p for v/T, (7.6) becomes

$$ds = \frac{c_p}{T} dT - \frac{R}{p} dp$$

Therefore, when s is put equal to zero at the reference state (p_0, T_0),

$$s = \int_{T_0}^{T} \frac{c_p}{T} dT - R \ln \frac{p}{p_0}$$

If c_p is constant, this reduces to

$$s = c_p \ln \frac{T}{T_0} - R \ln \frac{p}{p_0}$$

And the change of entropy between states defined by (p_1, T_1) and (p_2, T_2) is

$$s_2 - s_1 = c_p \ln \frac{T_2}{T_1} - R \ln \frac{p_2}{p_1} \tag{7.36}$$

In this section, and in Chapter 8, we have introduced the perfect gas by defining it as a substance which has the equation of state $pv = RT$. It then follows that u and h are functions only of T. When approaching the subject in this way, we are assuming that the absolute thermodynamic temperature T can be measured independently of the concept of a perfect gas. Now it is true that this can be done in principle by using a Carnot engine, and even in practice by making use of the Clausius-Clapeyron equation (see section 7.7). Or we can adopt the argument that all this is a matter of history and that the International Temperature Scale (ITS-90, see section 8.1) on which our instruments are calibrated is essentially equivalent to the thermodynamic scale. But it is a fact that, over a wide range of temperature, thermodynamic temperatures used for fixed points on the International Temperature Scale have been measured by gas thermometry. It is therefore instructive to see how the procedure can be justified without involving a circular argument. What we have to do is *to define a perfect gas independently of the concept of thermodynamic temperature, and to show that an empirical temperature measured by a thermometer using such a gas is identical with the thermodynamic temperature.* This we can do as follows.

Real gases are known to approximate asymptotically to two laws as their pressures are lowered. First, they obey *Boyle's law*

$$pv = \text{constant}]_{\theta = \text{constant}} \tag{7.37}$$

Secondly, they follow the *Joule-Thomson law*

$$h = h(\theta) \tag{7.38}$$

which can be established from the Joule-Thomson porous plug experiment described in section 7.4.4. Here θ denotes empirical temperature measured on any arbitrary scale, and the function $h(\theta)$ depends on the scale used as well as on the particular gas considered.

Boyle's law enables us to define a gas temperature θ_G which is a linear function of pv, i.e.

$$pv = A\theta_G \tag{7.39}$$

where A is an arbitrary constant. Extrapolating the product pv to zero provides us with an absolute zero for the perfect gas temperature scale. This, as yet, cannot imply that this zero coincides with that of the absolute thermodynamic scale. Furthermore, we have to show that θ_G is identical with the absolute thermodynamic temperature T.

From a combination of the first and second laws we can write

$$ds = \frac{dh}{T} - \frac{v\,dp}{T} = \frac{1}{T}\left\{ \frac{\partial h(\theta)}{\partial T} \right\} dT - \left(\frac{v}{T} \right) dp$$

But because s is a property and therefore ds is a perfect differential, it follows from equation (7.4) that

$$\frac{\partial}{\partial p}\left\{ \frac{1}{T} \frac{dh(\theta)}{dT} \right\}_T = -\left\{ \frac{\partial}{\partial T}\left(\frac{v}{T} \right) \right\}_p \tag{7.40}$$

the derivative within braces on the LHS being total in view of equation (7.38). The LHS of equation (7.40) must be zero, as the term inside braces is merely some function of temperature, and hence from the RHS it follows that

$$\left\{ \frac{\partial}{\partial T}\left(\frac{v}{T} \right) \right\}_p = 0$$

and therefore

$$\frac{v}{T} = \phi(p) \tag{7.41}$$

From equations (7.39) and (7.41) we can write

$$v = T\phi(p) = \frac{A\theta_G}{p}$$

or

$$p\phi(p) = \frac{A\theta_G}{T} \qquad (7.42)$$

Equation (7.42) can only be true for all values of the independent variables p and T if each side is equal to a constant, say K, and hence

$$T = \frac{A}{K}\theta_G \qquad (7.43)$$

From equation (7.39) it is clear that A can be chosen arbitrarily, and thus A/K can be made equal to unity. Thus we have established that the perfect gas temperature θ_G and the absolute thermodynamic temperature T can be made identical, and that they have a common zero datum.

To end the discussion on the equivalence $\theta_G \equiv T$, we can conclude the following:

(a) From equation (7.38) it follows that $h = h(T)$, and furthermore, because $u = h - pv = h(T) - RT$, it also follows that $u = u(T)$.

(b) From (a) it follows that $c_p = (\partial h/\partial T)_p$ and $c_v = (\partial u/\partial T)_v$ for a perfect gas are functions of temperature only. To assume that they are constant is a convenience, approximately true over limited ranges of temperature, and is in no way relevant to the main virtue of the concept of the perfect gas, namely that $\theta_G \equiv T$.

(c) By following a procedure similar to the one used in proving the identity $\theta_G \equiv T$, it is possible to show that for a gas which obeys the Boyle and Joule-Thomson laws, $1/\theta_G$ is an integrating factor for the energy equation $dQ = du + p\,dv = dh - v\,dp$, *without recourse to the Second Law*. It is thus possible to arrive at the limited concept of gas entropy $ds_G = dQ/\theta_G$ using the First Law only. In fact any differential which is a function of two independent variables must have an integrating·factor, but any differential in more variables has an integrating factor only if it possesses certain special characteristics. The Second Law's contribution, in the mathematical sense, consists in implying first that the integrating factor of dQ is the same, namely $1/T$, for all systems whose state is determined by two independent properties, and secondly that it still exists and is the same, namely $1/T$, for more complex systems requiring more than two properties to fix the state.

7.6.2 *The van der Waals gas*

The characteristic equation first suggested by van der Waals is one of a class of such equations in which v is not expressed as an explicit function of p and T. It can be recast, however, with p expressed explicitly as a function of v and T, i.e.

$$p = \frac{RT}{v - b} - \frac{a}{v^2}$$

110

In this case it will obviously be more suitable to consider v and T as the independent properties defining the state of the gas.

An expression for entropy in terms of v and T can be found as follows:

$$ds = \left(\frac{\partial s}{\partial T}\right)_v dT + \left(\frac{\partial s}{\partial v}\right)_T dv$$

Using (7.23) and the Maxwell relation (7.15), this becomes

$$ds = \frac{c_v}{T} dT + \left(\frac{\partial p}{\partial T}\right)_v dv \qquad (7.44)$$

This is the equivalent of equation (7.30). For the van der Waals gas,

$$\left(\frac{\partial p}{\partial T}\right)_v = \frac{R}{v-b}$$

So (7.44) becomes

$$ds = \frac{c_v}{T} dT + \frac{R}{v-b} dv$$

and on integration,

$$s = s_0 + \int_{T_0}^{T} \frac{c_v}{T} dT + R \ln \frac{v-b}{v_0-b} \qquad (7.45)$$

And if c_v can be assumed constant,

$$s = s_0 + c_v \ln \frac{T}{T_0} + R \ln \frac{v-b}{v_0-b}$$

When an equation of state has the form $p = p(v, T)$, it is easier to find the internal energy first and then deduce the enthalpy. Treating u as a function of v and T,

$$du = \left(\frac{\partial u}{\partial T}\right)_v dT + \left(\frac{\partial u}{\partial v}\right)_T dv$$

But $(\partial u/\partial T)_v = c_v$, and from (7.32) we have

$$\left(\frac{\partial u}{\partial v}\right)_T = T\left(\frac{\partial p}{\partial T}\right)_v - p = \frac{RT}{v-b} - p = \frac{a}{v^2}$$

Therefore

$$du = c_v dT + \frac{a}{v^2} dv$$

Integrating, we get

$$u = u_0 + \int_{T_0}^{T} c_v dT + a\left(\frac{1}{v_0} - \frac{1}{v}\right) \qquad (7.46)$$

For any state defined by (v, T), the value of u is given by (7.46), p is given by the equation of state, and consequently the enthalpy can be determined from $(u + pv)$. It is apparent that the van der Waals equation, unlike the perfect gas equation, implies that the internal energy and enthalpy vary with both v and T.

To find whether c_v also varies with v, we may derive a suitable expression for $(\partial c_v / \partial v)_T$. Differentiating (7.23) we get

$$\left(\frac{\partial c_v}{\partial v} \right)_T = T \left(\frac{\partial^2 s}{\partial T \partial v} \right)$$

Using the Maxwell relation (7.15), this becomes

$$\left(\frac{\partial c_v}{\partial v} \right)_T = T \left(\frac{\partial^2 p}{\partial T^2} \right)_v$$

From the van der Waals equation,

$$\left(\frac{\partial p}{\partial T} \right)_v = \frac{R}{v - b} \quad \text{and} \quad \left(\frac{\partial^2 p}{\partial T^2} \right)_v = 0$$

Therefore

$$\left(\frac{\partial c_v}{\partial v} \right)_T = 0$$

and hence c_v is independent of v. We may again infer that c_v is also independent of p and that it can therefore be a function only of T. It is evident that even this more accurate equation of state implies that c_v is independent of p and v, and this is not true for any real gas.

7.7 Change of phase

While a substance is undergoing a change of phase, the temperature and pressure are not independent variables. At any given pressure the change takes place at a definite temperature — the saturation temperature T_{sat}. The field of equilibrium states covering a change of phase from liquid to vapour is represented by the series of constant pressure lines on the T–v diagram of Fig. 7.8. An important

Fig. 7.8

Change of phase and the Clausius–Clapeyron equation

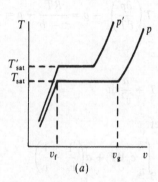

(a)

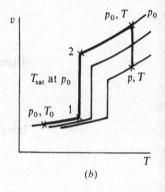

(b)

expression for the rate of change of p with T_{sat} can be deduced with the aid of the Gibbs function. From equation (7.8) we have

$$dg = v\,dp - s\,dT$$

Since p and T are constant during the change of phase, dg is zero, i.e. the Gibbs function is constant. Equating the values of g at the two extreme conditions we have

$$g_f = g_g$$

where subscripts f and g refer to the saturated liquid and vapour states. If the pressure is changed by an infinitesimal amount from p to $(p + dp)$, the saturation temperature will change from T_{sat} to $(T + dT)_{sat}$, and the Gibbs function from g to $(g + dg)$. At this new pressure we must also have

$$(g + dg)_f = (g + dg)_g$$

It follows that

$$dg_f = dg_g$$

$$v_f\,dp - s_f\,dT_{sat} = v_g\,dp - s_g\,dT_{sat}$$

or

$$(v_g - v_f)\,dp = (s_g - s_f)\,dT_{sat}$$

Now the change of state from f to g occurs at constant temperature and pressure, and thus

$$s_g - s_f = \frac{h_g - h_f}{T_{sat}}$$

The previous equation therefore becomes

$$\frac{dp}{dT_{sat}} = \frac{h_g - h_f}{T_{sat}(v_g - v_f)} \tag{7.47}$$

This is known as the *Clausius-Clapeyron equation*; it applies equally to changes from the solid to the liquid phase (fusion, i → f) and from the solid to the vapour phase (sublimation, i → g).

For a small change of pressure Δp, the latent enthalpy $(h_g - h_f)$ and difference of specific volumes $(v_g - v_f)$ can be considered constant, and the average rate of change of pressure with saturation temperature can be written as $(\Delta p/\Delta T_{sat})$. In this form the Clausius-Clapeyron equation permits the latent enthalpy to be estimated from measurements of v_f, v_g and the saturation temperatures at two nearby pressures.

The Clausius-Clapeyron equation also points to one possible way of measuring thermodynamic temperature. Equation (7.47) can be rewritten as

$$\frac{dT_{sat}}{T_{sat}} = \frac{v_{fg}}{h_{fg}}\,dp$$

and integrated between (T_0, p_0), defined by some fixed point, and (T, p), at which the temperature is to be measured. (T_0, p_0) may, for example, be the triple point of water, discussed in section 8.2. This integration yields

$$\ln\left(\frac{T}{T_0}\right)_{\text{sat}} = \int_{p_0}^{p} \frac{v_{\text{fg}}}{h_{\text{fg}}} \, dp$$

Measurements of h_{fg} and v_{fg} over the range p_0 to p can be made independently of temperature, and T can thus be found. By using solid–vapour, solid–liquid and liquid–vapour changes of phase, as well as different substances, a continuous and wide range of T can be covered. This method of measuring absolute thermodynamic temperature is not used in practice because gas thermometry is more accurate.

At the end of section 7.5 it was pointed out that equations (7.26) and (7.29) cannot be applied directly if a change of phase occurs between the reference state and the state at which the entropy and enthalpy are required. When a change of phase occurs, the p–v–T data in Fig. 7.5 will appear as in the v–T diagram of Fig. 7.8b. When the reference state lies within one phase region, and the second state lies within another, the changes in entropy and enthalpy may be found by adding the changes associated with each of four steps, e.g. (a) from state (p_0, T_0) to state 1, (b) from state 1 to state 2, (c) from state 2 to state (p_0, T), and (d) from state (p_0, T) to state (p, T). The changes of entropy and enthalpy during processes (a), (c) and (d) can be found in the way already described. During the constant pressure process (b), however, c_p is infinite since the temperature remains constant. For this step the latent enthalpy at p_0 must be known. The value of this quantity may be found by a calorimetric experiment, or by using the Clausius-Clapeyron equation as already explained. The change of enthalpy between state 1 and state 2 is then known, since it is equal to h_{fg}, and the change of entropy can be found from

$$s_2 - s_1 = \frac{h_2 - h_1}{T_1}$$

The derivation of the Clausius-Clapeyron equation has been given here as an example of the use of the Gibbs function. Another example of interest to engineers is provided by the following. We have seen that the Gibbs function has a unique value at any given pressure (or temperature) providing two phases are present. This fact can be used to simplify the calculation of the change of enthalpy during an isentropic process when the final state is in the two-phase region. Such calculations are frequently made when analysing the performance of steam turbine plant.

By definition $g = h - Ts$, so that the change of enthalpy during the process can be written as

$$h_2 - h_1 = (g_2 + T_2 s_2) - h_1 \tag{7.48}$$

Since the process is isentropic, $s_2 = s_1$, and assuming the initial state of the substance is known, the values of h_1 and s_1 can be found from tables of properties. If the final pressure is given, both T_2 and g_2 can also be found from the tables, and consequently (7.48) enables $(h_2 - h_1)$ to be calculated. Values of h in the two-phase region are not given directly in tables because they depend upon the relative amounts of liquid and vapour in the mixture. The somewhat lengthier method of calculating the enthalpy change when values of g are not available is given in section 10.2.

7.8   Processes undergone by solids and liquids

In a study of heat engines we are primarily concerned with processes undergone by a gas, or a vapour in contact with its liquid, and Part II is devoted to the consideration of such systems. Some processes undergone by solids or liquids will be considered briefly in this section, however, as they provide simple examples of the use of the general thermodynamic relations. Only *reversible* non-flow processes are considered, but the equations deduced apply equally to solids and liquids — with the proviso mentioned in the introduction to this chapter that for solids the stress must be uniform in all directions.

7.8.1   Constant volume process

It was pointed out in section 7.4 that the specific heat at constant volume of a solid or liquid is not easy to measure because of the large pressure required to maintain the substance at constant volume. The rise of pressure consequent upon an increase of temperature at constant volume can be found as follows.
   Equation (7.21) states that

$$\left(\frac{\partial p}{\partial T}\right)_v = \frac{\beta}{\kappa}$$

For solids and liquids the variations of β and κ with pressure and temperature are small. These properties may be assumed constant for many purposes, and mean values $\bar{\beta}$ and $\bar{\kappa}$ can be used. With this approximation, the above relation can be integrated for a constant volume process to give

$$(p_2 - p_1) \approx \frac{\bar{\beta}}{\bar{\kappa}}(T_2 - T_1) \tag{7.49}$$

7.8.2   Isothermal process

The change of volume accompanying a change of pressure during an isothermal process can be found from the compressibility of a substance. Thus from equation (7.20),

$$-\frac{1}{v}\left(\frac{\partial v}{\partial p}\right)_T = \kappa$$

Since the volume of a solid or liquid changes only slightly with pressure, a mean value $\bar{v}$ may be chosen. This, together with a mean value of κ, enables the expression to be integrated. Since T is constant for an isothermal process,

$$dv = -v\kappa\,dp$$

and

$$v_2 - v_1 \approx -\bar{v}\bar{\kappa}(p_2 - p_1) \tag{7.50}$$

The work done during an isothermal process is given by

$$W = -\left(\int p\,dv\right)_T \approx \bar{v}\bar{\kappa}\int_{p_1}^{p_2} p\,dp \approx \frac{\bar{v}\bar{\kappa}}{2}(p_2^2 - p_1^2) \tag{7.51}$$

The heat supplied during the isothermal process can be found by using equation (7.30), namely

$$ds = \frac{c_p}{T}\,dT - \left(\frac{\partial v}{\partial T}\right)_p dp$$

From (7.19), $(\partial v/\partial T)_p$ is equal to βv, and for an isothermal process dT is zero. Hence

$$ds = -\beta v\,dp$$

or

$$dQ = T\,ds = -T\beta v\,dp$$

Again assuming constant mean values $\bar{\beta}$ and $\bar{v}$, this can be integrated to give

$$Q \approx -T\bar{\beta}\bar{v}(p_2 - p_1) \tag{7.52}$$

The change in internal energy can be found from the energy equation, i.e. by substituting (7.51) and (7.52) in

$$u_2 - u_1 = Q + W$$

7.8.3 Isentropic process

During an isentropic process, the change in pressure, temperature or volume, accompanying a given change in any one of these properties, can be found as follows. Using equation (7.30) again, and rewriting it as

$$T\,ds = c_p\,dT - \beta vT\,dp$$

we have, when ds is zero,

$$c_p\,dT = \beta vT\,dp$$

Since the temperature rise will be small, a mean value of T can be used in the right-hand side of the equation, so that

$$(T_2 - T_1) \approx \frac{\bar{\beta}\bar{v}\bar{T}}{\bar{c}_p}(p_2 - p_1) \tag{7.53}$$

Similarly, to find T in terms of v, equation (7.44) can be rewritten as

$$T\,ds = c_v\,dT + T\left(\frac{\partial p}{\partial T}\right)_v dv$$

But from (7.21), $(\partial p/\partial T)_v = \beta/\kappa$, and therefore when ds is zero,

$$c_v\,dT = -\frac{T\beta}{\kappa}\,dv$$

And hence on integration,

$$(T_2 - T_1) \approx -\frac{\bar{T}\bar{\beta}}{\bar{c}_v\bar{\kappa}}(v_2 - v_1) \tag{7.54}$$

Finally, eliminating $(T_2 - T_1)$ between (7.53) and (7.54),

$$(p_2 - p_1) \approx -\frac{1}{\bar{v}\bar{\kappa}}\frac{\bar{c}_p}{\bar{c}_v}(v_2 - v_1) \tag{7.55}$$

The work done during an isentropic process is

$$W = -\left(\int p\,dv\right)_s$$

Using the differential form of equation (7.55), it follows that

$$W\frac{\bar{\kappa}\bar{v}\bar{c}_v}{\bar{c}_p} \int_{p_1}^{p_2} p\,dp$$

$$\approx \frac{\bar{\kappa}\bar{v}}{2}\frac{\bar{c}_v}{\bar{c}_p}(p_2^2 - p_1^2) \tag{7.56}$$

From the energy equation it follows that this must be equal to the change in internal energy.

7.9 Exergy and the Gibbs function

We close this chapter with an introduction to the concept of exergy, and a further discussion of the use of the Gibbs function. *Exergy* (sometimes known as *availability*) is a measure of the maximum useful work that can be done by a system interacting with an environment which is at a constant pressure p_0 and temperature T_0. The simplest case to consider is that of a heat reservoir (i.e. a heat source of infinite capacity and therefore invariable temperature) of temperature T. We have seen that the maximum efficiency with which heat withdrawn from a reservoir may be converted into work is the Carnot efficiency. Thus the exergy of a reservoir at T providing a heat transfer Q, in surroundings at T_0, is $Q(T - T_0)/T$.

The case of greatest interest in engineering is that of a system undergoing a non-cyclic process while doing work. Any power plant, even if part of it involves a secondary working fluid being taken through a cycle, when considered as a whole, is a system undergoing a non-cyclic process (e.g. see Fig. 11.1). Such a system can be considered to undergo the process while interacting ultimately with a single reservoir, namely the atmosphere at p_0 and T_0, and the fluid will be incapable of producing any further work when it has reached a state of equilibrium with the surroundings. A comparison of the actual work performed with the maximum possible, starting from a given initial state, is an indication of the effectiveness of the plant used. It will be convenient to consider closed systems and steady-flow open systems separately.

In what follows we shall consider systems whose initial states are such that they do work on the surroundings when degenerating to state (p_0, T_0). Similar arguments can be pursued for systems requiring work done on them in order to bring them to state (p_0, T_0), but for simplicity only the former type of system will be considered.

7.9.1 Exergy in closed systems

Let us consider a cylinder containing a compressed fluid at (p_1, T_1), the cylinder being closed by a piston. We shall calculate the useful work done when the system has reached a state which is in equilibrium with the surroundings and which therefore can be denoted by subscript 0. The initial and final internal energies U_1 and U_0 are fixed by the end states (p_1, T_1) and (p_0, T_0), and the work done by the fluid during the expansion, from the First Law, is

$$|W| = -(U_0 - U_1) + Q \tag{7.57}$$

The *useful* work done by the fluid on the piston is less than this, because work $p_0(V_0 - V_1)$ is done on the surrounding medium which is at a constant pressure p_0.* Thus the useful work W' is

$$|W'| = -(U_0 - U_1) + Q - p_0(V_0 - V_1) \tag{7.58}$$

The principle of increasing entropy states that the sum of the changes of entropy of the surroundings ΔS_0 and of the system ΔS is greater than or equal to zero. Now the change of entropy of the surroundings which are at a constant temperature T_0, when Q units of heat are transferred from them to the system, is $-Q/T_0$. We can therefore write

$$\Delta S + \left(-\frac{Q}{T_0}\right) \geqslant 0$$

or

$$Q \leqslant T_0 \Delta S$$

---

* When calculating the work done on a piston elsewhere in the book, we do not subtract the work $p_0(V_0 - V_1)$ because we always consider the boundary of the system to be the face of the piston, thus ignoring the question of whether this work is entirely transferred to a shaft linked to the piston or whether some of it is transferred to the atmosphere behind the piston. When we are concerned with a sequence of processes constituting a *machine* cycle, the net work done on the atmosphere in this way is zero, and the total work and the useful work over the machine cycle are equal.

and hence

$$|W'| \leqslant -(U_0 - U_1) + T_0(S_0 - S_1) - p_0(V_0 - V_1)$$

The maximum value is obtained when the process is reversible and the equality holds, and thus the exergy of the system can be written

$$|W|_{max} = (U_1 + p_0 V_1 - T_0 S_1) - (U_0 + p_0 V_0 - T_0 S_0)$$

$$= A_1 - A_0 \tag{7.59}$$

$A = (U + p_0 V - T_0 S)$ is called the *non-flow exergy function*. It is seen to be a composite property — composite because it is a property not only of the system but also of its surroundings.

In general it will be possible to think of an infinite variety of paths linking states (p_1, T_1) and (p_0, T_0), both irreversible and reversible; equation (7.59) implies that of these, *the reversible paths will all yield the same useful work*, namely $|W|_{max}$. Because the surroundings are at the invariable temperature T_0, the process can be conceived reversible only if either (a) all the heat is transferred when the system is at T_0 (e.g. during process $i - 0$ in Fig. (7.9a), or (b) the heat exchange with the surroundings is via appropriate reversible Carnot engines working between the system and the surroundings (e.g. during process $i - 0$ in Fig. 7.9b).

It is interesting to note that when the system is in state 0, A is identical with the Gibbs function G defined in section 7.1. Thus $G = H - TS$ which, when expanded and referred to state 0, becomes

$$G_0 = H_0 - T_0 S_0 = U_0 + p_0 V_0 - T_0 S_0 = A_0 \tag{7.60}$$

Let us now consider what appears to be a trivial case, namely when the identity $(p_1, T_1) \equiv (p_0, T_0)$ applies. When the closed system contains a gas, this identity also implies identical *states* and would yield zero work if, say, we compress and expand the gas isentropically. Less obvious is the case of a fluid changing phase isothermally, say from saturated liquid f to saturated vapour g. This still is in accord with the identity, although the *states* initially and finally are not the same. It would be meaningful to ask what useful work could be produced.

Fig. 7.9
Achieving maximum work
from a closed system in
surroundings at constant p_0
and T_0

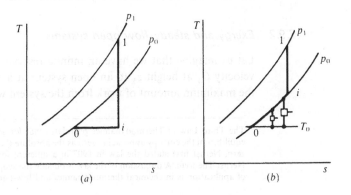

(a)   (b)

Applying equation (7.59),

$$|W|_{max} = (U_{f0} + p_0 V_{f0} - T_0 S_{f0}) - (U_{g0} + p_0 V_{g0} - T_0 S_{g0})$$
$$= -(H_{fg0} - T_0 S_{fg0}) \tag{7.61}$$

or, using equation (7.60),

$$|W|_{max} = G_{f0} - G_{g0}$$

Since $H_{fg} = TS_{fg}$, it must be concluded that no useful work can be derived from this process, and all the work done resulting from the absorption of latent heat from the surroundings is expended in doing useless work $p_0(V_{g0} - V_{f0})$ against the pressure p_0. It follows that $G_f = G_g$, a result already derived in section 7.7.

Another case where the initial and final values of p and T are the same, but where the states are different, is when a chemical reaction occurs and reactants R at (p_0, T_0) change to products P at (p_0, T_0). Then we have for the maximum useful work

$$|W|_{max} = (U_{R0} + p_0 V_{R0} - T_0 S_{R0}) - (U_{P0} + p_0 V_{P0} - T_0 S_{P0})$$
$$= (H_{R0} - H_{P0}) + T_0(S_{P0} - S_{R0}) = -\Delta H_0 + T_0(S_{P0} - S_{R0}) \tag{7.62}$$

or

$$|W|_{max} = (G_{R0} - G_{P0}) = -\Delta G_0 \tag{7.63}$$

ΔH_0 is the *enthalpy of reaction* discussed in section 15.8 (and in sections 15.4 to 15.6 under the less general title of enthalpy of combustion). It is thus seen that the maximum magnitude of the useful work that can be derived from a closed system containing reactants at (p_0, T_0) in surroundings at (p_0, T_0) is not in general equal to $-\Delta H_0$, because $T_0(S_{P0} - S_{R0})$ usually differs from zero. In calculating the entropy difference $(S_{P0} - S_{R0})$, the entropies of the reactants and products must be known relative to a common datum. Such information is available as a result of the *Third Law of Thermodynamics*,* which defines the absolute entropy of substances at absolute zero and thus provides the required common datum. 'Products' in this context must be further qualified as constituents which are in chemical equilibrium taking account of dissociation, and this is discussed more fully in section 7.9.3.

7.9.2 Exergy and steady-flow open systems

Let us imagine that we have an infinite reservoir feeding fluid at (p_1, T_1) with velocity C_1 at height z_1 to an open system at a steady rate. In order to derive the maximum amount of work from the system when discharging the fluid into

---

* The Third Law of Thermodynamics postulates that for any pure substance in thermodynamic equilibrium the entropy approaches zero as the absolute thermodynamic temperature approaches zero. Nernst first stated the law in 1907 in a different form, and it is often referred to as the Nernst Theorem. A discussion of the law is outside the scope of this book; the law's main sphere of application is in chemical thermodynamics and low-temperature physics.

surroundings at (p_0, T_0), the fluid must leave at (p_0, T_0) with zero velocity and at the lowest possible datum level z_0. Then from the steady-flow energy equation we get

$$|\dot{W}| = -(\dot{m}h_0 + \dot{m}gz_0 - \dot{m}h_1 - \tfrac{1}{2}\dot{m}C_1^2 - \dot{m}gz_1) + \dot{Q}$$

$$= \{\dot{H}_1 + \dot{m}(\tfrac{1}{2}C_1^2 + gz_1)\} - \{\dot{H}_0 + \dot{m}gz_0\} + \dot{Q} \qquad (7.64)$$

In practice, particularly when doing an overall analysis of plant such as boilers, turbines or condensers, the kinetic and potential energy terms can be omitted because they are insignificant. When analysing say a turbine, stage by stage in detail, the kinetic energy terms are significant and have to be carried throughout the analysis. For simplicity we shall omit the kinetic and potential energy terms in what follows.

With open systems the whole of $|\dot{W}|$ is useful work, the work done by and on the surroundings as the fluid enters and leaves the system being included in the enthalpy terms. We can use the same argument as before to establish $\dot{Q}$ in terms of entropy, and we therefore have

$$|\dot{W}| \leqslant -(\dot{H}_0 - \dot{H}_1) + T_0(\dot{S}_0 - \dot{S}_1) \qquad (7.65)$$

Again the maximum work will be done when the process is reversible and the equality holds. Thus the exergy of the fluid in state 1 is

$$|\dot{W}|_{\text{max}} = (\dot{H}_1 - T_0\dot{S}_1) - (\dot{H}_0 - T_0\dot{S}_0) = \dot{B}_1 - \dot{B}_0 \qquad (7.66)$$

where the quantity $B = (H - T_0 S) = (U + pV - T_0 S)$ is called the *steady-flow exergy function*. B differs from the non-flow exergy function $A = (U + p_0 V - T_0 S)$ in the pressure term. At state 0, $A \equiv B \equiv G$.

When a system works between states 1 and 2, where 2 is intermediate between 1 and 0, the maximum useful work quantities associated with the end states are

$$(|\dot{W}|_{\text{max}})_1 = \dot{B}_1 - \dot{B}_0 \quad \text{and} \quad (|\dot{W}|_{\text{max}})_2 = \dot{B}_2 - \dot{B}_0$$

and thus the maximum work available between states 1 and 2 is

$$(|\dot{W}|_{\text{max}})_{1-2} = \dot{B}_1 - \dot{B}_2 \qquad (7.67)$$

As an illustration of the use of B, let us consider a gas expanding in a turbine from state (p_1, T_1) to a pressure p_0. Since state 1 is an arbitrary state, the temperature reached after isentropic expansion will not necessarily be T_0; let us say it will be T_i' as in Fig. 7.10a. The rate of work attainable during the isentropic expansion, *per unit mass flow*, is

$$|\dot{W}|_{\text{isen}} = -(h_i' - h_1) = -c_p(T_i' - T_1) \qquad (7.68)$$

whereas during an actual adiabatic expansion the work will be

$$|\dot{W}| = -c_p(T_i - T_1) \qquad (7.69)$$

The isentropic efficiency of the turbine is then conventionally expressed as

$$\eta_{\text{isen}} = \frac{\dot{W}}{\dot{W}_{\text{isen}}} \qquad (7.70)$$

Fig. 7.10
Achieving maximum work
from a steady-flow open
system in surroundings at
constant p_0 and T_0

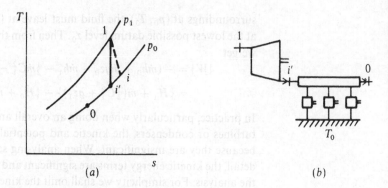

(a) (b)

Now the maximum useful work per unit mass flow, as derived from the specific
exergy function $b = B/m$, is

$$|\dot{W}|_{max} = b_1 - b_0 = (h_1 - h_0) - T_0(s_1 - s_0)$$

$$= c_0(T_1 - T_0) - c_p T_0 \ln \frac{T_1}{T_0} + R T_0 \ln \frac{p_1}{p_0}$$

$$= c_p(T_1 - T_i') + c_p(T_i' - T_0) - c_p T_0 \ln \left(\frac{T_1}{T_i'} \frac{T_i'}{T_0} \right) + R T_0 \ln \frac{p_1}{p_0}$$

$$= c_p(T_1 - T_i') + c_p T_0 \left\{ \left(\frac{T_i'}{T_0} \right) - 1 - \ln \frac{T_i'}{T_0} \right\} \qquad (7.71)$$

We may call the ratio $|\dot{W}|/|\dot{W}|_{max}$ the effectiveness ε of the process. It is clear
that $\eta_{isen} \neq \varepsilon$ except when $c_p T_0 [(T_i'/T_0) - 1 - \ln(T_i'/T_0)] = 0$, and this is
possible only in the special case when $T_i' = T_0$. Thus the isentropic efficiency
is a measure not of the fraction of the maximum useful work actually utilised,
but merely of the fraction of work available from a particular type of process,
i.e. from an adiabatic expansion. Fig. 7.10b illustrates how, in principle, the
exhaust gas at T_i' from an isentropic turbine could supply heat to a series of
Carnot engines in order to obtain $|\dot{W}|_{max}$ as calculated from the exergy function.

7.9.3 The Gibbs function and the steady-flow system

A steady-flow system of particular importance is one in which the fluid enters
and leaves at (p_0, T_0). In this case $B = G$ at both entry and exit. When the fluid
is also identical in *state* at entry and exit, this leads to the trivial case
$|\dot{W}|_{max} = \dot{G}_0 - \dot{G}_0 = 0$. Even when the *state* is not the same, e.g. when the fluid
changes phase from saturated liquid f to saturated vapour g, we again have
zero work, $|\dot{W}|_{max} = \dot{G}_{f0} - \dot{G}_{g0} = 0$, because the Gibbs function is constant
during a change of phase at constant temperature.

A case of practical importance, where (p, T) but not the state is identical at
entry and exit, arises when considering systems in which chemical reactions
occur as in external combustion power plant (see Figs 11.1 and 12.3). For such
plant the maximum amount of work would appear as

$$|\dot{W}|_{max} = \dot{G}_{RO} - \dot{G}_{PO} = -\Delta \dot{G}_0 \qquad (7.72)$$

or, in terms of the enthalpies and entropies,

$$|\dot{W}|_{max} = (\dot{H}_{R0} - T_0\dot{S}_{R0}) - (\dot{H}_{P0} - T_0\dot{S}_{P0}) = -\Delta\dot{H}_0 + T_0(\dot{S}_{P0} - \dot{S}_{R0}) \qquad (7.73)$$

That the above expressions are similar to the equivalent equations (7.62) and (7.63) applying to a closed system is not surprising; here we are neglecting the kinetic and potential energy terms, and for the closed system we subtracted the $p_0\Delta V$ work from $|W|$. It is of course only under the special conditions of $(p_1, T_1) \equiv (p_0, T_0)$ that the two expressions for $|W|_{max}$ and $|\dot{W}|_{max}$ are similar.

Equations (7.72) and (7.73) have to be qualified in two respects. First, if the products leaving at (p_0, T_0) can still react with the atmosphere, further work could still be done. In combustion, excess air is normally one of the reactants and such further reaction is then negligible, but with other reactions this point may be of importance. Secondly, strictly speaking additional work could still be derived from the products by letting each expand isothermally and reversibly to the partial pressure at which the particular constituent in the products exists in the atmosphere, perhaps by using devices with semipermeable membranes (see sections 14.3 and 15.7). For example, the partial pressure of CO_2 in the atmosphere is quite low, while its partial pressure in common products is quite high. Because such processes are impracticable at present, they will be ignored in evaluating $|\dot{W}|_{max}$.

If we define the effectiveness of a combustion power plant as $|\dot{W}|/|\dot{W}|_{max}$, where $|\dot{W}|_{max}$ is given by equation (7.73), it is a matter of indifference whether $\Delta\dot{H}_0$ is the value with water in the products as a liquid of a vapour, because the difference between using the one or the other is automatically compensated by the change in the value of the entropy term. That this must be so can be deduced from a comparison of equations (7.72) and (7.73) and the fact that the Gibbs function does not vary during an isothermal change of phase. The need to specify the phase of the water in the products when using *conventional* definitions of power plant efficiency was[*] emphasised in sections 15.6 and 17.5.

When discussing in section 17.5 the possibility of using $|\dot{W}|/|\dot{W}|_{max}$ in preference to conventional thermal efficiencies for assessing the performance of combustion power plant, we made use of the result of section 15.7.2 for the purpose of evaluating $|\dot{W}|_{max}$. In that section we derived $|\dot{W}|_{max}$ by considering a van't Hoff equilibrium box operating in surroundings at $p_0 = p^\ominus$ (where $p^\ominus$ is the standard state pressure, 1 bar) and at some arbitrary temperature T_0. We took the simple reaction $CO + \frac{1}{2}O_2 \rightarrow CO_2$ as a specific example, and showed that the maximum work attainable from this reaction in surroundings at $(p^\ominus, T_0)$ is

$$|\dot{W}|_{max} = \dot{n}\tilde{R}T_0 \ln K_0^\ominus \qquad (7.74)$$

where $\dot{n}$ is the molar rate of flow of CO. $K^\ominus$ is the equilibrium constant given by

$$K^\ominus = \frac{(p_{CO_2}/p^\ominus)}{(p_{CO}/p^\ominus)(p_{O_2}/p^\ominus)^{1/2}}$$

---

[*] As stated at the beginning of this chapter, the authors' intention is that it should be left until a preliminary study of the book has been completed, and we underline this here by using the past tense.

In principle, $K^\ominus$ could be a function of two independent properties, say p and T, determining the state in the equilibrium box. It was proved in section 15.7.2 that $K^\ominus$ was independent of that pressure. However, $K^\ominus$ could be a function of the temperature T which is kept equal to the temperature T_0 of the surroundings. It is in fact found by experiment that $K^\ominus$ varies markedly with T $(= T_0)$. The subscript on $K^\ominus$ refers to the temperature of the reaction, i.e. $K_0^\ominus$ is $K^\ominus$ at T_0. The form of the relation (7.74) for $|\dot{W}|_{\max}$ is quite general for all chemical reactions between perfect gases.

The remainder of this section is devoted to a discussion of the implications of equating the two expressions for $|\dot{W}|_{\max}$, namely (7.72) and (7.74). It follows immediately that

$$\tilde{R} \ln K_0^\ominus = -\frac{\Delta \tilde{g}_0^\ominus}{T_0} \qquad (7.75a)$$

and, as we can select T_0 arbitrarily, in general

$$\tilde{R} \ln K^\ominus = -\frac{\Delta \tilde{g}^\ominus}{T} \qquad (7.75b)$$

$\Delta \tilde{g}^\ominus$ is the change of molar Gibbs function at $(p^\ominus, T)$, namely $(\tilde{g}_P^\ominus - \tilde{g}_R^\ominus)$. It should be remembered that $K^\ominus$ could, for example, refer to the equation $CO + \frac{1}{2}O_2 \rightarrow CO_2$ or to the equation $2CO + O_2 \rightarrow 2CO_2$, giving numerically different equilibrium constants

$$\frac{(p_{CO_2}/p^\ominus)}{(p_{CO}/p^\ominus)(p_{O_2}/p^\ominus)^{1/2}} \quad \text{and} \quad \frac{(p_{CO_2}/p^\ominus)^2}{(p_{CO}/p^\ominus)^2(p_{O_2}/p^\ominus)}$$

It is important to evaluate $K^\ominus$ and $\Delta \tilde{g}^\ominus$ in equations (7.75) for the same form of chemical equation. As stated above, $K^\ominus$ is a function of T, and equations (7.75) imply that this must be true of $\Delta \tilde{g}^\ominus$.

The relation between $K^\ominus$ and $\Delta \tilde{g}^\ominus$ implies that a relation between $K^\ominus$ and $\Delta \tilde{h}^\ominus$ can also be derived, and such a relation can prove particularly useful. Let us proceed by finding $(\partial \ln K^\ominus/\partial T)_p$, first at T_0, and then by varying the reference temperature T_0. The partial notation can be omitted because $K^\ominus$ has been found to be independent of the total pressure p of the mixture. From equation (7.12), then, we can write

$$\tilde{s}_{P0}^\ominus = -\frac{d\tilde{g}_{P0}^\ominus}{dT} \quad \text{and} \quad \tilde{s}_{R0}^\ominus = -\frac{d\tilde{g}_{R0}^\ominus}{dT}$$

and substituting in equation (7.73) we obtain

$$-\frac{\Delta \tilde{g}_0^\ominus}{T_0} = -\frac{\Delta \tilde{h}_0^\ominus}{T_0} - \left(\frac{d\tilde{g}_{P0}^\ominus}{dT} - \frac{d\tilde{g}_{R0}^\ominus}{dT}\right) = -\frac{\Delta \tilde{h}_0^\ominus}{T_0} - \frac{d(\Delta \tilde{g}_0^\ominus)}{dT}$$

or

$$\frac{1}{T_0}\frac{d(\Delta \tilde{g}_0^\ominus)}{dT} - \frac{\Delta \tilde{g}_0^\ominus}{T_0^2} = \frac{d}{dT}\left(\frac{\Delta \tilde{g}_0^\ominus}{T_0}\right) = -\frac{\Delta \tilde{h}_0^\ominus}{T_0^2}$$

Since, from equation (7.75a),

$$\frac{d}{dT}\left(\frac{\Delta \tilde{g}_0^{\ominus}}{T_0}\right) = -\tilde{R}\frac{d}{dT}(\ln K_0^{\ominus})$$

it follows that

$$\frac{d}{dT}(\ln K^{\ominus}) = \frac{\Delta \tilde{h}_0^{\ominus}}{\tilde{R}T_0^2} \tag{7.76}$$

or

$$\frac{d}{d(1/T)}(\ln K_0^{\ominus}) = -\frac{\Delta \tilde{h}_0^{\ominus}}{\tilde{R}} \tag{7.77}$$

Equation (7.76), or its equivalent form (7.77), is known as the *van't Hoff isobar*. It provides a relation between $K^{\ominus}$, temperature T and the enthalpy of reaction $\Delta \tilde{h}_0^{\ominus}$, which is itself a function of temperature.

The relation between $K^{\ominus}$ and T is difficult to obtain experimentally. However, relations between $\Delta \tilde{h}^{\ominus}$ and $\Delta \tilde{g}^{\ominus}$ on the one hand, and T on the other, can be obtained more easily, and values of $K^{\ominus}$ can then be derived from (7.75) or (7.77) over a range of temperature. Furthermore, just as $\Delta \tilde{h}^{\ominus}$ at any temperature T can be calculated from a single known value of $\Delta \tilde{h}_0^{\ominus}$ at T_0 together with specific heat capacity data over the range T_0 to T (see section 15.4), equation (7.77) makes it possible for the value of $K^{\ominus}$ to be calculated at any temperature T from that single value of $\Delta \tilde{h}_0^{\ominus}$ together with the same specific heat capacity data. This is explained in greater detail in section 15.8.

Equations (7.75) and (7.77) can serve a further purpose. Values of $K^{\ominus}$, $\Delta \tilde{h}^{\ominus}$ and $\Delta \tilde{g}^{\ominus}$ are often obtained from different sources using different experimental sources or methods. Such data can be checked for thermodynamic self-consistency using these equations.

To sum up: in this section we have introduced the concept of exergy; related two exergy functions to other thermodynamic functions; and indicated how the concept can provide the basis for less arbitrary definitions of the effectiveness of processes than those in common use. The reader can find a detailed discussion of the rational definition of efficiency of internal-combustion plant in Ref. 12, together with derivations of overall optimum working conditions for several types of external-combustion power plant. Furthermore, it is claimed that an 'exergy balance' is one of the best methods for pinpointing the processes which contribute most to the overall loss due to irreversibilities in complex plant (e.g. in regenerative steam power plant). Certainly it can contrast the relative effects of internal and external irreversibilities, which a mere consideration of cycle efficiency cannot do. To distinguish it from the simple energy balance, such an analysis is often called a *Second Law analysis*: for further details the reader may consult Ref. 13. Finally, we have employed the concept of maximum work to derive useful relations between the equilibrium constant $K^{\ominus}$, the enthalpy of reaction $\Delta \tilde{h}_0^{\ominus}$ and the corresponding change of Gibbs function $\Delta \tilde{g}_0^{\ominus}$.

Part II

Applications to Particular Fluids

Introduction

The principles of thermodynamics have been explained in Part I without reference to any particular fluid. In Part II we shall apply these principles to closed and open systems consisting of either (a) liquids and vapours whose properties are most conveniently related in tabular form, or (b) gases whose thermodynamic properties can be related by simple algebraic equations. We shall still be concerned only to relate the heat and work crossing the boundary with the changes in the properties of fluid; the detailed analyses of the ways in which the work and heat transfers are effected are dealt with in Parts III and IV respectively. For example, we shall calculate the theoretical work done when a fluid enters a turbine with a certain state and is expanded to a lower pressure, but we shall not stop to consider how the turbine blading should be designed so that the actual work is as near the theoretical value as possible.

Part II opens with a description of the characteristics of typical working fluids used in power plant. This is followed by examples of non-flow, steady-flow and nonsteady-flow processes undergone by water and steam, considered as an example of a liquid and vapour, and air, considered as an example of a gas. The performance of the more important thermodynamic cycles is then analysed; for example, it is shown how the cycle efficiency and work ratio can be calculated when the working fluid is taken through a given cycle of states. When engines of the same sort are being compared, the work ratio provides an indication of the size of plant required for a given total output and also an indication of how far the actual efficiency will fall short of the theoretical value.

Finally, there is a chapter showing how the behaviour of systems consisting of a chemically inert mixture of fluids can be deduced from a knowledge of the properties of the constituents, and a chapter which is devoted to the thermodynamic aspects of combustion.

8

Properties of Fluids

Before describing the way in which the properties of a real fluid are related, with the aid of numerical examples, some system of units must be adopted. Of the three primary properties — pressure, specific volume and temperature — the adoption of units for the first two presents little difficulty. Pressure will always be expressed in bars, and specific volume in cubic metres per kilogram (see Appendix A). A pressure gauge or manometer usually measures the pressure relative to atmospheric pressure. The absolute value, which we shall always imply by the symbol p, can easily be obtained by adding the barometric pressure to the gauge pressure.

The unit of temperature needs more careful attention, and the first section is devoted to this topic. This is followed by a description of the characteristics of a liquid and a vapour. The most convenient method of tabulating values of the thermodynamic properties is discussed, and the more important graphical representations are described. Finally, the special case of a gas is dealt with, and it is shown how the assumption of a simple equation of state can lead to an easy analytical treatment of the relations between the properties.

8.1 The unit of temperature and the International Temperature Scale

Temperature measurement is now a field of study by itself, and only the briefest outline can be given here.* Let us first consider the procedure for setting up any empirical state of temperature. As explained in section 1.2, temperature may be defined in terms of the variation of some thermometric property such as the length of a column of liquid in a tube, the pressure of a gas maintained at constant volume, the resistance of a wire, or the EMF produced by a thermocouple. Three items of information must be specified if a scale of temperature is to be reproducible:

(a) The particular thermometric substance and property used
(b) The numbers to be attached to two standard fixed points
(c) The relation between the temperature and the thermometric property

---

* A comprehensive survey of the whole field can be found in Ref. 22, and short summaries in Refs 23 and 32.

130

which is to be used for interpolating between the fixed points and extrapolating beyond them.

We shall discuss items (b) and (c) first.

Two reference points, called the upper and lower fixed points, may be located on the scale of the thermometer by bringing it into contact with two systems in turn, each at a definite and reproducible temperature. For example, the lower fixed point may be provided by a mixture of ice and water in equilibrium at standard atmospheric pressure, and the upper fixed point by a mixture of water and steam in equilibrium at standard atmospheric pressure. When in a state of equilibrium both these mixtures provide definite and reproducible temperatures. On the Celsius scale the ice and steam points are assigned the numbers 0 and 100 respectively, while on the Fahrenheit scale the corresponding numbers are 32 and 212. There are therefore 100 units or degrees of temperature between the fixed points on the Celsius scale, and 180 on the Fahrenheit scale.

We have now to decide how to interpolate between the fixed points and extrapolate beyond them. In the early days of thermometry the simplest procedure was adopted, i.e. the scale was divided into a number of equal parts. This implies that the temperature is defined as a linear function of the thermometric property. Thus, if θ and X are the numerical values of the temperature and thermometric property,

$$\theta = aX + b$$

The constants a and b are determined by the numbers allotted to the fixed points. On the Celsius scale, a and b can be found by solving the simultaneous equations

$$0 = aX_i + b, \qquad 100 = aX_s + b$$

where X_i and X_s are the numerical values of the thermometric property at the ice and steam points. The solution is

$$a = \frac{100}{X_s - X_i}, \qquad b = -\frac{100X_i}{X_s - X_i}$$

Substituting these values in the original equation for the temperature, we get

$$\theta_C = 100 \frac{X - X_i}{X_s - X_i}$$

If this procedure is repeated for the Fahrenheit scale we have

$$\theta_F = 32 + 180 \frac{X - X_i}{X_s - X_i}$$

It follows that the relation between the numerical values of temperature on the two scales is

$$\theta_F = 32 + 1.8\theta_C$$

Provided the same thermometric substance and property are used, there is no fundamental difference between the two scales we have been considering. A temperature measured on one scale can always be converted into a temperature measured on the other with mathematical precision. For the moment then, let us assume we are using the Celsius system of numbering, and consider what happens when the substance or property is changed. For example, we might construct the following two scales. For a liquid-in-glass thermometer we could write

$$\theta_C = 100 \frac{l - l_i}{l_s - l_i}$$

where l is the length of the column of liquid. And for a constant-volume gas thermometer, where p is the pressure, we would have

$$\theta_C = 100 \frac{p - p_i}{p_s - p_i}$$

If linear interpolation is used in this way, we find that when any two thermometers using either different thermometric properties or substances are brought into contact with the same heat reservoir, *the readings will not be identical except at the fixed points*. For example, if the temperature measured by a constant-volume hydrogen thermometer is 40 °C, the temperature recorded by a typical mercury-in-glass thermometer will be 40.11 °C and by a platinum resistance thermometer 40.36 °C. If one thermometric property does not vary linearly with the other, the two temperature scales, defined linearly in terms of these properties, cannot be identical except at the fixed points. Unfortunately there is nothing in the foregoing method of setting up a temperature scale to suggest why we should adopt one type of thermometer rather than another as a standard instrument. Moreover the scales are not absolute, because the zero is assigned to some arbitrary point fixed only by convention.

Now we have seen (section 6.2) that an absolute scale of temperature arises as a consequence of the Second Law, and that this thermodynamic scale is independent of any particular thermometric substance or property. Also, the temperature defined in this way enables us to introduce the useful concept of entropy. This theoretical scale is clearly a good candidate for adoption as the ultimate standard. It will be recalled that the thermodynamic temperature T must satisfy the relation

$$T = T_0 \frac{Q}{Q_0} \tag{8.1}$$

where Q and Q_0 are the quantities of heat absorbed and rejected by a reversible engine operating between reservoirs at T and T_0. But this relation does not completely determine the scale; we have still to fix the size of the interval or unit of temperature. It was pointed out in section 6.2 that this could be varied by altering the number of engines in the series shown in Fig. 6.3, and there are two ways of approaching the problem.

First, we may choose two fixed points, such as the ice point T_i and the steam point T_s, and define the number of degrees between them. For example, we can write $T_s - T_i = 100$ units. This is equivalent to placing 100 reversible engines in the series between the fixed points. When used in conjunction with the equation $T_s/T_i = Q_s/Q_i$, this arbitrary choice fully defines a linear thermodynamic scale. Q_s/Q_i has a unique value because the efficiencies ($= 1 - Q_i/Q_s$) of all reversible engines operating between T_s and T_i are the same, and thus the two simultaneous equations yield unique values of T_s and T_i. The main advantage of this approach to the definition of the thermodynamic scale is that it provides a scale which coincides exactly at the fixed points with all empirical scales based on the same fixed points.

The second approach, adopted internationally in 1954, is the more obvious one of assigning an arbitrary number to T_0 at one easily reproducible fixed point. Then any other temperature is uniquely defined by $T = T_0(Q/Q_0)$ for the reason just discussed. This approach is equivalent to fixing the number of engines in Fig. 6.3 between the fixed point and absolute zero. *The fixed point chosen for the definition of the thermodynamic scale is the triple point of pure water.* A detailed discussion of this state is given in the next section; here it suffices to say that it is the state at which the solid, liquid and vapour phases can coexist in equilibrium and it is easily reproducible. The pressure of the triple point is very low, i.e. 0.006 112 bar, but the temperature is only slightly above that of the ice point at atmospheric pressure. The internationally agreed number for the triple point T_0 is 273.16, and thus:

The unit of thermodynamic temperature is the fraction $1/273.16$ of the thermodynamic temperature of the triple point of water.

The unit is called the *kelvin*, denoted by the unit symbol K.

It is pertinent to ask why such an odd number has been chosen. The reason lies in the fact that with this method of definition no *exact* value can now be attached to $T_s - T_i$ and it becomes a matter of experiment. The choice of 273.16 K for T_0, however, makes $T_s - T_i \approx 100$ K within 0.005 K, and thus the new unit is still for many practical purposes the same size as on all previous empirical Celsius scales.

The kelvin is not the only thermodynamic unit in use. The other thermodynamic unit, rapidly falling into disuse, is the *rankine*, which is the fraction $1/(1.8 \times 273.16) = 1/491.688$ of the thermodynamic temperature of the triple point of water. Thus the kelvin is 1.8 times as large as the rankine (unit symbol R).

Non-absolute versions of the thermodynamic scales are obtained by shifting the zero datum of the scales. For example, the *Celsius thermodynamic scale* employs the same size of unit or interval as the Kelvin scale, but has its datum at 273.15 K, i.e. at a temperature 0.01 K below the triple point. It should be noted that, although the temperature unit on the thermodynamic Celsius scale is identical with the kelvin, it is customary to denote temperatures measured relative to the 273.15 K datum by the symbol °C. Thus we can write

$$0\,°\mathrm{C} = 273.15\,\mathrm{K}\quad\text{exactly}$$

Fig. 8.1
Relations between
thermodynamic scales of
temperature

	T_K	T_C	T_R	T_F
$T_K =$	T_K	$T_C + 273.15\,K$	$\dfrac{1}{1.8}T_R$	$\dfrac{1}{1.8}(T_F + 459.67\,R)$
$T_C =$	$T_K - 273.15\,K$	T_C	$\dfrac{1}{1.8}(T_R - 491.67\,R)$	$\dfrac{1}{1.8}(T_F - 32\,R)$
$T_R =$	$1.8\,T_K$	$1.8\,T_C + 491.67\,R$	T_R	$T_F + 459.67\,R$
$T_F =$	$1.8\,T_K - 459.67\,R$	$1.8\,T_C + 32\,R$	$T_R - 459.67\,R$	T_F

By choosing this datum we find that

$$0\,°C \approx \text{ice point}, \quad 100\,°C \approx \text{steam point} \quad \text{(both at 1 atm)}$$

and therefore have a scale directly comparable with empirical Celsius scales described at the beginning of this section. Similarly, the *Fahrenheit thermodynamic scale* has the zero datum moved to 459.67 R, i.e. 32.018 R below the triple point, thereby yielding ice and steam points of approximately 32 °F and 212 °F. By shifting the zero we do not alter the fact that the scales are based on the laws of thermodynamics and not on the characteristics of a particular substance, but it does mean that the temperatures are no longer absolute. The relations between the temperatures on the four scales are summarised in Fig. 8.1. In this book, Fahrenheit and Rankine scales will never be used, and it will be clear from the context (or unit notation K and °C) whether an absolute or Celsius temperature is being referred to. Temperature will therefore always be denoted simply by T.

It should be realised that the unit Celsius (°C) is anomalous in that it fulfils two functions: it tells us that (a) the unit used is the kelvin (K), and (b) the datum is at the absolute temperature of 273.15 K. No other unit symbol serves a dual function like this. And no other quantity is given two symbols for the same unit, namely °C and K. Difficulties arise when subtracting Celsius temperatures, and when multiplying or dividing physical quantities whose units involve a mixture of °C and K. The problem is discussed in Appendix A.3, but the procedures to be adopted can be summarised as follows:

(a) The symbol °C should be used only for *temperature scale values*, for which the datum is the absolute temperature 273.15 K.

(b) When subtracting two Celsius temperatures, the unit for the difference is always K, e.g. $T_2 - T_1 = 56\,°C - 34\,°C = 22\,K$.

(c) When multiplying and dividing quantities whose units involve a mixture of °C and K, the °C and K can be cancelled because they are the same *unit*.

The foregoing is a logical account of the *definition* of a thermodynamic unit of temperature; the *determination* of a temperature by using a reversible engine and measuring Q/Q_0 is of course a practical impossibility. Various indirect methods have been devised of which some details can be found in Ref. 20. These methods usually involve the use of an elaborate type of gas thermometer and are the province of the physicist rather than the engineer. The measurement of a single temperature requires months of careful scientific work and the procedures are too intricate for the direct calibration of even precision instruments. For this reason a procedure for establishing a practical scale was adopted, originally at the Seventh General Conference of Weights and Measures in 1927; it was then called the International Practical Temperature Scale 1927 or IPTS-27 for short. The latest revision was agreed under the name of *International Temperature Scale* 1990 or ITS-90.

Apart from the greater practicality of the instruments used for establishing the ITS-90 — namely platinum resistance thermometers over most of the range — there is a further reason for its adoption: the accuracy with which thermodynamic temperatures can be measured by gas thermometry is relatively modest, whereas the reproducibility of measurements on the ITS-90 is very great. (No figures for accuracy and reproducibility are given here because they vary over the temperature scale.) Thus two experimenters can agree very closely indeed when measuring a temperature on the ITS-90, but they would both be uncertain to a greater degree how far they are from the equivalent thermodynamic temperature. When a distinction needs to be drawn between thermodynamic and ITS-90 temperatures, the latter are marked by a subscript 90, i.e. T_{90}.

The procedure for constructing the ITS-90 is, very briefly, as follows. The thermodynamic temperatures of various easily reproducible states — the triple, melting, freezing and boiling points of very pure substances — have been measured to the best accuracy available by gas thermometry. These temperatures range from the triple point of hydrogen (13.8033 K) to the freezing point of copper (1357.77 K), and they provide a skeleton of fixed points treated as exact values for the purpose of the ITS-90. The complete scale is defined by five overlapping ranges, with closely specified instruments (e.g. purity of platinum), and elaborate non-linear interpolating equations whose constants are calculated from measurements at an appropriate number of intermediate fixed points. The ranges and instruments are as follows:

(a) For 0.65 K to 5 K: vapour pressure of ^{3}He and ^{4}He
(b) For 3 K to 24.5561 K: constant-volume gas thermometer
(c) For 13.8033 K to 273.16 K: platinum resistance thermometer of specified purity
(d) For 273.15 K to 1234.93 K; platinum resistance thermometer of specified purity, but using different fixed points and interpolating equations from those used in (c)
(e) For 1234.93 K and above: instrument using a black-body cavity in conjunction with the Planck law of radiation (see equation (23.11)).

Further details can be found in Refs 25 and 32.

The ITS-90 is used by standards laboratories for calibrating scientific instruments. Direct reference to the thermodynamic scale is unnecessary, because the fixed points and interpolation formulae are chosen in such a way that the temperature measured on ITS-90 closely approximates the thermodynamic temperature; the difference is within the limits of the present accuracy of measurement. It will be assumed in the following chapters that all temperatures are measured by instruments calibrated to read the ITS-90; they are thereby virtually thermodynamic temperatures and the symbol T, not T_{90}, will be used.

8.2 Properties of liquids and vapours

We noted in section 1.1 that a knowledge of two independent properties suffices to determine the thermodynamic state of a fluid when it is in equilibrium, and therefore that any other thermodynamic property is a function of the chosen pair of independent properties. We shall consider first the relation between the primary properties p, v and T; the equation expressing this relation for any particular fluid is called the *equation of state** or *characteristic equation* of the fluid. Except for so-called perfect gases, considered in sections 8.5 and 8.6, no simple algebraic equation can be found which will cover all possible states, and the relation is best expressed in either graphical or tabular form.

It must be emphasised that the equation of state is essentially an *empirical* relation; it cannot be deduced by thermodynamic reasoning. Assumptions as to the microscopic structure of a liquid or vapour can lead to a prediction of the form of the equation, but there still remain constants which must be determined by experiment for each substance. We shall refer to this type of prediction again when we consider the behaviour of real gases; for the moment we will consider only the graphical expression of $p–v–T$ relations obtained by direct measurement. Although we are concerned mainly with liquids and vapours it will be necessary to refer briefly to the solid phase also, because of the adoption of the triple point of water as a standard fixed point.

8.2.1 *p–v–T data*

Since we have three variables to consider, the obvious procedure is to measure the variation of one with another while the third is kept constant, and to repeat this for a range of values of the third variable. Imagine unit mass of ice below freezing point, enclosed in a cylinder by a piston under a constant load such that the pressure is one atmosphere ($1 \text{ atm} = 1.01325 \text{ bar}$). Let us follow the events which occur as heat is transferred to the cylinder while the pressure is kept constant. The temperature rises and the ice expands until a temperature of 273.15 K (0 °C) is reached, as indicated by the full line AB in Fig. 8.2. Further heating does not continue to raise the temperature of the ice, but causes a change to the liquid phase (BC). The change of phase occurs at constant temperature and is accompanied by a reduction in specific volume. The heat required for this process is called the *latent heat of fusion*; because the pressure is constant, the heat transfer is equal to the change of enthalpy (a property change), which is consequently called the *latent enthalpy of fusion*. With the system of units used in this book, this enthalpy will be measured in kJ/kg. In contrast to latent enthalpy, the enthalpy change of a substance while its

---

* The relation between p, v and T is sometimes called the 'thermal' or 'temperature' equation of state to distinguish it from 'caloric' equations of state such as $u = u(v, T)$ or $h = h(p, T)$. When using the term 'equation of state' on its own, we shall imply the relation between p, v and T.

Fig. 8.2
Isobars on $T - v$ diagram

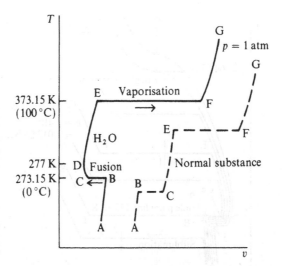

temperature changes is sometimes referred to as *sensible enthalpy*. Further heating, of what is now a liquid, results in a rise of temperature, a contraction in volume until the temperature is about 4 °C (point D), and subsequent expansion until a temperature of 373.15 K (100 °C) is reached (E). At this point a second phase change occurs at constant temperature with a large increase in volume until the liquid has been vaporised (F). The heat required in this case is called the *latent heat of vaporisation* and the associated enthalpy change is called the *latent enthalpy of vaporisation*. When vaporisation is complete, the temperature rises once more (FG). Water behaves in an anomalous way compared with other substances, in that it contracts on melting and also contracts before it expands when its temperature is raised above the melting point. The dashed curve in Fig. 8.2 shows the behaviour of normal pure substances. Constant pressure lines such as those in Fig. 8.2 are sometimes called *isobars*. It must be emphasised that in this and subsequent property diagrams the change in volume of the solid and liquid has been greatly exaggerated in comparison with the volume changes due to the liquid–vapour phase change or the heating of the vapour; the diagrams are not to scale.

Let us now consider what happens to water when the same sequence of events is followed through at a lower pressure (Fig. 8.3a). First, there is a slight rise in the melting point (as predicted by the Clausius-Clapeyron equation (7.47)). Secondly, there is a marked drop in the boiling point and a marked increase in the change of volume which accompanies evaporation. When the pressure is reduced to 0.006 112 bar, the melting and boiling temperatures become equal and the change of phase, ice–water–steam, is represented by a single horizontal line (bcf). As explained in the previous section, the temperature at which this occurs has been accepted internationally as a fixed point for the absolute temperature scale and is *by definition* 273.16 K. Only at this temperature, and the pressure of 0.006 112 bar, can ice, water and steam coexist in thermodynamic equilibrium in a closed vessel, and bcf is called the *triple point line*. If the pressure is reduced still further the ice, instead of melting, *sublimates* directly into steam.

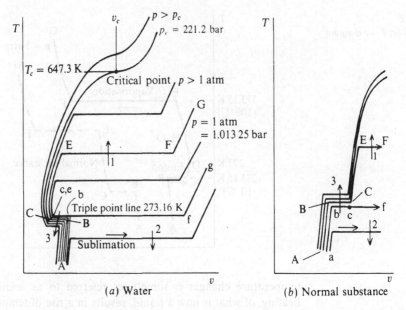

Fig. 8.3
Families of isobars on T–v
diagram: (a) water;
(b) normal substance

$p > p_c$
v_c
$p_c = 221.2$ bar

$T_c = 647.3$ K

Critical point, $p > 1$ atm

G

$p = 1$ atm
$= 1.013\ 25$ bar

E   F

1

g

c,e b
Triple point line 273.16 K
C
B   f
3
Sublimation   2

A

(a) Water

T

E F
1
3
C
B   b c   f
2
A   a

(b) Normal substance

Consider now the behaviour at pressures above atmospheric. The shape of the curves is similar to that of the atmospheric isobar, but there is a marked reduction in the change of volume accompanying evaporation. At a sufficiently high pressure this change of volume falls to zero, and the horizontal portion of the curve reduces to a point of inflexion. This is referred to as the *critical point*, and the properties at this state are known as the critical pressure p_c, critical temperature T_c and critical volume v_c, The values for water are

$$p_c = 221.2\ \text{bar}, \qquad T_c = 647.3\ \text{K}, \qquad v_c = 0.003\ 17\ \text{m}^3/\text{kg}$$

At pressures above critical, there is no definite transition from liquid to vapour and the two phases cannot be distinguished visually. The latent enthalpy of vaporisation falls to zero at the critical pressure, and at higher pressures the term has no meaning.

Fig. 8.3b shows the corresponding behaviour of normal substances. As the only difference is in the behaviour near the triple point line, only the left-hand portion of the diagram has been shown. It is apparent that normally both the melting and boiling points rise with increase in pressure and that liquids expand on heating at all pressures and temperatures.

It is instructive to show graphically how the sublimation, melting and boiling temperatures vary with pressure as in Fig. 8.4, because the origin of the term 'triple point' lies in this method of presenting the information. The boiling point curve is obtained by following arrow 1 in Fig. 8.3 from the triple point line to the critical point, and the sublimation point curve by following arrow 2 as the pressure is reduced below the triple point value. Two melting point curves are shown, the full line being for water and the dashed line for normal substances. These are obtained by following arrow 3 in Figs 8.3a and b respectively. The numerical values in Fig. 8.4 refer only to water.

In the foregoing we have considered how T varies with v at constant p, and

Fig. 8.4
Triple point of water

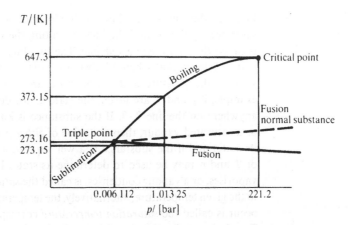

for the purpose of introducing the pattern of behaviour of the three phases this is very convenient. We have seen, however, that a $p-v$ diagram is more useful for depicting practical processes. By following a succession of constant temperature (i.e. horizontal) lines in Fig. 8.3, it may be seen that the corresponding $p-v$ diagram of Fig. 8.5 is obtained (the points E, F, G and c, f, g correspond to those in Fig. 8.3a). Alternatively, each of the isothermals can be imagined to be obtained by allowing a liquid to expand isothermally behind a piston. Since we shall have no need in practice to refer to behaviour in the solid phase, only the portion referring to a liquid and vapour is shown and it is unnecessary to distinguish between water and other substances in what follows. Various terms have been introduced to characterise the different states through which the substance passes during the expansion 1–2–3–4. From 1 to 2 the substance is an *unsaturated liquid*, while at 2 it is a *saturated liquid*. Between 2 and 3 it is a *two-phase mixture* of liquid and vapour or *wet vapour*. At 3 it is a *saturated vapour*, and from 3 to 4 an *unsaturated vapour*. If all the points representing saturated liquid and vapour states are joined to form a curve, i.e. cNf in

Fig. 8.5
$p-v$ diagram for water

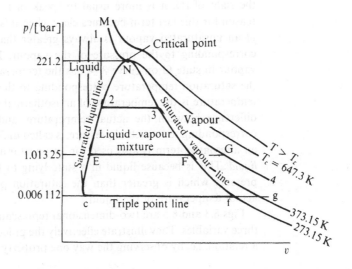

Fig. 8.5, the line separating the liquid and two-phase regions is called the *saturated liquid line*, and the line separating the vapour and two-phase regions is called the *saturated vapour line*. The two lines meet at the critical point N.

It is evident that when a substance exists in a saturated state, or as a wet vapour, the pressure and temperature are not independent properties. For example, if p and T are given, the state is not determined because it might lie anywhere on the line 2–3. If the substance is known to be a saturated liquid, or a saturated vapour, then the value of *either p or T* is sufficient to determine its state; and if the substance is a wet vapour, a knowledge of either p and v, or T and v, may be used to determine its state. The pressure at which a liquid vaporises, or a vapour condenses, is called the *saturation pressure* corresponding to the given temperature; alternatively, the temperature at which these phenomena occur is called the *saturation temperature* corresponding to the given pressure. The choice of phrasing depends on whether the temperature or pressure is being used as one of the independent variables.

Substances referred to as gases are those which lie in the region above the critical isothermal T_c at ordinary pressures and temperatures, i.e. they are substances which have a very low critical temperature. This should not be regarded as a rigid definition, however, and the terms 'gas' and 'vapour' are often used synonymously. A substance in a state lying above T_c cannot be liquefied by isothermal compression; it must first be cooled below the critical temperature. This explains why some substances, e.g. oxygen and hydrogen, were originally called 'permanent gases'. The critical temperatures of these substances are far below the temperature of any freezing mixture that was available in the early days of the science, and more sophisticated methods of liquefaction had not then been devised.

A vapour in a state lying along the saturated vapour line fN on Fig. 8.5 is sometimes called a *dry saturated vapour*, although the additional adjective 'dry' is superfluous in this instance. The term *dry vapour* may refer to a saturated or an unsaturated vapour. When the vapour is unsaturated, i.e. in a state lying to the right of fN, it is more usual to speak of it as a *superheated vapour*. The reason for this last term becomes clear when it is realised that the temperature of an unsaturated vapour is always greater than the saturation temperature corresponding to the pressure of the vapour. For example, an unsaturated vapour in state G on curve 3–4 has the temperature T_G, which is higher than the saturation temperature corresponding to the pressure p_G. This saturation temperature is the temperature of an isothermal passing through point F. The difference between the actual temperature, and the saturation temperature corresponding to the actual pressure, is called the *degrees of superheat*. Similarly, an alternative term is also used for an unsaturated liquid, namely *compressed liquid*. This is because liquid in a state lying to the left of cNM always has a pressure which is greater than the saturation pressure corresponding to the actual temperature of the liquid.

Figs 8.3 and 8.5 are two-dimensional representations of the relation between three variables. They illustrate effectively the practical method of obtaining such a relation, i.e. by observing the way one property varies with another while the

Fig. 8.6
$p-v-T$ surface for water

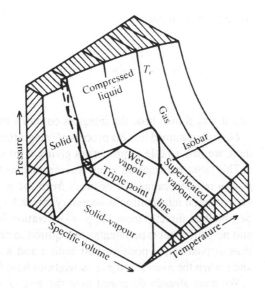

third is kept constant. A three-dimensional model, however, gives a clearer picture of the fact that only two properties need to be fixed to determine the state of the substance. If p, v and T are plotted along three mutually perpendicular axes as in Fig. 8.6, all possible equilibrium states lie on a surface called the $p-v-T$ surface. Any reversible process, i.e. succession of equilibrium states, can be represented by a line on the surface. A minor qualification is necessary: under certain conditions it is possible for a substance to be in a state of equilibrium represented by a point not on the surface. But such a state is not one of *stable* equilibrium; it must be either an *unstable* or a *metastable* state. If it is unstable, any infinitesimal disturbance causes the substance to undergo a spontaneous irreversible process which returns it to a state of stable equilibrium lying on the $p-v-T$ surface. If the state is metastable, a finite disturbance is necessary; an example of this kind of phenomenon is discussed in greater detail in section 18.2.

Having found the empirical relation between the properties p, v and T, the problem that remains is the determination of the internal energy, enthalpy and entropy in terms of the two primary properties chosen to describe the state of the substance. The procedure is somewhat complicated because u, h and s are not directly measurable properties. A proper analysis of the procedure is given in Chapter 7 for advanced students; all that is attempted in the next section is an indication of one possible method in simple terms.

8.2.2　$u-h-s$ data and specific heat capacities

A method of computing the value of the entropy s at any state defined by (p, v), relative to the value at some reference state (p_0, v_0) has been described in section 6.5.1. The equations expressing the First and Second Laws were combined

141

to yield the equation

$$s_1 - s_0 = \int_0^1 \frac{1}{T} \, du + \int_0^1 \frac{p}{T} \, dv \tag{8.2}$$

and it was shown how the integrals could be evaluated graphically.

Now we assumed for this process of integration that, in addition to the p–v–T data, we had a table of properties giving u for various pairs of values of p and v. This latter information is just as empirical as the p–v–T data. Moreover, the p–v–u relation cannot be deduced from the p–v–T relation; some additional experimental information is necessary. Since $h = u + pv$, values of enthalpy can be obtained directly from the p–v–u relation for ranges of values of p and v, and no additional experiments are required to determine this property. We have thus arrived at the position that both s and h can be expressed in terms of p and v when the p–v–T and p–v–u relations have been determined experimentally.

We have already described how the p–v–T data can be obtained; it is the determination of p–v–u data that we have now to discuss. A method of measuring changes of internal energy is suggested by the application of the non-flow energy equation to a constant-volume process, i.e. $Q = (u_2 - u_1)$. We can imagine unit mass of the liquid being heated in a closed container of volume v_0. The heat required to raise the pressure from p_0 to p_1, p_2, p_3 etc. can be measured, and these quantities of heat will be equal to the changes of internal energy between state (v_0, p_0) and the various states $(v_0, p_1), (v_0, p_2)$ etc. This procedure can be repeated for other values of v and, if the value of u at state (p_0, v_0) is put equal to zero, we shall have a series of values of u for a range of states defined by values of p and v. We can then proceed to calculate values of h and s in the manner suggested.

It is not essential that the empirical information required to supplement the p–v–T data be in the form of p–v–u data. In Chapter 7 we show how data on specific heat capacity can be used for the purpose. Chapter 7 also describes a method of calculating values of s which only requires sufficient supplementary information to cover a single line of reference states, e.g. a series of states at constant pressure, instead of the whole field of possible states. This method obviously requires much less experimental work to be performed. We shall not pursue this matter here, but since we shall find the idea of specific heat capacity particularly useful when dealing with the properties of gases, we will end this section with a discussion of this concept.

Originally the specific heat capacity was defined as the heat required to raise the temperature of unit mass of substance one degree. Since the quantity of heat depends upon the process employed to raise the temperature, and an infinite number of processes are possible, there is an infinite number of specific heat capacities. However, only two came to be used in practice: that at constant volume (c_v) was defined as the heat required to raise the temperature of unit mass one degree during a reversible constant volume process, and that at constant pressure (c_p) as the heat required to raise unit mass one degree during

Fig. 8.7
Determination of c_v from
u–T data

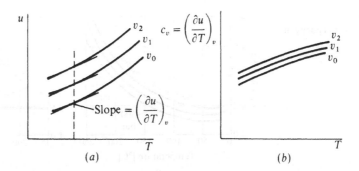

a reversible constant pressure process.* Now the quantities of heat added during these two processes are equal to the changes in internal energy and enthalpy respectively. The foregoing definitions can therefore be written as

$$c_v = \frac{Q_v}{\Delta T} = \frac{\Delta u}{\Delta T}, \qquad c_p = \frac{Q_p}{\Delta T} = \frac{\Delta h}{\Delta T} \tag{8.3}$$

The values of c_v and c_p, defined in this way, are found to vary with the value of ΔT, i.e. with the range of temperature used in the experiment, and also with the state of the substance at the beginning of the heating process. To make the definitions yet more precise, it is the practice in thermodynamics to use the following definitions:

$$c_v = \left(\frac{\partial u}{\partial T}\right)_v \tag{8.4a}$$

$$c_p = \left(\frac{\partial h}{\partial T}\right)_p \tag{8.4b}$$

These definitions are the limit of the original definitions (8.3) as ΔT approaches zero. c_v and c_p can each be seen to be the rate of change of one property with another while a third is kept constant. This is why in general the partial notation is necessary. Being defined solely in terms of properties, c_v and c_p must themselves be properties; they are therefore a function of any two independent properties that can be used to define the state of the substance. This will be made clear if we outline a method for their measurement.

c_v can easily be found by carrying out the experiment already described for the purpose of obtaining the p–v–u data. If the temperature is measured instead of the pressure, the results can be expressed on a u–T diagram, as in Fig. 8.7a. The slopes of the constant volume lines can be measured at various temperatures to give values of c_v corresponding to various values of v and T. These may be plotted as in Fig. 8.7b. Note that the arbitrary choice of a reference state, at which u is put equal to zero, does not affect the values of c_v. The choice of

---

* It is only necessary that the constant volume process be internally reversible, i.e. that there should be no paddle work, because then the quantity of heat is quite definite and depends only on the equilibrium end states (see section 3.2). However, the constant pressure process must be carried out slowly to make the effect of friction negligible during the expansion, and this implies a slow rate of heat addition.

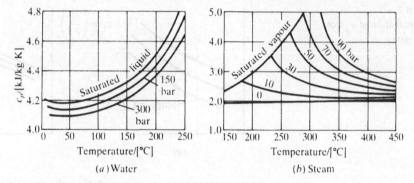

Fig. 8.8
Specific heat capacity at constant pressure

(a) Water

(b) Steam

reference state merely fixes the origin of the coordinates in relation to the family of curves in Fig. 8.7a, and does not affect the slope of the curves at any given state defined by values of T and v.

A similar plot of c_p versus T, this time for various constant values of the pressure, can be obtained by heating the substance at constant pressure, plotting h versus T for various values of p, and measuring the slopes of these curves. The actual variation of c_p with T and p, for water and steam, is depicted in Figs 8.8a and b. It will be noticed that the curves only cover a range of states up to the line of saturation states. This is because the concept of specific heat capacity is meaningful only when the substance exists in a single phase. When more than one phase is present, as in the case of a wet vapour, a substance undergoes a change in enthalpy without any change of temperature during a constant pressure process. c_p would therefore be infinite.

The difference between c_p and c_v for liquids is very small. Liquids have a low coefficient of expansion, i.e. the change of volume with temperature during a constant pressure process is negligible. Such a process is therefore effectively also a constant volume process, and we can write

$$\left(\frac{\partial h}{\partial T}\right)_p \approx \left(\frac{\partial h}{\partial T}\right)_v$$

Also, when p is constant the increase of enthalpy is effectively equal to the increase of internal energy because

$$dh = du + d(pv) = du + p\,dv \approx du$$

Therefore for liquids,

$$\left(\frac{\partial h}{\partial T}\right)_p \approx \left(\frac{\partial h}{\partial T}\right)_v \approx \left(\frac{\partial u}{\partial T}\right)_v \quad \text{or} \quad c_p \approx c_v$$

It is also worth noting that over normal ranges of temperature and pressure the variation of c_p and c_v is small: this applies to both liquids and vapours. In general, temperature has a greater effect than pressure, but even the variation with temperature can often be neglected for approximate calculations. Thus when the range of temperature and pressure is not too large in any process considered, mean values of c_p and c_v can be chosen and assumed constant for that particular process. As we shall show later, this procedure considerably simplifies many calculations.

Finally, a word about units. In the SI the coherent unit of c_p and c_v is the J/kg K, and the multiple we shall normally use is the kJ/kg K. When calorimetric heat units are used, it is evident from their definition (see footnote in section 2.3) that the value of the specific heat capacity will be the same in any system, e.g.

$$1 \text{ kcal/kg K} = 1 \text{ Chu/lb K} = 1 \text{ Btu/lb R}$$

and that all such units of specific heat capacity are 4.1868 times greater than the kJ/kg K.

8.3 Tables of properties

We are now in a position to describe the most convenient way of setting out the relations between p, v, T, u, h and s in a tabular form. The simple type of table illustrated in Fig. 1.1 is not used in practice because, by adopting the following method, the necessary information can be presented in a much more condensed form. All the properties for the whole fluid of Fig. 8.5 can be given in three tables, and for many purposes sufficiently accurately in only two.

8.3.1 Saturation table

We have noted that when a substance is known or specified to be either a saturated liquid or a saturated vapour, its state is completely determined when the value of one property is given. If pressure is chosen to be the independent variable, the corresponding saturation values of all other properties of the liquid and vapour can be set out as in Fig. 8.9. The subscripts f and g refer to saturated liquid and saturated vapour respectively. The subscript s is added to temperature because this is the same for both phases in the saturated state; when temperature is chosen to be the argument of the table, p carries the subscript s and these two columns are interchanged.

Sometimes, for brevity, the internal energy is not listed because it can easily

Fig. 8.9 Table for saturated water and steam

p [bar]	T_s [°C]	v_f $\left[\dfrac{\text{m}^3}{\text{kg}}\right]$	v_g $\left[\dfrac{\text{m}^3}{\text{kg}}\right]$	u_f $\left[\dfrac{\text{kJ}}{\text{kg}}\right]$	u_g $\left[\dfrac{\text{kJ}}{\text{kg}}\right]$	h_f $\left[\dfrac{\text{kJ}}{\text{kg}}\right]$	h_g $\left[\dfrac{\text{kJ}}{\text{kg}}\right]$	s_f $\left[\dfrac{\text{kJ}}{\text{kg K}}\right]$	s_g $\left[\dfrac{\text{kJ}}{\text{kg K}}\right]$
0.006 112	0.01	0.001 000 2	206.1	0	2375	0.0006	2501	0	9.155
0.010	7.0	0.001 000 1	129.2	29	2385	29	2514	0.106	8.974
↓									
1.013 25	100.0	0.001 044	1.673	419	2507	419	2676	1.307	7.355
↓									
220	373.7	0.002 69	0.003 68	1949	2097	2008	2178	4.289	4.552
221.2	374.15	0.003 17	0.003 17	2014	2014	2084	2084	4.430	4.430

be obtained from the values of p, v and h, i.e.

$$u_f = h_f - pv_f \quad \text{and} \quad u_g = h_g - pv_g$$

The values of v_f may also be omitted, or given in a separate shorter table, because the specific volume of a liquid varies so little with pressure. Thus, for water, v_f varies only from $0.001\,00\,\text{m}^3/\text{kg}$ at the triple point to $0.001\,29\,\text{m}^3/\text{kg}$ at a pressure of 50 bar, whereas when the liquid is transformed into saturated vapour the respective specific volumes become $206.1\,\text{m}^3/\text{kg}$ and $0.0394\,\text{m}^3/\text{kg}$. Indeed it is often sufficiently accurate to assume a constant value for v_f, and for water at moderate pressures the value of $0.001\,\text{m}^3/\text{kg}$ is frequently used.

On the other hand, where brevity is not important, the differences $(h_g - h_f)$ and $(s_g - s_f)$ are allotted columns in the table because they are so frequently required. For convenience they are denoted by the symbols h_{fg} and s_{fg}. Since the heat added in a reversible constant pressure process is equal to the increase of enthalpy, the latent heat of vaporisation must be equal to h_{fg}.

It will be appreciated that the tables only give the difference between the internal energy, enthalpy or entropy at any state and the value of the respective property at a reference state. The internal energy and enthalpy cannot be zero at the *same* reference state, however, because they are related by $h = u + pv$. Thus if u is put equal to zero at a state defined by (p_0, v_0), the value of h at this state is $p_0 v_0$. For steam tables, based on the International Skeleton Tables 1963, the liquid at the triple point is chosen as the datum state and both u_f and s_f are put equal to zero at this state.* The value of the enthalpy at this state is therefore

$$h_f = u_f + pv_f$$

$$= 0 + 0.006\,112[\text{bar}] \times 10^5 \left[\frac{\text{N/m}^2}{\text{bar}} \right] \times 0.001\,000\,2 \left[\frac{\text{m}^3}{\text{kg}} \right]$$

$$\times 10^{-3} \left[\frac{\text{kN m}}{\text{N m}} \text{ or } \frac{\text{kJ}}{\text{J}} \right]$$

$$= 0 + 0.006\,112 \times 0.001\,000\,2 \times 10^2 \text{ kJ/kg} = 0.000\,611\,2 \text{ kJ/kg} \qquad (8.5)$$

The saturation table for steam extends from the triple point pressure of 0.006 112 bar to the critical pressure of 221.2 bar. At the critical pressure the properties with subscript f become equal to the corresponding properties with subscript g, i.e. u_{fg}, h_{fg} and s_{fg} are all zero.

A knowledge of the properties along the saturation line enables the properties at any state in the wet region to be easily computed, and no separate table is required. The reason is that a wet vapour is a mixture of saturated liquid and saturated vapour. When two masses of the same substance, at the same pressure

---

* In earlier steam stables the datum state used was saturated liquid at $0\,^\circ\text{C}$, whereas the lowest temperature at which saturated liquid can exist is $0.01\,^\circ\text{C}$ (see the boiling curve in Fig. 8.4). Thus the datum state was an unstable state arrived at by extrapolation. Furthermore, it was h_f and not u_f which was put equal to zero at the datum state. The shift to the new datum has little effect on numerical values, amounting only to -0.0416 kJ/kg for enthalpy and $-0.000\,15 \text{ kJ/kg K}$ for entropy.

and temperature, are brought together, they will be in equilibrium with one another and there will be no change in pressure or temperature. The same argument can be applied to any *intensive* property, i.e. to any property whose value is independent of the mass of the system. It cannot be applied to *extensive* properties, such as V, U, H and S, whose values depend upon the amount of substance under consideration. An extensive property of a combination of the two masses is equal to the sum of the corresponding extensive properties of the individual masses. For example, if two masses m_1 and m_2 at the same pressure and temperature have specific volumes v_1 and v_2, the total volume on combination is given by

$$V_3 = V_1 + V_2 = m_1 v_1 + m_2 v_2$$

It will be meaningful to speak of the specific volume of the combination if the two masses are homogeneously mixed. Then we have

$$v_3 = \frac{V_3}{m_3} = \frac{m_1 v_1 + m_2 v_2}{m_1 + m_2}$$

All the specific properties, which are derived from extensive properties, can be treated in this way.

The foregoing provides the clue to the treatment of a wet vapour. Unit mass of wet vapour can be regarded as a mixture of x kg of saturated vapour and $(1 - x)$ kg of saturated liquid, each having different specific properties denoted by subscripts g and f respectively but the same pressure and temperature. These specific properties can be read from the saturation table when the pressure or temperature of the wet vapour is known. Any specific property of the wet vapour can then be found by adding the corresponding extensive properties of the two constituents which together make up unit mass of wet vapour. Thus

$$u = (1 - x)u_f + xu_g$$

$$h = (1 - x)h_f + xh_g$$

$$s = (1 - x)s_f + xs_g$$

When the difference columns are given in the tables, i.e. properties denoted by the subscript fg, less arithmetic is required if the equations are expressed in the form

$$u = u_f + xu_{fg} \tag{8.6}$$

$$h = h_f + xh_{fg} \tag{8.7}$$

$$s = s_f + xs_{fg} \tag{8.8}$$

The physical interpretation of (8.7), say, is that the enthalpy of unit mass of wet vapour is equal to the enthalpy of unit mass of saturated liquid plus the increase of enthalpy entailed by the evaporation of a proportion x at constant pressure.

The specific volume of the wet vapour is similarly given by

$$v = (1 - x)v_f + xv_g \tag{8.9}$$

p/[bar] (Tₛ/[°C])			T [°C]	200	250	300	350	400	450
15 (198.3)	v_g	0.1317	v	0.1324	0.1520	0.1697	0.1865	0.2029	0.2191
	u_g	2595	u	2597	2697	2784	2868	2952	3035
	h_g	2792	h	2796	2925	3039	3148	3256	3364
	s_g	6.445	s	6.452	6.711	6.919	7.102	7.268	7.423
20 (212.4)	v_g	0.0996	v		0.1115	0.1255	0.1386	0.1511	0.1634
	u_g	2600	u		2681	2774	2861	2946	3030
	h_g	2799	h		2904	3025	3138	3248	3357
	s_g	6.340	s		6.547	6.768	6.957	7.126	7.283
30 (233.8)	v_g	0.0666	v		0.0706	0.0812	0.0905	0.0993	0.1078
	u_g	2603	u		2646	2751	2845	2933	3020
	h_g	2803	h		2858	2995	3117	3231	3343
	s_g	6.186	s		6.289	6.541	6.744	6.921	7.082
40 (250.3)	v_g	0.0498	v/[m³/kg]			0.0588	0.0664	0.0733	0.0800
	u_g	2602	u/[kJ/kg]			2728	2828	2921	3010
	h_g	2801	h/[kJ/kg]			2963	3094	3214	3330
	s_g	6.070	s/[kJ/kg K]			6.364	6.584	6.769	6.935

NB: The entries throughout are regarded as pure numbers, and therefore the symbols for the physical quantities should be *divided* by the appropriate units as shown at p/[bar] = 40 and explained in Appendix A, section A.1. Because of lack of space, this has not been done for the other pressures in Fig. 8.10 or for any of the pressures in Fig. 8.11.

Fig. 8.10 Table for superheated steam

but this time the expression is modified in a different way. The term containing v_f can often be neglected, and in this case

$$v = xv_g \tag{8.10}$$

This simplification cannot be employed when the fraction x is small or the pressure high, but equation (8.10) will always be used unless otherwise stated.

The quantity of saturated vapour in unit mass of wet vapour, denoted by x, is referred to as the *dryness fraction*, or *quality*, of the vapour. The dryness fraction increases from 0 to 1 as the state of the substance changes from E to F in Fig. 8.5. It is a quantity which depends only on the state of the wet vapour, and it is therefore a property. In effect we have chosen to define the state of a wet vapour by (p, x).* If p and v are known, however, it is a simple matter to find x from (8.9) or (8.10) and then use (8.6), (8.7) and (8.8) to calculate the remaining properties.

8.3.2 Superheat table

When the vapour is superheated, the two properties usually chosen as the independent variables for the table are pressure and temperature. At any given pressure a superheated vapour may have any temperature greater than the saturation value. Fig. 8.10 illustrates one method of tabulation which enables the values of v, u, h and s to be found at any state defined by a pair of values

---

* One practical reason for doing this is that in many circumstances the dryness fraction is more easily measured than the specific volume. A method of measuring the dryness fraction is described in section 10.3.

	$T/[°C]$	0.01	100	200	300	350	374.15
$p/[bar]$ ($T_s/[°C]$)	p_s $v_f/10^{-2}$ h_f s_f	0.006112 0.1000 0 0	1.01325 0.1044 419 1.307	15.55 0.1157 852 2.331	85.92 0.1404 1345 3.255	165.4 0.1741 1671 3.779	221.2 0.317 2084 4.430
100 (311.0)	$(v-v_f)/10^{-2}$ $(h-h_f)$ $(s-s_f)$	−0.0005 +10 0.000	−0.0006 +7 −0.008	−0.0009 +4 −0.013	−0.0007 −2 0.007		
221.2 (374.15)	$(v-v_f)/10^{-2}$ $(h-h_f)$ $(s-s_f)$	−0.0011 +22 +0.001	−0.0012 +17 −0.017	−0.0020 +9 −0.031	−0.0051 −12 −0.053	−0.0107 −34 −0.071	0 0 0
500	$(v-v_f)/10^{-2}$ $(h-h_f)$ $(s-s_f)$	−0.0023 +49 0.000	−0.0024 +38 −0.037	−0.0042 +23 −0.068	−0.0117 −21 −0.134	−0.0298 −94 −0.235	−0.161 −269 −0.670
1000	$(v-v_f)/10^{-2}$ $(h-h_f)$ $(s-s_f)$	−0.0044 +96 −0.007	−0.0044 +76 −0.070	−0.0075 +51 −0.124	−0.0191 −17 −0.235	−0.0427 −119 −0.385	−0.180 −415 −0.853

NB: See note to Fig. 8.10.

Fig. 8.11 Table for compressed water

(p, T). The properties of superheated steam have been obtained for pressures up to 1000 bar and temperatures up to 800 °C. It will be noticed that the numbers in any vertical column cease when the saturation temperature corresponding to the pressure becomes greater than the value of the temperature at the head of the column. In abridged tables, where space saving is important, these columns are sometimes headed with 'degrees of superheat' rather than with the actual temperature of the vapour. There will then be no vacant spaces in the table.

Owing to the need for two independent variables, the superheat table is inevitably much more lengthy than the saturation table. For this reason the internal energy is often not included and must be found from $(h - pv)$.

8.3.3 Compressed liquid table

When the pressure of a liquid is higher than the saturation pressure corresponding to the temperature of the liquid, the state lies in the region to the left of MNc in Fig. 8.5. The pressure and temperature can be varied independently, and can therefore be considered to be the independent variables as in the case of a superheated vapour. Consequently the properties may be tabulated in the same way, i.e. as in Fig. 8.10. In fact it is possible to combine the compressed liquid and superheat tables by entering the compressed liquid data in the vacant spaces of Fig. 8.10. It is found, however, that the properties of a liquid change very little with pressure and it is often more convenient to list the compressed liquid values as deviations from the corresponding saturation values taken at the same temperature. Such a table is shown in Fig. 8.11. At ordinary pressures, say below 50 bar, deviations are very small and the properties v, u, h and s can be assumed to equal the saturation values v_f, u_f, h_f and s_f at the *temperature* of

149

the compressed liquid. This is equivalent to assuming that curves such as 1–2 in Fig. 8.5 are vertical straight lines (i.e. that the liquid is incompressible), and that the internal energy of a compressed liquid is a function only of temperature. We shall usually make this assumption in subsequent chapters.

The properties of water in its liquid and vapour phases have been investigated more thoroughly than those of any other substance. They are of particular interest to engineers owing to the extensive use of steam as a working fluid in heat engines. Several international conferences have been held to correlate the results obtained in various countries and by various experimental techniques.* At the Sixth International Conference on the Properties of Steam (1963), agreement was reached on a set of values to each of which was attached a tolerance indicating the agreed margin of experimental error. These values comprise the International Skeleton Tables 1963. (There have been only relatively minor revisions to these tables since.) The tolerances are well within the degree of accuracy required for any engineering calculations. The National Engineering Laboratory, Scotland, has used these values in computing the full set of *NEL Steam Tables* 1964 (Ref. 1), which employ sufficiently small intervals to make accurate interpolation a simple matter. For student use, an abridged set of steam tables is included in *Thermodynamic and Transport Properties of Fluids* (Ref. 17). The numbers appearing in subsequent examples are taken from these abridged tables and, where interpolation is necessary, linear interpolation is always used.

It should be noted that several sources provide computer programs of properties for various fluids from which data can be extracted. These programs can be particularly useful in repetitive calculations such as occur when optimising the design of process and power plant, or when evaluating experimental results. From a didactic point of view, it is important that a student familiarises himself with the handling of properties via tables and charts before plunging into the black-box treatment provided by computers.

8.4 Diagrams of properties

The characteristics of a liquid and a vapour have already been described by referring to diagrams using p and v, or T and v, as coordinates. Diagrams with other pairs of properties as coordinates will be shown to be useful for various purposes in later chapters, and three such diagrams are described in this section, namely the T–s, h–s and p–h diagrams. Property charts do not entirely take the place of tables because values of the properties cannot be read from them with as great an accuracy as they are given in tables.

8.4.1 Temperature–entropy diagram

When analysing the characteristics of heat engine cycles it is often helpful to plot the cycle on a diagram having temperature and entropy as the coordinates.

---

* An interesting account of this work may be found in Ref. 21.

Fig. 8.12
Temperature–entropy
diagrams

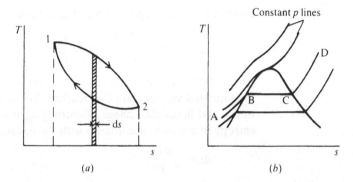

(a)   (b)

Fig. 8.12a illustrates this. If the processes in the cycle are reversible, the heat supplied during the cycle is given by

$$Q_{12} = \int_1^2 T\,ds$$

and the heat rejected by

$$Q_{21} = \int_2^1 T\,ds$$

These quantities are represented by the areas under the curves 1–2 and 2–1. It follows that the area enclosed by a reversible cycle represents the net heat supplied and hence, from the First Law, the net work done *by* the system *on* the surroundings.

In its simplest form the T–s diagram consists of a series of constant pressure lines and the saturation curve. The general shape of the curves can be deduced from the general property relation (6.13):

$$T\,ds = dh - v\,dp$$

Noting that the $v\,dp$ term is zero when p is constant, the equation reduces to

$$ds = \frac{dh}{T}$$

From equation (8.4b) dh can be expressed in terms of c_p as $c_p\,dT$, and it follows that

$$ds = c_p \frac{dT}{T}$$

We have been able to drop the partial notation of equation (8.4b), because we have no longer a second independent variable along the chosen path, namely a path at constant p. The value of c_p can still be a function of T, but if we can assume it to be constant, or take a mean value over the temperature range T_A to T_B at the particular pressure p, we can find the approximate shape of the curve. Integrating the expression for ds between an arbitrary value T_A and the saturation value T_B ($T_A < T_B$) we obtain, for the shape of the constant pressure

151

curve in the liquid region (AB in Fig. 8.12b),

$$s_B - s_A = c_p \int_A^B \frac{dT}{T} = c_p \ln \frac{T_B}{T_A}$$

As the enthalpy rise continues, the temperature remains constant at T_B until the saturated vapour state C is reached. The enthalpy of vaporisation is equal to h_{fg}, and hence the change of entropy s_{fg} is equal to h_{fg}/T_B. Thereafter the entropy increases in accordance with the equation

$$ds = c_p \frac{dT}{T}$$

where c_p is for the superheated vapour. The constant pressure line therefore continues from C to D with much the same shape as in the liquid region but of steeper slope. The slope of a curve on the T–s diagram is dT/ds, which for a constant pressure line equals T/c_p, and $(c_p)_{vap} < (c_p)_{liq}$.

Since h_{fg} falls with increase of pressure, the length BC decreases, and the family of constant pressure lines appears as in Fig. 8.12b. With water, the line representing a constant pressure of 0.006 112 bar cuts the temperature axis at 273.16 K, because this is the reference state at which the entropy is put equal to zero. Fig. 8.12b is out of proportion, because at any given temperature the change of entropy with pressure in the liquid region is in fact negligible. On any reasonable scale the constant pressure lines are so close together in the liquid region as to be indistinguishable, and for practical purposes they may be assumed to coincide with the saturated liquid line. Fig. 8.13 shows the T–s diagram for steam drawn to scale.

In view of the fact that the dryness fraction is used as one of the parameters

Fig. 8.13
Temperature–entropy
diagram for steam

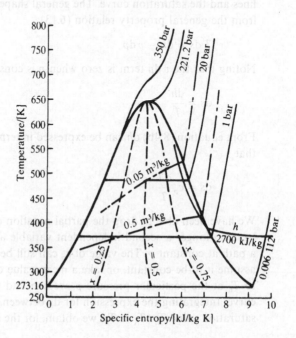

defining the state of a wet vapour, it is useful to have lines of constant dryness fraction superimposed on the diagram. From equation (8.8) we have $x = (s - s_f)/s_{fg}$. Therefore points on the constant dryness fraction line of value x can be obtained by marking off, on each horizontal constant pressure line such as BC in Fig. 8.12b, a length equal to $x(BC)$ from the saturated liquid end. The line of constant quality x is then found by joining up the points so obtained, as in Fig. 8.13.

It is also useful to have a general idea of the shape of constant volume and constant enthalpy lines in the wet and superheat regions. In the superheat region a constant volume line will be of similar shape to a constant pressure line, because, using equation (6.12) and a similar argument to that used for the constant pressure path, we have for a constant volume path

$$ds = c_v \frac{dT}{T}$$

Because c_v is always less than c_p (see section 7.4.3 for a formal demonstration), at any given state the constant volume line is always steeper than the constant pressure line. In the wet region a constant volume line, of value v say, can be plotted in the following way. At any given temperature or pressure, v_f and v_g can be found from the saturation table. Using the chosen value v, the corresponding value of the dryness fraction x can be found from equation (8.9). With x and either p or T known, it is possible to locate the point on the diagram. If this is repeated for other temperatures, the series of points representing states having the volume v can be joined to form a constant volume line. Such lines are found to be concave downwards in the wet region.

Finally, the general shape of a constant enthalpy line has been indicated in Fig. 8.13. In the wet region it may be located by the method already described for a constant volume line, except that equation (8.7) is used instead of (8.9). In the superheat region, points of constant enthalpy can be located by finding the pressure, at various temperatures, which corresponds to the chosen value of h. This may be done by interpolation from the superheat table. The fact that the resulting curve tends towards the horizontal as the amount of superheat increases can be deduced from a knowledge of the behaviour of a perfect gas. The more a vapour is superheated the more closely does it behave like a perfect gas, and we shall show in section 8.5 that the enthalpy of a perfect gas is a function only of temperature. Thus if the enthalpy remains constant so must the temperature, and hence the tendency of the curve to flatten out at high degrees of superheat. It is worth noting the fact that as the pressure falls at constant enthalpy, a wet vapour eventually becomes drier and if it is not too wet originally it becomes superheated; section 10.3 describes how this fact may be used in the measurement of the dryness fraction of a wet vapour.

8.4.2   Enthalpy–entropy diagram

The diagram in which the enthalpy and entropy are used as coordinates is known as the *Mollier diagram* after its proposer. It is very useful when analysing the performance of adiabatic steady-flow processes, such as occur in nozzles,

Fig. 8.14
Enthalpy–entropy diagram
for steam

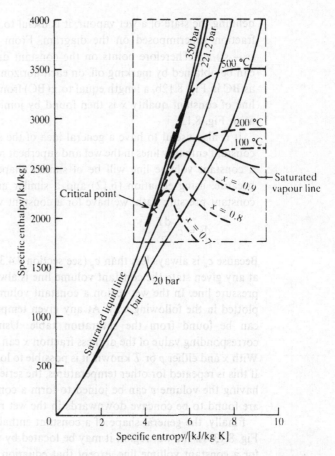

diffusers, turbines and compressors, and a glance at equations (4.5) and (4.6) will show why. For example, the work done by a fluid flowing through a turbine is equal to the drop in enthalpy between inlet and outlet (assuming no change in kinetic energy). Consequently, if the thermodynamic state of the fluid at inlet and outlet can be located as points on the h–s diagram, the vertical distance between the two points is proportional to the work done. Adiabatic processes which are also reversible, i.e. isentropic processes, are represented by vertical lines on the diagram.

The Mollier diagram is shown in Fig. 8.14. It may be seen to be a distorted form of the T–s diagram—distorted in such a way that the constant enthalpy lines become straight and horizontal. The constant pressure lines in the liquid region merge into the saturated line as before, and are straight in the wet region for the following reason. The increase of enthalpy from a saturated liquid state to any state of quality x at the same pressure is xh_{fg}. Since this is equal to the heat added in a reversible constant pressure process, the increase of entropy is xh_{fg}/T, where T is the saturation temperature corresponding to the given pressure. Thus the increase of entropy is directly proportional to the increase of enthalpy in the wet region, the slope of the constant pressure line $(dh/ds)_p$ being equal to T. The slope of successive constant pressure lines increases, because the saturation temperature increases with pressure. In the superheat region, the slope at any state is also equal to the temperature T at that state, because the increase of entropy is given by $ds = dh/T$. There is therefore no discontinuity at the saturation vapour line; the constant pressure lines start with a slope determined by the saturation temperature and curve upwards as the temperature increases.

Constant dryness fraction lines can be added by dividing each straight line in the wet region in the ratio x to $(1 - x)$ as before, and they are shown by the dashed curves in Fig. 8.14. Constant temperature lines are usually added in the superheat region; in the wet region they coincide with the constant pressure lines. As already explained in connection with the T–s diagram, the enthalpy becomes more nearly dependent on temperature alone as the amount of superheat increases. It follows, therefore, that on the h–s diagram constant temperature lines must tend towards the horizontal as shown in the figure. It should be noted that lines of constant degrees of superheat are sometimes used instead of lines of constant temperature, and that large-scale charts for practical use only show the most useful part of the diagram, enclosed by the dashed rectangle.

The fact already mentioned, that a reduction of pressure at constant enthalpy eventually results in the drying and superheating of a wet vapour, is clearly seen on the h–s diagram because the process is represented by a horizontal line.

8.4.3 Pressure–enthalpy diagram

A diagram showing the properties of a fluid on a pressure–enthalpy basis is of somewhat limited use, but as we shall refer to it later when considering refrigeration problems it deserves a brief mention here. Since pressure is one of the coordinates of this diagram, the main family of curves comprises those of constant temperature. In the liquid region they are substantially vertical (see Fig. 8.15) because the effect of pressure on the enthalpy is negligible. They then run horizontally across the saturated vapour line since they are also lines of constant pressure in the wet region. In the superheat region they fall steeply

Fig. 8.15
Pressure–enthalpy diagram

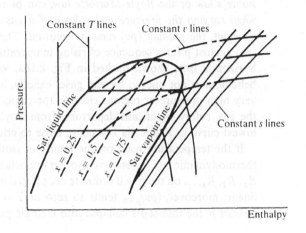

155

and approach the vertical for the same reason that they approach the horizontal on the enthalpy–entropy diagram. It is usual to add lines of constant volume in the wet and superheat regions, lines of constant dryness fraction in the wet region, and lines of constant entropy in the superheat region; these have the shape shown in Fig. 8.15.

8.5 Properties of a perfect gas

At pressures and temperatures usually obtaining in engineering applications, many substances are to be found in a state lying to the right of curve MNf in Fig. 8.5. In this section we shall restrict our attention to two regions in this field: (a) the region of high temperature, where the temperature is in excess of twice the absolute critical temperature; and (b) the region of low pressure, where the pressure is one atmosphere or less. The so-called 'permanent' gases, oxygen, hydrogen, nitrogen etc., all lie in the first region at ordinary working temperatures (the critical temperatures of the specified gases being 154.8 K, 33.99 K and 126.2 K respectively). The water vapour in the atmosphere lies in the second region, and is in fact superheated steam at very low pressure. The behaviour of substances in these two regions of states approximates very closely to that of a hypothetical substance known as a *perfect gas*. The perfect gas is a particularly useful concept because the properties are related by very simple equations. As before, we shall start by considering the relation between the primary properties p, v and T.

8.5.1 Equation of state of a perfect gas

The relation between p, v and temperature was first investigated by Robert Boyle in England, and somewhat later by Edme Mariotte in France, in the middle of the seventeenth century. The conclusion reached at the time, called *Boyle's law* or the *Boyle-Mariotte law*, can be recast into the following form: *when varying the pressure and volume of a gas while keeping the temperature constant, the product (pv) remains constant.* Therefore, if we plot products of (pv) against p for a sequence of rising temperatures, we should obtain a set of horizontal lines shown dashed in Fig. 8.16a. We now know that such ideal behaviour is not obeyed by real gases exactly, but we have to enter ranges of very high pressure or regions close to the critical pressure and temperature of the gas, before significant departures from Boyle's law can be observed. The lowest curve in Fig. 8.16a is a curve close to critical conditions.

If the temperature used on the family of isothermal curves is the absolute thermodynamic one, we observe another important fact. When the (pv) intercepts $R_1, R_2, R_3, \ldots$ on the $p = 0$ ordinate are plotted against T, the relation is exactly linear; moreover, $(pv)_{p=0}$ tends to zero at $T = 0$. Therefore, if we plot pv/T against p, the intercepts collapse into a single point R as shown in Fig. 8.16b.

Fig. 8.16
p–v–T data for gases

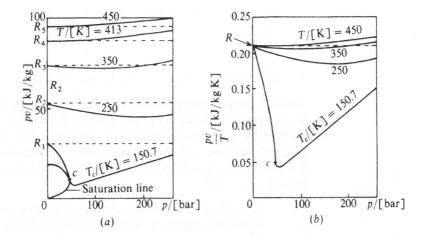

(a)

(b)

Mathematically this conclusion can be stated as*

$$\left.\frac{pv}{T}\right]_{p\to0} = R$$

It is clear from Fig. 8.16 that any equation relating p, v and T which will express the relation accurately will be complicated, particularly at high pressure and near critical conditions. Fortunately, for gases over a wide range of p and T, it is sufficiently accurate for most purposes to use the simple equation of state

$$pv = RT \tag{8.11}$$

If this equation were valid for all pressures and temperatures, the results depicted in Fig. 8.16b would collapse on to the single dashed line. The hypothetical substance which obeys the equation of state in this way is called a *perfect gas* or an *ideal gas*. The lower the pressure and the higher the temperature. the more nearly does a real gas approximate to a perfect gas. This can be explained on the basis of a theory as to the microscopic structure of a gas (see section 8.6). The constant R is called the *specific gas constant*, or often simply the *gas constant*.

If a mass m of gas is considered, the equation of state for a perfect gas becomes

$$pV = mRT$$

The product pV has the dimensions of energy, and in our system of units should be expressed in kJ. It is shown in equation (8.5) that when p is measured in bars (1 bar = 10^5 N/m^2 = 10^5 Pa) and V in m^2, pV must be multiplied by

---

* The perceptive student will note a possible logical flaw in the argument. What is this flaw? The clue lies in the fact that we have assumed that the thermodynamic temperature T can be measured independently of the notion of a perfect gas. In fact, except at extremely low and very high temperatures, the gas thermometer provides the only practical means of measuring an absolute thermodynamic temperature. The circularity in the argument can be avoided by proving that a perfect gas temperature θ_G defined by $pv = R\theta_G$ is identical with the absolute thermodynamic temperature T, and this is done formally at the end of section 7.6.1.

$10^5/10^3 = 100$ to obtain a result in kJ. The units of R which we shall employ are kJ/kg K.

8.5.2 Amount-of-substance and the molar gas constant

Although the gas constant differs for different gases, the equation of state can be generalised to include all perfect gases by making use of an important law of chemistry. Before doing so, however, we must introduce another measure of a quantity of matter: it is the *amount-of-substance*, symbolised by n, and its unit is the *mole*.* This was defined in 1971 as one of the base units of the SI by the following statement:

> *The mole is the amount-of-substance of a system which contains as many elementary entities as there are atoms in 0.012 kilogram of carbon 12. (When the mole is used, the elementary entities must be specified and may be atoms, molecules, ions, electrons, other particles, or specified groups of such particles.)*

In this book the entities will always be groups of identical atoms or molecules, or groups of specified mixtures of atoms and/or molecules (as with 'air'), as will be clear from the context. Furthermore, it will always be convenient to work in *kilomoles*, the unit symbol being *kmol*.

The number of entities in 1 kmol of carbon 12, each of mass $m(^{12}C)$, or by definition in 1 kmol of any other substance X having entities of mass $m(X)$, is

$$N_A = \frac{12\,kg}{m(^{12}C)}\,kmol^{-1}$$

The mass per kmol of any substance, called the *molar mass* $\tilde{m}$, is therefore given by

$$\tilde{m} = N_A m(X) = \left\{\frac{12\,kg}{m(^{12}C)}\,kmol^{-1}\right\}m(X) = \left\{\frac{m(X)}{\frac{1}{12}m(^{12}C)}\right\}\frac{kg}{kmol}$$

(The tilde (˜) will be used throughout this book to denote quantities per unit amount-of-substance, namely so-called *molar quantities*.) Several important points can be made as follows:

(a) N_A is the *Avogadro constant* which, according to the latest measurements, is equal to $6.022\,137 \times 10^{26}\,kmol^{-1}$

(b) The ratio $m(X)/\frac{1}{12}m(^{12}C)$ will be recognised as the definition of *relative atomic mass* A_r or *relative molecular mass* M_r, depending upon whether X is an atomic or a molecular species.

(c) The denominator $\frac{1}{12}m(^{12}C)$ is the unit of measurement on the 'atomic weight' scale. It is called the *unified atomic mass unit* and is symbolised by u.

(d) u is numerically equal to $1/N_A$, and hence $1\,u = 1.660\,565\,5 \times 10^{-27}\,kg$.

---

* At present the authors may be alone in hyphenating the term 'amount-of-substance', but the reasons for doing so are discussed in Appendix A. It will be interesting to see if it becomes standard practice.

(e) $\tilde{m}$, when measured in kg/kmol (or g/mol), is numerically equal to A_r or M_r but it is not dimensionless.

(f)   It follows from (e) that the mass m of an amount-of-substance n becomes

$$m = n\tilde{m} \tag{8.12}$$

Equation (8.11) can now be applied to a molar mass $\tilde{m}$, the volume of which is called the *molar volume* $\tilde{v}$, to yield

$$p\tilde{v} = \tilde{m}RT \tag{8.13a}$$

The fundamental law of chemistry required to generalise this equation of state is known as *Avogadro's law*. To explain the empirical fact that gases combine in simple integral ratios of volumes, Avogadro (1811) suggested that equal volumes of all gases contain the same number of molecules, when the volumes are measured under the same conditions of temperature and pressure. His argument can be found in any elementary textbook on chemistry. It is not exact in practice but, as with the equation of state, the accuracy of the law improves as the pressure of the gas is reduced. Now since a molar mass $\tilde{m}$ contains the same number of molecules whatever the gas (i.e. the Avogadro constant), $\tilde{v}$ must be the same for all gases at the same p and T. It follows from equation (8.13a) that the product $\tilde{m}R$ must be the same for all gases. This product is known as the *molar* (or *universal*) *gas constant*, and it will be symbolised by $\tilde{R}$. Equation (8.11) can therefore be written in a form which applies to all perfect gases, and approximately to all real gases, as

$$p\tilde{v} = \tilde{R}T \tag{8.13b}$$

Or, if V is the volume of an amount-of-substance n,

$$pV = n\tilde{R}T$$

Experiment shows that an average value for the volume of 1 kmol of the 'permanent' gases is 22.4141 m³ at standard atmospheric pressure (1 atm = 1.013 25 bar) and 0 °C. The value of $\tilde{R}$ is thus found to be

$$\tilde{R} = \frac{p\tilde{v}}{T} = \frac{100 \times 1.013\,25 \times 22.4141}{273.15}\ \frac{\text{kJ}}{\text{kmol K}} = 8.3145\frac{\text{kJ}}{\text{kmol K}}$$

The gas constant for any particular gas can be obtained from

$$R = \frac{\tilde{R}}{\tilde{m}}$$

For example, for oxygen O_2,

$$R = \frac{8.3145\ \text{kJ/kmol K}}{32\ \text{kg/kmol}} = 0.260\ \text{kJ/kg K}$$

8.5.3   *Other property relations for a perfect gas*

We have already noted in section 8.2.2 that a knowledge of the equation of state is not, by itself, sufficient to enable the other thermodynamic properties

159

to be determined. Some additional experimental data are necessary before u, h or s can be expressed in terms of two of the measurable properties p, v and T. It is possible to show that this is so for the perfect gas without difficulty. We have seen that the combination of the First and Second Laws gives rise to equation (6.12), i.e.

$$ds = \frac{1}{T}du + \frac{p}{T}dv$$

This is a general relation between thermodynamic properties which must be satisfied by any substance. If we now apply this general equation to a perfect gas, the equation of state enables p to be eliminated to give

$$ds = \frac{1}{T}du + \frac{R}{v}dv \qquad (8.14)$$

The expression for enthalpy is obtained more simply. From the definition of enthalpy we have

$$h = u + pv$$

which for a perfect gas becomes

$$h = u + RT \qquad (8.15)$$

It is evident from (8.14) and (8.15) that we require an expression for u in terms of v and T; when this is known, u can be eliminated from each of these equations to give expressions for s and h in terms of T and v.

It so happens that there is very simple expression for the internal energy of a perfect gas. First, we may note that the internal energy is a function only of temperature, i.e.

$$u = u(T) \qquad (8.16)$$

This can be shown to be a direct consequence of the equation of state of a perfect gas, but the proof is somewhat difficult and it has been dealt with at the beginning of section 7.6.1. Strictly, in view of that proof, experimental verification of equation (8.16) is superfluous, but it is worth while to record briefly the experiments of Gay-Lussac followed up by Joule in the first half of the nineteenth century. The principle followed is illustrated in Fig. 8.17, which shows two vessels which may be put into communication with one another by opening a valve. One vessel contains the pressurised gas under investigation, and the other is evacuated. The temperature of the gas is measured both before opening the valve, and after allowing the gas to reach equilibrium having

Fig. 8.17
The Joule experiment

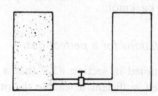

expanded freely into the evacuated vessel. If the vessels are perfectly insulated on the inside surfaces, we may conclude from the non-flow energy equation that the internal energies initially and finally are the same.

The internal energy u is a function of two independent properties, e.g. $u = u(T, v)$ or $u = u(T, p)$. Both p and v have changed in the expansion. If the temperature is found not to change, as was indeed observed by Joule, then it may be concluded that *the internal energy must be a function of temperature only*, as stated in equation (8.16); this conclusion is called *Joule's law*.

The weakness of Joule's experiments was that he surrounded his vessels by a water bath to serve as a detector of any temperature changes. Even if he had insulated the vessels themselves, their heat capacity would have masked even significant changes of gas temperature and therefore departures from Joule's law. For reasons which will be discussed in section 8.6.1, a gas in the so-called 'Joule free expansion' should display a small drop in temperature. If Joule's law is taken as valid, however, it follows that, in view of the equation of state $pv = RT$,

$$h = u + pv = u(T) + RT = h(T) \tag{8.17}$$

That is, *the enthalpy also must be a function of temperature only*. Subsequently, Joule and Thomson (Lord Kelvin) carried out steady-flow throttling experiments to verify this relation directly, and these did not suffer from the masking effects of heat capacity and defective insulation. The experiments, discussed in section 7.4.4, indeed revealed departures from the Joule-Thomson law $h = h(T)$, and consequently from Joule's law $u = u(T)$. The departures, however, were significant only in those regions of state in which departures from $pv = RT$ were significant also.

An important simplification follows from Joule's law, namely that a change of specific internal energy Δu can be expressed as a product of a temperature rise ΔT and c_v, *irrespective of whether the process is one at constant volume or not*. From equation (8.4a),

$$c_v = \left(\frac{\partial u}{\partial T}\right)_v$$

However, we can drop the partial notation and the subscript v because for the perfect gas u is a function only of T. Hence we obtain the result that

$$c_v = \frac{du}{dT} = f(T) \tag{8.18a}$$

It follows directly that

$$du = c_v\,dT \tag{8.18b}$$

and that the important simplification suggested above is indeed valid.

A similar simplification for enthalpy is obtained from equations (8.4b) and (8.17), from which it follows that the general expression

$$c_p = \left(\frac{\partial h}{\partial T}\right)_p$$

becomes for a perfect gas

$$c_p = \frac{\mathrm{d}h}{\mathrm{d}T} = \mathrm{f}(T) \tag{8.19a}$$

It follows again directly that

$$\mathrm{d}h = c_p \, \mathrm{d}T \tag{8.19b}$$

irrespective of whether the process is one at constant pressure or not.*

That c_p and c_v are related by a very simple expression can be deduced as follows. From the definition of enthalpy, $h = u + pv$, we can write

$$\mathrm{d}h = \mathrm{d}u + \mathrm{d}(pv)$$

which combined with equations (8.11), (8.18b) and (8.19b) becomes

$$c_p \, \mathrm{d}T = c_v \, \mathrm{d}T + R \, \mathrm{d}T$$

or

$$c_p - c_v = R \tag{8.20}$$

Equation (8.20) yields the important result that for any gas having the equation of state $pv = RT$, although c_v and c_p may each be functions of temperature, *their difference must always be constant and equal to the specific gas constant R.* Furthermore, because R is a positive quantity, c_p is always greater than c_v.

We may now recall that at the beginning of this sub-section we stated that a knowledge of the equation of state is not, by itself, sufficient for the calculation of the properties u, h or s. It should now be clear that the experimental data required for this purpose can be values of *either* c_v *or* c_p as functions of T; they are alternatives in view of the relation (8.20).

Although the variations of c_v and c_p with T are too large to be ignored completely, for many calculations it is sufficiently accurate to use a mean value over the temperature range of interest and treat it as a constant. Then, for example, equations (8.18) and (8.19) can be easily integrated to give

$$u_2 - u_1 = c_v(T_2 - T_1) \quad \text{and} \quad h_2 - h_1 = c_p(T_2 - T_1) \tag{8.21}$$

These equations are relations between properties and are valid for *any* process undergone by a perfect gas for which c_v and c_p can be regarded as constant. In certain non-flow processes, each side of the respective equations is equal to

---

* For the somewhat more advanced reader having some knowledge of partial differentials, the following way of looking at Joule's law, $u = u(T)$, and the equivalent Joule-Thomson law, $h = h(T)$, may be useful. Consider an infinitesimal process undergone by a real gas having two independent properties; then $u = u(T, v)$ and $h = h(T, p)$. It follows that

$$\mathrm{d}u = \left(\frac{\partial u}{\partial T}\right)_v \mathrm{d}T + \left(\frac{\partial u}{\partial v}\right)_T \mathrm{d}v \quad \text{and} \quad \mathrm{d}h = \left(\frac{\partial h}{\partial T}\right)_p \mathrm{d}T + \left(\frac{\partial h}{\partial p}\right)_T \mathrm{d}p$$

Joule's law implies that $(\partial u/\partial v)_T = 0$, and that $(\partial u/\partial T)_v$ can therefore be written as $(\mathrm{d}u/\mathrm{d}T)$, dropping the partial notation. The coefficient $(\mathrm{d}u/\mathrm{d}T)$ will be recognised as the specific heat capacity at constant volume, c_v, introduced in section 8.2.2, but with the Joule's law constraint that c_v is a function only of T. From the Joule-Thomson law, by a similar argument, we have $c_p = (\mathrm{d}h/\mathrm{d}T) = \mathrm{f}(T)$.

the heat transferred. More explicitly, when W is zero in a constant volume non-flow process, $Q = (u_2 - u_1)$ and therefore $Q_v = c_v(T_2 - T_1)$; and likewise for a reversible constant pressure non-flow process, $Q = (h_2 - h_1)$ and therefore $Q_p = c_p(T_2 - T_1)$. The expressions for Q_v and Q_p are seen to be consistent with the primitive definitions of c_v and c_p given in equation (8.3).

Unless otherwise stated we shall always assume that it is sufficiently accurate to use mean values of c_v and c_p, and in effect we shall be considering a perfect gas to be defined as one obeying the two equations

$$pv = RT \quad \text{and} \quad c_v \text{ (or } c_p) = \text{constant} \tag{8.22}$$

Furthermore, when taking a mean value of c_v or c_p from tables over a temperature range T_1 to T_2, we will adopt a simple approximate method as follows:

$$\text{mean } c = c \text{ at mean } T, \text{ where } \bar{T} = \tfrac{1}{2}(T_2 + T_1)$$

Another approximate method would be

$$\text{mean } c = \tfrac{1}{2}(c \text{ at } T_1 + c \text{ at } T_2)$$

These two mean values would only be equal, and identical with the true weighted mean value given by

$$\text{true mean } c = \frac{1}{T_2 - T_1} \int_1^2 c \, dT$$

if c varied linearly with T. Note that this expression for the true mean value is equivalent to the equally correct equations

$$\text{true mean } c_v = \frac{u_2 - u_1}{T_2 - T_1} \quad \text{and} \quad \text{true mean } c_p = \frac{h_2 - h_1}{T_2 - T_1}$$

To complete this section on the property relations of a perfect gas, we have to deduce expressions for the entropy in terms of any two of the measurable properties p, v and T. From equations (8.14) and (8.18) we have

$$ds = \frac{c_v}{T} dT + \frac{R}{v} dv$$

and hence

$$s_2 - s_1 = c_v \ln \frac{T_2}{T_1} + R \ln \frac{v_2}{v_1} \tag{8.23}$$

Unlike the internal energy and enthalpy, the entropy is a function of both temperature and volume. The relations between the entropy and the other two combinations of primary properties, p and T or p and v, can easily be obtained as follows. From the equation of state,

$$\frac{p_1 v_1}{T_1} = \frac{p_2 v_2}{T_2}$$

Substituting for v_2/v_1 in (8.23) we have

$$s_2 - s_1 = c_v \ln \frac{T_2}{T_1} + R \ln \left(\frac{p_1}{p_2} \frac{T_2}{T_1} \right)$$

$$= (c_v + R) \ln \frac{T_2}{T_1} - R \ln \frac{p_2}{p_1}$$

and using (8.20) this reduces to

$$s_2 - s_1 = c_p \ln \frac{T_2}{T_1} - R \ln \frac{p_2}{p_1} \qquad (8.24)$$

Similarly, by substituting for T_2/T_1 in (8.23) we get finally

$$s_2 - s_1 = c_v \ln \frac{p_2}{p_1} + c_p \ln \frac{v_2}{v_1} \qquad (8.25)$$

It may be helpful if the characteristics of a perfect gas are summarised as follows:

(a) The equation of state is $pv = RT$.

(b) A consequence of (a) is that $u = u(T)$.

(c) From (b) and the definition of c_v it follows that $c_v = \phi(T)$ or is constant, and that $du = c_v dT$ for any infinitesimal process.

(d) From (b) and the definition of enthalpy it follows that $h = h(T)$.

(e) From (d) and the definition of c_p it follows that $dh = c_p dT$ for any infinitesimal process, and that $c_p - c_v = R$.

(f) If a perfect gas is defined as also having constant specific heats, the following relations are valid irrespective of the process joining the end states 1 and 2:

$$u_2 - u_1 = c_v(T_2 - T_1)$$

$$h_2 - h_1 = c_p(T_2 - T_1)$$

$$s_2 - s_1 = c_v \ln \frac{T_2}{T_1} + R \ln \frac{v_2}{v_1}$$

$$= c_p \ln \frac{T_2}{T_1} - R \ln \frac{p_2}{p_1}$$

$$= c_v \ln \frac{p_2}{p_1} + c_p \ln \frac{v_2}{v_1}$$

8.5.4 Temperature–entropy diagram for a perfect gas

A T–s diagram showing the properties of a perfect gas usually consists simply of a family of constant pressure lines, as in Fig. 8.18. It may be constructed in the following manner. First a reference state is chosen for which the entropy is considered to be zero, e.g. a state defined by (p_0, T_0). The increase of entropy from this state to any other state at p_0, but at some other temperature T, can be found from equation (8.24). Thus in general

$$s_2 - s_1 = c_p \ln \frac{T_2}{T_1} - R \ln \frac{p_2}{p_1}$$

Fig. 8.18
Temperature–entropy
diagram for a perfect gas

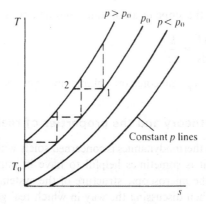

which in our case reduces to

$$s = c_p \ln \frac{T}{T_0} \tag{8.26}$$

The value of s can be found for several values of T, and the points so obtained can be joined up to form the constant pressure line p_0 on Fig. 8.18.

Now consider the isothermal compression process denoted by 1–2 on Fig. 8.18. The pressure increases from p_0 to p and, since T is constant, equation (8.24) reduces to

$$s_2 - s_1 = -R \ln \frac{p}{p_0}$$

It is evident that $(s_2 - s_1)$ is the same at any temperature. This suggests that any constant pressure line p can be found by stepping off horizontal distances from the line p_0, each equal to $R \ln(p/p_0)$. In this way a series of constant pressure lines can be rapidly constructed. It should be noticed that although the horizontal distance between any two constant pressure lines is the same at any temperature, the vertical distance increases with increase of temperature. This is due to the curvature of the constant pressure lines, and is clearly indicated by the dashed lines in the figure.

Constant volume lines could be added to the diagram, using equation (8.23). The general shape of the curves is the same except that they have a slightly steeper slope than the constant pressure lines at any given point. The slope of a constant pressure line can be found from the differential form of (8.26), i.e.

$$ds = \frac{c_p}{T} dT$$

and hence

$$\frac{dT}{ds} = \frac{T}{c_p}.$$

Similarly the slope of a constant volume line is

$$\frac{dT}{ds} = \frac{T}{c_v}$$

Since $c_v < c_p$, the constant volume line must have the steeper slope.

8.6   Kinetic theory and the properties of real gases

Although thermodynamics is concerned solely with the behaviour of macroscopic systems, it is sometimes helpful to have in mind a mechanical model which exhibits the microscopic structure of the system. Such a model is particularly helpful when discussing the way in which real gases differ from a perfect gas.

8.6.1   Kinetic theory of gases

On the kinetic theory of gases, a gas is conceived as a large number of minute hard particles, i.e. molecules, moving about at random with very high velocities. The pressure and temperature, which are terms used to describe the observed macroscopic phenomena, can then be explained in terms of the microscopic behaviour of the molecules. Thus pressure is regarded as the average force per unit area on the walls of the container due to bombardment by the molecules, and the absolute temperature is regarded as being proportional to the mean of the squares of the velocities of the molecules, i.e. to their average kinetic energy of translation. Any problem concerning the behaviour of gases is thereby reduced to one of mechanics. The kinetic theory has been developed to the point where most of the observed phenomena can be explained and predicted with the use of classical mechanics.* At points where the theory apparently breaks down, the difficulties can be resolved by the use of quantum mechanics.

The concept of a perfect gas can be shown to be a consequence of making the simplest assumptions about the molecules, and this part of the kinetic theory can be found in any elementary textbook on physics. The main assumptions are as follows:

(a)   The molecules are perfectly elastic and perfectly rigid, implying that no momentum or time is lost during collisions with the wall of the containing vessel.

(b)   The volume occupied by the molecules is negligible compared with the total volume.

(c)   The attractive forces between adjacent molecules are negligible.

The first assumption seems reasonable because no loss of pressure is observed when a gas is kept in a closed vessel over a long period, and one can only conclude that no loss of momentum occurs as the result of a vast number of collisions with the wall. The second assumption seems reasonable because a gas can be so easily compressed, and the last because a gas readily expands to

---

* For a clear account of the theory, see Ref. 14.

fill any space into which it is introduced. With these assumptions and the ordinary laws of mechanics, the characteristics of a perfect gas can be predicted quite simply; for example, we can obtain the form of the equation of state, Joule's law and Avogadro's law.

If assumptions (b) and (c) are not strictly true, it is easy to see why real gases behave more like a perfect gas as the pressure is reduced and the temperature raised. At the lower pressures the molecules are on the average further apart, so that the volume occupied by the molecules is a smaller proportion of the total volume and the attractive forces are less. At the higher temperatures the molecules are moving past one another with higher velocities; they are near one another for a shorter period, and consequently the attractive forces have less effect.

By making more realistic assumptions, the behaviour of real gases can also be predicted. For example, more accurate forms of the equation of state can be deduced by allowing for the volume occupied by the molecules and the attractive forces between them. The van der Waals equation provides a simple example, i.e.

$$\left(p + \frac{a}{v^2}\right)(v - b) = RT$$

Here R, a and b are constants which differ for different gases. The a/v^2 term takes account of the attractive forces, while b takes care of the volume of the molecules.

The departure from Joule's law is also easily explained by modifying assumptions (b) and (c). We know that the internal energy of a real gas depends slightly on a volume as well as on temperature, and that a slight drop of temperature must accompany a free expansion under adiabatic conditions. Let us see if this is to be expected of a van der Waals gas. An expression for the internal energy of a gas obeying the van der Waals equation of state is derived in Chapter 7 (equation (7.46)); in differential form it is

$$du = c_v \, dT + \frac{a}{v^2} \, dv$$

For an adiabatic free expansion the change in internal energy is zero, so that for this process we have

$$c_v \, dT = -\frac{a}{v^2} \, dv$$

The constant a, indicating the forces of attraction between the molecules, is always positive for gases. Therefore, since dv is positive in an expansion, dT must be negative. The physical explanation becomes clear when it is remembered that the internal energy includes both the kinetic energy of the molecules and the potential energy due to the attractive forces (section 2.4). If the analogy of a stretched spring is borne in mind, it is evident that the potential energy is increased by the expansion because the molecules are further apart. Since the internal energy is unchanged, the kinetic energy of the molecules must have decreased, and this is reflected in a drop of temperature.

Properties of Fluids

Fig. 8.19
Variation of c_v with
temperature for nitrogen at
ordinary pressures

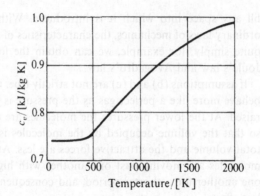

Before leaving the kinetic theory, it is worth noting the behaviour which it predicts for the specific heat capacities of perfect gases. According to this theory, c_v should be constant and equal to the increase in the total kinetic energy of the molecules per degree rise of temperature. The value predicted for c_v varies with the complexity of the molecules; for example, c_v is $3R/2$ for a monatomic gas and $5R/2$ for a diatomic gas. This difference is explained by the fact that monatomic gases possess translational kinetic energy only, whereas more complex molecules possess energy of rotation also, and all forms of energy are increased as the temperature is raised. For any given type of molecule, however, there is nothing in the simple kinetic theory to suggest why the increase in total energy per degree rise should be different at different temperatures.

For helium, of molar mass 4 kg/kmol, c_v becomes $(3/2)(8.3145/4)$ kJ/kg K = 3.118 kJ/kg K, and this prediction is in excellent agreement with observation at all temperatures. For nitrogen, a diatomic gas of molar mass 28 kg/kmol, c_v should be $(5/2)(8.3145/28)$ kJ/kg K = 0.742 kJ/kg K, which agrees with observation over a wide range of temperature up to about 400 K (Fig. 8.19). Above this temperature, however, c_v gradually increases owing to the fact that the molecules acquire vibrational energy as well as translational and rotational kinetic energy. This gradual rise cannot be predicted by the theory based on classical mechanics, although quantum theory does provide a satisfactory explanation. Quantum theory also suggests that at very low temperatures c_v for polyatomic gases should gradually drop to the value $3R/2$ valid for monatomic gases, implying thereby that rotational motion of the molecules ceases at such temperatures. This has in fact been confirmed for hydrogen at 40 K, but for heavier molecules this is expected to happen much closer to absolute zero and experimental evidence is lacking.

Finally, it is worth noting the physical meaning which the concept of entropy acquires when a model based on the microscopic structure of the system is considered. We have seen that any irreversibility results in an increase in the entropy of an adiabatic system; this is the important 'principle of increasing entropy'. On the microscopic view, an irreversibility is always associated with an increase in the disorderly motion of the molecules. For example, during an adiabatic expansion of a gas, internal viscous friction will result in a reduction in work done by the gas because the internal energy, i.e. random molecular energy, is higher in the final state than it would otherwise have been. Similarly, in an adiabatic expansion through a nozzle, viscous effects convert directional kinetic energy of a stream, which is fully available for doing work on say a turbine blade, into such random energy. Or again, two gases when mixed represent a higher degree of disorder than when they are separated, and we shall see in section 14.3 that there is an increase in entropy involved in an irreversible mixing process. In all natural processes irreversibilities are present, and there is a tendency to proceed towards a state of greater disorder. It is possible to establish a quantitative measure of disorder—in terms of a particular definition of the concept of probability—and then to derive a relation between entropy and this concept of probability. We are then led to a statistical interpretation of the Second Law and to a branch of the subject known as *statistical thermodynamics*.

8.6.2   Properties of real gases

Accurate equations of state are inconvenient for everyday calculations because they lead to unwieldy expressions. They are mostly used for the preparation of tables and diagrams of properties. When tables are not available, and for conditions where the perfect gas laws are too inaccurate, correction factors may be applied to the perfect gas relations. Thus the equation of state, for example, can be written as

$$pv = ZRT \tag{8.27}$$

where Z is the *compressibility factor*. The value of this factor depends upon the gas, and it is also a function of the pressure and temperature. The combination of $Z = \phi(p, T)$ and equation (8.27) is the complete equation of state. Charts have been prepared for the more common gases, showing Z plotted against pressure for various temperatures. Fig. 8.20 shows the compressibility chart for nitrogen. The advantages of plotting $Z = \phi(p, T)$ directly, are that (a) a much smaller range of values is required and (b) it shows at once how far the gas deviates from a perfect gas. The disadvantage is that, when v is one of the known parameters of state, a method of successive approximation is required to obtain the unknown property. For example, when v and T are given, p must be found from the perfect gas equation and a first approximation to Z obtained

Fig. 8.20
Compressibility factor for nitrogen

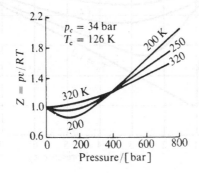

from the chart. Using this value of Z, a new value of p can be calculated from (8.27), a better approximation to Z obtained from the chart, and so on.

It so happens that the shape of the curves in the region to the right of the critical isothermal T_c in Fig. 8.5 is much the same for all gases, although the scales are different. This suggests that the scales might be brought into line if the properties were quoted as fractions of the critical values, i.e. as

$$p_R = \frac{p}{p_c}, \qquad v_R = \frac{v}{v_c}, \qquad T_R = \frac{T}{T_c}$$

p_R, v_R and T_R are referred to as the *reduced properties*. If the experimental p_R–v_R–T_R data for all gases were found to lie on the same set of curves, we could conclude that *any two gases at the same p_R and T_R have the same value of v_R*. This statement is known as the *law of corresponding states*. It can be expressed by saying that there is a functional relation

$$v_R = \phi(p_R, T_R)$$

which holds for all gases. It can be shown as follows that, if the law of corresponding states were true, it would be possible to compile a single set of curves expressing the variation of Z/Z_c with p_R and T_R which would hold for all gases. Thus since

$$Z = \frac{pv}{RT} = \frac{p_c v_c}{RT_c} \frac{p_R v_R}{T_R} = Z_c \left(\frac{p_R v_R}{T_R} \right)$$

then if $v_R = \phi(p_R, T_R)$ with ϕ the same for all gases, Z/Z_c must be a unique function of p_R and T_R. Unfortunately such a set of curves could not yield the necessary result that $Z \to 1$ as $p_R \to 0$ for all gases, because it is an experimental fact that Z_c differs for different gases. This is simply a way of saying that the law of corresponding states is not true.

Although too inaccurate to be used in this way, a modified form of the law is sometimes useful. The modified form asserts that $Z = f(p_R, T_R)$, with the function f the same for all gases. The *generalised compressibility chart* of Fig. 8.21 expresses the function f. Note that the chart implies that $Z_c = 0.22$ for

Fig. 8.21
Generalised compressibility
chart

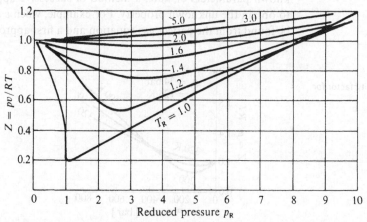

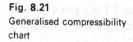

all gases, which is not the case, but at least it expresses the fact that $Z \rightarrow 1$ when $p_R \rightarrow 0$. Furthermore its use only involves a knowledge of p_c and T_c, and not of v_c which in general is not known accurately. (Critical data can be found from any tables of physical constants; see Ref. 33, for example.) Values of Z taken from the chart may deviate by as much as 10 per cent from the experimental value for a particular gas, but the chart is useful when very little experimental data are available for a substance, and also for showing when the assumption of perfect behaviour $(Z = 1)$ is no longer sufficiently accurate for a given purpose. Its use suffers from the disadvantage previously mentioned in relation to Fig. 8.20, that when v is one of the known parameters of state, successive approximation is necessary to determine the unknown property.

We have briefly indicated the method of dealing with the properties of real gases by referring to the p–v–T relation as an example. We cannot here go into the equivalent method for determining values of the other thermodynamic properties. This whole topic is of particular concern to chemical engineers, and a much fuller treatment can be found in textbooks on chemical engineering thermodynamics.*

At the beginning of section 8.5 we suggested that a gas can be treated as perfect when the temperature is more than twice the critical temperature, or the pressure is one atmosphere or less. Fig. 8.21 shows the latter criterion to be valid at all temperatures, since for most gases a pressure of one atmosphere corresponds to a reduced pressure of under 0.1. The first of these rough guides $(T_R > 2)$ is apparently not valid for all pressures. and ceases to be true for a reduced pressure greater than about 5. For most gases, however, this corresponds to a much higher pressure than is generally encountered in engineering applications, e.g. the corresponding pressure for nitrogen is 170 bar. For our purposes we shall always be in a position to assume that a gas has the characteristic equation $pv = RT$.

The second part of the definition of a perfect gas—that the specific heat capacities are constant—is not nearly such a good approximation. The slight variation of the specific heats with pressure can usually be neglected; indeed, in view of the decision to use the perfect gas equation of state, the specific heats must be treated as pure functions of temperature if we wish to be consistent (see section 8.5.2). Fig. 8.19 shows the variation of c_v with temperature for nitrogen. The corresponding curve for c_p can easily be obtained by using the relation (8.20) between the specific heats and the gas constant. If the approximate procedure of using a mean specific heat is not sufficiently accurate, some form of equation can be used such as

$$c_p = a + bT + cT^2$$

where a, b and c are constants. The change of enthalpy, for example, can then be obtained analytically as

$$h_2 - h_1 = \int_{T_1}^{T_2} (a + bT + cT^2)\,dT$$

---

* See Ref. 4, Chapter 4, and also Ref. 15.

Although air is strictly speaking a mixture of gases, its composition is sufficiently invariable for it to be treated as a single gas. Tables of properties of air which take account of the variation of c_p are available (Refs 12 and 9). The tables of Keenan and Kaye cover the range for which the $p-v-T$ data can be accurately represented by the perfect gas equation of state, so that the tables of internal energy and enthalpy require only one independent parameter— namely temperature. The internal energy and enthalpy are arbitrarily put equal to zero for all states at absolute zero of temperature.

The entropy of a perfect gas, however, has been shown to be a function of two independent properties. To avoid complicating the table by introducing a second independent parameter, the entropy is not given directly for all states, but a new variable ϕ is tabulated in its place. The differential form of equation (8.24) is

$$ds = \frac{c_p}{T} dT - \frac{R}{p} dp$$

When the reference state is chosen at absolute zero and some pressure p_0, the entropy at any state defined by (p_1, T_1) is given by

$$s_1 = \int_0^{T_1} \frac{c_p}{T} dT - R \int_{p_0}^{p_1} \frac{dp}{p}$$

$$= \int_0^{T_1} \frac{c_p}{T} dT - R \ln \frac{p_1}{p_0}$$

The change of entropy between any two states 1 and 2 is therefore given by

$$s_2 - s_1 = \int_0^{T_2} \frac{c_p}{T} dT - \int_0^{T_1} \frac{c_p}{T} dT - R \ln \frac{p_2}{p_1}$$

Finally, if we write

$$\phi = \int_0^T \frac{c_p}{T} dT$$

the change of entropy becomes

$$s_2 - s_1 = \phi_2 - \phi_1 - R \ln \frac{p_2}{p_1} \tag{8.28}$$

The variable ϕ is a function of temperature only and may therefore be tabulated in the same way as the internal energy and enthalpy. Equation (8.28) is used when the change of entropy between two states is required. We shall not make use of such tables in subsequent chapters; for our purpose it will be sufficiently accurate to use a mean c_p.

9

Non-Flow Processes

Non-flow processes have been classified and analysed in general terms in Chapter 3. The processes were characterised by (a) the volume, pressure or temperature remaining constant; (b) the heat transfer being zero; or (c) the pressure and volume varying in such a way that pv^n is constant. Most non-flow processes of practical interest approximate to one, or a succession, of these processes.

In this chapter we shall apply the analysis to closed systems consisting of particular fluids. Each process will be dealt with assuming the fluid to be (a) a vapour and (b) a perfect gas with constant specific heat capacities. Tables of properties must be used in the first case, but in the second the analysis can be carried out using algebraic relations. Steam is used as an example of a vapour, and we shall make use of the abridged tables of Ref. 17. Air is considered as an example of a perfect gas, and the following values will be used for c_p and R:

$$c_p = 1.005 \text{ kJ}/\text{kg K}, \qquad R = 0.287 \text{ kJ}/\text{kg K}$$

It follows from equation (8.20) that

$$c_v = 0.718 \text{ kJ}/\text{kg K}$$

For a summary of the relations between the properties of a perfect gas, which are valid for any process whether reversible or irreversible, the reader is referred to the end of section 8.5.3.

9.1   Constant volume process

If there is no paddle work, the energy equation for unit mass of any fluid undergoing a constant volume process is

$$Q = u_2 - u_1$$

When the fluid is a perfect gas this becomes

$$Q = c_v(T_2 - T_1)$$

For a perfect gas we also have the following relations between properties which are valid for any two states of the same volume. From the equation of state,

$$\frac{p_1}{T_1} = \frac{p_2}{T_2}$$

and from the definition of entropy,

$$s_2 - s_1 = \int_1^2 \left(\frac{dQ}{T}\right)_{rev} = \int_1^2 \frac{c_v}{T} dT = c_v \ln \frac{T_2}{T_1}$$

The latter equation can also be obtained by putting $v_2 = v_1$ in the general expression for the entropy change, equation (8.23).

Example 9.1 A fluid in a closed vessel of fixed volume $0.14 \, \text{m}^3$, exerts a pressure of $10 \, \text{bar}$ at $250 \, °\text{C}$. If the vessel is cooled so that the pressure falls to $3.5 \, \text{bar}$, determine the final temperature, heat transfer and change of entropy.

(a) *Steam* (Fig. 9.1a)
The first step is to find the mass of fluid in the system. Since T_1 is greater than the saturation temperature corresponding to p_1, the vapour is initially superheated. Using the superheat table we find $v_1 = 0.2328 \, \text{m}^3/\text{kg}$.
Since $V = 0.14 \, \text{m}^3$,

$$m = \frac{V}{v_1} = \frac{0.14}{0.2328} = 0.6014 \, \text{kg}$$

The vapour must be wet in its final state because mv_g is $0.6014 \times 0.5241 = 0.3152 \, \text{m}^3$, which is greater than $0.14 \, \text{m}^3$. The temperature must therefore be the saturation temperature corresponding to p_2, i.e. $t_2 = 138.9 \, °\text{C}$.
The dryness fraction can be found from equation (8.10), i.e.

$$x_2 = \frac{V}{mv_{g2}} = \frac{0.14}{0.3152} = 0.444$$

NB: If the accurate equation (8.9) is used, x_2 because 0.443.
From the superheat table:

$$u_1 = 2711 \, \text{kJ/kg}$$

From the saturation table:

$$u_2 = u_{f2} + x_2 u_{fg2} = 584 + 0.444(2549 - 584) = 1457 \, \text{kJ/kg}$$

Fig. 9.1a

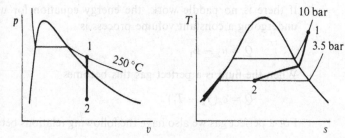

174

Fig. 9.1b

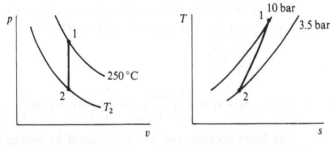

Heat transfer:

$$Q = m(u_2 - u_1) = 0.6014(1457 - 2711) = -754 \text{ kJ}$$

From the superheat table $s_1 = 6.926 \text{ kJ/kg K}$, and from the saturation table:

$$s_2 = s_{f2} + x_2 s_{fg2} = 1.727 + (0.444 \times 5.214) = 4.042 \text{ kJ/kg K}$$

Change of entropy:

$$S_2 - S_1 = m(s_2 - s_1) = 0.6014(4.042 - 6.926) = -1.734 \text{ kJ/K}$$

(b) *Air* (Fig. 9.1b)
Mass of gas:

$$m = \frac{p_1 V}{RT_1} = \frac{100 \times 10 \times 0.14}{0.287(250 + 273)} = 0.933 \text{ kg}$$

Final temperature:

$$T_2 = \frac{p_2}{p_1} T_1 = \frac{3.5}{10} 523 = 183 \text{ K}$$

Heat transfer:

$$Q = mc_v(T_2 - T_1) = 0.933 \times 0.718(183 - 523) = -228 \text{ kJ}$$

Change of entropy:

$$S_2 - S_1 = mc_v \ln \frac{T_2}{T_1} = 0.933 \times 0.718 \ln \frac{183}{523} = -0.703 \text{ kJ/K}$$

9.2 Constant pressure process

For a reversible constant pressure process undergone by unit mass of any fluid,

$$W = -p \int_1^2 dv = -p(v_2 - v_1)$$

$$Q = (u_2 - u_1) - W = (u_2 - u_1) + p(v_2 - v_1) = h_2 - h_1$$

When the fluid is a perfect gas,

$$W = -R(T_2 - T_1)$$

$$Q = c_p(T_2 - T_1)$$

For a perfect gas we also have the following relations between properties which are valid for any two states of the same pressure:

$$\frac{v_1}{T_1} = \frac{v_2}{T_2}$$

$$s_2 - s_1 = \int_1^2 \left(\frac{dQ}{T}\right)_{rev} = \int_1^2 \frac{c_p}{T} dT = c_p \ln \frac{T_2}{T_1}$$

The latter equation can also be obtained by putting $p_2 = p_1$ in the general expression for the entropy change, equation (8.24).

Example 9.2 A mass of 0.2 kg of fluid, initially at a temperature of 165 °C, expands reversibly at a constant pressure of 7 bar until the volume is doubled. Find the final temperature, work and heat transfers in two cases: (a) when the fluid is steam with an initial dryness fraction of 0.7, (b) when the fluid is air.

(a) *Steam* (Fig. 9.2a)
Initial specific volume:

$$v_1 = x_1 v_{g1} = 0.7 \times 0.2728 = 0.191 \text{ m}^3/\text{kg}$$

Final specific volume:

$$v_2 = 2v_1 = 0.382 \text{ m}^3/\text{kg}$$

Since $v_2 > v_{g2}$, the vapour must be superheated in its final state. From the superheat table by interpolation, the final temperature is

$$T_2 = 300 + \frac{0.382 - 0.3714}{0.4058 - 0.3714} 50 = 315 \,^\circ\text{C}$$

Work transfer:

$$W = -mp(v_2 - v_1) = -0.2 \times 100 \times 7(0.382 - 0.191) = -26.7 \text{ kJ}$$

From the saturation table:

$$h_1 = h_{f1} + x_1 h_{fg1} = 697 + (0.7 \times 2067) = 2144 \text{ kJ/kg}$$

From the superheat table, by interpolation:

$$h_2 = 3060 + \frac{15}{50}(3164 - 3060) = 3091 \text{ kJ/kg}$$

Fig. 9.2a

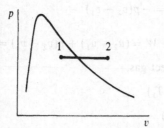
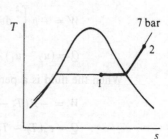

Fig. 9.2b

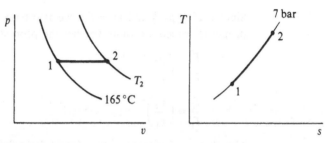

Heat transfer:

$$Q = m(h_2 - h_1) = 0.2(3091 - 2144) = 189 \text{ kJ}$$

(b) *Air* (Fig. 9.2b)
Initial volume:

$$V_1 = \frac{mRT_1}{p_1} = \frac{0.2 \times 0.287 \times 438}{100 \times 7} = 0.035\,92 \text{ m}^3$$

Final volume:

$$V_2 = 2V_1 = 0.071\,84 \text{ m}^3$$

Final temperature:

$$T_2 = \frac{V_2}{V_1} T_1 = 876 \text{ K}$$

Work transfer:

$$W = -p(V_2 - V_1) = -100 \times 7 \times 0.035\,92 = -25.1 \text{ kJ}$$

Heat transfer:

$$Q = mc_p(T_2 - T_1) = 0.2 \times 1.005 \times 438 = 88.0 \text{ kJ}$$

9.3 Polytropic process

When a polytropic process is reversible, the work transfer is given by
equation (3.12), i.e.

$$W = \frac{(p_2 v_2 - p_1 v_1)}{n - 1} \tag{9.1}$$

Therefore, from the energy equation,

$$Q = (u_2 - u_1) - \frac{(p_2 v_2 - p_1 v_1)}{n - 1}$$

When the fluid is a perfect gas, these expressions can be written as

$$W = \frac{R}{n - 1}(T_2 - T_1)$$

$$Q = c_v(T_2 - T_1) - \frac{R}{n - 1}(T_2 - T_1) = \left(c_v - \frac{R}{n - 1}\right)(T_2 - T_1)$$

Since $p_1 v_1^n = p_2 v_2^n$ and $pv = RT$, we also have the following relations between properties which are valid whether the process is reversible or irreversible:

$$\frac{T_2}{T_1} = \left(\frac{p_2}{p_1}\right)^{(n-1)/n} \tag{9.2}$$

$$\frac{T_2}{T_1} = \left(\frac{v_2}{v_1}\right)^{1-n} \tag{9.3}$$

The change of entropy is best found from first principles as in the following example.

Example 9.3 A mass of 0.9 kg of fluid, initially at a pressure of 15 bar and a temperature of 250°C, expands reversibly and polytropically to 1.5 bar. Find the final temperature, work and heat transfers, and change of entropy, if the index of expansion is 1.25.

(a) *Steam* (Fig. 9.3a)
From the superheat table:

$$v_1 = 0.152 \, \text{m}^3/\text{kg}$$

Final specific volume:

$$v_2 = v_1 \left(\frac{p_1}{p_2}\right)^{1/n} = 0.1520 \times 10^{1/1.25} = 0.959 \, \text{m}^3/\text{kg}$$

v_{g2} is $1.159 \, \text{m}^3/\text{kg}$ so that the vapour is wet in the final state, and the temperature is the saturation value corresponding to 1.5 bar, i.e. $T_2 = 111.4°C$.
Dryness fraction:

$$x_2 = \frac{v_2}{v_{g2}} = \frac{0.959}{1.159} = 0.827$$

Work transfer:

$$W = \frac{m}{n-1}(p_2 v_2 - p_1 v_1)$$

$$= \frac{100 \times 0.9}{0.25}\{(1.5 \times 0.959) - (15 \times 0.152)\} = -303 \, \text{kJ}$$

Fig. 9.3a

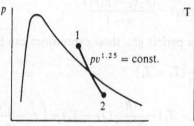

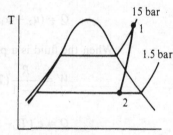

From the superheat table:

$$u_1 = 2697 \text{ kJ/kg}$$

From the saturation table:

$$u_2 = u_{f2} + x_2 u_{fg2} = 467 + 0.827(2519 - 467) = 2164 \text{ kJ/kg}$$

Heat transfer:

$$Q = m(u_2 - u_1) - W = 0.9(2164 - 2697) + 303 = -177 \text{ kJ}$$
$$s_1 = 6.711 \text{ kJ/kg K}$$
$$s_2 = s_{f2} + x_2 s_{fg2} = 1.434 + (0.827 \times 5.789) = 6.222 \text{ kJ/kg K}$$

Change of entropy:

$$S_2 - S_1 = m(s_2 - s_1) = 0.9(6.222 - 6.711) = -0.440 \text{ kJ/K}$$

(b) *Air* (Fig. 9.3b)
Final temperature:

$$T_2 = T_1\left(\frac{p_2}{p_1}\right)^{(n-1)/n} = 523\left(\frac{1}{10}\right)^{0.25/1.25} = 330 \text{ K}$$

Work transfer:

$$W = \frac{mR}{n-1}(T_2 - T_1) = \frac{0.9 \times 0.287}{0.25}(330 - 523) = -199 \text{ kJ}$$

Heat transfer:

$$Q = mc_v(T_2 - T_1) - W$$
$$= \{0.9 \times 0.718(330 - 523)\} + 199 = 74.3 \text{ kJ}$$

Change of entropy, from first principles:

$$ds = \left(\frac{dQ}{T}\right)_{\text{rev}} = \frac{1}{T}du + \frac{p}{T}dv = \frac{c_v}{T}dT + \frac{R}{v}dv \quad \text{(for perfect gas)}$$

$$s_2 - s_1 = c_v \ln\frac{T_2}{T_1} + R\ln\frac{v_2}{v_1}$$

$$= c_v \ln\frac{T_2}{T_1} - \frac{R}{n-1}\ln\frac{T_2}{T_1} \quad \text{(using (9.3))}$$

Fig. 9.3b

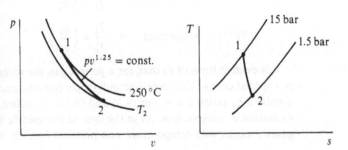

$$= \left(c_v - \frac{R}{n-1} \right) \ln \frac{T_2}{T_1}$$

$$S_2 - S_1 = 0.9 \left(0.718 - \frac{0.287}{0.25} \right) \ln \frac{330}{523} = 0.178 \text{ kJ/K}$$

9.4 Adiabatic process

For a fluid undergoing an adiabatic process the energy equation per unit mass reduces to

$$W = (u_2 - u_1)$$

When the fluid is a perfect gas,

$$W = c_v (T_2 - T_1)$$

For a perfect gas undergoing a reversible adiabatic (i.e. isentropic) process, we can deduce the following relations between properties:

$$0 = c_v \, dT + p \, dv \quad \text{(First Law)}$$

$$R \, dT = p \, dv + v \, dp \quad \text{(equation of state)}$$

Eliminating dT from these two equations, we obtain

$$0 = \left(1 + \frac{c_v}{R} \right) p \, dv + \frac{c_v}{R} v \, dp$$

$$= c_p p \, dv + c_v v \, dp \quad \text{(since } R = c_p - c_v\text{)}$$

Writing $c_p/c_v = \gamma$, this reduces to

$$\gamma \frac{dv}{v} + \frac{dp}{p} = 0$$

and on integration,

$$\gamma \ln v + \ln p = \text{constant}$$

$$pv^\gamma = \text{constant} \tag{9.4}$$

Since we also have $pv/T = \text{constant}$, we can eliminate v and p in turn to give

$$Tp^{(1-\gamma)/\gamma} = \text{constant} \quad \text{or} \quad \frac{T_2}{T_1} = \left(\frac{p_2}{p_1} \right)^{(\gamma-1)/\gamma} \tag{9.5}$$

$$Tv^{\gamma-1} = \text{constant} \quad \text{or} \quad \frac{T_2}{T_1} = \left(\frac{v_2}{v_1} \right)^{1-\gamma} \tag{9.6}$$

It is evident from (9.4) that, for a perfect gas, the reversible adiabatic process is a special case of the reversible polytropic process, and (9.5) and (9.6) can be obtained by putting $n = \gamma$ in (9.2) and (9.3). γ is called the *index of isentropic expansion* or *compression*. As in the case of the specific heat capacities, for real gases γ varies with temperature and pressure (mainly with the former), but a mean value can be used for most purposes. If we put $n = \gamma$ in the expression for the work transfer in a polytropic process, we have

$$W = \frac{R}{\gamma - 1}(T_2 - T_1)$$

This can easily be shown to be identical with the expression already derived, as follows:

$$\frac{R}{\gamma - 1}(T_2 - T_1) = \frac{c_p - c_v}{c_p/c_v - 1}(T_2 - T_1) = c_v(T_2 - T_1)$$

In a reversible adiabatic process $s_2 = s_1$, and equation (9.4) could have been obtained by putting this result in the general expression (8.25). If this is done we have

$$c_p \ln\frac{v_2}{v_1} + c_v \ln\frac{p_2}{p_1} = 0$$

and hence

$$\frac{p_2}{p_1} = \left(\frac{v_1}{v_2}\right)^{\gamma}$$

Since the process is reversible, the foregoing relation applies to any pair of states between the end states, and consequently throughout the process

$$pv^{\gamma} = \text{constant}$$

Example 9.4   Assuming the process in Example 9.3 is isentropic (instead of polytropic with index 1.25), find the final temperature and the work done.

(a)   *Steam* (Fig. 9.4a)
To find the final state we make use of the fact that $s_2 = s_1$, and from the superheat table, $s_1 = 6.711$ kJ/kg K. Since $s_1 = s_2 < s_{g2}$, the vapour must be wet in the final state, and therefore $T_2 = 111.4\,°C$ (i.e. T_s at p_2).
From

$$s_1 = s_2 = s_{f2} + x_2 s_{fg2}$$

we have

$$x_2 = \frac{s_2 - s_{f2}}{s_{fg2}} = \frac{6.711 - 1.434}{5.789} = 0.912$$

Fig. 9.4a

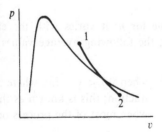

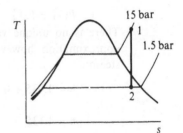

Fig. 9.4b

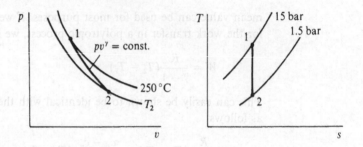

From the superheat table:

$$u_1 = 2697 \text{ kJ/kg}$$

From the saturation table:

$$u_2 = u_{f2} + x_2 u_{fg2} = 467 + (0.912 \times 2052) = 2338 \text{ kJ/kg}$$

Work transfer:

$$W = m(u_2 - u_1) = 0.9(2338 - 2697) = -323 \text{ kJ}$$

(b) *Air* (Fig. 9.4b)

For air,

$$\gamma = \frac{c_p}{c_v} = \frac{1.005}{0.718} = 1.40$$

Final temperature:

$$T_2 = T_1 \left(\frac{p_2}{p_1}\right)^{(\gamma-1)/\gamma} = 523\left(\frac{1}{10}\right)^{1/3.5} = 271 \text{ K}$$

Work transfer:

$$W = mc_v(T_2 - T_1) = 0.9 \times 0.718(271 - 523) = -163 \text{ kJ}$$

For a vapour, there is no simple and unique relation between p and v which applies to every isentropic expansion and compression. Nevertheless it is sometimes convenient to assume an approximate relation of the polytropic form $pv^n = $ constant; n then becomes the index of isentropic expansion or compression, although it is not necessarily equal to the ratio c_p/c_v. Indeed, if part of the process occurs in the wet region, where $c_p = \infty$, this ratio has no meaning. The value of n can be found, as in the following example, by substituting the values of p and v at the end states in the expression

$$p_1 v_1^n = p_2 v_2^n$$

There is no unique value for n; it varies with the end states. As a rough approximation, however, the following average values of n may be used for steam:

$$n = 1.035 + 0.1x \quad \text{when } 0.7 < x < 1.0, \text{ where } x \text{ is the initial dryness fraction; this is known as the } \textit{Zeuner's equation}$$

$$n = 1.135 \quad \text{when most of the process occurs in the wet region}$$

with the steam initially saturated or slightly superheated

$n = 1.30$ when the process occurs mostly in the superheat
region

Example 9.5   Steam, initially dry saturated, expands isentropically from a pressure of 15 bar
to 0.15 bar. Find the index of isentropic expansion.

We have (Fig. 9.5)

$$s_2 = s_1 = s_{g1} = 6.445 \text{ kJ/kg K}$$

$$x_2 = \frac{s_2 - s_{f2}}{s_{fg2}} = \frac{6.445 - 0.755}{7.254} = 0.784$$

$$v_1 = v_{g1} = 0.1317 \text{ m}^3/\text{kg}$$

$$v_2 = x_2 v_{g2} = 0.784 \times 10.06 = 7.887 \text{ m}^3/\text{kg}$$

If we can write $p_1 v_1^n = p_2 v_2^n$, then

$$15 \times 0.1317^n = 0.15 \times 7.887^n$$

from which $n = 1.125$.

Fig. 9.5

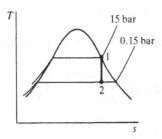

This approximate method of treating the isentropic expansion or compression
of a vapour as polytropic will be found useful in Chapter 18. Although it must
be remembered that the isentropic process is only strictly polytropic when the
fluid is a perfect gas with constant specific heats, when the vapour is *steam* and
superheated throughout the process the approximation is very close to actual
behaviour, as is indicated by the following. It has been found that over a wide
field in the superheat region the u-p-v data are related by the simple equation

$$u - B = \frac{1}{n-1} p(v - C) \tag{9.7}$$

where the empirical constants n, B and C are

$$n = 1.3, \qquad B = 1943 \text{ kJ/kg}, \qquad C = -0.000\,175 \text{ m}^3/\text{kg}$$

This equation was originally proposed by H. L. Callendar. By inspection of the
superheat table it can be seen that, at pressures below 100 bar, C is always less

than 1 per cent of v. For many engineering purposes C can be ignored, and thus

$$u - B = \frac{1}{n-1}pv \tag{9.8}$$

From equation (9.8) it is possible to deduce rigorously* that the following set of relations must hold for an *isentropic* process:

$$
\begin{aligned}
pv^n &= \text{constant}, && p/T^{n/(n-1)} = \text{constant} \\
Tv^{(n-1)} &= \text{constant}, && pv/T = \text{constant}
\end{aligned}
\tag{9.9}
$$

n is the constant having the value 1.3, and in this context is the index of isentropic expansion or compression. The last equation in (9.9) does not imply that the perfect gas equation is applicable, because it only applies to an isentropic process and the constant pv/T is different for different isentropic processes (i.e. it depends on the value of s).

Finally we may note that since $h = u + pv$, equation (9.8) can be written

$$h - B = \frac{n}{n-1}pv \tag{9.10}$$

It follows that for superheated steam any change in enthalpy is given very closely by

$$h_2 - h_1 = \frac{n}{n-1}(p_2 v_2 - p_1 v_1)$$

And for an *isentropic* process, for which we have seen that $p_2 v_2^n = p_1 v_1^n$, this becomes

$$h_2 - h_1 = \frac{n}{n-1}p_1 v_1 \left\{ \left(\frac{p_2}{p_1} \right)^{(n-1)/n} - 1 \right\}$$

$$= (h_1 - B) \left\{ \left(\frac{p_2}{p_1} \right)^{(n-1)/n} - 1 \right\} \tag{9.11}$$

Relations (9.9) and (9.11) are particularly useful when dealing with supersaturated states, discussed in section 18.2, which are not covered by steam tables.

9.5 Isothermal process

For unit mass of any fluid undergoing a reversible isothermal process,

$$Q = T(s_2 - s_1)$$

and hence from the energy equation,

$$W = (u_2 - u_1) - Q = (u_2 - u_1) - T(s_2 - s_1)$$

When the fluid is a perfect gas (for which u is a function only of temperature),

---

* This is a useful exercise for students who have studied Chapter 7; the main equations required are (7.13), (7.14), (7.23) and (7.24).

$u_2 = u_1$ and it follows from the energy equation that

$$Q = -W$$

Making use of the equation of state, we can find W from $\int p\,dv$ if the process is reversible. Thus for a reversible isothermal process undergone by a perfect gas,

$$Q = -W = \int_1^2 p\,dv = RT\int_1^2 \frac{dv}{v} = RT\ln\frac{v_2}{v_1} \qquad (9.12)$$

For a perfect gas we also have the following relations between properties which are valid for any two states of the same temperature:

$$p_1 v_1 = p_2 v_2$$

$$s_2 - s_1 = \frac{1}{T}\int_1^2 (dQ)_{rev} = R\ln\frac{v_2}{v_1} \quad \text{(from equation (9.12))}$$

The latter equation can also be obtained by putting $T_2 = T_1$ in the general expression for the entropy change. Since $p_1 v_1 = p_2 v_2$, equation (9.12) can be written alternatively as

$$Q = -W = -RT\ln\frac{p_2}{p_1} \qquad (9.13)$$

and hence also

$$s_2 - s_1 = -R\ln\frac{p_2}{p_1}$$

It is evident that for a perfect gas the reversible isothermal process is another special case of a reversible polytropic process, i.e. one for which $n = 1$. Note that we cannot put $n = 1$ in equation (9.1) to obtain the work transfer—the reason being that the integral of dv/v^n is $\ln v$ when $n = 1$.

Example 9.6   A fluid, initially at 155.5 °C and 1 bar, is compressed reversibly and isothermally to a state where the specific volume is 0.28 m³/kg. Find the change of internal energy, change of entropy, and heat and work transfers, per kg of fluid.

(a) *Steam* (Fig. 9.6a)
From the superheat table, by interpolation:

$$u_1 = 2583 + \frac{5.5}{50}\,76 = 2591\ \text{kJ/kg}$$

Since $v_2 = 0.28\ \text{m}^3/\text{kg}$ is less than the specific volume of saturated vapour at 155.5 °C, the vapour must be wet in its final state. Hence

$$x_2 = \frac{v_2}{v_{g2}} = \frac{0.28}{0.3427} = 0.817$$

$$u_2 = u_{f2} + x_2 u_{fg2} = 655 + (0.817 \times 1910) = 2215\ \text{kJ/kg}$$

185

Fig. 9.6a

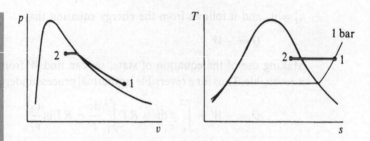

Change of internal energy:

$$u_2 - u_1 = 2215 - 2591 = -376 \text{ kJ/kg}$$

From the superheat table, by interpolation:

$$s_1 = 7.614 + \frac{5.5}{50} 0.220 = 7.638 \text{ kJ/kg K}$$

Also:

$$s_2 = s_{f2} + x_2 s_{fg2} = 1.897 + (0.817 \times 4.893) = 5.895 \text{ kJ/kg K}$$

Change of entropy:

$$s_2 - s_1 = 5.895 - 7.638 = -1.743 \text{ kJ/kg K}$$

Heat transfer:

$$Q = T(s_2 - s_1) = 428.5(-1.743) = -747 \text{ kJ/kg}$$

Work transfer:

$$W = (u_2 - u_1) - Q = -376 + 747 = 371 \text{ kJ/kg}$$

(b) *Air* (Fig. 9.6b)

Change of internal energy is zero.

   Initial specific volume:

$$v_1 = \frac{RT}{p_1} = \frac{0.287 \times 428.5}{100 \times 1.0} = 1.230 \text{ m}^3/\text{kg}$$

Change of entropy:

$$s_2 - s_1 = R \ln \frac{v_2}{v_1} = 0.287 \ln \frac{0.28}{1.23} = -0.425 \text{ kJ/kg K}$$

Fig. 9.6b

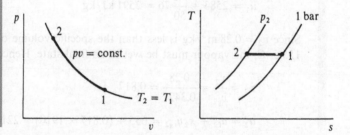

Heat transfer:

$$Q = T(s_2 - s_1) = 428.5(-0.425) = -182 \, \text{kJ/kg}$$

Work transfer:

$$W = -Q = 182 \, \text{kJ/kg}$$

9.6 Irreversibility and the free expansion

We noted in section 5.4.1 that most practical non-flow processes can be assumed reversible. Nevertheless it is worth reviewing our position when the processes we have considered are irreversible:

(a) Constant volume, constant pressure, polytropic and isothermal processes: when these are irreversible we must know either W or Q in addition to the end states before the unknown can be determined.

(b) Adiabatic process: when this is irreversible the work transfer can be predicted if the end states are known, but when it is reversible only *one* property in the final state need be known. The adiabatic process differs from the others in that only one property in the final state can be varied independently; the final state then depends upon the amount of irreversibility present.

To illustrate the principle of increasing entropy, we shall consider as a final example the Joule free expansion for a perfect gas (see section 8.5.3). In this case both Q and W are zero and the entropy of the gas must increase because the process is irreversible and adiabatic.

Example 9.7 Air, initially at a pressure and temperature of 3.5 bar and 15 °C, is enclosed in a vessel 0.06 m³ in volume. The air is allowed to expand into an evacuated vessel also 0.06 m³ in volume. If the process is adiabatic, find the change in entropy of the air.

The mass of air in the system (Fig. 9.7) is given by

$$m = \frac{p_1 V_1}{R T_1} = \frac{100 \times 3.5 \times 0.06}{0.287 \times 288} = 0.254 \, \text{kg}$$

From the energy equation, since $W = Q = 0$, $u_2 - u_1 = 0$. If air can be treated as a perfect gas, $T_2 - T_1 = 0$ also. To find the change of entropy,

Fig. 9.7

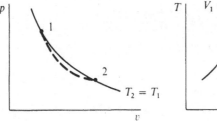
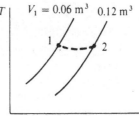

either we can use the general expression (8.23), or, if we wish to work directly from the equation defining entropy, $ds = (dQ/T)_{rev}$, we can adopt the following procedure. The irreversible process can be 'replaced' by any suitable reversible path which joins the two given states defined by ($V_1 = 0.06\,\text{m}^3$, $T_1 = 288$ K) and ($V_2 = 0.12\,\text{m}^3$, $T_2 = 288$ K) and for which Q can be easily calculated. The obvious choice is a reversible isothermal path; then using equation (9.12) we have

$$s_2 - s_1 = \frac{1}{T}\int_1^2 (dQ)_{rev} = R \ln \frac{v_2}{v_1}$$

Since $v_2/v_1 = V_2/V_1 = 2$, we get finally

$$S_2 - S_1 = mR \ln \frac{v_2}{v_1} = 0.254 \times 0.287 \ln 2 = 0.0505\,\text{kJ/K}$$

10

Flow Processes

In Chapter 4 it was shown how the heat and work crossing the boundary during a steady-flow process can be related to the properties of the fluid at the inlet and outlet of an open system. This relation, the steady-flow energy equation (4.2), was applied to some important open systems but without reference to any particular fluid. As in Chapter 9, we shall again consider the fluid to be either steam or air and illustrate the applications with numerical examples. As pointed out in section 5.4.1, the irreversibility due to viscous friction cannot be neglected unless the velocity of flow is very small. In many cases it is necessary to calculate the unknown quantity assuming the process to be reversible, and multiply the result by a *process efficiency*. Various process efficiencies are introduced in the following examples. A second artifice for dealing with irreversibility in adiabatic steady-flow processes is also mentioned: this involves treating the process as a polytropic process.

Finally, this chapter ends with the consideration of multistream processes and nonsteady-flow processes.

10.1 Boiler and condenser

Since the work done in a boiler or condenser is zero, the steady-flow energy equation reduces to

$$\dot{Q} = \dot{m}\{(h_2 - h_1) + \tfrac{1}{2}(C_2^2 - C_1^2)\}$$

The velocity of flow in the inlet and outlet pipes is small, and, as the following example will show, the change in kinetic energy can be neglected. The velocity in the boiler or condenser itself is even smaller, so that the effect of friction can be neglected and the process can be regarded as internally reversible. This implies that there is no pressure drop due to friction, and the pressure can be assumed constant throughout the system.

In the following example of a steam boiler plant, it is assumed that before the steam leaves the system it is passed through a separate bank of tubes, the *superheater*, situated in the stream of furnace gases. Fig. 4.4 shows a boiler without a superheater.

Example 10.1 1500 kg of steam is to be produced per hour at a pressure of 30 bar with 100 K of superheat. The feed water is supplied to the boiler at a temperature of 40 °C. Find the rate at which heat must be supplied, assuming typical values for the velocity at inlet and outlet: 2 m/s in the feed pipe and 45 m/s in the steam main.

In Section 8.3.3 we agreed to assume that the enthalpy of a compressed liquid is equal to the enthalpy of saturated liquid at the same temperature. Therefore, from the saturation table at 40 °C, $h_1 = 167.5$ kJ/kg. The saturation temperature at 30 bar is 233.8 °C, and the outlet temperature is therefore 333.8 °C. From the superheat table, by interpolation,

$$h_2 = 2995 + \frac{33.8}{50} 122 = 3077.5 \text{ kJ/kg}$$

The rate of heat transfer required is

$$\dot{Q} = \dot{m}\{(h_2 - h_1) + \tfrac{1}{2}(C_2^2 - C_1^2)\}$$

$$= \frac{1500}{3600}\left[\frac{\text{kg}}{\text{s}}\right]\left\{(3077.5 - 167.5)\left[\frac{\text{kJ}}{\text{kg}}\right]\right.$$

$$+ \frac{1}{2}(45^2 - 2^2)\left[\frac{1}{\text{kg}} \frac{\text{kg m}^2}{\text{s}^2} \text{ or } \frac{\text{N m}}{\text{kg}}\right]\frac{1}{10^3}\left[\frac{\text{kJ}}{\text{N m}}\right]\right\}$$

$$= (1212.5 + 0.42)\left[\frac{\text{kJ}}{\text{s}}\right] = 1213 \text{ kW}$$

It is easy to see that the change of kinetic energy of 0.42 kW can be neglected.

10.2 Adiabatic steady-flow processes

For the reasons given in sections 4.2.2 and 4.2.3, the processes in a nozzle, diffuser, turbine and rotary compressor can be assumed adiabatic. The energy equation for the nozzle or diffuser, where $W = 0$, becomes

$$\tfrac{1}{2}(C_2^2 - C_1^2) = (h_1 - h_2)$$

And for the turbine or rotary compressor, when the velocity at inlet is approximately the same as that at outlet, the energy equation reduces to

$$\dot{W} = \dot{m}(h_2 - h_1)$$

The state of the fluid is usually known at the inlet of these systems, but only one property, e.g. the pressure, can be arbitrarily fixed at the outlet. To fix the final thermodynamic state of the fluid, and hence determine h_2, it is necessary to assume the process to be reversible; the flow is then isentropic and we can use the fact that $s_2 = s_1$. This has been explained in section 6.6, and the subsequent examples should make the point clear.

When the fluid is a perfect gas, the foregoing special forms of the energy equation become:

Nozzle and diffuser: $\qquad\qquad\qquad\qquad\qquad\frac{1}{2}(C_2^2 - C_1^2) = c_p(T_1 - T_2)$

Turbine and rotary compressor: $\qquad\qquad\quad\dot{W} = \dot{m}c_p(T_2 - T_1)$

Also, from equation (8.24) we have, for a perfect gas,

$$s_2 - s_1 = c_p \ln\frac{T_2}{T_1} - R \ln\frac{p_2}{p_1}$$

This equation relates the difference in entropy between states 1 and 2 to the pressure and temperature of the gas at these states. The fact that the gas is flowing during any process has no effect on relations between its *thermodynamic* properties, and the equation can therefore be applied to the thermodynamic states of a perfect gas at the inlet and outlet of an open system. For any isentropic steady-flow process $(s_2 - s_1)$ is zero, and we shall arrive at the same relation between p and T that we deduced for the isentropic non-flow process, i.e. equation (9.5):

$$\frac{T_2}{T_1} = \left(\frac{p_2}{p_1}\right)^{(\gamma - 1)/\gamma}$$

This, together with $p_1 v_1 / T_1 = p_2 v_2 / T_2$, yields

$$p_1 v_1^\gamma = p_2 v_2^\gamma \quad \text{and} \quad \frac{T_2}{T_1} = \left(\frac{v_2}{v_1}\right)^{1-\gamma}$$

Thus the relations between the thermodynamic properties of a perfect gas in its initial and final states are the same for both isentropic steady-flow and isentropic non-flow processes.

Since the velocity of flow is very high in a nozzle, diffuser, turbine or rotary compressor, the effect of friction cannot be neglected. Nevertheless the laws of thermodynamics do not enable quantitative predictions to be made for irreversible processes. One method of accounting for the effect of viscous friction is to calculate the unknown quantity assuming the process to be reversible and then to multiply the result by a *process efficiency* to obtain a more realistic estimate. The value of the process efficiency must be determined from tests carried out on a similar system. For nozzles it is usual to define the efficiency in terms of the outlet kinetic energy as

$$\text{nozzle efficiency } \eta_N = \frac{C_2^2}{(C_2')^2} \qquad\qquad\qquad\qquad (10.1)$$

C_2 is the actual outlet velocity, while C_2' is the outlet velocity which would have been achieved had the final pressure been reached isentropically. A prime will always be used to denote the result obtained by assuming the process to be isentropic.

Diffusers are designed to obtain the maximum possible pressure rise at the expense of a given reduction in velocity, and the process efficiency is often defined by

$$\text{diffuser efficiency } \eta_D = \frac{p_2 - p_1}{p_2' - p_1} \tag{10.2}$$

Here p_2 is the actual outlet pressure, p_2' is the pressure which would result from an isentropic process leading to the same outlet velocity.

Note that process efficiencies are always defined in such a way that they are positive numbers less than unity. This explains the different ways of defining process efficiencies for turbines and rotary compressors, namely

$$\eta_T = \frac{W}{W'} \quad \text{and} \quad \eta_C = \frac{W'}{W} \tag{10.3}$$

When the fluid can be treated as a perfect gas, and the change in kinetic energy between inlet and outlet can be ignored, these become

$$\eta_T = \frac{T_1 - T_2}{T_1 - T_2'} \quad \text{and} \quad \eta_C = \frac{T_2' - T_1}{T_2 - T_1}$$

The way in which process efficiencies are used will be illustrated in the following examples. Apart from the fact that these efficiencies are always defined in such a way that they are numerically less than unity, their definitions are quite arbitrary; they should be regarded merely as empirical correction factors. Since all the foregoing process efficiencies are defined by comparing the actual process with an isentropic process, they may be called *isentropic efficiencies*.

Example 10.2 A fluid expands from 3 bar to 1 bar in a nozzle. The initial velocity is 90 m/s, the initial temperature 150 °C, and from experiments on similar nozzles it has been found that the isentropic efficiency is likely to be 0.95. Estimate the final velocity.

(a) *Steam* (Fig. 10.1a)
From the superheat table,

$$h_1 = 2762 \text{ kJ/kg}, \qquad s_2' = s_1 = 7.078 \text{ kJ/kg K}$$

Since $s_2' < s_{g2}$, the vapour must be wet on leaving the nozzle after a reversible

Fig. 10.1a

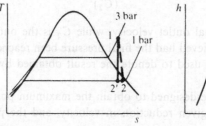
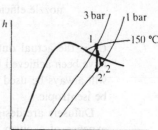

Fig. 10.1b

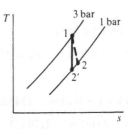

expansion. Hence

$$x'_2 = \frac{s'_2 - s_{f2}}{s_{fg2}} = \frac{7.078 - 1.303}{6.056} = 0.954$$

$$h'_2 = h_{f2} + x'_2 h_{fg2} = 417 + (0.954 \times 2258) = 2571 \text{ kJ/kg}$$

From the energy equation,

$$\frac{(C'_2)^2/[m^2/s^2] - 90^2}{2 \times 10^3} = (2762 - 2571)$$

$$(C'_2)^2 = 0.390 \times 10^6 \text{ m}^2/\text{s}^2$$

$$C_2^2 = \eta_N (C'_2)^2 = 0.95 \times 0.390 \times 10^6 \text{ m}^2/\text{s}^2$$

$$C_2 = 609 \text{ m/s}$$

(b)   *Air* (Fig. 10.1b)

After a reversible expansion the final temperature would be

$$T'_2 = T_1 \left(\frac{p_2}{p_1}\right)^{(\gamma - 1)/\gamma}$$

Assuming $\gamma = 1.40$, we have

$$T'_2 = 423 \left(\frac{1}{3}\right)^{0.4/1.4} = 309 \text{ K}$$

From the energy equation,

$$\frac{(C'_2)^2/[m^2/s^2] - 90^2}{2 \times 10^3} = 1.005(423 - 309)$$

$$(C'_2)^2 = 0.237 \times 10^6 \text{ m}^2/\text{s}^2$$

$$C_2^2 = 0.95 \times 0.237 \times 10^6 \text{ m}^2/\text{s}^2$$

$$C_2 = 475 \text{ m/s}$$

Example 10.3   A fluid enters a turbine at the rate of 14 kg/s with an initial pressure and temperature of 3 bar and 150 °C. If the final pressure is 1 bar and the isentropic efficiency of the turbine is 0.85, find the power developed and the change of entropy between inlet and outlet. p_1, T_1 and p_2 are the same as in the previous example, and Figs 10.1a and b, which show changes in the *thermodynamic* properties only, also apply to this case.

(a) *Steam*

Using the results of Example 10.2, we have

$$h_1 = 2762 \text{ kJ/kg}, \qquad x_2' = 0.954, \qquad h_2' = 2580 \text{ kJ/kg}$$

From the energy equation,

$$\dot{W}' = \dot{m}(h_2' - h_1) = 14 \times (-182) = -2548 \text{ kJ/s or kW}$$

$$\dot{W} = \eta_T \dot{W}' = 0.85 \times (-2548) = -2170 \text{ kW}$$

To find the change of entropy we must first determine the actual final state, i.e. state 2:

$$h_1 - h_2 = \eta_T(h_1 - h_2') = 0.85 \times 182 = 154.7 \text{ kJ/kg}$$

$$h_2 = 2762 - 154.7 = 2607 \text{ kJ/kg}$$

$$x_2 = \frac{h_2 - h_{f2}}{h_{fg2}} = \frac{2607 - 417}{2258} = 0.970$$

$$s_2 = s_{f2} + x_2 s_{fg2} = 1.303 + (0.970 \times 6.056) = 7.177 \text{ kJ/kg K}$$

Since $s_2 = 7.078$ kJ/kg K, the change of entropy is

$$\dot{S}_2 - \dot{S}_1 = \dot{m}(s_2 - s_1) = 14 \times 0.099 = 1.39 \text{ kJ/s K}$$

(b) *Air*

From Example 10.2b, $T_2' = 309$ K.

The actual work transfer is given by

$$\dot{W} = \eta_T \dot{m} c_p(T_2' - T_1) = 0.85 \times 14 \times 1.005(309 - 423) = -1363 \text{ kW}$$

The actual final temperature can be found from

$$T_1 - T_2 = \eta_T(T_1 - T_2')$$

$$T_2 = 423 - (0.85 \times 114) = 326 \text{ K}$$

The values of p_1, T_1, p_2 and T_2 can be substituted in the appropriate general expression (8.24) for the change of entropy. Alternatively, we can replace the irreversible path 1–2 in Fig. 10.1b by a reversible path consisting of the isentropic process 1–2' and the reversible constant pressure process 2'–2. We then have

$$\dot{S}_2 - \dot{S}_1 = \dot{S}_2 - \dot{S}_2' = \int_{2'}^{2} \left(\frac{d\dot{Q}}{T}\right)_{rev} = \dot{m} c_p \ln \frac{T_2}{T_2'}$$

$$= 14 \times 1.005 \ln \frac{326}{309} = 0.753 \text{ kW/K}$$

It is worth mentioning one other method of accounting for irreversibility in an adiabatic flow process. The actual thermodynamic path of all these adiabatic processes may be regarded as being approximately polytropic in form, i.e. we may assume that

$$pv^n = \text{constant}$$

The polytropic expression can only have a meaning if p and v are regarded as average values at any point in the process because, although we normally assume that every elemental mass of fluid has the same properties at inlet and outlet of an open system, not all elements necessarily pass through exactly the same series of states between inlet and outlet.

The value of the index of an irreversible adiabatic expansion or compression is not equal to γ even when the fluid is a perfect gas; n is an empirical constant depending on the amount of friction. If n is known from previous experiments on a similar system, an unknown final state can then be predicted by making use of the equation

$$p_1 v_1^n = p_2 v_2^n$$

Or, when the fluid is a gas, we can also use

$$\frac{T_2}{T_1} = \left(\frac{p_2}{p_1}\right)^{(n-1)/n}$$

Once the final state has been determined, the energy equation, which applies to both reversible and irreversible processes, can then be used in the usual way.

10.3 Throttling process

The throttling process is an adiabatic steady-flow process, but it was not included in the previous section because this was concerned with adiabatic processes which ideally should be isentropic. The throttling process is *essentially* irreversible: it is a means of reducing the pressure of a fluid by intentionally introducing friction into the flow.

In section 4.2.4 we noted that the throttling process was such that

$$h_1 = h_2$$

When the fluid is a perfect gas, it follows that

$$T_1 = T_2$$

The fact that a slight change of temperature is observed when the fluid is a real gas has been noted in section 7.4.4, and it indicates that the enthalpy of a real gas is not a function only of temperature.

When a gas or vapour is throttled, the specific volume downstream of the restriction is greater than it is upstream, i.e. $v_2 > v_1$. If the restriction is in a pipe of uniform diameter, the continuity equation (4.3) implies that $C_2 > C_1$. Nevertheless, the following example shows that for ordinary flow velocities the kinetic energy terms in the energy equation are negligible and for practical purposes $h_2 = h_1$.

Example 10.4 Air flows at the rate of 2.3 kg/s in a 15 cm diameter pipe. It has a pressure of 7 bar and a temperature of 95 °C before it is throttled by a valve to 3.5 bar. Find the velocity of the air downstream of the restriction,

Fig. 10.2

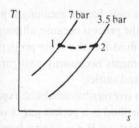

and show that the enthalpy is essentially the same before and after the throttling process. Also find the change of entropy.

Fig. 10.2 illustrates the process. The temperature actually falls as the fluid velocity increases through the restriction, and then rises because most of this increase in kinetic energy is dissipated by friction. The initial specific volume is

$$v_1 = \frac{RT_1}{p_1} = \frac{0.287 \times 368}{100 \times 7} = 0.151 \text{ m}^3/\text{kg}$$

and the initial velocity, from the continuity equation, is

$$C_1 = \frac{mv_1}{A} = \frac{2.3 \times 0.151 \times 4}{\pi(0.15)^2} = 19.65 \text{ m/s}$$

Similarly, the final velocity is

$$C_2 = \frac{m R T_2}{A \ p_2} = \frac{2.3}{(\pi/4)(0.15)^2} \frac{0.287}{100 \times 3.5} \left[\frac{m}{s}\right] \frac{T_2}{[K]} = 0.1067 \left[\frac{m}{s}\right] \frac{T_2}{[K]}$$

Since Q and W are zero, the energy equation for a perfect gas reduces to

$$c_p T_2 + \tfrac{1}{2} C_2^2 = c_p T_1 + \tfrac{1}{2} C_1^2$$

or

$$1.005 \frac{T_2}{[K]} + \frac{\tfrac{1}{2}(0.1067)^2}{10^3} \frac{T_2^2}{[K^2]} = 1.005 \frac{T_1}{[K]} + \frac{\tfrac{1}{2}(19.65)^2}{10^3}$$

and hence

$$\frac{T_2}{[K]} + 5.66 \times 10^{-6} \frac{T_2^2}{[K^2]} = \frac{T_1}{[K]} + 0.192$$

Without further calculation it is evident that the kinetic energy terms can be ignored and T_2 is effectively equal to T_1. Hence the final velocity is

$$C_2 = 0.1067 \times 368 = 39.3 \text{ m/s}$$

Since the process is adiabatic and irreversible, the fluid must undergo an increase of entropy as it flows through the system. The initial and final thermodynamic states could be joined by a reversible non-flow isothermal process, and hence

$$s_2 - s_1 = \int_1^2 \left(\frac{dQ}{T}\right)_{\text{rev}} = -R \ln \frac{p_2}{p_1} = -0.287 \ln \frac{3.5}{7} = 0.199 \text{ kJ/kg K}$$

$$\dot{S}_2 - \dot{S}_1 = \dot{m}(s_2 - s_1) = 2.3 \times 0.199 = 0.458 \text{ kJ/s K}$$

Fig. 10.3
Throttling calorimeter

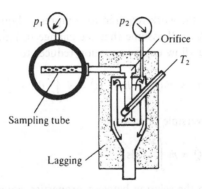

Before leaving the throttling process, we may note how use is made of it in the *throttling calorimeter* for the determination of the dryness fraction of a wet vapour. Normally the state of a fluid is most conveniently determined by measuring the intensive properties p and T, but for a wet vapour these are not independent properties. The throttling calorimeter, illustrated in Fig. 10.3, enables a wet state 1 to be determined by measuring p and T alone. A steady stream of wet vapour is sampled from the main flow and passed through a small orifice in a well-lagged chamber. The vapour pressure, initially p_1, falls to some value p_2 as a result of the throttling process. Since $h_2 = h_1$, it is evident from the h–s diagram (Fig. 8.14) that if the pressure drop is sufficient and the vapour not too wet, the sampled vapour will be superheated after the expansion. The thermodynamic state can therefore be determined by measuring the independent properties p_2 and T_2. The enthalpy h_2 can then be found from the superheat table. If the initial pressure p_1 is also measured, and the corresponding values of h_f and h_{fg} are taken from the saturation table, the dryness fraction is found from

$$x_1 = \frac{h_1 - h_{f1}}{h_{fg1}} = \frac{h_2 - h_{f1}}{h_{fg1}}$$

The process must of course be continued long enough for the calorimeter to reach a steady temperature before readings are taken. The chief difficulty is in ensuring that the sample is representative of the main flow: unfortunately the liquid accumulates on the wall of the pipe, and the sample tends to be drier than the main stream as a whole.

10.4   Reversible steady-flow process

An expression for the work transfer in a reversible steady-flow process, whether adiabatic or not, which is equivalent to the expression

$$dW = -p\,dv$$

that applies to a non-flow process, can often be very useful. This will be particularly apparent in Chapter 16. We will develop the basic equation here, however, because we shall want to use a special version of it in Chapter 11 to calculate the work required to compress a liquid passing through a boiler feed pump. We will assume that the change in kinetic energy is negligible, so that the steady-flow energy equation reduces to

$$\dot{W} = \dot{m}(h_2 - h_1) - \dot{Q} = \dot{m}\int_1^2 dh - \dot{Q}$$

For a reversible process,

$$\dot{Q} = \dot{m}\int_1^2 T\,ds$$

and from the relation between properties, equation (6.13),

$$\int_1^2 T\,ds = \int_1^2 (dh - v\,dp)$$

The equation for $\dot{W}$ then becomes

$$\dot{W} = \dot{m}\int_1^2 dh - \dot{m}\int_1^2 (dh - v\,dp) = \dot{m}\int_1^2 v\,dp \qquad (10.4)$$

Equation (10.4) applies to adiabatic or non-adiabatic processes, provided that they are reversible and that changes in kinetic energy are negligible. To evaluate $\dot{W}$ we need to know the relation between v and p along the path 1–2. For example, if the reversible process is adiabatic and the fluid is a perfect gas, $pv^\gamma = $ constant. If the fluid is a liquid which can be assumed incompressible, $v = $ constant and

$$\dot{W} = \dot{m}v\int_1^2 dp = \dot{m}v(p_2 - p_1) \qquad (10.5)$$

This is the special case which we shall need to use in Chapter 11.

10.5 Isothermal steady-flow process

It was pointed out in section 4.2.5 that a reciprocating compressor (or expander) can be regarded as an open system undergoing a steady-flow process, provided that a receiver is included between the cylinder and the measuring section to damp out the pulsations. The fluid flows through a reciprocating machine at a comparatively slow rate and there is time for an appreciable amount of heat to be exchanged with the surroundings. It is possible to imagine a limiting case in which the temperature of the fluid remains constant throughout its passage through the system. This is the case considered here.

Since we have postulated low velocities, the energy equation reduces to

$$\dot{Q} + \dot{W} = \dot{m}(h_2 - h_1)$$

When the fluid is a perfect gas, $(h_2 - h_1)$ is zero because the enthalpy is a function only of temperature. For the isothermal expansion or compression of a perfect gas we therefore have

$$\dot{Q} = -\dot{W}$$

If the process is assumed reversible, these equations can be evaluated to find the work done when the states of the fluid are known at inlet and outlet. Thus, when the fluid is a vapour, $(h_2 - h_1)$ and $(s_2 - s_1)$ can be found from tables of properties and, since the temperature T is constant, $\dot{Q}$ can be calculated from $\dot{m}T(s_2 - s_1)$. Hence $\dot{W}$ can be found from the energy equation. When the fluid is a perfect gas, a simple expression for $\dot{W}$ can be deduced in terms of the temperature T and the inlet and outlet pressures p_1 and p_2. Thus putting $T = $ constant in (8.24),

$$s_2 - s_1 = -R \ln \frac{p_2}{p_1}$$

and hence

$$\dot{W} = -\dot{Q} = \dot{m}RT \ln \frac{p_2}{p_1} \tag{10.6}$$

Equation (10.6) is in fact the same expression that was obtained for the work transfer when a perfect gas undergoes a reversible *non-flow* isothermal process (section 9.5). The same equality of work does not hold when the fluid is a vapour because in a non-flow process

$$\dot{Q} + \dot{W} = \dot{m}(u_2 - u_1)$$

Only when the fluid is a perfect gas are the flow and non-flow isothermal work transfers the same, because only then does $(u_2 - u_1) = (h_2 - h_1)$, both being zero.

Owing to the comparatively low fluid velocities, the effect of *fluid* friction in a reciprocating machine is small. Hence the question of introducing a process efficiency to take account of irreversibility in this type of process has not arisen in practice. There remain the questions of how to predict the work transfer when the heat exchanged is not sufficient to maintain the temperature constant, and how *mechanical* friction is taken into account. These matters will be dealt with in Chapter 16.

Example 10.5   Recalculate the work and heat transfers per unit mass for Example 9.6, assuming that the isothermal compression occurs in a steady-flow process.

The thermodynamic states before, during and after compression are identical with those of the non-flow process of Example 9.6. The processes for steam and air are therefore depicted respectively by Figs 9.6a and b, and some of the required property values can be taken from that example.

(a) *Steam*
The heat transferred is the same as for the non-flow process, i.e. $Q = T(s_2 - s_1) = -747 \text{ kJ/kg}$. From the energy equation the work done is

$$W = (h_2 - h_1) - Q$$

From the superheat table, by interpolation,

$$h_1 = 2777 + \frac{5.5}{50} 99 = 2788 \text{ kJ/kg}$$

x_2 has been found to be 0.817, and thus

$$h_2 = h_f + x_2 h_{fg} = 417 + (0.817 \times 2258) = 2262 \text{ kJ/kg}$$

Hence

$$W = (2262 - 2788) + 747 = 221 \text{ kJ/kg}$$

(b) *Air*

The heat transferred is the same as for the non-flow process, i.e. $Q = -182 \text{ kJ/kg}$. Also, since $(h_2 - h_1) = (u_2 - u_1)$, both being zero, the magnitudes of the work and heat transfers are equal as for the non-flow process.

10.6 Multistream steady-flow processes

Reference to section 4.1 will show that, provided the streams do not react chemically with one another, there is nothing inherent in the derivation of the steady-flow energy equation (4.2) to prevent its application to an open system in which more than one stream of fluid enters and leaves the system. The enthalpy, kinetic energy and potential energy terms associated with each stream can be summed at the inlet and outlet respectively, to give the following equation:

$$\dot{Q} + \dot{W} = \sum_{\text{out}} \dot{m}(h + \tfrac{1}{2}C^2 + gz) - \sum_{\text{in}} \dot{m}(h + \tfrac{1}{2}C^2 + gz)$$

Also, for conservation of mass we have the equation

$$\sum_{\text{out}} \dot{m} = \sum_{\text{in}} \dot{m}$$

One simple example of a multistream system is given here, but other more important cases can be found in Chapter 14.

Example 10.6 Steam is to be condensed by direct injection of cold water. The steam enters the condenser at a rate of 450 kg/h with a dryness fraction 0.9 and a pressure 1 atm. The estimated heat loss from the condenser to the surroundings is 8500 kJ/h. If the cold water enters with a temperature of 15 °C, and the mixture of condensate and cooling water is to leave at 95 °C, determine the rate of flow of cooling water required.

Fig. 10.4 illustrates the system. The energy equation, neglecting the kinetic and potential energy terms, becomes

$$\dot{Q} = \dot{m}_3 h_3 - (\dot{m}_1 h_1 + \dot{m}_2 h_2)$$

and for conservation of mass,

$$\dot{m}_3 = \dot{m}_1 + \dot{m}_2$$

Fig. 10.4

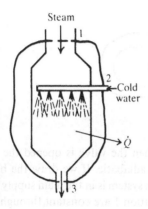

Steam

Cold water

$\rightarrow \dot{Q}$

From the saturation table,

$$h_1 = h_{f1} + x_1 h_{fg1} = 419.1 + (0.9 \times 2256.7) = 2450 \, \text{kJ/kg}$$

$$h_2 = 62.9 \, \text{kJ/kg}, \qquad h_3 = 398.0 \, \text{kJ/kg}$$

Therefore

$$-8500 = (450 + \dot{m}_2)398 - \{(450 \times 2450) + \dot{m}_2 62.9\}$$

$$\dot{m}_2 = 2730 \, \text{kg/h}$$

10.7 Nonsteady-flow processes

The only nonsteady-flow processes we shall consider are those undergone by the fluid in an open system as it changes from one equilibrium state to another. The appropriate energy equation has been derived in section 4.3, namely equation (4.9). If we neglect the potential energy terms, as we have done with the steady-flow processes, the equation becomes

$$Q + W = (m''u'' + m'u') + \Sigma \delta m_2 (h_2 + \tfrac{1}{2}C_2^2) - \Sigma \delta m_1 (h_1 + \tfrac{1}{2}C_1^2)$$

Q and W refer to the quantities of heat and work crossing the boundary of the open system during the time it takes for the system to change from one equilibrium state to another. The term $(m''u'' - m'u')$ refers to the change of internal energy of the system between these two equilibrium states, and the remaining two terms refer to the summation of the quantities of enthalpy and kinetic energy leaving and entering the system with each element of fluid. We shall now apply this equation to two particular cases.

10.7.1   Filling a reservoir from an infinite source of fluid

Fig. 10.5 illustrates the system. An air bottle of volume V contains air at pressure p' and temperature T'. It is to be filled from a compressed air line maintained at a constant pressure p_1 and temperature T_1. We require to find the mass and temperature of the air in the bottle after the valve has been opened to allow the pressure in the bottle to rise to the supply pressure p_1.

Fig. 10.5

Filling a compressed air bottle

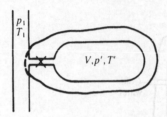

We may assume that when the valve is opened the air enters the bottle so rapidly that the process is adiabatic. If we draw the boundary in such a way that the entrance to the open system is in the main supply line, the thermodynamic properties of the fluid at station 1 are constant throughout the process, and C_1 is negligible. The velocity will be high in the locality of the valve—but local transformations of energy within the open system do not concern us. Also, no fluid leaves the system, and W is zero. The energy equation therefore reduces to

$$(m''u'' - m'u') = h_1 \Sigma \delta m_1$$

Since mass is conserved,

$$(m'' - m') = \Sigma \delta m_1$$

and hence

$$(m''u'' - m'u') = h_1(m'' - m') \tag{10.7}$$

In our example the fluid is air, which can be treated as a perfect gas. Consequently (10.7) can be written as

$$c_v(m''T'' - m'T') = c_p T_1(m'' - m')$$

Moreover, we also have

$$\frac{m''}{m'} = \frac{p''V/RT''}{p'V/RT'} = \frac{p''/T''}{p'/T'} \quad \text{and} \quad p'' = p_1$$

Substituting these in the energy equation, we get

$$c_v\left(\frac{p_1/T''}{p'/T'}T'' - T'\right) = c_p T_1\left(\frac{p_1/T''}{p'/T'} - 1\right)$$

Since p', T', p_1 and T_1 are given, this equation can be used to find T''. Having found T'' we can find m'' from

$$m'' = \frac{p_1 V}{RT''}$$

Note that in the foregoing treatment we have assumed the internal energy to be zero at absolute zero. The reference state chosen can be important for the following reason. By rewriting equation (10.7) explicitly in terms of an internal energy u, relative to the internal energy u_0 at some arbitrary reference state 0, we have

$$m''(u''_r + u_0) - m'(u'_r + u_0) = h_1(m'' - m')$$

and hence, since $h_1 = h_{r1} + h_0 = h_{r1} + u_0 + p_0 v_0$, we get

$$(m''u''_r - m'u'_r) + u_0(m'' - m') = (h_{r1} + p_0 v_0)(m'' - m') + u_0(m'' - m')$$

Although the terms involving u_0 cancel, there remains the $p_0 v_0$ term which arises because the enthalpy and internal energy cannot normally both be zero at the same reference state. The exception is when the fluid is a perfect gas and the reference temperature is absolute zero, because then $p_0 v_0 = R T_0 = 0$. In the following numerical example which deals with steam, the $p_0 v_0$ term is not zero but can be neglected because it is equal to only 0.000 611 2 kJ/kg in the reference state used in the tables, namely saturated liquid at the triple point.

Example 10.7 A vessel of volume 0.085 m³ contains steam at 1 bar and 0.8 dryness fraction. The vessel is momentarily connected to a steam main in which the steam is at 20 bar and 260 °C. If the pressure in the vessel is allowed to rise to the main pressure, estimate the final state and mass of the steam in the vessel.

Making the appropriate assumptions, the energy equation (10.7) can be used, i.e.

$$(m''u'' - m'u') = h_1(m'' - m')$$

From the superheat table, by interpolation,

$$h_1 = 2904 + \left(\frac{10}{50} \times 121\right) = 2928 \text{ kJ/kg}$$

From the saturation table,

$$u' = 417 + (0.8 \times 2089) = 2088 \text{ kJ/kg}$$

$$m' = \frac{V}{x'v'_g} = \frac{0.085}{0.8 \times 1.694} = 0.0627 \text{ kg}$$

$$m'' = \frac{V}{v''} = \frac{0.085[\text{m}^3]}{v''}$$

Substituting these values in the energy equation we get

$$\left(\frac{0.085[\text{m}^3]}{v''}u'' - 0.0627[\text{kg}] \times 2088\left[\frac{\text{kJ}}{\text{kg}}\right]\right)$$

$$= 2928\left[\frac{\text{kJ}}{\text{kg}}\right]\left(\frac{0.085[\text{m}^3]}{v''} - 0.0627[\text{kg}]\right)$$

or

$$\frac{u''/v''}{[\text{kJ/m}^3]} = \frac{2928}{v''/[\text{m}^3/\text{kg}]} - 620$$

The final pressure p'' is 20 bar, but no exact algebraic relation between

Fig. 10.6

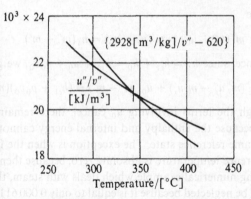

u'', v'' and p'' is known. A graphical method can be used to solve the equation as follows:

20 bar and °C	300	350	400
$v''/[\text{m}^3/\text{kg}]$	0.1255	0.1386	0.1511
$u''/[\text{kJ}/\text{kg}]$	2 744	2 861	2 946
$(u''/v'')/[\text{kJ}/\text{m}^3]$	21 900	20 600	19 500
$\{2928[\text{m}^3/\text{kg}]/v'' - 620\}$	22 700	20 500	18 800

By plotting the last two lines of figures against temperature as in Fig. 10.6, it is found that the steam has a temperature of 343 °C in the final state. That the final temperature in the vessel is higher than the temperature in the steam main is due to the fact that the steam is recompressed adiabatically in the vessel after being throttled.

The final mass of steam in the vessel can now be found. At 20 bar and 343 °C, by interpolation from the superheat table,

$$v'' = 0.1255 + \frac{43}{50}0.0131 = 0.1368 \text{ m}^3/\text{kg}$$

Hence

$$m'' = \frac{V}{v''} = \frac{0.085}{0.1368} = 0.621 \text{ kg}$$

NB: If the approximate relation between p, v and u given by equation (9.7) is used, $v'' = 0.135 \text{ m}^3/\text{kg}$ and $m'' = 0.63 \text{ kg}$.

10.7.2 Maximum work attainable by allowing a reservoir of fluid to discharge via a turbine

This example has already been introduced in general terms in section 4.3, and Fig. 4.10 illustrates the system. By making suitable assumptions, the energy equation was shown to reduce to

$$-W = (m'u' - m''u'') - \Sigma\delta m_2 h_2$$

The maximum work will be obtained when the expansion through the turbine is reversible. Since we are assuming the process to be adiabatic, the additional assumption of reversibility implies that the process is isentropic. In the following numerical example we shall consider the fluid to be air.

Example 10.8 A tank of volume 0.3 m³ is filled with air at a pressure and temperature of 35 bar and 40 °C. The air is allowed to discharge through a turbine into the atmosphere, until the pressure in the tank has fallen to the atmospheric level of 1 bar. Find the maximum amount of work that could be delivered by the turbine.

The air in the tank progressively decreases in pressure and temperature from p' and T' to p'' and T''. But since the pressure p_2 at the outlet is constant, i.e. atmospheric, and the expansion is isentropic, the temperature T_2 at the outlet must also remain constant during the process. This can be made clear by the following argument. Consider the mass of air which remains in the tank at the end of the expansion and treat it as a closed system. This mass, originally occupying only a fraction of the volume of the tank, expands isentropically during the process. If at any instant the pressure and temperature is p and T, then we have

$$\frac{T}{T'} = \left(\frac{p}{p'}\right)^{(\gamma-1)/\gamma}$$

But p and T must also represent the pressure and temperature of the air as it enters the turbine at this particular instant, and since the expansion through the turbine is also isentropic,

$$\frac{T_2}{T} = \left(\frac{p_2}{p}\right)^{(\gamma-1)/\gamma}$$

Multiplying this pair of equations we get

$$\frac{T_2}{T'} = \left(\frac{p_2}{p'}\right)^{(\gamma-1)/\gamma}$$

T' and p' are the given initial conditions in the tank, and p_2 is constant, i.e. atmospheric pressure. Therefore T_2 must be constant also. Moreover, since $p'' = p_2$, the final temperature of the air in the tank must be equal to T_2.

From the conservation of mass, and the fact that T_2 is constant, the energy equation becomes

$$-W = c_v(m'T' - m''T'') - c_p T_2(m' - m'')$$

where

$$T'' = T_2 = T'\left(\frac{p_2}{p'}\right)^{(\gamma-1)/\gamma} = 313\left(\frac{1}{35}\right)^{0.4/1.4} = 113\ \text{K}$$

$$m' = \frac{p'V}{RT'} = \frac{100 \times 35 \times 0.3}{0.287 \times 313} = 11.68\ \text{kg}$$

$$m'' = \frac{p''V}{RT''} = \frac{100 \times 1 \times 0.3}{0.287 \times 113} = 0.925\ \text{kg}$$

Hence

$$W = -0.718\{(11.68 \times 313) - (0.925 \times 113)\}$$

$$+ \{1.005 \times 113(11.68 - 0.925)\} = -1330\ \text{kJ}$$

11

Vapour Power Cycles

One common method of producing mechanical power employs the transfer of heat from a reservoir to a working fluid which is taken through a thermodynamic cycle. The cycles considered in this chapter have two characteristics in common: (a) the working fluid is a condensable vapour which is in the liquid phase during part of the cycle, and (b) the cycle consists of a succession of steady-flow processes, with each process carried out in a separate component specially designed for the purpose. Each component constitutes an open system, and all the components are connected in series so that, as the fluid circulates through the power plant, each fluid element passes through a cycle of mechanical and thermodynamic states (see section 4.4).

To simplify the analysis, we shall assume that the change in kinetic and potential energy of the fluid between entry and exit of each component is negligible compared with the change of enthalpy. Also, when evaluating the work and heat transfers during the various processes in a cycle, it will normally be convenient to consider the steady-flow energy equation *per unit mass* rather than for a rate of flow $\dot{m}$ as was done in equation (4.2). The energy equation for our present purpose therefore becomes

$$Q + W = h_2 - h_1$$

We shall also assume, in the main, that the processes are reversible. Cycles composed of reversible processes are called *ideal cycles*.

After a discussion of suitable criteria for comparing their effectiveness, various ideal cycles are analysed in turn. The Carnot cycle is considered first, and the Rankine cycle is then presented as a logical modification of this to meet certain practical considerations. Finally, other modifications used in modern power plant are described.

Although the working fluid usually employed is steam, because it is cheap and chemically stable, the principles presented here apply equally to any condensable vapour. The characteristics of an ideal working fluid are discussed, and a possible power plant where steam would be quite unsuitable is described.

The chapter ends with a section on economic assessment. This is to remind the student that, although this book is almost solely concerned with technical matters, one should never forget that economic factors usually determine which of alternative technical solutions are adopted in practice.

11.1 Criteria for the comparison of cycles

The choice of power plant for a given purpose is determined largely by considerations of operating cost and capital cost. The former is primarily a function of the overall efficiency of the plant, while the latter depends mainly on its size and complexity. In general the efficiency can always be improved by adding to the complexity of the plant, so that a suitable compromise between low operating and low capital costs must be reached.

Consider first the efficiency of the plant. Fig. 11.1 illustrates essential features of the type of power plant considered here. Until the 1950s the high-temperature reservoir had always been a stream of hot gases produced by the continuous combustion of a hydrocarbon fuel in air. Since then a large number of nuclear power plant have been built wherein the source of heat is nuclear fission. On a more modest scale, plant using solar heat sources are being used in suitable locations (see Ref. 28). These new sources of energy do not affect the main discussion here, which is concerned with factors which govern the performance of the vapour cycles themselves. Whatever the source of energy, the *overall thermal efficiency* of a vapour cycle plant is suitably assessed by the proportion of latent energy in the fuel, or more generally of the energy available in the source, which is converted into useful mechanical work. This overall efficiency can be expressed as the product of two efficiencies: (a) the *combustion efficiency* or *source efficiency*, which expresses the proportion of the available energy transferred as heat to the working fluid; and (b) the *cycle efficiency*, which expresses the proportion of this heat which is converted into mechanical work. In this chapter we are concerned with the comparison of various cycles and with the calculation of cycle efficiency. (Calculation of combustion efficiency requires a knowledge of the thermodynamics of mixtures and chemical reactions, and must be left until Chapter 15 and in particular section 15.6.) One should always be aware, however, that modifications to a cycle to improve its cycle efficiency may incur a penalty in reduced combustion or source efficiency unless steps are taken to avoid it. Situations where such interaction of cycle and source efficiency is significant are considered in sections 11.6 and 11.7.

Let us now recapitulate briefly the reasons why the cycle efficiency is not zero:

Fig. 11.1
The essential elements of a vapour power plant

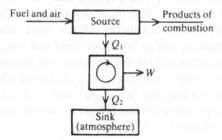

Thermodynamic The Second Law expresses the fact that even in the best power cycle some heat must be rejected. This best form of cycle was shown in section 6.1 to be one in which: (a) all the heat supplied is transferred while the working fluid is at a constant upper temperature T_a, and all the heat rejected leaves while the working fluid is at a constant lower temperature T_b; and (b) all the processes are reversible. The efficiency of such a cycle is $(T_a - T_b)/T_a$, irrespective of the working fluid. If the cycle, even though reversible, is such that the temperature of the working fluid changes during a heat transfer process, the cycle efficiency will be less than $(T_a - T_b)/T_a$, where T_a and T_b now refer to the maximum and minimum temperatures reached by the working fluid (section 6.3).

Practical All real processes are irreversible, and irreversibilities reduce the cycle efficiency (section 5.5).

It is a simple matter to calculate the efficiency of a cycle when all the processes are assumed to be reversible. The result is known as the *ideal cycle efficiency*. By introducing process efficiencies as defined in Chapter 10, it is also possible to estimate the actual cycle efficiency. The ratio of the actual cycle efficiency to the ideal cycle efficiency is called the *efficiency ratio*.

Some cycles are more sensitive to irreversibilities than others. That is, two cycles may have the same ideal cycle efficiencies, but after allowing for the same process efficiencies we find that their actual cycle efficiencies are markedly different. A high ideal cycle efficiency is not therefore by itself a good indication of whether or not the cycle will provide a power plant of high overall efficiency. An additional criterion which indicates the cycle's sensitivity to irreversibilities is required. Such a criterion is furnished by the *work ratio* r_w. Any power cycle consists of one or more processes where work is done by the working fluid and others where work is absorbed. The work ratio is defined as the ratio of the *net work output* to the *gross work output*. Irreversibilities, accounted for by process efficiencies, always have the effect of decreasing work outputs and increasing work inputs. Thus if the ideal gross output is only slightly greater than the ideal work input, i.e. if r_w is only slightly greater than zero, quite a small amount of process inefficiency is sufficient to reduce the net output to zero and the actual cycle efficiency will drop to zero. On the other hand, as the work ratio approaches unity, the same amount of process inefficiency will have a much smaller effect on the net work output and hence on the actual cycle efficiency. This point is illustrated in Fig. 11.2, by taking two ideal cycles involving work output W_T from a turbine and work input W_C to a compressor. The cycles have the same heat input Q_{in} and cycle efficiency η, and thus the same net work W, but have radically different work ratios. It is seen that when process efficiencies η_T and η_C for the turbines and compressors are taken into account (see equation (10.3)), the efficiency η of the cycle having a low work ratio drops much more than that for a cycle having a high work ratio.

Summarising, we may say that a *high ideal cycle efficiency together with a high work ratio provide a reliable indication that the real power plant will have a good overall efficiency.*

Fig. 11.2
The effect of work ratio

	Ideal		With $\eta_T = \eta_C = 0.9$	
	Cycle 1	Cycle 2	Cycle 1	Cycle 2
Q_{in}	120	120	120	120
W_T	100	40	90	36
W_C	61	1	67.8	1.1
net W	39	39	22.2	34.9
r_w	0.390	0.975	0.247	0.969
η	0.325	0.325	0.185	0.291

The next consideration is some criterion which will indicate the relative size of plant for a given power output; the complexity of the plant will be obvious from inspection of the ideal cycle. Here again the work ratio sometimes serves as a useful criterion. The component producing the work output has to provide the power for the component requiring the work input, and therefore a work ratio approaching unity indicates that these components will be of least possible size for a given net power output. Most practical vapour cycles, however, have work ratios very near unity; the work ratio is then not very informative and a more direct criterion for size is necessary.

In general, the size of the components will depend on the amount of working fluid which has to be passed through them. A more direct indication of relative sizes of steam plant is therefore provided by the *specific steam consumption* (SSC), i.e. the mass flow of steam required per unit power output.* It is usually expressed in kg/kW h. If the magnitude of the net work output per unit mass flow is $|W|/[kJ/kg] = |W|/[kW s/kg]$, the SSC can be found from

$$SSC = \frac{1}{|W|} = \left(\frac{1}{|W|/[kJ/kg]} \right) \left[\frac{kg}{kW\,s} \right] \times 3600 \left[\frac{s}{h} \right]$$

$$= \left(\frac{3600}{|W|/[kJ/kg]} \right) \frac{kg}{kW\,h}$$

11.2 Carnot cycle

One ideal cycle in which the heat is taken in at a constant upper temperature (T_a) and rejected at a constant lower temperature (T_b) is that suggested by Sadi Carnot (Ref. 2). It consists of two reversible isothermal processes at T_a and T_b respectively, connected by two reversible adiabatic (isentropic) processes. When the working fluid is a condensable vapour, the two isothermal processes are easily obtained by heating and cooling at constant pressure while the fluid is a wet vapour. The cycle is represented on the T–s diagram for steam in Fig. 11.3, and a diagrammatic sketch of the plant accompanies it.

Saturated water in state 1 is evaporated in a boiler at constant pressure to

---

* If the effect of different working fluids is being investigated, account must be taken of their different densities because it is strictly the volume flow which is relevant.

Fig. 11.3
The Carnot cycle

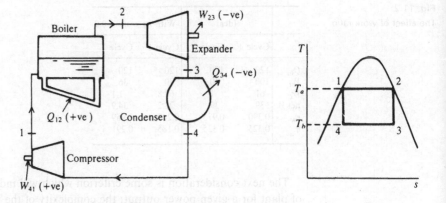

form saturated steam in state 2, the heat added being

$$Q_{12} = h_2 - h_1$$

The steam is expanded isentropically to state 3 while doing work in a turbine or reciprocating engine.* The work transfer is

$$W_{23} = (h_3 - h_2)$$

After expansion the steam is then partially condensed at constant pressure while heat

$$Q_{34} = h_4 - h_3$$

is rejected. Condensation is stopped at state 4, where $s_4 = s_1$. Finally the steam is compressed isentropically in a rotary or reciprocating compressor to state 1, the work transfer being

$$W_{41} = (h_1 - h_4)$$

The calculation of the work and heat transfers in the separate processes can be carried out by the methods given in Chapter 10.

Example 11.1 Calculate the heat and work transfers, cycle efficiency, work ratio and specific steam consumption of a Carnot cycle (Fig. 11.3), using steam between pressures of 30 and 0.04 bar.

From tables we find that at 30 bar $T_1 = T_2 = 507.0$ K and

$$h_1 = h_f = 1008 \text{ kJ/kg}, \qquad h_2 = h_g = 2803 \text{ kJ/kg}$$

Putting $s_4 = s_1$ and $s_3 = s_2$ (see section 10.2), we find that at the condenser pressure of 0.04 bar, at which $T_3 = T_4 = 302.2$ K,

$$x_3 = 0.716 \quad \text{and} \quad x_4 = 0.276$$

---

* For the remainder of this chapter we shall refer to this component as a turbine. The operation of turbines and reciprocating engines is described in detail in Chapters 19 and 16, and the circumstances in which one or the other is preferable are mentioned in section 16.4.

210

Hence from $h = h_f + xh_{fg}$ we have

$$h_3 = 121 + x_3 2433 = 1863 \text{ kJ/kg}$$

$$h_4 = 121 + x_4 2433 = 793 \text{ kJ/kg}$$

The turbine work is

$$W_{23} = (h_3 - h_2) = -940 \text{ kJ/kg}$$

and the compressor work is

$$W_{41} = (h_1 - h_4) = 215 \text{ kJ/kg}$$

The heat transfers in the boiler and condenser respectively are

$$Q_{12} = (h_2 - h_1) = 1795 \text{ kJ/kg}$$

$$Q_{34} = (h_4 - h_3) = -1070 \text{ kJ/kg}$$

The net work for the cycle is therefore

$$W = W_{23} + W_{41} = -725 \text{ kJ/kg}$$

and this is equal to $-(Q_{12} + Q_{34})$ as expected from the First Law.
The cycle efficiency, as defined by equation (5.2), is

$$\eta = \frac{|W|}{Q_{12}} = \frac{725}{1795} = 0.404$$

This must, of course, also be given by

$$\eta = \frac{T_1 - T_3}{T_1} = \frac{507.0 - 302.2}{507.0} = 0.404$$

The work ratio is

$$r_w = \frac{W}{W_{23}} = \frac{725}{940} = 0.771$$

and the specific steam consumption is

$$SSC = \frac{1}{|W|} = \frac{3600}{725} = 4.97 \text{ kg/kW h}$$

The wider the range of temperature, the more efficient becomes the cycle. The lowest possible temperature of the condensing steam is governed by two factors. The first is the temperature of the sink of heat—atmosphere, ocean or river—for which an average figure of 15 °C may be assumed. (Only natural sinks of heat need be considered; the additional work obtained by using a refrigerated sink could never be greater than the work required for the refrigeration, and with real irreversible processes would always be less.) The second is the temperature difference required for the heat transfer process. The rate of heat transfer is approximately proportional to the surface area across which heat flows, and the temperature difference between the condensing steam and the cooling fluid (see Part IV). In practice, the required rate of heat transfer can be obtained

Fig. 11.4
Variation of Carnot
efficiency with condenser
pressure

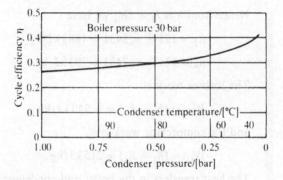

with a reasonable size of condenser only if a temperature difference of 10 K to
15 K is provided. The lowest practical condensing temperature in a cycle is
therefore 25 °C to 30 °C, the corresponding pressure being 0.032 bar to 0.042 bar.
The condenser pressure of 0.04 bar used in Example 11.1, for which the saturation
temperature is 29.0 °C, will be used in all the other examples in this chapter.
To show how important it is to keep the condenser pressure as low as possible,
the variation of cycle efficiency with condenser pressure has been calculated for
a constant boiler pressure of 30 bar and the results are presented in Fig. 11.4.

The maximum possible temperature of the working fluid, in power plants
of the kind considered in this chapter, is governed by the strength of the
materials available for the highly stressed parts of the plant, e.g. boiler
tubes or turbine blades. This *metallurgical limit* may be assumed to be
600 °C to 650 °C for steam plant at present, the exact figure depending upon
the life required of the plant. For a Carnot cycle operating with steam in the
wet region, the highest possible temperature is that corresponding to the
critical state: $T_c = 374.15$ °C and $p_c = 221.2$ bar. Modern materials cannot,
therefore, be used to their best advantage with this cycle when steam is the
working fluid. Fig. 11.5 shows the variation of cycle efficiency and steam
consumption with boiler pressure, for a constant condenser pressure of 0.04 bar.
It is evident that in the higher pressure range there is only a small gain in cycle
efficiency for increased boiler pressure. The cost of the boiler, pipe lines and
turbine casing increases with boiler pressure. Moreover the specific steam
consumption, and hence the size of plant, increases after a certain pressure is

Fig. 11.5
Variation of Carnot
efficiency and *SSC* with
boiler pressure

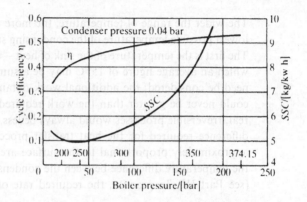

reached. Evidently the most economic pressure must be determined by reaching a compromise between low operating cost and low capital cost.

In the previous section we pointed out that the ideal cycle efficiency is not by itself a good guide to the probable overall efficiency of the actual plant. The work ratio for the cycle in Example 11.1 is, by comparison with other types of vapour cycle, quite low (0.771), and we must expect irreversibilities to have an appreciable effect on the cycle efficiency and steam consumption. The following example shows the effect of assuming values less than unity for the process efficiencies of the turbine and compressor when the boiler and condenser pressures are 30 bar and 0.04 bar as before.

Example 11.2   Recalculate Example 11.1 with isentropic efficiencies of 0.80 for the compression and expansion processes (Fig. 11.6), to estimate the actual cycle efficiency and steam consumption.

The actual turbine work is

$$W_{23} = (h_3 - h_2) = 0.80(h'_3 - h_2) = -752 \text{ kJ/kg}$$

and the actual compressor work is

$$W_{41} = (h_1 - h_4) = \frac{(h'_1 - h_4)}{0.80} = 269 \text{ kJ/kg}$$

The net work is therefore

$$W = W_{23} + W_{41} = -483 \text{ kJ/kg}$$

The enthalpy in state 1 is

$$h_1 = h_4 + W_{41} = 1062 \text{ kJ/kg}$$

and hence the heat transfer to the boiler is

$$Q_{12} = (h_2 - h_1) = 1741 \text{ kJ/kg}$$

The thermal efficiency is

$$\eta = \frac{|W|}{Q_{12}} = 0.277$$

and the specific steam consumption is

$$SSC = \frac{1}{|W|} = \frac{3600}{483} = 7.45 \text{ kg/kW h}$$

Fig. 11.6

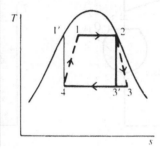

The previous examples show that the cycle efficiency is reduced by irreversibilities from 0.404 to 0.277, and that the steam consumption is increased from 4.97 kg/kW h to 7.45 kg/kW h. We shall show that more practical forms of steam cycle have work ratios nearer unity and so are much less affected by irreversibilities.

11.3 Rankine cycle

There are two major reasons why the Carnot cycle is not used in practice: first, because it has a low work ratio; and secondly, because of practical difficulties associated with the compression. It would be difficult to control the condensation process so that it stopped at state 4, and then carry out the compression of a very wet vapour efficiently. The liquid tends to separate out from the vapour and the compressor would have to deal with a non-homogeneous mixture. Moreover the volume of the fluid is high and the compressor would be comparable in size and cost with the turbine. It is comparatively easy, on the other hand, to condense the vapour completely, and compress the liquid to boiler pressure in a small feed pump. The resulting cycle, shown in Fig. 11.7, is known as the *Rankine cycle*.

It is evident without calculation that the efficiency of this cycle will be less than that of the Carnot cycle operating between the same temperatures, because all the heat supplied is not transferred at the upper temperature. Some heat is added while the temperature of the liquid varies from T_5 to T_1. It is also evident, from the comparative areas of the two cycles, that the net work output per unit mass of steam is greater in the Rankine cycle (in section 8.4.1 it was shown that the area $= \oint (T \, ds)_{rev} = \oint dQ = |W|$). It follows that the steam consumption is less and the work ratio is greater. Thus, in spite of a lower ideal cycle efficiency, the actual cycle efficiencies may not be so different, and the size of the Rankine plant will certainly be much smaller. The following example verifies these deductions.

Fig. 11.7
The Rankine cycle

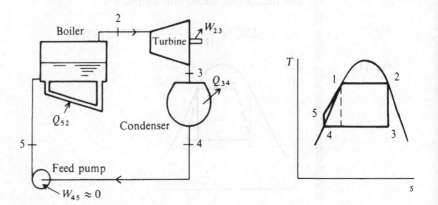

Example 11.3   Calculate the cycle efficiency, work ratio, and steam consumption of the Rankine cycle in Fig. 11.7, working between the same pressures as the Carnot cycle in Example 11.1. Estimate the actual cycle efficiency and specific steam consumption when the isentropic efficiencies of the expansion and compression processes are each 0.80.

(a) *Ideal cycle*
As in Example 11.1,

$$h_2 = 2803 \text{ kJ/kg} \quad \text{and} \quad h_3 = 1863 \text{ kJ/kg}$$

And the turbine work is, as before,

$$W_{23} = (h_3 - h_2) = -940 \text{ kJ/kg}$$

Using equation (10.5), the feed pump work of compression W_{45} is given by

$$W_{45} = v_f(p_5 - p_4) = 0.001(30 - 0.04) \times 100 = 3 \text{ kJ/kg}$$

And since the process is adiabatic, we have directly from the steady-flow energy equation

$$W_{45} = (h_5 - h_4)$$

Now $h_4 = h_f = 121 \text{ kJ/kg}$, and hence

$$h_5 = W_{45} + h_4 = 3 + 121 = 124 \text{ kJ/kg}$$

The heat supplied is then

$$Q_{52} = (h_2 - h_5) = 2803 - 124 = 2679 \text{ kJ/kg}$$

Therefore

$$\eta = \frac{|W|}{Q_{52}} = \frac{940 - 3}{2679} = 0.350$$

$$r_w = \frac{W}{W_{23}} = \frac{940 - 3}{940} = 0.997$$

$$SSC = \frac{1}{|W|} = \frac{3600}{940 - 3} = 3.84 \text{ kg/kW h}$$

(b) *Actual cycle* (Fig. 11.8)
Actual expansion work is

$$W_{23} = -0.80 \times 940 = -752 \text{ kJ/kg}$$

and the actual compression work is

$$W_{45} = \frac{3}{0.80} = 4 \text{ kJ/kg}$$

The enthalpy at state 5 now becomes

$$h_5 = h_4 + W_{45} = 125 \text{ kJ/kg}$$

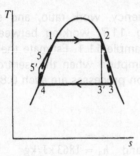

Fig. 11.8

and the heat supplied is

$$Q_{52} = (h_2 - h_5) = 2803 - 125 = 2678 \, \text{kJ/kg}$$

Therefore

$$\eta = \frac{|W|}{Q_{52}} = \frac{752 - 4}{2678} = 0.279$$

$$SSC = \frac{1}{|W|} = \frac{3600}{752 - 4} = 4.81 \, \text{kg/kW h}$$

The first point to note from the previous example is that the compressor work, or *feed pump term*, is very small compared with the other energy transfers. When the boiler pressure is comparatively low, a good approximation to the ideal cycle efficiency will be obtained if it is neglected. The approximate calculation yields the following results for the ideal cycle of the previous example:

$$W \approx W_{23} = -940 \, \text{kJ/kg}, \qquad Q_{52} \approx (h_2 - h_4) = 2682 \, \text{kJ/kg}$$

$$\eta \approx 0.350, \qquad SSC \approx 3.83 \, \text{kg/kW h}$$

This confirms the fact that the points representing states 4 and 5 almost coincide on the T–s diagram if it is drawn to any reasonable scale (see section 8.4.1).

The second point worth noting is that the difference between the performance of the ideal and actual cycles is much smaller than in the case of the Carnot cycle working between the same pressures and with the same process efficiencies. This is emphasised by the following table, in which the actual cycle performances are compared with the ideal values. For the assumed operating conditions the actual cycle efficiency of the Rankine plant (0.279) is slightly greater than that of the Carnot plant (0.277).

Cycle	r_W	Efficiency ratio	$\dfrac{\text{Actual } SSC}{\text{Ideal } SSC}$
Carnot	0.771	0.686	1.50
Rankine	0.997	0.797	1.25

Fig. 11.9 shows the results of a series of ideal cycle calculations with various boiler pressures and a constant condenser pressure of 0.04 bar. The cycle efficiency does not increase continuously with boiler pressure up to the critical

Fig. 11.9

Variation of Rankine cycle
efficiency and *SSC* with
boiler pressure

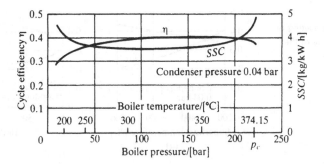

pressure, but reaches a maximum when the pressure is about 160 bar. The
reason is that the latent heat, and therefore the proportion of the heat supplied
which is transferred at the upper temperature, becomes smaller as the pressure
increases. Sooner or later the effective average temperature at which the heat
is added starts to decrease and the efficiency falls.

For a high efficiency it is essential to keep the condenser pressure as low as
possible. However, where space is restricted as in a steam locomotive, or where
no cooling water is available, the condenser is omitted and an open cycle is
used (see section 4.4). When the boiler feed water temperature is 100 °C, the
ideal cycle efficiency is then identical with that of a closed cycle plant condensing
at 1 atm. The condition of the fluid is the same at entry to the boiler in the two
cases, and the fact that the fluid entering the boiler is not the same as that
leaving the turbine makes no difference. If the boiler feed water temperature is
less than 100 °C, the efficiency will be reduced because more 'sensible heat'
must be added in the boiler.

It has already been remarked that the metallurgical limit cannot be approached
when the steam leaves the boiler in a saturated condition. But by placing in
the combustion gases a separate bank of tubes (the superheater) leading
saturated steam away from the boiler, it is possible to raise the steam temperature
without at the same time raising the boiler pressure. The Rankine cycle then
appears as in Fig. 11.10, from which it is evident that the average temperature
at which heat is supplied is increased by superheating and hence the ideal cycle

Fig. 11.10

The Rankine cycle with
superheat

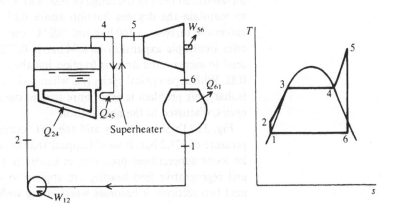

Fig. 11.11
Effect of superheating on
the performance of the
Rankine cycle

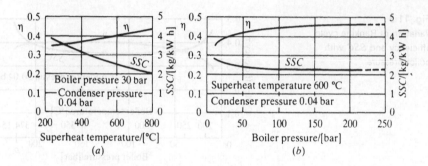

efficiency is increased. There is very little change in susceptibility to irreversibilities, the work ratio being so very near unity in the unsuperheated Rankine cycle that the slight increase obtained by superheating makes very little difference. Nevertheless, the specific steam consumption is markedly reduced, the net work per unit mass of steam being much greater, so that the added complexity of a superheater is compensated by a reduction in the size of other components. Fig. 11.11a shows the variation of ideal cycle efficiency and specific steam consumption with superheat temperature up to 800 °C. There is evidently still much to be gained by improving high-temperature materials. Unlike the efficiency of the unsuperheated cycle, the efficiency of the superheated cycle increases continuously with pressure. Fig. 11.11b illustrates this for a cycle with 0.04 bar condenser pressure and superheating to 600 °C—the metallurgical limit for long-life plant.

There is an additional reason why superheating is always used in practice. In the unsuperheated cycle of Example 11.3 the dryness fraction at the turbine exhaust is 0.716. Inspection of the T–s diagram shows that with higher boiler pressures the turbine exhaust would become even wetter. This is a very undesirable feature, because droplets in the steam erode the blading and reduce the turbine isentropic efficiency; see section 19.2.4. In practice the dryness fraction at the turbine exhaust is not allowed to fall below about 0.88. Superheating increases the dryness fraction, although with the present metallurgical limit in the range of 600–650 °C it is not always by itself sufficient to maintain the dryness fraction above 0.88. For example, when the steam enters the turbine at 160 bar and 600 °C, the turbine exhaust dryness fraction after isentropic expansion to 0.04 bar is 0.772; irreversibilities in the turbine tend to increase the dryness fraction but they would not bring the value up to 0.88. With supercritical cycles (i.e. when 2–3–4–5 in Fig. 11.10 is a supercritical isobar) this problem is even more severe; the remedy lies in the use of reheat cycles, discussed in the next section.

Fig. 11.11b shows the η and the SSC curves extended beyond the critical pressure of 221.2 bar. It would appear that the use of pressures beyond 160 bar, let alone supercritical pressures, is hardly justified. However, when reheating and regenerative feed heating are applied to such cycles, as described in the next two sections, it becomes worth using such extreme pressures.

Fig. 11.12
The reheat cycle

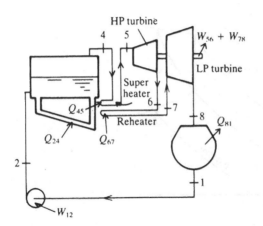

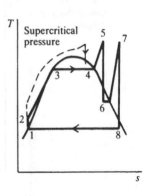

11.4   Reheat cycle

With the reheat cycle the expansion takes place in two turbines. The steam expands in the high-pressure turbine to some intermediate pressure, and is then passed back to yet another bank of tubes in the boiler where it is reheated at constant pressure, usually to the original superheat temperature.* It then expands in the low-pressure turbine to the condenser pressure. The cycle appears as in Fig. 11.12, and the following example shows the effect of reheating on the ideal cycle efficiency and specific consumption. A boiler pressure of 30 bar has been assumed for the sake of comparison with the other examples in this chapter, although this is well below the most economical pressure for which to design a reheat cycle plant.

Example 11.4   Find the ideal cycle efficiency and specific steam consumption of a reheat cycle (Fig. 11.12) operating between pressures of 30 and 0.04 bar, with a superheat temperature of 450 °C. Assume that the first expansion is carried out to the point where the steam is dry saturated and that the steam is reheated to the original superheat temperature. The feed pump term may be neglected.

From tables,

$$h_2 \approx h_1 = 121 \text{ kJ/kg}, \qquad h_5 = 3343 \text{ kJ/kg},$$

$$s_5 = 7.082 \text{ kJ/kg K}$$

To find the intermediate reheat pressure p_6, we find from the saturation table the pressure at which $s_g = s_5$. This gives

$$p_6 = p_7 = 2.3 \text{ bar} \quad \text{and hence} \quad h_6 = 2713 \text{ kJ/kg}$$

---

* It has been suggested that as an alternative to the conventional reheat scheme, it is better to reheat the steam near the turbine via a liquid metal circulating between the boiler and reheater. The appreciable pressure drop in the lengthy conventional reheat circuit is avoided, but this gain is partially offset by the extra temperature drop required for the liquid metal circuit.

Fig. 11.13
Use of the *h*–*s*
diagram

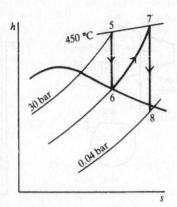

From the superheat table,

$$h_7 = 3381 \text{ kJ/kg} \quad \text{and} \quad s_7 = 8.310 \text{ kJ/kg K}$$

At the turbine outlet,

$$x_8 = 0.980 \quad \text{and} \quad h_8 = 2505 \text{ kJ/kg}$$

The total quantity of heat transferred to the steam in the boiler is

$$Q_{25} + Q_{67} = (h_5 - h_2) + (h_7 - h_6) = 3222 + 668 = 3890 \text{ kJ/kg}$$

and the total turbine work is

$$W_{56} + W_{78} = (h_6 - h_5) + (h_8 - h_7)$$
$$= -630 - 876 = -1506 \text{ kJ/kg}$$

The cycle efficiency is therefore

$$\eta = \frac{|(W_{56} + W_{78})|}{Q_{25} + Q_{67}} = \frac{1506}{3890} = 0.387$$

and the specific steam consumption is

$$SSC = \frac{1}{|W|} = \frac{3600}{1506} = 2.39 \text{ kg/kW h}$$

This example, as well as the other examples in this chapter, can be solved more quickly by means of an *h*–*s* chart. This is illustrated in Fig. 11.13. The chart usually covers only the superheat region and the two-phase region near the saturated vapour line, and it cannot therefore be used for finding h_1, h_2 and h_3. It enables one, however, to find h_5, h_6, h_7 and h_8 more quickly than by means of tables.

Comparing the foregoing results with those of Examples 11.1 and 11.3, and the appropriate values from Fig. 11.11a (all cycles with a boiler pressure of 30 bar and a condenser pressure of 0.04 bar), we arrive at the following table for *ideal* cycles:

	Carnot	Rankine (no superheat)	Rankine (super-heat to 450 °C)	Reheat (to 450 °C)
η	0.404	0.350	0.375	0.387
$SSC/[\text{kg}/\text{kW h}]$	4.97	3.84	2.98	2.39

It can be seen that reheating reduces the steam consumption appreciably, as might be expected from consideration of the area of the cycle on the $T–s$ diagram which equals the magnitude of the net work output per unit mass of steam. This reduction is a particularly important consideration in higher-pressure cycles because it implies a smaller boiler—an expensive item in high-pressure plant. However, this decrease in size cannot completely offset the disadvantage of the added complexity, and it must be stressed that the main reason for reheating is to avoid too wet a condition in the turbine.

It is clear that reheating makes only a little difference to the ideal cycle efficiency. Whether it increases or decreases the efficiency, in comparison with the Rankine cycle having the same conditions in the boiler and condenser, depends upon the point in the expansion at which reheating is carried out. The reheat cycle can be regarded as a combination of the Rankine cycle and the cycle abcd (or a'b'c'd) in Fig. 11.14. If the latter has a lower efficiency than the Rankine cycle, the efficiency of the combination will be lower also. The effective average temperature at which the heat is added in the cycle abcd may well be lower than that in the Rankine cycle if the intermediate pressure is too low.

Cycles using supercritical pressures have been coming into operation in recent years. With such cycles the problem of moisture in the turbine is even more severe, and the use of reheating is essential. So far, it has been possible to avoid the additional complication of reheating at more than one point in the expansion, although double-reheat units are now being considered. Typical modern supercritical and subcritical ideal cycles are compared in the following table, where reheating is assumed to occur when the steam is just saturated ($x_a = 1$

Fig. 11.14
The effect of reheat pressure on the cycle efficiency

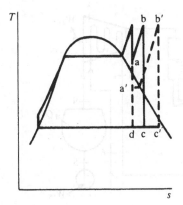

in Fig. 11.14):

	Superheat to 600 °C		Superheat and reheat to 600 °C	
	160 bar	350 bar	160 bar	350 bar
η	0.453	0.486	0.468	0.485
$SSC/[\text{kg}/\text{kW h}]$	2.31	2.37	1.76	1.80
x_{exit}	0.772	0.708	0.954	0.871

Although the increase in efficiency resulting from the use of supercritical pressures seems small, it should not be discounted. A 1 per cent increase in efficiency for a cycle which has an actual efficiency of say 40 per cent is equivalent to $1/0.4 = 2.5$ per cent saving in fuel—a saving well worth having. Nevertheless it is true to say that a marked improvement in efficiency of the reheat cycle cannot be obtained by using higher pressures; it can be achieved only by developing new high-temperature alloys or other materials for turbine blading and superheater tubing and thereby raising the metallurgical limit.

11.5 Regenerative cycle

The efficiency of the unsuperheated cycle (Fig. 11.7) is less than the Carnot efficiency $(T_a - T_b)/T_a$, because some of the heat supplied is transferred while the temperature of the working fluid varies from T_5 to T_1. If some means could be found to transfer this heat *reversibly* from the working fluid in another part of the cycle, then all the heat supplied from an *external* source would be transferred at the upper temperature and the Carnot cycle efficiency would therefore be achieved. A cycle in which this artifice is used to raise the efficiency is called a *regenerative cycle*.

One method which is theoretically possible is indicated in Fig. 11.15. The feed water, at T_6, is passed into passages in the turbine casing at the point where the expanding steam has a temperature only infinitesimally greater than T_6. The water flows in a direction opposite to that of the expanding steam, and

Fig. 11.15
A hypothetical
regenerative cycle

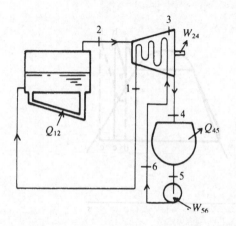
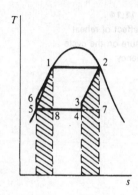

is thereby heated to a temperature only infinitesimally smaller than T_2 before it passes into the boiler. At all points the heat transfer is effected by an infinitesimal temperature difference and the process is therefore reversible. Most of the expansion in the turbine is no longer an adiabatic process, but follows the path 2–3–4. Since the heat rejected in process 2–3 equals that supplied in process 6–1, the shaded areas on the T–s diagram of Fig. 11.15 must be equal. The heat supplied from the external source is equal to the area under line 1–2, and the heat rejected to the external sink equals the area under line 4–5. Inspection of the areas involved shows that not only are the efficiencies of the regenerative cycle and the Carnot cycle 1–2–7–8 equal, but the steam consumptions also. On the other hand the work ratio of the regenerative cycle, requiring the negligible pump work $(h_6 - h_5)$, is very much higher than that of the Carnot cycle and is comparable with that of the Rankine cycle.

Such a regenerative cycle is impractical for two reasons. First, it would be impossible to design a turbine which would operate efficiently as both turbine and heat exchanger. Secondly, the steam expanding through the turbine would reach an impracticably low dryness fraction. For these reasons the basic idea of regeneration is applied in a somewhat different way: instead of the feed water being taken to the turbine, some of the turbine steam is taken to the feed water.

The simplest approximation to a practical regenerative cycle is shown in Fig. 11.16. Consider 1 kg of steam in state 2 passing from the boiler into the turbine. This steam is expanded to an intermediate state 3, at which point a quantity y kg is bled off and taken to a *feed water heater*. The remaining $(1-y)$ kg is expanded to condenser pressure and leaves the turbine in state 4. After condensation to state 5, the $(1-y)$ kg of water is compressed in the first feed pump to the bleeding pressure $(p_6 = p_3)$. It is then mixed in the feed water heater with y kg of bled steam in state 3, and the 1 kg of mixture leaves the heater in state 7. A second feed pump compresses the water to boiler pressure, state 1. In this cycle the *average* temperature at which the heat is added from an *external source* is higher than in the Rankine cycle, and therefore the efficiency is increased. The cycle is not a true ideal cycle, because the mixing process between steam at state 3 and water at state 6 is irreversible. In the limit, as the number of bleedings and feed water heaters is increased to infinity, the mixing processes

Fig. 11.16
A simple regenerative
cycle using one feed
water heater

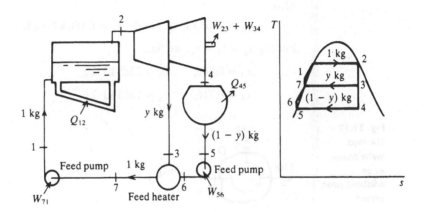

become reversible, all the heat from the external source is supplied at the upper temperature, and the cycle will therefore have the Carnot efficiency.

Since a regenerative cycle of this kind is really a combination of cycles undergone by different quantities of fluid, there is some difficulty in portraying it on a T–s diagram. Fig. 11.16 must be interpreted as implying that $(1 - y)$ kg is carried through cycle 5–6–7–1–2–3–4–5, while y kg follows the path 7–1–2–3–7.

Example 11.5 Find the cycle efficiency and specific steam consumption of a regenerative cycle with one feed heater, if the steam leaves the boiler dry saturated at 30 bar and is condensed at 0.04 bar (Fig. 11.16). Neglect the feed pump work.

It is first necessary to select the pressure p_3 at which the steam is to be bled off. It is shown later that the cycle efficiency is a maximum when the temperature T_3 is approximately halfway between T_2 and T_4, i.e.

$$T_3 = \frac{T_2 + T_4}{2} = \frac{233.8 + 29.0}{2} = 131.4\,°C$$

and hence

$$p_3 = 2.8 \text{ bar}$$

We can now calculate the correct mass y kg to be bled off at p_7. Consider the heater as an adiabatic open system (Fig. 11.17). No work is done and the energy equation reduces to

$$0 = 1h_7 - yh_3 - (1 - y)h_6$$

Putting $h_6 = h_5$, we find that

$$y = \frac{h_7 - h_5}{h_3 - h_5}$$

From tables,

$$h_5 = 121 \text{ kJ/kg} \quad \text{and} \quad h_7 = 551 \text{ kJ/kg}$$

Also,

$$h_2 = 2803 \text{ kJ/kg} \quad \text{and} \quad s_2 = 6.186 \text{ kJ/kg K}$$

Putting $s_2 = s_3 = s_4$, we find

$$x_3 = 0.846, \qquad h_3 = 2388 \text{ kJ/kg}$$

$$x_4 = 0.716, \qquad h_4 = 1863 \text{ kJ/kg}$$

Fig. 11.17
The feed water heater as an adiabatic open system

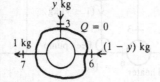

Hence

$$y = \frac{551 - 121}{2388 - 121} = 0.1897$$

The heat transferred in the boiler is

$$Q_{12} = (h_2 - h_1) = 2803 - 551 = 2252 \text{ kJ/kg}$$

The turbine work is

$$W_{23} + W_{34} = 1(h_3 - h_2) + (1 - y)(h_4 - h_3)$$
$$= -415 - 425 = -840 \text{ kJ/kg}$$

Therefore

$$\eta = \frac{|(W_{23} + W_{34})|}{Q_{12}} = \frac{840}{2252} = 0.373$$

and the specific steam consumption is

$$SSC = \frac{1}{|W|} = \frac{3600}{840} = 4.29 \text{ kg/kW h}$$

In Fig. 11.18 the cycle efficiency is plotted against bleed temperature, all the other conditions remaining constant. It can be seen that the cycle efficiency is a maximum when the bleed temperature is approximately equal to the mean of the boiler and condenser temperatures, and that a slight deviation from this value does not affect the efficiency significantly.

Comparing the results of Example 11.5 with those of the ideal unsuperheated Rankine cycle in Example 11.3, the efficiency has been increased from 0.350 to 0.373 with the use of only one feed heater. On the other hand the specific consumption has been increased from 3.84 kg/kW h to 4.29 kg/kW h. In practice the best return for the additional capital cost is obtained with several feed heaters, the exact number depending on the steam conditions. The proper choice of the bleed pressures is a matter of lengthy optimisation calculations which cannot be entered into here. The *open heater*, in which the bled steam is freely mixed with the feed water, is not often used because of the large number

Fig. 11.18
Effect of bleed temperature
on the cycle efficiency

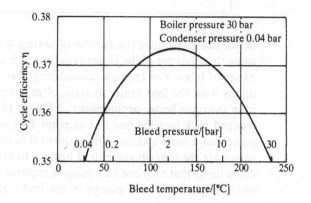

225

Fig. 11.19
A regenerative cycle with
three feed water heaters

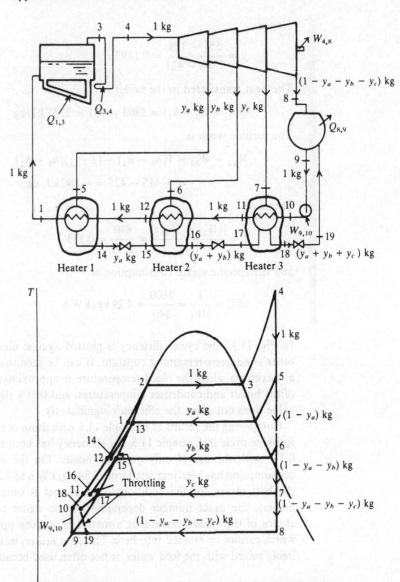

of feed pumps required (i.e. number of heaters + 1). Fig. 11.19 illustrates a plant
using three heaters of the *closed* type, in which the heat is transferred through
banks of tubes. For example, considering heater 1, the bled steam in state 5
drains from the feed heater in state 14 as a separate stream; this is different
from the open heater arrangement of Fig. 11.16. The drain in state 14 can be
pumped back into the feed line at point 1 by means of a small drain or drip
pump, but a more common arrangement is to cascade it back through throttle
valves, via the lower-pressure feed heaters, to the condenser. The advantage of
doing this is that only one feed pump is required; a similar train of open heaters
would require four feed pumps in the feed water line. The throttling of the

drains is accompanied in practice by the formation of some steam, and this can lead to rapid erosion in the cascade line. To avoid this erosion, the drains are throttled into large flash chambers (not shown) which reduce the velocity and therefore the erosion.

Considering the T–s diagram in Fig. 11.19, the feed water leaving the feed pump in state 10 is successively heated to temperatures T_{11}, T_{12} and T_1 which, ideally, are equal to the saturation temperatures T_{17}, T_{15} and T_{13}* respectively. In practice $T_{11} < T_{17}$, $T_{12} < T_{15}$, $T_1 < T_{13}$, the differences usually being referred to as the *terminal temperature differences* of the heaters. Similarly the condensed bled steam should drain at temperatures $T_{14} = T_{12}$, $T_{16} = T_{11}$ and $T_{18} = T_{10}$. Such ideal conditions can only be achieved with closed heaters having infinitely large heat exchange areas. The following example, which is concerned with the ideal cycle, assumes such limiting conditions to exist.

Example 11.6   Calculate the ideal cycle efficiency and specific steam consumption of a regenerative cycle using three closed heaters as shown in Fig. 11.19. The steam leaves the boiler at 30 bar superheated to 450 °C, and the condenser pressure is 0.04 bar. Choose the bleed pressures so that the temperature difference $(T_2 - T_c)$ is divided into approximately equal steps. (Such a choice of bleed pressures makes the efficiency of the ideal cycle approximately a maximum.)

Making the temperature differences $(T_2 - T_{13})$, $(T_{13} - T_{15})$, $(T_{15} - T_{17})$, $(T_{17} - T_9)$ approximately equal, the bleed pressures become 11, 2.8 and 0.48 bar. All the relevant enthalpies in the plant can now be found. Before during and after expansion in the turbine these are

$$h_4 = 3343 \text{ kJ/kg}, \qquad h_5 = 3049 \text{ kJ/kg}$$

$$h_6 = 2749 \text{ kJ/kg}, \qquad h_7 = 2458 \text{ kJ/kg}, \qquad h_8 = 2133 \text{ kJ/kg}$$

In finding the enthalpies in the feed line, the following assumptions will be made:

(a)   The feed pump term is negligible, i.e. $h_9 \approx h_{10}$.

(b)   In throttling the condensed bled steam, which is a process of equal initial and final enthalpy, the state after throttling lies approximately on the saturation line; e.g. in throttling from 14 to 15, $h_{14} = h_{15}$ will be identical with h_f corresponding to pressure p_6.

(c)   The enthalpy of the compressed liquid in the feed line is approximately equal to that of saturated liquid at the same temperature, e.g. $h_{12} \approx h_{15}$.

---

* It might appear feasible, where the bled steam is initially superheated and condensed in a counter-flow heater, for the exit temperature of the feed water to attain the superheat temperature, e.g. $T_1 = T_5$ in heater 1. This ideal cannot be achieved, however, because the difference between the sensible enthalpy capacities of the bled superheated steam and the feed water would necessitate heat transfer from colder steam to hotter feed water over the temperature range $T_{13} \rightarrow T_5$. Although the condition $T_1 = T_5$ is impossible, the heater could be designed so that the ideal feed temperature T_1 is slightly above T_{13}, but this possibility will be neglected in what follows.

With these assumptions we can write

$$h_{10} = h_{18} = h_{19} = h_9 = 121 \text{ kJ/kg}$$

$$h_{11} = h_{16} = h_{17} = 336 \text{ kJ/kg}$$

$$h_{12} = h_{14} = h_{15} = 551 \text{ kJ/kg}$$

$$h_1 = h_{13} = 781 \text{ kJ/kg}$$

To determine the correct amounts of steam to be held for each heater per kg of steam leaving the boiler, an energy equation can be written down for each heater.

First heater: $\quad 1h_1 + y_a h_{14} - y_a h_5 - 1h_{12} = 0$

$$y_a = \frac{h_{13} - h_{15}}{h_5 - h_{15}} = 0.0921$$

Second heater: $\quad 1h_{12} + (y_a + y_b)h_{16} - y_b h_6 - 1h_{11} - y_a h_{15} = 0$

$$y_b = (1 - y_a)\frac{h_{15} - h_{17}}{h_6 - h_{17}} = 0.0809$$

Third heater: $\quad 1h_{11} + (y_a + y_b + y_c)h_{18} - y_c h_7 - (y_a + y_b)h_{17}$
$$- 1h_{10} = 0$$

$$y_c = (1 - y_a - y_b)\frac{h_{17} - h_9}{h_7 - h_9} = 0.0761$$

(Always start with the highest-pressure heater so as to have only one unknown at each step in the calculation.)

We can now calculate the heat and work transfers for the cycle. The heat added in the boiler is

$$Q_{1,4} = (h_4 - h_1) = 2562 \text{ kJ/kg}$$

and the heat rejected in the condenser is

$$Q_{8,9} = 1h_9 - (1 - y_a - y_b - y_c)h_8 - (y_a + y_b + y_c)h_{19}$$
$$= -1511 \text{ kJ/kg}$$

The work done in the turbine is

$$W_{4,8} = 1(h_5 - h_4) + (1 - y_a)(h_6 - h_5) + (1 - y_a - y_b)(h_7 - h_6)$$
$$+ (1 - y_a - y_b - y_c)(h_8 - h_7) = -1051 \text{ kJ/kg}$$

(As a check, $W_{4,8}$ must also be given by $W_{4,8} = -(Q_{1,4} + Q_{8,9}) = -1051 \text{ kJ/kg}$.)
The cycle efficiency is

$$\eta = \frac{|W_{4,8}|}{Q_{1,4}} = 0.410$$

and the specific consumption is

$$SSC = \frac{1}{|W|} = \frac{3600}{1051} = 3.43 \text{ kg/kW h}$$

The ideal efficiency and steam consumption for the Rankine cycle corresponding to the cycle 9–2–4–8–9 in Fig. 11.19 can be found from Fig. 11.11a to be 0.375 and 2.98 kg/kW h. For the regenerative cycle these become 0.410 and 3.43 kg/kW h. Apart from the marked improvement in cycle efficiency, regeneration has the advantage of easing the difficulties in the design of the blading at the low-pressure end of the turbine. With the Rankine cycle this blading has to pass a very large volume flow and the blades must be undesirably long. By bleeding, the volume flow at the low-pressure end is considerably reduced; this is indicated by the stepped outline of the turbine in Fig. 11.19. The size of the condenser is also reduced, which partially compensates for the additional feed heating components.

It is necessary to point out that if the isentropic efficiency of the turbine is not unity, points 5, 6, 7, 8 on the *T–s* diagram will not be vertically below point 4. To estimate the actual cycle efficiency with an irreversible expansion it is necessary to know the path of the expansion (i.e. *line of condition*), and this is considered in section 19.2.5.

With modern steam conditions the best compromise between additional capital costs and improved efficiency is obtained when a train of about eight feed heaters is used. It is common to include one open heater at a moderate pressure which incorporates a de-aerator, because dissolved air leads to corrosion in the boiler, and is detrimental to heat transfer and the maintenance of a high vacuum in the condenser. There will normally be two closed heaters at pressure below the open heater, with the condensed bleed cascading back into the condenser. At pressures above the open heater there will be about three closed heaters whose condensate cascades back into the open heater. A description of modern plant and a more detailed thermodynamic analysis of regenerative cycles can be found in Refs 18 and 34 respectively.

The observant student may have noticed that to call the 'open feed heater' a heater is a misnomer. The component is an adiabatic mixing chamber, and no 'heat' in the thermodynamic sense is involved in the process.

11.6 Economiser and air preheater

So far we have been comparing the performance of the various cycles on the basis of cycle efficiency, and have assumed in effect that the combustion process can be carried out with equal efficiency in all plants. This is not, in fact, the case. Without discussing combustion efficiency in detail, it can be appreciated that if the combustion gases leave the boiler plant at a temperature higher than atmospheric, some of the latent energy in the fuel is being wasted. Useful work could still be obtained by operating a cycle between the exhaust gas temperature and atmospheric temperature. With the Carnot cycle, the lowest temperature at which the exhaust gases can leave the plant is the upper temperature of the cycle. With the Rankine cycle, on the other hand, the exhaust gases could be reduced, ideally, to the temperature of the water leaving the feed pump. A reduction in exhaust gas temperature is accomplished in practice by passing the feed water through a bank of tubes, the *economiser*, situated in the chimney.

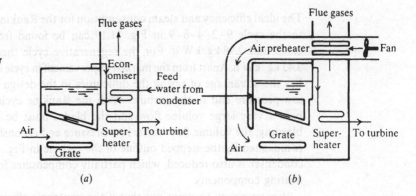

Fig. 11.20
Diagrammatic sketch of a
boiler plant with (a) an
economiser and (b) an air
preheater

The flow is in the direction indicated in Fig. 11.20a, so that the hottest gases are transferring heat to the hottest water, and the temperature difference between the fluids is kept to a minimum throughout the process. One limitation is that the products of combustion should not normally be cooled below their dew point (see section 14.5), otherwise condensation containing corrosive acids may cause serious damage to the economiser tubes. The dew point of sulphuric acid vapour is at a higher temperature than that of pure water vapour, and in practice 150 °C is considered the safe lower limit. For small commercial and domestic boilers burning natural gas which is free of sulphur, it is economical to use stainless steel components and this limit is unnecessary; these are called *condensing boilers.*

It would appear that the advantage of higher ideal efficiency possessed by the Carnot cycle is at least partly diminished by its inability to abstract all the energy available in the products of combustion—a further argument in favour of the practical superiority of the Rankine cycle. The regenerative cycle suffers from the same disadvantage as the Carnot cycle in this respect. If an economiser is added to the cycle shown in Fig. 11.19, the minimum temperature to which the combustion gases can be cooled is T_1. When a large number of feed heaters is used, the feed water entering the boiler is nearly at boiling point and an economiser becomes superfluous.

An alternative method of reducing the temperature of the combustion gases, which can be used with all the cycles, is known as *air preheating.* The air preheater is a bank of tubes in the chimney through which the combustion air passes before reaching the grate, as in Fig. 11.20b. The combustion gases are cooled while the temperature of the air is increased prior to combustion. Since the reactants start with a higher temperature, less fuel need be burnt to arrive at the same products temperature. The net result is an increase in combustion efficiency comparable with that obtained with an economiser. Air preheating is often used in conjunction with an economiser in Rankine and reheat plants, but the degree of preheating cannot be carried as far as in the regenerative plant where no economiser is fitted. (It is worth noting that the most common type of air preheater is not a fixed bank of tubes, but a rotating matrix of the type illustrated schematically in Fig. 24.5.)

One practical consequence of cooling the combustion gases is that only a small amount of natural draught can be obtained in the chimney. The heat exchanging banks of tubes, grate and chimney require a fair pressure gradient to maintain the necessary air flow for combustion. For this reason a forced draught, produced by a fan, is always used in modern boiler plant. The power expended on driving the fan is small compared with the advantage gained by improving the combustion efficiency.

Enough has been said to indicate that a complete evaluation of an external-combustion power cycle must take account of the interdependence between the combustion and cycle efficiencies. The adoption of means to improve one efficiency may easily lead to the reduction of the other. A formal analysis of the plant as a whole is possible using the concept of exergy introduced in section 7.9, and Refs 12 and 13 of Part I provide a good introduction to this approach.

11.7 Steam cycles for nuclear power plant

Nuclear power plant have been developed mainly on what can be called conventional lines, by using the nuclear reactor as a source of heat for a steam cycle. Some effort is being directed towards the direct conversion of nuclear energy into electrical energy, e.g. via the magnetohydrodynamic generator briefly described in Chapter 20, but these efforts still have to bear fruit. Here we shall discuss briefly some of the consequences arising from the application of nuclear energy sources to steam cycles. Although the principles discussed in the preceding sections apply also to nuclear plant, there exist a number of difficulties peculiar to such plant. They arise largely from present restrictions on the maximum permissible temperature which 'fuel' elements in a reactor are allowed to reach, and from the use of a secondary fluid to transfer energy from them to the steam. There is every prospect that further development of reactor materials will ease these restrictions and therefore remove at least some of these peculiar difficulties.

Fig. 11.21a shows diagrammatically a simple scheme employing a secondary fluid which circulates through the reactor and transfers heat to the steam boiler.

Fig. 11.21
Simple nuclear power plant

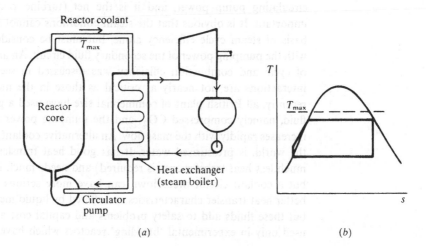

(a)   (b)

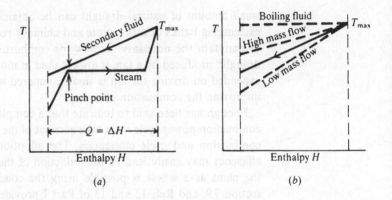

Fig. 11.22
An application of the
temperature–enthalpy
diagram

In early reactors the permissible maximum temperature T_{max} of the secondary fluid leaving the reactor was below the critical temperature of steam, and it might appear that the cycle shown in Fig. 11.21b would have been the obvious choice. However, quite apart from the difficulty of excessive moisture in the turbine which such a choice would entail, it should be remembered that the secondary fluid falls in temperature as it flows through the heat exchanger, and therefore the saturation temperature of the steam must be well below T_{max}. This is most easily appreciated on the T–H diagram of Fig. 11.22a, where H is the product of mass flow and specific enthalpy of the respective fluids. ΔH must be the same for the two curves, it being equal to the total quantity of heat transferred. The saturation temperature is chosen so that at the so-called *pinch point* the secondary fluid temperature is marginally higher than the saturation temperature, and it can be seen that under these conditions a certain amount of superheating is possible. The use of such T–H diagrams, and the significance of pinch points, will be illustrated in examples in sections 11.9 and 12.5.

The secondary fluid temperature drop, for a specified heat transfer, can be varied by varying the mass flow as indicated in Fig. 11.22b. A higher mass flow enables a higher saturation temperature to be used for the power cycle and thus a higher steam cycle efficiency to be obtained, but it also entails a higher circulating pump power, and it is the net (turbine–pump) work which is important. It is obvious that the steam conditions cannot be optimised on the basis of steam cycle efficiency alone, but must be considered in conjunction with the pumping power of the secondary fluid circuit. An analogous interaction of cycle and combustion efficiency was discussed in section 11.6, but such interactions are not nearly as critical as those in the nuclear reactor. Until recently, all British plant of commercial size have used a gas as the secondary fluid, namely compressed CO_2, and the pumping power for gas is large and increases rapidly with the mass flow. An alternative coolant, widely used around the world, is pressurised water. It has good heat transfer characteristics (i.e. much less heat transfer area is required) and needs much less pumping power, but a coolant circuit breakdown can have more serious consequences. Even better heat transfer characteristics are offered by liquid metals such as sodium, but these fluids add to safety problems and capital cost and so far have been used only in experimental 'breeding' reactors which have exceptionally small

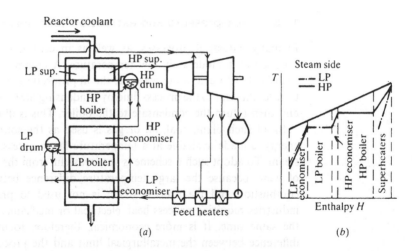

Fig. 11.23
Dual-pressure cycle

reactor cores and consequently very restricted heat transfer surface area. It should be appreciated that the number of possible secondary fluids is limited because, as with any material in the reactor core, the nuclear characteristics play an overriding role. In particular, materials must have only a very weak capacity for absorbing neutrons—unless of course they are put there specifically for that purpose in the form of control rods.

A secondary fluid which changes phase (e.g. boiling water) undergoes no temperature drop as it condenses in the heat exchanger and would enable the highest possible saturation temperature to be used for the steam cycle. But it carries the risk of 'burn-out' of the reactor fuel elements (see section 22.8.2) and it requires from the designer a precise knowledge of boiling heat transfer which until recently has been lacking. A further difficulty which arises with a boiling fluid in a reactor derives from the fact that the nuclear reactions in the fuel elements are appreciably affected by the ratio of vapour to liquid surrounding the elements, and very close control of the boiling process is essential. One attraction of using boiling heat transfer to steam is that the secondary fluid circuit can be dispensed with by passing the steam directly into the turbine, although care has to be taken to avoid steam leakage from any part of the circuit because it may be contaminated with radioactivity.

Nothing very final can be said about the best choice of cycle, because reactor materials and metallurgical limits are still changing rapidly. With gas cooling, British practice has been to use a *dual-pressure* cycle, a simplified version of which is shown in Fig. 11.23. It is seen to incorporate regenerative feed heating to improve cycle efficiency, and other refinements (not shown) are mainly concerned with the reduction of moisture by reheating, moisture extraction or some method of steam drying. Comparing Figs 11.22a and 11.23b, it can be seen that the dual-pressure cycle improves the cycle efficiency by reducing the average temperature difference between the secondary fluid and steam, or in other words by increasing the average temperature at which heat is supplied to the working fluid in the cycle. Further information on steam cycles for nuclear power plant can be found in Ref. 35.

233

11.8 Back-pressure and extraction turbines, and cogeneration

In many industrial processes, as well as in central heating, heat has to be supplied at a moderately low temperature. A common method of supplying such heat is to evaporate water at the appropriate temperature and pressure, transfer the heat to the process fluid by condensing the steam in a heat exchanger, and then return the condensate to the boiler. This is illustrated in Fig. 11.24.

In all such plant, coal, oil or gas is used as the source of energy, and the energy is made available at a temperature far in excess of that of the process steam. To adopt such a scheme is very wasteful from the thermodynamic point of view, because the large temperature difference between the products of combustion and the process steam is not used to produce work. In most industries requiring process heat, electrical or mechanical power is required at the same time. It is more economical, therefore, to utilise the temperature difference between the metallurgical limit and the process steam temperature for the production of work, and obtain the process heat from the heat rejected in the steam condenser. Such a plant is illustrated in Fig. 11.25. A turbine exhausting into a condenser at a relatively high pressure, in which the rejected heat is employed usefully, is called a *back-pressure turbine*.

It is clear that, apart from the thermodynamic economy achieved in combining the power and heating plant, the capital cost is also reduced. A single boiler serves two purposes, and the usual condenser of the power plant becomes superfluous as it is replaced by the process heat exchanger.

The use of a back-pressure turbine is practical if the power and heat requirements are fairly steady and well matched. When the power requirements are larger than those that can be obtained from a simple back-pressure turbine,

Fig. 11.24
A simple heating plant

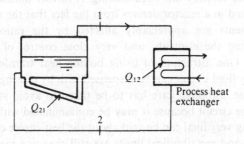
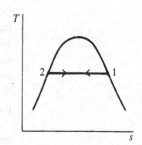

Fig. 11.25
A back-pressure turbine plant

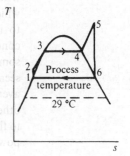

Fig. 11.26
A pass-out or extraction
turbine plant

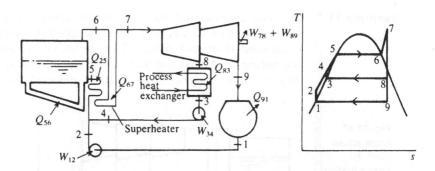

an *extraction* or *pass-out turbine* can be used. In this alternative scheme some
of the steam is expanded to the lowest possible temperature of about 29 °C, the
remainder being extracted from the turbine at the correct intermediate temperature
(Fig. 11.26). The extracted steam is condensed in the process heat exchanger
and finally returned to the boiler. This scheme enables variations in power and
heat requirements to be at least partly accommodated by controlling the amount
of extracted steam.

Schemes involving the *combined production of heat and power* are variously
known as CHP plant, *cogeneration* plant, or *total energy* plant. Some at least
of the heat requirement is seasonal, e.g. the part concerned with building heating,
and it is not always easy to match the heat and power demands. The economic
viability of CHP plant for industry often rests upon the financial terms under
which excess power can be sold to the country's electricity network, or the
price at which the network is prepared to sell shortfalls to the industry. In the
past, developments in this area were often inhibited by satutory regulations or
legislation designed to protect existing technologies.

With the new emphasis on energy conservation, both for economic reasons
and because of increasing concern with environmental damage (atmospheric
pollution, acid rain, greenhouse effect etc.), serious consideration is being given
to the use of back-pressure or pass-out turbines in large power stations located
near cities. The rejected heat would be conveyed to buildings by hot water
mains. Inevitably some electricity production capacity is lost and must be made
up from other power stations in the generating network. A useful criterion of
performance is provided by a ratio Φ given by

$$\Phi = \frac{\text{heat produced for district heating}}{\text{extra heat used in network to replace lost electricity}}$$

The denominator could be evaluated on the basis of the average efficiency of
base-load power stations in the network. The ratio Φ might be termed the
thermal advantage and is a crude measure of the saving in fuel consumption.
Up to now, when capital and maintenance costs are included, the economic
advantage over heating appliances in individual buildings has been marginally
against such schemes in the UK. The saving in fuel consumption and reduction
in environmental damage, however, would be very considerable: see Ref. 38 for
an example.

Example 11.7 The low-pressure turbine of a power station is to be replaced by a pass-out turbine so that heat can be supplied to a town. Two schemes are considered, illustrated in Fig. 11.27. In both cases the inlet conditions for the turbine are 11 bar and 560 °C, and the condenser pressure is 0.04 bar. The isentropic efficiency of the turbine expansion can be taken as 0.90, and

Fig. 11.27
Cogeneration plant for district heating scheme

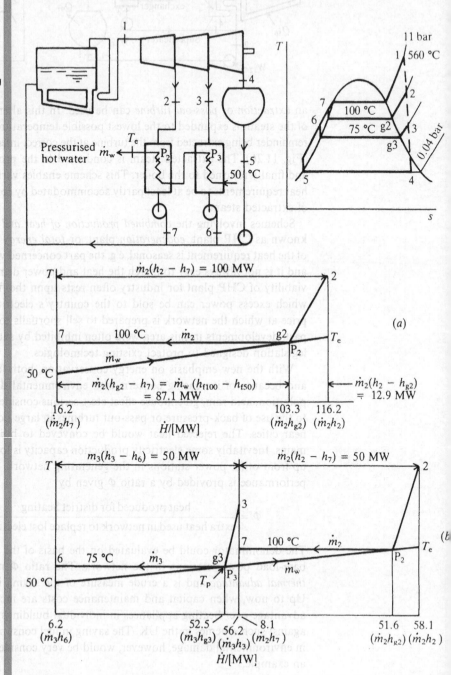

the average base-load power station efficiency is $\eta_{bl} = 0.36$. Heat at the rate of 100 MW is to be provided to pressurised water circulating to dwellings in the town. Compare the thermal advantage Φ of the following schemes:

(a)   A single bleed point is used at a pressure which provides steam with a saturation temperature of 100 °C for the district heating.

(b)   The district-heating hot water is to be heated in two stages, with half the heat provided by steam bled as in scheme (a), and half by steam bled at a pressure corresponding to a saturation temperature of 75 °C.

In both schemes the bled steam is condensed without subcooling before being returned to the boiler. The effect of feed pump work can be neglected.

Sketch the processes undergone by the steam and hot water on a $T-\dot{H}$ diagram and determine the minimum rate of flow of hot water in each of the schemes, assuming that the return temperature of the water for both schemes is 50 °C and that the water enthalpy increases linearly with temperature. Finally, calculate the temperature of the pressurised water leaving the plant in each case.

From the steam $h-s$ chart, assuming a straight line of condition (see sections 11.5 and 19.2.5),

$$h_2 = 3010 \text{ kJ/kg}, \qquad h_3 = 2825 \text{ kJ/kg}, \qquad h_4 = 2498 \text{ kJ/kg}$$

and from tables,

$$h_6 = 314 \text{ kJ/kg}, \qquad h_7 = 419 \text{ kJ/kg}$$

Let $\dot{m}_2$ be the pass-out steam at $p_2 = 1.013\,25$ bar, and $\dot{m}_3$ be the pass-out steam at $p_3 = 0.3855$ bar.

Thermal advantages

For scheme (a), the heat transfer to pressurised hot water is

$$\dot{Q} = \dot{m}_2(h_2 - h_7), \qquad \dot{m}_2 = \frac{100\,000}{(3010 - 419)} = 38.60 \text{ kg/s}$$

The loss of electric power is

$$\Delta\dot{W} = \dot{m}_2(h_2 - h_4)$$

Hence

$$\Phi = \frac{\dot{Q}}{\Delta\dot{W}/\eta_{bl}} = \frac{(3010 - 419)}{(3010 - 2498)/0.36} = 1.822$$

For scheme (b), for equal contributions of heat to the pressurised water,

$$\dot{m}_2 = \frac{\tfrac{1}{2}\dot{Q}}{(h_2 - h_7)} = \frac{50\,000}{(3010 - 419)} = 19.30 \text{ kg/s}$$

$$\dot{m}_3 = \frac{\tfrac{1}{2}\dot{Q}}{(h_3 - h_6)} = \frac{50\,000}{(2825 - 314)} = 19.91 \text{ kg/s}$$

$$\Delta \dot{W} = \dot{m}_2(h_2 - h_4) + \dot{m}_3(h_3 - h_4)$$

$$= 19.30(3010 - 2498) + 19.91(2825 - 2498)$$

$$= 9882 + 6511 = 16\,393\,\text{kW}$$

$$\Phi = \frac{100\,000}{16\,393/0.36} = 2.196$$

Flow rates

Fig. 11.27a shows the T-$\dot{H}$ diagram for scheme (a). The enthalpy values on the abscissa are the products of the specific enthalpies of the *steam*, and its flow rate $\dot{m}_2$ determined by the 100 MW heat specification. The minimum water flow rate $\dot{m}_w$ is prescribed by the line starting at the return temperature of 50 °C which just touches the pinch point P_2: lower flows imply a water temperature which lies above P_2, and heat then cannot flow from the steam to the water. Hence

$$(\dot{m}_w)_{\min} = \frac{87\,100\,[\text{kW}]}{(h_{f100} - h_{f50})} = \frac{87\,100\,[\text{kW}]}{(419 - 209)\,[\text{kJ/kg}]} = 415\,\text{kg/s}$$

Fig. 11.27b shows the T-$\dot{H}$ diagram for scheme (b). It is not immediately obvious whether the value $(\dot{m}_w)_{\min}$ should be deduced from the water T-$\dot{H}$ line when it just touches P_2 or P_3. We shall assume that the minimum flow is governed by P_2. Let us check that, with this assumption, the water temperature T_P falls below P_3. As the water T-$\dot{H}$ line is straight,

$$\frac{T_P/[°C] - 50}{(52.5 - 6.2)} = \frac{100 - 50}{(51.6 - 8.1) + (56.2 - 6.2)}$$

and hence $T_P = 74.8\,°C$, i.e. just below the temperature of the steam of 75 °C at P_3. The reader can easily verify that if we were to make $T_P = 75\,°C$, the water temperature at P_2 would lie slightly above 100 °C, namely at 100.6 °C.

We can now calculate $(\dot{m}_w)_{\min}$ for scheme (b). With the water T-$\dot{H}$ line just touching P_2,

$$(\dot{m}_w)_{\min} = \frac{\{(56.2 - 6.2) + (51.6 - 8.1)\}\,10^3\,[\text{kW}]}{(419 - 209)\,[\text{kJ/kg}]} = 445.2\,\text{kg/s}$$

In practice, a design will specify a temperature difference of several degrees at all the pinch points, and the values of $(\dot{m}_w)_{\min}$ calculated here are limiting values only.

Exit temperatures

The exit temperature T_e for the pressurised water for scheme (a) will be given by

$$\frac{T_e/[°C] - 50}{100 - 50} = \frac{100}{103.3 - 16.2}$$

and hence $T_e = 107.4\,°C$.

For scheme (b), T_e will be given by

$$\frac{T_e/[^\circ C] - 50}{100 - 50} = \frac{50 + 50}{(56.2 - 6.2) + (51.6 - 3.1)}$$

and hence $T_e = 103.5\,^\circ C$.

We have seen that of the two schemes in Example 11.7, scheme (b) is better from the thermodynamic point of view. This is not surprising because the average temperature difference between steam and water is less in scheme (b), and hence the effect of this cause of irreversibility is lower. The transfer of heat in the two schemes is typical of the kind of situations encountered in the process industries, where it is also important to optimise the thermodynamic performance of plant by reducing temperature differences in heat transfer. When one fluid changes phase, an attempt to reduce temperature difference may lead to the kind of pinch point problem outlined in the foregoing example, namely the danger of wasting heat exchanger area by not completing the desired heat transfer process. Once the temperature difference drops to zero in a heat exchanger, all heat transfer ceases. It is relatively easy to avoid this situation arising under design point conditions as we have seen, but in practice it is essential to see that it cannot happen under off-design, or part-load, operating conditions also. This can be done by what is called *pinch point analysis*, which is described in Refs 41 and 42. Such an analysis is also used to optimise the thermodynamic performance of complex multistream process plant by so arranging heat exchanges between the streams that a minimum of heat is required from an external source. In essence one is trying to minimise the effect of irreversibilities due to temperature differences.

Although we have chosen to introduce the idea of cogeneration schemes in this chapter, and hence their realisation via steam turbine driven plant, it should be appreciated that the waste heat from any combustion power plant can be used for such schemes. Any small-scale CHP plant for an individual factory, hospital complex, or large leisure centre with swimming pool and ice rink, is more likely to use an electric generator driven by a reciprocating internal-combustion engine or gas turbine. In such applications the low-grade heat and electrical power requirements are often roughly constant through the year and in a ratio suited to these power plants. A few simple case studies with economic assessment can be found in Ref. 42.

11.9 Low-temperature power cycles

Much of this chapter has been concerned with various modifications to the simple Rankine cycle to make the best possible use of energy sources which are at a high temperature. In this section we will consider vapour power plant for electricity generation which make use of low-temperature sources such as waste heat from a factory process, hot water from a geothermal reservoir, or solar radiation absorbed in a shallow lake or 'solar pond'. Because of the small temperature drop available, only the simple Rankine cycle can be used and the

Fig. 11.28

Comparative performance
of low-temperature cycles
with alternative working
fluids

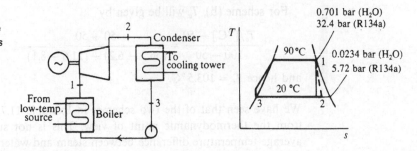

Working fluid	x_2	η	$\dot{m}$ [kg/s]	v_{g1} [m³/kg]	$\dot{V_1}$ [m³/s]	$\dot{V_2}$ [m³/s]	$\dfrac{\dot{V_2}}{\dot{V_1}}$	Boiler duty [MW]	Condenser duty [MW]
Steam	0.877	0.164	2.36	2.361	5.58	120	21.5	6.08	5.08
R134a	0.934	0.140	36.0	0.00462	0.166	1.21	7.29	7.13	6.13

cycle efficiency will be low. This is not serious, however, because the 'fuel' is free. The cost of electricity generated by such plant will depend on the capital cost, the effective life of the plant (i.e. the period over which the capital cost must be written off), and the maintenance cost. A low efficiency does imply large components for a given power output, and hence inevitably a high capital cost.

As might be expected, the type of working fluid used in refrigerators and heat pumps (see section 13.2) is much more suitable than steam for low-temperature power plant. The main reason, as we will see, is that the specific volume of such vapours at low temperature is much less than that of steam, with the consequence that the turbine can be much smaller and less expensive. Turbogenerator units, sealed to avoid loss of working fluid, and suitable for use with a variety of low-temperature sources, are available in modules of up to 1 MW of electrical output.

To illustrate the significance of the specific volume of the vapour, the cycle in Fig. 11.28 has been evaluated for two working fluids—steam and Refrigerant 134a (or R134a). The turbine output is 1 MW in each case. A turbine isentropic efficiency of 90 per cent was assumed, the feed pump term was neglected, and the fluid properties were taken from Ref. 17. The salient results are given in the table incorporated in Fig. 11.28. The main points to be noted, where the R134a has the advantage over steam, are as follows:

(a) The dryness fraction at outlet from the turbine is appreciably higher (0.934 versus 0.877), so that there should be no serious problems arising from droplets impinging on the turbine blades (discussed at the end of section 19.2.4).

(b) Although a much higher mass flow is required for the given power output (36.0 kg/s versus 2.36 kg/s), this is not significant. The specific volume of R134a vapour is so much less than that of steam that the *volume* flow rates $\dot{V_1}$ and $\dot{V_2}$, upon which the size of the turbine depends, are some 30 and 100 times smaller. Moreover, the *ratio* of the outlet to inlet volume flows is also very much less (7.29 versus 21.5). This means that all the design problems arising from the need to accomodate the vast volume flow at the low-pressure end of steam turbines are avoided (see section 19.2).

(c) From the pressures shown on the *T*–s diagram, it is clear that the pressure in the R134a plant is nowhere less than atmospheric. There are no problems associated with the vacuum that is required in steam condensers, as discussed in sections 14.4 and 22.8.1.

The only points at which steam seems to have the advantage over R134a are as follows:

(a) The efficiency of the R134a cycle is lower — but we have already pointed out that this is not directly of importance when the 'fuel' is free.

(b) An indirect effect of the lower efficiency is a larger boiler duty ($|\dot{W}|/\eta$) and condenser duty ($|\dot{W}|/\eta + |\dot{W}|$). Whether the boiler and condenser would actually be larger for the R134a plant depends on the relative heat transfer characteristics of the vaporising liquids and condensing vapours (see section 22.8).

Before leaving the subject of low-temperature vapour cycles, it is worth mentioning one particular scheme which makes use of a source which is virtually at atmospheric temperature—namely the ocean. We refer to what is called an *ocean thermal energy conversion* (OTEC) plant, which makes use of the temperature difference existing between the surface of the ocean and its deeper levels. In certain tropical locations, a temperature difference of about 20 K is available without having to use water from a depth much over 300 m. Fig. 11.29 includes a diagrammatic representation of such a plant, showing typical values of inlet and outlet temperatures of the sea water: 28 °C and 26 °C for the boiler, and 7 °C and 10 °C for the condenser. Assuming minimum temperature differences of 2 K between sea water and working fluid, the maximum and minimum temperatures of the Rankine cycle will be 24 °C and 12 °C, as indicated on the *T*–$\dot{H}$ diagram. This time taking the working fluid to be ammonia, again using the properties given in Ref. 17, and assuming turbine and feed pump isentropic efficiencies of 90 per cent, the cycle efficiency is readily found to be 0.0354. With such a very low efficiency it is not surprising that the plant turns out to be extremely large. Thus for a plant of 100 MW turbine output, the boiler and condenser heat capacities would be

$$\dot{Q}_1 = \frac{|\dot{W}|}{\eta} = \frac{100}{0.0354} = 2825 \text{ MW} \quad \text{and} \quad |\dot{Q}_2| = (\dot{Q}_1 + \dot{W}) = 2725 \text{ MW}$$

The capacities of the corresponding components of a fossil-fuel steam power plant of 0.40 cycle efficiency would be 250 MW and 150 MW. Thus for the same work output, the OTEC boiler and condenser would be about 11 times and 18 times larger than the corresponding components in conventional plant. It is not surprising that OTEC plant turn out to have a high capital cost.

As discussed in section 11.8 and illustrated in Example 11.7, we have plotted the ammonia cycle, and the processes undergone by the warm and cold sea

Fig. 11.29

An ocean thermal energy
conversion (OTEC) plant

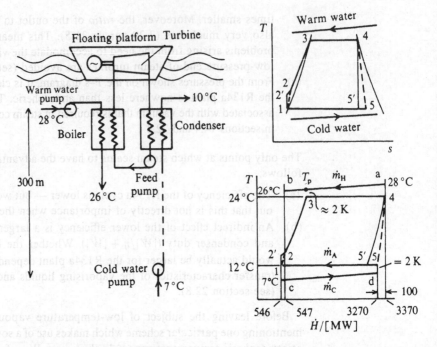

water flows $\dot{m}_H$ and $\dot{m}_C$, on a T–$\dot{H}$ diagram. The enthalpy values on the abscissa
are the products of the specific enthalpies of the ammonia, and its flow rate $\dot{m}_A$
required to provide 100 MW of power output. The sea water rates of flow must
satisfy the enthalpy balances:

$$-\dot{m}_H(h_b - h_a) = \dot{m}_A(h_4 - h_2)$$

$$\dot{m}_C(h_d - h_c) = -\dot{m}_A(h_1 - h_5)$$

If the flow rates of sea water are reduced below those so calculated, the
temperature at b would drop below 26 °C and at d it would rise above 10 °C;
it is seen that problems could arise at pinch points 3 and 5, as explained in
Example 11.7.

So far, apart from an early short-lived French experimental plant, OTEC
schemes have remained as paper studies. Like many proposals for utilising
renewable resources for electricity generation, such as solar, wind, tidal and
wave energy, the capital and maintenance costs turn out to be too large for
widespread adoption at present. Although the 'fuel' costs nothing, such schemes
are likely to remain uneconomic as long as plentiful supplies of traditional fuels
exist. Increasing concern with the environmental side-effects of burning fossil
fuels and of nuclear waste disposal may soon bring neglected hidden costs into
the balance sheet, to the advantage of renewable resources. One should
remember, however, that energy sources of low concentration or 'space density',
as the renewable sources tend to be, inevitably entail the use of very large plant,
and sheer size can have its own undesirable effects upon the environment. For
example, rain is the most widely used renewable resource and some large
hydroelectric schemes, such as the Aswan High Dam, have had very serious

repercussions. The tides can provide another renewable resource, but the proposed tidal power plant for the Severn Estuary, for example, will have ecological consequences which must be taken into account.

In assessing implications of 'low-density' power plant, it must also be borne in mind that large quantities of material would be necessary for the construction of such plant, and engineering materials are energy intensive; that is, their production involves a large expenditure of energy. There is normally little point in proposing power plant which use up nearly as much energy in their construction as will be produced in the lifetime of the plant. A form of energy accounting, called *energy analysis*, has been introduced as a supplement to economic analysis to make sure that this kind of mistake is avoided. A brief commentary on energy analysis can be found in Ref. 40.

11.10 The ideal working fluid and binary cycles

Apart from the Carnot cycle, which was shown to be impractical, all the cycles discussed in this chapter have efficiencies and specific consumptions which are dependent upon the properties of the working fluid. Although for reasons of cost and chemical stability, steam is almost always used as the working fluid in vapour power cycles, its behaviour is far from ideal. It is worth considering briefly the characteristics that would be desirable in an ideal working fluid. A T–s diagram for one such fluid is sketched in Fig. 11.30a, and its main features are as follows:

(a) The critical temperature is well above the metallurgical limit. Superheating is therefore superfluous and most of the heat can be added at the upper temperature. The saturation pressure at the metallurgical limit is moderate to reduce the capital and maintenance costs of the plant.

(b) The specific heat capacity of the liquid is small, i.e. the saturation line is steep. The heat required to bring the liquid to boiling point is then also small, again increasing the proportion added at the upper temperature.

(c) The latent enthalpy is high, implying a low specific consumption and therefore smaller plant for a given power output. The size of plant is also reduced if the fluid has a high density.

Fig. 11.30
Ideal fluids for a vapour power cycle.

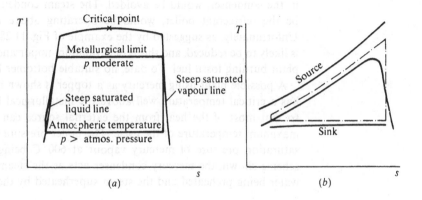

(d) The saturated vapour line is very steep, so that the dryness fraction after the expansion can be maintained above 0.9 without recourse to superheating.

(e) The saturation pressure at the lower temperature of about 29 °C is slightly higher than atmospheric, so that no vacuum is needed in the condenser. This avoids leakage of air into the system, the undesirability of which is discussed in sections 14.4 and 22.8.1.

No single fluid has been found which possesses all these desirable thermodynamic characteristics, and yet at the same time is cheap, chemically stable, non-toxic and non-corrosive.

It will be apparent from what was said about cycles for nuclear power plant in section 11.7 that the desirable characteristics of the working fluid will depend to some extent on the nature of the source of heat. The foregoing ideal working fluid is desirable only if the source is of essentially constant temperature. When the source is a hot gas undergoing a marked drop in temperature as it gives up its energy, the desirable T–s diagram of the working fluid is as shown in Fig. 11.30b. A cycle using a supercritical pressure, shown by the chain dotted lines, then enables the external irreversibility due to the temperature difference between source and working fluid to be reduced to a minimum. In this case it would be desirable for the critical temperature of the working fluid to be *below* the metallurgical limit. A more comprehensive discussion of the desirable characteristics of working fluids can be found in Ref. 39. (A quantitative assessment of the effect of external irreversibilities can best be made using the concept of exergy discussed in section 7.9.)

Because no single substance possesses all the desirable characteristics listed above, attention has been paid to the benefits which might follow from using different fluids for different parts of the temperature range of a cycle. Systems with more than two fluids are thought to be impractical. Cycles with two fluids are referred to as *binary* cycles. The primary fluid is usually assumed to be steam. When the second fluid is used at the high-temperature end of the cycle it is called a 'topper', and when at the low-temperature end it is called a 'bottomer'. From the discussion of low-temperature cycles in section 11.9, it might be thought that a binary cycle using a refrigerant as bottomer would be attractive. All the problems associated with low dryness fraction and very high volume flow at the low-pressure end of the steam turbine, and with a vacuum in the condenser, would be avoided. The steam condenser, which would also be the refrigerant boiler, would be operating above atmospheric pressure. Unfortunately, as suggested by the example of Fig. 11.28, the overall efficiency is likely to be reduced, and this is of paramount importance in high-temperature plant burning fossil fuel. To date, no suitable bottomer has been found.

A possible plant using mercury as a topper is shown in Fig. 11.31. Mercury has a critical temperature well above the metallurgical limit of about 600 °C, so that most of the heat from the external source can be transferred at the maximum temperature of the cycle. The boiler pressure would be modest, the saturation pressure of mercury vapour at 600 °C being only 23 bar. In the scheme shown, the mercury condenser acts as the steam boiler, with the feed water being preheated and the steam superheated by the combustion gases of

Fig. 11.31
A binary vapour cycle

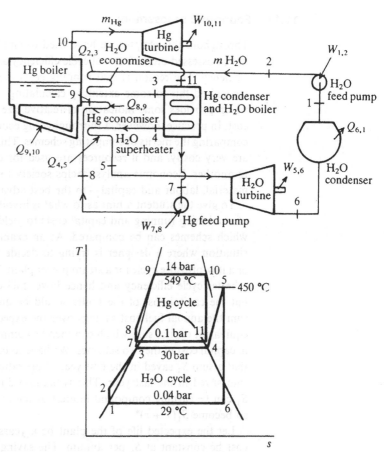

the mercury boiler. The two cycles shown superimposed on the same T–s diagram are linked by the equation

$$m_{Hg}(h_{11} - h_7) = m_{H_2O}(h_4 - h_3)$$

For the operating conditions stated on the diagram, and using the properties of mercury from Ref. 17, it is readily found that a mercury flow of 8.36 kg/s is required per 1 kg/s of steam, and that the ideal efficiency of the combined cycle is 0.518. This is a temptingly high value, and one or two experimental plants were built before the Second World War. Unfortunately, mercury is very expensive and highly toxic, and attacks most metals in common use. Moreover its inability to 'wet' boiler and condenser surfaces leads to difficulties in the design of these components. While the use of liquid metals may well be justified in a nuclear breeding reactor programme, designed to increase the utilisable fraction of the world's resources of uranium, it is unlikely to be economic in a fossil fuel plant. This is certainly the case now with the advent of the gas turbine. The principle of the binary cycle is being increasingly used in the form of a combined gas and steam cycle, where energy in the exhaust gas from the gas turbine is used to produce steam for a Rankine cycle plant. This is described in section 12.5.

11.11   Economic assessment

Throughout this chapter we have tried to emphasise that power plant should not be assessed on the basis of cycle efficiency alone, or even by overall thermal efficiency. The reason is that running costs are only part of the picture.* We recognised this to some extent by calculating the specific steam consumption, which provides some indication of relative size and hence comparative capital cost. In practice, however, a thoroughgoing economic analysis is essential when comparing the merits of competing schemes. This is because engineering projects are very costly, and if resources are used for one project they will be denied to another. Economic analysis helps society to use its overall resources—raw material, labour and capital—to the best advantage.

To give the student a hint as to what is involved, we will present one method of combining running and capital costs to yield a single economic criterion by which schemes can be compared. As an example, we shall have in mind the situation where a designer is trying to decide whether to use a high-pressure or a low-pressure cycle for a steam power plant. The higher pressure would yield a better cycle efficiency and hence lower fuel costs over the life of the plant, but the capital cost of the boiler would be greater. A simple approach is to sum the annual fuel cost savings over the expected life of the plant to yield an equivalent capital sum which can then be compared directly with the difference in capital cost of the two schemes. We have to take account of the fact, however, that a sum S_1 saved in the first year of operation is worth more than the same sum saved in the last year. This is because during the period of n years, say, S_1 can be earning compound interest at the rate of r per cent per annum and so become $S_1(1 + r)^n$.

Let the expected life of the plant be n years and the annual saving in fuel cost be constant at S_a per annum. The saving S_a in year x will earn interest over $(n - x)$ years. The *total* sum saved by the end of year n is then

$$S = S_a(1 + r)^{n-1} + S_a(1 + r)^{n-2} + \ldots + S_a$$

Multiplying throughout by $(1 + r)$ and subtracting the original equation we get

$$S = S_a\{(1 + r)^n - 1\}/r$$

This is the sum in the bank at the end of year n as a result of fuel saving. This sum must now be discounted back to the beginning of the first year of operation to enable it to be compared directly with the increase in capital cost incurred in that year by the use of a higher boiler pressure. The whole process is referred to as 'present value (PV) discounting procedure'. The present value of S will be

$$S_{PV} = \frac{S}{(1 + r)^n} = S_a\left\{\frac{(1 + r)^n - 1}{r(1 + r)^n}\right\}$$

The term in braces is the reciprocal of what is called the 'annuity present worth

---

* And this fact is why relatively little use is made in practice of the additional refinements possible through the use of the more rigorous Second Law analyses, using such concepts as exergy, referred to at the end of section 7.9.

factor', f_{AP}, and the equation can be written

$$S_{PV} = s_a / f_{AP}$$

Continuing with our example, let us suppose that a particular 100 MW steam turbine plant would cost an additional £350 000 if the design boiler pressure was increased by 50 bar. Cycle calculations show that the efficiency would be increased from 30 to 31.5 per cent. The load factor of the plant (i.e. the fraction of a year during which the plant is operating) is 0.5, the heating value of the fuel (coal) is 30 000 kJ/kg, and the fuel cost is £30 per tonne. The annual saving in fuel cost will be

$$S_a = \frac{0.5 \times 100\,000 \times 8760 \times 3600 \times 30}{30\,000 \times 1000}\left(\frac{1}{0.30} - \frac{1}{0.315}\right) = £250\,000$$

Assuming a discount rate r of 10 per cent, and a life of 30 years,

$$f_{AP} = (0.1 \times 1.1^{30})/(1.1^{30} - 1) = 0.106$$

$$S_{PV} = 250\,000/0.106 = £2\,360\,000$$

On this basis the use of the higher boiler pressure would be justified because the increase in capital cost is only about one-seventh of the saving in fuel cost.

The real situation is much more complex than outlined here because maintenance costs, depreciation charges and the effect of inflation have not been taken into account. But if this brief excursion into economics encourages the student of engineering to take courses in that subject seriously it will have served its purpose.

Finally, in a world where the population is still increasing exponentially, and a larger fraction is expecting to enjoy an ever-increasing standard of living, even a complete economic analysis is not enough by itself. *Homo sapiens* is proving to have such a devastating effect on the planet that, in future, no assessment of a new engineering project or technology will be complete without an investigation into the likely environmental impact of its widespread adoption.

12

Gas Power Cycles

This chapter is concerned with cycles which form the basis of power plant in which the working fluid is a gas. The gas is normally air, or the products of combustion of fuel and air. Such power plant may be classified into two main groups—gas turbine engines and reciprocating engines. The former are analogous to steam plant in that the individual processes are steady-flow processes carried out in separate components. The latter involve non-flow processes accomplished in a cylinder fitted with a reciprocating piston.

With few exceptions, only the ideal cycles which form the basis of these engines will be discussed in this chapter. Gas turbine cycles follow on naturally from the previous discussion of vapour power cycles; they are therefore considered first, although in a historical survey the order of presentation would be reversed.

12.1 Internal-combustion engines and air-standard cycles

In the previous chapter it was seen that a practical vapour power cycle can be devised consisting of two isentropic processes and two constant pressure processes, i.e. the Rankine cycle. This cycle has a good ideal efficiency, since most of the heat supplied is transferred at the upper temperature and the whole of the heat rejected is transferred at the lower temperature. Furthermore the work ratio is very near unity, and therefore the efficiency is not greatly affected by irreversibilities. Let us now consider the probable effect on the performance of the cycle of using a gas as the working fluid; the cycle is then known as the *Joule* (or *Brayton*) cycle. The p–v and T–s diagrams for the cycle appear as in Fig. 12.1. A diagrammatic sketch of the plant—known as a closed-cycle gas turbine—is also shown. The steady-flow constant pressure processes during which heat is transferred are no longer constant temperature processes and the ideal efficiency must therefore be appreciably less than the Carnot efficiency based upon the maximum and minimum temperatures of the cycle, i.e. $\eta < (T_3 - T_1)/T_3$. Also, the magnitude of the compressor work, $c_p(T_1 - T_2)$, is an appreciable proportion of that of the expansion work, $c_p(T_3 - T_4)$, so that the work ratio is considerably less than unity. The cycle has therefore a lower ideal efficiency than the Rankine cycle, and it is also much more susceptible to

Fig. 12.1
The Joule cycle applied
to the closed-cycle gas
turbine

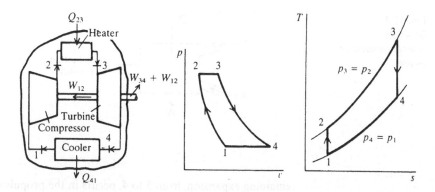

irreversibilities. Clearly, if such a cycle is to find favour it must do so on other grounds.

Bearing in mind the fact that the source of energy is normally provided by the combustion of fuel in air, it can be seen that there is an advantage to be gained by using a gas cycle if the gas is air, since the fuel can be burnt directly in the working fluid. This idea of *internal combustion* leads to the open-cycle gas turbine plant of Fig. 12.2, in which the heater of the closed cycle is replaced by an internal-combustion chamber, and the cooler becomes superfluous because the turbine exhaust gases are rejected to the atmosphere. The plant is thus much less bulky and expensive than an equivalent vapour plant with its large boiler and condenser. These are very important advantages in the case of power plant for transport, where small size and low weight are important requirements, or for peak-load generating sets where the capital cost is more important than the running cost.

The internal-combustion turbine is particularly suitable for aircraft propulsion when used in conjunction with either an airscrew or a propelling nozzle (see section 18.4.1). When a propeller turbine (Fig. 18.15b) is used, the net shaft work ($W_{34} + W_{12}$) in Fig. 12.2 is simply supplied to the airscrew. If propulsion is by jet, the turbine is required to supply merely the compressor work and it uses only part of the expansion to atmospheric pressure, from 3 to 5 say. The

Fig. 12.2
The internal-combustion
gas turbine

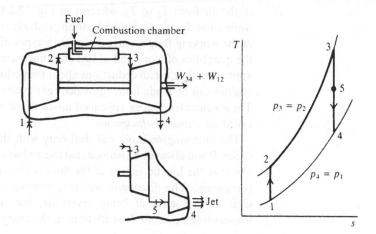

Fig. 12.3
Schematic
internal-combustion
engine

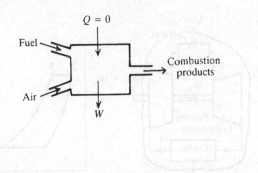

remaining expansion, from 5 to 4, occurs in the propulsion nozzle, and the exit velocity can be calculated by the method of Example 10.2b.

It should be appreciated that an open-cycle plant with internal combustion departs considerably from the conventional thermodynamic idea of a heat engine. In the thermodynamic sense no heat is involved at all, and the cycle is replaced by a continuous, adiabatic, steady-flow process during which the chemical energy in the fuel is converted into work in a more direct way. Power plant of this kind are called *internal-combustion engines*, and Fig. 12.3 illustrates the essential features common to all such plant (cf. Fig. 11.1). The combustion process is now an integral part of the whole, and it is no longer possible to treat the overall efficiency of the plant as the product of a cycle efficiency and a combustion efficiency as was done in the previous chapter. A full analysis of the performance of internal-combustion engines is therefore complex, and it involves consideration of the combustion process itself (see Chapters 15 and 17). Fortunately a great deal of useful information can be obtained from a simplified treatment.

Let us compare the closed and open gas turbine plants of Fig. 12.1 and Fig. 12.2 a little more closely. First, the net work outputs differ mainly because the specific heat capacities and mass flows of the gases passing through the turbines are not the same; in the closed plant the fluid is air, and in the open plant the fluid consists of products of combustion. Secondly, in Fig. 12.1 the fuel is consumed externally while heat is transferred to raise the temperature of the air from T_2 to T_3, whereas in Fig. 12.2 the fuel is consumed internally while air at T_2 changes to combustion products at T_3. Since the major proportion of the working fluid is nitrogen in both types of plant, it is not surprising that the quantities of work and of fuel consumed are not widely different. As a first approximation, useful deductions about the performance of internal-combustion engines can be made from equivalent gas cycles using air as the working fluid. These equivalent cycles are called *air-standard cycles*, and their efficiencies are called *air-standard efficiencies*.

The following sections will deal only with the performance of air-standard cycles. It will always be assumed that the air has constant specific heat capacities, and that the kinetic energy of the fluid is the same at inlet and outlet of each component. The discussion will not, however, be limited to cycles which are *ideal* in the sense of being reversible, but will also include the effect of irreversibilities, i.e. of fluid friction, in the compressor and the turbine.

12.2 Simple gas turbine cycle

Expressions for the efficiency and work ratio of the Joule cycle shown in Fig. 12.1 can be found in the following way. The compressor and turbine work transfers, per unit mass, are respectively

$$W_{12} = (h_2 - h_1) = c_p(T_2 - T_1)$$

$$W_{34} = (h_4 - h_3) = c_p(T_4 - T_3)$$

The heat supplied during the cycle is

$$Q_{23} = (h_3 - h_2) = c_p(T_3 - T_2)$$

and the cycle efficiency is therefore

$$\eta = \frac{|W_{34}| - |W_{12}|}{Q_{23}} = \frac{(T_3 - T_4) - (T_2 - T_1)}{(T_3 - T_2)} \tag{12.1}$$

The cycle temperatures can be related to the *pressure ratio* $r_p = p_2/p_1 = p_3/p_4$. For isentropic compression and expansion,

$$T_2 = T_1 r_p^{(\gamma - 1)/\gamma} \quad \text{and} \quad T_3 = T_4 r_p^{(\gamma - 1)/\gamma}$$

Inserting these values in (12.1), the ideal air-standard efficiency of the Joule cycle is found to be

$$\eta = 1 - \left(\frac{1}{r_p}\right)^{(\gamma - 1)/\gamma} \tag{12.2}$$

The work ratio is

$$r_w = \frac{W_{12} + W_{34}}{W_{34}} = \frac{(T_2 - T_1) + (T_4 - T_3)}{(T_4 - T_3)}$$

On introducing the pressure ratio r_p, this expression can be reduced to

$$r_w = 1 - \frac{T_1}{T_3} r_p^{(\gamma - 1)/\gamma} \tag{12.3}$$

The efficiency of the ideal cycle is a function of the pressure ratio only, while the work ratio, and therefore the cycle's susceptibility to irreversibilities, depend also upon T_1 and T_3. The efficiency of the real plant will therefore depend on these temperatures as well as the pressure ratio. Evidently T_1 should be as low as possible and T_3 as high as possible. In practice T_1 is limited to atmospheric temperature (say 288 K at sea level). T_3 is fixed by the metallurgical limit, i.e. the maximum temperature which the highly stressed parts of the turbine can withstand. The value depends upon the life required of the plant and the heat-resistant alloy available, but for the purpose of the present discussion we may assume a limit of 1000 K. This is rather higher than the conservative figure chosen for steam plant in the previous chapter, but for many applications of gas turbines a somewhat shorter working life is acceptable and it is possible to employ alloys which are too expensive to use in a large boiler.

Fig. 12.4
Effect of pressure ratio on
work output and efficiency

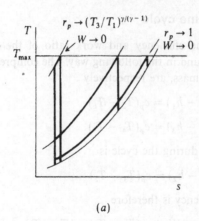
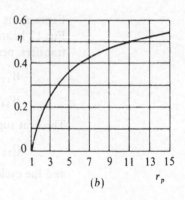

(a) (b)

Having fixed T_1 and T_3, the maximum pressure ratio theoretically possible is given by

$$(r_p)_{max} = \left(\frac{T_3}{T_1}\right)^{\gamma/(\gamma-1)} \tag{12.4}$$

A glance at Fig. 12.4a shows that this is not a practical value, because at this pressure ratio the compressor and turbine works are equal and there is no net work output. The net output is also zero at a pressure ratio of unity, so that there will be some intermediate pressure ratio at which the work output is a maximum. The net output per unit mass, i.e. the *specific work output*,* is given by

$$|W| = -c_p(T_2 - T_1) - c_p(T_4 - T_3)$$

$$= -c_p T_1\{r_p^{(\gamma-1)/\gamma} - 1\} - c_p T_3\left\{\frac{1}{r_p^{(\gamma-1)/\gamma}} - 1\right\} \tag{12.5}$$

Treating T_1 and T_3 as constant, differentiating with respect to r_p, and equating dW/dr_p to zero, it can be shown that for maximum work output

$$r_p = \left(\frac{T_3}{T_1}\right)^{\gamma/2(\gamma-1)} \quad \text{or} \quad r_p = \sqrt{(r_p)_{max}} \tag{12.6}$$

With T_1 at 288 K and T_3 at 1000 K, the optimum pressure ratio is 8.8, and with this value the mass flow of air for a given power output, and hence the size of plant, becomes a minimum. Fig. 12.4b shows the variation of ideal efficiency with pressure ratio obtained from equation (12.2). Evidently the gain in efficiency obtained by using a pressure ratio greater than 8.8 is not very large, and would probably not be worth the accompanying increase in size of plant.

As soon as compressor and turbine inefficiencies are introduced, as indicated in Fig. 12.5, the importance of a high work ratio becomes obvious. With a low

---

* In gas turbine practice it is usual to use the specific work output as a criterion of plant size, rather than its reciprocal which would be the equivalent of the specific steam consumption used in the previous chapter.

Fig. 12.5
Effect of losses in turbine
and compressor

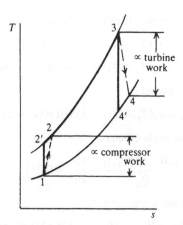

value of T_3, the difference between the turbine work and the compressor work
becomes very small, and a slight decrease in the former and an increase in the
latter is sufficient to reduce the work output, and cycle efficiency, to zero.
General expressions for cycle efficiency and specific work output become rather
unwieldy when isentropic process efficiencies are taken into account, and to
show the effect of variation of r_p and T_3 on the performance it is easier to make
a series of calculations of the type shown in the following example.

Example 12.1   Calculate the efficiency and specific work output of a simple gas turbine
plant operating on the Joule cycle. The maximum and minimum temperatures
of the cycle are 1000 K and 288 K respectively, the pressure ratio is 6, and
the isentropic efficiencies of the compressor and turbine are 85 and
90 per cent respectively.

The isentropic temperature changes in the compressor and turbine are found
from

$$T'_2 = T_1 r_p^{(\gamma - 1)/\gamma} = 288 \times 6^{0.4/1.4} = 288 \times 1.6685 = 481 \text{ K}$$

$$T'_4 = \frac{T_3}{r_p^{(\gamma - 1)/\gamma}} = \frac{1000}{6^{0.4/1.4}} = \frac{1000}{1.6685} = 599 \text{ K}$$

Hence the actual temperature after compression is given by

$$T_2 - T_1 = \frac{T'_2 - T_1}{\eta_C} = \frac{481 - 288}{0.85} = 227 \text{ K}$$

or

$$T_2 = 515 \text{ K}$$

The actual temperature after expansion is given by

$$T_3 - T_4 = \eta_T(T_3 - T'_4) = 0.90(1000 - 599) = 361 \text{ K}$$

or

$$T_4 = 639 \text{ K}$$

The compressor and turbine works are

$$W_{12} = c_p(T_2 - T_1) = 1.005(515 - 288) = 288 \text{ kJ/kg}$$

$$W_{34} = c_p(T_4 - T_3) = 1.005(639 - 1000) = -363 \text{ kJ/kg}$$

and the heat added is

$$Q_{23} = c_p(T_3 - T_2) = 1.005(1000 - 515) = 487 \text{ kJ/kg}$$

Therefore the cycle efficiency is

$$\eta = \frac{|(W_{12} + W_{34})|}{Q_{23}} = \frac{135}{487} = 0.277$$

and the specific work output is

$$|W| = |(W_{12} + W_{34})| = 135 \text{ kJ/kg} \quad \text{or} \quad \text{kW per kg/s of air}$$

The results of calculations similar to the foregoing, but for different values of r_p and T_3, are given in Fig. 12.6. The efficiency of the irreversible cycle is a function not only of r_p but also of T_3. There is an optimum pressure ratio for maximum cycle efficiency as well as an optimum pressure ratio for maximum specific work output, although these optimum pressure ratios are not the same. The latter pressure ratio would probably be adopted in an actual plant, because it results in the smallest plant and the efficiency curve is fairly flat in this region. The ideal efficiency curve is also shown in Fig. 12.6, to emphasise the marked reduction in efficiency caused by irreversibilities in the compressor and turbine. The following section deals with the more important modifications to the simple cycle which may be adopted to improve both the ideal efficiency and work ratio.

12.3 Gas turbine cycles with heat exchange, intercooling and reheating

12.3.1 Simple cycle with heat exchanger

With normal values of the pressure ratio and turbine inlet temperature, the turbine outlet temperature is always above the compressor outlet temperature.

Fig. 12.6
The simple cycle with
$T_1 = 288 \text{ K}$, $\eta_C = 0.85$,
$\eta_T = 0.90$

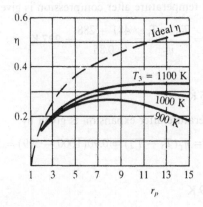
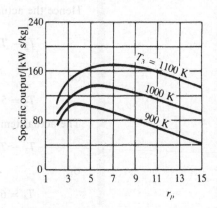

ig. 12.7
imple cycle with heat
xchange

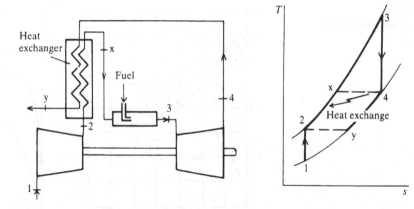

An improvement in performance can therefore be effected by the addition of a *heat exchanger* which transfers heat from the gases leaving the turbine to the air before it enters the combustion chamber. The equivalent air-standard cycle then appears as in Fig. 12.7. By arranging for the heat exchange to occur in a counter-flow heat exchanger (see section 24.1), it is theoretically possible for the temperature of the compressed air to be raised from T_2 to $T_x = T_4$, while the gas leaving the turbine is cooled from T_4 to $T_y = T_2$. At each point in the heat exchange process the heat is being transferred over an infinitesimal temperature difference, so that the process can be regarded as reversible and the cycle as ideal.

The effect of the heat exchanger is to reduce the amount of heat required from an external source to

$$Q_{x3} = c_p(T_3 - T_x) = c_p(T_3 - T_4) \tag{12.7}$$

The net work output and work ratio are unchanged, but it can easily be shown that the ideal air-standard efficiency now becomes

$$\eta = 1 - \frac{T_1}{T_3} r_p^{(\gamma - 1)/\gamma} \tag{12.8}$$

In this case, the lower the pressure ratio the higher the efficiency, the maximum value being $(T_3 - T_1)/T_3$ when $r_p = 1$. This is the Carnot efficiency based upon the maximum and minimum temperatures of the cycle. This result is not surprising because, as r_p is reduced to unity, the external heat transfers tend to take place more nearly at the upper and lower temperatures (see Fig. 12.4a). The efficiency curves, shown in Fig. 12.8a, meet the curve for the simple cycle where the pressure ratio is such that $T_2 = T_4$, because at this point the heat exchanger becomes superfluous. Equating (12.8) and (12.2), it is apparent that this occurs when

$$r_p = \left(\frac{T_3}{T_1}\right)^{\gamma/2(\gamma - 1)}$$

i.e. at the optimum pressure ratio for maximum work output (see equation

255

Fig. 12.8
Effect of heat exchange on
efficiency

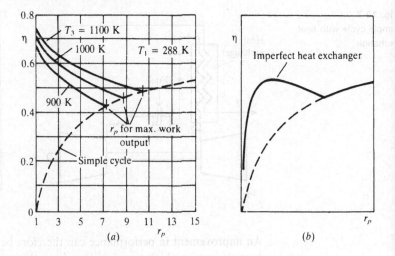

(12.6)). Clearly, if a heat exchanger is to be used, a pressure ratio somewhat less than the optimum must be adopted. Fig. 12.8a emphasises a fact which is obvious from the $T-s$ diagram, which is that the higher the value of T_3, the greater is the advantage to be obtained from the addition of a heat exchanger.

In practice the heat exchanger is never 'perfect', and the actual temperature T_x reached by the compressed air is always less than T_4. This results in a major change in the shape of the efficiency curves because, as r_p tends to unity and the net work output tends to zero, the external heat supplied no longer tends to zero. The result is that at $r_p = 1$ the efficiency has a value of zero, instead of the Carnot efficiency as with the ideal heat exchanger. An actual efficiency curve therefore appears as shown in Fig. 12.8b.

12.3.2 Intercooling and reheating

The addition of a heat exchanger improves the ideal efficiency but does not improve the work ratio. The latter may be increased by either reducing the compressor work input or increasing the turbine work output.

Consider the compression work first. The curvature of the constant pressure lines on the $T-s$ diagram is such that the vertical distance between them decreases in the direction of the arrow in Fig. 12.9a. Therefore the further to the left the compression 1-2 takes place, the smaller is the work required to drive the compressor. State 1 is determined by the atmospheric pressure and temperature, but if the compression is carried out in two stages, 1-3 and 4-5, with the air cooled at constant pressure p_i between the stages, some reduction in compression work can be obtained. The sum of the temperature rises $(T_3 - T_1)$ and $(T_5 - T_4)$ is clearly less than the temperature rise $(T_2 - T_1)$.

Ideally, it is possible to cool the air to atmospheric temperature, i.e. $T_4 = T_1$, and in this case the intercooling is said to be *complete*. With isentropic

Fig. 12.9
Intercooling and reheating

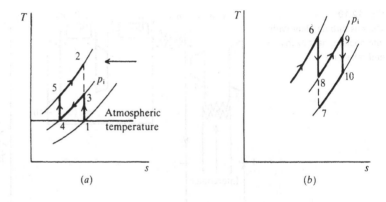

(a)   (b)

compression and complete intercooling the compression work is

$$W = c_p(T_3 - T_1) + c_p(T_5 - T_4)$$

$$= c_p T_1 \left\{ \left(\frac{p_i}{p_1} \right)^{(\gamma - 1)/\gamma} - 1 \right\} + c_p T_1 \left\{ \left(\frac{p_2}{p_i} \right)^{(\gamma - 1)/\gamma} - 1 \right\}$$

The saving in work will depend on the choice of the intercooling pressure p_i. By equating dW/dp_i to zero, the condition for minimum work is found to be

$$p_i = \sqrt{(p_1 p_2)} \tag{12.9}$$

Hence

$$\frac{p_i}{p_1} = \frac{p_2}{p_i} = r_{pi} \quad \text{or} \quad r_{pi} = \sqrt{\left(\frac{p_2}{p_1} \right)} = \sqrt{r_p} \tag{12.10}$$

Thus for minimum compressor work, the compression ratios and work inputs for the two stages are equal.

The compression work can be reduced further by increasing the number of stages and intercoolers, but the additional complexity and cost make more than two or three stages uneconomic. It is possible to generalise the expression for the minimum compression work to cover n stages and to show that the pressure ratios in all stages must be equal.

From here it is only a small step to the idea of *reheating* during the expansion. The principle of reheating has been mentioned previously in section 11.4, but there the main object was to avoid excessive moisture in the steam turbine, and the work ratio, already near unity in the Rankine cycle, is practically unaffected. Reheating is employed in gas turbine plant principally to increase the work ratio, and so increase the specific work output and decrease the effect of component losses. Fig. 12.9b illustrates the relevant part of the cycle showing an expansion in two stages with reheating to the metallurgical limit, i.e. $T_9 = T_6$. The magnitude of the turbine work is increased from $|W_{67}|$ to

$$|W_{6,8}| + |W_{9,10}| = c_p(T_6 - T_8) + c_p(T_9 - T_{10})$$

It is possible to show that with isentropic expansion the optimum intermediate

257

Fig. 12.10
The gas turbine plant with intercooling, heat exchange and reheating

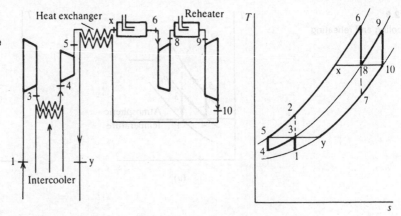

pressure, this time for *maximum* work output, is given by

$$p_i = \sqrt{(p_6 p_7)} \quad \text{or} \quad r_{pi} = \sqrt{r_p} \tag{12.11}$$

Reheating can also be extended to more than two stages, although this is seldom done in practice, and with open-cycle plant a limit is set by the oxygen available for combustion.

Although intercoolers and reheaters improve the work ratio, these devices by themselves can lead to a decrease of ideal cycle efficiency. This is because the heat supplied is increased as well as the net work output. The full advantage is only realised if a heat exchanger is also included in the plant, as shown in Fig. 12.10. The additional heat required for the colder air leaving the compressor can then be obtained from the hotter exhaust gases, and there is a gain in ideal cycle efficiency as well as work ratio.

It is worth considering briefly what happens if the idea of multistage compression and expansion, with intercooling, reheating and heat exchange, is carried to its logical conclusion. Fig. 12.11 shows a cycle with a large number of such stages. It is evident that with an infinite number of stages this cycle would have all its heat addition at the upper temperature T_3, and all its heat

Fig. 12.11
The Ericsson cycle

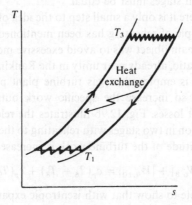

rejection at the lower temperature T_1. The compression and expansion processes become isothermals, and the efficiency of the cycle equals the Carnot efficiency, i.e. $(T_3 - T_1)/T_3$. This cycle is called the *Ericsson cycle*.

12.4 Closed-cycle gas turbine

In section 12.1 it was implied that a gas turbine working on a closed cycle (Fig. 12.1) had little to commend it in comparison with the equivalent steam plant. Nevertheless several closed-cycle plants have been built and the type deserves a brief mention here. Some features favouring the closed-cycle gas turbine are as follows:

(a)   The system may be pressurised, i.e. the general pressure level of the cycle may be raised, so that the size of all the components can be reduced for the same mass flow.

(b)   With a pressurised system it is possible to accommodate changes in load by varying the mass flow of fluid in the circuit instead of by reducing the turbine inlet temperature as in an open-cycle gas turbine. The efficiency at part load will then be closer to the value obtained when running at the design condition.

(c)   Coal, or oil of poor quality, can be used as a fuel because the combustion gases do not pass through the turbine.

(d)   It is possible to use a gas having more favourable properties than air. A simple calculation with the aid of equation (12.2) shows that the cycle efficiency is improved if the value of γ is increased from 1.4 to 1.67, which is the value for all monatomic gases such as helium and argon. Helium, because of its lower relative molecular mass, possesses much better heat transfer characteristics than air; that is, it has a higher thermal conductivity, and it permits the use of higher fluid velocities for the same pressure loss. The net result is that the size of the heat exchangers would be appreciably smaller than that of equivalent components designed for use with air.

All closed-cycle plants built so far have used air as the working fluid. If the high-temperature nuclear reactor ever came to fruition, closed-cycle gas turbines using helium would be an appropriate choice of power plant. Helium could be passed directly through the reactor core and there would be no need for a secondary fluid with all the wasteful temperature drops that this entails.

12.5 Combined gas and steam cycles

The advantage of a binary cycle in making the best use of the available temperature difference between source and sink was pointed out in section 11.10. Because the exhaust gases leave a gas turbine at a moderately high temperature (about 600 K) it is possible to use the energy therein to form steam for a Rankine cycle plant. Such combined power plants are often referred to as COGAS plant, and an increasing number are being built for base-load electricity generation. A dual-pressure steam cycle might be used to make the best use of the low-grade heat, as explained in section 11.7 on cycles for nuclear power plant and depicted in Fig. 11.23. The only change is that the turbine exhaust gases replace the reactor coolant in the figure.

Because of the restriction on the maximum temperature which the turbine blades can withstand, gas turbines operate with a very high air/fuel ratio. One consequence is that additional fuel can be burnt in the ample oxygen remaining in the exhaust gases. An alternative to using the complex dual-pressure steam cycle, therefore, is to burn fuel in the steam boiler and use a higher-pressure simple steam cycle. Low-grade fuel can be used for this part of the cycle. The solution to be preferred in practice depends upon the effect of the relative capital cost of the different types of boiler upon the cost of the electricity produced. Combined cycle plant efficiencies of about 45 per cent are possible.

At present most COGAS plant are designed by taking a well-tried gas turbine and designing a steam turbine to suit it. The practice is echoed in the following example, where we make use of the gas turbine data of Example 12.1.

Example 12.2 A simple Rankine cycle using superheated steam at 16 bar and condensing at 0.04 bar is to be added to the gas turbine plant of Example 12.1. From the cycle calculations of that example it can be seen that the gas turbine exhaust temperature is 639 K = 366 °C, the specific work output is 135 kW per kg/s of air, and the heat input is 487 kW per kg/s of air. The gas turbine engine is to be of such a size as to produce 100 MW of power. Making the following assumptions, determine the power delivered by the Rankine plant and the overall efficiency of the combined cycle, neglecting the feed pump work:

(a) The minimum temperature difference between gas and steam or water is to be 20 K.

(b) The isentropic efficiency of the steam turbine is 0.85.

(c) The temperature of the gas leaving the steam boiler should be at least 170 °C to avoid corrosion due to condensation of water vapour in the products of combustion.

Fig. 12.12 shows the h–s diagram for the steam turbine expansion and the T–$\dot{H}$ diagram for the gas turbine exhaust products and the steam cycle. State 4 corresponds to the gas turbine exit state on Fig. 12.5. The air

Fig. 12.12

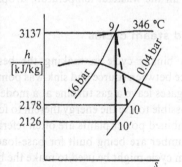

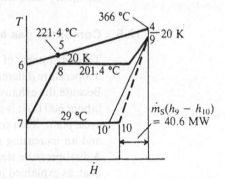

mass flow rate required for the gas turbine is

$$\dot{m}_G = \frac{|\dot{W}|}{135\,\text{kW}/(\text{kg/s})} = \frac{100\,000\,\text{kW}}{135\,\text{kW}/(\text{kg/s})} = 740.7\,\text{kg/s}$$

The gas enthalpy change between turbine exit state 4 and the pinch point state 5 is

$$\dot{H}_5 - \dot{H}_4 = \dot{m}_G c_p (T_5 - T_4)$$

$$= 740.7 \times 1.005(221.4 - 366) = -107\,600\,\text{kW}$$

This must be equal to the magnitude of the enthalpy change of the steam:

$$\dot{H}_9 - \dot{H}_8 = \dot{m}_S(h_9 - h_8) \quad \text{and} \quad \dot{m}_S = \frac{107\,600}{3137 - 859} = 47.23\,\text{kg/s}$$

The isentropic enthalpy drop in the turbine from the h–s chart is

$$h_9 - h'_{10} = 3137 - 2126 = 1011\,\text{kgJ/kg}$$

The steam turbine power is

$$|\dot{W}_S| = \dot{m}_S \eta_T (h_9 - h'_{10}) = 47.23 \times 0.85 \times 1011 = 40\,600\,\text{kW}$$

and

$$\text{combined cycle efficiency} = \frac{\text{total power output}}{\text{heat input to gas turbine}}$$

$$= \frac{100\,000 + 40\,600}{740.7 \times 487} = 0.390$$

The efficiency of the gas turbine plant alone, from Example 12.1, was 0.277, so this represents a substantial increase in efficiency.

We have yet to check the temperature of the gas leaving the boiler, namely the value of T_6. An enthalpy balance between 5–6 and 7–8 is

$$\dot{m}_S(h_8 - h_7) = \dot{m}_G c_p (T_5 - T_6)$$

As $h_7 \approx h_f = 121\,\text{kJ/kg}$ at 0.04 bar,

$$47.23(859 - 121) = 740.7(221.4 - T_6/[^\circ\text{C}])$$

It follows that $T_6 = 174.3\,^\circ\text{C}$. Had T_6 been below the required minimum temperature of $170\,^\circ\text{C}$, it would have been necessary to have modified the steam pressure and repeated the whole calculation.

It should be obvious from the foregoing remarks about COGAS cycles that gas turbines can also be used in conjunction with waste heat boilers to produce process steam or hot water for use in factories; this is yet another form of cogeneration (or CHP) plant, discussed in section 11.8.

Before leaving the subject of gas turbines, it is worth emphasising that the processes are carried out in separate components which can be multiplied and linked together in a variety of ways to suit different applications. No attempt has been made here to indicate the actual diversity which is possible. For this

261

kind of information, and for methods of estimating the performance of actual gas turbine plant as opposed to air-standard cycles, the reader is referred to more specialised books such as Refs 3 and 10. The remaining sections in this chapter will be devoted to a survey of air-standard cycles which form the basis of reciprocating internal-combustion engines.

12.6 Reciprocating engine cycles

So far in the discussion of vapour and gas power cycles we have thought of the cycle as a series of steady-flow processes, each being carried out in a separate component. The turbine has therefore always been regarded as the natural power producing component. As will be seen in Chapter 19, the turbine becomes very small for low power outputs, i.e. for small mass flows of working fluid, and the effect of viscous friction becomes relatively great. Consequently, for a small plant the process efficiency of the turbine is very low. It is usually only practicable to think in terms of a turbine plant if the power required is at least several hundred kilowatts.

The combination of steady-flow components into a power plant is not the only method of obtaining mechanical power from the combustion of fuel. For small powers it is usually preferable to employ a cycle consisting of a succession of non-flow processes. A given mass of working fluid can be taken through a series of processes in a cylinder fitted with a reciprocating piston. Such non-flow processes are much more nearly reversible than the rapid flow processes occurring in a turbine or a rotary compressor (see section 5.4.1).

A second advantage of the reciprocating engine is that the maximum permissible temperature of the working fluid is much higher than it is in a turbine plant ($\approx 2800 \, \text{K}$ compared with $\approx 1000 \, \text{K}$ in a gas turbine). This is because the cylinder of the intermittently working reciprocating engine is only exposed to the peak temperature of the fluid for a small fraction of the duration of a complete cycle. The cylinder temperature therefore never even approaches this peak value. It follows that metallurgical considerations are much less stringent in a reciprocating engine. The chief disadvantage of a reciprocating engine is the comparatively low rate at which it can handle the working fluid. This feature makes it excessively bulky and heavy when large power outputs are required. There is of course a range of power output where reciprocating and turbine plant are competitive, and their relative merits will be more fully appreciated after a reading of Chapters 17 and 19.

Like the normal type of gas turbine plant, the practical reciprocating engine does not use an external heat source or employ a true thermodynamic cycle, but derives its energy from the direct combustion of fuel in the working fluid. The engine takes in air and fuel and rejects products of combustion as depicted in Fig. 12.3. The actual processes occurring in reciprocating engines will be described in Chapter 17, and here we shall consider only the equivalent air-standard cycles with external heat addition and rejection taking the place of internal combustion and rejection of hot exhaust gases. There are three important air-standard cycles which form the basis of all practical reciprocating

Fig. 12.13
The Otto and Diesel cycles

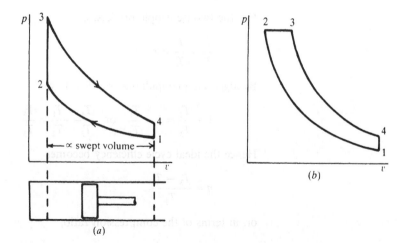

(a)

(b)

engines; they are the Otto, Diesel, and dual or mixed cycles. A few other cycles have been used and will be mentioned briefly, but so far they have not attained any importance.

12.7 Otto, Diesel and mixed cycles

The *Otto cycle* forms the basis of spark-ignition and high-speed compression-ignition engines. The four non-flow processes comprising a complete cycle are shown in Fig. 12.13a. They may be imagined to occur in a cylinder fitted with a reciprocating piston having a swept volume equal to $m(v_1 - v_2)$, where m is the mass of fluid in the cylinder. The processes are as follows:

1–2   Air is compressed isentropically through a volume ratio v_1/v_2, known as the *compression ratio* r_v.
2–3   A quantity of heat Q_{23} is added at constant volume until the air is in state 3.
3–4   The air is expanded isentropically to the original volume.
4–1   Heat Q_{41} is rejected at constant volume until the cycle is completed.

The efficiency of the cycle is

$$\eta = \frac{|W|}{Q_{23}} = \frac{Q_{23} + Q_{41}}{Q_{23}}$$

Assuming constant specific heat capacities for the air, and considering unit mass of fluid, the heat transfers are

$$Q_{23} = c_v(T_3 - T_2), \qquad Q_{41} = c_v(T_1 - T_4)$$

Consequently

$$\eta = 1 - \frac{T_4 - T_1}{T_3 - T_2}$$

For the two isentropic processes,

$$\frac{T_2}{T_1} = \frac{T_3}{T_4} = r_v^{\gamma - 1}$$

By algebraic manipulation we then have

$$1 - \frac{T_2}{T_3} = 1 - \frac{T_1}{T_4} \quad \text{or} \quad \frac{T_4 - T_1}{T_3 - T_2} = \frac{T_4}{T_3}$$

Hence the ideal cycle efficiency becomes

$$\eta = \frac{T_3 - T_4}{T_3} \tag{12.12}$$

or, in terms of the compression ratio,

$$\eta = 1 - \frac{1}{r_v^{\gamma - 1}} \tag{12.13}$$

The maximum possible efficiency based upon the maximum and minimum temperatures of the cycle, i.e. the Carnot efficiency, is $(T_3 - T_1)/T_3$. Equation (12.12) indicates that the cycle efficiency is less than this, since $T_4 > T_1$. This result is to be expected because the heat addition and rejection do not take place at the upper and lower temperatures. Equation (12.13) emphasises the important fact that the efficiency depends only on the compression ratio and not upon the peak temperature T_3. The specific work output, on the other hand, does increase with increase of T_3.

In the *Diesel cycle** the heat addition occurs at constant pressure instead of constant volume. The cycle is shown in Fig. 12.13b, and consists of the following processes:

1–2 Air is compressed isentropically through the compression ratio $r_v = v_1/v_2$.
2–3 Heat Q_{23} is added while the air expands at constant pressure to volume v_3. At state 3 the heat supply is cut off and the volume ratio v_3/v_2 may conveniently be called the *cut-off ratio* r_c.
3–4 The air is expanded isentropically to the original volume.
4–1 Heat Q_{41} is rejected at constant volume until the cycle is completed.

The heat transfers in this cycle are

$$Q_{23} = c_p(T_3 - T_2), \qquad Q_{41} = c_v(T_1 - T_4)$$

Hence the efficiency is

$$\eta = \frac{Q_{23} + Q_{41}}{Q_{23}} = 1 - \frac{T_4 - T_1}{\gamma(T_3 - T_2)}$$

---

* The name is strictly speaking a misnomer, because Diesel's efforts were originally directed towards building an engine which would have the Carnot cycle as its equivalent air-standard cycle. Ackroyd Stuart was the first to build a successful engine working on the so-called Diesel cycle.

The efficiency can be expressed in terms of r_v and r_c in the following way:

$$\frac{T_2}{T_1} = r_v^{\gamma-1} \quad \text{and hence} \quad T_1 = T_2\left(\frac{1}{r_v}\right)^{\gamma-1}$$

For the constant pressure process,

$$\frac{T_3}{T_2} = r_c \quad \text{and hence} \quad T_3 = T_2 r_c$$

Also

$$\frac{T_4}{T_3} = \left(\frac{v_3}{v_4}\right)^{\gamma-1} = \left(\frac{v_3 v_2}{v_2 v_4}\right)^{\gamma-1} = \left(\frac{r_c}{r_v}\right)^{\gamma-1}$$

and hence

$$T_4 = T_2 r_c \left(\frac{r_c}{r_v}\right)^{\gamma-1}$$

Substituting for T_1, T_3 and T_4 in the expression for the efficiency, we have

$$\eta = 1 - \frac{1}{r_v^{\gamma-1}}\left\{\frac{r_c^{\gamma} - 1}{\gamma(r_c - 1)}\right\} \tag{12.14}$$

Evidently the efficiency of the Diesel cycle depends upon r_c, and hence upon the quantity of heat added, as well as on the compression ratio r_v. Since the term in braces is always greater than unity (except for the trivial case where $r_c = 1$ and there is no heat addition), the Diesel cycle always has a lower efficiency than the Otto cycle of the same compression ratio (Fig. 12.14). This is not a very significant result because, as will be explained in Chapter 17, practical engines based upon the Diesel cycle can employ higher compression ratios than those based on the Otto cycle.

The behaviour of many reciprocating engines is more adequately represented by the *dual* or *mixed cycle* shown in Fig. 12.15. In this cycle part of the heat

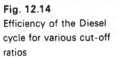

Fig. 12.14
Efficiency of the Diesel
cycle for various cut-off
ratios

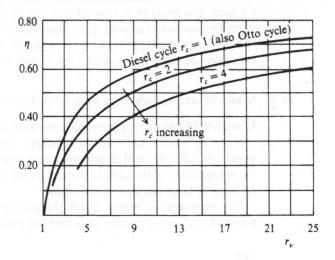

Fig. 12.15
The mixed or dual cycle

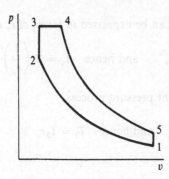

Fig. 12.16
Comparison of cycles

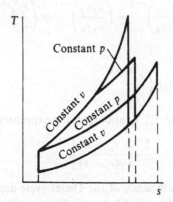

addition occurs during a constant volume process and the remainder during a constant pressure process. Writing $r_v = v_1/v_2$, $r_c = v_4/v_3$ and $r_p = p_3/p_2$, it is possible to show that the efficiency is given by

$$\eta = 1 - \frac{1}{r_v^{\gamma-1}} \frac{r_p r_c^{\gamma} - 1}{(r_p - 1) + \gamma r_p (r_c - 1)} \tag{12.15}$$

Fig. 12.16 shows the three cycles on the T–s diagram. They have been drawn for the case where both the compression ratios and the heat inputs are the same for each. The quantity of heat rejected can be seen from the areas to be least in the Otto cycle and greatest in the Diesel cycle. Without recourse to equations (12.13), (12.14) and (12.15), therefore, it can be seen that the air-standard cycle efficiencies decrease in the order Otto, mixed, Diesel.

12.8 Mean effective pressure as a criterion of performance

In section 11.1 it was explained that the ideal cycle efficiency is not the only criterion by which a cycle should be judged. The work ratio was shown to be another useful criterion of the performance of steady-flow cycles, since it indicates the susceptibility of the cycle to irreversibilities and also whether the plant will be small or large per unit power output.

In a reciprocating engine, where the processes are carried out in a single component, it is not so easy to isolate the positive and negative work in the

Fig. 12.17
Mean effective pressure

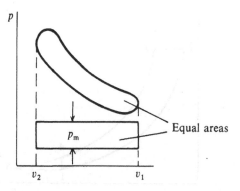

cycle. For this reason another criterion, called the *mean effective pressure*, is usually preferred to the work ratio when comparing air-standard cycles of reciprocating engines. The mean effective pressure p_m is defined as the height of a rectangle on the p–v diagram having the same length and area as the cycle. This is illustrated in Fig. 12.17, from which it is apparent that

$$p_m(v_1 - v_2) = \oint p \, dv = -W \tag{12.16}$$

where $-W$ is the net work output per unit mass of fluid. p_m can be regarded as that constant pressure which, by acting on the piston over one stroke, can produce the net work of the cycle. The mean effective pressure, unlike the work ratio, is not dimensionless, and it will here be expressed in bars. A method of evaluating the mean effective pressures of actual engines is described in section 16.2.

From equation (12.16) it is evident that a cycle with a large mean effective pressure will produce a large work output per unit swept volume, and hence an engine based on this cycle will be small for a given work output. Irreversibilities due to viscous friction are usually small in non-flow processes, unless a considerable amount of turbulence is artificially introduced as in certain types of compression-ignition engine. What is of considerable significance in reciprocating engines is *mechanical* friction, which results in the useful shaft power being appreciably less than the work done by the fluid on the piston. Since mechanical friction decreases with decrease in engine size, a large mean effective pressure implies that a smaller fraction of the net work of the cycle will be dissipated in this manner.*

It follows that the mean effective pressure is a useful criterion for the comparison of reciprocating engine cycles in that it indicates relative engine size, and also how far the actual engine efficiency will depart from the ideal cycle efficiency. As an illustration of this, consider the modification to the Diesel

---

* Mechanical friction also depends to some extent on the peak pressure and the average absolute pressure level during the cycle; higher pressures lead to greater bearing losses, particularly if lubrication is imperfect. It has been suggested that a better criterion for susceptibility to mechanical friction loss is provided by the ratio of mean effective pressure to peak pressure. This criterion, which is dimensionless, is truly analogous to the work ratio.

Fig. 12.18
Effect of complete
expansion on the
performance of the Diesel
cycle

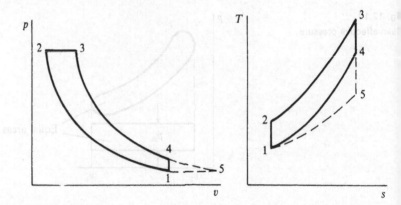

cycle shown in Fig. 12.18. In this case the rejection of heat occurs during a constant pressure process instead of a constant volume process. The cycle efficiency is improved because the heat rejection occurs at a lower average temperature (T_5 being lower than T_4). The additional work resulting from this modification, however, is obtained at the expense of a disproportionate increase in piston stroke, i.e. the mean effective pressure is reduced. The actual engine based upon this cycle would therefore not necessarily have a higher efficiency than one based upon the Diesel cycle, and it would certainly be a larger engine. The modified cycle is in fact the Joule cycle, described previously in section 12.1, which has found acceptance only as a basis for gas turbine plant. The following example shows the relative magnitudes of the mean effective pressure of the Diesel and Joule cycles.

Example 12.3   A mass of 1 kg of air is taken through a Diesel cycle (Fig. 12.13b) and a Joule cycle (Fig. 12.1). Initially the air is at 288 K and 1 atm. The compression ratio v_1/v_2 for both cycles is 15, and the heat added is 1850 kJ in each case. Calculate the ideal cycle efficiency and mean effective pressure for each cycle.

For both cycles
The initial volume of the air is

$$v_1 = \frac{RT_1}{p_1} = \frac{0.287 \times 288}{1.013\,25 \times 100} = 0.816 \, \text{m}^3$$

After compression,

$$T_2 = T_1\left(\frac{v_1}{v_2}\right)^{\gamma-1} = 288 \times 15^{0.4} = 851 \, \text{K}$$

$$v_2 = \frac{0.816}{15} = 0.054 \, \text{m}^3$$

The temperature rise during heat addition is given by

$$Q_{23} = c_p(T_3 - T_2) = 1.005(T_3 - 851) = 1850 \, \text{kJ/kg}$$

and hence

$$T_3 = 2692 \text{ K}$$

For the Diesel cycle

$$\frac{v_4}{v_3} = \frac{v_4 \, v_2}{v_2 \, v_3} = 15 \times \frac{851}{2692} = 4.742$$

and hence

$$T_4 = T_3 \left(\frac{v_3}{v_4} \right)^{\gamma - 1} = 2692 \left(\frac{1}{4.742} \right)^{0.4} = 1444 \text{ K}$$

The heat rejected is

$$Q_{41} = c_v(T_1 - T_4) = 0.718(288 - 1444) = -830 \text{ kJ/kg}$$

and the net work output is

$$|W| = Q_{23} + Q_{41} = 1020 \text{ kJ/kg}$$

Therefore the efficiency is

$$\eta = \frac{|W|}{Q_{23}} = \frac{1020}{1850} = 0.551$$

The mean effective pressure is

$$P_m = \frac{|W|}{v_1 - v_2} = \frac{1020}{(0.816 - 0.054)100} = 13.4 \text{ bar}$$

For the Joule cycle
We have

$$T_4 = T_3 \left(\frac{v_3}{v_4} \right)^{\gamma - 1} = 2692 \left(\frac{1}{15} \right)^{0.4} = 911 \text{ K}$$

$$v_4 = \frac{RT_4}{p_4} = \frac{0.287 \times 911}{1.013\,25 \times 100} = 2.580 \text{ m}^3$$

The heat rejected is

$$Q_{41} = c_p(T_1 - T_4) = 1.005(288 - 911) = -626 \text{ kJ/kg}$$

and the net work is

$$|W| = Q_{23} + Q_{41} = 1224 \text{ kJ/kg}$$

The efficiency is therefore

$$\eta = \frac{|W|}{Q_{23}} = \frac{1224}{1850} = 0.662$$

The mean effective pressure is

$$p_m = \frac{|W|}{v_4 - v_2} = \frac{1224}{(2.580 - 0.054)100} = 4.85 \text{ bar}$$

Note that the net work outputs could have been calculated from $\oint p\,dv$, and the efficiencies from equations (12.14) and (12.2) respectively.

12.9 Cycles having the Carnot efficiency

The Otto, Diesel and mixed cycles all have efficiencies less than the Carnot efficiency based upon the maximum and minimum temperatures in the cycle. The Carnot cycle itself is quite unsuitable as a basis for a reciprocating engine using a gas as a working fluid because the mean effective pressure of the cycle is very small. This should be apparent from the thin appearance of the cycle on the $p–v$ diagram in Fig. 12.19. There are other cycles having the Carnot efficiency which do not suffer from this defect and, although they are of little practical significance at present, they are worthy of a brief mention here.

Consider the cycle shown in Fig. 12.20 consisting of two constant volume processes and two isothermals; it is called the *Stirling cycle*. The heat supplied during process 2–3 is equal in quantity to the heat rejected during process 4–1. Furthermore, the temperature of the fluid varies between the same limits during these two processes. It is therefore theoretically possible for the heat rejected, Q_{41}, to be returned to the working fluid as Q_{23}. Ideally, this heat transfer can be accomplished reversibly in a *regenerator*, which consists essentially of a matrix of wire gauze or small tubes. Fig. 12.21 illustrates the principle of operation. A temperature gradient from T_a to T_b is maintained along the matrix. The working fluid enters the matrix in state 4, transfers heat to the matrix, and

Fig. 12.19
The Carnot cycle

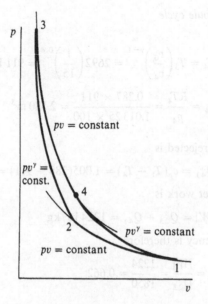

p

3

$pv = \text{constant}$

$pv^\gamma = $ const.

4

2

$pv^\gamma = \text{constant}$

$pv = \text{constant}$

1

v

Fig. 12.20
The Stirling cycle

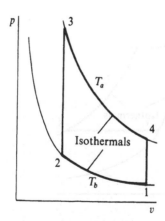

Fig. 12.21
The regenerator

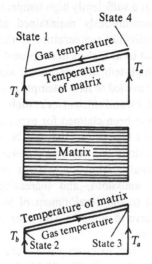

leaves in state 1; each element of the matrix is raised in temperature by an infinitesimal amount. Then working fluid in state 2 passes in the reverse direction, cooling each element of the matrix by an infinitesimal amount, and leaving in state 3. At no time need the working fluid and matrix differ more than infinitesimally in temperature, so that the entire heat transfer process is carried out reversibly.

With a perfect regenerator, the only heat added from an external source during the cycle is that which is transferred during the isothermal process 3–4 (i.e. at T_a), and the only heat rejected to an external sink is the quantity transferred during the isothermal process 1–2 (i.e. at T_b). It follows that the efficiency of the cycle is $(T_a - T_b)/T_a$. The mean effective pressure of this cycle is much greater than that of the Carnot cycle, and is in fact comparable to that of the Otto cycle. Engines which have been built to operate on the Stirling cycle are in fact heat engines in the sense of Fig. 12.1, with external combustion. The main reason why such engines have had little success is the difficulty of designing an efficient regenerator of reasonable size (air being a poor conductor of heat)

Fig. 12.22
The Ericsson cycle

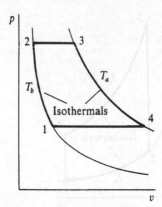

which can operate at a sufficiently high temperature. One end of the regenerator matrix must be continuously maintained at the upper temperature, and the maximum permissible temperature is therefore subject to metallurgical limitations; it cannot be as high as in reciprocating internal-combustion engines. Developments in high-temperature alloys, and improved knowledge of heat transfer processes, have led to new attempts to construct a Stirling engine. These are described in Ref. 24, and efficiencies as high as those achieved in compression-ignition engines have been claimed for experimental engines.* Since there are no restrictions on the type of fuel that can be used, such engines may be useful for military applications and for small power plant in developing countries. Furthermore, external combustion systems can be designed to give exhausts with low noxious emissions, and increasing concern with environmental pollution may lead to the development of Stirling engines for road vehicles. They would then have to compete with attempts to build Rankine cycle plant for the same purpose.

A similar cycle—the *Ericsson cycle*—consists of two constant pressure processes and two isothermals (Fig. 12.22). In this case the heat rejected during one constant pressure process is returned via a regenerator to the working fluid during the other constant pressure process, and again the cycle has the Carnot efficiency. This is in fact the same cycle as that depicted in Fig. 12.11—and it was originally proposed as a basis for a reciprocating engine. The Ericsson cycle suffers from the same drawbacks as the Stirling cycle.

---

* A very successful air liquefaction plant working on the reversed Stirling cycle has also been developed and is now widely used.

13

Heat Pump and Refrigeration Cycles

In a power cycle, heat is received by the working fluid at a high temperature and rejected at a low temperature, while a net amount of work is done *by* the fluid. Cycles can be conceived in which the reverse happens, heat being received at a low temperature and rejected at a high temperature, while a net amount of work is done *on* the fluid. The latter are called *heat pump* or *refrigeration* cycles. The term 'heat pump' is usually applied to a machine whose principal purpose is to supply heat at an elevated temperature, and the term 'refrigerator' to one whose purpose is the extraction of heat from a cold space. This distinction in terminology is arbitrary because a heat pump and a refrigerator are identical in principle and it is possible to use one machine to fulfil the function of a heat pump and a refrigerator simultaneously. For example, one machine can provide a cold space for food storage and also supply heat to a domestic hot water tank. When no distinction is necessary we shall refer to the cycle as a refrigeration cycle.

Practical refrigeration cycles are composed of flow processes, each process being carried out in a separate component. As in Chapter 11, we shall again assume that changes in potential and kinetic energy between the inlet and outlet of each component are negligible. The working fluids are almost always in the liquid or vapour phase. Air is occasionally used, but only in air-conditioning plant where the air fulfils the dual function of the refrigerating fluid and air-conditioning medium.

13.1 Reversed Carnot cycle and performance criteria

If the series of processes which make up a reversible power cycle are plotted on a p–v or T–s diagram, the enclosed area is traced out in a clockwise sense, indicating that the net work done is negative. The positive net work of a reversible refrigeration cycle is proportional to an area traced out by processes in an anticlockwise sense. A reversed Carnot cycle, using a wet vapour as a working fluid, is shown in Fig. 13.1. Vapour is compressed isentropically from a low pressure and temperature (state 1) to a higher pressure and temperature (state 2), and is passed through a condenser in which it is condensed at constant pressure to state 3. The fluid is then expanded isentropically to its original pressure (state 4), and is finally evaporated at constant pressure to state 1.

Fig. 13.1

The refrigeration or heat pump cycle

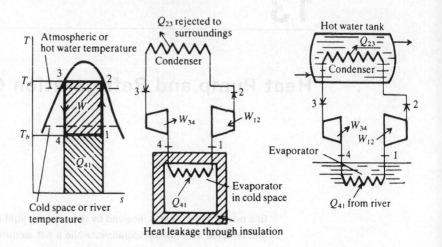

The criterion of performance of the cycle, expressed as the ratio output/input, depends upon what is regarded as the output. In a refrigerator we endeavour to extract the maximum amount of heat Q_{41} in the evaporator for a net expenditure of work W. Therefore the *coefficient of performance* of a refrigerator is defined as

$$CP_{ref} = Q_{41}/W \qquad (13.1)$$

In a heat pump we are concerned to obtain the maximum amount of heat Q_{23} from the condenser for the net expenditure of work W, and therefore the coefficient of performance of a heat pump is defined by

$$CP_{hp} = -Q_{23}/W \qquad (13.2)$$

The minus sign is necessary because Q_{23} is negative, and it is conventional to define a coefficient of performance as a positive quantity as we do with the efficiency of an engine.

The relation between these two coefficients of performance can be established by applying the First Law. Thus

$$(Q_{41} + Q_{23}) + W = 0$$

and hence

$$CP_{hp} = CP_{ref} + 1 \qquad (13.3)$$

Inspection of the areas representing Q_{41}, Q_{23} and W on the T–s diagram (Fig. 13.1) shows that CP_{ref} may be greater than unity, and that CP_{hp} must always be greater than unity; this is the reason the term 'efficiency' is not employed.

From equation (13.2) it is evident that CP_{hp} is the reciprocal of the efficiency of a power cycle. The CP_{hp} of a reversed Carnot cycle, operating between an upper temperature T_a and a lower temperature T_b, must therefore be equal to $T_a/(T_a - T_b)$. Equation (13.3) then shows that the CP_{ref} of a reversed Carnot cycle is $T_b/(T_a - T_b)$.

Both coefficients become smaller as the temperature range of the cycle is increased. The upper cycle temperature must be 10 K or so above the temperature of the atmosphere (refrigerator) or hot water tank (heat pump), so that the required rate of heat transfer can be accomplished in a condenser of economic size. Similarly the lower cycle temperature must be below the temperature of the cold space (refrigerator) or surroundings (heat pump) to enable the evaporator to be of economic size. Evidently these necessary temperature differences (i.e. external irreversibilities) place a limit on the coefficient of performance attainable.

A typical temperature range over which the working fluid of a heat pump might operate is from 5 °C to 60 °C. The ideal coefficient of performance of a heat pump operating on a reversed Carnot cycle under these conditions is therefore $333/(60 - 5) = 6.05$. That is, 6.05 times the quantity of work supplied is delivered as heat at the required temperature. If the heat pump is driven by a power plant operating with an actual overall efficiency of about 0.30, the heat delivered at the required temperature is twice the heat supplied from the high-temperature source of the power cycle. This ratio might be termed the *thermal advantage* of the combined plant. It would appear that there is much to be gained by burning fuel in a heat engine coupled to a heat pump, instead of using the combustion as a direct source of heat for warming a building. This is only to be expected; the latter procedure involves a considerable degradation of energy, because the quantity of heat is allowed to flow through a large temperature range without producing work. To arrive at the advantage of about 2, however, we have assumed the use of a perfect heat pump. In practice the ideal cycle used has a lower coefficient of performance than the reversed Carnot cycle, and irreversibilities reduce the coefficient of performance still further. The real advantage of such a plant would therefore be smaller than 2. Whether in any proposed installation the advantage will be worth the outlay in plant must be determined by careful economic analysis of fuel, capital and maintenance costs.

13.2   Practical refrigeration cycles

Using arguments similar to those in Chapter 5, it is possible to show that all reversible cycles operating between the same two reservoirs have the same coefficient of performance, i.e. that of the reversed Carnot cycle. One has only to assume the opposite to be true and show that this contradicts the Second Law. Practical refrigerators, however, use a different form of cycle which, although having a lower ideal *CP*, has other features to commend it.

A major simplification in the plant is achieved by dispensing with an expansion machine and using a simple throttle valve to obtain the reduction in pressure (Fig. 13.2). Thus the end states 3 and 4 of the expansion process lie on a constant enthalpy line instead of an isentropic. The effect of this modification can be seen by comparing the T–s diagrams of Figs 13.1 and 13.2. The net work required is now equal to the compression work, because no work is obtained from the expansion process. The heat transfer in the condenser is unaffected,

Fig. 13.2
A refrigeration cycle
incorporating a throttle
valve

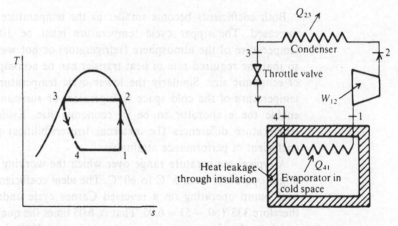

but the heat extracted in the evaporator is diminished. Both CP_{ref} and CP_{hp} are therefore reduced by the modification. Also, the rate of flow of working fluid is increased *when the cycle is used for refrigeration*, because the heat extracted per unit mass of refrigerant (Q_{41}) is reduced. Q_{41}, known as the *refrigeration effect*, is a useful criterion for comparing cycles on the basis of size of plant required for a given *duty* (heat extracted per unit time).

Although the heat transfers still take place at the upper and lower temperatures of the cycle, the throttling process introduces an irreversibility which makes the cycle irreversible as a whole. The coefficient of performance is then no longer independent of the working fluid as it is for the reversed Carnot cycle. By and large, the properties required of an ideal working fluid for heat pumps and refrigerators are similar to those required for an engine fluid and listed in section 11.10. The principal modifications are that: (a) the critical temperature need only be above atmospheric temperature (or hot water temperature) and not above the metallurgical limit, and (b) the saturation pressure should be above atmospheric pressure at the lowest evaporator temperature likely to be required. The latter is desirable so that any leak in the circuit will lead to an efflux of refrigerant (easily detectable), and not an influx of atmospheric air. The latter contains moisture which would ice up the throttle valve.

Fluids most commonly used in recent years have been ammonia (NH_3) for large industrial plant, and chlorofluorocarbons (CFCs) for commercial and domestic refrigeration. CFCs were tailor-made by the chemical industry for a variety of purposes, not only as refrigerants. Unfortunately, they are so stable that when discharged to atmosphere the molecules diffuse to the stratosphere before being ultimately decomposed by ultraviolet radiation. It has now been found that the liberated chlorine atoms attack the ozone layer which protects the Earth from that radiation—and moreover by a chain reaction wherein every chlorine atom breaks up about 10^5 ozone molecules. International agreement has been reached to phase out the use of CFCs in favour of a tetrafluoroethane (HFC) that does not contain the offending chlorine atom. The HFC chosen was refrigerant 134a ($CH_2F - CF_3$). Recently, however, it has been shown that if released to atmosphere it acts as a 'greenhouse gas' contributing to *global warming*. The major contributor to global warming is the carbon dioxide produced by burning fossil fuel. Although the quantity of HFC released when refrigeration plant are scrapped is small compared with this CO_2, HFC is several thousand times worse, per unit mass, than CO_2, so that its contribution to global warming cannot be ignored (Refs 43 and 44). The search is on to find another refrigerant that has neither defect.

Comprehensive tables of properties of refrigerants can be found in Ref.27. The author's abridged tables (Ref.17) have always contained properties of ammonia, and of dichlorodifluoromethane CF_2Cl_2 referred to as R12. Some examples and Problems involving R12, in previous impressions of this book, have now been reworked using the HFC tetrafluoroethane (R134a). Properties of this new, environmentally more acceptable refrigerant have been included in the fifth edition of Ref.17.

Example 13.1 Calculate the refrigeration effect and coefficient of performance for the refrigeration cycle shown in Fig. 13.2, when the fluid is ammonia and the upper and lower temperatures are 30 °C and −15 °C respectively. Find also the corresponding values for a reversed Carnot cycle operating between the same temperatures.

From the ammonia tables we have

$$h_4 = h_3 = h_f = 323.1 \text{ kJ/kg}, \qquad h_2 = h_g = 1468.9 \text{ kJ/kg},$$

$$s_2 = 4.984 \text{ kJ/kg K}$$

From $s_1 = s_2$ we have $x_1 = 0.889$, and hence

$$h_1 = h_f + x_1 h_{fg} = 1280.7 \text{ kJ/kg}$$

The refrigeration effect is

$$Q_{41} = (h_1 - h_4) = 957.6 \text{ kJ/kg}$$

and the net work expended is

$$W = W_{12} = (h_2 - h_1) = 188.2 \text{ kJ/kg}$$

As a refrigerator the coefficient of performance is

$$CP_{ref} = \frac{957.6}{188.2} = 5.09$$

For the reversed Carnot cycle,

$$CP_{ref} = \frac{(273 - 15)}{30 - (-15)} = 5.73$$

$s_3 = 1.204 \text{ kJ/kg K}$, and from $s_4 = s_3$ we have $x_4 = 0.147$, and hence $h_4 = 305.6 \text{ kJ/kg}$. The refrigeration effect is therefore

$$Q_{41} = (h_1 - h_4) = 975.1 \text{ kJ/kg}$$

The foregoing example shows that the refrigeration effect is not significantly altered by replacing the expansion machine with a throttle valve, but that the coefficient of performance is noticeably reduced—from 5.73 to 5.09. The work

Fig. 13.3
A practical simple
refrigeration cycle

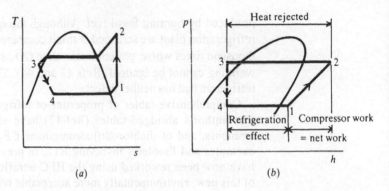

(a)   (b)

recovered in the expander of the reversed Carnot plant is, however, quite small compared with the compression work, e.g. -17.5 versus $+188.2\,kJ/kg$. In an actual plant using this ideal cycle, much of the expansion work would be dissipated by mechanical friction. The substitution of a throttling expansion does not therefore result in a significant change in the performance of the real cycle, and it constitutes a worthwhile mechanical simplification of the plant.

A practical ideal cycle differs in two other respects from the reversed Carnot cycle. First, the compression is usually carried out in the superheat region. Not only would it be difficult to arrange for the evaporation to cease at state 1 (Fig. 13.2), but any liquid refrigerant passing into the compressor would tend to wash away the lubricating oil. This is obviously undesirable if, as is usual, the compressor is a reciprocating or positive displacement rotary type with rubbing surfaces. Moreover the oil would be carried to the evaporator where it might form a film on the tube surfaces and impair the heat transfer process. It is usual, therefore, to transfer a saturated or slightly superheated vapour to the inlet of the compressor. The second modification is that the condensed liquid is often subcooled before entering the throttle valve. As already observed, most of the heat transferred in the condenser must be rejected by virtue of an appreciable temperature difference, to keep the size of condenser within reasonable limits. It is therefore possible to subcool the liquid after condensation to within a few degrees of the surrounding temperature.

Both these modifications are illustrated in Fig. 13.3a, and it is clear that they both tend to increase the refrigeration effect. The former also increases the compression work, $(h_2 - h_1)$, and the net effect is a slight decrease in the coefficient of performance, as illustrated by the following example. It was suggested in section 8.4.3 that a p–h chart is a useful aid when considering refrigeration cycles. Fig. 13.3b shows the cycle on such a diagram, from which it appears that the refrigeration effect, heat rejected, and work required can be read directly from the h-axis. This method is used in the example.

Example 13.2 The cycle in Example 1.3.1 is modified so that the refrigerant enters the compressor as a saturated vapour, and is subcooled to $18\,°C$ before entering the throttle valve. Find the refrigeration effect and CP_{ref}. What would the result be if R134a were the refrigerant instead of ammonia?

Fig. 13.4

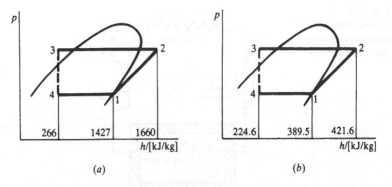

(a)   (b)

Fig. 13.4a shows the cycle located on the $p–h$ chart for ammonia, from which the following values are obtained:

$$h_1 = 1427 \text{ kJ/kg}, \qquad h_2 = 1660 \text{ kJ/kg},$$

$$h_3 = h_4 = 266 \text{ kJ/kg}$$

The refrigeration effect is

$$Q_{41} = (h_1 - h_4) = 1161 \text{ kJ/kg}$$

The net work required is

$$W = (h_2 - h_1) = 233 \text{ kJ/kg}$$

and the coefficient of performance is

$$CP_{\text{ref}} = \frac{Q_{41}}{W} = \frac{1161}{233} = 4.98$$

Similarly, Fig. 13.4b shows the cycle on a $p–h$ chart for R134a, from which we obtain the refrigeration effect

$$Q_{41} = 389.5 - 224.6 = 164.9 \text{ kJ/kg}$$

and the coefficient of performance

$$CP_{\text{ref}} = \frac{164.9}{32.1} = 5.14$$

From the previous example we see that R134a gives a slightly higher CP than ammonia. On the other hand the refrigeration effect *per unit mass* for ammonia is about 7 times larger than that for R134a. A comparison of refrigeration effects per unit *volume* of refrigerant is more useful, because the displacement of the compressor and the size of the plant in general depends mainly on this value. R134a is about 4 times denser than ammonia, so that the advantage of ammonia in this respect is less than 2. Other factors also govern the choice of refrigerant. Ammonia, for example, attacks many common metals and is very hygroscopic — two disadvantages from which R134a does not suffer.

Comparing the results of Examples 13.1 and 13.2, it can be seen that the dry compression and subcooling increase the refrigeration effect of ammonia from

279

Fig. 13.5
A refrigerator with
two-stage compression
and flash chamber

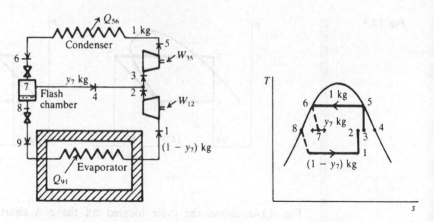

958 to 1161 kJ/kg, while only reducing the coefficient of performance from 5.09 to 4.98.

All the values in the examples have been calculated on the assumption that the cycles are composed of ideal processes. The adjective 'ideal' here does not imply that a process is reversible, for the throttling process is essentially irreversible; it simply means that there are no unintended effects. In practice the compression is neither adiabatic nor reversible; the throttling process is not perfectly adiabatic; and the processes of condensation and evaporation are accompanied by small pressure drops due to friction in the pipes. Such deviations from the ideal lead to a reduction in the coefficient of performance, and the values obtained here must be regarded only as an indication of the best that can be achieved with the given cycle conditions and given refrigerant.

As with power cycles, a better performance can always be obtained at the expense of additional complexity. Only one example of a more complex cycle will be mentioned here: the multicompression system with flash chamber, shown in Fig. 13.5. The object of this layout is to reduce the disadvantageous effect of the useless vaporisation which occurs in the throttling expansion. In the simple plant, this flash vapour passes through the evaporator without extracting any heat from the cold source, and work must be supplied to compress this vapour, together with the 'useful' vapour, through the full range of pressure. In the two-stage plant, the liquid is expanded to an intermediate pressure in the flash chamber, and the useless flash vapour is passed to the inlet of the second-stage compressor. The liquid in the flash chamber is expanded in a second throttle valve to the final pressure and passes to the evaporator in the usual way. Less work is required, because the flash vapour removed at the intermediate pressure need only be compressed over a part of the pressure range of the cycle. For a given amount of heat rejection, a reduction of work implies an increase in heat extraction (First Law), and therefore the coefficient of performance, whether as a heat pump or a refrigerator, is improved.

13.3 Water refrigerator

So far no mention has been made of water as a refrigerant. It is quite unsuitable

Fig. 13.6

Application of an ejector
pump to a steam
refrigeration cycle

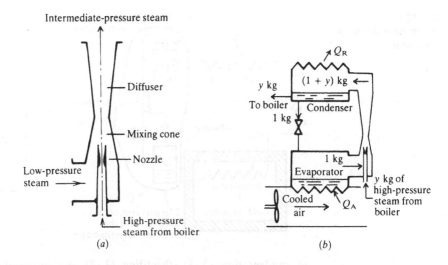

(a)   (b)

for use in the type of plant we have been discussing because of its very low vapour pressure and high specific volume at low temperatures. At temperatures encountered in air-conditioning plant, however, it is possible to maintain the degree of vacuum required. Even so, at $7\,^{\circ}C$ the vapour pressure is about 0.01 bar, and the corresponding specific volume is about $129\ m^3/kg$. The large volume flow implied by this has led to the use of an ejector pump in place of the usual compressor for this type of plant. The ejector pump is illustrated in Fig. 13.6a. Steam is expanded in a nozzle to form a high-speed jet at low pressure, which entrains the vapour to be extracted from the vacuum chamber. The combined steam from the mixing chamber is then diffused in the divergent part of the venturi until the required exhaust pressure is reached. Such a pump has no moving parts, but it has a very low isentropic efficiency.

Fig. 13.6b shows how the pump is used in the refrigeration plant. Water in the evaporator at low pressure vaporises and is pumped, together with the motive steam, into the condenser. A portion of the condensate is throttled into the evaporator, and the remainder is pumped back to the steam boiler. If waste steam is available from an existing boiler plant, the poor efficiency of the ejector pump is of no consequence, and the refrigeration plant itself is cheap to construct and operate.

13.4 Absorption refrigerators

The type of plant we have considered in previous sections is known as *vapour compression plant*, and in such plant the work of compression is comparable in magnitude with the other energy transfers in the cycle. The compression work can be reduced considerably, however, if the vapour is dissolved in a suitable liquid before compression. After compression the vapour can be drawn off, and then throttled and evaporated in the usual way. This principle is employed in *absorption refrigerators*.

An ammonia absorption refrigerator is illustrated in Fig. 13.7. The processes

281

Fig. 13.7
An ammonia absorption
refrigerator

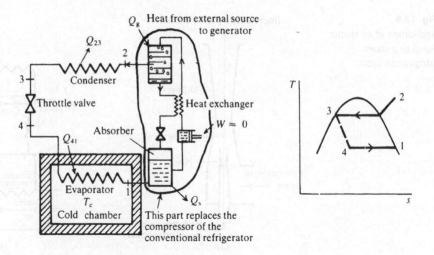

of condensation (2–3), throttling (3–4) and evaporation (4–1) occur in conventional components. After evaporation to state 1, the vapour is first passed into an absorber and dissolved in water. The water temperature is only a little above atmospheric, and at such a temperature the solubility of ammonia vapour is very high. The process of solution is accompanied by a rejection of heat Q_s to the surroundings (just as the process of driving off the vapour from the solution requires heat absorption). The liquid solution is then compressed to the required pressure and heated, first in a heat exchanger, and then in the generator which is maintained at a temperature T_g. At the higher temperature the solubility of ammonia in water is appreciably smaller, and the heat received Q_g results in the removal of vapour from solution. The generator may be heated by steam coils, gas or electricity. The ammonia vapour is passed to the condenser to complete the main cycle, while the remaining weak solution is returned to the absorber via a throttle valve. The heat exchanger is merely used to reduce the quantities of heat Q_g and Q_s.

The work required to compress the liquid solution is very much smaller than that required for compressing a corresponding amount of ammonia vapour, but on the other hand heat has to be supplied to the generator from an external source. The analysis of the compression process requires a knowledge of the thermodynamic properties of ammonia-in-water solutions and cannot be given here.* Nevertheless, by concentrating on the essential nature of the cycle, simple thermodynamic principles can be applied to show that there is a limit to the coefficient of performance which can be achieved with any given set of temperature levels.

Energy is transferred in the form of heat at three temperature levels: the atmospheric temperature T_a at which heat is rejected in the condenser and absorber; the temperature T_c at which heat is taken from the cold chamber; and the temperature T_g at which heat is received in the generator. A small quantity of energy is also transferred as work in the pump, but this is negligible

---

* An example of such an analysis can be found in Ref. 11.

Fig. 13.8
A 'reversible equivalent' of
an absorption refrigerator

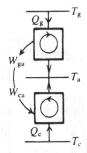

compared with the other energy transfers. It is possible to imagine an arrangement of reversible machines (Fig. 13.8) performing a function equivalent to that of the absorption plant. First, a reversible heat engine receives a quantity of heat Q_g at T_g and rejects heat at T_a while producing a quantity of work W_{ga} with an efficiency

$$\frac{|W_{ga}|}{Q_g} = \frac{T_g - T_a}{T_g}$$

Secondly, a reversible refrigerator receives a quantity of heat Q_c at T_c and rejects heat at T_a while absorbing a quantity of work W_{ca}. The coefficient of performance of the refrigerator is

$$\frac{Q_c}{W_{ca}} = \frac{T_c}{T_a - T_c}$$

If $|W_{ga}|$ is made equal to W_{ca}, this plant will be equivalent to an absorption refrigerator for which the pump work is zero. The coefficient of performance of the combined plant acting as a refrigerator can be defined as Q_c/Q_g, which on combining the previous two equations becomes

$$CP_{ref} = \frac{Q_c}{Q_g} = \frac{T_c(T_g - T_a)}{T_g(T_a - T_c)} \qquad (13.4)$$

Although this limiting coefficient is greater than unity with normal operating temperatures, the properties of ammonia-in-water solutions are such that an ammonia absorption refrigerator has a coefficient of performance less than unity. These refrigerators are rarely used unless waste heat is available from some existing source.

A special form of ammonia absorption refrigerator, in which the pump is dispensed with entirely, is widely used for domestic purposes where the power consumption (electricity or gas) is so small that efficiency is not a prime consideration.* Having no moving parts at all, the refrigerator requires little maintenance. Its operation depends on the principle that if a liquid is exposed

---

* The refrigerator described here was invented by B. von Platen and C. G. Munters when studying at the Royal Institute of Technology in Stockholm. It is often called the Electrolux refrigerator, after the firm who first developed it commercially.

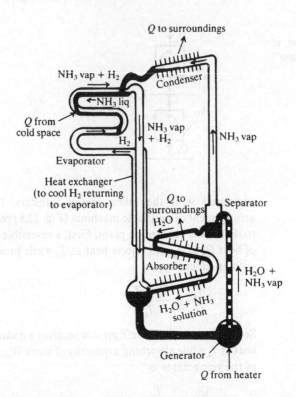

Fig. 13.9
Absorption refrigerator with
no moving parts

Q to surroundings

NH₃ vap + H₂

Condenser

←NH₃ liq

Q from
cold space

NH₃ vap
+ H₂

H₂

NH₃ vap

Evaporator

Heat exchanger
(to cool H₂ returning
to evaporator)

Q to
surroundings

Separator

H₂O

Absorber

H₂O +
NH₃ vap

H₂O + NH₃
solution

Generator

Q from heater

to an inert atmosphere, which is not saturated with the vapour of the liquid, some of the liquid will evaporate and so produce a cooling effect. The total pressure is effectively uniform throughout the plant, but the partial pressure of the ammonia vapour varies, being high in the condenser and low in the evaporator. This variation is accomplished by concentrating a gas (hydrogen) in the parts of the circuit where the ammonia vapour pressure ·is required to be low. There being no material change in total pressure during the cycle, circulation of the fluid can be maintained by convection currents set up by density gradients.

A diagrammatic sketch of the more essential components of this type of absorption refrigerator is shown in Fig. 13.9. The ammonia-in-water solution is boiled in the generator and rises to the separator. From here the water, while cooling, returns to the absorber through a liquid trap, and the ammonia vapour rises further to the condenser. There it loses heat to the surroundings, and the ammonia condensate flows through a liquid trap into the evaporator coils. In the evaporator there is some hydrogen present, and the ammonia evaporates at a low temperature corresponding to its low partial pressure. The mixture of hydrogen and ammonia flows down through a heat exchanger to the absorber, and the ammonia vapour returns into the cold water solution. From the absorber the hydrogen rises back to the evaporator, while the ammonia-in-water solution flows into the generator to complete the cycle. Thus there are three essential circuits to this plant: (a) the main ammonia circuit, (b) the subsidiary water circuit, and (c) the subsidiary hydrogen circuit. The actual plant is in fact rather more complicated than Fig. 13.9 suggests, and the thermodynamic analysis of the cycle is difficult.

As discussed in section 13.3, water can be used as a refrigerant in a vapour compression refrigerator at the temperature levels which prevail in air-conditioning plant and heat pumps. There is no reason why water should not be the refrigerant in an absorption refrigerator designed for such temperatures. The most common absorbent in this case is lithium bromide. It is a particularly good absorber because, unlike the water in ammonia systems, lithium bromide does not evaporate at the temperature used to drive off the water vapour from solution. This means that there is no need for a rectification column in the generator to separate the liquid and vapour phases of the absorbent, as there is in ammonia-in-water systems. Water-in-lithium bromide systems are therefore simpler, and in addition the properties of lithium bromide solutions are such that CP_{ref} is higher.

13.5   Gas cycles

When a gas is used as a refrigerating fluid it is essential to employ an expander because the temperature remains substantially unchanged by throttling. The processes in the cooler and heater, which replace the condenser and evaporator of a vapour compression machine, are usually constant pressure, but not constant temperature, processes. The ideal cycle is in fact a reversed Joule cycle, as shown in Fig. 13.10. For a refrigerator, the temperature at state 3 must be somewhat above atmospheric temperature, and at state 1 somewhat below the cold space temperature. Consequently a refrigerator using a gas as a working fluid is less efficient than one using a vapour, because its operating temperature range is very much wider, i.e. from T_4 to T_2 instead of from T_1 to T_3. It is also much bulkier than a vapour plant of the same duty, because a gas requires relatively larger surface areas for a given heat transfer. For these reasons gases are never used nowadays as working fluids for refrigerators, when the sole object is refrigeration.

When cool air is required for air-conditioning, however, it is sometimes more convenient to cool the air directly than by the means indicated in section 13.3. The air then combines the function of refrigerating fluid and air-conditioning medium. A typical modern application is illustrated by the following example.

Fig. 13.10
A simple refrigeration cycle using air

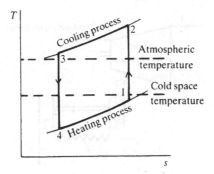

Example 13.3 An air-conditioning unit of a pressurised aircraft receives its air from the jet engine compressor at a pressure of 1.22 bar. The atmospheric pressure and temperature are 0.227 bar and 217 K respectively. The air-conditioning unit consists of a freewheeling compressor and turbine mounted on one shaft (Fig. 13.11). The air coming into the unit is compressed to a pressure p, cooled at constant pressure, and expanded in the turbine to a pressure of 1 bar and temperature of 280 K. Assuming that all processes are reversible, calculate the pressure p and the temperature of the air at exit from the cooler.

The engine compressor intake state 1 is

$$p_1 = 0.227 \text{ bar}, \qquad T_1 = 217 \text{ K}$$

and the air bleed state 2 is

$$p_2 = 1.22 \text{ bar},$$

$$T_2 = T_1 \left(\frac{p_2}{p_1}\right)^{(\gamma-1)/\gamma} = 217 \left(\frac{1.22}{0.227}\right)^{0.4/1.4} = 315 \text{ K}$$

The freewheeling compressor outlet temperature is

$$T_3 = T_2 \left(\frac{p}{p_2}\right)^{0.4/1.4}$$

and hence this compressor work is

$$W_{23} = (h_3 - h_2) = c_p(T_3 - T_2) = c_p T_2 \left\{ \left(\frac{p}{p_2}\right)^{0.4/1.4} - 1 \right\}$$

The required turbine outlet state 5 is

$$p_5 = 1 \text{ bar}, \qquad T_5 = 280 \text{ K}$$

The cooler outlet temperature is therefore

$$T_4 = T_5 \left(\frac{p}{p_5}\right)^{0.4/1.4}$$

Fig. 13.11
An aircraft air-conditioning unit

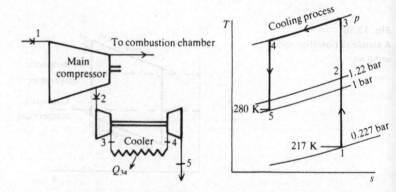

and the turbine work is

$$W_{45} = (h_5 - h_4) = c_p(T_5 - T_4) = c_p T_5 \left\{ 1 - \left(\frac{p}{p_5} \right)^{0.4/1.4} \right\}$$

Since the turbine is only to produce sufficient work to drive the compressor,

$$W_{23} = -W_{45}$$

and hence the equation from which the unknown pressure p can be found is

$$c_p T_2 \left\{ \left(\frac{p}{p_2} \right)^{0.4/1.4} - 1 \right\} = -c_p T_5 \left\{ 1 - \left(\frac{p}{p_5} \right)^{0.4/1.4} \right\}$$

By trial and error the cooler pressure is found to be

$$p = 3.06 \text{ bar}$$

The required cooler exit temperature is

$$T_4 = T_5 \left(\frac{3.06}{1} \right)^{0.4/1.4} = 385 \text{ K}$$

Another circumstance in which a gas cycle is used is when the object is to liquefy the gas. The simplest liquefaction process was first developed by Linde for liquefying air, and it is illustrated in Fig. 13.12. Air at atmospheric pressure, state 1, is compressed to state 2, and is then cooled at constant pressure back to atmospheric temperature, state 3, in a water cooler. The air is cooled further to state 4 in a heat exchanger before being throttled to state 5. In this state the liquid portion 5_f is drained off and the vapour portion 5_g is taken to the heat exchanger and back to the compressor. To keep the mass of air in the system

Fig. 13.12

A simple gas liquefaction plant

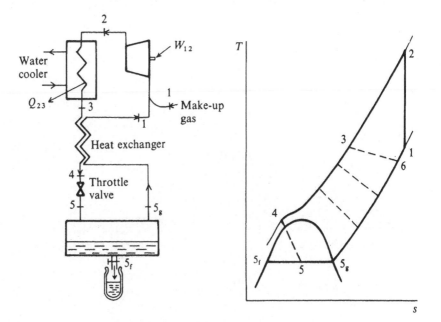

constant, make-up air, equal in mass to the liquid air drained off, is introduced into the system in state 1.

It is evident that when starting such a plant there is no cold gas in the system, and the throttling process will follow path 3–6. But provided that the gas is below its inversion temperature (see section 7.4.4), a little cooling will occur. This cooling effect is cumulative, as it is utilised in the heat exchanger, and the throttling curve 3–6 will shift towards path 4–5. The ultimate steady position of state 4 depends on the rate at which liquid is drained off, and on the rate at which heat leaks into the system.

When the gas to be liquefied has an inversion temperature below atmospheric, it is necessary to precool the gas below its inversion temperature with a conventional refrigerator, or to replace the throttle valve with an expansion machine. The reason why a throttle valve was originally preferred to an expansion machine like a turbine is that it was difficult to construct one which would work satisfactorily at very low temperatures. Using new materials, suitable expanders have been developed and much better plant efficiencies can now be obtained. The subject of low-temperature engineering—called *cryogenics*—is of increasing importance but it is outside the scope of this book. A survey of work in this field can be found in Ref. 13.

14

Properties of Mixtures

Any homogeneous mixture of gases can be regarded as a single substance if the constituents do not react chemically with one another and are in a fixed proportion by mass. The properties of such a mixture can be determined experimentally just as for a single substance, and they can be tabulated or related algebraically in the same way. The composition of air can be assumed invariable for most purposes, and air is usually treated as a single substance. As air is such a common fluid, its properties have been determined by direct measurement. For less common mixtures, however, it is necessary to have some method of deducing the properties of the mixture from those of its constituents. This chapter describes how this can be done for mixtures of perfect gases, and for mixtures of gases and vapours at low pressure. More refined methods, for use when the gases or vapours cannot be assumed to be perfect, are given in textbooks on chemical thermodynamics (e.g. Ref. 4).

Steam condensers, air-conditioning plant and cooling towers provide suitable examples of systems involving mixtures of gases and vapours at low pressure, and the thermodynamic analysis of the processes which occur in these systems is given here. The special nomenclature associated with the study of moist atmospheric air (hygrometry) is introduced, and the chapter ends with a brief description of the hygrometric chart.

14.1 An empirical law for mixtures of gases

Any mixture of gases can be imagined to be separated into its constituents in such a way that each occupies a volume equal to that of the mixture and each is at the same temperature as the mixture. An important empirical law can then be stated as follows:

> *The pressure and internal energy of a mixture of gases are respectively equal to the sums of the pressures and internal energies of the individual constituents when each occupies a volume equal to that of the mixture at the temperature of the mixture.*

When stated with reference to pressure alone, this is the proposition known as *Dalton's law*. The extended law has been referred to as the *Gibbs-Dalton law*, and we shall adopt this usage.

As an immediate deduction from the Gibbs-Dalton law it may be shown that an equivalent statement can be made about the enthalpy of a mixture. Thus the Gibbs-Dalton law can be expressed symbolically by

$$p = \sum p_i]_{V,T} \quad \text{and} \quad U = \sum U_i]_{V,T} \tag{14.1}$$

Subscript i refers to a typical constituent i, and subscripts V and T outside the square brackets indicate that the property must be evaluated when the constituent alone occupies the volume V of the mixture at the temperature T of the mixture. By definition the enthalpy H is $(U + pV)$ and therefore, using (14.1), the enthalpy of a mixture becomes

$$H = \sum U_i]_{V,T} + V \sum p_i]_{V,T}$$

But

$$H_i]_{V,T} = (U_i + p_i V)]_{V,T} = U_i]_{V,T} + V p_i]_{V,T}$$

and therefore

$$H = \sum H_i]_{V,T} \tag{14.2}$$

The Gibbs-Dalton law has been determined from experiments on mixtures of gases. It has been found that the accuracy of the law improves as the pressure of the mixture is decreased, and consequently it may be inferred that it is strictly true for mixtures of perfect gases. This inference is confirmed by the fact that the law can be deduced from the postulates of the simple kinetic theory of gases. Briefly, if the size of the molecules is negligible compared with their distance apart and there are no attractive forces between them, each constituent will contribute its share of pressure and internal energy as if it were the only gas in the vessel; and this in fact is what the law implies.

In the following section we shall deduce the consequences of the Gibbs-Dalton law for a mixture of perfect gases, and show how the properties of such a mixture can be determined from the properties of the constituents. Arguments based on the kinetic theory can tell us what to expect. According to this theory the perfect gas relations (8.18) to (8.25) are theoretical deductions based only on the laws of mechanics and thermodynamics. Although the values of the constants R, c_v and c_p depend upon the particular gas, i.e. on the mass and structure of the molecules, the *form* of the relations is the same for all perfect gases. For any mixture of perfect gases, therefore, we may also expect to be able to write:

$$pv = RT \tag{14.3}$$

$$u - u_0 = c_v(T - T_0) \tag{14.4}$$

$$h - h_0 = c_p(T - T_0) \tag{14.5}$$

$$s - s_0 = c_p \ln \frac{T}{T_0} - R \ln \frac{p}{p_0} \tag{14.6}$$

In this case R, c_v and c_p are specific constants for the particular mixture. The problem of determining the behaviour of a mixture of perfect gases then reduces to one of obtaining expressions for R, c_v and c_p in terms of the gas constants and specific heat capacities of the constituents. Once the mixture constants have been determined, the analysis of both non-flow and flow processes can be carried out just as though the fluid were a single gas.

14.2   Mixtures of perfect gases

First we shall show formally that equations (14.3) to (14.6) follow from the application of the Gibbs-Dalton law to mixtures of perfect gases. If a mixture occupies a volume V at a temperature T, the pressure p_i of any constituent when it alone occupies the volume V at temperature T is given by

$$p_i V = n_i \tilde{R} T$$

p_i is known as the *partial pressure* of the constituent i, and n_i is the *amount-of-substance* of the constituent in the volume V (here measured in kmol). By writing an equation of the above form for each constituent and summing the equations, we have

$$V \sum p_i = \tilde{R} T \sum n_i$$

Remembering that the amount-of-substance is proportional to the number of molecules, and that the number of molecules remains unchanged during any process which does not involve a chemical reaction, the amount-of-substance of mixture n is given by

$$n = \sum n_i$$

Also, from Dalton's law we have

$$p = \sum p_i]_{V,T}$$

Consequently for the mixture we can write

$$pV = n\tilde{R} T$$

The molar mass $\tilde{m}$ of the mixture, from equation (8.12), is

$$\tilde{m} = \frac{m}{n} \tag{14.7}$$

where m is the mass of the mixture. We therefore have

$$pV = \frac{m}{\tilde{m}} \tilde{R} T = mRT$$

where $R = \tilde{R}/\tilde{m}$ is the specific gas constant for the mixture. Per unit mass of mixture this becomes equation (14.3), namely

$$pv = RT$$

Thus the equation of state of the mixture has the same form as that for any individual gas.

An expression for the specific gas constant of a mixture, in terms of the gas constants of the constituents, can now be found:

$$R = \frac{\tilde{R}}{\tilde{m}} = \frac{n}{m}\tilde{R}$$

Substituting $n = \Sigma n_i = \Sigma(m_i/\tilde{m}_i)$ and $\tilde{m}_i = (\tilde{R}/R_i)$, this becomes

$$R = \frac{\tilde{R}}{m}\sum m_i \frac{R_i}{\tilde{R}} = \sum \frac{m_i}{m} R_i \qquad (14.8)$$

m_i/m is the *mass fraction* of the constituent i having the gas constant R_i.

It has been stated in section 8.5.3, and proved in section 7.6.1, that the internal energy of any substance having the equation of state of a perfect gas must be a function only of temperature. Having shown that (14.3) holds for a mixture, it follows that the internal energy of the mixture must be a function only of the temperature of the mixture. We can therefore apply the equation

$$dU = mc_v\, dT$$

to the mixture as well as to each constituent. But from the Gibbs-Dalton law (14.1) we have

$$U = \sum U_i]_{V,T}$$

Since the internal energy depends only on temperature, the subscript V can be omitted when applying the law to perfect gases. In differential form the equation therefore becomes

$$mc_v\, dT = \sum m_i c_{vi}\, dT$$

and hence c_v for the mixture is given by

$$c_v = \sum \frac{m_i}{m} c_{vi} \qquad (14.9)$$

If the specific heat capacities of the constituents can be treated as constants, then c_v for the mixture is constant also and we arrive at (14.4),

$$u - u_0 = c_v(T - T_0)$$

Another consequence of the equation of state of a perfect gas is that

$$c_p - c_v = R$$

and this relation must also hold for the mixture. The specific heat capacity at constant pressure of a mixture of perfect gases is therefore given by

$$c_p = \sum \frac{m_i}{m} R_i + \sum \frac{m_i}{m} c_{vi} = \sum \frac{m_i}{m} c_{pi} \qquad (14.10)$$

The expected equation (14.5) then follows from the definition of enthalpy, and (14.6) from the laws of thermodynamics, just as in the case of a single gas, and there is no need to repeat the argument here.

From the foregoing paragraphs it is evident that for any process from some reference state 0 to some other state, the changes in u, h and s can be found by calculating R, c_v and c_p for the mixture using equations (14.8), (14.9) and (14.10), and then substituting these values in equations (14.4), (14.5) and (14.6). Another approach, which is particularly useful when dealing with mixtures of gases and vapours, follows more immediately from the Gibbs-Dalton law. Thus from equation (14.1) we can write

$$U - U_0 = \sum U_i]_T - \sum U_i]_{T_0}$$

or

$$m(u - u_0) = \sum m_i u_i]_T - \sum m_i u_i]_{T_0} = \sum m_i c_{vi}(T - T_0) \qquad (14.11)$$

Similarly, from equation (14.2) we get

$$m(h - h_0) = \sum m_i h_i]_T - \sum m_i h_i]_{T_0} = \sum m_i c_{pi}(T - T_0) \qquad (14.12)$$

These two equations express the fact that the changes in internal energy and enthalpy of a mixture can be calculated from the sum of the changes in internal energy and enthalpy of the constituents.

The equivalent equation for the change in entropy cannot be deduced in such a direct manner because there is no explicit reference to entropy in our statement of the Gibbs-Dalton law. We may proceed by substituting (14.8) and (14.10) in (14.6) to give

$$m(s - s_0) = \sum m_i c_{pi} \ln \frac{T}{T_0} - \sum m_i R_i \ln \frac{p}{p_0} \qquad (14.13)$$

Now for each constituent

$$p_i V = m_i R_i T$$

and for the mixture

$$pV = mRT$$

By division it is evident that p_i/p is constant during any process for which the composition (i.e. each mass fraction) remains constant. Hence

$$\frac{p_i}{p} = \frac{p_{i0}}{p_0} \quad \text{or} \quad \frac{p}{p_0} = \frac{p_i}{p_{i0}}$$

Substituting this result in (14.13), we get

$$m(s - s_0) = \sum m_i \left(c_{pi} \ln \frac{T}{T_0} - R_i \ln \frac{p_i}{p_{i0}} \right) \qquad (14.14)$$

Equation (14.14) is akin to (14.11) and (14.12), merely differing in form because, unlike u or h, s is a function of both temperature *and* pressure.

Remembering that p_i is the pressure of a constituent at the volume and temperature of the mixture, (14.14) can be written alternatively as

$$m(s - s_0) = \sum m_i s_i]_{V,T} - \sum m_i s_i]_{V_0, T_0}$$

If the entropy of each constituent is put equal to zero at the state (V_0, T_0), then we can say that

$$ms = \sum m_i s_i]_{V,T} \quad \text{or} \quad S = \sum S_i]_{V,T} \qquad (14.15)$$

Evidently the Gibbs-Dalton law implies that:

> The entropy of a mixture of perfect gases is the sum of the entropies of the constituents evaluated when each occupies alone the volume of the mixture at the temperature of the mixture.

Example 14.1 A mixture of gases has the following composition by mass:

$$N_2\ 60\%,\ O_2\ 30\%,\ CO_2\ 10\%.$$

A mass of 0.9 kg of mixture, initially at 1 bar and 27 °C, is compressed to 4 bar. The compression can be assumed to be a reversible non-flow polytropic process with a polytropic index of 1.2. Find the work and heat transfers and change of entropy. The values of c_p for the constituents are

$$N_2\ 1.040,\ O_2\ 0.918,\ CO_2\ 0.846\ kJ/kg\ K.$$

The constants for the mixture are

$$R = \sum \frac{m_i}{m} R_i = 0.60 \frac{8.314}{28} + 0.30 \frac{8.314}{32} + 0.10 \frac{8.314}{44} = 0.275 \ \text{kJ/kg K}$$

$$c_p = \sum \frac{m_i}{m} c_{pi} = (0.60 \times 1.04) + (0.30 \times 0.918) + (0.10 \times 0.846)$$

$$= 0.984 \ \text{kJ/kg K}$$

$$c_v = c_p - R = 0.984 - 0.275 = 0.709 \ \text{kJ/kg K}$$

The final temperature is given by

$$T_2 = T_1 \left(\frac{p_2}{p_1} \right)^{(n-1)/n} = 300 \left(\frac{4}{1} \right)^{0.2/1.2} = 378 \ \text{K}$$

The work done is

$$W = \frac{mR(T_2 - T_1)}{n - 1} = \frac{0.9 \times 0.275(378 - 300)}{0.2} = 96.5 \ \text{kJ}$$

The heat transferred is

$$Q = mc_v(T_2 - T_1) - W = 0.9 \times 0.709(378 - 300) - 96.5 = -46.7 \ \text{kJ}$$

The change of entropy is

$$S_2 - S_1 = m \left(c_p \ln \frac{T_2}{T_1} - R \ln \frac{p_2}{p_1} \right)$$

$$= 0.9 \left(0.984 \ln \frac{378}{300} - 0.275 \ln \frac{4}{1} \right) = -0.138 \ \text{kJ/K}$$

It is worth noting another empirical law, variously known as the *law of partial volumes, Amagat's law* or *Leduc's law*, which states that:

> The volume of a mixture of gases is equal to the sum of the volumes of the individual constituents when each exists alone at the pressure and temperature of the mixture.

For perfect gases this law will now be shown to be a consequence of Dalton's law, although for real gases both laws are only approximately true and one cannot be deduced from the other. If a constituent i is placed in an empty vessel having the volume of the mixture V, at the mixture temperature T, it will exert the partial pressure p_i. Keeping the temperature constant and increasing the pressure to the pressure of the mixture p, the volume of this constituent reduces to

$$V_i = \frac{p_i}{p} V$$

V_i is the *partial volume* of the constituent by definition. If all such equations, for each constituent, are added, we have

$$\sum V_i = \frac{V}{p} \sum p_i$$

But $\sum p_i = p$, from Dalton's law, and hence

$$V = \sum V_i]_{p,T} \tag{14.16}$$

Sometimes problems concerning mixtures are simplified if the analysis is carried through in terms of *mole fractions* rather than mass fractions. The following relations are then useful. However, before embarking on the remainder of this section, the reader is well advised to reread section 8.5.2 and remember the conclusion that the molar mass $\tilde{m}$, when measured in kg/kmol (or g/mol), is numerically equal to A_r or M_r.

For each constituent we can write

$$p_i V = n_i \tilde{R} T$$

and for the mixture

$$pV = n\tilde{R}T$$

By division, and writing $n_i/n = x_i$ for the mole fraction of the constituent i, we have

$$p_i = x_i p \tag{14.17}$$

We also have

$$pV_i = n_i \tilde{R} T$$

and by a similar argument

$$V_i = x_i V \tag{14.18}$$

The molar mass of the mixture is given by $\tilde{m} = m/n$, and hence

$$\tilde{m}n = \sum m_i = \sum \tilde{m}_i n_i$$

or

$$\tilde{m} = \sum x_i \tilde{m}_i \tag{14.19}$$

If required, the gas constant for the mixture can then be found from $R = \tilde{R}/\tilde{m}$.

The concept of *molar heat capacity*, i.e. specific heat capacity per unit amount-of-substance, is also useful and widely used. A molar heat capacity will be denoted by $\tilde{c}$ to distinguish it from the specific heat capacity c, and the unit used here will be kJ/kmol K. Since by definition $\tilde{c} = \tilde{m}c$, an expression for $\tilde{c}_v$ equivalent to (14.9) can be found by combining this equation (14.7). Thus

$$\tilde{c}_v = \tilde{m}\sum\frac{m_i}{m}c_{vi} = \sum\tilde{m}\frac{m_i}{m}\frac{\tilde{c}_{vi}}{\tilde{m}_i}$$

$$= \sum\frac{n_i}{n}\tilde{c}_{vi} \quad\text{or}\quad \sum x_i\tilde{c}_{vi} \tag{14.20}$$

Similarly it can be shown that

$$\tilde{c}_p = \sum x_i\tilde{c}_{pi} \tag{14.21}$$

Further, from the definition of $\tilde{c}$,

$$\tilde{c}_p - \tilde{c}_v = \tilde{m}(c_p - c_v) = \tilde{m}R = \tilde{R} \tag{14.22}$$

When an analysis of a gas mixture is carried out experimentally, e.g. by using an Orsat apparatus (section 15.3), the analysis by volume is usually obtained. The volume V of a sample of gas is first measured at some fixed pressure and temperature, usually atmospheric. Then each constituent is absorbed in turn by a suitable chemical reagent and the reduction in volume is voted. The volumes are always measured at the same pressure and temperature, so that any reduction in volume will be equal to the partial volume V_i of the constituent in the original sample. The result is expressed as a volumetric analysis, i.e. a set of values of V_i/V, and it follows from equation (14.18) that this is also an analysis by mole fractions. The mass fractions, and hence the gravimetric analysis, can be deduced from the volumetric analysis if the molar masses of the constituents are known. Thus

$$\frac{m_i}{m} = \frac{n_i\tilde{m}_i}{\sum n_i\tilde{m}_i} = \frac{(n_i\tilde{m}_i/n)}{\sum(n_i\tilde{m}_i/n)} = \frac{x_i\tilde{m}_i}{\sum x_i\tilde{m}_i}$$

And finally, substituting V_i/V for x_i from equation (14.18) we have

$$\frac{m_i}{m} = \frac{(V_i/V)\tilde{m}_i}{\sum(V_i/V)\tilde{m}_i} \tag{14.23}$$

Example 14.2 A mixture of gases at a temperature of 150 °C has a pressure of 4 bar. A sample is analysed and the volumetric analysis is found to be

CO_2 14%, O_2 5%, N_2 81%.

Determine the gravimetric analysis and partial pressures of the gases in the mixture.

If 2.3 kg of mixture are cooled at constant pressure to 15 °C, find the final volume.

Using equation (14.23), the procedure for finding the gravimetric analysis can be set out as follows:

i	V_i/V	$\dfrac{\tilde{m}_i}{[kg/kmol]}$	$\dfrac{(V_i/V)\tilde{m}_i}{[kg/kmol]}$	m_i/m
CO_2	0.14	44	6.16	0.202
O_2	0.05	32	1.60	0.053
N_2	0.81	28	22.68	0.745
	1.00		30.44	1.000

The gravimetric analysis appears in the last column. Note that according to (14.18) the second column also gives the mole fractions, and according to (14.19) the final result 30.44 in the fourth column is the molar mass of the mixture. From (14.17) the partial pressures are

CO_2 $p_i = 0.14 \times 4 = 0.56$ bar

O_2 $p_i = 0.05 \times 4 = 0.20$ bar

N_2 $p_i = 0.81 \times 4 = 3.24$ bar

The amount-of-substance in 2.3 kg is

$$n = \frac{2.3}{30.44} = 0.0756 \text{ kmol}$$

and the final volume of the mixture is

$$V = \frac{n\tilde{R}T}{p} = \frac{0.0756 \times 8.3145 \times 288}{100 \times 4} = 0.453 \text{ m}^3$$

14.3 The mixing process

So far we have considered methods of dealing with gases which are already mixed; in this section we shall consider the mixing process itself. The simplest case is the adiabatic mixing of perfect gases which are initially at the same pressure and temperature.

Imagine an insulated vessel in which two gases are separated by a partition, as in Fig. 14.1. The pressure and temperature of each gas is p and T, and the masses are m_a and m_b. On removing the partition, the gases diffuse into one another and each gas expands to fill the total volume. No work is done, and we are considering an adiabatic mixing process, so that the internal energy must remain unchanged. It follows that the temperature of the mixture will be the same as the original temperature of the constituents. The volumes initially occupied by the gases are, by definition, the partial volumes associated with a mixture of them at pressure p and temperature T. Conversely, from the law of

Fig. 14.1
The mixing of two gases

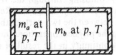
m_a at p, T | m_b at p, T

partial volumes and the fact that the temperature T is unchanged, the pressure of the mixture must be the same as the initial pressure of the constituents. Both the pressure and the temperature of the mixture are therefore the same as the original pressure and temperature of the constituents, although the pressure which each gas exerts is now reduced to the corresponding partial value p_a or p_b. Each gas behaves as though the other were not present, and can be considered to have undergone a free expansion. Evidently this diffusion process is irreversible, and it follows from the principle of increasing entropy that the entropy of this isolated system must have increased. The initial entropies of the separate gases, each reckoned from the same datum state (p_0, T_0), are given by equation (8.24) as

$$S_a = m_a c_{pa} \ln \frac{T}{T_0} - m_a R_a \ln \frac{p}{p_0}$$

$$S_b = m_b c_{pb} \ln \frac{T}{T_0} - m_b R_b \ln \frac{p}{p_0}$$

As expressed by equation (14.15), the entropy of the mixture is equal to the sum of the entropies of the constituents, evaluated at the volume and temperature of the mixture. These entropies, from equation (14.14), are

$$S'_a = m_a c_{pa} \ln \frac{T}{T_0} - m_a R_a \ln \frac{p_a}{p_0}$$

$$S'_b = m_b c_{pb} \ln \frac{T}{T_0} - m_b R_b \ln \frac{p_b}{p_0}$$

The total change of entropy for the whole system is therefore

$$(S'_a + S'_b) - (S_a + S_b) = -m_a R_a \ln \frac{p_a}{p} - m_b R_b \ln \frac{p_b}{p}$$

Since p_a and p_b are each less than p, this is a positive quantity indicating an increase of entropy.*

If the temperatures of the gases are initially different, there will be an additional increase of entropy due to the irreversible redistribution of internal energy which occurs within the system. The following example illustrates this more general case, and also the use of molar heat capacities.

---

* It is interesting to note that if the two gases become more and more alike, the change of entropy on mixing does not reduce to zero in the limiting case of two identical gases. Yet there is no change of entropy when a mass $(m_a + m_b)$ of gas exists in a closed vessel at fixed p and T, although the molecules are continuously 'diffusing' through the volume. This contradiction is known as the *Gibbs paradox*. It has been resolved by Bridgman (Ref. 2 in Part I) in terms of our inability even in principle to distinguish between the two parts of the gas when the molecules are identical; and if there is a discontinuity in the physical operations implicit in the description of the problem, it is reasonable to expect a discontinuity in the result of the analysis.

Example 14.3   Two containers, each 1.4 m^3 in volume, are isolated from one another by a valve. One contains oxygen at 7 bar and 150°C, and the other carbon dioxide at 2 bar and 15°C. The valve is opened and the gases are allowed to mix. Assuming the process is adiabatic, determine the equilibrium temperature and pressure of the mixture, and the change of entropy associated with the system as a whole. The values of $\tilde{c}_v$ for the constituents are O$_2$ 21.0, CO$_2$ 28.3 kJ/kmol K.

For convenience let the oxygen be denoted by subscript a and the carbon dioxide by subscript b. Since $n = pV/\tilde{R}T$, the amount-of-substance of each gas is

$$n_a = \frac{100 \times 7 \times 1.4}{8.3145 \times 423} = 0.279 \text{ kmol},$$

$$n_b = \frac{100 \times 2 \times 1.4}{8.3145 \times 288} = 0.117 \text{ kmol}$$

The total amount-of-substance in the mixture is

$$n = n_a + n_b = 0.396 \text{ kmol}$$

Since W and Q are zero, the total internal energy of the system must remain constant. Initially the internal energy, reckoned from zero at T_0, is

$$n_a \tilde{c}_{va}(T_a - T_0) + n_b \tilde{c}_{vb}(T_b - T_0)$$

and finally it is $n\tilde{c}_v(T - T_0)$, where T is the equilibrium temperature and $\tilde{c}_v$ refers to the mixture. But according to equation (14.20),

$$n\tilde{c}_v = n_a \tilde{c}_{va} + n_b \tilde{c}_{vb}$$

Hence, on equating the initial and final internal energy, we get

$$(n_a \tilde{c}_{va} + n_b \tilde{c}_{vb})(T - T_0) = n_a \tilde{c}_{va}(T_a - T_0) + n_b \tilde{c}_{vb}(T_b - T_0)$$

or

$$n_a \tilde{c}_{va}(T - T_a) + n_b \tilde{c}_{vb}(T - T_b) = 0$$

$$\{0.279 \times 21.0(T/[K] - 423)\} + \{0.117 \times 28.3(T/[K] - 288)\} = 0$$

$$T = 374 \text{ K}$$

The equilibrium pressure of the mixture is

$$p = \frac{n\tilde{R}T}{V} = \frac{0.396 \times 8.3145 \times 374}{100 \times 2.8} = 4.40 \text{ bar}$$

The change in entropy can be found by summing the changes associated with each constituent. Thus the change in entropy of oxygen, in terms of T and V, is

$$\Delta S_a = n_a \left(\tilde{c}_{va} \ln \frac{T}{T_a} + \tilde{R} \ln \frac{V}{V_a} \right)$$

$$= 0.279 \left(21.0 \ln \frac{374}{423} + 8.3145 \ln \frac{2.8}{1.4} \right) = 0.886 \text{ kJ/K}$$

And similarly for carbon dioxide,

$$\Delta S_b = 0.117 \left(28.3 \ln \frac{374}{288} + 8.3145 \ln \frac{2.8}{1.4} \right) = 1.540 \text{ kJ/K}$$

The total change in entropy is an increase of

$$\Delta S = \Delta S_a + \Delta S_b = 2.426 \text{ kJ/K}$$

It should not be supposed from the foregoing that it is impossible *in principle* for gases to be mixed in a reversible manner. To see how this can be done it is necessary first to introduce the concept of a *semipermeable membrane*, i.e. a membrane which is permeable to one gas only and impermeable to the other gases in the mixture. This is an idealised piece of apparatus, like the frictionless pulley or the non-conducting wall. A membrane of palladium foil which, at red heat, is permeable to hydrogen but practically impermeable to all other common gases, is an example which closely approximates to the ideal. The gas to which the membrane is permeable will continue to pass through it until the partial pressure of that gas is the same on each side; *membrane equilibrium* is then said to exist.

Consider the imaginary device of Fig. 14.2, suggested by Planck. A cylinder is divided into two compartments of equal volume by a membrane permeable to gas *a*, but impermeable to a second gas *b*. Two pistons are coupled together, of which one is impermeable to both gases and the other is permeable only to gas *b*. The initial configuration is as shown in Fig. 14.2a, with the pistons to the right and the gases in separate compartments at the same temperature. As the pistons are moved to the left the gases diffuse through the semipermeable membranes until eventually the two gases are mixed in the left-hand compartment, leaving a vacuum in the other. It remains to show that this mixing process is reversible.

We shall suppose first that the motion of the pistons is infinitely slow, so that membrane equilibrium exists throughout the process, and secondly that the whole system is maintained at constant temperature. Under these conditions the volumes and temperatures of the separate gases, which are initially equal, are also the same as the volume and temperature of the final mixture. Therefore if p_a and p_b are the initial pressures of the gases, they will also be the partial pressures of the gases when mixed. At any intermediate point in the process, if the piston area is A, the net force acting on the left-hand piston is

$$A\{(p_a + p_b) - p_b\} = Ap_a$$

Fig. 14.2
A reversible mixing process

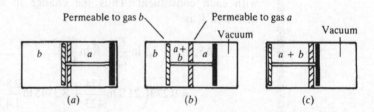

Permeable to gas *b*   Permeable to gas *a*

Vacuum   Vacuum

b   *a*   *b* | a+b | *a*   a + b

(a)   (b)   (c)

tending to move it to the left. And the net force on the other piston is

$$A(p_a - 0) = Ap_a$$

tending to move it to the right. It follows that the piston combination is always acted upon by balanced forces. Since only an infinitesimal force is required to set the pistons in motion in either direction, the process is reversible. No work is done, there is no change in temperature and therefore in internal energy, and so according to the First Law no heat crosses the boundary. Thus the surroundings are not affected by the process. We shall have occasion to refer again to the concept of the semipermeable membrane and the reversible mixing process in section 15.7.1.

14.4   Gas and saturated vapour mixtures

When a liquid is introduced into an evacuated vessel of greater volume than the liquid, some of it will evaporate. The more rapidly moving molecules of liquid escape from the surface to the space above, and at first few of these return to the liquid. As more and more molecules fill the vacant space and the vapour pressure increases, so a greater proportion find their way back into the liquid. If the vessel is maintained at a constant temperature, eventually equilibrium will be established between the rates of evaporation and condensation, and the pressure will remain constant. The space above the liquid then contains the maximum possible amount of vapour at the given temperature. The vessel is filled with saturated liquid and saturated vapour, and the pressure is the saturation vapour pressure corresponding to the given temperature. At any instant, only the behaviour of the molecules in the immediate vicinity of the surface governs the rates of evaporation and condensation. Therefore the saturation pressure is independent of the relative masses of liquid and vapour present and depends solely on the temperature. An increase of temperature permits more molecules to overcome the attractive forces of the liquid molecules, and a new equilibrium is established at a higher pressure. If the temperature is increased sufficiently, all the liquid evaporates and the vapour becomes superheated.

We have already seen that, provided the pressure is not too high, each gas in a gaseous mixture can be considered to behave as though the others were not present. This is also approximately true if one of the constituents is a vapour. Thus in the case we have been considering, if the vessel is filled with a gas prior to the introduction of the liquid, the gas will have a negligible effect on the final state of equilibrium between the liquid and its vapour. The presence of the gas molecules will retard the establishment of equilibrium, but eventually the vapour will exert the saturation vapour pressure corresponding to the temperature of the mixture. This saturation pressure is the partial pressure of the vapour in the mixture, and the total pressure in the vessel is the sum of the partial pressures of the vapour and the gas. Under these conditions the gas (or mixture of gases) is said to be 'saturated with vapour', although strictly speaking it is the vapour which is saturated. Note that the liquid is subjected to the vapour *and* gas pressure and so is strictly speaking a compressed liquid. However, as pointed out in section 8.3.3, the properties of a compressed liquid are nearly the same as those of saturated liquid at the same temperature. For practical purposes, therefore, both the liquid and the vapour may be regarded as saturated.

Example 14.4   A closed vessel contains 0.1 kg of wet steam having a dryness fraction of 0.1, and 0.15 kg of nitrogen. The temperature of the mixture is 95 °C. Find the volume of the vessel and the pressure of the mixture. Also find the temperature to which the mixture must be raised for all the water to be evaporated, and the corresponding pressure of the mixture.

There are 0.01 kg of saturated steam and 0.09 kg of saturated water in the vessel. It is immaterial whether the liquid is a single mass or is distributed through the vapour as droplets. Hitherto we have treated such a mixture as wet steam, but it is more convenient here to consider the two phases separately. When considering mixtures in general, we use subscripts to denote the substances involved. In this chapter we shall use s for steam (the vapour phase in the mixture, saturated in this example because liquid is present) and w for water (the liquid phase, saturated because vapour is present). From the saturation table at 95 °C, $p_s = 0.8453$ bar and $v_s = 1.982$ m^3/kg, and p_s is the partial pressure of the steam in the mixture. The volume of the vessel must be equal to the volume of the water plus the volume of the mixture of steam and nitrogen. But the volume of the mixture of steam and nitrogen can be found from the volume of the steam alone at the partial pressure of the steam and the temperature of the mixture. Therefore the volume of the vessel is

$$V = m_w v_w + m_s v_s = (0.09 \times 0.001) + (0.01 \times 1.982)$$

$$= 0.000\,09 + 0.019\,82 = 0.0199 \text{ m}^3$$

The volume of the steam itself, i.e. 0.019 82 m^3, is equal to the volume of the nitrogen at the partial pressure of the nitrogen p_N and the temperature of the mixture. Therefore

$$p_N = \frac{m_N R_N T}{V_s} = \frac{0.15(8.3145/28)368}{100 \times 0.019\,82} = 8.28 \text{ bar}$$

The pressure of the mixture is

$$p = p_s + p_N = 9.125 \text{ bar}$$

When the water is completely evaporated,

$$v_s = \frac{V}{m_s} = \frac{0.0199}{0.1} = 0.199 \text{ m}^3/\text{kg}$$

From the saturation table, the corresponding vapour pressure is, by interpolation,

$$p_s = 10 - \frac{0.199 - 0.1944}{0.2149 - 0.1944} 1 = 9.78 \text{ bar}$$

and similarly the temperature required is found to be 179 °C or 452 K. The volume occupied by the nitrogen is now 0.0199 m^3, and therefore the corresponding partial pressure is

$$p_N = \frac{m_N R_N T}{V} = \frac{0.15(8.3145/28)452}{100 \times 0.0199} = 10.11 \text{ bar}$$

The final pressure of the mixture is

$$p = p_s + p_N = 9.78 + 10.11 = 19.9 \text{ bar}$$

We have seen that for perfect gases the internal energy, enthalpy and entropy of a mixture are respectively equal to the sums of the internal energies, enthalpies and entropies of the constituents, evaluated when each exists alone at the volume and temperature of the mixture. This result holds well for real gases, and with somewhat less accuracy for mixture of gases and saturated vapours. When a liquid phase is present the internal energy, for example, of a mixture of liquid, vapour and gas can be found by considering the system in two parts: (a) the saturated vapour and gas mixture, and (b) the saturated liquid. The internal energy of the vapour–gas mixture can be determined by applying the Gibbs-Dalton law, and the internal energy of the liquid can be found from tables in the usual way. The total internal energy of the system is equal to the sum of the internal energies of the two parts. Such an approach can always be adopted when dealing with extensive properties.

Example 14.5 Find the heat that must be added during the process of evaporating the water in Example 14.4. Assume that for nitrogen $c_v = 0.747 \text{ kJ/kg K}$.

Applying the non-flow energy equation to this constant volume process, we have

$$Q = U_2 - U_1$$

The initial internal energy of the mixture is

$$U_1 = m_{w1} u_{w1} + m_{s1} u_{s1} + m_N u_{N1}$$

where u_{w1} and u_{s1} are found from the saturation tables of u_f and u_g at T_1. Similarly the final internal energy is

$$U_2 = m_{s2} u_{s2} + m_N u_{N2}$$

where $m_{s2} = m_{w1} + m_{s1}$ and u_{s2} is u_g at T_2. It follows that

$$Q = (m_{s2} u_{s2} - m_{w1} u_{w1} - m_{s1} u_{s1}) + m_N c_{vN}(T_2 - T_1)$$

Now the initial and final temperatures are $T_1 = 95\,°\text{C}$ and $T_2 = 179\,°\text{C}$; and the masses are $m_{s1} = 0.01 \text{ kg}$, $m_{w1} = 0.09 \text{ kg}$, $m_N = 0.15 \text{ kg}$. Using the saturation table, we find that the heat transferred is

$$Q = \{(0.1 \times 2583) - (0.09 \times 399) - (0.01 \times 2500)\}$$
$$+ \{0.15 \times 0.747(179 - 95)\} = 207 \text{ kJ}$$

The higher the pressure, the less accurate does the foregoing treatment become, but in a great many applications of practical interest to engineers the pressure is atmospheric or less and the results are sufficiently accurate. The steam condenser provides an important example of such a case and is worth considering in some detail. We shall consider the most common type—the *shell-and-tube condenser*—where steam flows over a bank of tubes through which cold water is pumped continuously. We have seen in section 11.2 that the temperature of the condensing steam may be as low as 25 °C. At this temperature the corresponding saturation pressure is 0.032 bar, i.e. a vacuum of 736 mm of mercury. With a pressure of this order in the low-pressure side of the plant, it is impossible to prevent some air from leaking into the system through glands, or air dissolved in the boiler feed water from coming out of solution. The condenser is therefore always filled with a mixture of water, steam and air.

We may now consider the effect of the air on the design and performance of the condenser. First, it might be thought that because the back pressure on the turbine is increased (it is equal to the saturation pressure of the steam plus the partial pressure of the air), the work output of the turbine will be reduced. As the subsequent numerical example will show, this effect is negligible for normal rates of air leakage. Secondly, for the reasons given at the end of section 22.8.1, the air reduces the rate of heat transfer per unit area per unit temperature difference between steam and cooling water. Thus either the surface area of tubing or the temperature difference must be increased for a given condenser duty. The most obvious consequence of air leakage is the need for a pump of sufficient capacity to extract the air continuously and so maintain the vacuum in the condenser. Since the air cannot be separated from the steam with which it is mixed, this entails a loss of potential condensate. Furthermore, the presence of air results in undercooling, i.e. the condensate is cooled below the saturation temperature of the incoming steam. As the condensate is usually returned to the boiler, a reduction of condensate temperature necessitates an increased supply of heat in the boiler.

To see how undercooling can arise, suppose that steam enters the condenser in a dry saturated condition and that with every kilogram of steam there is a mass m_a of air; m_a is of course a small fraction. Consider the behaviour of a mass of steam–air mixture occupying a volume equal to the volume of 1 kg of steam. The pressure at entry is equal to the sum of the partial pressure of the air and the saturation pressure of the steam entering the condenser. Since the velocity of steam flow is small, the pressure may be assumed constant throughout the condenser. As the mass of mixture we are considering flows through the condenser, some of the steam condenses and the volume that each kilogram occupies is reduced. Since the volume of the remaining vapour is also the volume occupied by the mass of air m_a, the partial pressure of the air increases. But the total pressure is constant, and an increase in the partial pressure of the air must be accompanied by a decrease in the saturation pressure, and hence temperature, of the steam. The temperature of the condensate therefore falls progressively below that of the incoming steam as condensation proceeds. The following example should help to make this clear.

Example 14.6   A condenser is to deal with steam of dryness fraction 0.95 and temperature 38 °C, at the rate of 5000 kg/h. If the estimated air leakage is 5 kg/h, determine the amount of vapour carried away with the air for condensate temperatures of 37, 35, 32 and 28 °C. Find also the capacity of the air extraction pump in each case.

The pressure in the condenser is first found from the inlet conditions. At 38 °C, from the saturation table,

$$p_s = 0.066\,24\ \text{bar} \quad \text{and} \quad v_s = 21.63\ \text{m}^3/\text{kg}$$

There are 5 kg of air to $0.95 \times 5000 = 4750$ kg of vapour, and therefore the mass of air m_a in a mass of mixture having a volume of $21.63\ \text{m}^3$ is $5/4750 = 1/950$ kg. Hence the partial air pressure is given by

$$p_a = \frac{m_a R_a T}{v_s} = \frac{(1/950)0.287 \times 311}{100 \times 21.63} = 0.000\,04\ \text{bar}$$

The partial pressure of the air at entry is therefore negligible, and the total condenser pressure p is 0.0662 bar. At 37 °C, by interpolation from the saturation table,

$$p_s = 0.0628\ \text{bar} \quad \text{and} \quad v_s = 22.8\ \text{m}^3/\text{kg}$$

$$p_a = p - p_s = 0.0662 - 0.0628 = 0.0034\ \text{bar}$$

The mass of air per kg of vapour is

$$m_a = \frac{p_a v_s}{R_a T} = \frac{100 \times 0.0034 \times 22.8}{0.287 \times 310} = 0.087\,13\ \text{kg}$$

Consequently the mass of vapour per kg of air is $1/m_a = 11.48$ kg. Since 5 kg of air must be extracted per hour, this result implies that 57.4 kg of steam are extracted per hour with the air. Each kg of steam occupies $22.8\ \text{m}^3$, so that the capacity required of the air pump is

$$57.4 \times 22.8 = 1310\ \text{m}^3/\text{h}$$

Similar calculations made for other condensate temperatures yield the following results:

Condensate temperature/[°C]	37	35	32	28
m_s/m_a	11.5	3.52	1.59	0.828
Air pump capacity/[m³/h]	1310	447	235	152

In the foregoing example, the water flow lost from the feed circuit varies from 57.4 to 4.14 kg/h as the condensate temperature is reduced from 37 °C to 28 °C. Neglecting the effect of the change in quantity of condensate, the additional heat which must be applied in the boiler as a result of the reduced temperature of the feed water is $5000 \times 4.19(37 - 28) = 189\,000$ kJ/h (taking the specific heat of water as 4.19 kJ/kg K). Evidently a compromise must be reached between the conflicting requirements of low feed water loss and high condensate temperature. When plotted as in Fig. 14.3, the results show that in our example

Fig. 14.3
Effect of undercooling

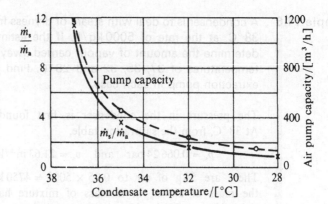

there is little to be gained in this respect by designing for a lower condensate temperature than about 32 °C. The size of air pump required is also relatively unaffected by a further reduction of temperature.

It is possible, by special design, to reduce the feed water loss and air pump capacity without excessive undercooling. For example, before leaving the condenser the air–steam mixture can be drawn over a section of tubes, the *air cooler*, which is shielded from the main flow of steam and condensate. Most of the condensing process occurs with very little undercooling and the remainder is carried out in the air cooler at a lower temperature. The effect of the small amount of low-temperature feed water upon the temperature of the hot well is negligible, little vapour is lost, and a smaller air pump can be used. Further improvement in performance is obtained with the 'regenerative' condenser. Fig. 14.4 illustrates a central-flow condenser of this type wherein some of the steam is allowed to pass unimpeded to the bottom, and in passing upwards meets the cooler condensate falling through the nest of tubes. The condensate is thereby reheated to a temperature approaching that of steam at inlet. The air, saturated with steam, is withdrawn from the centre of one end of the condenser, after passing over the air-cooling section of tubes.

The shell-and-tube condenser is evidently an example of the multistream open system introduced in section 10.6. To determine the mass flow of cooling water

Fig. 14.4
Cross-section of a
central-flow condenser

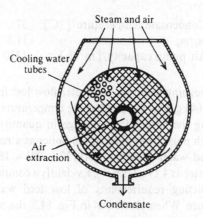

required, the steady-flow energy equation may be applied as in the following example.

Example 14.7   A condensate temperature of 37 °C is to be adopted for the condenser considered in the previous example. Separate condensate and air pumps are to be employed and an air-cooling section of tubes is to reduce the temperature of the air pump suction to 32 °C. Calculate the mass flow of cooling water required if the temperature rise of the cooling water is to be restricted to 11 K, from an initial temperature of 15 °C.

Fig. 14.5 illustrates the system. From the previous example we have

$$\dot{m}_{a1} = m_{a3} = 5 \text{ kg/h}, \qquad \dot{m}_{s1} = 4750 \text{ kg/h}, \qquad \dot{m}_{w1} = 250 \text{ kg/h}$$

The amount of steam extracted with the air is 1.59 kg per kg of air at 32 °C. Therefore $\dot{m}_{s3} = 7.95$ kg/h. Also

$$\dot{m}_{w2} = (\dot{m}_{s1} + \dot{m}_{w1}) - \dot{m}_{s3} = 4992 \text{ kg/h}$$

The energy equation, neglecting kinetic energy terms, becomes

$$\dot{Q} = (\dot{m}_{a3} h_{a3} + \dot{m}_{s3} h_{s3} + \dot{m}_{w2} h_{w2}) - (\dot{m}_{a1} h_{a1} + \dot{m}_{s1} h_{s1} + \dot{m}_{w1} h_{w1})$$

$$= \dot{m}_a c_{pa}(T_3 - T_1) + (\dot{m}_{s3} h_{s3} - \dot{m}_{s1} h_{s1}) + (\dot{m}_{w2} h_{w2} - \dot{m}_{w1} h_{w1})$$

Using the saturation table, and taking $c_{pa} = 1.005$ kJ/kg K,

$$\dot{Q} = 5 \times 1.005(32 - 38) + \{(7.95 \times 2559.3) - (4750 \times 2570.1)\}$$

$$+ \{(4992 \times 154.9) - (250 \times 159.1)\} = -11.46 \times 10^6 \text{ kJ/h}$$

Therefore, for a temperature rise from 15 °C to 26 °C, the cooling water flow is

$$\dot{m}_{cw} = \frac{\dot{Q}}{h_{f26} - h_{f15}} = \frac{11.46 \times 10^6}{108.9 - 62.9} = 0.249 \times 10^6 \text{ kg/h}$$

Fig. 14.5

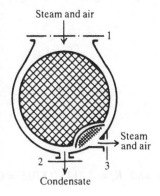

Steam and air

Steam and air

Condensate

What may be called the 'thermodynamic analysis' of a condenser has now been completed. Such an analysis cannot yield any information about the actual size, i.e. surface area of tubing, required for a given duty. Before this can be estimated, a study of the actual mechanism of heat transfer processes is necessary. Part IV is devoted to this topic.

14.5 Hygrometry (or psychrometry)

The previous section described a method of dealing with a mixture of saturated vapour and gas. If the vapour is superheated, however, the procedure can be simplified. When the pressure is sufficiently low for the Gibbs-Dalton law to be valid, a superheated vapour can be treated as a perfect gas. A mixture of superheated vapour and gas can then be regarded as a mixture of perfect gases and the method of section 14.2 is applicable. Humid atmospheric air is an example of a mixture which can be treated in this way.

Normally the atmosphere is not saturated with water vapour but is a mixture of air and superheated vapour. Many industrial processes, in the paper and textile industries for example, require close control of the vapour content of the atmosphere as well as its temperature. So too, in many regions of the world, do the comfort of human beings and the operation of their computers. Knowledge of the properties of humid air is essential for the science of meteorology and for the design of such plant as air-conditioning systems and cooling towers. So important is the subject that it has been given a special name—*hygrometry* (or *psychrometry*). Hygrometry makes use of certain technical terms which arise either from the need to specify the composition of the mixture or from the method of measuring the composition. These technical terms must now be introduced.

Specific humidity (or *moisture content*) ω is the ratio of the mass of water vapour m_s to the mass of *dry* air m_a in any given volume V of mixture. Thus

$$\omega = \frac{m_s}{m_a} = \frac{m_s/V}{m_a/V} = \frac{v_a}{v_s} \tag{14.24}$$

where v_a and v_s are the specific volumes of the dry air and vapour in the mixture. Treating the water vapour as a perfect gas, and writing p_s for the partial pressure of the vapour, we have

$$p_s V = m_s R_s T$$

Similarly for the dry air,

$$p_a V = m_a R_a T$$

It follows that

$$\omega = \frac{R_a p_s}{R_s p_a}$$

Now $R_a = 0.2871 \text{ kJ/kg K}$ and $R_s = 8.3145/18.015 = 0.4615 \text{ kJ/kg K}$. Also

$p_a = p - p_s$, where p is the barometric pressure. Therefore

$$\omega = 0.622 \frac{p_s}{p_a} = 0.622 \frac{p_s}{p - p_s} \tag{14.25}$$

Relative humidity ϕ is the ratio of the actual partial pressure p_s of the vapour to the partial pressure p_g of the vapour when the air is saturated at the same temperature.* Thus

$$\phi = \frac{p_s}{p_g} \tag{14.26}$$

and it is often expressed as a percentage. The case with which the atmosphere takes up moisture from any surface depends on how far the air is short of being saturated rather than the specific humidity when industrial drying processes or air-conditioning problems are being considered. Alternative expressions for ϕ can be found if the vapour is treated as a perfect gas. Thus, multiplying the numerator and denominator of equation (14.26) by $V/R_s T$, we have

$$\phi = \frac{p_s V/R_s T}{p_g V/R_s T} = \frac{m_s}{(m_s)_{sat}} \tag{14.27a}$$

And, dividing m_s and $(m_s)_{sat}$ by V, we have

$$\phi = \frac{m_s/V}{(m_s)_{sat}/V} = \frac{v_g}{v_s} \tag{14.27b}$$

where v_s is the actual specific volume of the vapour in the mixture, and v_g is the specific volume of the vapour when the air is saturated at the same temperature.

In air-conditioning the concept of *degree of saturation* μ is often used as an alternative to relative humidity ϕ. It is defined as

$$\mu = \frac{m_s}{(m_s)_{sat}}$$

It is evident from the derivation of equation (14.27a) that ϕ and μ are equal if both air and vapour behave like perfect gases. The difference between ϕ and μ can be up to 2 per cent in some ranges of pressure and temperature encountered in air-conditioning practice. Such departure is principally due to the vapour constituent not obeying perfect gas laws near its saturation line.

Dew point is the temperature to which unsaturated air must be cooled at constant pressure for it to become saturated (or for condensation to begin). For the vapour in the mixture at temperature T we have

$$p_s = \frac{m_s R_s T}{V}$$

---

* Since in this chapter subscript s is used to denote the constituent 'steam', we shall use subscript g to refer to the saturated state.

Fig. 14.6
Dew point temperature

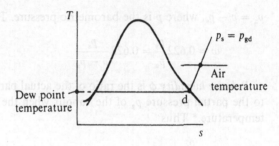

and for the mixture

$$p = \frac{mRT}{V}$$

Therefore

$$\frac{p_s}{p} = \frac{m_s R_s}{mR}$$

Since the ratio m_s/m remains unchanged as the unsaturated mixture is cooled at constant pressure, p_s must remain constant. The cooling process undergone by the vapour constituent is illustrated in Fig. 14.6. The partial pressure of the vapour at the dew point is the saturation pressure p_{gd} corresponding to the dew-point temperature, and hence $p_s = p_{gd}$. Once the dew point has been determined, for example by cooling a metal surface and observing its temperature when dew begins to form on it, the relative humidity can be found from equation (14.26), i.e.

$$\phi = \frac{p_{gd}}{p_g}$$

An alternative way of finding the relative humidity is by means of the *wet- and dry-bulb temperatures*. If a stream of unsaturated air flows past a thermometer having a wetted sleeve of cotton or linen around the bulb, the temperature recorded will be less than the actual temperature of the air. The temperature falls owing to evaporation from the wetted sleeve, and as a result there will be a transfer of heat from the air to the wetted sleeve. The thermometer reading reaches a steady value, called the wet-bulb temperature, when the rate of heat transfer balances the loss of energy due to vaporisation. The actual temperature of the air is sometimes called the dry-bulb temperature to emphasise the distinction. When the air is unsaturated, the wet-bulb temperature lies between the dry-bulb temperature and the dew-point. The lower the relative humidity of the air, the more rapid is the evaporation from the wet-bulb and the larger becomes the *wet-bulb depression*, i.e. the difference between the dry- and wet-bulb temperatures. When the air is saturated, the wet-bulb, dry-bulb and dew-point temperatures are identical.

Since the evaporation, and therefore the wet-bulb temperature, depend on the equilibrium established between the heat and mass transfer rates to and

Fig. 14.7
Wet and dry bulb
hygrometer

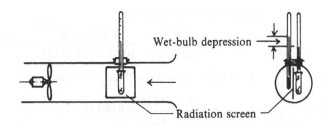

from the wetted sleeve, any slight draught increases the wet-bulb depression. It is found, however, that although the wet-bulb temperature falls as the air velocity is increased to about 2 m/s, it thereafter remains sensibly constant for velocities up to about 40 m/s. Provided that the air velocity is kept within this range, it is possible to relate the relative humidity to the wet- and dry-bulb temperatures alone. The equations are complicated and the relation is best expressed in the form of tables as in Ref. 29. Fig. 14.7 illustrates a simple form of wet- and dry-bulb hygrometer, in which the air stream is produced by a small fan. The sling hygrometer is a commonly used portable type, and this consists of wet- and dry-bulb thermometers mounted on a frame which can be whirled through the air by hand. A brief description of these and other methods of measuring humidity can be found in Ref. 31.

We have seen that the relative humidity can be deduced from measurements of either the dew point or the wet- and dry-bulb temperatures. If required, the specific humidity can be determined from equations relating it to the relative humidity. Thus, by combining (14.24) and (14.27b), we have

$$\phi = \omega \frac{v_g}{v_a} \tag{14.28}$$

or by combining (14.25) and (14.26),

$$\phi = \frac{\omega(p - p_s)}{0.622 p_g} \tag{14.29}$$

Example 14.8   The pressure and temperature of the air in a room are 1 bar and 28 °C. If the relative humidity is found to be 30 per cent, find the partial pressure of the water vapour and the dew point, the specific volume of each constituent, and the specific humidity.

From the saturation table, at 28 °C $p_g = 0.03778$ bar. Since $\phi = (p_s/p_g)$, $p_s = 0.3 \times 0.037\,78 = 0.011\,33$ bar. But $p_s = p_{gd}$ (Fig. 14.6), and the saturation temperature corresponding to 0.011 33 bar is 8.8 °C: this temperature is the dew point. (When dealing with saturated steam at very low pressures the temperature table of Ref. 17 will be used because the intervals are smaller than in the pressure table and linear interpolation more accurate.) For the vapour,

$$v_s = \frac{R_s T}{p_s} = \frac{0.462 \times 301}{100 \times 0.011\,33} = 122.7 \,\text{m}^3/\text{kg}$$

311

Similarly for the dry air,

$$v_a = \frac{R_a T}{(p - p_s)} = \frac{0.287 \times 301}{100(1.0 - 0.0113)} = 0.874 \, \text{m}^3/\text{kg}$$

The specific humidity is therefore, from equation (14.24),

$$\omega = \frac{v_a}{v_s} = \frac{0.874}{122.7} = 0.007\,12$$

The application of hygrometric principles to processes which occur in air-conditioning plant and cooling towers may now be considered.

14.5.1 Air-conditioning plant

Air-conditioning* involves a regulated supply of air at some desired temperature and relative humidity. A typical plant is illustrated in Fig. 14.8. In winter, heating coils are in operation to warm the air. If this reduces the relative humidity to an uncomfortably low level, water is sprayed into the air at a controlled rate. In summer, when the air is cooled, the relative humidity increases unless some form of dehumidifying process is introduced. The combined cooling and dehumidifying is conveniently accomplished by the process illustrated in Fig. 14.9, which shows what happens to the vapour in the mixture. Cooling coils reduce the temperature of the incoming air to the dew point and condensation commences. Sufficient cooling surface is provided for the temperature to fall to the dew point corresponding to the required *exit* condition of the air. The air

Fig. 14.8
Typical air-conditioning plant

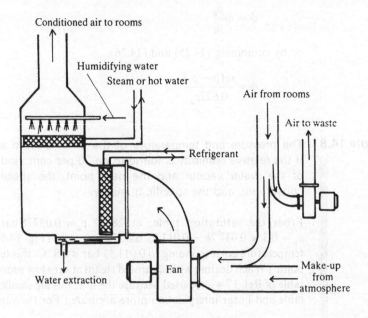

Conditioned air to rooms

Humidifying water

Steam or hot water

Air from rooms

Air to waste

Refrigerant

Water extraction

Fan

Make-up from atmosphere

---

* See Refs 5, 11 and 27 for detailed treatments of this subject.

Fig. 14.9
Combined cooling and
dehumidifying

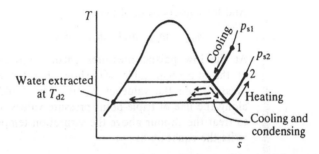

leaving the cooling coils is therefore saturated and at a lower temperature than
is required finally. Simple heating at constant pressure to the final temperature
will then reduce the relative humidity to the desired value. This is best explained
by a numerical example.

Example 14.9   On a summer's day the air has a pressure of 1 bar, a temperature of 35 °C,
and a relative humidity of 90 per cent. An air-conditioning plant is to deliver
30 m³/min at a temperature of 20 °C and with a relative humidity of 55 per
cent. This is to be accomplished by cooling the air to the dew point of the
delivery air and reheating it. An axial-flow fan, situated before the cooler,
absorbs 1.1 kW. Find the temperature to which the air must be cooled by
the cooling coils, and the heat transfer rates required in the cooler and
heater. Assume that the whole of the intake consists of atmospheric air, and
that the pressure remains constant throughout the process at 1 bar.

The temperature of the air leaving the cooler, at plane 2 in Fig. 14.10,
can be found by considering the process which occurs in the heater. Here the
composition of the mixture remains unchanged, so that the partial pressure of
the vapour must be constant between planes 2 and 3. Hence

$$p_{s2} = p_{s3} = \phi_3 p_{g3} = 0.55 \times 0.023\,37 = 0.012\,85 \text{ bar}$$

At plane 2 the air has just left the cooler where condensation has occurred and
the air is saturated with vapour. The temperature must therefore be the
saturation temperature corresponding to p_{s2}, i.e. $T_2 = 10.7\,°C$.
   The energy equation may be applied between planes 2 and 3 to find
the rate of heat transfer in the heater. Neglecting changes in kinetic energy, we
have

$$\dot{Q}_{23} = (\dot{m}_{a3}h_{a3} + \dot{m}_{s3}h_{s3}) - (\dot{m}_{a2}h_{a2} + \dot{m}_{s2}h_{s2})$$

Fig. 14.10

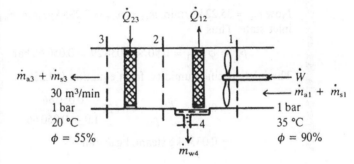

313

And for conservation of mass,

$$\dot{m}_{a3} = \dot{m}_{a2} \quad \text{and} \quad \dot{m}_{s3} = \dot{m}_{s2}$$

At the low partial pressures encountered in hygrometric work, a glance at the superheat table will show that the enthalpy is not a function of pressure and the value of h_{s3} at $20\,°C$ could be obtained by interpolating along the line of triple-point pressure values. It is more convenient, however, to treat the vapour above the saturation temperature T_2 as a perfect gas, and write the equation as

$$\dot{Q}_{23} = \dot{m}_{a3}c_{pa}(T_3 - T_2) + \dot{m}_{s3}c_{ps}(T_3 - T_2)$$

Over the range of temperature met in air-conditioning plant, an average value for c_{ps} is $1.86\,kJ/kg\,K$ and for c_{pa} is $1.005\,kJ/kg\,K$ (see Ref. 17). The mass of vapour in $30\,m^3/min$ of mixture is

$$\dot{m}_{s3} = \frac{p_{s3}\dot{V}}{R_s T} = \frac{100 \times 0.01285 \times 30}{0.462 \times 293} = 0.285\,kg/min$$

Similarly, the mass of air is

$$\dot{m}_{a3} = \frac{(p - p_{s3})\dot{V}}{R_a T} = \frac{100(1.0 - 0.01285)30}{0.287 \times 293} = 35.22\,kg/min$$

The heat transferred in the heater is therefore

$$\dot{Q}_{23} = \{35.22 \times 1.005(20 - 10.7)\}$$
$$+ \{0.285 \times 1.86(20 - 10.7)\}$$
$$= 329.2 + 4.9 = 334.1\,kJ/min$$

To find the heat $\dot{Q}_{12}$ transferred in the cooler, the energy equation is applied to the open system bounded by planes 1–2–4. Thus

$$\dot{Q}_{12} = (\dot{m}_{a2}h_{a2} + \dot{m}_{s2}h_{s2} + \dot{m}_{w4}h_{w4}) - (\dot{m}_{a1}h_{a1} + \dot{m}_{s1}h_{s1}) - \dot{W}$$

This equation can be rearranged, remembering from conservation of mass that $\dot{m}_{a3} = \dot{m}_{a2} = \dot{m}_{a1} = \dot{m}_a$ and $\dot{m}_{s1} = \dot{m}_{s2} + \dot{m}_{w4}$, to give either

$$\dot{Q}_{12} = \dot{m}_a c_{pa}(T_2 - T_1) + (\dot{m}_{s2}h_{s2} + \dot{m}_{w4}h_{w4} - \dot{m}_{s1}h_{s1}) - \dot{W} \quad \text{(a)}$$

or

$$\dot{Q}_{12} = \dot{m}_a c_{pa}(T_2 - T_1) + \dot{m}_{s2}c_{ps}(T_2 - T_1) + \dot{m}_{w4}(h_{w4} - h_{s1}) - \dot{W} \quad \text{(b)}$$

Now $\dot{m}_a = 35.22\,kg/min$, $\dot{m}_{s2} = \dot{m}_{s3} = 0.285\,kg/min$. $\dot{m}_{s1}$ can be found from the inlet state. Thus

$$p_{s1} = \phi_1 p_{g1} = 0.90 \times 0.05629 = 0.05066\,bar$$

The inlet specific humidity, from equation (14.25), is

$$\omega_1 = 0.622\frac{p_{s1}}{p_1 - p_{s1}} = 0.622\frac{0.05066}{1.0 - 0.05066}$$
$$= 0.0332\,kg\,steam/kg\,dry\,air$$

and hence

$$\dot{m}_{s1} = \omega_1 \dot{m}_a = 0.0332 \times 35.22 = 1.169 \text{ kg/min}$$

$$\dot{m}_{w4} = \dot{m}_{s1} - \dot{m}_{s2} = 1.169 - 0.285 = 0.884 \text{ kg/min}$$

The apparent advantage of using the second expression (b) for $\dot{Q}_{12}$ is that the enthalpy term involving $\dot{m}_{s2}$ can be easily calculated from the perfect gas approximation for steam (as was indeed done when calculating $\dot{Q}_{23}$). But when some of the steam or water changes phase in the process, there is very little saving in labour and the use of expression (a) reduces the chance of errors from algebraic manipulation. All enthalpies must then be calculated relative to the triple point datum of the steam tables. This approach will be adopted here.

The temperature of the condensed vapour will be equal to T_2, and hence $h_{w4} = 44.9 \text{ kJ/kg}$ from the h_f column of the saturation table. The enthalpy $h_{s2} = (h_g \text{ at } 10.7\,°C) = 2519.8 \text{ kJ/kg}$. The enthalpy h_{s1} can be found from

$$h_{s1} = (h_g \text{ at } p_{s1}) + c_{ps}(T_1 - T_g \text{ at } p_{s1})$$

$$= 2561.3 + 1.86(35 - 33.1) = 2565 \text{ kJ/kg}$$

Alternatively, h_{s1} can be found interpolating along any low-pressure line in the superheat table, because h is almost independent of p. Choosing the closest pressure to p_{s1}, namely 0.05 bar,

$$h_{s1} = 2561 + \frac{35 - 32.9}{50 - 32.9}(2594 - 2561) = 2565 \text{ kJ/kg}$$

The energy equation for the cooler therefore becomes

$$\dot{Q}_{12} = 35.22 \times 1.005(10.7 - 35) + \{(0.285 \times 2519.8)$$

$$+ (0.884 \times 44.9) - (1.169 \times 2565)\} - 1.1 \times 60$$

$$= -3166 \text{ kJ/min}$$

Here again, as we noted at the end of our analysis of condensers, the thermodynamic analysis only enables the required rates of heat transfer to be found. Further information is required before the necessary size of the cooling and heating coils can be determined. To reduce the quantities of heat involved, and therefore the size of the heat transfer surfaces, and yet maintain the freshness in the room, it is usual to draw about one-third of the total air supply from the atmosphere and to recirculate the remainder from the rooms (see Fig. 14.8).

14.5.2 Cooling towers

Steam power stations, refrigerating plant and many other industrial processes require large quantities of cooling water. If the plant is not situated near a natural source such as a river, it is necessary to cool the water after use and recirculate it. One of the most effective methods is to use the principle of evaporative cooling in a cooling tower. The warm water is sprayed into the tower near the top and allowed to fall through a packing of slats which break

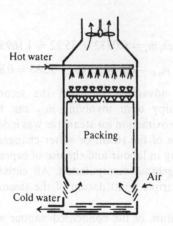

Fig. 14.11
Induced-draught cooling
tower

Hot water

Packing

Air

Cold water

up the stream and provide a large wetted surface to facilitate evaporation. A current of air passes up the tower, either naturally as in a chimney, or induced by a fan as shown in Fig. 14.11. The warm water is cooled, mainly by evaporation, while the air is raised in temperature and saturated, or nearly saturated, with water vapour. The water may be cooled to a temperature below that of the air entering the tower—ideally to the wet-bulb temperature of the air. The rate of cooling falls off as this equilibrium condition is approached, and the increase in height of tower which would be required to obtain the last possible few degrees of cooling is uneconomic. Generally, the tower is designed for the outlet water temperature to be about 8 K greater than the wet-bulb temperature of the atmosphere.

The cooling towers described above are a form of *direct-contact* heat exchanger. The advantages of this type over the conventional one, where the two fluids are separated by a solid wall, are twofold: first, the heat exchanger can be much smaller; and secondly, the water can be cooled to a lower temperature. (It can be cooled to within only a few degrees of the *dry*-bulb temperature in the conventional type.) The disadvantages are also twofold. First, some of the cooling water is lost by evaporation and has to be replaced continuously by expensively treated fresh water. Secondly, a group of large cooling towers can have an undesirable effect on the local environment. The vapour condenses above the towers and, if it is not cooled sufficiently rapidly, clouds can be formed some distance away which throw dense shadows over agricultural crops. These disadvantages have led to the development of the so-called *hybrid* tower in which initial cooling is performed in a conventional heat exchanger, followed by evaporative cooling towards the wet-bulb temperature in a direct-contact heat exchanger.

For an introduction to the theory of design of cooling towers, and further references, the reader may turn to Refs 16 and 11. The design is a problem in both heat and mass transfer from droplets and liquid films, and the detailed analysis to determine the volume of packing required for a given cooling duty is outside the scope of this book.

Example 14.10   Air enters the base of a natural-draught cooling tower at the rate of 1100 m³/min with a pressure of 1 bar, a temperature of 15 °C, and a relative humidity of 65 per cent. The water enters the tower at 38 °C and leaves at 17 °C. If the air leaves the tower at 32 °C in a saturated condition, find the mass flow of water entering the tower and the percentage loss of water by evaporation.

Fig. 14.12 illustrates the system. At the air inlet section 1 we have

$$p_{s1} = \phi_1 p_{g1} = 0.65 \times 0.017\,04 = 0.011\,08 \text{ bar}$$

$$\dot{m}_{s1} = \frac{p_{s1}\dot{V}}{R_s T} = \frac{100 \times 0.011\,08 \times 1100}{0.462 \times 288} = 9.16 \text{ kg/min}$$

$$\dot{m}_{a1} = \frac{(p - p_{s1})\dot{V}}{R_a T} = \frac{100(1.0 - 0.011\,08)1100}{0.287 \times 288} = 1316 \text{ kg/min}$$

At the air outlet section 2 we have

$$p_{s2} = p_{g2} = 0.047\,54 \text{ bar}$$

$$\omega_2 = 0.622 \frac{p_{s2}}{p - p_{s2}} = \frac{0.622 \times 0.047\,54}{(1.0 - 0.047\,54)} = 0.031\,05$$

Since $\dot{m}_{a2} = \dot{m}_{a1}$,

$$\dot{m}_{s2} = \omega_2 \dot{m}_{a1} = 0.031\,05 \times 1316 = 40.86 \text{ kg/min}$$

Water is lost by evaporation at the rate of

$$\dot{m}_{s2} - \dot{m}_{s1} = 40.86 - 9.16 = 31.7 \text{ kg/min}$$

Neglecting changes of kinetic energy and heat loss from the tower to atmosphere, the energy equation is

$$(\dot{m}_{a2} h_{a2} + \dot{m}_{s2} h_{s2} + \dot{m}_{w4} h_{w4}) - (\dot{m}_{a1} h_{a1} + \dot{m}_{s1} h_{s1} + \dot{m}_{w3} h_{w3}) = 0$$

Or in more convenient form,

$$\dot{m}_a c_{pa}(T_2 - T_1) + (\dot{m}_{s2} h_{s2} - \dot{m}_{s1} h_{s1}) + (\dot{m}_{w4} h_{w4} - \dot{m}_{w3} h_{w3}) = 0$$

Fig. 14.12
Natural-
draught
cooling
tower

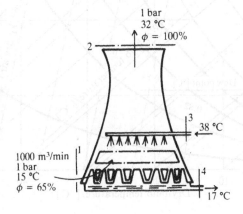

317

From conservation of mass,

$$\dot{m}_{s2} + \dot{m}_{w4} = \dot{m}_{s1} + \dot{m}_{w3} \quad \text{and hence} \quad \dot{m}_{w4} = \dot{m}_{w3} - 31.7 \, \text{kg/min}$$

From the saturation table, since T_{g1} at p_{s1} is 8.48 °C,

$$h_{s1} = h_{g1} + c_{ps}(T_1 - T_{g1}) = 2516 + 1.86(15 - 8.48) = 2528 \, \text{kJ/kg}$$

and

$$h_{s2} = h_{g2} = 2559.3 \, \text{kJ/kg}, \qquad h_{w3} = h_{f3} = 159.1 \, \text{kJ/kg}$$

$$h_{w4} = h_{f4} = 71.3 \, \text{kJ/kg}$$

Finally, taking $c_{pa} = 1.005 \, \text{kJ/kg K}$, we get

$$1316 \times 1.005(32 - 15) + \{(40.86 \times 2559) - (9.16 \times 2528)\}$$
$$+ \{(\dot{m}_{w3} - 31.7)71.3 - \dot{m}_{w3} 159.1\} = 0$$

The water flow at inlet $\dot{m}_{w3}$ is consequently 1160 kg/min. The percentage loss by evaporation is

$$\frac{\dot{m}_{s2} - \dot{m}_{s1}}{\dot{m}_{w3}} 100 = 2.7 \text{ per cent}$$

14.6 Hygrometric chart

Calculations involved in the type of problem considered in section 14.5 can be considerably simplified if use is made of the hygrometric chart, Fig. 14.13. This chart enables the enthalpy of humid atmospheric air, of any relative humidity,

Fig. 14.13
The hygrometric chart

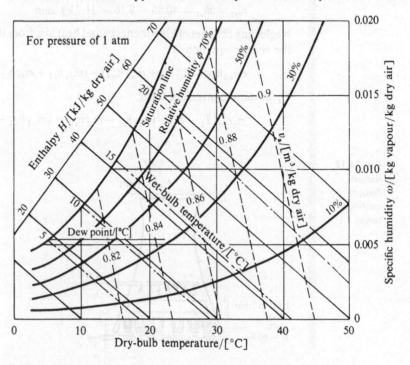

to be read off directly. The enthalpy of the mixture is expressed as kJ per kg of *dry* air in the mixture. If this quantity is denoted by H, then

$$H = h_a + \omega h_s$$

Although h_a is fixed solely by the temperature of the air (dry-bulb temperature T), the value of ωh_s depends upon the specific humidity and both the pressure and the temperature of the air. Thus equation (14.25) indicates that when ω and p are known, the partial pressure of the vapour p_s is determined. If in addition the temperature T is known, then h_s is fixed. The chart is drawn for a fixed barometric pressure so that ω and T can be regarded as the only independent variables. These form the ordinate and abscissa scales respectively, and lines of constant enthalpy H are plotted on the diagram.

Equation (14.29) shows that, for a given barometric pressure, the relative humidity ϕ is a function of ω, p_s and p_g. p_g is the saturation pressure corresponding to the dry-bulb temperature T, and we have already seen that p_s is a function of ω for a fixed barometric pressure. It follows that ϕ is also a function of ω and T, and therefore lines of constant relative humidity can be added to the diagram. Since humidity measurements are so often made in terms of wet- and dry-bulb temperatures, lines of constant wet-bulb temperature are also included. Note that the wet-bulb temperature at any state along the saturation line ($\phi = 100$ per cent) is equal to the dry-bulb temperature, and also the dew point, at that state. Lines of constant dew point are horizontal because they are also lines of constant specific humidity. The constant wet-bulb temperature lines slope down towards the right of the diagram and follow very closely the lines of constant enthalpy.

Finally, lines of constant specific volume v_a of the dry air in the mixture are usually included. v_a is a function of the dry-bulb temperature T and the partial pressure of the air ($p - p_s$). But we have seen that p_s is a function of ω and p, and so, for a given barometric pressure p, v_a is a function of T and ω.

The way in which the hygrometric chart can be used to simplify the solution of a problem will be indicated briefly by referring to the air-conditioning plant of Fig. 14.10. The process undergone by the mixture can be represented as in Fig. 14.14, points 1 and 3 being located from the given values of T and ϕ at the inlet and outlet of the system. The temperature T_2 to which the air must

Fig. **14.14**
Use of hygrometric chart

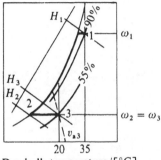

Dry-bulb temperature/[°C]

be cooled can be read directly from the chart. Before applying the energy equation, the next step must be to find the mass flow of dry air because all the 'specific' quantities on the chart refer to unit mass of dry air. Thus v_{a3} is read from the chart, and hence $\dot{m}_a$ can be found from $\dot{V}_3/v_{a3}$, where $\dot{V}_3$ is the volume flow of mixture delivered.

The energy equation for the heating process, i.e. between planes 2 and 3 in Fig. 14.10, can be written in the convenient form

$$\dot{Q}_{23} = \dot{m}_a(H_3 - H_2)$$

since the values of H are in kJ/kg of dry air in the mixture, and $\dot{m}_a$ does not change between planes 2 and 3. Both H_3 and H_2 can be read from the chart, and so $\dot{Q}_{23}$ can be determined directly.

Similarly, the energy equation for the cooling and condensing process can be written as

$$\dot{Q}_{12} = \dot{m}_a(H_2 - H_1) + \dot{m}_{w4} h_{w4} - \dot{W}$$

H_2 and H_1 can be read from the chart, $\dot{W}$ is given, and h_{w4} can be found from the saturation table in the usual way; it remains to find $\dot{m}_{w4}$. For conservation of mass,

$$\dot{m}_{s1} = \dot{m}_{s2} + \dot{m}_{w4} \quad \text{or} \quad \dot{m}_{w4} = \dot{m}_a(\omega_1 - \omega_2)$$

Both ω_1 and ω_2 can be read from the chart, and therefore $\dot{m}_{w4}$ and thence $\dot{Q}_{12}$ can be rapidly calculated.

Although a hygrometric chart is drawn for a particular barometric pressure, it can be used without much loss of accuracy for any reasonable variation in this pressure. For example, the chart of Ref. 6 is drawn for a pressure of 1 atm, but it can be used without sensible error between 0.9 and 1.1 bar. All the information conveyed by the chart can also be obtained in the form of tables such as those of Ref. 29.

15

Combustion Processes

Previous chapters have been wholly concerned with the behaviour of fluids which remain in the same chemical state throughout the processes considered. Here we shall deal with the thermodynamic aspects of a particular type of process involving chemical reactions, namely combustion. The term 'combustion' refers to the fairly rapid reaction, usually accompanied by a flame, which occurs between a fuel and an oxygen carrier such as air. The molecules of fuel and air have a certain amount of energy stored in the bonds between their constituent atoms, a form of internal energy which we have not had to consider hitherto because it remains constant for all processes not involving chemical reactions. In the new molecules formed by a reaction this 'chemical' energy is at a lower level, and the energy thus released can be transferred to the surroundings in the form of heat. Combustion is therefore said to be an *exothermic* reaction.

After the relevant combustion equations which relate the masses of reactants and products are discussed, methods of applying the energy equation to the combustion process are examined and the efficiency of such a process is defined. The idea of a reversible combustion process is introduced, and a method of estimating the effect of dissociation is described.

Many properties required for the analysis of chemical reactions cannot be measured directly and have to be derived from others. The interrelation between the various properties, the method of their tabulation, and tests for self-consistency are discussed. Some important aspects of combustion cannot be handled by thermodynamic reasoning alone; the rate at which a reaction proceeds and the stability of flames are two examples of great importance in the design of internal combustion engines. The chapter concludes with a brief discussion of the limitations of thermodynamic analysis.

15.1 Fuels

Most common fossil fuels consist mainly of hydrogen and carbon, whether the fuel be solid (e.g. coal), liquid (e.g. petroleum) or gaseous (e.g. natural gas). We

Fig. 15.1

Typical ultimate analyses of coals

Coal	C	H	O	N + S	Ash
Anthracite	90.27	3.00	2.32	1.44	2.97
Bituminous	74.00	5.98	13.01	2.26	4.75
Lignite	56.52	5.72	31.89	1.62	4.25

shall assume that the chemical analysis of the fuel is known.* For solid and liquid fuels the analysis is usually quoted as a percentage by mass of each chemical *element* in the fuel; it is termed an *ultimate* analysis. The analysis of a gaseous fuel, on the other hand, is usually given in terms of the percentage by volume of each gas or type of hydrocarbon present.

In coal, the combustible elements are chiefly carbon (C) and hydrogen (H) with a minor quantity of sulphur (S); the incombustibles are nitrogen (N), moisture (H_2O) and small quantities of minerals which form the ash after combustion. Typical ultimate analyses of the three main types of coal—anthracite, bituminous coal and lignite—are given in Fig. 15.1. Since there are numerous varieties of each type of coal, the figures can only serve as a rough guide. Moreover the analyses refer to dry coals; the moisture content is as low as 1 per cent in anthracite, varies from 2 to 10 per cent in the bituminous coals, and is as high as 15 per cent in lignite.

Petroleum oils are complex mixtures of a large number of different hydrocarbons. These hydrocarbons have been classified into groups, the most common being paraffins (having a molecular formula of the form C_nH_{2n+2}), olefins and naphthenes (C_nH_{2n})† and aromatics (typically C_nH_{2n-6}). Although analysis in terms of actual compounds is difficult and sometimes impossible, the ultimate analysis is a simple matter and Fig. 15.2 gives typical examples. The analyses are very similar and the choice of fuel for a particular application depends mainly on other characteristics such as viscosity, ignition temperature, knocking tendency (in petrol engines), coking tendency (in gas turbines) and so on.

Most hydrocarbons in petroleum deposits occur naturally as a liquid, but a few exist in the gaseous phase at atmospheric temperature. At present, North Sea gas fields meet most of the UK's commercial and domestic needs for gaseous fuel. Methane (a paraffin, CH_4), known as 'marsh gas' and 'fire-damp' when occurring naturally, is produced by the decay of organic matter. Sewage works

Fig. 15.2

Typical ultimate analyses of petroleum oils

	Motor petrol	Vaporising oil	Kerosene	Diesel oil (gas oil)	Light fuel oil	Heavy fuel oil
C	85.5	86.8	86.3	86.3	86.2	86.1
H	14.4	12.9	13.6	12.8	12.4	11.8
S	0.1	0.3	0.1	0.9	1.4	2.1

* See Ref. 19 for complete data on typical fuels.
† Although olefins and naphthenes have the same C/H ratio, they are distinguished by an important difference in molecular structure.

Fig. 15.3
Typical volumetric
analyses of gaseous fuels

	H_2	CO	'CH$_4$'	C_nH_m	O_2	N_2	CO_2
Coal gas	49.4	18.0	20.0	C_4H_8 2.0	0.4	6.2	4.0
Producer gas	12.0	29.0	2.6	C_2H_4 0.4	—	52.0	4.0
Blast furnace	2.0	27.0	—	—	—	60.0	11.0
North Sea gas	—	—	93.0	C_2H_6 4.8	—	2.0	0.2

Fig. 15.3
Typical volumetric
analyses of gaseous fuels

and biodigesters on farms can supply methane for local use as a supplementary fuel. Prior to the Second World War, the most widely used gaseous fuels were formed by heating coal in various ways. Typical compositions of three forms—coal (or town) gas, producer gas, and blast furnace gas—are given in Fig. 15.3, with that of North Sea gas for comparison. Hydrogen and carbon monoxide are easily isolated, but the various hydrocarbons are usually grouped into two types representing respectively an average composition of the paraffins in the gas (assumed to have the formula CH_4) and an average of the remainder (C_nH_m).

In the following sections concerned with typical combustion calculations, we shall neglect the effect of minor elements, such as sulphur, in the fuel. Although for the purpose of setting out mass and energy balances this is permissible, it should not be thought that the presence of a small quantity of a substance is always unimportant. Thus sulphur in fossil fuels is the principal cause of 'acid rain'. Less well known are the effects of such impurities as sodium and vanadium. These produce corrosive compounds which attack engine components. Vanadium compounds, for example, break down the protective oxide layer on turbine blades and effectively prevent the use of the cheaper oils as fuel for gas turbines. The presence (or absence) of an impurity may well determine the choice of fuel for a particular application.

15.2   Chemical equations and conservation of mass

The first step in the description of a combustion process is the formulation of the chemical equation which shows how the atoms of the reactants are rearranged to form the products. Before the chemical equation can be written it is necessary to know the number of atoms of each element in the molecules of the reactants and products. In any purely chemical, as opposed to nuclear, reaction the process is simply one of rearrangement of the atoms to form new molecules, and the total number of atoms of each element is unchanged. A chemical equation expresses the principle of the conservation of mass in terms of the conservation of atoms.

Consider the simple chemical equation expressing the complete combustion of carbon and oxygen to carbon dioxide:

$$C + O_2 \rightarrow CO_2 \tag{15.1}$$

This equation states that one atom of carbon will combine with one molecule of oxygen (2 atoms of O) to produce one molecule of carbon dioxide (1 atom of C + 2 atoms of O). The number of atoms of each element is the same on either side of the equation, and the arrow represents the direction of the reaction.

Equation (15.1) can also represent the *amount-of-substance* involved in the reaction and be written as

$$1 \text{ kmol C} + 1 \text{ kmol O}_2 \rightarrow 1 \text{ kmol CO}_2 \qquad (15.2)$$

Since the *molar masses* of the substances are numerically equal to the *relative atomic* or *molecular masses*,* equation (15.2) can be converted into a mass equation as follows:

$$12 \text{ kg C} + 32 \text{ kg O}_2 \rightarrow 44 \text{ kg CO}_2 \qquad (15.3)$$

Now all gases occupy equal volumes *per kmol* when reduced to the same pressure and temperature. Although this is strictly true only for perfect gases, it is substantially true for all gases and dry vapours at moderate pressures. If any of the reactants or products are in the solid or liquid phase, the volume occupied by them can be neglected in comparison with the volume of the gases present. It follows that equation (15.2) is also equivalent to

$$0 \text{ vol. C} + 1 \text{ vol. O}_2 \rightarrow 1 \text{ vol. CO}_2 \qquad (15.4)$$

Equation (15.4) implies that the volume of the products is equal to the volume of the reactants, when measured at the same pressure and temperature.

If insufficient oxygen is present for all the carbon to burn to carbon dioxide, some will burn to carbon monoxide. The reaction is then symbolised by

$$C + \tfrac{1}{2}O_2 \rightarrow CO \qquad (15.5)$$

Carbon monoxide can be subsequently burnt to carbon dioxide, the appropriate equation being

$$CO + \tfrac{1}{2}O_2 \rightarrow CO_2 \qquad (15.6)$$

It is for this reason that the combustion of carbon to carbon monoxide is said to be 'incomplete', and to carbon dioxide 'complete'.

Equations similar to (15.1) to (15.4) can be written for the combustion of hydrogen, the other main constituent of a hydrocarbon fuel:

$$H_2 + \tfrac{1}{2}O_2 \rightarrow H_2O$$
$$1 \text{ kmol H}_2 + \tfrac{1}{2} \text{ kmol O}_2 \rightarrow 1 \text{ kmol H}_2O$$
$$2 \text{ kg H}_2 + 16 \text{ kg O}_2 \rightarrow 18 \text{ kg H}_2O$$
$$1 \text{ vol. H}_2 + \tfrac{1}{2} \text{ vol. O}_2 \rightarrow 1 \text{ vol. H}_2O \text{ (vap)}$$
$$\rightarrow 0 \text{ vol. H}_2O \text{ (liq)} \qquad (15.7)$$

---

* For a discussion of the relation between amount-of-substance, molar mass and relative atomic or molecular mass, see section 8.5.2. Various 'atomic weight' scales have been used in the past. A chemical scale was fixed when the existence of three isotopes of oxygen of differing mass was not known; it was formed by allotting the number 16 to a 'mean' oxygen atom. This proved unsatisfactory because the proportions of oxygen isotopes vary in nature. When nuclear studies became important a physical scale was adopted in which the number 16 was attached to the most common isotope of oxygen (^{16}O). In 1961 a new scale was adopted by both chemists and physicists based on a particular isotope of carbon (^{12}C) which was assigned the value 12. Values on the old chemical scale and new ^{12}C scale differ only by about 0.004 per cent. For combustion calculations, whole number values (e.g. C 12, O 16, H 1, N 14) are sufficiently accurate, and thus these changes in the basis of the relative atomic mass scale are insignificant.

The abbreviation (vap) or (liq) must be included when the phase of a reactant or product is in doubt.

In most engineering combustion systems the necessary oxygen is obtained by mixing the fuel with air.* For our purposes it will be sufficiently accurate to use the following figures for the composition of air:

	O_2	N_2
Volumetric analysis %	21	79
Gravimetric analysis %	23.3	76.7

Here the symbol N is used to denote not only the nitrogen, but all the inert gases present in air which remain unchanged throughout the reaction. The molar mass of N_2 can be taken as 28 kg/kmol, and that of air as 29 kg/kmol. (A more precise composition of air is given in Ref. 17.)

The following two examples, concerning a liquid and a gaseous fuel respectively, show how chemical equations may be used (a) to predict the analysis of the products of combustion when the composition of the fuel and the air/fuel ratio are known, and (b) to determine the *stoichiometric* (or *correct*) air/fuel ratio. A stoichiometric mixture is one in which there is theoretically just sufficient oxygen to burn all the combustible elements in the fuel completely. In practical combustion systems the time available for the reaction is limited and excess air must be provided to ensure complete combustion. This is not only because of imperfect mixing of the fuel and air, but also because the inert gas molecules obstruct the reaction between the active molecules of fuel and oxygen.

The analysis of the products of combustion may be quoted on a volume or a mass basis. In either case, if the water vapour is assumed to be present as it is in the hot exhaust gases from an engine, the analysis is called a *wet* analysis. When the vapour is assumed to be condensed and removed, it is called a *dry* analysis.

Example 15.1   Determine the stoichiometric air/fuel ratio for a petrol approximating to hexane C_6H_{14}. Hence deduce the chemical equation if the petrol is burnt in 20 per cent excess air, and the wet volumetric analysis of the products (a) if all the water vapour is present, and (b) if the products are cooled to an atmospheric pressure and temperature of 1 bar and 15 °C. Determine also the dry volumetric analysis.

Finally, estimate the chemical equation if only 80 per cent of the air required for stoichiometric combustion is provided.

Chemical equation
Since the combustion is theoretically complete with a stoichiometric mixture, the products will consist only of CO_2, H_2O and the N_2 brought in with the air. The amount of oxygen required can be found by first balancing the carbon

---

* The chief exception is the rocket motor, described in section 18.4.2. In this case the necessary oxygen is obtained from liquid oxygen, liquid ozone, or some oxygen carrier such as hydrogen peroxide or nitric acid.

and hydrogen atoms on each side of the equation and then summing the number of atoms of oxygen in the products:

$$C_6H_{14} + 9\tfrac{1}{2}O_2 \rightarrow 6CO_2 + 7H_2O$$

$$86 \text{ kg } C_6H_{14} + 304 \text{ kg } O_2 \rightarrow 264 \text{ kg } CO_2 + 126 \text{ kg } H_2O$$

Since air contains 23.3 per cent by mass of oxygen, we have

$$\text{stoichiometric air/fuel ratio} = \frac{304 \times 100}{86 \times 23.3} = 15.17$$

If there is 20 per cent excess air, the equation, including the nitrogen, becomes

$$C_6H_{14} + 1.2\left\{9\tfrac{1}{2}O_2 + \left(\frac{79}{21}\right)9\tfrac{1}{2}N_2\right\} \rightarrow$$

$$6CO_2 + 7H_2O + (0.2)9\tfrac{1}{2}O_2 + 1.2\left(\frac{79}{21}\right)9\tfrac{1}{2}N_2$$

Wet volumetric analysis

(a) The amount-of-substance of the products is

$$6(CO_2) + 7(H_2O) + 1.9(O_2) + 42.89(N_2) = 57.79 \text{ kmol}$$

Now the mole fraction of a constituent equals the volume fraction (equation (14.18)). The wet volumetric analysis if all the water vapour is present is therefore

$$CO_2 \quad \frac{6 \times 100}{57.79} = 10.38\%; \qquad H_2O \quad \frac{7 \times 100}{57.79} = 12.11\%$$

$$O_2 \quad \frac{1.9 \times 100}{57.79} = 3.29\%; \qquad N_2 \quad \frac{42.89 \times 100}{57.79} = 74.22\%$$

(b) The partial pressure of saturated water vapour at 15 °C is 0.017 04 bar. The mole fraction of the water vapour in the mixture, from equation (14.17), is

$$x_s = \frac{0.017\,04}{1.0} = 0.017\,04$$

If y is the amount-of-substance of water vapour remaining in the products after cooling, the total amount-of-substance becomes $\{(57.79 - 7)[\text{kmol}] + y\}$, and therefore

$$\frac{y}{50.79\,[\text{kmol}] + y} = 0.017\,04$$

from which $y = 0.88$ kmol. The total amount-of-substance of products under these conditions is 51.67 kmol in the vapour state, and the volumetric analysis becomes

$$CO_2 \ 11.61\%; \quad H_2O \ 1.70\%; \quad O_2 \ 3.68\%; \quad N_2 \ 83.01\%$$

Dry volumetric analysis

Merely cooling the products does not remove the water vapour entirely. If all the vapour is assumed to be removed, say by a drying agent, the total amount of substance is 50.79 kmol. The dry analysis is

$$CO_2 \; 11.81\%; \quad O_2 \; 3.74\%; \quad N_2 \; 84.45\%$$

Chemical equation with insufficient air

When insufficient air is supplied for complete combustion, some of the carbon will burn to carbon monoxide, and there may also be some free hydrogen. Insufficient information is given for the determination of the chemical equation. Hydrogen, however, has a greater affinity for oxygen than has carbon, and if the mixture is not too rich in fuel it is reasonable to assume that all the hydrogen will be burnt.* We can then write, for the rich mixture,

$$C_6H_{14} + 0.8\left\{9\tfrac{1}{2}O_2 + \left(\frac{79}{21}\right)9\tfrac{1}{2}N_2\right\} \rightarrow$$

$$aCO_2 + bCO + 7H_2O + 0.8\left(\frac{79}{21}\right)9\tfrac{1}{2}N_2$$

From the carbon balance,

$$6 = a + b$$

From the oxygen balance,

$$0.8 \times 9\tfrac{1}{2} = a + b/2 + 7/2$$

Solving these simultaneous equations, we get $a = 2.2$ and $b = 3.8$. The chemical equation is therefore

$$C_6H_{14} + 7.6O_2 + 28.6N_2 \rightarrow 2.2CO_2 + 3.8CO + 7H_2O + 28.6N_2$$

Example 15.2   A gaseous fuel has the following percentage composition by volume:

$$CO \; 12.6\%; \quad H_2 \; 41.6\%; \quad CH_4 \; 26.6\%; \quad O_2 \; 1.9\%;$$

$$CO_2 \; 2.6\%; \quad N_2 \; 14.7\%$$

Find the wet volumetric and gravimetric analyses of the products of combustion when 10 per cent excess air is provided.

The solution can be set out in tabular form. The first table determines the oxygen required for stoichiometric combustion, and the amounts of CO_2 and H_2O produced thereby, per mole of fuel burnt. Note that the amount of oxygen in the fuel is taken into account when estimating the oxygen required from the air.

---

* An accurate prediction of the products analysis for a mixture lacking sufficient oxygen for complete combustion can only be obtained by the method outlined in section 15.7.2. This makes use of additional information in the form of equilibrium constants for the various reactions.

Reactants	$\dfrac{kmol}{kmol\ fuel}$	Reaction	O_2 required	Products CO₂		Products H₂O

Reactants	$\dfrac{\text{kmol}}{\text{kmol fuel}}$	Reaction	O_2 required	CO_2	H_2O
CO	0.126	$CO + \frac{1}{2}O_2 \rightarrow CO_2$	0.063	0.126	—
H₂	0.416	$H_2 + \frac{1}{2}O_2 \rightarrow H_2O$	0.208	—	0.416
CH₄	0.266	$CH_4 + 2O_2 \rightarrow CO_2 + 2H_2O$	0.532	0.266	0.532
O₂	0.019	—	−0.019	—	—
CO₂	0.026	—	—	0.026	—
N₂	0.147	—	—	—	—
	1.000		0.784	0.418	0.948

So 0.784 kmol of oxygen is required, per kmol of fuel burnt, for stoichiometric combustion. Since 10 per cent excess air is provided, 0.0784 kmol of oxygen is additionally present and remains unchanged throughout the process. The total amount of nitrogen in the products is

$$1.1\left(\frac{79}{21}\right)0.784 + 0.147 = 3.392\ \text{kmol/kmol of fuel}$$

The analyses of the products by volume and by mass (see equation (14.23)) are therefore as in the following table:

Products	$\dfrac{\text{kmol}}{\text{kmol fuel}}$ (a)	% by volume	$\tilde{m}^*$ [kg/kmol]	$\dfrac{\text{kg}}{\text{kmol fuel}}$ $m \times (a)$	% by mass
CO₂	0.418	8.6	44	18.39	13.8
H₂O	0.948	19.6	18	17.06	12.8
O₂	0.078	1.6	32	2.50	1.9
N₂	3.392	70.2	28	94.98	71.5
	4.836	100.0		132.93	100.0

* Note from section 8.5.2 that $\tilde{m}$, when measured in kg/kmol (or g/mol), is numerically equal to A_r or M_r but is not dimensionless.

15.3 Experimental products analysis

When investigating the effectiveness of combustion plant it is often necessary to analyse the products experimentally. By taking samples at different stages of a reaction the combustion process can be studied, and the analyses can be used to discover lack of uniformity in fuel–air distribution. A products analysis also enables the air/fuel ratio to be computed in cases where direct measurement of the rate of air flow is not easily accomplished.

A brief description of various exhaust gas analysers can be found in Ref. 8. The most common method is by successive absorption of the CO_2, O_2 and CO as in the Orsat apparatus (Fig. 15.4). The sample of exhaust gas is drawn into the measuring burette by lowering the levelling bottle containing water. This known volume of sample at atmospheric temperature and pressure is forced in succession into each of the reagent bottles which contain the absorbents. The

Fig. 15.4
Orsat apparatus for
exhaust gas analysis

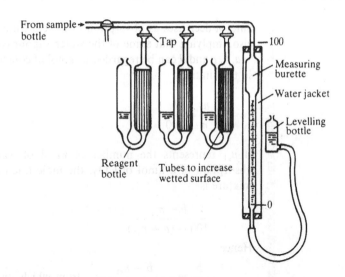

volume is measured after each absorption process by returning the sample to the burette and bringing it to atmospheric pressure with the aid of the levelling bottle. The change in volume after a particular constituent has been absorbed is then the partial volume of that constituent in the original sample (see section 14.2). The gas which remains is assumed to be nitrogen.

The resulting analysis is by volume and is on a dry basis. Although most of the water vapour is condensed when the sample is first cooled to atmospheric temperature, the sample is nevertheless saturated with water vapour at this temperature throughout the analysis because the sample is contained in the measuring burette over water. The reason why the Orsat apparatus yields a true dry analysis is therefore not obvious, and it is left to the following example to show that this is so. A second example shows how the analysis can be used to compute the air/fuel ratio when the percentage by mass of carbon in the fuel is known.

Example 15.3   A sample of exhaust gases, when cooled to atmospheric temperature, has the following percentage composition by volume:

$$CO_2 \; a; \quad H_2O \; b; \quad O_2 \; c; \quad N_2 \; d$$

Show that the Orsat analysis yields the true *dry* analysis, which is evidently

$$CO_2 \; \frac{100a}{100 - b}; \quad O_2 \; \frac{100c}{100 - b}; \quad N_2 \; \frac{100d}{100 - b}$$

Since the sample is in contact with water at a constant temperature throughout the analysis, the partial pressure p_s of the water vapour must remain constant at the saturation value. But from equation (14.17),

$$\frac{p_s}{p} = \frac{n_s}{n}$$

and the pressure p of the mixture is atmospheric. It follows that n_s/n is constant.

329

Since n decreases as absorption of the constituents proceeds, n_s must decrease also, implying that some of the water vapour condenses.

a, b, c and d can be regarded as kmol of constituent per 100 kmol of mixture, so that initially

$$\frac{n_s}{n} = \frac{b}{100}$$

If n_{s1} represents the number of kmol of water vapour condensed during absorption of a kmol of CO_2, the mole fraction of vapour in the remaining mixture is

$$\frac{b - n_{s1}}{100 - (a + n_{s1})}$$

Hence

$$\frac{b}{100} = \frac{b - n_{s1}}{100 - (a + n_{s1})} \quad \text{from which} \quad n_{s1} = \frac{ab}{100 - b}$$

The first percentage contraction of volume noted from the Orsat apparatus is therefore

$$a + n_{s1} = \frac{100a}{100 - b}$$

which is the percentage by volume of CO_2 in a *dry* sample.

Similarly, if n_{s2} is the number of kmol of water vapour condensed on absorption of the O_2 we have

$$\frac{b}{100} = \frac{b - (n_{s1} + n_{s2})}{100 - (a + n_{s1} + c + n_{s2})}$$

After substituting for n_{s1}, this gives

$$n_{s2} = \frac{bc}{100 - b}$$

The second contraction noted from the Orsat apparatus is therefore

$$c + n_{s2} = \frac{100c}{100 - b}$$

which is the percentage by volume of O_2 in a dry sample.

The remaining volume, consisting of N_2 and water vapour, is

$$100 - (a + n_{s1} + c + n_{s2})$$

After substituting for n_{s1} and n_{s2}, this reduces to

$$\frac{100d}{100 - b}$$

which is the percentage by volume of N_2 in a dry sample.

Example 15.4   A petrol has the following ultimate analysis:

C 83.7%;   H 16.3%

If the dry products analysis by volume is

CO_2 11.8%; O_2 3.7%; N_2 84.5%

determine the air/fuel ratio used.

Carbon balance method
Treating the volume fractions as mole fractions, 1 kmol of dry products contains 0.845 kmol of N_2. Now 0.845 kmol of N_2 are brought in with

$$0.845 \times 28\left(\frac{100}{76.7}\right) = 30.85 \text{ kg of air}$$

1 kmol of dry products contains 0.118 kmol of CO_2, which in turn contain 0.118×12 kg of carbon. This amount of carbon implies the combustion of

$$\frac{0.118 \times 12}{0.837} = 1.692 \text{ kg of petrol}$$

Thus 1 kmol of dry products is produced when 30.85 kg of air are burnt with 1.692 kg of petrol, i.e.

$$\text{air/fuel ratio} = \frac{30.85}{1.692} = 18.2$$

The foregoing method, using a carbon balance between reactants and products, is the most satisfactory when carbon is the predominant element in the fuel. The result may be inaccurate, however, if the exhaust gases are smoky, indicating unburnt carbon not included in the products analysis. An oxygen–hydrogen balance can be made as a check, although since the relevant quantities are relatively small the result is more open to error from inaccuracies of measurement.

Oxygen–hydrogen balance method
First, 1 kmol of dry products contains

$$32(0.118 + 0.037) = 4.960 \text{ kg of } O_2$$

But the oxygen accompanying the nitrogen is

$$0.845 \times 28\left(\frac{23.3}{76.7}\right) = 7.187 \text{ kg}$$

Hence $(7.187 - 4.960) = 2.227$ kg of O_2 have combined with the hydrogen in the fuel to form water vapour. It follows from equation (15.7) that 2.227/8 kg of H_2 are involved, which corresponds to

$$\frac{2.227}{8 \times 0.163} = 1.708 \text{ kg of petrol}$$

Therefore 30.85 kg of air are associated with 1.708 kg of fuel, i.e.

$$\text{air/fuel ratio} = \frac{30.85}{1.708} = 18.1$$

With coal-burning appliances there is an additional complication because some of the combustion products will be in solid form. The analysis of the refuse is easily accomplished by heating a sample above its ignition temperature in a stream of oxygen. The loss of weight is measured and assumed to be carbon, while the remainder is the ash. The following example shows how a complete mass balance can be compiled for a combustion process if the composition of the fuel, gaseous products and refuse are measured. In general the air will have a certain moisture content, which can be found by wet- and dry-bulb temperature measurements (sections 14.5 and 14.6), and this is also taken into account in the example.

Example 15.5 Determine the complete mass balance for a combustion process, on the basis of 1 kg of coal burnt, given the following data:

Fuel consumption (fractions by mass):

C 0.69; H 0.03; O 0.04; N 0.01; H_2O 0.10; ash 0.13

Dry exhaust gas analysis (fractions by volume):

CO_2 0.146; CO 0.020; O_2 0.055; N_2 0.779

Refuse analysis (fractions by mass):

C 0.40; ash 0.60

Air: dry-bulb temperature 22.8 °C, wet-bulb temperature 15.5 °C.

(a) The mass of refuse m_R per kg of fuel burnt can be found from an ash balance, i.e. $0.6 m_R = 0.13$ kg and hence $m_R = 0.217$ kg.

(b) The mass of dry gaseous products can be found from a carbon balance. Basis: 1 kg of fuel.

Carbon in fuel   = 0.69 kg   or   0.0575 kmol
Carbon in refuse = 0.4×0.217 = 0.087 kg   or   0.0072 kmol
Carbon in gaseous products   = 0.603 kg   or   0.0503 kmol
Basis: 1 kmol of dry gaseous products.
Carbon in CO_2 = 0.146 kmol
Carbon in CO   = 0.020 kmol
Carbon in gaseous products = 0.166 kmol
Ratio of dry gaseous products to fuel = $0.0503/0.166 = 0.303$ kmol/kg.
The dry gaseous products per kg of fuel are therefore:

CO_2 = $0.146 \times 0.303 = 0.0442$ kmol   or $\times 44 = 1.95$ kg
CO = $0.020 \times 0.303 = 0.0061$ kmol   or $\times 28 = 0.17$ kg
O_2 = $0.055 \times 0.303 = 0.0167$ kmol   or $\times 32 = 0.53$ kg
N_2 = $0.779 \times 0.303 = 0.236$ kmol   or $\times 28 = 6.61$ kg
                                           Total = 9.26 kg

(c) The mass of dry air can be found from a nitrogen balance.
Basis: 1 kg of fuel.
    Nitrogen in gaseous products = 0.236 kmol (from (b))
    Nitrogen in fuel = 0.01/28   = negligible
    Nitrogen required from air   = 0.236 kmol
    Dry air supplied = 0.236/0.79 = 0.299 kmol
                    or × 29 = 8.67 kg

(d) The mass of water vapour in the air, found from the hygrometric chart
or tables, is specific humidity = 0.0081 kg/kg of dry air. Therefore the
mass of water vapour in the air per kg of fuel = 0.0081 × 8.67 = 0.07 kg.

(e) The water vapour in the gaseous products can be found from a hydrogen
balance.
Basis: 1 kg of fuel.
    H_2O entering with air   = 0.07 kg
    H_2O in fuel   = 0.10 kg
    H_2O from combustion of H_2 = 0.03 × 9 = 0.27 kg
                                    Total = 0.44 kg

Mass balance summary

	Reactants			Products	
Fuel	1.00 kg		Dry gases	9.26 kg
Dry air	8.67 kg		Moisture	0.44 kg
Moisture	0.07 kg		Refuse	0.22 kg
	9.74 kg			9.92 kg

The degree of balance obtained is an indication of the accuracy of the analyses
of fuel and products of combustion.

15.4 First Law applied to combustion processes

The First Law of Thermodynamics applies to any system, and the non-flow and
steady-flow energy equations deduced from this law must be applicable to
systems undergoing combustion processes. Before these equations can be used,
however, data must be available from which we can find the change of internal
energy or enthalpy when the chemical composition of the system changes as
well as the thermodynamic properties. As we shall see, we shall need to develop
two new concepts for this purpose, namely *internal energy of combustion* and
enthalpy of combustion. To develop these concepts we shall consider a hypothetical
sequence of processes undergone by a stoichiometric mixture of a fuel and air
which involves a chemical reaction going to completion. Although we shall
have combustion in mind, the ideas apply to any chemical reaction. Let us first
consider the change of internal energy.

15.4.1 Internal energy of combustion $\Delta \tilde{u}_0^{\ominus}$

Since the internal energy is a function of state, a change of internal energy is independent of the path of the process. Consider a non-flow combustion process, starting with a stoichiometric mixture of the fuel and air in an arbitrary state (p_1, T_1) and ending with the products in another arbitrary state (p_2, T_2). The process can conveniently be regarded as consisting of three successive processes via intermediate reference or so-called *standard states*, as shown in Fig. 15.5. The reactants are brought to a standard state (p_0, T_0) by some process a–b not involving a chemical reaction; the reaction b–c is then brought about in such a way that the products are at the standard state (p_0, T_0); and finally the products are brought to the final state (p_2, T_2) by some process c–d. We may write

$$(U_{P2} - U_{R1}) = (U_{P2} - U_{P0}) + (U_{P0} - U_{R0}) + (U_{R0} - U_{R1}) \qquad (15.8)$$

where subscripts R and P refer to reactants and products respectively, and subscripts 1 and 2 refer to the initial and final states. The first and third terms on the right-hand side represent changes of internal energy in processes not involving a chemical reaction, which can be evaluated by the methods applying to mixtures presented in Chapter 14. The middle term has to be obtained from additional experimental information because it involves a chemical reaction. However, by choosing a path which always involves the same pair of standard states at (p_0, T_0), only one piece of information is required for any given chemical reaction.

The standard pressure p_0 agreed by international convention is $p^{\ominus} = 1$ bar, the superscript $\ominus$ denoting this reference pressure. The corresponding difference in internal energy, denoted by $\Delta U_0^{\ominus}$, is equal to

$$\Delta U_0^{\ominus} = U_{P0}^{\ominus} - U_{R0}^{\ominus}$$

where the superscript $\ominus$ refers to $p^{\ominus}$ and the subscript 0 to the standard temperature T_0. Again by international agreement, T_0 is chosen to be $298.15 \text{ K} = 25\,^{\circ}\text{C}$. Furthermore, it is usual to associate $\Delta U_0^{\ominus}$ with the combustion of 1 kmol of fuel and to use the molar symbol $\Delta \tilde{u}_0^{\ominus}$. This is the quantity called the *internal energy of combustion*.

Two important points must be noted here. First, the volume V_0 at state c is not necessarily equal to the volume V_0 at state b. From the discussion in section 15.2 it should be clear that only when the amount-of-substance of the *gaseous* products in state c, n_P, is equal to that of the *gaseous* reactants in state b, n_R,

Fig. 15.5
Imaginary path linking the end states of a combustion process

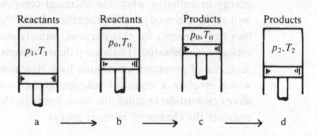

are the volumes equal (as they are in the reaction of equation (15.4) and are not in that of equation (15.7)). This point is of some importance because of the way in which $\Delta \tilde{u}_0^{\ominus}$ is determined experimentally for solid and liquid fuels, a problem discussed more fully in section 15.5. Here it suffices to say that $\Delta \tilde{u}_0^{\ominus}$ is deduced from the heat Q released in a constant volume process, and that the magnitude of Q is very nearly equal to the magnitude of $\Delta \tilde{u}_0^{\ominus}$.

The second point to be made is that to return the system to its original temperature T_0 after an exothermic reaction, as combustion is, some heat must be transferred to the surroundings. Q is thus negative, and it must be concluded that there has been a reduction of internal energy of the system even though the temperature is the same for the reactants and the products. The explanation is that each molecule possesses potential energy stored in the bonds between the constituent atoms, and this energy—which we may term *chemical energy*—is smaller for the molecules of the products than it is for the molecules of the reactants. In the process b–c this energy is normally released to the surroundings as heat (although a small quantity could be transferred as work if $V_{0b} \neq V_{0c}$). It follows that for an exothermic reaction $\Delta \tilde{u}_0^{\ominus}$ must be a negative quantity.

Let us now rewrite equation (15.8) for the molar quantity of the fuel involved, namely

$$(U_{P2} - U_{R1}) = (U_{P2} - U_{P0}) + \Delta \tilde{u}_0^{\ominus} + (U_{R0} - U_{R1}) \tag{15.9}$$

where the first and third terms on the right-hand side relate to quantities associated with 1 kmol of fuel reacting. In combustion processes the mixtures of reactants and products normally consist of gases and vapours at low pressure which can be assumed to behave as perfect gases, and possibly some liquid and solid substances. In all such cases the internal energy can be taken as a function only of temperature, so that subscripts 0, 1 and 2 in equation (15.9) can be taken to refer to T_0, T_1 and T_2. It has also been found that at normal pressures $\Delta \tilde{u}_0^{\ominus}$, though it depends on the choice of T_0, depends only insignificantly on $p^{\ominus}$. Therefore we can often dispense in practice with the superscript $\ominus$, and frequently there is no need to refer to pressure at all when applying equation (15.9). (Important exceptions are dealt with in sections 15.7 and 15.8.)

Using known u or c_v data, and assuming that no changes of phase occur during the processes a–b and c–d, the first and third terms on the right-hand side of equation (15.9) can therefore be found from an appropriate choice of the following equations:

$$U_{P2} - U_{P0} = \sum_P n_i(\tilde{u}_{i2} - \tilde{u}_{i0}) = \sum_P n_i \tilde{c}_{vi}(T_2 - T_0)$$

$$\text{or} \quad = \sum_P m_i(u_{i2} - u_{i0}) = \sum_P m_i c_{vi}(T_2 - T_0)$$

$$U_{R0} - U_{R1} = \sum_R n_i(\tilde{u}_{i0} - \tilde{u}_{i1}) = \sum_R n_i \tilde{c}_{vi}(T_0 - T_1)$$

$$\text{or} \quad = \sum_R m_i(u_{i0} - u_{i1}) = \sum_R m_i c_{vi}(T_0 - T_1)$$

$$\tag{15.9a}$$

335

Here n_i and m_i are the amount-of-substance and the mass of constituent i (per kmol of fuel reacting), and $\tilde{c}_{vi}$ and c_{vi} are its molar and specific heat capacities. If any constituent undergoes a change of phase in the temperature range $T_1 \rightarrow T_0$ or $T_0 \rightarrow T_2$, the U_{fg} data must also be known and included in the summation.

15.4.2 Enthalpy of combustion and its relation to $\Delta \tilde{u}_0^\ominus$

Considerations similar to those raised in relation to internal energy in the previous subsection also apply when establishing the change of enthalpy between reactants in state 1 and products in state 2. Thus the change of enthalpy can be broken down into three steps:

$$(H_{P2} - H_{R1}) = (H_{P2} - H_{P0}) + \Delta \tilde{h}_0^\ominus + (H_{R0} - H_{R1}) \qquad (15.10)$$

This equation is equivalent to (15.9), i.e. it applies to 1 kmol of fuel. The *enthalpy of combustion* $\Delta \tilde{h}_0^\ominus$ is explicitly given by

$$\Delta \tilde{h}_0^\ominus = (H_P \text{ at } p^\ominus, T_0) - (H_R \text{ at } p^\ominus, T_0)$$

As with $\Delta \tilde{u}_0^\ominus$, $\Delta \tilde{h}_0^\ominus$ is only very slightly dependent on the choice of the standard pressure, and in practice the superscript $\ominus$ can often be omitted: *this we will do until the end of section 15.6.* The standard temperature T_0 is, as before, $298.15 \text{ K} = 25\,^\circ\text{C}$. The first and third terms in equation (15.10) can be calculated from one pair of equations below, the choice depending upon what data are available:

$$H_{P2} - H_{P0} = \sum_P n_i(\tilde{h}_{i2} - \tilde{h}_{i0}) = \sum_P n_i \tilde{c}_{pi}(T_2 - T_0)$$

$$\text{or} \qquad = \sum_P m_i(h_{i2} - h_{i0}) = \sum_P m_i c_{pi}(T_2 - T_0)$$

$$\qquad\qquad\qquad\qquad\qquad\qquad\qquad\qquad\qquad (15.10a)$$

$$H_{R0} - H_{R1} = \sum_R n_i(\tilde{h}_{i0} - \tilde{h}_{i1}) = \sum_R n_i \tilde{c}_{pi}(T_0 - T_1)$$

$$\text{or} \qquad = \sum_R m_i(h_{i0} - h_{i1}) = \sum_R m_i c_{pi}(T_0 - T_1)$$

The set of equations (15.10a) is equivalent to that of (15.9a).

Direct experimental determination of $\Delta \tilde{h}_0$ is carried out in a steady-flow gas calorimeter, which is described briefly in section 15.5. When quoting values of $\Delta \tilde{u}_0$ or $\Delta \tilde{h}_0$, it is necessary to specify the phase of any individual reactant or product which may be in doubt. The magnitude of $\Delta \tilde{h}_0$ for a liquid hydrocarbon, for example, is less than the magnitude for the same hydrocarbon in gaseous form; and it is less by an amount equal to the latent enthalpy of vaporisation at the standard temperature T_0. Or to take another example, when the fuel contains hydrogen, the resulting H_2O in the products may be in the vapour or the liquid phase. This point will be considered again in the next section. The conventional way of conveying the data is to give the combustion equation to which the value of $\Delta \tilde{u}_0$ or $\Delta \tilde{h}_0$ is applicable. For example, the enthalpy of combustion at the standard temperature $T_0 = 25\,^\circ\text{C}$ for hydrogen burning to water vapour is

$$H_2 + \tfrac{1}{2}O_2 \rightarrow H_2O(\text{vap}); \quad \Delta \tilde{h}_0 = -241\,830 \text{ kJ/kmol of } H_2$$

It may sometimes be more convenient to work in terms of mass units, and in such cases we find Δu_0 and Δh_0 are quoted per unit mass of fuel. Taking the exact value for molar mass of H_2, $\tilde{m} = 2.016$ kg/kmol, then for the above reaction $\Delta h_0 = -119\,960$ kJ/kg of H_2.

It is usual to make direct experimental determinations of $\Delta \tilde{u}_0$ for solid and liquid fuels, and of $\Delta \tilde{h}_0$ for gaseous fuels. Once either $\Delta \tilde{u}_0$ or $\Delta \tilde{h}_0$ has been determined experimentally, the other quantity can be calculated by making use of the following relation:

$$\Delta \tilde{h}_0 = H_{P0} - H_{R0} = (U_{P0} + p_{P0} V_{P0}) - (U_{R0} + p_{R0} V_{R0})$$

$$= \Delta \tilde{u}_0 + (p V_{P0} - p V_{R0})$$

For gaseous reactants and products we can write $pV = n\tilde{R}T$, and for solid and liquid constituents the pV terms are negligible compared with the internal energy term. The relation between $\Delta \tilde{h}_0$ and $\Delta \tilde{u}_0$ can therefore be written as

$$\Delta \tilde{h}_0 = \Delta \tilde{u}_0 + \tilde{R} T_0 (n_P - n_R)_{\text{gas}} \tag{15.11}$$

where n_R and n_P are the amounts-of-substance of *gaseous* reactants and products respectively. It follows that when n_R for gaseous reactants is equal to n_P for the gaseous products, then $\Delta \tilde{u}_0$ and $\Delta \tilde{h}_0$ are equal. For most fuels the difference is quite small, as will be shown in the particular case dealt with in Example 15.8.

It is evident from equations (15.9) and (15.10) that, in addition to values of $\Delta \tilde{u}_0$ or $\Delta \tilde{h}_0$, we require a knowledge of the internal energies or enthalpies of the various reactants and products, or of heat capacities, as functions of temperature. Ref. 17 contains tables of molar internal energies and enthalpies, namely values of $\tilde{u}$ and $\tilde{h}$, for most common gases and a representative selection of hydrocarbon fuels. These are tabulated against absolute temperature, and their use will be illustrated in Example 15.7. Ref. 17 also contains values of c_p tabulated against absolute temperature, and their use will be illustrated in Example 15.6. Attention is drawn to the discussion in section 8.5.3 of the evaluation of mean specific heat capacities over a range of temperature T_1 to T_2. There it is explained that using a value at, say, $\tfrac{1}{2}(T_1 + T_2)$ will lead to inaccuracies unless c_p varies linearly with T. Since the temperature ranges met with in combustion processes are often large, c_p tables used in this way can be much less accurate than $\tilde{u}$ and $\tilde{h}$ tables.

It is worth emphasising that in tables of internal energy or enthalpy, one or other value must be put equal to zero at some arbitrary value of temperature. In Ref. 17 it is the enthalpy which is put equal to zero at $T_0 = 298.15$ K. The tables can be used to find changes of internal energy and enthalpy only along paths which do *not* involve a chemical reaction, because no account is taken of the particular form of internal energy which changes when a reaction occurs.

Example 15.6 When all the products of the gaseous hydrocarbon engine (C_2H_6) are in the gaseous phase, the enthalpy of combustion at 25 °C is $-47\,590$ kJ/kg. Find (a) the corresponding internal energy of combustion, and (b) the enthalpy of combustion at 540 °C.

Calculate the heat transferred when 0.2 kg of ethane is burnt at constant pressure in a cylinder containing 4.0 kg of dry air, the temperature of the reactants and products being 40 °C and 54 °C respectively.

The relevant mean specific heat capacities at constant pressure, for the range 25 °C to 540 °C, are found from Ref. 17 at the mean temperature 555 K to be

C_2H_6 2.800; O_2 0.989; CO_2 1.049; H_2O(vap) 1.987; N_2 1.066 kJ/kg K

And for the range 25 °C to 40 °C,

C_2H_6 1.788; O_2 0.919; N_2 1.040 kJ/kg K

(a) *Internal energy of combustion at 25 °C*
The stoichiometric combustion equation is

$$C_2H_6 + 3\tfrac{1}{2}O_2 \rightarrow 2CO_2 + 3H_2O(\text{vap})$$

There are $4\tfrac{1}{2}$ kmol of reactants and 5 kmol of products per kmol of ethane, so that in equation (15.11) we have

$$(n_P - n_R) = \tfrac{1}{2} \text{ kmol}$$

Since Δh_{25} is given in kJ/kg, and 1 kmol of ethane is equivalent to a mass of 30 kg,

$$\Delta u_{25} = -47\,590 - \frac{8.3145 \times 298}{2 \times 30} = -47\,630 \text{ kJ/kg of } C_2H_6$$

(b) *Enthalpy of combustion at 540 °C*
From equation (15.10) we have

$$\Delta h_{540} = (H_{P540} - H_{R540})$$

$$= (H_{P540} - H_{P25}) + \Delta h_{25} + (H_{R25} - H_{R540})$$

In terms of mass, the combustion equation is

$$30 \text{ kg } C_2H_6 + 112 \text{ kg } O_2 \rightarrow 88 \text{ kg } CO_2 + 54 \text{ kg } H_2O$$

On the basis of 1 kg of C_2H_6, we have

$$(H_{P540} - H_{P25}) = \sum_P m_i c_{pi}(540 - 25)$$

$$= \frac{515}{30}\{(88 \times 1.049) + (54 \times 1.987)\}$$

$$= 3247 \text{ kJ/kg of } C_2H_6$$

Similarly,

$$(H_{R25} - H_{R540}) = \sum_R m_i c_{pi}(25 - 540)$$

$$= -\frac{515}{30}\{(30 \times 2.80) + (112 \times 0.989)\}$$

$$= -3345 \text{ kJ/kg of } C_2H_6$$

$$\Delta h_{540} = 3427 - 47590 - 3345 = -47510 \text{ kJ/kg of } C_2H_6$$

From (a) and (b) it should be noted that *the difference between Δh_0 and Δu_0 is small, and that the values are not greatly affected by a change of reference temperature.*

Constant pressure combustion

In the constant pressure combustion, the products are not returned to the initial temperature and we must take account of the change in enthalpy of the non-reacting substances. The heat transferred is equal to the change of enthalpy if the expansion work can be regarded as $\int p\,dv$. Therefore

$$Q = (H_{P540} - H_{R40})$$
$$= (H_{P540} - H_{P25}) + \Delta h_{25} + (H_{R25} - H_{R40})$$

The stoichiometric combustion equation for 0.2 kg of ethane is

$$0.2 \text{ kg } C_2H_6 + 0.747 \text{ kg } O_2 \rightarrow 0.587 \text{ kg } CO_2 + 0.360 \text{ kg } H_2O$$

But 4 kg of air are provided, consisting of

$$(4 \times 0.233 \text{ kg } O_2) + (4 \times 0.767 \text{ kg } N_2) = 0.932 \text{ kg } O_2 + 3.068 \text{ kg } N_2$$

Evidently there is some excess air, and the combustion equation for the specified mixture is

$$0.2 \text{ kg } C_2H_6 + 0.932 \text{ kg } O_2 + 3.068 \text{ kg } N_2 \rightarrow$$

$$0.587 \text{ kg } CO_2 + 0.360 \text{ kg } H_2O + 0.185 \text{ kg } O_2 + 3.068 \text{ kg } N_2$$

On the basis of 0.2 kg of ethane:

$$(H_{P540} - H_{P25}) = 515\{(0.587 \times 1.049) + (0.360 \times 1.987)$$

$$+ (0.185 \times 0.989) + (3.068 \times 1.066)\} = 2464 \text{ kJ}$$

$$(H_{R25} - H_{R40}) = -15\{(0.2 \times 1.788) + (0.932 \times 0.919)$$

$$+ (3.068 \times 1.040)\} = -66 \text{ kJ}$$

Therefore

$$Q = 2464 - (0.2 \times 47590) - 66 = -7120 \text{ kJ}$$

15.4.3 U–T and H–T diagrams

We have already noted that, during changes of state involving no chemical reaction (see the first and third terms on the right-hand sides of equations (15.9) and (15.10)), the internal energies and enthalpies can be taken as functions of temperature only. Under these circumstances, U and H for the reactants and products can be plotted as *single lines* on $U–T$ and $H–T$ diagrams as shown in Fig. 15.6.* The only constraint is that the two lines must be separated by the correct amount. The vertical separation must, at T_0, be equal to $\Delta \tilde{u}_0$ in Fig. 15.6a and to $\Delta \tilde{h}_0$ in Fig. 15.6b. For an exothermic reaction the products line must lie below the reactants line. The location of the two lines on the graph is otherwise arbitrary, because the datum state for either reactants or products can be chosen arbitrarily.

During any combustion process 1–2 in a closed system, both work and heat may be transferred across the boundary in accordance with the non-flow energy equation

$$Q + W = U_{P2} - U_{R1}$$

There are two combustion processes of special interest. One is often referred to as the *calorimeter process*, 1–3, carried out at constant volume and with $T_3 = T_1$. In this process the work is zero and the heat transferred is effectively equal to the internal energy of combustion at T_1. This process yields the maximum possible transfer of energy to surroundings at T_1. The second process of special interest is *adiabatic combustion* at constant volume. Since both the heat and work transfers are zero, the internal energy remains constant. There is merely a redistribution of internal energy resulting in a rise of temperature, i.e. we may say that *chemical energy* is transformed into *sensible internal energy*. This process, 1–4 in Fig. 15.6a, results in the maximum possible rise of temperature for any given air/fuel ratio.

Fig. 15.6
U–T and *H–T* diagrams
for combustion processes

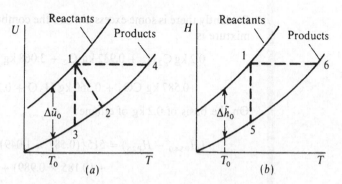

---

* One reservation must be mentioned: if the mixtures of reactants and products contain constituents that can change phase, then the ratio of vapour to liquid of such constituents must not change along 1–0 or 0–2. Otherwise a family of lines would be required to describe the $U–T$ or $H–T$ relations.

When considering steady-flow processes, it is appropriate to depict these on an $H-T$ diagram (Fig. 15.6b). The steady-flow calorimeter process, in which the heat transferred is equal to the enthalpy of combustion, is represented by 1–5. Steady-flow adiabatic combustion, with zero work and no change of kinetic energy, is represented by 1–6; this process yields the maximum possible temperature rise for steady-flow combustion.

In solving combustion problems, great care must always be taken with signs. Intelligent use of the diagrams, as illustrated in Example 15.7, can save one from this source of error.

Example 15.7   Liquid heptane (C_7H_{16}) has an enthalpy of combustion of $-4\,465\,300\ \text{kJ}/$ kmol at 298 K when the water in the products is in the vapour phase. This fuel is to be burnt adiabatically in a steady-stream of air in stoichiometric proportions. If the initial temperature of the fuel and air is 288 K, estimate the temperature of the products. For liquid heptane $\tilde{c}_p = 230\ \text{kJ}/\text{kmol K}$.

The stoichiometric combustion equation, including the nitrogen introduced with the air, is

$$C_7H_{16}(\text{liq}) + 11O_2 + \frac{79}{21}11N_2 \rightarrow 7CO_2 + 8H_2O(\text{vap}) + \frac{79}{21}11N_2$$

The steady-flow energy equation reduces to $H_{PT} - H_{R288} = 0$, where T refers to the products' absolute temperature. Expanding the equation, following the path of calculation indicated in Fig. 15.7,

$$(H_{PT} - H_{P298}) + \Delta\tilde{h}_{298} + (H_{R298} - H_{R288}) = 0$$

or

$$\sum_P n_i(\tilde{h}_{PT} - \tilde{h}_{P298}) + \Delta\tilde{h}_{298} + \sum_R n_i(\tilde{h}_{R298} - \tilde{h}_{R288}) = 0$$

The evaluation of this equation involves successive approximations because the values of $\tilde{h}_{PT}$ of the constituents of the products depend upon the unknown temperature T. Guessing initially that $T = 2200$ K, it is possible to extract the

Fig. 15.7
Path of
calculation

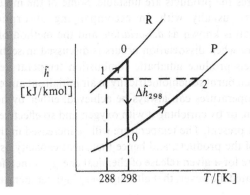

following table of molar enthalpies $\bar{h}/[\text{kJ/kmol}]$ from Ref. 17:

	O_2	N_2	CO_2	$H_2O(\text{vap})$
$T_1 = 288$ K	-296	-296	-353	-339
$T_0 = 298$ K	0	0	0	0
$T = 2200$ K	66 802	63 371	103 570	83 036

Hence we can write, per kmol of C_7H_{16},

$$7(103\,570 - 0) + 8(83\,036 - 0) + \frac{79}{21}11(63\,371 - 0)$$

$$+ (-4\,465\,300) + \{1 \times 230(298 - 288)\}$$

$$+ 11\{0 - (-296)\} + \frac{79}{21}11\{0 - (-296)\} = -435\,865\,\text{kJ}$$

Clearly, the guess $T = 2200$ K was not correct, because the result is not equal to zero. Repeating with enthalpy values for $T = 2400$ K, the imbalance in the enthalpy equation becomes $+35\,473$ kJ. Linear interpolation between the imbalance terms of $-435\,865$ kJ and $+35\,473$ kJ yields a value for T of 2385 K. The temperature intervals in the molar tables of Ref. 17 are 200 K, while those in the original *Janaf Thermochemical Tables* [Ref. 37] from which they were abstracted are 100 K. The denser table would yield a somewhat more accurate result when the variation of $\bar{h}$ with T is not linear in the relevant temperature interval.

The adiabatic temperature rise can also be obtained directly from special charts, such as the *Diagram of Temperature Rise versus Fuel–Air Ratio* published in association with Ref. 17. This chart provides adiabatic temperature rises for any initial temperature of reactants and any air/fuel ratio. However, it applies strictly for only one particular fuel, in this instance one with a mass ratio of hydrogen to carbon of 13.92/86.08 and an enthalpy of reaction of $-43\,100$ kJ/kg.

The actual temperature of the products from the adiabatic combustion of a stoichiometric mixture would not be as high as the value calculated in the manner of the previous example. The combustion would in fact be incomplete, partly for the reasons already given in section 15.2, and partly because at high temperatures the products are unstable. Some of the molecules split into their constituents, usually with an accompanying absorption of energy. This phenomenon is known as *dissociation*, and the method of estimating the final temperature when dissociation occurs is discussed in section 15.7.

Most fuels produce adiabatic combustion temperatures between 2200 and 2700 K when burnt stoichiometrically in air initially at atmospheric temperature. Higher temperatures can always be achieved, either by heating the air before combustion, or by enriching it with oxygen and so effectively reducing the mass of nitrogen present. The temperature will be increased in the latter case because the mass of the products, and hence their heat capacity, is reduced. The rise in temperature for a given release of chemical energy is therefore greater. It should be appreciated, however, that although very high temperatures may be desirable from a thermodynamic point of view, they cannot always be employed in power plant. In a gas turbine, for example, where the highly stressed parts of the turbine are in a continuous stream of hot gaseous products, serious overheating would occur unless a large quantity of excess air were provided to reduce the temperature at exit from the combustion chamber.

15.5 Experimental determination of $\Delta \tilde{u}_0$ and $\Delta \tilde{h}_0$ and calorific values

For *solid* and *liquid* fuels it is the value of $\Delta \tilde{u}_0$ with water in the products in the liquid phase which is found from experiments: we shall denote the value by $\Delta \tilde{u}_0(\text{liq})$. Values of $\Delta \tilde{u}_0$ with water in the vapour phase, namely $\Delta \tilde{u}_0(\text{vap})$, and corresponding values of $\Delta \tilde{h}_0$ with water in either liquid or vapour phase, must be found by calculation from the value of $\Delta \tilde{u}_0(\text{liq})$ and from the ultimate analysis of the fuel. Thus

$$\Delta \tilde{u}_0(\text{vap}) - \Delta \tilde{u}_0(\text{liq}) = n_{\text{H}_2\text{O}} \tilde{u}_{\text{fg}} \qquad (15.12\text{a})$$

$$\Delta \tilde{h}_0(\text{vap}) - \Delta \tilde{h}_0(\text{liq}) = n_{\text{H}_2\text{O}} \tilde{h}_{\text{fg}} \qquad (15.12\text{b})$$

The amount-of-substance of H_2O formed per unit amount-of-substance of fuel, $n_{\text{H}_2\text{O}}$, can be deduced from the fuel analysis. The internal energy and enthalpy of evaporation, $\tilde{u}_{\text{fg}}$ and $\tilde{h}_{\text{fg}}$, must be taken at the standard temperature of 25 °C. The relation between $\Delta \tilde{u}_0$ and $\Delta \tilde{h}_0$ has already been derived in section 15.4.2, equation (15.11). Calculations of the kind described above are illustrated, in mass units, in Example 15.8.

The experimental value of $\Delta \tilde{u}_0$ is found by burning a measured quantity of fuel in a *bomb calorimeter*. This consists essentially of a gas-tight steel vessel, the 'bomb', which is immersed in a conventional water calorimeter. The 'water equivalent' of the calorimeter and bomb is found by conducting a preliminary experiment using an electrical resistance method of heating (or benzoic acid, whose value of $\Delta \tilde{u}_0(\text{liq})$ is accurately known). The bomb is then charged with the fuel sample, and with oxygen at a high pressure to ensure complete combustion. A small quantity of water is placed in the bomb initially to saturate the volume, and any water formed by the combustion will therefore condense. Thus the value obtained will be that with water in the liquid phase. After ignition, the final steady temperature of the calorimeter is noted; it is arranged to be not more than about 3 K above an initial temperature of about 23.5 °C. Although the temperature of the products is not exactly equal to that of the reactants, or equal to the standard temperature of 25 °C, the value of $\Delta \tilde{u}_0$ so obtained should be very close to that demanded by the definition. Example 15.6 showed that a large change in T_0 had a small effect on $\Delta \tilde{h}_0$, and this is true also of $\Delta \tilde{u}_0$.

The concept of internal energy of combustion was explained and defined in section 15.4 with the help of a 'paper' experiment involving a stoichiometric mixture of fuel and *air*. In the experiment just described pure oxygen is supplied, and moreover in excess of stoichiometric requirements. Does this matter? In principle it does not, because the initial and final temperatures are ideally the same and there will therefore be no net change in internal energy of any non-reacting substance present. For example, excess oxygen and water in the bomb should have no effect other than to ensure complete combustion of the fuel and complete condensation of the water vapour in the products respectively. The presence (or in this case absence) of inert constituents of air should likewise have no effect on $\Delta \tilde{u}_0(\text{liq})$. Because in the actual experiment the temperature of the products is not exactly equal to that of the reactants, corrections have to be applied when obtaining precise values of $\Delta \tilde{u}_0(\text{liq})$ from the experimental results.

Other corrections may also have to be made. For example, there may be heat released or absorbed when some of the gaseous products dissolve in the water in the bomb. A more fundamental correction, not necessarily larger in magnitude, arises from the fact that the pressure in the reaction vessel is not the standard pressure $p^{\ominus}$. We are seeking an internal energy change

$$(\tilde{u} \text{ at } p^{\ominus}, T_0)_\text{P} - (\tilde{u} \text{ at } p^{\ominus}, T_0)_\text{R}$$

while what we obtain from experiment, after all the above corrections have been applied, is

$$(\tilde{u} \text{ at } p_1, T_0)_\text{P} - (\tilde{u} \text{ at } p_2, T_0)_\text{R}$$

Here p_1 is the pressure to which the bomb is charged, and this is very high; so too is the final pressure p_2. In fact, $p_2 = p_1(n_\text{P}/n_\text{R})_\text{gas}$. The corrections are of two kinds: those due to departures from perfect gas behaviour at high pressure, and those due to any difference between n_P and n_R. (The reader should satisfy himself that the second correction, obtainable from equation (9.13), is equal to $n_\text{P} \tilde{R} T_0 \ln(n_\text{P}/n_\text{R})$.

For gaseous fuels it is the value of $\Delta \tilde{h}_0(\text{liq})$ which is found from experiment; $\Delta \tilde{u}_0(\text{liq})$, $\Delta \tilde{u}_0(\text{vap})$ and $\Delta \tilde{h}_0(\text{vap})$ should be found by calculation from $\Delta \tilde{h}_0(\text{liq})$ and the ultimate analysis of the fuel. The value of $\Delta \tilde{h}_0(\text{liq})$ is most conveniently measured by burning a mixed stream of gas and air at atmospheric pressure and temperature, under steady-flow conditions in a gas calorimeter. The gas–air mixture is saturated with water vapour. After burning, the hot products of combustion flow over cooling coils through which water flows steadily in the opposite direction. With this counter-flow arrangement the products leave the calorimeter at approximately atmospheric temperature and all the water vapour produced is condensed. An approximate value of $\Delta \tilde{h}_0(\text{liq})$ of the gas can be readily calculated from the mass flow and temperature rise of the cooling water. Certain corrections have to be applied to the results obtained, as had to be done to the results for $\Delta \tilde{u}_0(\text{liq})$ from the bomb calorimeter. However, because the experiment is carried out at a pressure approximately equal to $p^{\ominus}$, and the pressures at inlet to and exit from the calorimeter are very nearly equal, corrections for effects due to high pressure and changes in amounts-of-substance do not arise.

Example 15.8 The value of $\Delta u_0(\text{liq})$ for liquid kerosene was found by experiment to be $-46\,890 \text{ kJ/kg}$. The ultimate analysis of the kerosene was 86 per cent carbon and 14 per cent hydrogen. Calculate the value of $\Delta u_0(\text{vap})$, and the corresponding values of $\Delta h_0(\text{liq})$ and $\Delta h_0(\text{vap})$.

First, 1 kg of fuel produces $0.86(44/12) = 3.15$ kg of CO_2
and $0.14(18/2) = 1.26$ kg of H_2O.
At 25 °C, $u_{fg} = 2304$ kJ/kg and $h_{fg} = 2442$ kJ/kg. So that

$$\Delta u_0(\text{vap}) = \Delta u_0(\text{liq}) + m_{H_2O} u_{fg}$$
$$= -46\,890 + (1.26 \times 2304) = -43\,987 \text{ kJ/kg}$$

The combustion equation can be written as

$$1 \text{ kg fuel} + 3.41 \text{ kg } O_2 \rightarrow 1.26 \text{ kg } H_2O + 3.15 \text{ kg } CO_2$$

The relation between $\Delta h_0(\text{liq})$ and $\Delta u_0(\text{liq})$ can be obtained from equation (15.11). Remembering that only gaseous reactants and products should be included, and given that the fuel is in liquid form, the equation becomes

$$\Delta h_0(\text{liq}) = \Delta u_0(\text{liq}) + \tilde{R}T_0 \left(\sum_P \frac{m_i}{\tilde{m}_i} - \sum_R \frac{m_i}{\tilde{m}_i} \right)_{\text{gas}}$$

$$= -46\,890 + \left\{ 8.3145 \times 298.15 \left(\frac{3.15}{44} - \frac{3.41}{32} \right) \right\}$$

$$= -46\,890 - 87 = -46\,977 \text{ kJ/kg}$$

$$\Delta h_0(\text{vap}) = \Delta h_0(\text{liq}) + m_{H_2O} h_{fg}$$

$$= -46\,977 + (1.26 \times 2442) = -43\,900 \text{ kJ/kg}$$

As a check, we can find $\Delta h_0(\text{vap})$ from $\Delta u_0(\text{vap})$ using equation (15.11):

$$\Delta h_0(\text{vap}) = \Delta u_0(\text{vap}) + \tilde{R}T_0 \left(\sum_P \frac{m_i}{\tilde{m}_i} - \sum_R \frac{m_i}{\tilde{m}_i} \right)_{\text{gas}}$$

$$= -43\,987 + \left\{ 8.3145 \times 298.15 \left(\frac{1.26}{18} + \frac{3.15}{44} - \frac{3.41}{32} \right) \right\}$$

$$= -43\,900 \text{ kJ/kg}$$

Note that the difference between $\Delta u_0(\text{liq})$ and $\Delta u_0(\text{vap})$ is 6.2 per cent, whereas $\Delta u_0(\text{liq})$ and $\Delta h_0(\text{liq})$ differ only by about 0.2 per cent. In any applications of combustion data, it is evidently more important to decide whether the H_2O in the products should be regarded as liquid or vapour than whether Δu_0 or Δh_0 data are appropriate.

When dealing with energy transfers in combustion processes, engineers have in the past commonly related these transfers to some *calorific value* of the fuel rather than to the properties Δu_0 and Δh_0. Calorific values refer directly to quantities of heat liberated when unit mass of fuel is burnt completely in a calorimeter under specified conditions. Because calorific values are *defined* in terms of quantities of heat, the definition must specify not merely the end states but also the details of the process connecting these end states. Provided standardised equipment is used and the specific conditions are adhered to, the results obtained will be accurately reproducible. The fact that the quantities are not identical with the more rigorously defined properties Δu_0 and Δh_0 is not important for such purposes as comparing the efficiency of power plant, or meeting statutory requirements for the heating value of a gas supply.

The four calorific values that have been in common use are as follows, together with the values of Δu_0 and Δh_0 to which they correspond most closely:

Gross (or higher) calorific value at constant volume: $\quad Q_{gr,v} \equiv -\Delta u_{25}(\text{liq})$

Net (or lower) calorific value at constant volume: $\quad Q_{net,v} \equiv -\Delta u_{25}(\text{vap})$

Gross (or higher) calorific value at constant pressure: $\quad Q_{gr,p} \equiv -\Delta h_{25}(\text{liq})$

Net (or lower) calorific value at constant pressure: $\quad Q_{net,p} \equiv -\Delta h_{25}(\text{vap})$

Two points should be noted. First, while values of Δu_0 and Δh_0 for an exothermic reaction in accord with our sign convention are negative numbers, calorific values are always quoted as positive numbers. Secondly, gross (or higher) and net (or lower) refer to the phase of H_2O in the products, the former to liquid and the latter to vapour.

15.6   Efficiency of power plant and of combustion processes

The cycle efficiency of a heat engine is calculated without reference to the source of heat. When considering the efficiency of the power plant as a whole, however, we are also concerned with the efficiency of the means of producing the heat, i.e. whether the fuel is in fact being completely burnt under the most advantageous conditions. The *overall thermal efficiency* of a power plant can be suitably defined as the ratio of the work produced to the latent energy in the fuel supplied. The question arises as to how this latent energy should be assessed.

Any power plant, considered as a whole, is an open system undergoing a steady-flow process—with air and fuel entering the system, and the products of combustion leaving it, at a steady rate. This is illustrated in Fig. 15.8a. The fuel and air enter at atmospheric temperature, and the largest quantity of energy that can be transferred to the surroundings will be produced if (a) the fuel is burnt completely, (b) the products leave at atmospheric temperature, and (c) any water in the products is in the liquid phase. The energy transferred under

Fig. 15.8
Schematic combustion
power plant

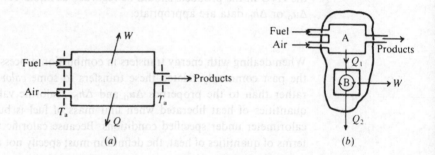

these conditions, per unit mass of fuel burnt, is $\Delta h_a^{atm}(liq)$, where 'a' and 'atm' refer to the ambient reference temperature and pressure respectively. To all intents and purposes $\Delta h_a^{atm}(liq) = \Delta h_0(liq)$. If $\Delta h_0(liq)$ is regarded as the effective latent energy in the fuel, the efficiency of the power plant is suitably defined by

$$\eta = \frac{W}{\Delta h_0(liq)} \qquad (15.13)$$

where W is the work transfer per unit mass of fuel.

Now the temperature of the products is never reduced to atmospheric temperature in practice, for this would entail an infinitely large heat exchange surface somewhere in the plant (e.g. in the economiser of a steam plant). Moreover, this condition is not even approached, if for no other reason than the undesirability of allowing water vapour to condense. Combustion products usually include a small quantity of sulphur dioxide which would dissolve in the water and form corrosive sulphuric acid (but note the reference to so-called 'condensing boilers' in section 11.6). Considerations of this type have led many engineers to prefer to define thermal efficiency in terms of $\Delta h_0(vap)$, i.e.

$$\eta = \frac{W}{\Delta h_0(vap)} \qquad (15.14)$$

This definition yields slightly higher values for the thermal efficiency because $\Delta h_0(vap)$ is smaller in magnitude than $\Delta h_0(liq)$.

It is clear that power plant efficiencies are process efficiencies and, like all such efficiencies, they are comparisons between an achieved result and some arbitrary standard. It is most important always to state clearly which standard, $\Delta h_0(liq)$ or $\Delta h_0(vap)$, is being used. A more rational definition of power plant efficiency is discussed in section 17.5, from which it is apparent that, of the two arbitrary definitions presented here, definition (15.14) is to be preferred.

It must be emphasised that the foregoing discussion applies equally to steam power plant and internal-combustion engines. For the former, Fig. 15.8a can be analysed further as in Fig. 15.8b; part A of the system is regarded as the boiler furnace and part B as the working fluid which is taken through a thermodynamic cycle. Most of the heat rejected Q_2 passes out in the condenser cooling water. When the combustion process itself can be isolated from the rest of the plant, as in a steam boiler or gas turbine combustion chamber, it is necessary to have some measure of its efficiency so that the performance of different combustion systems can be compared. Combustion efficiency is most generally defined as the fraction of the latent energy input which is effectively utilised in the desired manner. The detailed definition will depend upon the method of designating the latent energy input and the effectively used output.

In the case of a steam boiler, for example, the combustion is used to produce heat and so transform water into steam. The combustion efficiency can therefore be alternatively defined as

$$\eta = \frac{Q}{-\Delta h_0(liq)} \quad \text{or} \quad \frac{Q}{-\Delta h_0(vap)} \qquad (15.15)$$

where Q is the heat transferred to the water, i.e. the increase in enthalpy of the water per unit mass of fuel supplied.

To take a second example, the object of the adiabatic combustion in a gas turbine combustion chamber is to increase the *sensible* enthalpy of the fluid flowing through it—so that this can be used to produce work in the turbine. The efficiency may be defined, therefore, as the ratio of the actual increase of sensible enthalpy per kilogram of fuel to the increase obtained when each kilogram of fuel is burnt completely. The energy equation is

$$(H_{P2} - H_{R1}) = (H_{P2} - H_{P0}) + \Delta h_0 + (H_{R0} - H_{R1}) = 0$$

With complete combustion, the increase in sensible enthalpy is given by

$$(H_{P2} - H_{P0}) - (H_{R1} - H_{R0}) = -\Delta h_0$$

With incomplete combustion, the increase in sensible enthalpy will be

$$\{(H_{P2} - H_{P0}) - (H_{R1} - H_{R0})\}_{\text{actual}} = -\Delta h_0 - \sum_i m_i(-\Delta h_{0i})$$

The summation is of unburnt or partially burnt constituents; m_i is the mass of constituent i per unit mass of fuel, and Δh_{0i} is its enthalpy of combustion. The choice of reference temperature T_0 has little effect on the efficiency, but the phase of the H_2O in the products must be specified. The expression for combustion efficiency becomes

$$\eta = \frac{\{(H_{P2} - H_{P0}) - (H_{R1} - H_{R0})\}_{\text{actual}}}{-\Delta h_0} \tag{15.16}$$

The enthalpy of combustion can be taken as either $\Delta h_0(\text{liq})$ or $\Delta h_0(\text{vap})$ according to convention.

The numerator in equation (15.16) is best determined from the results of an experimental analysis of the products. A second definition of efficiency frequently employed is the fraction of the actual fuel used which would have been sufficient to achieve the actual products temperature with complete combustion. Further discussion of these and other ways of expressing gas turbine combustion efficiencies can be found in Ref. 26.

Example 15.9 Find the efficiency of the combustion process of Example 15.5 on the basis of $\Delta h_0(\text{vap})$ and the percentage of complete combustion attained. The following data can be assumed:

$$\Delta h_0(\text{vap}) \text{ of the coal} = -24\,490 \text{ kJ/kg}$$
$$\Delta h_0 \text{ of solid carbon} = -32\,790 \text{ kJ/kg}$$
$$\Delta h_0 \text{ of carbon monoxide} = -10\,110 \text{ kJ/kg}$$

The efficiency may be expressed by

$$\eta = \frac{-\Delta h_0(\text{vap}) - \sum m_i(-\Delta h_0)_i}{-\Delta h_0(\text{vap})}$$

From the solution of Example 15.5, the unburnt and partially burnt constituents in the products, per kg of coal burnt, are

0.17 kg of CO in the gaseous products

$0.4 \times 0.217 = 0.0868$ kg of C in the refuse

Therefore

$$\sum m_i(-\Delta h_0)_i = (0.17 \times 10\,110) + (0.0868 \times 32\,790) = 4565 \text{ kJ/kg}$$

$$\eta = \frac{24\,490 - 4565}{24\,490} = 0.814$$

15.7 Dissociation

It was pointed out in section 15.4 that the maximum temperature reached in an adiabatic combustion process is limited by the phenomenon of dissociation. Consider, for example, the reaction

$$CO + \tfrac{1}{2}O_2 \to CO_2$$

When it proceeds in the direction indicated by the arrow it is accompanied by a release of energy. The reaction can be made to proceed in the reverse direction, however, if sufficient energy is supplied to molecules of CO_2. Some of the CO_2 molecules in the combustion products do receive sufficient energy in collision for this to occur, i.e. some of the molecules undergo the reaction

$$CO_2 \to CO + \tfrac{1}{2}O_2$$

This possibility is symbolised by writing the equation as

$$CO + \tfrac{1}{2}O_2 \rightleftharpoons CO_2$$

The reversed reaction is accompanied by an absorption of energy, and it is termed an *endothermic* reaction. It is found that at any particular temperature and pressure the proportions of CO_2, CO and O_2 adjust themselves until the two reactions proceed at the same rate, i.e. until the number of CO_2 molecules being formed is equal to the number dissociating. A state of stable chemical equilibrium is then said to exist. The state of equilibrium is not a static one, because the two reactions are going on continuously and simultaneously. It is only at high temperatures, above about 1500 K, that a significant proportion of the CO_2 molecules must dissociate to provide an equilibrium mixture.

The preceding remarks apply equally to H_2O molecules in combustion products. It is now possible to appreciate why the adiabatic combustion temperature is less than that predicted by the simple calculation of Example 15.7. Evidently the products contain an equilibrium mixture of CO_2, CO and O_2, and an equilibrium mixture of H_2O, H_2 and O_2. The presence of CO and H_2 indicates that not all the chemical energy in the fuel is released. The question arises as to how the states of chemical equilibria can be predicted. We shall proceed to show that a condition for equilibrium can be deduced from the Second Law of Thermodynamics. The first step is to visualise how a thermodynamically reversible chemical reaction can be achieved, and the argument suggested by van't Hoff in 1887 will be used here.

15.7.1   The van't Hoff equilibrium box

Consider a stoichiometric reaction between CO and O_2, each initially at the standard pressure $p^\ominus$ and a temperature T, to form CO_2 at the same pressure and temperature. This reaction can be carried out in many ways. In the gas calorimeter, for example, all the energy released is transferred as heat and the reaction is irreversible. When the reaction is made reversible, however, we shall find that some of the energy is transferred as work. Fig. 15.9 illustrates one conceivable steady-flow open system in which the reaction can proceed reversibly. The reaction itself occurs in the reaction chamber, or 'equilibrium box', which contains CO_2, CO and O_2 in such proportions that the reactions

$$CO + \tfrac{1}{2}O_2 \rightarrow CO_2 \quad \text{and} \quad CO_2 \rightarrow CO + \tfrac{1}{2}O_2$$

are proceeding simultaneously at equal rates. The box is maintained at a constant temperature T by surrounding it with a reservoir at T. Any heat exchanges will therefore take place reversibly. The total pressure in the box may have any arbitrary value p, which may be greater or smaller than $p^\ominus$, determined by the total mass of gas present. The CO, O_2 and CO_2 enter or leave the box through semipermeable membranes, the mass flows at entry and exit being equal. If these mass transfers are to take place reversibly (see section 14.3), the pressure of each constituent outside the box must be equal to its partial pressure inside the box (i.e. p_{CO}, p_{O_2} or p_{CO_2}), and the temperature of each constituent outside the box must be equal to T. Since the pressure and temperature of the CO, O_2 and CO_2 are $p^\ominus$ and T at the boundary, reversible isothermal compressors and expanders must be included in the system to maintain the respective pressures at p_{CO}, p_{O_2} and p_{CO_2} outside the semipermeable membranes.

Imagine that CO and O_2 are transported slowly into the reaction box at the steady molar flow rates of $\dot{n}$ and $\dot{n}/2$ respectively, and that the reaction proceeds

Fig. 15.9
The van't Hoff equilibrium box

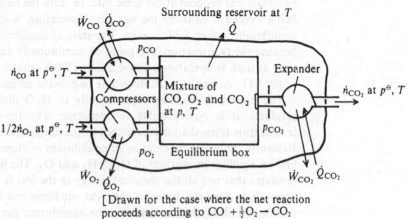

[Drawn for the case where the net reaction proceeds according to $CO + \tfrac{1}{2}O_2 \rightarrow CO_2$ and any partial pressure $> p^\ominus$]

in the normal direction. The equilibrium mixture will remain unchanged if CO_2 is discharged at the steady molar flow rate of $\dot{n}$. Only an infinitesimal change in the external conditions is needed to reverse the expanders and compressors and to cause the reaction to proceed in the opposite direction. All the quantities of heat and work transferred across the boundary then have the same magnitude but are reversed in sign. The whole isothermal steady-flow process can therefore be regarded as reversible.

We shall proceed to show that the power output from this hypothetical reversible plant is the maximum attainable from this chemical reaction in surroundings at the temperature T. In the course of so doing we shall find that the relative proportions of constituents in the equilibrium box, expressed in terms of mole fractions, depend upon a parameter K which is a function of T but not of p. For simplicity we shall assume here that the reaction involves only perfect gases, for which a mole fraction is proportional to the partial pressure, equation (14.17).

15.7.2 Maximum work of a chemical reaction and equilibrium constants

The rate of work transfer when a perfect gas undergoes a reversible isothermal steady-flow process is given by equation (10.6). When the gas flows at a molar rate of $\dot{n}$, it can be written as

$$\dot{W} = \dot{n}\tilde{R}T\ln\frac{p_2}{p_1}$$

The net power *output* from the system shown in Fig. 15.9 is therefore

$$|\dot{W}| = \dot{n}\tilde{R}T\left(\ln\frac{p_{CO_2}}{p^\ominus} + \ln\frac{p^\ominus}{p_{CO}} + \frac{1}{2}\ln\frac{p^\ominus}{p_{O_2}}\right)$$

$$= \dot{n}\tilde{R}T\ln\frac{(p_{CO_2}/p^\ominus)}{(p_{CO}/p^\ominus)(p_{O_2}/p^\ominus)^{1/2}} \tag{15.17a}$$

Now suppose that the pressure p in the reaction box is changed to p', but all other conditions remain unchanged. The new partial pressures will be p'_{CO}, p'_{O_2}, and p'_{CO_2} such that

$$p'_{CO} + p'_{O_2} + p'_{CO_2} = p'$$

and the net power output becomes

$$|\dot{W}'| = \dot{n}\tilde{R}T\ln\frac{(p'_{CO_2}/p^\ominus)}{(p'_{CO}/p^\ominus)(p'_{O_2}/p^\ominus)^{1/2}} \tag{15.17b}$$

Either $|\dot{W}| = |\dot{W}'|$ or $|\dot{W}| \neq |\dot{W}'|$. If the latter, the system producing the lesser power could be reversed and the two systems coupled together. The combined system will then operate in a cycle and produce a net amount of work while exchanging heat with a single reservoir of uniform temperature T. This contradicts the Second Law, and so $|\dot{W}|$ must be equal to $|\dot{W}'|$. The same argument would apply to any reversible system that can be conceived operating with the same boundary conditions of $p^\ominus$ and T, and the power $|\dot{W}|$ is therefore the *maximum that can be obtained from this chemical reaction*. When the process is irreversible, the power output will be less; in the calorimeter process it is zero.

Since $|\dot{W}| = |\dot{W}'|$, it follows that

$$\frac{(p_{CO_2}/p^\ominus)}{(p_{CO}/p^\ominus)(p_{O_2}/p^\ominus)^{1/2}} = \frac{(p'_{CO_2}/p^\ominus)}{(p'_{CO}/p^\ominus)(p'_{O_2}/p^\ominus)^{1/2}}$$

Thus the combination of pressure ratios $(p_i/p^\ominus)$ above is independent of the total pressure p in the equilibrium box. This combination, or parameter, is called the *standard* or *thermodynamic equilibrium constant* for the reaction considered. The symbol used is $K^\ominus$, the superscript indicating that all partial pressures are normalised by the standard pressure $p^\ominus$. Thus

$$K^\ominus = \frac{(p_{CO_2}/p^\ominus)}{(p_{CO}/p^\ominus)(p_{O_2}/p^\ominus)^{1/2}} \tag{15.18a}$$

It is sometimes useful to gather all $p^\ominus$ terms together and rewrite equation (15.18a) as

$$K^\ominus = \frac{(p_{CO_2})(p^\ominus)^{1/2}}{(p_{CO})(p_{O_2})^{1/2}} \tag{15.18b}$$

(as is done in the table headings of Ref. 17 to save space). Although $K^\ominus$ is dimensionless, its numerical value will depend on the choice of $p^\ominus$. It is independent of $p^\ominus$ only for reactions in which $n_P = n_R$, when the net exponent of the $p^\ominus$ term becomes zero.* In common with other chemical-thermodynamic data which have to be referred to a standard pressure (e.g. $\Delta u_0^\ominus$, $\Delta h_0^\ominus$), the standard pressure agreed upon internationally is 1 bar. There is nothing in the foregoing to suggest that $K^\ominus$ is independent of the temperature T of the mixture, and experiment shows that it varies strongly with temperature, as we shall see later.

As anticipated earlier, we have not only shown that $K^\ominus \neq f(p)$, but also derived the important result that equation (15.17a) expresses the maximum work $|\dot{W}|_{max}$ attainable from this particular reaction. The result can be generalised to apply to any other chemical reaction involving perfect gases for which the equilibrium constant $K^\ominus$ is known, and $|\dot{W}|_{max}$ can be related to $K^\ominus$ by

$$|\dot{W}|_{max} = \dot{n}\tilde{R}T \ln K^\ominus \tag{15.19}$$

This result is discussed further in section 17.7 and, for the more advanced student, in section 7.9.3.

In generalising the foregoing arguments to other chemical equations, let us

---

* It used to be common practice to define the equilibrium constant in terms of partial pressures, e.g. in the case considered here as $K_p = (p_{CO_2})/(p_{CO})(p_{O_2})^{1/2}$. The subscript p was added to imply the above mode of definition. K_p would then in general not be dimensionless unless $n_P = n_R$. Tables used to present values of $\log K_p$ (or $\ln K_p$), an inadmissible practice because arguments of logarithms, or of any transcendental function, should always be dimensionless quantities. Why did this breach not lead to errors? It is easy to show that if the unit in which the partial pressures are measured is equal to the standard pressure adopted (it used to be 1 atm), then *numerically* $K_p = K^\ominus$ and the breach is thus swept under the carpet.

consider any stoichiometric equation such as

$$\nu_1 \text{ kmol of A} + \nu_2 \text{ kmol of B} \rightleftharpoons \nu_3 \text{ kmol of C} + \nu_4 \text{ kmol of D}$$

where ν_1, ν_2, ν_3 and ν_4 are called the *stoichiometric coefficients*; the coefficients of the products are by convention taken as positive, and those of the reactants as negative. We would then arrive at the expression

$$K^\ominus = \frac{(p_C/p^\ominus)^{\nu_3}(p_D/p^\ominus)^{\nu_4}}{(p_A/p^\ominus)^{\nu_1}(p_B/p^\ominus)^{\nu_2}}$$

And this could be written even more generally as

$$K^\ominus = \prod_i (p_i/p^\ominus)^{\nu_i} \quad \text{or} \quad \ln K^\ominus = \sum_i \ln(p_i/p^\ominus)^{\nu_i} \tag{15.20}$$

where $\prod_i$ means the *product* for all constituents i, and $\sum_i$ is the *sum* of the logarithmic terms.

Applying equation (15.20) to the reaction $H_2 + \frac{1}{2}O_2 \rightleftharpoons H_2O$, for example, we get for the equilibrium constant

$$K^\ominus = \frac{(p_{H_2O}/p^\ominus)}{(p_{H_2}/p^\ominus)(p_{O_2}/p^\ominus)^{1/2}} = \frac{(p_{H_2O})(p^\ominus)^{1/2}}{(p_{H_2})(p_{O_2})^{1/2}} \tag{15.21}$$

It should be clear that when tabulating experimentally determined values of $K^\ominus$, it is *necessary to specify the reaction*. The equilibrium constant $K^\ominus$ would have different values if the reaction were written as, say, $2H_2 + O_2 \rightleftharpoons 2H_2O$ or $H_2O \rightleftharpoons H_2 + \frac{1}{2}O_2$. In the former case $K^\ominus$ would be the square of that given by equation (15.21), and in the latter it would be the reciprocal of it.

Remembering that the partial pressures are proportional to the mole fractions as given by equation (14.17), it is evident that $K^\ominus$ is a measure of the amount of dissociation. A high value implies that the mixture contains a large proportion of undissociated products and so there is little dissociation. For exothermic reactions, such as those we have been considering, we would expect $K^\ominus$ to decrease with increase of temperature because more molecules of products would

Fig. 15.10

Variation of equilibrium

constant with temperature

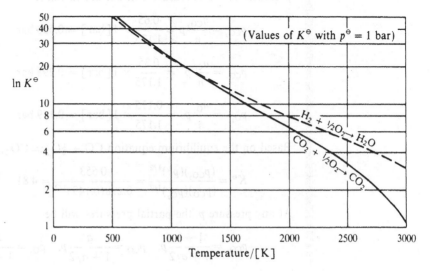

receive sufficient energy in collisions to dissociate. That $K^{\ominus}_{CO_2}$ and $K^{\ominus}_{H_2O}$ decrease strongly at very high temperatures is indicated in Fig. 15.10. It is usual to plot and tabulate values of $\ln K^{\ominus}$ rather than values of $K^{\ominus}$. This is because graphs plotted logarithmically cope more easily with the wide range of variation of $K^{\ominus}$, and linear interpolation from tables of $\ln K^{\ominus}$ provides values which are closer to the true values than would be obtained from linear interpolation between values of $K^{\ominus}$. Moreover, thermodynamic theory normally requires values of $\ln K^{\ominus}$ (see equation (15.19)). Values of $\ln K^{\ominus}$ for several reactions of importance in combustion are tabulated against temperature in Ref. 17.

The following example illustrates the method of calculating the equilibrium constant when the percentage dissociation has been obtained by a products analysis, and also how this equilibrium constant can then be used to predict the percentage dissociation in other circumstances.

Example 15.10   The products from the combustion of a stoichiometric mixture of CO and O_2 are at a pressure of 1 bar and a certain temperature. The products analysis shows that 35 per cent of each kmol of CO_2 is dissociated. Determine the equilibrium constant for this temperature, and thence find the percentage dissociation when the products are at the same temperature but compressed to 10 bar.

The combustion equation for the reaction to products in equilibrium is

$$CO + \tfrac{1}{2}O_2 \rightarrow (1 - a)CO_2 + aCO + \tfrac{1}{2}aO_2$$

where a is the fraction of CO_2 dissociated. At 1 bar the products consist of

$$0.65 \text{ kmol } CO_2 + 0.35 \text{ kmol } CO + 0.175 \text{ kmol } O_2$$

The total amount of substance of products is 1.175 kmol, and the partial pressures of the constituents in bar are therefore

$$p_{CO_2} = \frac{n_{CO_2}}{n}p = \frac{0.65}{1.175} \times 1[\text{bar}] = 0.553 \text{ bar}$$

$$p_{CO} = \frac{n_{CP}}{n}p = \frac{0.35}{1.175} \times 1[\text{bar}] = 0.298 \text{ bar}$$

$$p_{O_2} = \frac{n_{O_2}}{n}p = \frac{0.175}{1.175} \times 1[\text{bar}] = 0.149 \text{ bar}$$

Based on the equilibrium equation $CO + \tfrac{1}{2}O_2 \rightleftharpoons CO_2$,

$$K^{\ominus} = \frac{(p_{CO_2})(p^{\ominus})^{1/2}}{(p_{CO})(p_{O_2})^{1/2}} = \frac{0.553}{0.298(0.149)^{1/2}} = 4.81$$

At any pressure p, the partial pressures will be

$$p_{CO_2} = \frac{1 - a}{1 + a/2}p, \quad p_{CO} = \frac{a}{1 + a/2}p, \quad p_{O_2} = \frac{a/2}{1 + a/2}p$$

And the equilibrium constant will be

$$K^\ominus = \frac{\left(\dfrac{1-a}{1+a/2}\right)}{\left(\dfrac{a}{1+a/2}\right)\left(\dfrac{a/2}{1+a/2}\right)^{1/2}} \times \frac{p(p^\ominus)^{1/2}}{p \times p^{1/2}} \qquad (15.22)$$

Since the temperature is unchanged, $K^\ominus$ will still equal 4.81. At 10 bar, therefore,

$$4.81 = \frac{(1-a)(2+a)^{1/2}}{a^{3/2}} \times \frac{1}{10^{1/2}}$$

Squaring and simplifying, we have

$$230.4a^3 + 3a = 2$$

and the solution, by trial and error or graphical means, is $a = 0.185$. Thus the dissociation is 18.5 per cent of the CO_2.

The preceding example illustrates the important point that *although the equilibrium constant is independent of the pressure of the reacting mixture, the actual fraction of the dissociated product usually varies with pressure.* Inspection of equation (15.22) in the example shows that the term containing p only vanishes when the amount-of-substance of dissociating compound and of dissociated constituents is the same.

We may now see how a knowledge of the equilibrium constants enables the combustion equation to be established, and the adiabatic combustion temperature to be predicted, for the reaction of Example 15.7. The reactants are liquid heptane and air in stoichiometric proportions. Assuming that some of the CO_2 and H_2O molecules have dissociated, the combustion equation will be

$$C_7H_{16} + 11O_2 + \frac{79}{21}11N_2 \rightarrow aCO_2 + bH_2O + cCO + dO_2 + eH_2 + \frac{79}{21}11N_2$$

There are five unknowns: a, b, c, d and e. Three equations can be written down directly by equating the number of atoms of carbon, hydrogen and oxygen on each side of the equation:

$$a + c = 7$$
$$2b + 2e = 16$$
$$2a + b + c + 2d = 22$$

The remaining equations can be formulated with the aid of the equilibrium constants, which establish the proportions in which CO_2, CO and O_2, and H_2O, H_2 and O_2, can exist in equilibrium. If n is the total amount-of-substance of products, given by

$$n = a + b + c + d + e + \frac{79}{21}11$$

then the partial pressures are

$$p_{CO_2} = \frac{a}{n}p, \quad p_{CO} = \frac{c}{n}p, \quad \text{etc.}$$

The two equations are therefore

$$(CO + \tfrac{1}{2}O_2 \rightleftharpoons CO_2) \quad K_{CO_2}^{\ominus} = \frac{a}{c(d/n)^{1/2}}\left(\frac{p^{\ominus}}{p}\right)^{1/2}$$

$$(H_2 + \tfrac{1}{2}O_2 \rightleftharpoons H_2O) \quad K_{H_2O}^{\ominus} = \frac{b}{e(d/n)^{1/2}}\left(\frac{p^{\ominus}}{p}\right)^{1/2}$$

Since p appears in these equations, the pressure at which the reaction occurs must be known. (In Example 15.7 this was irrelevant because the enthalpies can be assumed to be independent of pressure.) Assuming the pressure is specified, there is still the difficulty that the dissociation constants are functions of the unknown temperature. The method of solution is to assume a final temperature, obtain the appropriate values of $K^{\ominus}$ from tables, e.g. Ref. 17, and then solve the five simultaneous equations for a, b, c, d and e. Once the composition of the products is known, the final temperature can be computed from the energy equation. If this does not agree with the assumed temperature, a better approximation to the values of $K^{\ominus}$ can be obtained and the calculation repeated until the desired agreement is reached.

The energy equation for the reaction in Example 15.7 must now be written more generally as

$$(H_{PT} - H_{P298}) + \Delta H_{298} + (H_{R298} - H_{R298}) = 0$$

ΔH_{298} replaces $\Delta \tilde{h}_{298}$ because, although we are still relating the solution to 1 kmol of heptane, $\Delta \tilde{h}_{298}$ must be modified to make allowance for the unburnt CO and H_2 in the products; that is, $|\Delta \tilde{h}_{298}|$ must be decreased by the magnitudes of the enthalpies of combustion of c kmol of CO and e kmol of H_2. The numerical solution of such a dissociation problem is too lengthy to be given here, but the reader can find some simple problems in Appendix B and a variety of worked examples in Ref. 7.

When the fuel/air mixture is appreciably richer than stoichiometric, it will be found that the amount-of-substance d of oxygen in the products is negligible. A somewhat simpler treatment involving only one equilibrium constant can then be used. The argument rests on the fact that the oxygen produced by the dissociation of CO_2 can be regarded as being wholly used in the combustion of H_2. The two reaction equations

$$CO + \tfrac{1}{2}O_2 \rightleftharpoons CO_2 \quad \text{and} \quad H_2 + \tfrac{1}{2}O_2 \rightleftharpoons H_2O$$

can then be combined to yield the so-called *water–gas reaction*

$$CO_2 + H_2 \rightleftharpoons CO + H_2O$$

With the O_2 eliminated from the products, one fewer equation is required, and the water–gas equilibrium constant is all that is needed for the solution of the simultaneous equations. Values of

$$K^\ominus = \frac{(p_{H_2O})(p_{CO})}{(p_{H_2})(p_{CO_2})}$$

are also given in Ref. 17.

The foregoing method of solution is for an adiabatic steady-flow process at a known constant pressure, such as occurs in a ram-jet combustion chamber. (This type of process also occurs in gas turbine combustion chambers, but the temperatures are too low for dissociation to be significant.) In the cylinders of many reciprocating internal-combustion engines the reaction occurs at substantially constant volume and the final pressure is unknown. The following example deals with this case, using carbon monoxide as the fuel for simplicity.

Example 15.11 The analysis of the products obtained from the adiabatic combustion of a stoichiometric mixture of CO and air at constant volume showed that there were 0.808 kmol of CO_2, 0.192 kmol of CO and 0.096 kmol of O_2, per kmol of CO in the reactants. The initial pressure and temperature of the reactants were 1 atm and 333 K, and the final temperature was found to be 2742 K. Check the accuracy of the results by an atom balance and by verifying that the equilibrium condition is satisfied.

The reactants for a stoichiometric mixture, per kmol of CO, are

$$CO + \tfrac{1}{2}O_2 + \left(\frac{79}{21}\right)\frac{1}{2}N_2$$

The combustion equation for the reaction is therefore

$$CO + 0.5\,O_2 + 1.881\,N_2 \rightarrow 0.808\,CO_2 + 0.192\,CO + 0.096\,O_2 + 1.881\,N_2$$

Checking the atom balance we have

(C) $0.808 + 0.192 = 1$

(O) $1.616 + 0.192 + 0.192 = 2$

The relevant partial pressures are

$$p_{CO_2} = \frac{0.808}{n}\,p, \quad p_{CO} = \frac{0.192}{n}\,p, \quad p_{O_2} = \frac{0.096}{n}\,p$$

Since the reactants and products are assumed to be perfect gases, and the reaction occurs at constant volume,

$$\frac{n_1\tilde{R}T_1}{p_1} = \frac{n\tilde{R}T}{p}$$

where subscript 1 refers to the initial conditions. The amount-of-substance of reactants is

$$n_1 = 1 + 0.5 + 1.881 = 3.381 \text{ kmol}$$

and $p_1 = 1\,atm = 1.013\,25\,bar$ and $T_1 = 333\,K$. Hence

$$\frac{p}{n} = \frac{p_1 T}{n_1 T_1} = \frac{1.013\,25[bar] \times 2742[K]}{3.381[kmol] \times 333[K]} = 2.468\,\frac{bar}{kmol}$$

The equilibrium constant is

$$K^{\ominus} = \frac{\left(\dfrac{p_{CO_2}}{p^{\ominus}}\right)}{\left(\dfrac{p_{CO}}{p^{\ominus}}\right)\left(\dfrac{p_{O_2}}{p^{\ominus}}\right)^{1/2}} = \frac{\left(\dfrac{n_{CO_2}}{n}p\right)}{\left(\dfrac{n_{CO}}{n}p\right)\left(\dfrac{n_{O_2}}{n}\dfrac{p}{p^{\ominus}}\right)^{1/2}}$$

$$= \frac{0.808[kmol]}{0.192[kmol]\left(2.468\dfrac{[bar]}{[kmol]}\dfrac{0.096[kmol]}{1[bar]}\right)^{1/2}} = 8.65$$

This is in good agreement with the linearly interpolated value obtained from Ref. 17, which is 8.64.

The check can be completed by showing that the energy equation is satisfied. For this adiabatic constant volume process, the energy equation will be

$$(U_{P2472} - U_{P298}) + \Delta U_{298} + (U_{R298} - U_{R333}) = 0$$

ΔU_{25} is the internal energy of combustion of 0.808 kmol of CO, per kmol of CO supplied in the reactants.

The treatment of the combustion of hydrocarbon fuels in air given here requires some qualification. First, at high temperatures nitrogen is not the inert gas we have hither supposed it to be; some of it combines with oxygen to form nitric oxide according to the equation $\frac{1}{2}O_2 + \frac{1}{2}N_2 \rightleftharpoons NO$. The combination is endothermic and causes a reduction in products temperature. Secondly, some of the molecules of water vapour dissociate not only into hydrogen and oxygen, but also into hydrogen and hydroxyl ($\frac{1}{2}H_2 + OH \rightleftharpoons H_2O$). And finally, some of the molecules of oxygen, nitrogen and hydrogen dissociate into their respective atoms. The dissociation constants for all these reactions are known, and their effect on the products temperature can be taken into account in more accurate calculations.

It must be emphasised that dissociation does not affect the internal energies and enthalpies of combustion, which are determined at about atmospheric temperature. In general, if the products of combustion of a hydrocarbon fuel–air mixture are cooled below 1500 K before leaving the system, the chemical energy liberated is not much affected by dissociation. As the products of combustion are cooled, the dissociated products recombine and the combustion is effectively complete below 1500 K.* The efficiency of the combustion process itself is therefore not affected by any dissociation that may occur due to a high temperature reached at some intermediate stage. The efficiency of a power plant

---

* When the products are cooled very rapidly, however, as when a sample is withdrawn through a water-cooled sampling tube, the reaction rates may be reduced to such an extent that very little recombination takes place.

in which the combustion process occurs may be affected, however, because the heat transferred to the working fluid is now transferred at a lower average temperature—the maximum temperature reached being reduced by the dissociation. In other words, the quantity of energy liberated is the same as if there were no dissociation, but its effectiveness for producing work is diminished. For steam or gas turbine plants this point is of no importance owing to the use of relatively low maximum temperatures imposed by the metallurgical limit. The discussions in sections 17.4 and 18.4.2, however, indicate that dissociation is an important factor limiting the efficiency of reciprocating internal-combustion engines and rocket motors.

15.8   Tabulation of thermodynamic reaction data

It is worth emphasising that although this chapter has been concerned with the particular class of chemical reaction known as combustion, most of the theory presented applies equally to chemical reactions in general. The enthalpy of combustion, for example, is then referred to as the *enthalpy of reaction*. In this wider context, it is impracticable to tabulate the enthalpies of all reactions which a chemical compound may undergo with other substances. Instead it is the enthalpy of formation $\Delta \tilde{h}_{f0}$ which is tabulated and, as will be shown, it is a simple matter to calculate the enthalpy of reaction $\Delta \tilde{h}_0$ in any particular case from the values of $\Delta \tilde{h}_{f0}$ of the substances taking part in the reaction.

The *enthalpy of formation* is defined as the increase in enthalpy when a compound is formed from its constituent elements in their natural forms and in a standard state. It is usually expressed in energy units per unit of amount-of-substance of compound, and is referred to the case where each of the reacting elements is at $p^{\ominus} = 1$ bar and $T_0 = 25\,°C = 298.15\,K$ and the product is at the same pressure and temperature. The qualification 'natural forms' implies that it is the enthalpy of formation of, say, gaseous hydrogen H_2, and not that of the dissociated monatomic gas H, which is put equal to zero. Of course some elements may exist in several 'natural forms' and only one can be used as a datum state; for example, for carbon it is graphite and not diamond which is used for this purpose.

The enthalpies of formation of three compounds at $T_0 = 25\,°C$ are as follows:

$$C(\text{graphite}) + 2H_2 \rightarrow CH_4; \quad (\Delta\tilde{h}_{f25})_{CH_4} = -74\,870\,kJ/kmol\ of\ CH_4$$

$$C(\text{graphite}) + O_2 \rightarrow CO_2; \quad (\Delta\tilde{h}_{f25})_{CO_2} = -393\,520\,kJ/kmol\ of\ CO_2$$

$$H_2 + \tfrac{1}{2}O_2 \rightarrow H_2O(\text{vap}); \quad (\Delta\tilde{h}_{f25})_{H_2O} = -241\,830\,kJ/kmol\ of\ H_2O$$

Since the change of enthalpy is independent of the process by which the end state is reached, we can view a reaction in two stages: a breaking up of the reactants into elements, followed by a recombination to form the products. Thus to find the enthalpy of reaction of methane and oxygen we can write

$$CH_4 + 2O_2 \rightarrow C + 2H_2 + 2O_2 \rightarrow CO_2 + 2H_2O(\text{vap})$$

and hence

$$\Delta \bar{h}_{25} = (\Delta \bar{h}_{f25})_{CO_2} + 2(\Delta \bar{h}_{f25})_{H_2O} - (\Delta \bar{h}_{f25})_{CH_4} - 2(\Delta \bar{h}_{f25})_{O_2}$$

$$= (-393\,520) + 2(-241\,830) - (-74\,870) - 0$$

$$= -802\,310\,kJ/kmol\ of\ CH_4$$

Two important points must be made here. First, the reader is reminded that Chapter 7 is intended to be studied on a second reading of the book. *The same applies to the remainder of this chapter which requires an understanding, in particular, of section 7.9.3.*

Secondly, near the end of section 15.4.1 it was suggested that the superscript $\ominus$, which refers to properties at the standard pressure $p^{\ominus} = 1$ bar, can safely be omitted. This was because we were going to assume that, in the absence of changes of phase, the properties U and H of reactants and products can be taken as independent of pressure. In the following we shall be dealing with two properties, namely the entropy S and the Gibbs function G (or their molar equivalents $\bar{s}$ and $\bar{g}$), and even for perfect gases these are strongly dependent on pressure. In view of this we shall revert to the more rigorous notation incorporating the superscript $\ominus$ for properties at standard pressure. For consistency the superscript will be attached not just to S and G, but also to U and H, although in the latter case we shall neglect variations with pressure where appropriate.

We have seen in section 7.9.3 that data for enthalpy of reaction $\Delta \bar{h}_0^{\ominus}$, change in Gibbs function $\Delta \bar{g}_0^{\ominus}$ and equilibrium constant $K_0^{\ominus}$ are interchangeable. Thus from equations (7.72), (7.73) and (7.75),

$$-\Delta \bar{g}_0^{\ominus} = -\Delta h_0^{\ominus} + T_0(\bar{s}_{P0}^{\ominus} - \bar{s}_{R0}^{\ominus}) \tag{15.23}$$

$$\ln K_0^{\ominus} = -\frac{\Delta \bar{g}_0^{\ominus}}{\tilde{R} T_0} \tag{15.24}$$

By virtue of the Third Law (see section 7.9.1), which enables absolute entropies to be determined for the reactants and products relative to a common datum at absolute zero of temperature, the entropy term in equation (15.23) can be calculated. The Gibbs function of formation $\Delta \bar{g}_{f0}^{\ominus}$ can then be defined in an analogous manner to the value of $\Delta \bar{h}_{f0}^{\ominus}$; and the values of $\Delta \bar{g}_0^{\ominus}$ for any reaction can be found by adding the formation values as for $\Delta \bar{h}_0^{\ominus}$. Consequently it follows from equation (15.24) that it is also possible to define logarithms of the equilibrium constant of formation $\ln K_{f0}^{\ominus}$, from which the logarithm of the equilibrium constant $K_0^{\ominus}$ for any reaction can be calculated from a similar summation procedure.* A short compilation of various chemical-thermodynamic data from Refs 36 and 37 is given in Fig. 15.11; it contains values of $\Delta \bar{h}_{f0}^{\ominus}$, $\Delta \bar{g}_{f0}^{\ominus}$,

---

* Because values of $\ln K_0^{\ominus}$ can be found from additions of the appropriate values of $\ln K_{f0}^{\ominus}$, it follows that values of $K_0^{\ominus}$ can be found by multiplication of the $K_{f0}^{\ominus}$ values. This should also be clear from the definition of the equilibrium constant in section 15.7.2 since, by multiplication of suitable equilibrium constants and cancellation of partial pressure terms, any required equilibrium constant can be found.

Fig. 15.11
A selection of chemical
thermodynamic data

	$\tilde{m}$	at $p^{\ominus} = 1$ bar and $T_0 = 298.15$ K				
		$\Delta\tilde{h}_{f0}^{\ominus}$	$\Delta\tilde{g}_{f0}^{\ominus}$		$\tilde{c}_{p0}^{\ominus}$	$\tilde{s}_0^{\ominus}$
	$\left[\dfrac{kg}{kmol}\right]$	$\left[\dfrac{kJ}{kmol}\right]$	$\left[\dfrac{kJ}{kmol}\right]$	$\ln K_{f0}^{\ominus}$	$\left[\dfrac{kJ}{kmol\ K}\right]$	$\left[\dfrac{kJ}{kmol\ K}\right]$
C (graphite)	12.011	0	0	0	8.53	5.69
C (diamond)	12.011	1 900	2 870	−1.157	6.06	2.44
C (gas)	12.011	714 990	669 570	−270.098	20.84	158.10
CH_4 (gas)	16.043	−74 870	−50 810	20.498	35.64	186.26
C_2H_4 (gas)	28.054	52 470	68 350	−27.573	42.89	219.33
CO (gas)	28.0105	−110 530	−137 160	55.331	29.14	197.65
CO_2 (gas)	44.010	−393 520	−394 390	159.093	37.13	213.80
H (gas)	1.008	217 990	203 290	−82.003	20.79	114.71
H_2 (gas)	2.016	0	0	0	28.84	130.68
OH (gas)	17.005	39 710	35 010	−14.122	29.99	183.61
H_2O (liq)	18.0155	−285 820	−237 150	95.660	75.32	70.00
H_2O (vap)	18.0155	−241 830	−228 590	92.207	33.58	188.83
N (gas)	14.0065	472 650	455 500	−183.740	20.79	153.30
N_2 (gas)	28.013	0	0	0	29.21	191.61
NO (gas)	30.006	90 290	86 600	−34.933	29.84	210.76
O (gas)	15.9995	249 170	231 750	−93.481	21.91	161.06
O_2 (gas)	31.999	0	0	0	29.37	205.14

$\ln K_{f0}^{\ominus}$ and also of the molar heat capacity $\tilde{c}_{p0}^{\ominus}$ and the absolute molar entropy $\tilde{s}_0^{\ominus}$, all in the standard state of $p^{\ominus} = 1$ bar and $T_0 = 298.15$ K.

Both the enthalpy and the equilibrium constant for perfect gases are independent of pressure, and in practice the data for $\Delta\tilde{h}_{f0}^{\ominus}$ and $\ln K_{f0}^{\ominus}$ can be assumed to be constant for real gases and vapours over wide ranges of pressure. Similarly, these values are very nearly independent of pressure for liquids and solids. The Gibbs function, however, involves an entropy term which varies appreciably with pressure for gaseous substances (although not for liquids and solids), and this variation must be taken into account when any gaseous reactants or products are not at the standard pressure of 1 bar.

A particular difficulty appears with regard to substances which cannot exist at the standard state. Thus H_2O vapour cannot exist at 1 bar at 25 °C, and H_2O in the standard state can exist only as a compressed liquid. The tables make use of a fictitious vapour at the standard state, obtained by assuming that the substance behaves as a perfect gas between the saturated vapour state at 25 °C (0.031 66 bar in the case of H_2O) and the standard state. This is permissible because we are interested only in using tabulated data to calculate *changes* in $\tilde{h}$ or $\tilde{g}$. As an example, let us consider the differences between the tabulated liquid and vapour values for water. For the enthalpy of formation, omitting the subscript 25 for brevity, we have

$$(\Delta\tilde{h}_f^{\ominus})_{vap} \text{ at } 1 \text{ bar} - (\Delta\tilde{h}_f^{\ominus})_{liq} \text{ at } 1 \text{ bar}$$

$$= \{(\Delta\tilde{h}_f^{\ominus})_{vap} \text{ at } 1 \text{ bar} - (\Delta\tilde{h}_f)_{vap} \text{ at } 0.031\ 66 \text{ bar}\}$$

$$+ \{(\Delta\tilde{h}_f)_{vap} \text{ at } 0.031\ 66 \text{ bar} - (\Delta\tilde{h}_f)_{liq} \text{ at } 0.031\ 66 \text{ bar}\}$$

$$+ \{(\Delta\tilde{h}_f)_{liq} \text{ at } 0.031\ 66 \text{ bar} - (\Delta\tilde{h}_f^{\ominus})_{liq} \text{ at } 1 \text{ bar}\}$$

$$= 0 + \tilde{h}_{fg} + 0 = 43\ 990 \text{ kJ/kmol of } H_2O$$

The first and third terms are zero because the enthalpy of vapour and of liquid is taken as independent of pressure; the middle term represents the latent enthalpy of vaporisation per kmol of H_2O. Considering the Gibbs function of formation, again at 25 °C, we have

$$(\Delta \tilde{g}_f^{\ominus})_{vap} \text{ at 1 bar} - (\Delta \tilde{g}_f^{\ominus})_{liq} \text{ at 1 bar}$$

$$= \{(\Delta \tilde{g}_f^{\ominus})_{vap} \text{ at 1 bar} - (\Delta \tilde{g}_f)_{vap} \text{ at 0.031 66 bar}\}$$

$$+ \{(\Delta \tilde{g}_f)_{vap} \text{ at 0.031 66 bar} - (\Delta \tilde{g}_f)_{liq} \text{ at 0.031 66 bar}\}$$

$$+ \{(\Delta \tilde{g}_f)_{liq} \text{ at 0.031 66 bar} - (\Delta \tilde{g}_f^{\ominus})_{liq} \text{ at 1 bar}\}$$

$$= 8.3145 \times 298.15 \left[\frac{kJ}{kmol} \right] \ln \frac{1}{0.031\,66} + 0 + 0 = 8559 \text{ kJ/kmol of } H_2O$$

The first term represents extrapolation to the fictitious vapour state using (15.23) and assuming that the vapour behaves as a perfect gas over that range. The second term is zero because the Gibbs function remains constant in an isothermal change of phase (see sections 7.7 and 7.9.1), and the third term is zero because the Gibbs function of a liquid is taken as independent of pressure.

Finally, considering the entropy at 25 °C we can write

$$(\tilde{s}^{\ominus})_{vap} \text{ at 1 bar} - (\tilde{s}^{\ominus})_{liq} \text{ at 1 bar}$$

$$= \{(\tilde{s}^{\ominus})_{vap} \text{ at 1 bar} - (\tilde{s})_{vap} \text{ at 0.031 66 bar}\}$$

$$+ \{(\tilde{s})_{vap} \text{ at 0.031 66 bar} - (\tilde{s})_{liq} \text{ at 0.031 66 bar}\}$$

$$+ \{(\tilde{s})_{liq} \text{ at 0.031 66 bar} - (\tilde{s}^{\ominus})_{liq} \text{ at 1 bar}\}$$

$$= -8.3145 \left[\frac{kJ}{kmol\,K} \right] \ln \frac{1}{0.031\,66} + \frac{43\,990[kJ/kmol]}{298.15[K]} + 0$$

$$= (-28.71 + 147.54)[kJ/kmol\,K] = 118.83 \text{ kJ/kmol K}$$

Or, since $\tilde{g} = \tilde{h} - T\tilde{s}$ and the temperature is constant at T_0, the change in entropy can also be found from

$$\frac{\Delta \tilde{h}^{\ominus}}{T_0} - \frac{\Delta \tilde{g}^{\ominus}}{T_0} = \frac{(43\,990 - 8559)[kJ/kmol]}{298.15[K]} = 118.83 \text{ kJ/kmol K}$$

We conclude this brief explanation of the way thermodynamic reaction data are presented with an example illustrating their use to calculate the values of $\Delta \tilde{h}$, $\Delta \tilde{g}$ and K for a reaction at a specified temperature and pressure which differs from the standard state.

Example 15.12 Calculate $\Delta \tilde{h}$, $\Delta \tilde{g}$ and $\ln K^{\ominus}$ at 298.15 K for the reaction

$$CO_2 + H_2 \rightarrow CO + H_2O \text{ (vap)}$$

where the *total* pressure of the reactants and products is 1 bar each. Use the data on Fig. 15.11 and check them for consistency.

Also calculate the value of $\ln K^{\ominus}$ at $T = 400$ K, using first equation

(15.24) and secondly equation (7.77); assume in each case that the molar heat capacities $\tilde{c}_p$ are constant over the temperature range considered.

Enthalpy, Gibbs function and equilibrium constant at 298.15 K
The enthalpy of reaction $\Delta h_{298}^{\ominus}$ when each constituent is at 1 bar is

$$\Delta \tilde{h}_{298}^{\ominus} = \{(-110\,530) + (-241\,830) - (-393\,520) - 0\}[\text{kJ}]$$

$$= +41\,160\,\text{kJ}$$

This will also be equal to $\Delta \tilde{h}_{298}$ for the specified pressure of each reactant and product (in this case 0.5 bar each), because the enthalpy can be taken as independent of pressure.
   The change of Gibbs function $\Delta \tilde{g}_{298}^{\ominus}$ is given by

$$\Delta \tilde{g}_{298}^{\ominus} = \{(-137\,160) + (-228\,590) - (-394\,390) - 0\}[\text{kJ}]$$

$$= +28\,640\,\text{kJ}$$

To find the change of Gibbs function for the reactants and products each at 0.5 bar, the Gibbs function of each term will have to be modified by $n\tilde{R}T_0 \ln(p^{\ominus}/p)$, where $p^{\ominus} = 1$ bar and $p = 0.5$ bar. It is obvious that these modifications (with appropriate signs) will cancel in this case and $\Delta \tilde{g}_{298} = \Delta \tilde{g}_{298}^{\ominus}$; there will be a net effect only when the reaction is such that the amount-of-substance of the gaseous products differs from that of the gaseous reactants.
   The equilibrium constant is

$$\ln K^{\ominus} = 55.331 + 92.207 - 159.093 - 0 = -11.555$$

To check for consistency, let us first apply equation (15.23);

$$-\Delta \tilde{h}_{298} = -\Delta \tilde{g}_{298} - T_0 \left(\sum_P n_i \tilde{s}_{i298} - \sum_R n_i \tilde{s}_{i298} \right)$$

$$= -28\,640[\text{kJ}] - 298.15[\text{K}]\{(1 \times 197.65)$$

$$+ (1 \times 188.83) - (1 \times 213.80) - (1 \times 130.68)\}\left[\frac{\text{kJ}}{\text{K}}\right]$$

$$= \{-28\,640 - (298.15 \times 42.00)\}[\text{kJ}] = -41\,160\,\text{kJ}$$

Also, from equation (15.24),

$$\ln K^{\ominus} = -\frac{\Delta \tilde{g}_{298}}{\tilde{R}T_0} = -\frac{28\,640}{8.3145 \times 298.15} = -11.553$$

Equilibrium constant at 400 K
To calculate the value of $\ln K_T^{\ominus}$ at $T = 400$ K using equation (15.24), we will first write equations for $\Delta \tilde{h}_T$ and $(S_{PT} - S_{RT})$ at T, taking the values of $\tilde{c}_p$ from Fig. 15.11. From equation (15.10),

$$\Delta \tilde{h}_T = \{(1 \times 29.14) + (1 \times 33.58)\}\left[\frac{\text{kJ}}{\text{K}}\right](T - 298.15[\text{K}]) + 41\,160[\text{K}]$$

$$+ \{(1 \times 37.13) + (1 \times 28.84)\}\left[\frac{kJ}{K}\right](298.15[K] - T)$$

$$= \left\{41\,160 - 3.25\left(\frac{T}{[K]} - 298.15\right)\right\}[kJ] = \left(42\,130 - 3.25\frac{T}{[K]}\right)kJ$$

and remembering that the pressure terms cancel in this case,

$$(S_{PT} - S_{RT}) = \sum_P n_i \tilde{c}_{pi} \ln\frac{T}{T_0} + \left(\sum_P n_i \tilde{s}_{i298} - \sum_R n_i \tilde{s}_{i298}\right) + \sum_R n_i \tilde{c}_{pi} \ln\frac{T_0}{T}$$

$$= \left(42.00 - 3.25\ln\frac{T}{298.15[K]}\right)\frac{kJ}{K}$$

At $T = 400\,K$,

$$\Delta \tilde{g}_T = \Delta \tilde{h}_T - T(S_{PT} - S_{RT})$$

$$= \{42\,130 - (3.25 \times 400)\} - 400\left(42.00 - 3.25\ln\frac{400}{298.15}\right)[kJ]$$

$$= +24\,410\,kJ$$

and from (15.24),

$$\ln K_T^\ominus = -\frac{24\,410}{8.3145 \times 400} = -7.340$$

Alternatively, using equation (7.77) and treating $\Delta \tilde{h}$ as a variable between T_0 and T,

$$\int_{T_0}^T d(\ln K^\ominus) = \frac{1}{\tilde{R}}\int_{T_0}^T \Delta \tilde{h}\,d\left(\frac{1}{T}\right)$$

and hence, using the intermediate result for $\Delta \tilde{h}_T$ above,

$$\ln K_{400}^\ominus - \ln K_{298}^\ominus = -\frac{1}{8.3145}\int_{T_0}^T \left(42\,130 - \frac{3.25}{[K]/T}\right)d\left(\frac{[K]}{T}\right)$$

$$= -\left\{\frac{1}{8.3145}\frac{42\,130}{T/[K]} - 3.25\ln\left(\frac{[K]}{T}\right)\right\}_{T_0}^T$$

$$= -\frac{1}{8.3145}\left(\frac{42\,130}{400} - \frac{42\,130}{298.15} - 3.25\ln\frac{298.15}{400}\right) = +4.213$$

Thus, using $\ln K^\ominus = -11.555$ at $298.15\,K$ from the first part of the example,

$$\ln K_{400}^\ominus = 4.213 - 11.555 = -7.342$$

which agrees closely with the result obtained above.

15.9 Limitations of the thermodynamic analysis

In the previous chapter it was emphasised that the thermodynamic analysis of the processes occurring in condensers and air-conditioning plant is limited to the prediction of final states and energy transfers from a knowledge of the initial states and certain operating conditions. A more detailed analysis of the way in which heat is transferred must be undertaken before an actual plant can be designed.

The thermodynamic analysis of combustion processes, given in this chapter, is limited in a similar way: it does not enable us to specify the conditions under which the process can actually be carried out in practice. For example, it cannot be used to predict the air/fuel ratio and initial temperature necessary for self-ignition to occur. Nor has the simple thermodynamic treatment anything to say about the rate at which the process can be carried out; for example, it cannot predict flame speeds, or the conditions under which a stable flame is possible, or the delay periods experienced in internal-combustion engines.

A great deal of empirical data has been amassed over the years to explain the detailed phenomena encountered in practical combustion systems such as coal and oil fired furnaces, gas burners, reciprocating engines, gas turbines, ram-jets and rocket motors. The concepts necessary for a synthesis of this mass of data are now being formulated with the growth of the fundamental sciences of combustion kinetics and combustion wave theory. Quantitatively there is still a wide gap to be bridged before these sciences can be applied directly so that new combustion systems can be designed on the drawing board, but even now they can be used to aid consistent thinking and to reduce the amount of *ad hoc* development which is still required before a new design can be made to work efficiently. Ref. 30 provides an introduction to combustion kinetics and combustion wave theory.

Part III

Work Transfer

Introduction

So far in this book we have been concerned mainly with relations between fluid properties and the quantities of work and heat which accompany changes of state. Before it is possible to design plant which will effect the desired changes of state, it is necessary to analyse the mechanisms of work and heat transfer in some detail; the former mode of energy transfer is discussed here and the latter in Part IV. This division is easily justified in such cases as steam plant, refrigeration plant and air-conditioning plant, because the work and heat transfers are carried out in separate components. It is not so easily justified when considering reciprocating air compressors or internal-combustion engines. To cover these latter examples it may be said that Part III deals with those systems whose main purpose is the transfer of work and for which exchanges of heat with the surroundings are only incidental.

Fundamentally, there are two types of machine used to perform the process of work transfer: (a) positive displacement machines, and (b) non-positive displacement machines. The former comprise all reciprocating expanders and compressors and also some types of rotary compressor such as the Roots blower and the vane pump. The features common to class (a) are: these machines possess members (e.g. pistons and valves) which ensure positive admission and delivery of the working fluid and prevent any undesired reversal of flow within the machine; their operation is intermittent and they subject the fluid to non-flow processes; and work is transferred by virtue of a hydrostatic pressure force exerted on a moving boundary. In non-positive displacement machines, which comprise axial-flow and radial-flow turbines and compressors, there are no means for preventing a reversal of flow in the machine; the processes are steady-flow processes; and work is transferred by virtue of the change in momentum of a stream of fluid flowing at a high speed over blades or vanes attached to a rotor.

In all practical power plant, work is done during successive compressions and expansions of the working fluid. To obtain a net amount of work, it is essential to change the stage of the working fluid between the compression and expansion processes. So far we have mainly considered plant in which this change of state is brought about by external heat addition, e.g. steam power plant and closed-cycle gas turbine plant. The one exception in Part II has been the open-cycle gas turbine wherein the change of state is effected by a chemical reaction. In Part III we shall describe the reciprocating internal-combustion engine, where the compression, change of state by combustion, and subsequent expansion are all performed in a single component—the engine cylinder. Reciprocating internal-combustion engines fall within the class of positive displacement machines, as does the newer rotary type known as the Wankel engine which is also described briefly.

The scheme of Part III may now be outlined. Chapter 16 deals with positive displacement compressors and expanders, with the reciprocating air compressor and steam engine discussed as important examples of each type. The following chapter describes the processes in positive-displacement internal-combustion engines. The knowledge of non-flow processes already gained from a study of Parts I and II is adequate for the purposes of these two chapters. For a study of non-positive displacement machines, however, the treatment of steady-flow processes given so far is insufficiently detailed; we need to know something about the nature of the flow *within* the open system. Chapter 18 analyses the simplest type of flow—one-dimensional steady flow—and the results are then applied in Chapter 19 to the processes which occur in non-positive displacement machines.

When dealing with stationary power plant, the useful net work is always delivered by the engine as a torque in a rotating shaft. When the power plant is used for propelling a vehicle, this need not necessarily be the case. Admittedly in rail, road and ship propulsion the power is usually delivered via a shaft, but in the more recent developments of aircraft propulsion the force required to move an aircraft against atmospheric drag or gravitational pull is derived without the intermediary of shaft work. The analysis of the behaviour of jet power plant is basically a problem of one-dimensional flow, and as such it is treated in Chapter 18.

Finally, it should be realised that the major fraction of the total mechanical work produced by the world's power plant is utilised in the production of electrical power, i.e. it is used to drive electric generators. If the primary source of energy—whether chemical or nuclear—could be converted directly into electricity, both a higher efficiency and an overall simplification of plant might be attained. Part III closes with a chapter describing briefly the main devices which are being developed for direct conversion. The excuse for including this topic in a part entitled 'Work Transfer' is that in principle electrical and mechanical work are mutually convertible without loss and in this sense are equivalent.

16

Reciprocating Expanders and Compressors

The function of a compressor is to admit fluid from a low-pressure region, compress it, and deliver it to a high-pressure region. An expander carries out the reverse processes with the object of producing work.

Although this chapter is mainly concerned with reciprocating macnines, of which the air compressor and steam engine are considered as typical examples, the last section deals with rotary positive displacement compressors. These are more akin to their reciprocating equivalent than they are to the non-positive displacement compressors described in Chapter 19, even though the letter are rotary machines. The essential feature common to all positive displacement machines is that the fluid is prevented by a solid boundary from flowing back in the direction of the pressure gradient. All the compressors described here are therefore capable of producing large pressure ratios.

As already pointed out, reciprocating machines can be regarded as open systems being steadily supplied with working fluid and transferring work and heat between the fluid and its surroundings at a uniform rate. Nevertheless the internal processes are intermittent, and this fact imposes an important limitation on reciprocating machines—the comparatively low rate at which machines of reasonable size can handle the working fluid.

16.1 Work transfer in reversible reciprocating machines

A reciprocating machine consists essentially of a cylinder and a piston, with the piston connected to a rotating shaft by a connecting rod and crank as shown in Fig. 16.1. Valves permit the fluid to flow into and out of the cylinder at appropriate times. The total piston travel is called the *stroke*, and the volume displaced is called the *swept volume*. There is always some minimum volume, the *clearance volume*, when the piston is at the end of the stroke. This is necessary to accommodate the valves and avoid contact of piston and cylinder head.

The succession of events can best be explained with the aid of a diagram (Fig. 16.2a) showing how the pressure in the cylinder varies during one revolution of the crankshaft, i.e. during one complete *machine cycle*. The change in state of the fluid as it passes through the machine will be depicted on a $p-v$ diagram (Fig. 16.2b). We shall refer explicitly to the operation of an expander, and bear

Fig. 16.1
The reciprocating
expander or compressor

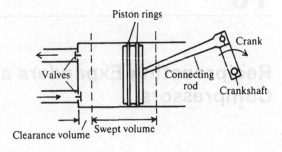

Fig. 16.2
$p–V$ and $p–v$ diagrams
for an ideal expander

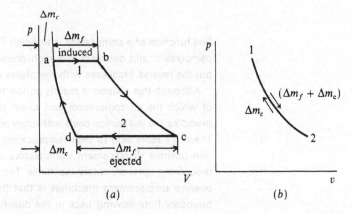

in mind the fact that in a compressor the machine cycle is traversed in the reverse direction. The following analysis refers to an idealised machine in which the processes are reversible, the state of the fluid at inlet and outlet remains constant with respect to time, and the kinetic energy at inlet and outlet is negligible.

a–b　The inlet valve is open, and a mass of fluid Δm_f in state 1 enters the cylinder without change of state. It mixes reversibly with a mass Δm_c already present in the clearance volume in the same state 1.

b–c　Both valves are closed and the mass $(\Delta m_f + \Delta m_c)$ changes its state during the expansion to pressure p_2.

c–d　The exhaust valve is open and a mass Δm_f is ejected from the cylinder without further change of state.

d–a　Both valves are closed and a mass Δm_c is compressed to the original state 1.

It is important to note that *although Fig. 16.2a represents the events during a machine cycle, it does not represent a thermodynamic cycle.* Admittedly the mass Δm_c is carried through a thermodynamic cycle, although it consists merely of the traversing and retraversing of a single path of states as shown on the $p–v$ diagram of Fig. 16.2b. But the mass Δm_f is not carried through a cycle at all, and simply has its state changed from state 1 to state 2.

Before the work done can be estimated, the processes of expansion and compression between states 1 and 2 must be defined. Since the speed of flow through the machine is not very great, these processes cannot be assumed to be adiabatic. A better approximation is to assume that they are polytropics, i.e. of the form pV^n = constant. An expression for the work done can be derived in two ways: either by considering the forces on the piston during a complete machine cycle, or by applying the steady-flow energy equation between inlet and outlet of the machine. The same assumption of constant inlet and outlet conditions has to be made in both cases. That is, it must be assumed that there is sufficient intake and receiver volume for the intermittent working of the machine to make a negligible difference to the fluid properties at inlet and outlet.

16.1.1   Machine cycle analysis

The net work done per machine cycle is the algebraic sum of the work transfers in the four processes, each of which can be found from $\int pA \, dL$ or $\int p \, dV$. A is the area of the piston and L is the distance moved. Referring to Fig. 16.2,

$$\oint dW = -\int_a^b p \, dV - \int_b^c p \, dV - \int_c^d p \, dV - \int_d^a p \, dV = -\oint p \, dV$$

The magnitude of $\oint dW$ is evidently equal to the area of the p–V diagram. Carrying out the integration, making use of equation (3.12), we have

$$\oint dW = -p_1(V_b - V_a) + \frac{(p_2 V_c - p_1 V_b)}{n-1} - p_2(V_d - V_c) + \frac{(p_1 V_a - p_2 V_d)}{n-1}$$

$$= \frac{n}{n-1}\{p_1(V_a - V_b) + p_2(V_c - V_d)\}$$

The work done can be expressed in terms of the fluid properties at inlet and outlet by noting that

$$V_a = \Delta m_c v_1, \qquad V_b = (\Delta m_f + \Delta m_c)v_1$$
$$V_c = (\Delta m_f + \Delta m_c)v_2, \quad V_d = \Delta m_c v_2$$

We then have

$$\oint dW = \Delta m_f \frac{n}{n-1}(p_2 v_2 - p_1 v_1) \tag{16.1}$$

The rate of work done is obtained by multiplying the net work done during the machine cycle by the number of cycles N per unit time. If the mass flow per unit time $(N\Delta m_f)$ is denoted by $\dot{m}$, the rate of work done is

$$\dot{W} = \dot{m}\frac{n}{n-1}(p_2 v_2 - p_1 v_1) \tag{16.2}$$

Equation (16.2) can be recast in terms of the pressure ratio as follows:

$$\dot{W} = \dot{m} p_1 v_1 \frac{n}{n-1}\left(\frac{p_2 v_2}{p_1 v_1} - 1\right)$$

373

and since $v_2/v_1 = (p_1/p_2)^{1/n}$,

$$\dot{W} = \dot{m}p_1 v_1 \frac{n}{n-1}\left\{\left(\frac{p_2}{p_1}\right)^{(n-1)/n} - 1\right\} \qquad (16.3)$$

Identical expressions are obtained for the case where the machine cycle is carried out in the reverse direction as in a compressor; p_2 is then greater than p_1 and $\dot{W}$ becomes a positive quantity.

The exact path of the expansion and compression processes, i.e. the value of the polytropic index n, depends upon the heat flow through the cylinder walls. Ideally, heat is only transferred during the processes b–c and d–a, because processes a–b and c–d are merely mass transfers to and from the cylinder without change of state. The heat transferred during the compression of Δm_c along d–a is equal and opposite to the heat transferred during its expansion from b to c. The net heat transfer per machine cycle is therefore that associated with the expansion of Δm_f along b–c. Since the system is closed during this process, the appropriate energy equation is

$$\oint dQ = \Delta m_f(u_2 - u_1) + \Delta m_f \int_1^2 p\, dv$$

$$= \Delta m_f(u_2 - u_1) - \Delta m_f \frac{1}{n-1}(p_2 v_2 - p_1 v_1)$$

Since $u = h - pv$, this can also be written as

$$\oint dQ = \Delta m_f(h_2 - h_1) - \Delta m_f \frac{n}{n-1}(p_2 v_2 - p_1 v_1)$$

The rate of heat transfer per unit time is therefore

$$\dot{Q} = \dot{m}(h_2 - h_1) - \dot{m}\frac{n}{n-1}(p_2 v_2 - p_1 v_1) \qquad (16.4)$$

16.1.2 Steady-flow analysis

The foregoing expressions for the work and heat transfers can also be obtained by applying the steady-flow energy equation, without the necessity for such a detailed analysis of the events which take place within the cylinder. The energy equation, neglecting the kinetic energy terms, has been shown in section 10.4 to lead to

$$\dot{W} = \dot{m}\int_1^2 v\, dp \qquad (16.5)$$

Making the further assumption that the reversible process is polytropic, as before, we can perform the integration and obtain

$$\dot{W} = \dot{m}\frac{n}{n-1}(p_2 v_2 - p_1 v_1)$$

Fig. 16.3
Effect of polytropic index
on the work transfer

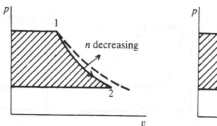
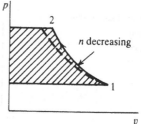

and hence also, from the steady-flow energy equation,

$$\dot{Q} = \dot{m}(h_2 - h_1) - \dot{m}\frac{n}{n-1}(p_2v_2 - p_1v_1)$$

These equations are identical with equations (16.2) and (16.4).

There are two important points to be noted from the analysis of the reversible reciprocating machine.

(a) If the machine is an expander then the magnitude of the work increases as the value of n decreases, while for a compressor it decreases as n decreases. There is no need to evaluate equation (16.2) to show this; it is evident from the $p-v$ diagrams of Fig. 16.3. Equation (16.2) is represented by ($\dot{m}$ × shaded area), i.e. by $\dot{m}\int_1^2 v\,dp$, and the negative slope of a polytropic curve decreases with decrease of n (section 3.4).

(b) Equation (16.1) indicates that the clearance volume has no effect on the work done *per unit mass flow*. The mass Δm_c in the clearance volume is expanded and recompressed along the same state path and no net work is done on or by it. The clearance volume does, however, affect the capacity of the machine, i.e. the mass Δm_f of fluid which a cylinder of given size can handle per machine cycle. The greater the clearance volume per unit swept volume, the smaller the amount of fluid that can be handled by the machine. This will be shown formally for an air compressor in section 16.3.

16.2 The indicator diagram

There is one important respect in which the actual $p-V$ diagram of all real reciprocating machines differs from the ideal diagram of a reversible machine. Owing to the fact that valves take a finite time to open and close, the corners of the diagram are rounded and ill defined. When a valve port is only partly open, throttling occurs and there is a considerable pressure drop in the direction of flow. Even when the port is fully open, some pressure drop is inevitable due to fluid friction. Thus the real $p-V$ diagrams for an expander and a compressor appear as in Fig. 16.4a and b. It must be remembered, too, that in the real machine the expansion and compression processes will not necessarily be exactly polytropic.

Since the real processes are not reversible, the actual work and heat transfers

Fig. 16.4
Effect of valve loss on the
p–V diagram:
(a) expander;
(b) compressor

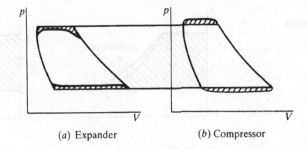

(a) Expander   (b) Compressor

Fig. 16.5
The mechanical indicator

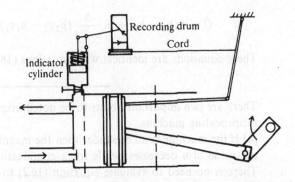

cannot be individually expressed in terms of the fluid properties at inlet and
outlet as in equations (16.2) and (16.4). Nevertheless a good approximation to
the actual work done can still be obtained from $\oint$ (force on piston $\times dL$) or
$\oint p\,dV$, provided the variation of average pressure in the cylinder is plotted during
the machine cycle. Strictly speaking it is the pressure on the piston face which
should be measured, but this presents too difficult a problem of measurement
for ordinary purposes. (The error can become significant when considerable
turbulence is present as in high-speed compression-ignition engines; see
section 17.3.2.)

The real p–V diagram is obtained by fitting an *indicator* to the machine.
Fig. 16.5 illustrates a simple *mechanical indicator* suitable for machines of low
rotational speed.* The main part of the indicator is itself a small cylinder and
piston which can be put into communication with the cylinder of the machine.
The volume of the indicator cylinder must be small compared with the clearance
volume of the machine cylinder, otherwise the diagram will be altered appreciably
when the indicator cock is opened. The indicator piston is spring loaded so
that its movement is directly proportional to the pressure, and this movement
is magnified by a link mechanism connecting the piston and a pencil. The spring
is calibrated, the *spring constant k* being expressed as the number of units of

---

* Descriptions of other indicators, e.g. electronic and optical types, can be found in the *Proceedings
of the Institution of Mechanical Engineers* and in the *Transactions of the Society of Automotive
Engineers*. Such indicators are more suitable for high-speed machines because the inertia of their
moving parts is much less than that of the mechanical indicator described here.

Fig. 16.6
Finding the mean effective
pressure

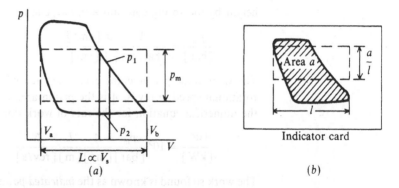

(a)   (b)

pressure required to move the pencil point vertically through unit distance. The
pencil point moves along the surface of a drum parallel to its axis, while the
drum is rotated by a cord connected, via a reducing linkage, to the piston of the
machine. Thus while the pencil moves along the drum a distance proportional
to the pressure, the drum surface moves past the pencil a distance proportional
to the engine piston stroke and in phase with it. In this way the $p-V$ diagram
can be recorded on an *indicator card* wrapped round the drum. When the chart
is unwrapped the area of the diagram can be measured with a planimeter, this
area being proportional to the net work transfer per machine cycle. In practice
the constant of proportionality is not evaluated, and the work done is usually
deduced by making use of the concept of mean effective pressure already
introduced in section 12.8.

Consider the $p-V$ diagram of Fig. 16.6a. The net work transfer per machine
cycle can be expressed by

$$\oint dW = -\int_{V_a}^{V_b} (p_1 - p_2)\, dV = -\int_0^L (p_1 - p_2) A\, dL$$

where A is the area of the piston and L is the stroke. This can be written as

$$\left| \oint dW \right| = p_m AL \tag{16.6}$$

where

$$p_m = \frac{1}{L} \int_0^L (p_1 - p_2)\, dL$$

Conventionally, p_m is always treated as a positive quantity. Thus p_m is the height
of a rectangle of the same area and length as the $p-V$ diagram. p_m is known
as the *indicated mean effective pressure*, and it can be regarded as that constant
pressure which, if it acted on the piston over one stroke, would do the same
amount of work as is done in one machine cycle. Since the actual indicator
card is drawn to a reduced scale (Fig. 16.6b), it is first necessary to find its
mean height a/l, say in cm, and then deduce p_m in bar by multiplying the mean

height by the spring constant k in bar/cm, i.e.

$$\frac{p_m}{[\text{bar}]} = \frac{k}{[\text{bar/cm}]} \frac{a/[\text{cm}^2]}{l/[\text{cm}]} \quad (16.7)$$

The work done per machine cycle can then be found from (16.6). If N is the rotational speed in rev/s, A is the piston area in m^2 and L is the stroke in m, the numerical equation for the rate of work done becomes

$$\frac{|\dot{W}|}{[\text{kW}]} = 10^2 \frac{p_m}{[\text{bar}]} \frac{A}{[\text{m}^2]} \frac{L}{[\text{m}]} \frac{N}{[\text{rev/s}]} \quad (16.8)$$

The work so found is known as the *indicated power* (*IP*). The power of machines is still sometimes expressed in horsepower units, and it is then referred to as the indicated horsepower (*IHP*). The British and metric horsepower units are related to the kilowatt by the following equation, to four significant figures:

$$1 \text{ kW} = \frac{1}{0.7457} \text{ British hp} = \frac{1}{0.7355} \text{ metric hp}$$

The actual power produced at the shaft of an expander will be less than the *IP* because some work is dissipated by friction between piston and cylinder and in the bearings. The *shaft power* (*SP*) is measured by some type of dynamometer,* of which the friction brake is a common example, and consequently it is often referred to as the *brake power* (*BP*). The ratio

$$\eta_{\text{mech}} = \frac{BP}{IP} \quad \text{or} \quad \frac{SP}{IP} \quad (16.9)$$

is called the *mechanical efficiency* of the expander. If the machine is a compressor, equation (16.8) gives the rate of work done *on* the fluid by the piston. In fact more work than this must be supplied to the shaft to overcome mechanical friction losses, and the mechanical efficiency is therefore defined in this case as

$$\eta_{\text{mech}} = \frac{IP}{SP} \quad (16.10)$$

For reasons similar to those given in section 12.8, a machine cycle yielding a high indicated mean effective pressure is likely to provide the basis for a compressor or expander having a high mechanical efficiency.

In this section we have concentrated on the essential differences which exist between all real and ideal reciprocating machines. There are other differences which are peculiar to particular types of machine and these will be brought out in the following sections. For brevity we shall consider one example of a compressor, the air compressor, and one example of an expander, the steam engine.

---

* A description of the more common types of dynamometer can be found in textbooks on mechanics of machines.

16.3 Reciprocating air compressors

One special feature of a compressor is the use of spring-loaded, non-return valves which open and close automatically (Fig. 16.7). This considerable mechanical simplification is made possible by the fact that the fluid is forced in the direction opposing the pressure gradient. In an expander it is necessary to use mechanically operated valves, timed to open and close by some linkage from the crankshaft. Automatic spring-loaded valves tend to be less positive in their action and lead to greater throttling losses than mechanically operated valves, but the mechanical simplification is considered to be worth the small amount of additional compression work entailed. A typical p–V diagram is shown in Fig. 16.7. The wavy lines during the suction and delivery processes are due to valve bounce, which arises because initially a rather large pressure difference is required across the valves to overcome their inertia. Apart from these peculiarities the actual indicator diagram follows the ideal p–V diagram closely, and for the remainder of this section only the ideal diagram will be considered.

When air is the working fluid, the equation of state for a perfect gas enables equations (16.2), (16.3) and (16.4) to be put in the following form:

$$\dot{W} = \dot{m}\frac{n}{n-1}R(T_2 - T_1) \tag{16.11}$$

$$\dot{W} = \dot{m}\frac{n}{n-1}RT_1\left\{\left(\frac{p_2}{p_1}\right)^{(n-1)/n} - 1\right\} \tag{16.12}$$

$$\dot{Q} = \dot{m}c_p(T_2 - T_1) - \dot{m}\frac{n}{n-1}R(T_2 - T_1)$$

Since $R = c_v(\gamma - 1)$, the last equation reduces to

$$\dot{Q} = \dot{m}\left\{\gamma c_v - \frac{n}{n-1}c_v(\gamma - 1)\right\}(T_2 - T_1)$$

$$= \dot{m}\frac{\gamma - n}{1 - n}c_v(T_2 - T_1) \tag{16.13}$$

Fig. 16.7
Self-acting valves for a compressor and their effect on the actual indicator diagram

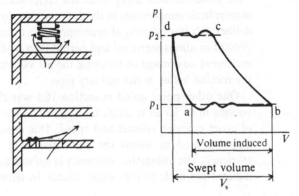

379

In section 16.1 it was pointed out that the work done *on* the air decreases as the value of n decreases. For this reason the compressor cylinder is either water cooled, or finned and air cooled. Even with good cooling the value of n is usually between 1.2 and 1.3, whereas the compression work is a minimum when $n = 1$, i.e. for an isothermal compression. (If $n < 1$ the air is cooled below the inlet temperature, implying the use of refrigeration on which work would have to be expended.) These considerations give rise to the practice of quoting the performance of a compressor in terms of an *isothermal efficiency* defined by

$$\eta_{\text{iso}} = \frac{\text{isothermal work}}{\text{actual indicated work}} \tag{16.14}$$

If the mechanical friction losses are included, we have the *overall isothermal efficiency* defined as the ratio of the isothermal work to the actual brake work.

The reversible isothermal work cannot be obtained by putting $n = 1$ in (16.11), since this would yield the indeterminate solution 0/0. The anomaly arises from the fact that $\int dv/v$ is a special case of $\int dv/v^n$, for which the solution is $\ln v$. A repetition of the derivation of equation (16.2) for the special case $n = 1$ can be shown to yield

$$\dot{W}_{\text{iso}} = \dot{m} p_1 v_1 \ln \frac{p_2}{p_1} = \dot{m} R T_1 \ln \frac{p_2}{p_1} \tag{16.15}$$

This is the quantity used as the numerator in the expression for the isothermal efficiency (16.14).

When the air is compressed non-isothermally, i.e. when $1 < n < \gamma$, the extra work expended is not necessarily wasted. If the high-pressure air were to be used directly in an expander with the same polytropic index as the compressor, all the extra work could ideally be recovered. There are two main reasons why recovery is not feasible in practical applications. First, for n to lie between 1 and γ during an expansion, heat has to be supplied *to* the air. But this heat cannot be drawn from the cooler surroundings, and some means would have to be provided for transferring the heat rejected during the compression directly to the expander in a reversible manner. Secondly, the compressed air is normally used some distance away from the reciprocating compressor and it cools to atmospheric temperature in the delivery pipe. In fact the air is sometimes cooled deliberately immediately after compression, to condense the water vapour always present in atmospheric air and permit it to be drained off. This cooling has the incidental advantage of reducing the air viscosity and volume flow and hence the friction losses in the delivery pipe.

One other point noted in section 16.1 was the importance of the clearance volume in so far as it limits the mass flow which can be passed by a machine of given cylinder volume and speed. This consideration gives rise to another quantity used to assess the performance of a compressor—the *volumetric efficiency*. The volumetric efficiency is defined as the ratio of the actual volume induced per cycle to the swept volume. In terms of easily measured quantities it is given by

$$\eta_{vol} = \frac{\dot{m}v_1}{NV_s}$$

The quantity $\dot{m}v_1$ is known as the *free air delivery*; it is the rate of volume flow measured at inlet (e.g. atmospheric) pressure and temperature.

An expression for the volumetric efficiency of a reversible compressor can be deduced as follows. With reference to Fig. 16.7,

$$\eta_{vol} = \frac{V_b - V_a}{V_s} = \frac{V_s + V_d - V_a}{V_s}$$

$$= 1 + \frac{V_d}{V_s} - \frac{V_d V_a}{V_s V_d} = 1 - \frac{V_d}{V_s}\left\{\left(\frac{p_2}{p_1}\right)^{1/n} - 1\right\} \qquad (16.16)$$

Evidently with a fixed value of V_d/V_s, called the *clearance ratio*, the volumetric efficiency decreases with increase of pressure ratio. This is also obvious from Fig. 16.8a. At some pressure ratio the flow will be zero, but even before this extreme value is reached it is more economical to split the compression into two or more stages, rather than simply increase the size of cylinder to obtain the desired flow.

The p–V diagram for a reversible two-stage machine is shown in Fig. 16.8b. Air is compressed to some intermediate pressure p_i in the low-pressure cylinder and is then transferred to the high-pressure cylinder for final compression to p_2. The intermediate pressure p_i is determined by the relative values of the swept volumes in the two stages and their respective clearance ratios (see Example 16.1). The volumetric efficiency is usually expressed in terms of the first-stage swept volume V_s, i.e. $(V_b - V_a)/V_s$. If the whole compression were accomplished in the low-pressure cylinder, the dashed curve in Fig. 16.8b indicates that the volumetric efficiency would be reduced to $(V_b - V_a')/V_s$.

An improvement in volumetric efficiency is not the only benefit to be obtained by compounding the compression. Equation (16.12) indicates that the work required decreases as the inlet temperature T_1 decreases. If an *intercooler* is fitted between the stages, cooling the air leaving the first stage to T_1 before it

Fig. 16.8
The effect of multistage compression on volumetric efficiency

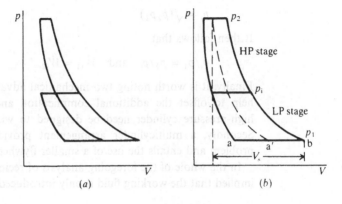

(a)   (b)

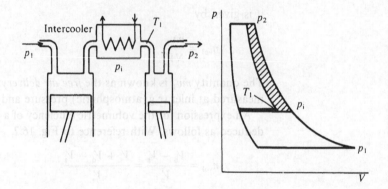

Fig. 16.9
The effect of intercooling
on the work of a
two-stage compressor

enters the second stage, the work required to drive the second stage is reduced. Fig. 16.9 illustrates this; the shaded area represents the saving in work. Intercooling brings the compression nearer to the ideal of isothermal compression. With an infinite number of stages this ideal would be reached, but in practice more than three stages are not used unless unusually high pressure ratios are required.

The actual saving in work depends on the choice of intermediate pressure. It is easy to show that in the case of reversible polytropic compression the total work required is a minimum when the work is divided equally between the stages. This applies to any number of stages, but here it will only be proved for the two-stage machine. With complete intercooling to T_1 at constant pressure, the total work required in the two stages is

$$\dot{W} = \dot{W}_{1i} + \dot{W}_{i2}$$

$$= \dot{m}\frac{n}{n-1}RT_1\left\{\left(\frac{p_i}{p_1}\right)^{(n-1)/n} - 1\right\} + \dot{m}\frac{n}{n-1}RT_1\left\{\left(\frac{p_2}{p_i}\right)^{(n-1)/n} - 1\right\}$$

Differentiating with respect to p_i and equating the zero,

$$\frac{n-1}{n}\left(\frac{1}{p_1}\right)^{(n-1)/n}\left(\frac{1}{p_i}\right)^{1/n} - \frac{n-1}{n}p_2^{(n-1)/n}p_i^{(1-2n)/n} = 0$$

or

$$p_i = \sqrt{(p_2 p_1)} \tag{16.17}$$

It then follows that

$$p_i/p_1 = p_2/p_i \quad \text{and} \quad \dot{W}_{1i} = \dot{W}_{i2} \tag{16.18}$$

Finally, it is worth noting two mechanical advantages of compounding which help to offset the additional complication and cost. First, only the small high-pressure cylinder need be designed to withstand the delivery pressure. Secondly, a multicylinder arrangement provides a less difficult balancing problem and entails the use of a smaller flywheel.

In the whole of the foregoing analysis of reciprocating machines it has been implied that the working fluid is only introduced to one side of the piston. The

Fig. 16.10
The double-acting
compressor

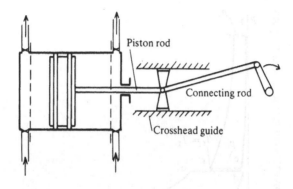

work capacity of the machine can be very nearly doubled if both sides of the piston are used; the machine is then said to be *double acting*. The chief difference in construction between a single- and a double-acting machine is that the latter requires the addition of a piston rod and crosshead, as depicted in Fig. 16.10, because it is necessary to seal the 'open' end of the cylinder with a gland. The piston performs two complete machine cycles per revolution. To determine the indicated power of a double-acting machine, it is necessary to take indicator diagrams from each end of the cylinder, and evaluate each diagram separately. It must be remembered that the effective piston area (A in equation (16.8)) is not the same in each case; the cross-sectional area of the piston rod must be subtracted from the piston area when evaluating the indicated power associated with the crosshead side of the piston.

Example 16.1   A single-acting two-stage compressor with complete intercooling delivers 6 kg/min of air at 16 bar. Assuming an intake state of 1 bar and 15 °C, and that the compression and expansion processes are reversible and polytropic with $n = 1.3$, calculate the power required, the isothermal efficiency and the free air delivery. Also calculate the net heat transferred in each cylinder and in the intercooler. If the clearance ratios for the low- and high-pressure cylinders are 0.04 and 0.06 respectively, calculate the swept and clearance volumes for each cylinder. The speed is 420 rev/min. (See Fig. 16.11.)

The pressure ratio per stage is

$$r_p = \frac{p_i}{p_1} = \frac{p_2}{p_i} = \sqrt{\left(\frac{16}{1}\right)} = 4$$

The work done in the two stages is

$$\dot{W} = \dot{W}_1 + \dot{W}_2 = 2\dot{m}\frac{n}{n-1}RT_1\{r_p^{(n-1)/n} - 1\}$$

$$= 2 \times \frac{6}{60} \times \frac{1.3}{0.3} \times 0.287 \times 288(4^{0.3/1.3} - 1) = 2 \times 13.50 = 27.00 \text{ kW}$$

Fig. 16.11

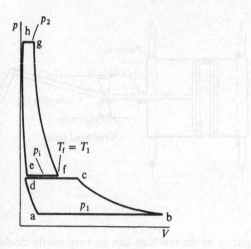

The isothermal work is

$$\dot{W}_{iso} = \dot{m}RT_1 \ln \frac{p_2}{p_1} = \frac{6}{60} \times 0.287 \times 288 \ln \frac{16}{1} = 22.92 \text{ kW}$$

and the isothermal efficiency is

$$\eta_{iso} = \frac{\dot{W}_{iso}}{\dot{W}} = \frac{22.92}{27.00} = 84.9 \text{ per cent}$$

The free air delivery is

$$\dot{V} = \dot{m}\frac{RT_1}{p_1} = 6 \times \frac{0.287 \times 288}{100 \times 1} = 4.96 \text{ m}^3/\text{min}$$

The temperature at the exit of each stage is

$$T_c = T_g = T_1 r_p^{(n-1)/n} = 288 \times 4^{0.3/1.3} = 397 \text{ K}$$

Hence the net heat rejected from each cylinder is found from the energy equation

$$\dot{Q} = \dot{m}c_p(T_c - T_1) - \dot{W}_1 = \dot{m}c_p(T_g - T_1) - \dot{W}_2$$

$$= \frac{6}{60} \times 1.005(397 - 288) - 13.50 = -2.55 \text{ kW}$$

and from the intercooler

$$\dot{Q} = \dot{m}c_p(T_1 - T_c) = \frac{6}{60} \times 1.005(288 - 397) = -10.95 \text{ kW}$$

The volumetric efficiency for each stage is found from (16.16) as

$$\eta_{vol,1} = 1 - 0.04(4^{1/1.3} - 1) = 0.924$$

$$\eta_{vol,2} = 1 - 0.06(4^{1/1.3} - 1) = 0.887$$

384

Hence for the first stage the swept volume is

$$V_b - V_d = \frac{\text{free air delivery}}{\text{speed} \times \eta_{\text{vol},1}} = \frac{4.96}{420 \times 0.924} = 0.012\,78 \text{ m}^3$$

and the clearance volume is

$$V_d = 0.04(V_b - V_d) = 0.000\,51 \text{ m}^3$$

For the second stage the swept volume is

$$V_f - V_h = \frac{1}{r_p} \frac{\text{free air delivery}}{\text{speed} \times \eta_{\text{vol},2}} = \frac{1}{4} \times \frac{4.96}{420 \times 0.887} = 0.003\,33 \text{ m}^3$$

and the clearance volume is

$$V_h = 0.06(V_f - V_h) = 0.000\,20 \text{ m}^3$$

It must be noted that points d and e need not coincide on the indicator diagram because they represent different states and different clearance masses Δm_{c1} and Δm_{c2}. In this particular case

$$V_e = V_h r_p^{1/n} = 0.000\,20 \times 4^{1/1.3} = 0.000\,58 \text{ m}^3$$

16.4   The steam engine

The reciprocating steam engine is a particular type of expander designed to produce work from steam expanding from a high to a low pressure. It is used as an alternative to a turbine in small steam plant (up to a few hundred kilowatts) where a turbine would be very inefficient, and where the inherent intermittent working of a reciprocating machine, which allows only moderate rates of flow and rotational speeds, is no disadvantage. (The reasons for the inefficiency of small turbines will become apparent after a reading of Chapter 19.) The range of expansion for the engine is governed by considerations of the thermodynamic cycle, and it will be remembered from Chapter 11 that a very wide range of pressure is required if a steam cycle is to be efficient. This requirement leads to multistage expansion in successive cylinders, but only the single-cylinder steam engine is described here in any detail.

There are two features peculiar to the steam engine which result in its ideal indicator diagram being different from the ideal diagram of an expander shown in Fig. 16.2a. The first lies in the fact that the temperature of the working fluid is always much greater than the surroundings. Thus, although the work done increases as the index of expansion n decreases, the best that can be hoped for in practice is that the expansion shall be isentropic. An index of expansion less than the isentropic index would imply heat reception from the surroundings. The second peculiarity arises because with steam at low pressures there is a very rapid increase of specific volume as the pressure is decreased isentropically, i.e. $-(dv/dp)_s$ is very large. With the pressure ranges employed in practice, this implies that a very long stroke would be required if the steam were to be expanded reversibly down to condenser pressure inside the engine cylinder. Such a long stroke is undesirable not only for structural reasons, but also

Fig. 16.12
A double-acting steam
engine cylinder with an
ideal p–V diagram

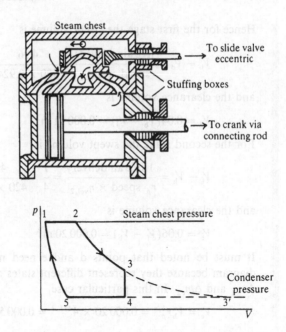

because it would reduce the mean effective pressure of the machine cycle and so increase the proportion of the indicated power expended in overcoming mechanical friction. That complete expansion entails a decrease in mean effective pressure should be evident from the p–V diagram of Fig. 16.12, the mean effective pressure of the additional area 4–3–3' being so small.

Fig. 16.12 shows a sketch of a double-acting steam engine fitted with a simple slide valve which is actuated by an eccentric on the crankshaft. As with all expanders, mechanically operated valves are necessary, and this feature makes possible the opening and closing of ports at any desired point in the machine cycle. The events on one side of the piston are as follows, those on the other side being similar but displaced in time by half a revolution of the crankshaft:

1–2 *Admission* When the piston is at outer dead centre the inlet port is opened, and a mass Δm_f of high-pressure steam is admitted by the time the inlet port is closed at the point of *cut-off*. The steam admitted mixes with a mass Δm_c which remained in the clearance volume after completion of the previous cycle.

2–3 *Expansion* The steam expands isentropically until the exhaust port is opened at the end of the stroke.

3–4 *Blow-down* The pressure at the end of the expansion stroke p_3 is higher than the condenser pressure p_4. When the exhaust port opens, some of the steam 'blows down' into the condenser until the pressure in the cylinder is p_4.

4–5 *Exhaust* On its return stroke the piston displaces the steam left in the cylinder after the blow-down until the exhaust port closes at point 5.

5–1 *Compression or 'cushioning'* The steam Δm_c left in the cylinder is compressed isentropically during the remainder of the stroke. Point 5

Fig. 16.13
State path of steam in the
cylinder

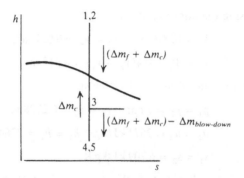

may be so chosen that the final pressure is equal to p_1, when Δm_c will mix reversibly with the next charge Δm_f.

The state path of the steam in the cylinder is depicted in Fig. 16.13. Admission 1–2 occurs ideally with no change in state, and the ensuing expansion follows an isentropic path 2–3 up to the blow-down. Although the blow-down is an irreversible expansion process, it may be imagined to consist of two parts, one reversible and the other irreversible. First, the steam in the cylinder expands isentropically, displacing some steam into the condenser; the expelled steam acquires some kinetic energy in the process. The state of the steam remaining in the cylinder is represented by point 4. Secondly, the kinetic energy of the expelled steam is dissipated irreversibly in the condenser; this part of the process is not shown on the h–s diagram. During the exhaust process 4–5 the state of the steam in the cylinder is unchanged, though the displaced steam will mix with steam in the condenser irreversibly. Finally, the mass Δm_c in state 4,5 is returned isentropically to state 1,2.

Owing to the blow-down, as well as for other reasons elaborated below, the expansion of the mass Δm_f passing through the cylinder is not isentropic. The overall enthalpy drop $\Delta m_f(h_1 - h_6)$ is less than the isentropic drop $\Delta m_f(h_1 - h_5)$, if h_6 denotes the enthalpy of the exhaust steam in the condenser space before it has rejected any heat to the cooling water. The ratio between the actual and the isentropic enthalpy drops is the *isentropic efficiency* of the engine. Example 16.2 shows how the effect of blow-down on the isentropic efficiency can be estimated.

Example 16.2 A steam engine cylinder has a swept volume of 0.03 m³ and a clearance volume of 0.001 m³. Cut-off is at 0.4 of the stroke. Saturated steam is admitted at 7 bar and expands isentropically to the blow-down. The mass which expands *inside* the cylinder during the blow-down may be assumed to do so isentropically. Cushioning is timed so that isentropic compression brings the clearance steam to the admission state. Calculate the work done per machine cycle and the isentropic efficiency when the engine exhausts at atmospheric pressure.

Using the notation of Fig. 16.12,

$$V_1 = 0.001 \text{ m}^3, \quad V_3 = V_4 = 0.031 \text{ m}^3,$$

$$V_2 = V_1 + 0.4(V_3 - V_1) = 0.013 \text{ m}^3$$

During the admission 1–2 the state is

$$p_1 = p_2 = 7 \text{ bar}, \quad v_1 = v_2 = 0.2728 \text{ m}^3/\text{kg}$$

$$u_1 = u_2 = 2573 \text{ kJ/kg}, \quad h_1 = h_2 = 2764 \text{ kJ/kg},$$

$$s_1 = s_2 = 6.709 \text{ kJ/kg K}$$

During exhaust 4–5 the pressure is 1.013 bar, and the dryness fraction is found from $s_1 = s_5 = s_4$ to be 0.893. Then

$$v_4 = v_5 = 1.494 \text{ m}^3/\text{kg}, \quad u_4 = u_5 = 2283 \text{ kJ/kg},$$

$$h_4 = h_5 = 2434 \text{ kJ/kg}$$

At the beginning of the blow-down, state 3, the specific volume is

$$v_3 = v_2\left(\frac{V_3}{V_2}\right) = 0.2728 \times \frac{0.031}{0.013} = 0.6505 \text{ m}^3/\text{kg}$$

By trial and error from tables, or more quickly from the h–s chart, we find that in state 3, defined by $v_3 = 0.6505 \text{ m}^3/\text{kg}$ and $s_3 = s_2 = 6.709 \text{ kJ/kg K}$, $p_3 = 2.6 \text{ bar}$ and $x_3 = 0.939$. Hence $u_3 = 2417 \text{ kJ/kg}$.

The masses of steam in the cylinder at the points 1 to 5 are

$$m_1 = m_5 = V_1/v_1 = 0.0037 \text{ kg}$$

$$m_2 = m_3 = V_2/v_2 = V_3/v_3 = 0.0477 \text{ kg},$$

$$m_4 = V_4/v_4 = 0.0207 \text{ kg}$$

Cushioning must begin when

$$V_5 = m_5 v_5 = 0.0055 \text{ m}^3$$

The total work done per machine cycle can now be found from five non-flow processes:

$W_{12} = -p_1(V_2 - V_1) = -100 \times 7 \times 0.012 =$		-8.40 kJ
$W_{23} = m_2(u_3 - u_2) = -0.0477 \times 156 =$		-7.44 kJ
$W_{34} =$		$0 \quad \text{kJ}$
$W_{45} = -p_4(V_5 - V_4) = 100 \times 1.013 \times 0.0255 =$		$+2.58 \text{ kJ}$
$W_{51} = m_5(u_1 - u_5) = 0.0037 \times 290 =$		$+1.07 \text{ kJ}$
$W =$		-12.19 kJ

The isentropic work can be found in two ways. Assuming that full expansion is achieved by lengthening the stroke to 3′, corresponding to the exhaust state 4,5,

$$V_3' = m_3 v_4 = 0.0713 \text{ m}^3$$

Hence the total work is

$$W_{12} = \qquad\qquad\qquad\qquad\qquad\qquad\qquad -8.40\,\text{kJ}$$

$$W_{23'} = m_2(u_3' - u_2) = -0.0477 \times 290 = \qquad -13.83\,\text{kJ}$$

$$W_{3'5} = -p_3'(V_5 - V_3') = 100 \times 1.013 \times 0.0658 = \quad +6.67\,\text{kJ}$$

$$W_{51} = \qquad\qquad\qquad\qquad\qquad\qquad\qquad +1.07\,\text{kJ}$$

$$W_{\text{isen}} = \qquad\qquad\qquad\qquad\qquad\qquad\qquad -14.49\,\text{kJ}$$

We arrive at the same answer more easily using the steady-flow analysis. The flow steam per machine cycle is

$$\Delta m_f = m_2 - m_1 = 0.0477 - 0.0037 = 0.0440\,\text{kg}$$

and, because from the $h-s$ chart $(h_3' - h_1) = -330\,\text{kJ/kg}$,

$$W_{\text{isen}} = \Delta m_f(h_3' - h_1) = -0.0440 \times 330 = -14.52\,\text{kJ}$$

The isentropic efficiency is

$$\eta_{\text{isen}} = \frac{W}{W_{\text{isen}}} = \frac{-12.19}{-14.52} = 0.84$$

Note that the mean effective pressure for the complete reversible expansion is

$$(p_\text{m})_{\text{isen}} = \frac{|W|_{\text{isen}}}{V_3' - V_1} = \frac{14.52}{100 \times 0.0703} = 2.07\,\text{bar}$$

and for the irreversible expansion is

$$p_\text{m} = \frac{|W|}{V_4 - V_1} = \frac{12.19}{100 \times 0.030} = 4.06\,\text{bar}$$

Thus in practice, when mechanical friction is taken into account, the irreversible expansion would probably yield a greater brake power.

It has already been mentioned that the ports may be opened and closed at any desired point in the cycle. The point of cut-off and the point where cushioning begins require special comment. If the cut-off is too early in the expansion stroke the work done per cycle will be unduly small, and if it is too late the additional work will not be commensurate with the additional amount of steam admitted (see Fig. 16.14a). The work done per machine cycle can also be increased by delaying the onset of cushioning (Fig. 16.14b), but again this will be at the expense of an increase in steam consumption. This is because the pressure of the clearance steam after cushioning is then below the steam main pressure and, when the inlet port is opened, steam rushes in to raise the cylinder pressure in an irreversible manner.

The indicator diagram taken from an actual engine differs from the ideal diagram of Fig. 16.12 for a number of reasons. There are the usual differences already mentioned in section 16.3 associated with the finite time required for opening and closing valve ports and the pressure drops incurred by fluid friction as the steam enters and leaves the cylinder. There is another important difference

Fig. 16.14
The effect of varying
(a) cut-off and
(b) cushioning on the p–V
diagram

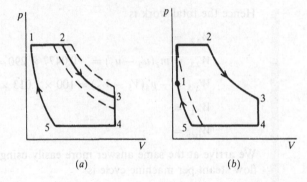

(a)   (b)

Fig. 16.15
Cyclic variation of
temperature

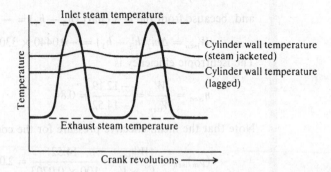

associated with the fact that it is not possible to eliminate heat transfers between
the steam and the cylinder. The steam undergoes a considerable change in
temperature during its passage through the machine but, owing to the resistance
to heat flow between fluid and cylinder, the cylinder temperature fluctuates
between much narrower limits; this is indicated in Fig. 16.15. Evidently the
temperature difference between the steam and the cylinder varies in such a way
that heat is rejected by the steam during admission and early expansion, while
heat is received during the latter part of the expansion and during the exhaust
process. Even if the cylinder is well lagged or steam jacketed, and the heat
rejected to the surrounding atmosphere is small, the cylinder itself acts
alternately as a sink and a source of heat.

The effect of the heat exchanges is not very marked if superheated steam is
being used, but it becomes very pronounced if the steam is only just dry at
entry. Heat rejection during admission is then manifested by condensation of
steam on the cylinder walls. Once condensation occurs there is a sudden and
very large increase in the rate of heat transfer,* and hence the condensation
process is accelerated. Heat transfer from the cylinder during the latter part of
the expansion and exhaust stroke re-evaporates some of the condensate, but
too late for the resulting vapour to do much work. The main effect of the
re-evaporation is an increase in exhaust pressure due to the increased specific

---

* A condensing vapour exchanges heat with a surface at a rate which may be several hundred
times larger than that for a dry vapour or gas; see Fig. 22.25.

volume of the steam flowing through the exhaust port. The net result of all these heat exchanges is an increase in steam consumption and a decrease of work output.

Both the loss of work associated with the failure to expand down to condenser pressure in the cylinder, and that due to the heat transfers, become more pronounced as the pressure range is increased. More efficient operation can then be achieved by compounding, i.e. by carrying out the expansion in two or more stages. The large volume of low-pressure steam can be handled in a large-diameter cylinder without the need for an excessively long stroke, and at the same time the range of temperature variation in each cylinder is only a fraction of the total temperature change of the steam. Sometimes, to keep the low-pressure cylinder within reasonable dimensions, the low-pressure steam is split between two cylinders in parallel. The expansion may be completed down to the condenser pressure if a turbine is added as a final stage. Even if the plant is of relatively low power output, a turbine can be quite efficient if it is called upon to deal with the steam at the low-pressure end where the volume flow is large. The combination of reciprocating engine and turbine was used for medium-size marine plant before the oil engine began to supplant the steam engine.

The power output of a steam engine can be controlled in one of two ways. From what has been said about the choice of the point of cut-off (Fig. 16.14a), it will be clear that one possibility is the use of a special valve gear which will permit the timing of the cut-off to be varied; this is called *cut-off governing*. The second method, *throttle governing*, consists of throttling the steam in a regulating valve before admission to the steam chest, thereby reducing the inlet pressure and effective enthalpy drop available from the expansion. The effect of both methods is illustrated in Fig. 16.16 for the simple case where the clearance volume is zero. In the cut-off governed engine the reduction in work is obtained by a reduction in the mass of steam admitted, and the *ideal* enthalpy drop per unit mass is unchanged. In the throttle governed engine the work is reduced by an irreversible reduction of steam chest pressure, which results in an appreciable reduction in available enthalpy drop per unit mass, and the mass of steam admitted is only slightly reduced by virtue of the fact that the specific volume of the steam is increased. The former is clearly the more efficient method of governing, and is always preferred for such applications as steam locomotives

Fig. 16.16
Cut-off and throttle governing

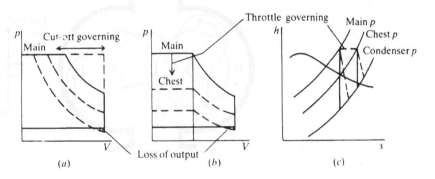

(a) (b) (c)

where the engine is not speed governed. The heavy valve gear required for varying the point of cut-off is unsuitable for use with the normal type of speed governor, and where constant speed is required (e.g. for pumping plant) the ease with which a simple throttle valve can be operated by a governor outweighs considerations of fuel economy. Reference to Fig. 16.16a will indicate another reason why cut-off governing is used for traction engines. By operating the engine non-expansively, a rectangular diagram is obtained. This provides the particularly large torques required for starting purposes, and the disproportionate increase in steam consumption is of no significance for such a short duration.

16.5 Rotary positive displacement compressors

In the type of compressor discussed earlier, the component which displaces the fluid from the low- to the high-pressure region performs a reciprocating motion. Here we shall discuss compressors in which the displacement is performed by a rotating component. The rotary machine can operate at high speeds and can therefore handle larger rates of flow than its reciprocating counterpart—or is smaller for a given flow. The processes are for this reason more nearly adiabatic than in reciprocating compressors, and the indicated isothermal efficiency will be lower. To some extent this is offset by the fact that the mechanical efficiency is usually higher than for reciprocating machines, thus giving similar *overall* isothermal efficiencies for both classes of compressor. Rotary compressors are particularly suitable as superchargers for internal-combustion engines and as vacuum pumps, and they are often arranged in stages.

There are several distinct designs of rotary compressor, and one of the simplest and best known is the *Roots blower* shown in Fig. 16.17. Its essential parts are two rotors, each rotor having two or more lobes with profiles formed by complete epicycloids and hypocycloids. This geometric form ensures that at all angular

Fig. 16.17
The Roots blower

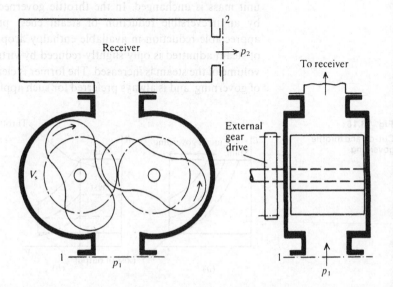

ig. 16.18
eciprocating analogue of
bots blower

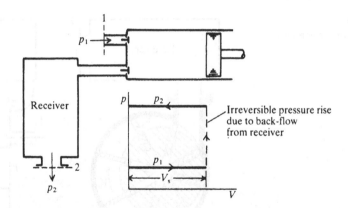

positions the high-pressure space is sealed from the low-pressure space. One rotor is coupled to the source of power, the other being driven from it by gears external to the casing (not through the lobes). There is always a slight clearance between the meshing lobes to avoid wear at the sealing surfaces.

The mode of action is as follows. In the position shown, a volume V_s of air, at atmospheric pressure say, is being trapped between the left-hand rotor and the casing. Assuming adiabatic conditions, this trapped volume does not change its state until the space V_s is opened to the high-pressure region. At that instant some high-pressure air will rush back from the receiver and mix irreversibly with the air in the lower until the pressure is equalised. The air is then displaced into the receiver. This happens four times per complete revolution, and the free air delivery of the compressor is thus $4V_s$ per revolution. The air flow into the receiver is intermittent, even though the rotors revolve with uniform speed.

To see how the work done in this irreversible flow process may be calculated, let us consider the reciprocating compressor of Fig. 16.18 with no clearance and a swept volume of V_s. After air at atmospheric pressure p_1 is drawn in, the inlet valve is closed and the delivery valve is opened immediately afterwards with the piston still at inner dead centre. Back-flow from the receiver will equalise the pressure in the receiver and the cylinder by an irreversible process. We shall consider the receiver to be of infinite volume compared with the volume V_s, i.e. that the equalised pressure will be p_2, which is the steady pressure of the air leaving at section 2. This compressor performs the same process as a Roots blower with an infinite receiver.[*] The work required per four revolutions of the reciprocating machine, equivalent to that required per revolution of the Roots blower is,

$$W = (p_2 - p_1)4V_s \qquad (16.19)$$

Note that this is greater than the work required to drive a reversible adiabatic compressor.

Fig. 16.19a shows a *vane pump*, whose mode of action differs slightly from that of the Roots blower. Volumes V_a, V_b, V_c, V_d are trapped between the vanes

---

[*] The analysis for the case of a finite receiver is complicated, and for this the reader is referred to Ref. 17.

Fig. 16.19

The rotary vane compressor

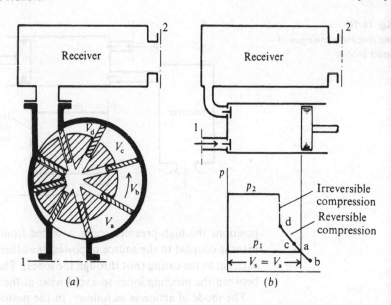

(a)   *(b)*

and the casing, the vanes sliding in slots in the eccentrically placed rotor. Consider the volume V_a of air which has just been trapped at atmospheric pressure p_1. When it reaches the position of volume V_d, which is on the verge of being uncovered, it will have been reduced in size owing to the asymmetrical placing of the inlet and outlet ports; thus $p_d > p_1$ assuming adiabatic conditions. In practical applications the pressure p_d is normally less than the delivery pressure p_2, and further compression is obtained by an irreversible back-flow of air from the receiver as in the Roots blower. An idealised equivalent reciprocating compressor of swept volume V_s equal to V_a is shown in Fig. 16.19b. The initial part of the compression from p_1 to p_d is reversible and, after the delivery valve is opened at d, further compression to p_2 is achieved irreversibly. The total work per N revolutions, being equivalent to the work required per revolution by a vane pump with N vanes, is

$$W = N\frac{\gamma}{\gamma - 1}p_1 V_a\left\{\left(\frac{p_d}{p_1}\right)^{(\gamma - 1)/\gamma} - 1\right\} + N(p_2 - p_d)V_d \qquad (16.20)$$

The vane compressor is said to have internal compression owing to the reduction in volume from V_a to V_d, a feature which is absent in the Roots blower. By comparing the $p-V$ diagrams in Figs 16.18 and 16.19, it is evident that internal compression reduces the work required. The *Lysholm compressor*, which is similar to the Roots blower but with helical lobes, possesses a high degree of internal compression: it is described fully in Ref. 9.

17

Reciprocating Internal-Combustion Engines

There are two principal classes of reciprocating internal-combustion (or IC) engine. They are distinguished mainly by whether the combustion is initiated by a spark, or spontaneously by virtue of the rise in temperature during the compression process. Petrol and gas engines are in the former class and they will be referred to here as *spark-ignition* (or SI) engines. The term *compression-ignition* (or CI) engine will be used to refer to the second class, although the terms 'Diesel engine' and 'oil engine' are also common.

After the modes of action of some typical SI and CI engines are described, suitable criteria of performance are discussed, and the factors which limit the performance of practical IC engines are outlined. This is followed by a comparison of the real processes of an IC engine with the equivalent air-standard cycle. The chapter ends with a brief discussion of the limits that are imposed by the laws of thermodynamics on the conversion of chemical energy into work.

17.1 The working of IC engines

Both SI and CI engines can be designed so that one complete cycle of events in the cylinder is completed during either four or two strokes of the piston. The main events occurring in a *four-stroke* petrol SI engine are illustrated in Fig. 17.1 and are as follows:

1–2 *Induction stroke* A mixture of air and petrol vapour is drawn into the cylinder, the pressure of the mixture being a little below atmospheric owing to friction in the induction pipe. The inlet valve closes just after the end of the stroke.

2–3 *Compression stroke* With both inlet and exhaust valves closed, the air–fuel mixture is compressed. Just before the piston reaches outer dead centre, ignition is effected by an electric spark. Combustion is not instantaneous, but occupies a finite period. Nevertheless much of it occurs at nearly constant volume because the piston is moving relatively slowly near dead centre.

3–4 *Expansion or working stroke* Combustion is *nominally* completed at the beginning of the expansion stroke, and the products expand until the

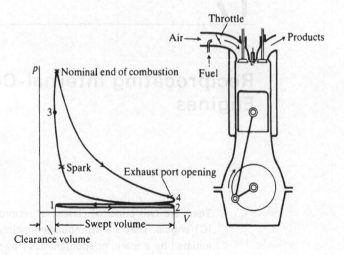

Fig. 17.1
The spark-ignition SI
engine

exhaust valve opens just before the end of the stroke. As the valve opens, the gases blow down the exhaust duct until the pressure in the cylinder has fallen to approximately atmospheric pressure.

4–1 *Exhaust stroke* The products which have not escaped from the cylinder during the blow-down are displaced by the piston. To provide the pressure difference necessary to overcome friction in the exhaust duct, the pressure in the cylinder is slightly above atmospheric. At the end of the stroke there will be some residual gases in the clearance volume, which will dilute the next charge drawn into the cylinder.

The events in a four-stroke CI engine, illustrated in Fig. 17.2, differ from those in the SI engine in the following manner:

1–2 *Induction stroke* Air alone is admitted to the cylinder.

2–3 *Compression stroke* The air is compressed, and towards the end of the stroke liquid fuel is sprayed into the cylinder. The temperature of the air at the end of compression is sufficiently high for the droplets of fuel to vaporise and ignite as they enter the cylinder.

3–4 *Expansion or working stroke* Since the fuel is sprayed into the cylinder

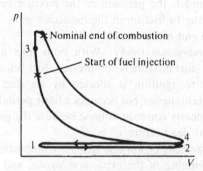

Fig. 17.2
Four-stroke SI engine
cycle

Fig. 17.3
The two-stroke engine

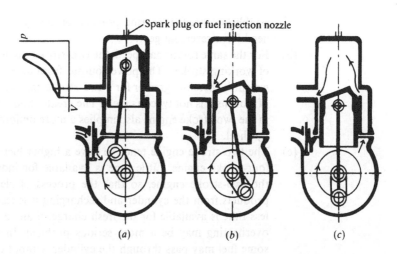

Spark plug or fuel injection nozzle

(a)   (b)   (c)

at a controlled rate, the pressure may remain fairly constant during combustion. In modern high-speed engines, however, there is often a rise in pressure during the initial stages of combustion. At some point in the expansion stroke the combustion is nominally complete and the pressure then falls steadily until the exhaust valve is opened and blow-down occurs.

4–1   *Exhaust stroke*   This follows as in the SI engine.

When the *two-stroke* cycle is employed, the induction and exhaust strokes are eliminated. The piston stroke must be longer, because part of the compression and expansion strokes are used for the processes of exhaust and induction. Fig. 17.3 shows a section of a common type of two-stroke engine. Apart from the self-acting spring-loaded valve on the crankcase, no valves are required, and the piston itself is used to open and close the inlet and exhaust ports. In Fig. 17.3a the piston is shown near the end of the compression stroke. The upward motion has decompressed the crank case and air has been admitted through the self-acting valve to the crankcase. During the expansion stroke the air in the crankcase is compressed, and near the end of this stroke the exhaust port is uncovered to allow the hot gases to blow down the exhaust duct. Further movement of the piston uncovers the inlet port, and compressed air from the crankcase flows into the cylinder. The exhaust and inlet ports are open simultaneously for a short period so that the incoming air can assist in clearing the cylinder of combustion products. The machine cycle is finally completed by compression of the air trapped in the cylinder. The two-stroke engine can be built as an SI engine, with petrol vapour and air being admitted to the crankcase, or as a CI engine.

A full discussion of the relative merits of two-stroke and four-stroke engines would be out of place here, but the following points are worth noting:

(a)   The two-stroke engine does not require any mechanically operated valves. This implies not only considerable mechanical simplification, but also that the engine can be run in either direction. The two-stroke CI engine has established itself in marine practice primarily because it eliminates the need for a reversing gear.

(b) For the same rotational speed, the two-stroke engine has twice the number of working strokes. The power output from an engine of given bulk and weight is therefore greater for a two-stroke engine, although for a number of reasons it is not twice as great. The greater frequency of working strokes in the two-stroke engine also implies a more uniform torque and a smaller flywheel.

(c) The two-stroke engine tends to have a higher fuel consumption than the four-stroke engine. Little time is available for induction and exhaust in the two-stroke engine, so that the process of clearing the combustion products from the cylinder and recharging it is less complete. Moreover, less time is available for the fresh charge of air to cool the cylinder, and overheating may be a more serious problem. In two-stroke SI engines some fuel may pass through the cylinder without combustion because of the necessary overlap of the periods when the inlet and exhaust ports are open.

A description of the general working of IC engines would not be complete without the mention of a rotary variant, a recent design of which is known as the *Wankel engine*. It is akin to the two-stroke engine in that it requires no valves. The diagrammatic sketch in Fig. 17.4 shows the principles of operation. The triangular rotor A, having internal teeth meshing with a central gear fixed to the engine casing, performs a planetary motion around this gear. An eccentric B, integral with the power output shaft, revolves in a recess of rotor A at three times its speed. The shape of the outer casing is such that the apexes of the triangular rotor seal off three distinct spaces 1, 2 and 3. The shape of the curved surfaces of rotor A is unimportant, except in so far as it determines the maximum and minimum volumes of the sealed spaces, and therefore the compression ratio. The curved surfaces are recessed as shown, mainly to avoid 'throttling' of the flame spreading from the spark plug through the combustion space.

The sequence of events is not difficult to follow. Fig. 17.4a shows the situation where a charge is being induced into space 1, the preceding charge is fully compressed in space 2, and the combustion products are being exhausted from space 3. Fig. 17.4b represents the situation a little later, with the new charge occupying the maximum volume and about to be compressed in space 1, combustion gases expanding in space 2 to provide the 'working stroke', and space 3 being reduced in volume and thus exhausting the products through the outlet port.

The rotary engine has one important feature in common with its reciprocating counterpart: it is a positive displacement machine, and the processes occur in a cyclic intermittent manner. We therefore consider it here for the same reason that the Roots blower and vane pump were considered in the chapter on reciprocating compressors. Its obvious advantages *vis-à-vis* the reciprocating engine are that it is capable of handling fairly large mass flows for its size and

Fig. 17.4
The Wankel engine

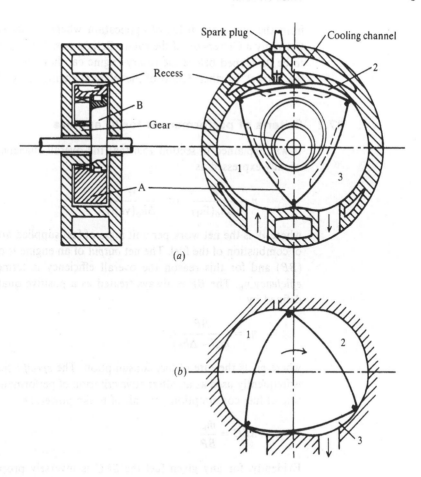

(a)

(b)

thus has a larger power/weight ratio, and also that its rotor can be perfectly balanced by the addition of appropriate masses.

Three disadvantages of the rotary design are apparent. First, because the processes occur in a sequence of positions around the casing, the surfaces near the spark plug are intermittently cooled by the *compressed* charge, whereas the reciprocating engine cylinder is intermittently cooled by the colder *uncompressed* charge. Furthermore, the casing surface adjacent to space 3 is permanently exposed to the expanding burnt gases. This implies the need for good local cooling arrangements. Although the problem is eased by the high surface/volume ratio of the combustion space, it does of course result in high heat losses. Secondly, the long narrow shape of the combustion space is not good from the point of view of using high compression ratios, as will become clear after the discussion of detonation in section 17.3.1. Thirdly—and this is the reason for the failure of many early attempts to develop a rotary engine—there is an inherently difficult sealing problem at the apexes and flat side faces of the rotor. After many years of development, and in spite of some degree of success, it now looks unlikely that the Wankel engine will displace the reciprocating engine

399

from the numerous fields of application where the latter is well established. Certainly a CI version of the rotary design, possible in principle, will also have to be developed before the rotary engine can hope to capture a major part of the market. Further details of the Wankel engine can be found in Ref. 22.

17.2 Criteria of performances for IC engines

It was explained in section 15.6 that the overall efficiency of a power plant is usually expressed as

$$\eta = \frac{W}{\Delta h_0(\text{liq})} \quad \text{or} \quad \frac{W}{\Delta h_0(\text{vap})}$$

where W is the net work per unit mass of fuel supplied and Δh_0 is the enthalpy of combustion of the fuel. The net *output* of an engine is called the *brake power* (*BP*) and for this reason the overall efficiency is termed the *brake thermal efficiency* η_b. The *BP* is always treated as a positive quantity, and hence η_b is defined by

$$\eta_b = \frac{BP}{\dot{m}_F(-\Delta h_0)} \tag{17.1}$$

where $\dot{m}_F$ is the rate of fuel consumption. The *specific fuel consumption* (*SFC*) is frequently used as an alternative criterion of performance. It is defined as the rate of fuel consumption per unit of brake power, i.e.

$$SFC = \frac{\dot{m}_F}{BP} \tag{17.2}$$

Evidently, for any given fuel the *SFC* is inversely proportional to η_b. Most common hydrocarbon fuels have very similar enthalpies of combustion, and the *SFC* can therefore be used when comparing the economy of engines using different fuels.

In a reciprocating engine an appreciable part of the loss is due to mechanical friction, and it is informative if the thermodynamic and mechanical friction losses are separated. The overall efficiency is therefore analysed as the product of the *indicated thermal efficiency* η_i and the *mechanical efficiency* η_{mech}. Thus

$$\eta_b = \left(\frac{IP}{\dot{m}_F(-\Delta h_0)}\right)\left(\frac{BP}{IP}\right) = \eta_i \eta_{\text{mech}} \tag{17.3}$$

The *indicated power* (*IP*) is the actual rate of work done by the working fluid on the piston, and the difference between the *IP* and the *BP* is the power absorbed by mechanical friction (piston, bearings etc.). As its name implies, the *IP* can be determined from an *indicator diagram*. The procedure has been explained in section 16.3. The only point of difference here is that with a four-stoke engine the area of the small anticlockwise loop (Fig. 17.5) must be subtracted from the area of the main diagram when determining the *indicated mean effective pressure* (*IMEP*) p_m. The work represented by the small loop is

Fig. 17.5
Effect of pumping loss on
he indicator diagram

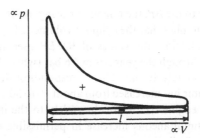

termed the *pumping loss*; it is the result of viscous friction in the induction and
exhaust strokes. The physical equation equivalent to (16.8) for the *IP* is

$$IP = p_m LAN \tag{17.4}$$

Here N is the number of machine cycles per unit time, namely half the rotational
speed for a four-stroke engine, and the rotational speed for a two-stroke engine.

When an engine is run at constant speed, the variation of η_b and η_{mech} with
load appears as in Fig. 17.6. At constant speed the power expended on mechanical
friction—termed the *friction power (FP)*—is approximately constant. Therefore,
as the *BP* is reduced the mechanical friction loss exercises an increasing influence
on the efficiencies. At zero *BP* all the fuel is consumed in overcoming friction,
and both η_b and η_{mech} are zero. With an engine of good mechanical design,
η_{mech} should be between 80 and 90 per cent at full load. η_b depends upon the
type of engine, but at full load it is usually 25–35 per cent for SI engines and
30–40 per cent for CI engines.

When discussing air-standard cycles for reciprocating engines it was suggested
that the mean effective pressure provides a useful guide to the relative size of
an engine. In practice it is usual to use the concept of *brake mean effective
pressure (BMEP)* for this purpose. The *BMEP*, which may be denoted by p_{mb},
is defined by an equivalent equation to (17.4), i.e.

$$BP = p_{mb} LAN \tag{17.5}$$

The *BMEP* may be regarded as that part of the *IMEP* which is imagined to

Fig. 17.6
Variation of efficiency with
load at constant speed

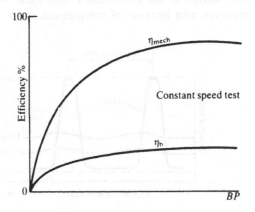

contribute to the *BP*, the remainder being used to overcome friction. An increase in *BMEP* implies that the cylinder volume *LA* can be smaller for a given output. As an illustration, the values of *BMEP* used in SI car engines have steadily increased through the years from 4.6 bar (when the RAC rating was introduced) to approximately 10 bar. The corresponding *BP* obtained per litre of cylinder swept volume has increased from about 10 to 30 kW. This considerable reduction of specific engine size is not due solely to the increase in *BMEP* but is partly due to a simultaneous increase in permissible engine speed. In the following section we shall discuss the more important factors which limit the efficiency and *BMEP* of SI and CI engines.

17.3 Factors limiting the performance of IC engines

When discussing gas turbine power plant in section 12.2 it was pointed out that the performance was limited by the maximum gas temperature that can be permitted in the engine. This 'metallurgical limit' is imposed because the turbine is continuously exposed to high temperatures under conditions of severe stress. Provided that proper attention is paid to the cooling of the cylinder (particularly the cylinder head) and exhaust valves, no such limitation is encountered in reciprocating engines where the working stresses are much lower. The reason for this is indicated in Fig. 17.7, which shows qualitatively the temperature variation of the gas in an engine cylinder. The peak gas temperature may be as high as 2800 K, but this temperature is reached in intermittent combustion and is not due to a transfer of heat through the cylinder wall. The metal temperature therefore fluctuates between much narrower limits. Moreover, owing to cylinder cooling, and the insulating properties of a gas boundary layer and a film of lubricating oil which are adhering to the wall, the mean metal temperature is well below the mean gas temperature.

There are several factors of a different nature limiting the performance of reciprocating engines and, as they differ for SI and CI engines, each type of engine will be considered separately.

17.3.1 *The SI engine*

The analysis of the air-standard Otto cycle showed that the cycle efficiency improves with increase of compression ratio. This is also true of the brake

Fig. 17.7
Cyclic variation of
temperature

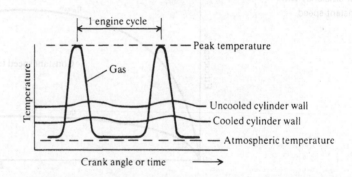

Fig. 17.8
Combustion in an SI
engine

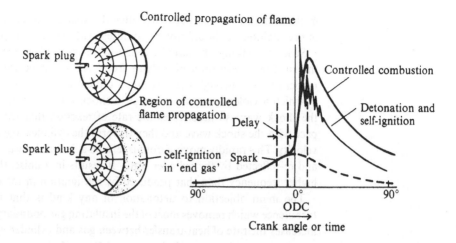

thermal efficiency of SI engines. There is an upper limit to the compression ratio that can be employed, however, which has its origin in the fact that the liquid compressed in the cylinder is a mixture of fuel vapour and air. The temperature of the combustible mixture increases on compression, and if the compression ratio is too high it is possible for self-ignition to occur before spark ignition. The onset of combustion at too early a point in the compression stroke would lead to a serious loss of power and must be avoided.

Even a compression ratio sufficiently low to avoid *pre-ignition* may be too high for efficient operation. This is due to the phenomenon of *detonation*. Although a considerable effort has been made to determine the exact nature of detonation in an engine cylinder, it is still a controversial topic. There are undoubtedly several phenomena involved, and such terms as 'knocking' and 'pinking' are often used in an attempt to distinguish between them. Here we can only give a very brief and oversimplified picture, with the aid of Fig. 17.8.

Under normal conditions combustion begins near the spark plug after a short delay following the formation of the spark, and the flame spreads through the mixture with a rapid but finite velocity. The energy released by the spark is only small, and it sets off a relatively slow flameless reaction which occupies the *delay period*. Further energy is released at an accelerating rate by the reaction, until a proper flame front develops. (The delay period is very short— approximately 0.002 second—but it may correspond to an appreciable movement of the crank in a high-speed engine. For example, at 3000 rev/min the crank turns through 36 degrees in 0.002 second. This is the reason why the point of ignition is always well in advance of outer dead centre (ODC).) As the flame front spreads in a uniform manner across the combustion space, it compresses the unburnt part of the mixture before it. The temperature of the unburnt portion is raised by intense radiation from the flame as well as by the compression. If the initial pressure and temperature are too high, the unburnt portion appears to reach a critical condition resulting in self-ignition at numerous points in the unburnt 'end gas'. A violent pressure rise is then produced which may result in a knocking noise. This phenomenon of self-ignition in the end gas, though occurring after the spark, is akin to the phenomenon of pre-ignition. It should not be confused with detonation proper.

Strictly speaking, the term 'detonation' refers to phenomena associated with the sudden acceleration of a flame front. As the flame front progresses at a moderate rate through the mixture, a critical condition is sometimes reached at which a violent pressure wave, i.e. a shock wave, is formed. The violence of the shock wave so accelerates the rate of reaction that the flame front keeps pace with the shock wave and they traverse the cylinder together at a very high velocity. This rapidly moving front is termed a *detonation wave*, and it is reflected and re-reflected by the cylinder walls. It results in a noise, though usually of a higher frequency than that produced by self-ignition in the end gas.*

The main objection to detonation of any kind is that it causes excessive turbulence which removes most of the insulating gas boundary layer. It therefore increases the rate of heat transfer between gas and cylinder wall and may result in serious overheating of the engine. Even if this is avoided, continuous detonation may cause the formation of local hot spots which eventually lead to pre-ignition. Excessive turbulence also results in a reduction of power output. From the mechanical point of view, detonation may cause deterioration of the bearing surfaces in a lightly built engine. Lastly, the appearance of carbon in the exhaust gases when detonation occurs indicates that it results in incomplete combustion. For all these reasons a compression ratio sufficiently high to cause detonation must be avoided.

Some fuels permit the use of a higher compression ratio than others,[†] and there are compounds ('dopes') which can be added to petrols to suppress the tendency to detonate. It is difficult to devise a measure of the detonating tendency of a fuel. One method is to compare the performance of a fuel with that of a heptane-octane mixture in a special variable compression-ratio engine. n-heptane (C_7H_{16}) is a fuel liable to give detonation at low compression ratios, while iso-octane (C_8H_{18}) detonates at much higher ratios; different mixtures of the two provide a continuous *octane number* scale from 0 to 100 per cent in octane content. The compression ratio of the engine is raised until the fuel under test detonates, and the highest percentage of octane in a heptane-octane mixture that produces detonation at the same compression ratio is called the octane number of the fuel. It should be emphasised, however, that the octane rating is an arbitrary measure, and it is possible to mix a fuel which is better than pure iso-octane and which therefore has an octane rating greater than 100. The need for a test engine of agreed design arises from the fact that the size and shape of the combustion space and the location of the spark plug are also important factors governing detonation, because they determine the length of time during which the end gas is exposed to the advancing flame front. For the same reason, in an engine of given size a large number of small cylinders is preferable to a small number of large cylinders. Over the last fifty years,

---

* A discussion of various theories can be found in Refs 10 and 21.
† Fuel oils have a marked tendency to detonate and therefore cannot be used in SI engines. Apart from this, oils do not evaporate as readily as petrols and homogeneous combustible mixtures are not easily obtained.

Fig. 17.9
Effect of mixture strength
on engine performance

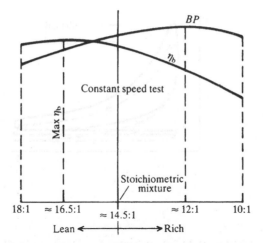

developments in 'doped' fuels and combustion chamber design (Ref. 12) have succeeded in raising the permissible compression ratio of ordinary car engines from about 4.5 to 9.

With the compression ratio fixed, the other factor limiting the performance is the rise in pressure obtainable during combustion. The *IMEP* increases with increase in peak pressure, and an increase in *IMEP* is desirable because it implies that the engine will be smaller for a given power output and that a relatively smaller share of the *IP* will be absorbed in overcoming mechanical friction. The peak pressure is fixed by the amount of fuel that can be burnt and hence by the amount of oxygen available. Theoretically it will be a maximum if a stoichiometric mixture is used. Stoichiometric air/fuel ratios by weight are nearly identical for all common liquid fuels, i.e. about 14.5:1. In practice, maximum brake thermal efficiency is achieved with a slightly weak mixture giving complete combustion of the fuel, and maximum power with a slightly rich mixture giving complete combustion of the oxygen (Fig. 17.9).

The variation of efficiency with load has already been mentioned in the previous section, and the method of regulating the power output deserves some mention here. At first sight it would seem that the work output could be reduced by weakening the mixture and thereby reducing the rise in pressure during combustion. Unfortunately, reliable ignition by a spark is only possible over a fairly narrow range of air/fuel ratio, 18:1 being about the weakest limit. It follows that variation of the air/fuel ratio is quite unsuitable as a method of governing SI engines. Instead, approximately stoichiometric ratios are used at all loads, and regulation is achieved by reducing the mass of mixture induced in each working cycle. This method is referred to as *throttle* or *quantity governing*. Throttling results in subatmospheric pressure in the cylinder during the induction stroke, and an increase in the 'pumping loss' (Fig. 17.10). Since the exhaust process always occurs at atmospheric pressure, the dilution of the fresh charge with residual products is more serious at part load. In fact, at very low loads, mixtures richer than stoichiometric must be supplied to ensure satisfactory

405

Fig. 17.10
Effect of throttle governing
on the indicator diagram

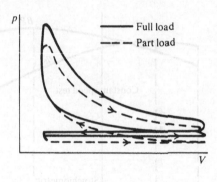

ignition. Evidently throttle governing is an inefficient method, and the part-load efficiency of SI engines is poor for this reason.

The normal method of achieving the appropriate mixture of air and fuel is by means of a *carburettor*, which consists of a venturi throat in the induction manifold, and one or more fuel jets through which petrol can be introduced into the air stream at this section. The pressure depression at the throat, whose magnitude depends on the air flow, causes petrol to be sucked from the jets into the air stream. From what has been said previously it is clear that the normal requirement from a carburettor is an approximately stoichiometric mixture at most speeds and throttle settings in order to work near the point of maximum efficiency. But in addition a rich mixture is required (a) at full throttle to attain maximum power, and (b) at very low throttle settings when there is marked dilution by residual products. Carburettors usually satisfy these requirements only moderately well, and moreover it is found that they produce non-homogeneous mixtures of air and fuel and uneven distribution to the various cylinders. Fitting a multicylinder engine with several carburettors may improve this situation, but such an arrangement requires frequent adjustment. Solutions giving more positive control have been sought, using injection pumps and nozzles capable of metering the correct amounts of petrol—preferably into individual cylinders. *Direct petrol injection* has been used successfully on several engines but, because of the high cost of injection equipment compared with that of carburettors, it has been restricted to the more expensive car engines.

One way of overcoming our apparent inability to govern an SI engine by weakening the mixture is by charging the cylinder with a controlled non-uniform mixture. Part of the cylinder is filled with a layer of ignitable mixture, while the remainder is filled with air. In this way ignition can be achieved with an *average* charge well below stoichiometric ratio. This method of filling a cylinder with a non-homogeneous air–fuel mixture is called *stratified charging*. Although engines have been successfully governed in this way under laboratory conditions, few commercial engines using this principle have been produced. A successful engine of this type would provide a major breakthrough in improving the part-load, and therefore overall, economy of SI engines.

17.3.2 The CI engine

Because the fuel is introduced into the cylinder of a CI engine only when combustion is required, i.e. towards the end of the compression stroke, pre-ignition cannot occur. Moreover, since the fuel is injected at a controlled rate, the simultaneous combustion of the whole quantity of fuel cannot occur, and the problem of detonation as in SI engines does not arise. It follows that the compression ratio can be much higher in CI engines, and in fact there is a lower limit of about 12:1 below which compression ignition of common fuel oils is not possible.

In a CI engine most of the combustion occurs at substantially constant pressure, and the maximum pressure reached in the cylinder is largely determined by the compression ratio employed. The upper limit of the compression ratio is therefore fixed by the strength of the cylinder, the bearings, and other parts whose stresses are determined by the peak pressure forces. Evidently the designer must reach a compromise between high efficiency and low weight and cost. From the analysis of the air-standard Diesel cycle, summarised in Fig. 12.14, it is evident that compression ratios in excess of 20:1 give diminishing returns, and this is in fact about the maximum value used in practical engines. A comparison of the air-standard efficiencies of the Diesel and Otto cycles (Fig. 12.14), when made at appropriate compression ratios, suggests that the CI engine will be the more efficient. This is borne out in practice, and in general CI engines are more efficient than SI engines.

We must next consider a factor limiting the *IMEP* of CI engines. It is evident from the *p–V* diagram that the mean effective pressure increases with increase in the change of volume which occurs during the combustion at constant pressure (Fig. 17.2). This change in volume is a maximum when all the fuel that can be burnt in the oxygen available is injected into the cylinder. At first sight it appears that this implies the use of a stoichiometric air/fuel ratio ($\approx 14.5:1$) as in SI engines. To see why this is not so, it is necessary to outline briefly the way in which combustion is accomplished in CI engines.

Although the fuel is injected as a deeply penetrating spray of fine droplets, the fact that it is in liquid form means that the delay period between injection and initiation of combustion is appreciably longer than in SI engines. Each droplet must first partially evaporate until sufficient vapour diffuses into the surrounding air to form a layer having an air/fuel ratio which is combustible. This vaporisation cools the droplet and surrounding layer, and time is required for the necessary temperature to be re-established. Combustion then begins simultaneously at many points in the combustion space, and there is an initial rapid and uncontrolled rise of pressure. As the cylinder fills with combustion products, the rate of reaction becomes more controlled and the pressure remains sensibly constant. If the delay period is too long, there is time for a large fraction of the charge to enter the cylinder and a rather violent initial combustion may occur, resulting in rough running and the so-called *Diesel knock*.

Diesel knock is thus seen to be a function of the fuel, and it also depends on droplet size, the rate at which droplets are introduced into the cylinder, and the heat transferred between droplets and their environment. If the latter

Fig. 17.11

Methods of improving the mixing of fuel droplets and air

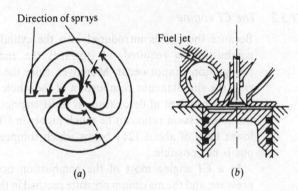

Direction of sprays

Fuel jet

(a)   (b)

parameters are kept substantially constant, by using a standard engine as is done when measuring octane numbers, the Diesel knock tendency can be measured by matching the fuel with a two-component fuel-oil mixture. For this purpose cetane ($C_{16}H_{34}$) and alpha-methyl-naphthalene ($C_{11}H_{10}$) are used to establish the so-called *cetane number scale*. It is found, not surprisingly, that a high octane number implies a low cetane number and vice versa, and this is one of the principal reasons why petrols are unsuitable for CI engines.

Apart from reducing the delay period to avoid Diesel knock, another difficulty, particularly in the later stages of injection, is to ensure that all the fuel molecules collide with oxygen molecules to complete the process of combustion. To assist the mixing process, some turbulence or swirl is deliberately stimulated by careful design of the inlet port and combustion chamber. The turbulence must not be excessive, otherwise the initial uncontrolled rise of pressure may be too violent, and the work in the expansion stroke may be reduced unduly. What is required, therefore, is a controlled movement of the bulk of the air, and not small-scale random turbulence. Ideally the spray of fuel should be carried with the air through one complete sector between successive sprays by the time combustion is completed (Fig. 17.11a). Unfortunately this approach requires several small fuel jets (which may become choked), and very high injection pressures to achieve good fuel 'atomisation'. Another way of solving this problem (Fig. 17.11b) is to have some kind of separate *swirl chamber* into which the fuel is sprayed in a relatively coarse spray. Break-up of the fuel and mixing with oxygen is achieved as a result of the intense vortex motion produced as the air is forced into the chamber during the compression stroke. In spite of much ingenuity expended on combustion chamber design (Ref. 14), it is not possible to burn all the fuel completely if stoichiometric ratios are used, and the minimum air/fuel ratio, corresponding to full load, usually lies between 18:1 and 25:1. Consequently the engine must be larger than would be the case were it to be capable of burning stoichiometric ratios. The swirl chamber design, while allowing the use of air/fuel ratios down to 18:1, also results in higher heat losses during combustion and a lower efficiency than direct injection.

When comparing the size and weight of CI and SI engines, three main factors must be borne in mind: utilisation of air, cylinder peak pressure and thermal efficiency. The CI engine, being incapable of using stoichiometric ratios and working with high peak pressures, tends to be larger and heavier than an equivalent SI engine, although the former has a higher thermal efficiency.

Turning to the question of governing, it is found that very weak mixtures can be ignited and burnt in a CI engine, so that it is possible to reduce the power output by reducing the fuel supply. Reduction of the fuel supply is equivalent to a reduction of the cut-off ratio r_c of the air-standard Diesel cycle, and Fig. 12.14 shows that this improves the cycle efficiency. In practice, although an improvement in the indicated thermal efficiency may be achieved at part load, the fall in mechanical efficiency more than outweighs this effect and the brake thermal efficiency always falls off. Nevertheless the reduction in efficiency with decrease of load is not so marked as in SI engines. Governing the power output by weakening the mixture is usually referred to as *quality governing*.

So far in our discussion of both SI and CI engines we have considered factors limiting the work done per complete cycle*—but the actual power output will also depend on the rotational speed. It would seem that, other things being equal, the power output of an engine can be raised by increasing the speed—at least up to the limit imposed by purely mechanical considerations of stress and piston sliding velocities. In practice, however, it is found that the maximum indicated work per engine cycle varies considerably with speed, and beyond a certain speed the *IP* may even fall with further increase in speed. Typical curves are shown in Fig. 17.12. The reduction in indicated work per cycle at high speeds is chiefly due to a reduction in the mass of the charge induced during each engine cycle. Theoretically, an unsupercharged engine should induce a mass equivalent to the swept volume at ambient pressure and temperature. As a result of fluid friction and expansion of the charge in the hot inlet manifold, considerably less is taken in at high engine speeds when gas velocities are high and the manifold is very hot. (This is only a rough generalisation, and whether or not the mass induced falls with increase in speed depends also upon the valve timing and the design of the inlet and exhaust manifolds.)

The 'breathing' capacity of an engine is expressed in terms of a *volumetric efficiency* defined as

$$\frac{\text{volume of induced charge per induction stroke}}{\text{swept volume of piston}} \text{ reckoned at a reference pressure and temperature} \tag{17.6}$$

The reference pressure and temperature should logically be taken as the ambient values prevailing when the volumetric efficiency is determined, but sometimes they are assumed to be at some arbitrary level such as $0\,°C$ and 1 atm. When comparing volumetric efficiencies care should be taken to ensure that they are based on the same definition.

Fig. 17.12 shows that the indicated work per engine cycle also falls at low

---

* The work done per engine cycle is, of course, proportional to the mean engine torque, i.e. it equals $4\pi \times$ torque for the four-stoke engine and $2\pi \times$ torque for the two-stroke engine.

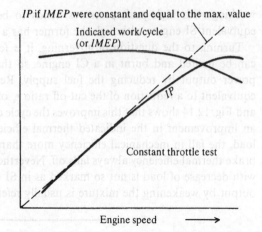

Fig. 17.12
Variation of indicated
work with engine speed

IP if *IMEP* were constant and equal to the max. value

Indicated work/cycle
(or *IMEP*)

IP

Constant throttle test

Engine speed ⟶

speeds. This is due partly to increased leakage past valves and piston for which more time is available at low speed. It is also due to reduced turbulence and the increased cooling time available, which make the combustion process less efficient. At very low speeds the combustion tends to be erratic, and below a certain speed the engine will not run at all.

Other things being equal, the total power developed in an engine cylinder depends upon the mass of the charge induced, and from the earlier remarks it might be supposed that this is limited by the prevailing ambient pressure and temperature of the air. In SI engines the induction temperature is lowered slightly by the evaporative cooling effect of liquid fuels. This is the reason for the superiority of alcohol over petrol as a fuel: its latent enthalpy of vaporisation is about three times that of petrol and the improved volumetric efficiency is sufficient to outweigh the disadvantage of the magnitude of the enthalpy of combustion being only about half that of petrol. Sometimes a liquid of high latent enthalpy, such as methanol, is injected into the induction manifold to lower the temperature still further; this device has been used in some aircraft piston engines for short periods of thrust boosting. Finally, by utilising resonance effects in the inlet and exhaust manifolds a certain amount of pressure charging can be achieved at selected speeds.

A much greater increase in charge density can be obtained, however, by pre-compressing the charge before induction with some type of *supercharger*. A Roots blower or a centrifugal compressor is commonly used for this purpose. The supercharger may be gear driven from the crankshaft, or its power may be derived from a turbine driven by the exhaust gases.

Although the net increase in power obtained by supercharging can be very considerable, it has little effect on the brake thermal efficiency. The reason is that the fuel supply must be increased in proportion to the increase in air charge in order to maintain the required air/fuel ratio. Owing to its greater mechanical complexity, a supercharged engine is not always preferred to its larger and heavier unsupercharged equivalent. Nevertheless, supercharging has become established practice in three important fields. First, a reciprocating aircraft engine must be supercharged at high altitudes, as otherwise the power falls off owing to reduced atmospheric pressure. Secondly, two-stroke CI engines are usually supercharged because there is the added advantage that the cylinders can be more effectively cleared—or *scavenged*—of combustion products. Thirdly, in recent years supercharging has established itself in CI engines for automobiles, enabling them, through sophisticated control systems, to achieve high thermal efficiencies throughout their power range. Engine mass can be kept low by this means, allowing such cars to compete in terms of acceleration with their SI counterparts.*

High thermal efficiency is important not only because it reduces running costs but also because it implies a reduction of noxious exhaust emissions. Urban pollution has become of paramount importance in the last decade or so as our cities have become choked with road traffic. The main pollutants from SI engines are carbon monoxide, unburnt hydrocarbons and oxides of nitrogen. The first two are strongly dependent on air/fuel ratio, and are much reduced in 'lean-burn' engines designed to run on a high air/fuel ratio over a wide range of power and speed. Another approach is to incorporate a 'catalytic converter' in the exhaust system. The main component is a ceramic honeycomb, or a bed of ceramic particles, impregnated with noble metals like platinum and palladium. Because lead attacks most catalysts of this kind, and is itself a toxic pollutant, the use of lead as a dope in petrol is being phased out. Although in general CI engines cause less pollution than SI engines, it should be remembered that *all* engines running on fossil fuel contribute to the increase in concentration of carbon dioxide in the atmosphere. This in turn may lead to a significant rise in ambient temperature owing to the 'greenhouse effect' (see section 23.5). There is little doubt that, as long as fossil fuel is used for road transport, when all forms of pollution are considered the only satisfactory solution is a reduction in the size of automobiles and a greater use of public transport.

Enough has been said to indicate the main factors which influence the design of an engine. In practice the design must be a compromise between thermodynamic and mechanical considerations which are closely interlinked, and for detailed discussions the reader is referred to specialised texts on the subject such as Refs 4, 21 and 27. A good discussion of combustion in SI and CI engines is presented in Ref. 19, and of pollution formation and control in Chapter 11 of Ref. 21.

17.4 Comparison of real IC engine processes with air-standard cycles

That an analogy exists between the processes in real IC engines and the equivalent air-standard Otto, Diesel or mixed cycles has been suggested in Chapter 12, but further explanation is required. The analogy rests on the fact that the $p-v$ diagram for the air-standard cycle is similar in shape to the $p-V$

---

* A useful survey of supercharging practice is given in Ref. 15, and more recent work specifically on *turbocharging* is described in Ref. 16.

diagram obtained from the engine, i.e. that the MEP of the cycle is approximately equal to the $IMEP$ of the engine. This implies that the indicated work W_i produced by an engine inducing a mass m of air is approximately equal to mW, where W is the net work per unit mass of air taken through the air-standard cycle. The energy of reaction made available for work, by burning a mass m_F of fuel, is approximately $m_F(-\Delta h_0)$. Ideally this is equal to the heat input $mc_v(T_3 - T_2)$ in the Otto cycle (see Fig. 12.13a) or $mc_p(T_3 - T_2)$ in the Diesel cycle (see Fig. 12.13b). It follows that the indicated thermal efficiency of the engine is approximately equal to the air-standard efficiency. For example, for the SI engine,

$$\eta_i = \frac{|W_i|}{m_F(-\Delta h_0)} = \frac{m|W|}{mc_v(T_3 - T_2)} = \text{Otto cycle efficiency}$$

In practice this analogy is far less close than the comparable analogy between the processes in the open-cycle gas turbine and the air-standard Joule cycle. The reasons for the poorer analogy in the case of the reciprocating engine are as follows:

(a) Since the processes are carried out intermittently in a single component they are not so clearly defined. For example, the corners of the p–V diagram are rounded owing to the time taken for valves to open and close, and combustion does not occur precisely at constant volume (or constant pressure as the case may be).

(b) The temperature changes involved in the expansion and compression are much larger than in gas turbines, and the consequent variation of specific heat capacities is appreciable.

(c) The air/fuel ratios used in reciprocating engines are much smaller, so that the properties of the working fluid are markedly different from those of air.

(d) The maximum temperature reached at the end of the combustion process is much higher than in gas turbines, and dissociation plays an important role. This implies that the chemical energy of the fuel is used much less effectively for the production of work.

(e) Owing to the use of cylinder cooling and the relatively low mass flow per unit surface area in a reciprocating machine, the compression and expansion processes cannot be so nearly described as adiabatic.

Nothing further need be said about item (a), but the remaining points require amplification. This will be done by considering the compression, combustion and expansion processes in turn.

Compression process

The ratio of specific heat capacities γ decreases with increase of temperature, and its mean value for the temperature range normally encountered in the compression process is appreciably less than 1.4 even if the gas is air. The mixing of the incoming charge with residual products of combustion results in a lower value for γ for the mixture because the products contain CO_2 and H_2O which individually have a relatively low value of γ. In SI engines the gas compressed is an air–fuel mixture, and this too has a lower value of γ than air. Finally, heat transfers from the cylinder to the gas in the early stages of the compression, and from the gas to the cylinder in the later stages, mean that the compression does not follow an isentropic path. The net result of all these effects is that the pressure and temperature at the end of the compression are appreciably less than the values predicted by air-standard calculations (see Example 17.1).

Combustion process

Owing to the high temperature reached in the combustion process there is an appreciable proportion of dissociated products at the nominal end of combustion. The result is that the full enthalpy of combustion of the fuel is not released and the actual temperature rise is less than would be predicted if dissociation were ignored. The calculation of the adiabatic temperature rise in a chemical reaction was discussed in sections 15.4 and 15.7.

Expansion process

As the temperature during the expansion falls, some of the dissociated molecules combine, and strictly speaking the combustion process still continues during the expansion. By the end of the expansion the temperature has fallen to a level where the proportion of dissociated products is very small, and the fuel can then be regarded as completely burnt. Evidently the unused part of the enthalpy of combustion is recovered to some extent, although the energy recovered in this way is not so effective for the production of work. This is because the increased pressures resulting from the completion of the reaction are available only over part of the stroke. The efficiency with which the chemical energy is converted into work is therefore decreased by the dissociation occurring in the early stages of combustion. The expansion is also markedly different from the isentropic expansion of air because the hot combustion products have a low value of γ and the expansion is far from adiabatic. An appreciable quantity of energy is rejected as heat, particularly during the period of intense chemical activity when radiation from the burning gases to the cylinder wall plays an important role.

The effect of all these factors on the p–V diagram of an SI engine is shown in Fig. 17.13. The net result is a considerable reduction in both mean effective

Fig. 17.13
Effect of variation of γ,
dissociation and heat loss
on the air-standard cycle

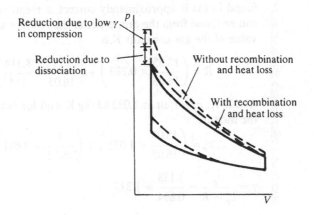

pressure and efficiency. It is possible to analyse the processes in IC engines taking the more important of these factors into account, and thermodynamic charts enabling this to be done have been produced by Hottel et al. (Ref. 3). The air-standard cycle is a simple model adequate only for predicting the effect of compression ratio on the performance of an engine. The more complex models can predict the effect of other parameters such as the air/fuel ratio. Nevertheless, such calculations are more useful in showing the relative importance of the various 'losses' than for the prediction of an actual engine's performance. This is because other variables, such as the design of the induction system, or those mentioned in the first of the five points listed earlier, also play an important part in determining the performance.

Example 17.1 A charge enters a SI engine at 330 K and 1 bar, and is compressed isentropically through a compression ratio of 7:1. Estimate the temperature and pressure at the end of compression, taking the charge to be (a) pure air with constant specific heat capacities, (b) a stoichiometric mixture of air and octane (C_8H_{18}) with variable specific heat capacities. (Neglect the effect of dilution with residual products of combustion.)

(a) With air, the temperature and pressure at the end of compression are given by

$$T_2 = T_1 r_v^{\gamma-1} = 330 \times 7^{0.4} = 719 \text{ K}$$

$$p_2 = p_1 \frac{v_1 T_2}{v_2 T_1} = 1 \times 7 \times \frac{719}{330} = 15.25 \text{ bar}$$

(b) The combustion equation for octane is

$$C_8H_{18} + 12.5O_2 + \frac{79}{21}12.5N_2 \rightarrow 8CO_2 + 9H_2O + 3.76 \times 12.5N_2$$

Hence the air/fuel ratio by mass is

$$\frac{(12.5 \times 32) + (3.76 \times 12.5 \times 28)}{114} = 15.05$$

The value of γ for the mixture will vary with temperature. Assuming that T_2 found in (a) is approximately correct, a mean value of γ for the compression can be found from the properties of the mixture at $(330 + 719)/2 \approx 525$ K. The value of the gas constant R is

$$R = \left(\frac{15.05}{16.05} \times 0.287\right) + \left(\frac{1}{16.05} \times \frac{8.314}{114}\right) = 0.274 \text{ kJ/kg K}$$

At 525 K, c_p for air is 1.035 kJ/kg K and for octane 2.691 kJ/kg K. Hence for the mixture

$$c_p = \left(\frac{15.05}{16.05} \times 1.035\right) + \left(\frac{1}{16.05} \times 2.691\right) = 1.138 \text{ kJ/kg K}$$

$$\gamma = \frac{c_p}{c_p - R} = \frac{1.138}{0.864} = 1.317$$

The temperature and pressure after compression are therefore

$$T_2 = 330 \times 7^{0.317} = 612 \text{ K}$$

$$\cdot p_2 = 1 \times 7 \times \frac{612}{330} = 13.0 \text{ bar}$$

A better estimate can now be obtained by taking the properties of the constituents at the mean temperature of $(330 + 612)/2 = 471$ K, when for the mixture $c_p = 1.115$ kJ/kg K and $\gamma = 1.326$. T_2 is then found to be 622 K and p_2 13.2 bar. Evidently a further approximation is not necessary.

17.5   Maximum work of a chemical reaction

It has been seen that there are practical limits to the work output which can be obtained from the combustion of a fuel in an internal-combustion engine in which the reaction is rapid and highly irreversible. Of rather more academic interest is the question of what is the maximum possible work that can be derived from any particular chemical reaction. Since the power is derived from a non-cyclic process while heat is exchanged with a single reservoir (i.e. the surrounding atmosphere), and not from a cycle working between two reservoirs, the Carnot efficiency cannot be a guide in answering this question.

In effect the question posed has been answered in section 15.7, but the following paragraphs discuss this problem more explicitly. For an efficient conversion of chemical energy into work it is essential for the reaction to be carried out reversibly. A hypothetical reversible IC plant has already been described in section 15.7.1—the van't Hoff equilibrium box. The particular van't Hoff box described therein performs the reaction $CO + \frac{1}{2}O_2 \rightarrow CO_2$ reversibly while exchanging heat with one reservoir. In doing so it produces the maximum possible amount of work, and hence it rejects the least possible amount of heat. The reaction proceeds isothermally, indicating that a high temperature at some point in a combustion process is not essential for maximum work output. The reason why the efficiency of a real IC engine increases with increase of compression ratio, and hence of peak temperature, is therefore not obvious. It lies in the fact that in the hypothetical reversible engine the chemical energy is transformed directly into work, which is not the case in a conventional IC engine. The rapid combustion occurring in the latter results in the chemical energy being first of all transformed into random molecular energy (i.e. sensible internal energy) as manifested by the rise in temperature accompanying the combustion process. Apart from the chemical change of some of the constituents, this irreversible combustion has the same effect of increasing the sensible internal energy of the gases (mainly nitrogen) as an external heat addition at the appropriate temperatures. Once the intermediate transformation into sensible internal energy is accepted as inevitable, the analogy between the real process and the equivalent air-standard cycle has shown that the practical IC engine efficiency will improve with increase of peak temperature (i.e. compression ratio). It should not be forgotten, however, that a reversible isothermal reaction would result in a much high proportion of the chemical energy being transformed into work.

A numerical example may be helpful. The expression for the maximum work which can be done in any reversible process by the reactants CO and O_2, exchanging heat with a single reservoir at temperature T, was found in section 15.7.2, to be given by equation (15.19). The maximum work, per kmol of CO, therefore becomes

$$|W|_{max} = \tilde{R}T \ln K^{\ominus}$$

The reactants are assumed to enter in stoichiometric proportions at standard pressure $p^{\ominus}$ and temperature T, with the product CO_2 leaving at the same pressure and temperature. For a temperature $T = 298.15$ K, the equilibrium constant is found from tables to be $\ln K^{\ominus} = 103.762$. Hence, per kmol of CO,

$$|W|_{max} = 8.3145 \times 298.15 \times 103.762 = 257\,220 \text{ kJ}$$

Since the enthalpy of reaction $\Delta \tilde{h}_{298}^{\ominus}$ is $-282\,990$ kJ per kmol of CO, it is evident that $|W|_{max}$ is nearly equal to $|\Delta \tilde{h}_{298}|$. Neglecting kinetic energy terms, the heat transferred to the surroundings can be found from the steady-flow energy equation

$$Q = \Delta \tilde{h}_{298}^{\ominus} + |W|_{max} = -282\,990 + 257\,220 = -25\,770 \text{ kJ}$$

The work $|W|_{max}$ need not necessarily be less than the negative of the enthalpy of reaction. If a similar calculation is carried out for the reversible combustion of a stoichiometric mixture of C and O_2, it can be shown than $|W|_{max}$ is greater than $(-\Delta \tilde{h}_{298}^{\ominus})$; in this case heat is received from the surroundings during the process. The definition of efficiency that is normally used for IC plant, whether $W/\Delta \tilde{h}_0^{\ominus}(\text{liq})$ of $W/\Delta \tilde{h}_0^{\ominus}(\text{vap})$, is therefore not logically sound because theoretically it can be greater than unity. A process efficiency should be defined as a ratio X/X_{max}, where X and X_{max} are the actual and maximum possible values of the physical quantities concerned in the process. A more rational definition therefore would be $|W|/|W|_{max}$.

It is found that for hydrogen and the usual hydrocarbon fuels $-\Delta \tilde{h}_0^{\ominus}(\text{vap})$ is numerically close to $|W|_{max}$, while $-\Delta \tilde{h}_0^{\ominus}(\text{liq})$ differs from $|W|_{max}$ by a much wider margin. Hence

$$\frac{|W|}{|W|_{max}} \approx \frac{|W|}{-\Delta \tilde{h}_0^{\ominus}(\text{vap})}$$

and this provides the principal argument in favour of defining thermal efficiencies by equation (15.14) rather than (15.13). It is interesting to note that the value of $|W|_{max}$, unlike that of $\Delta \tilde{h}_0^{\ominus}$, does not depend on the phase of H_2O in the products of the fuel, and this is proved formally in section 7.9.3.

One final comment: we have seen that there is no fundamental thermodynamic reason why the efficiency of an IC engine should not be 100 per cent, and therefore present-day utilisation of our fuel resources is far removed from the ultimate standard of perfection. Because an appreciable fraction of the work produced by the world's power plant is used for the production of electricity, an improvement in fuel utilisation would undoubtedly follow if we could convert chemical (and nuclear) energy directly into electrical energy in a reversible reaction. Although there are some chemical reactions which allow chemical → electrical energy conversions with a high degree of reversibility, as in the lead-acid accumulator and the hydrogen-oxygen fuel cell (see section 20.4), no equally efficient device has yet been developed for common fuels and air. Any such device would almost certainly not permit high *rates* of energy transformation; the advantage of irreversible combustion at high temperature is that very high power outputs can be produced by relatively small power plant.

18

One-Dimensional Steady Flow and Jet Propulsion

The steady-flow energy equation was deduced in Chapter 4 as a consequence of the First Law of Thermodynamics. The equation relates the heat and work transfers across the boundary of an open system, to the mechanical and thermodynamic properties of the fluid at the inlet and outlet where these properties can be assumed constant across the cross-section of flow. No assumption had to be made about whether the flow was frictionless or not, and the derivation did not require any knowledge of the flow *within* the open system. We have seen that this equation enables a useful range of problems to be solved. For example, when considering adiabatic flow in a nozzle, a knowledge of the initial enthalpy, initial velocity and final enthalpy enables the final velocity to be calculated. If the adiabatic flow is also assumed to be frictionless, the fact that the entropy is constant—a consequence of the Second Law of Thermodynamics—enables the final thermodynamic state to be predicted. The principle of conservation of mass—in the form of the continuity equation—then enables the inlet and outlet areas to be determined for any given mass flow.

The foregoing analysis, however, has nothing to say about how the cross-sectional area of the nozzle must change between inlet and outlet for the results to be physically possible. Before this kind of information can be obtained from the analysis, some knowledge of the flow within the open system is evidently necessary. This extension of the analysis is undertaken in the science of *fluid dynamics*.

With the advent of high-speed flight, turbo-jet engines, ram-jets and rockets, fluid dynamics has been enormously extended in recent years—particularly the branch dealing with compressible flow known as *gas dynamics*. Gas dynamics is now studied as a subject in its own right, and can no longer be adequately covered by a chapter in a book of this kind. All that will be attempted here is the consideration of a few special cases with the object of emphasising the point at which a simple thermodynamic analysis must be reinforced by a more complete treatment. Such a treatment (a) must involve some assumption about the flow within the open system, and (b) may involve *explicitly* Newton's Second Law of Motion. A case where item (a) is necessary and sufficient will be considered first before any attempt is made to explain what is meant by item (b).

18.1   Isentropic flow in a duct of varying area

When a fluid flows through a duct with no work or heat transfer, the only factors which can cause a change in fluid properties are (i) a change in flow area, and (ii) frictional forces. In this section we shall assume that frictional forces are absent. The effect of variation in the cross-sectional area of the duct may be determined if some assumption is made about the nature of the flow.

The simplest type of flow conceivable is *one-dimensional* steady flow. With reference to Fig. 18.1, the flow is said to be one-dimensional if the following conditions are fulfilled:

(a)   Changes in area and curvature of the axis are gradual.
(b)   Thermodynamic and mechanical properties are uniform across planes normal to the axis of the duct.

No real flow is truly one-dimensional, but provided that there are no sudden changes in direction or area, and that average values of the properties at any cross-section are used in the analysis, the one-dimensional treatment yields results which are sufficiently accurate for many purposes.

When the flow is one-dimensional, the properties are uniform over any cross-section of the flow within the open system—not merely at inlet and outlet. It is therefore possible to apply the energy equation to the flow between any two planes 1 and 2, and so, for given inlet conditions, to determine the properties at any section along the duct. Consider the case of isentropic flow in a nozzle (or diffuser). Given p_1 and T_1 (or x_1 if the fluid is a wet vapour), the thermodynamic properties at various values of p_2 can be found using the equation of state (or tables of properties) together with the fact that s_2 equals s_1. Given also the initial velocity C_1, corresponding values of C_2 can be found from the energy equation

$$h_2 + \frac{C_2^2}{2} = h_1 + \frac{C_1^2}{2}$$

Finally, given the inlet cross-sectional area A_1, corresponding values of A_2 can be found from the continuity equation

$$\frac{A_2 C_2}{v_2} = \frac{A_1 C_1}{v_1}$$

The variation of v_2, C_2 and A_2 with p_2 can then be represented by curves of the form shown in Fig. 18.2. Although the precise shape of the curves depends upon the equation of state of the fluid, all gases and vapours exhibit the same

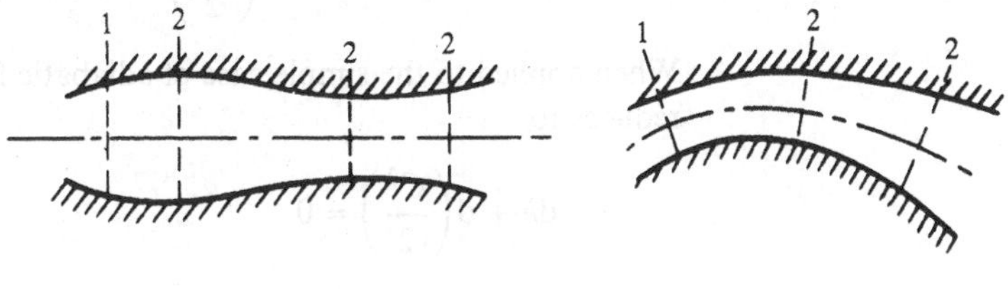

Fig. 18.1
One-dimensional' ducts

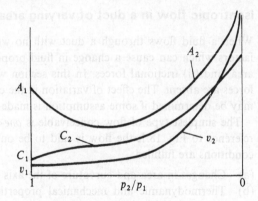

Fig. 18.2
Variation of v, C and A
with pressure along a duct

general behaviour under these conditions. One point of interest is the very gradual change in specific volume v at low velocities. For some analyses of low-speed gas flow it is possible to simplify the calculations without much loss of accuracy by assuming that the specific volume is constant. This realm of fluid dynamics is called *incompressible flow* and the treatment is then identical for liquids and gases.

Fig. 18.2 can be interpreted as applying to either a nozzle or a diffuser. Moving from left to right on the diagram, the pressure p_2 is falling and the duct acts as nozzle. Although both the specific volume and the velocity increase continuously during the expansion, the flow area decreases to a minimum and then increases. A glance at the continuity equation shows that this will happen if the rate of increase of specific volume is at first less than, and finally greater than, the rate of increase of velocity. Such behaviour is always exhibited by gases and vapours. The pressure ratio at which the minimum area is reached is called the *critical pressure ratio*; at this point the mass flow per unit area is a maximum.

18.1.1 Derivation of the basic equations

It is more informative if the foregoing step-by-step method of calculation is replaced by the analytical approach which follows. First it is necessary to arrive at equations expressing the First and Second Laws, and the principle of conservation of mass (continuity), in differential form. Applying the steady-flow energy equation between any two planes an infinitesimal distance apart, we arrive at the differential energy equation per unit mass:

$$dQ + dW = dh + d\left(\frac{C^2}{2}\right) \tag{18.1}$$

When applied to the simple case of adiabatic flow in a nozzle or diffuser, (18.1) reduces to

$$dh + d\left(\frac{C^2}{2}\right) = 0 \tag{18.2}$$

Applying the Second Law to the flow between planes an infinitesimal distance apart, we have the result that for a reversible process

$$dQ = T\,ds$$

We also have the general relation between properties, equation (6.13), which states that

$$T\,ds = dh - v\,dp$$

For an isentropic process, therefore,

$$dh = v\,dp \tag{18.3}$$

The differential form of the continuity equation is most easily obtained by logarithmic differentiation. Thus we have

$$\log A + \log C - \log v = \text{constant}$$

and differentiating,

$$\frac{dA}{A} + \frac{dC}{C} - \frac{dv}{v} = 0 \tag{18.4}$$

Equations (18.2) to (18.4) can be used to find expressions for the changes in velocity and area with pressure in an isentropic process. Thus, combining (18.2) and (18.3),

$$v\,dp + d\left(\frac{C^2}{2}\right) = 0 \tag{18.5}$$

For the flow between any two planes 1 and 2 we therefore have

$$\tfrac{1}{2}(C_2^2 - C_1^2) = -\int_1^2 v\,dp \tag{18.6}$$

For any given fluid there is a definite relation between p and v in an isentropic process, and when this is known in algebraic form the RHS of the equation can be evaluated.

To find the change in area required to accommodate the flow, equation (18.5) can be substituted in (18.4) to yield

$$\frac{dA}{A} = \frac{v}{C^2}\,dp + \frac{dv}{v} = v\,dp\left(\frac{1}{C^2} + \frac{1}{v^2}\frac{dv}{dp}\right) \tag{18.7}$$

It is shown in texts on fluid dynamics that the velocity of propagation of a small pressure wave through a fluid (i.e. a sound wave) is given by

$$a^2 = -v^2(\partial p/\partial v)_s \tag{18.8}$$

The bracketed term is the rate of change of pressure with specific volume at constant entropy.* Since equation (18.7) refers to isentropic flow, (18.8) may

---

* It is conventional to use the density ρ in place of v in fluid dynamics; the expression is therefore usually written as $a^2 = (\partial p/\partial \rho)_s$.

be used to substitute for dv/dp to give

$$\frac{dA}{A} = v\,dp\left(\frac{1}{C^2} - \frac{1}{a^2}\right) \qquad (18.9)$$

where a is the local velocity of sound in the fluid at the section in the flow where the pressure is p and the specific volume is v.

Equation (18.9) may be interpreted directly without integration. Considering accelerated flow, decelerated flow and constant velocity flow in turn, the most important consequences are as follows:

Accelerated flow (nozzle) dp must be negative so that:
(a) When $C < a$, dA is negative, i.e. the duct must converge.
(b) When $C > a$, dA is positive, i.e. the duct must diverge.

Decelerated flow (diffuser) dp must be positive so that:
(a) When $C < a$, dA is positive.
(b) When $C > a$, dA is negative.

Constant velocity flow dp is zero so that:
(a) Whether $C \gtrless a$, dA is zero.

It follows immediately that if the flow is to be continuously accelerated from a subsonic to a supersonic velocity the duct must have a throat between the two regions, at which dA is zero and the velocity C is equal to the local sonic velocity a, as in Fig. 18.3a. The same remarks apply to a flow continuously decelerating from a supersonic to a subsonic velocity, as depicted in Fig. 18.3b.

Fig. 18.3
Flow in a duct of varying area

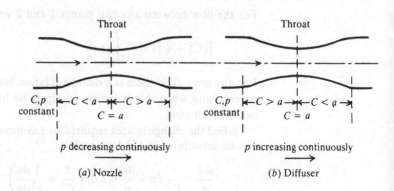

p decreasing continuously

(a) Nozzle

p increasing continuously

(b) Diffuser

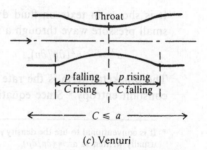

(c) Venturi

When there is not a continuous rise (or fall) of pressure, the presence of a throat does not necessarily imply that the velocity there is sonic: Fig. 18.3c illustrates the case of a venturi where a subsonic flow is accelerated and then decelerated without sonic velocity ever being reached. The condition at the throat is that of constant velocity flow with dp zero. One final point is worth noting from the foregoing analysis: it is that *the critical pressure ratio is that pressure ratio which will accelerate the flow to a velocity equal to the local velocity of sound in the fluid*, because this is the point in the flow where the area is a minimum and the mass flow per unit area a maximum.

All these deductions have been made without reference to any particular fluid, and they apply equally to liquids and gases. The reason why it is never necessary in practice to use convergent-divergent nozzles or diffusers for liquids is that the velocity of sound in a liquid is about 1500 m/s. Such a velocity is quite outside the range of practicable velocities of flow in view of the friction which would be involved.

The analysis can be carried further if we restrict our attention to certain types of fluid for which there is a simple algebraic relation between p and v in an isentropic process; equations (18.5) and (18.7) may then be integrated analytically. For a perfect gas we have the isentropic relation

$$pv^{\gamma} = \text{constant}$$

Although no such simple equation can be formulated for the isentropic expansion or compression of a vapour, it was pointed out in section 9.4 that a good approximation is provided by the same type of polytropic law, i.e.

$$pv^{n} = \text{constant}$$

When the vapour is steam, initially wet with a dryness fraction $0.7 < x < 1.0$, then for an isentropic expansion $n \approx 1.035 + 0.1x$ (see section 9.4). Thus with $x \approx 1.0$ and the whole expansion in the wet region, $n \approx 1.135$. When the steam is initially sufficiently superheated for the whole of the expansion to lie within the superheat region, $n \approx 1.30$. Consideration of what happens when the steam is initially only slightly superheated, so that condensation can be expected to occur inside the nozzle, must be left to section 18.2. To provide a uniform solution for gases and vapours, the symbol n will be used for the index of isentropic expansion. The resulting equations, however, will be exact only for perfect gases, i.e. for the case where $n = \gamma$.

To avoid obscuring the essentials by lengthy equations, we shall consider only the simple case of *a continuous expansion from an initial state where the velocity may be considered negligible*. Fig. 18.4 shows the nomenclature employed. Using the polytropic relation between p and v, and putting C_1 equal to zero, equation (18.6) gives the velocity at any plane 2, whether in the convergent or the divergent part of the duct, as

$$\tfrac{1}{2}C_2^2 = \frac{n}{1 - n}(p_2 v_2 - p_1 v_1)$$

Fig. 18.4
Convergent-divergent
nozzle

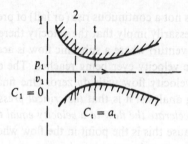

and hence

$$C_2 = \left[\frac{2n}{1-n} p_1 v_1 \left\{ \left(\frac{p_2}{p_1} \right)^{(n-1)/n} - 1 \right\} \right]^{1/2} \tag{18.10}$$

Note that, for any given initial state, there is a maximum possible velocity which is achieved when the fluid is expanded to zero pressure. This maximum velocity is

$$C_{max} = \left(\frac{2n}{n-1} p_1 v_1 \right)^{1/2} \tag{18.11}$$

The curve representing C_2 in Fig. 18.2 does not, therefore, proceed to infinity. The required area at any plane 2 can be found by integrating (18.7), but it is more easily obtained by computing C_2 and v_2 and using the continuity equation directly. Thus, if $\dot{m}$ is the mass flow, we have

$$\dot{m} = \frac{A_2 C_2}{v_2} \quad \text{or} \quad \frac{A_2}{\dot{m}} = \frac{v_2}{C_2} = \frac{v_1}{C_2 (p_2/p_1)^{1/n}} \tag{18.12}$$

An expression for the mass flow per unit area can be found by taking the reciprocal of (18.12) and substituting for C_2 from (18.10). This yields

$$\frac{\dot{m}}{A_2} = \left[\frac{2n}{1-n} \frac{p_1}{v_1} \left\{ \left(\frac{p_2}{p_1} \right)^{(n+1)/n} - \left(\frac{p_2}{p_1} \right)^{2/n} \right\} \right]^{1/2} \tag{18.13}$$

The mass flow per unit area is a maximum at the throat, and the pressure at the throat can therefore be found by differentiating (18.13) with respect to p_2 and equating to zero. The result is that $\dot{m}/A_2$ is a maximum when

$$\frac{p_2}{p_1} = \left(\frac{2}{n+1} \right)^{n/(n-1)}$$

In this equation p_2 is the throat pressure p_t, and it is also referred to as the critical pressure p_c. The critical pressure ratio is therefore

$$\frac{p_t}{p_1} = \frac{p_c}{p_1} = \left(\frac{2}{n+1} \right)^{n/(n-1)} \tag{18.14}$$

The following gives the critical pressure ratio for four values of n:

n	1.135	1.300	1.400	1.667
p_c/p_1	0.577	0.546	0.528	0.487

The value of the maximum mass flow per unit area can be found by substituting (18.14) in (18.13), giving

$$\frac{\dot{m}}{A_t} = \left\{ n \left(\frac{2}{n+1} \right)^{(n+1)/(n-1)} \frac{p_1}{v_1} \right\}^{1/2}$$

(18.15)

The general result, that the velocity at the throat will be sonic, has already been deduced from equation (18.9); it is easy to check this for the special case of fluids which expand isentropically according to the law $pv^n = $ constant. Thus substituting (18.14) in (18.10), the throat velocity is

$$C_t = \left(\frac{2n}{1+n} p_1 v_1 \right)^{1/2}$$

Using $p_1 v_1^n = p_t v_t^n$ in conjunction with (18.14), this can be transformed to

$$C_t = (n p_t v_t)^{1/2}$$

(18.16)

Sonic velocity at the throat can be found from (18.8), since by differentiating the isentropic relation $pv^n = $ constant we have

$$\left(\frac{\partial p}{\partial v} \right)_s = -\frac{np}{v}$$

and hence when $p = p_t$ and $v = v_t$,

$$a_t = (n p_t v_t)^{1/2}$$

The required identity between C_t and the local sonic velocity is thereby established.

It must be emphasised once again that this analysis is for a *continuous* expansion. The pressure p_t and velocity C_t, given by the foregoing equations, are the minimum and maximum values respectively which can be achieved at the throat with the given initial conditions p_1 and v_1. Higher values of p_t, and lower values of C_t, are possible in a venturi where the pressure increases after the throat.

When the fluid is a perfect gas, we may substitute $n = \gamma$ and $pv = RT$ in the previous equations to obtain

$$C_2 = \left[\frac{2\gamma}{1-\gamma} RT_1 \left\{ \left(\frac{p_2}{p_1} \right)^{(\gamma-1)/\gamma} - 1 \right\} \right]^{1/2}$$

(18.17)

$$\frac{\dot{m}}{A_2} = p_1 \left[\frac{2\gamma}{1-\gamma} \frac{1}{RT_1} \left\{ \left(\frac{p_2}{p_1} \right)^{(\gamma+1)/\gamma} - \left(\frac{p_2}{p_1} \right)^{2/\gamma} \right\} \right]^{1/2}$$

(18.18)

$$\frac{p_t}{p_1} = \frac{p_c}{p_1} = \left(\frac{2}{\gamma+1} \right)^{\gamma/(\gamma-1)}$$

(18.19)

$$C_t = a_t = (\gamma R T_t)^{1/2}$$

(18.20)

$$\frac{\dot{m}}{A_t} = p_1 \left\{ \frac{\gamma}{RT_1} \left(\frac{2}{\gamma+1} \right)^{(\gamma+1)/(\gamma-1)} \right\}^{1/2}$$

(18.21)

A simple expression for the ratio T_t/T_1 can also be formulated in this instance:

$$\frac{T_t}{T_1} = \left(\frac{p_t}{p_1}\right)^{(\gamma-1)/\gamma} = \frac{2}{\gamma+1} \tag{18.22}$$

Equations (18.17) to (18.22) can be deduced more easily and directly by using the energy equation in the form

$$c_p T_1 = c_p T_2 + \tfrac{1}{2} C_2^2$$

but this is left as an exercise for the student.

Much of the preceding analysis has only been necessary to obtain an expression for the critical pressure ratio, equation (18.14). Most calculations on the design of nozzles are easily made from first principles once (18.14) has been established. The following example illustrates this.

Example 18.1   Determine the throat area, exit area and exit velocity for a steam nozzle to pass a mass flow of 0.2 kg/s when the inlet conditions are 10 bar and 250 °C and the final pressure is 2 bar. Assume that the expansion is isentropic and that the inlet velocity is negligible.

Fig. 18.5 illustrates the process on an h–s diagram. Using $n = 1.3$ when finding the critical pressure ratio, we have from (18.14)

$$\frac{p_t}{p_1} = \left(\frac{2}{1.3 + 1}\right)^{1.3/0.3} = 0.546$$

and hence

$$p_t = 0.546 \times 10 = 5.46 \text{ bar}$$

Since the expansion is isentropic,

$$s_t = s_1 = 6.926 \text{ kJ/kg K}$$

The steam is still superheated at the throat because s_t is greater than the saturation value 6.794 kJ/kg K at the throat pressure of 5.46 bar. By a double interpolation in the superheat table, of which only the second step is

Fig. 18.5

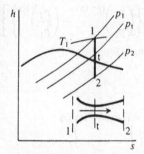

426

given here, the enthalpy and specific volume at the throat are found to be

$$h_t = 2753 + (2854 - 2753)\frac{6.926 - 6.794}{7.018 - 6.794} \quad \text{(at 5.46 bar)}$$

$$= 2813 \text{ kJ/kg}$$

$$v_t = 0.3476 + (0.3916 - 0.3476)\frac{6.926 - 6.794}{7.018 - 6.794} \quad \text{(at 5.46 bar)}$$

$$= 0.3735 \text{ m}^3/\text{kg}$$

Now from the energy equation with $C_1 = 0$,

$$C_t = \{2(h_1 - h_t)\}^{1/2}$$

$$= \{2 \times 10^3(2944 - 2813)\}^{1/2} = 511.9 \text{ m/s}$$

From the continuity equation, the required throat area is

$$A_t = \frac{\dot{m}v_t}{C_t} = \frac{0.2 \times 0.3735}{511.9}[\text{m}^2] = 1.46 \text{ cm}^2$$

The dryness fraction at exit may be found from

$$s_2 = s_1 = s_{f2} + x_2 s_{fg2}$$

$$x_2 = \frac{6.926 - 1.530}{5.597} = 0.964$$

Therefore

$$h_2 = 505 + (0.964 \times 2202) = 2628 \text{ kJ/kg}$$

$$v_2 = 0.964 \times 0.8856 = 0.8537 \text{ m}^3/\text{kg}$$

The exit velocity is therefore

$$C_2 = \{2 \times 10^3(2944 - 2628)\}^{1/2} = 795.0 \text{ m/s}$$

and the exit area required is

$$A_2 = \frac{0.2 \times 0.8537}{795.0}[\text{m}^2] = 2.15 \text{ cm}^2$$

Note that the approximate expression $pv^{1/3} = \text{constant}$ has been used only to determine the critical pressure ratio, and hence indirectly the throat area. The throat and exit velocities have been calculated from the correct isentropic enthalpy drop and not from $\int v\, dp$. Note also that such calculations are greatly simplified if values of the enthalpy drop and specific volume can be read directly from an h–s chart.

18.1.2 Phenomena in nozzles operating off the design pressure ratio

This section has so far been devoted to establishing the area changes necessary for a continuous isentropic expansion from a given initial state to a given final pressure. It is also of interest to know what happens to the flow in a nozzle of given dimensions when the downstream pressure differs from the value for which the nozzle is designed. In this respect the behaviour of convergent and convergent-divergent nozzles is different, and the two types must be considered separately.

Convergent nozzle

Consider the experimental set-up shown in Fig. 18.6. The inlet conditions are maintained constant and the downstream pressure p_e is gradually reduced from the inlet pressure p_1 by opening the valve.

When $p_e = p_1$ there is no pressure drop and no flow, shown by curve (i). As p_e is reduced, the axial pressure distribution takes the form of curve (ii), and the mass flow increases as shown in Fig. 18.6b. The pressure p_2 in the plane of the nozzle exit is always equal to p_e. This state of affairs continues until p_e/p_1 is reduced to the critical pressure ratio p_c/p_1, corresponding to curve (iii). At this operating condition the nozzle passes the maximum mass flow, given by equation (18.15), and $p_2 = p_e = p_c$.

Further reduction of p_e cannot produce any change in the flow within the nozzle because we have seen that p_2/p_1 *cannot be less than the critical pressure ratio unless there is a throat upstream of plane 2*. Consequently, for all values of p_e less than p_c, the pressure p_2 in the plane of the exit remains constant at the critical pressure p_c. There is therefore no further change in specific volume or velocity at plane 2 and no change in mass flow. The mass flow remains at the maximum value, as shown in Fig. 18.6b, and the nozzle is said to be *choked*. On leaving plane 2 the fluid undergoes an unrestrained and irreversible expansion to p_e, as illustrated by curve (iv), and the flow is no longer amenable to simple one-dimensional treatment. What happens is that the pressure

Fig. 18.6

Flow in a convergent nozzle with varying back pressure

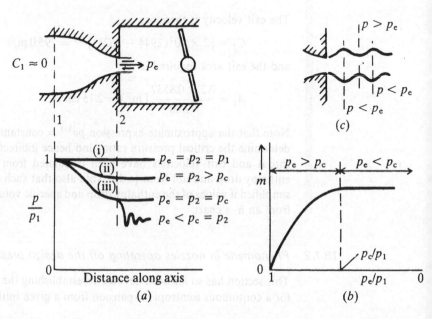

(a)

(b)

(c)

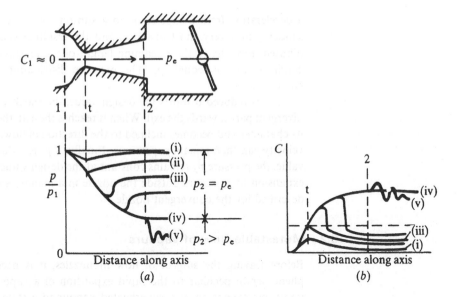

Fig. 18.7
Flow in a
convergent–divergent
nozzle with varying back
pressure

oscillates around p_e, as shown in Fig. 18.6c, and the supersonic velocity achieved in the initial divergence of the stream is rapidly reduced by viscous friction.

Convergent-divergent nozzle

Fig. 18.7 shows a similar set-up with a convergent-divergent nozzle. When operating at the design pressure ratio, appropriate to the throat and exit areas of the nozzle, the flow accelerates continuously from a subsonic to a supersonic velocity. The axial pressure and velocity distributions are then represented by curves (iv) in Figs 18.7a and b.

Now consider what happens as p_e is slowly reduced from p_1 to the design exit pressure. At first the duct acts as a subsonic nozzle followed by a subsonic diffuser, i.e. as a venturi, and the pressure distribution appears as curve (i). The mass flow increases during this range of p_e until the conditions are such that the throat pressure p_t is equal to the critical pressure p_c, shown by curve (ii). The mass flow is then a maximum and the nozzle is choked. Further reduction of p_e cannot alter the conditions at the throat and the mass flow thereafter remains constant.

If p_e is reduced below the value giving rise to curve (ii), the process of acceleration followed by diffusion can no longer continue in the same manner as before. This is because once the stream has acquired a supersonic velocity, a *converging* duct is necessary for an isentropic diffusion process. Evidently the normal type of continuous isentropic flow process can no longer exist under these conditions. Mathematically speaking, the equations expressing the constancy of energy, mass and entropy cannot be satisfied simultaneously in the given duct. The energy and continuity equations are fundamental and must be satisfied; it is the assumption of isentropic flow which must be discarded. What happens is that a discontinuity—known as a *shock wave*—is formed in the flow. A shock wave involves a rise of pressure, an increase of entropy, and

429

a deceleration from a supersonic to a subsonic velocity.* These events occur suddenly in a very short distance, and the resulting subsonic stream is then diffused normally in the remaining length of the divergent duct to satisfy the condition that p_2 equals p_e. The pressure distribution then corresponds to curve (iii).

As p_e is reduced towards the design value, the shock wave moves down the divergent part towards the exit. When it reaches the exit, the shock wave changes its character and becomes inclined to the direction of flow, and the downstream velocity can then remain supersonic. Finally, if p_e is reduced below the design value, the pressure p_2 remains constant at the design value and an uncontrolled expansion to p_e occurs outside the nozzle in a manner similar to that already described for the convergent nozzle.

18.2 Metastable flow of vapours

Before leaving the subject of flow in nozzles, it is necessary to describe a phenomenon peculiar to the rapid expansion of a vapour. The ideal case of isentropic expansion of a superheated vapour to a state in the wet region is depicted on the $T-s$ diagram in Fig. 18.8a. At the point in the expansion where the pressure is p_2 a change of phase should begin to occur. At this point the random kinetic energy of the molecules has fallen to a level which is insufficient to overcome the attractive forces of the molecules, and some of the slower moving molecules coalesce to form tiny droplets of condensate. Now this process, although rapid, does not have time to occur in a nozzle where the flow velocity is very great. The achievement of equilibrium between the liquid and vapour phases is therefore delayed, and the vapour continues to expand in a dry state.

If the constant pressure line p_3 in the superheat region is extended into the wet region, the final state could be represented by point 3 in Fig. 18.8b. Between pressures p_2 and p_3 the vapour is said to be *supersaturated* or *supercooled*. The latter term owes its origin to the fact that at any pressure between p_2 and p_3 the temperature of the vapour is always less than the saturation temperature corresponding to that pressure. The path of the process between 2 and 3 is shown dashed in Fig. 18.8b because these states are not states of stable equilibrium; they are called *metastable* states. The type of equilibrium established is certainly not stable because a disturbance, such as the introduction of a measuring instrument, can bring about condensation and a restoration of the stable state of equilibrium between liquid and vapour. Neither can the state be regarded as unstable, because this term is only applied to states for which any infinitesimal disturbance will cause a major change of state. An infinitesimal disturbance, such as the formation of a tiny droplet, is insufficient to bring about general condensation.

When designing steam nozzles, it may be assumed that the supersaturated vapour expands according to the laws of the superheated vapour. As steam

---

* A one-dimensional treatment can still be used to analyse flow involving some types of shock wave, but for this the student must turn to texts on fluid dynamics, e.g. Ref. 5 or the useful summary in Appendix A of Ref. 1.

Fig. 18.8
Metastable states

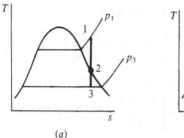
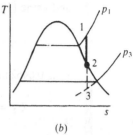

(a)   (b)

tables do not normally extend the stable superheat range into the metastable supersaturated region, extrapolation of property values is most easily carried out by reference to approximate property relations for superheated steam. The simplest equation which can be used for this purpose is equation (9.8), which led to the following two useful relations for an isentropic process:

$$pv^{1.3} = \text{constant} \quad \text{and} \quad p/T^{1.3/0.3} = \text{constant}$$

These equations enable the final state and the isentropic enthalpy drop to be predicted. Thus in practice, owing to the phenomenon of supersaturation, the value of 1.3 should be used for n even if the steam is only just superheated initially and most of the expansion occurs in the 'wet region'.

The following example shows that the mass flow through a nozzle is increased by supersaturation. In early experiments on nozzle flow it was noticed that the measured mass flow was often greater than the value estimated on the assumption of a normal expansion with phase equilibrium, and it was this fact that drew the attention of engineers to the phenomenon of supersaturation.

Example 18.2 Dry saturated steam at 2.8 bar is expanded in a simple convergent nozzle to a pressure of 1.7 bar. The throat area is 3 cm² and the inlet velocity is negligible. Estimate the exit velocity and mass flow (a) if phase equilibrium is assumed throughout the expansion and (b) if the steam is assumed to be supersaturated.

(a) Assuming isentropic expansion, the dryness fraction at the exit is given by

$$s_1 = s_2 = s_{f2} + x_2 s_{fg2}$$

$$7.015 = 1.475 + x_2 5.707 \quad \text{and hence} \quad x_2 = 0.971$$

Hence

$$h_1 - h_2 = 2722 - \{483 + (0.971 \times 2216)\} = 87 \text{ kJ/kg}$$

$$C_2 = \{2(h_1 - h_2)\}^{1/2} = (2 \times 10^3 \times 87)^{1/2} = 417 \text{ m/s}$$

$$v_2 = x_2 v_{g2} = 0.971 \times 1.031 = 1.001 \text{ m}^3/\text{kg}$$

$$\dot{m} = \frac{A_2 C_2}{v_2} = \frac{3 \times 417}{10^4 \times 1.001} = 0.125 \text{ kg/s}$$

(b) Assuming the supersaturated expansion to conform to $pv^{1.3} = $ constant,

431

and using (18.10), we have

$$C_2 = \left[\frac{2n}{1-n} p_1 v_1 \left\{ \left(\frac{p_2}{p_1} \right)^{(n-1)/n} - 1 \right\} \right]^{1/2}$$

v_1 is 0.6462 m^3/kg from tables, so that

$$C_2 = \left[\frac{2 \times 1.3}{0.3} 10^5 \times 2.8 \times 0.6462 \left\{ 1 - \left(\frac{1.7}{2.8} \right)^{0.3/1.3} \right\} \right]^{1/2} = 413 \text{ m/s}$$

$$v_2 = v_1 \left(\frac{p_1}{p_2} \right)^{1/n} = 0.6462 \left(\frac{2.8}{1.7} \right)^{1/1.3} = 0.949 \text{ m}^3/\text{kg}$$

$$\dot{m} = \frac{3 \times 413}{10^4 \times 0.949} = 0.131 \text{ kg/s}$$

Note that part (b) may be solved using equation (9.11) to find $(h_2 - h_1)$ and hence C_2, and (9.10) to find v_2.

Provided that the vapour remains supersaturated up to the outlet of the nozzle, the method used in the previous example is adequate because, in the absence of friction, the process within the nozzle can be considered reversible and therefore isentropic. The restoration of equilibrium is an irreversible process, however, and if this occurs at some point within the nozzle the prediction of the final state is difficult.

The supersaturated condition cannot continue indefinitely; the delay in condensation leads to a build-up of molecular cohesive forces which finally results in sudden condensation at many points in the vapour. Much work has been done to determine the minimum pressure to which steam may be expanded before condensation occurs, and a description of some of these experiments is given in Refs 7 and 8. It has been found that even if the steam is only just superheated at the beginning of the expansion, the condensation pressure is less than the critical pressure. Thus the irreversible restoration of stable equilibrium always occurs *after* the throat of a steam nozzle, and an estimate of the mass flow for a given throat area can always be made in the manner indicated by Example 18.2b.

The difficulty arises in predicting the conditions at the outlet of convergent-divergent nozzles of large pressure drop. Experiments have shown that the condensation occurs suddenly with an increase of both entropy and pressure.

Fig. 18.9
Restoration of equilibrium

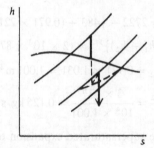

Fig. 18.9 illustrates a frictionless expansion of this kind on the $h–s$ diagram. When designing nozzles in practice, it is always necessary to introduce a 'coefficient' or 'efficiency' to allow for the increase of entropy due to friction, and this factor, being experimentally determined, will automatically take into account the increase in entropy due to the condensation process. The prediction of the final state by such means will be made clearer in the next section when the effects of friction are discussed.

18.3 The momentum equation

It is now appropriate to explain what was meant in the introduction to this chapter by the statement that it is sometimes necessary to invoke *explicitly* Newton's Second Law of Motion. It may seem surprising that we have been able to solve any problem concerned with motion without reference to this fundamental principle. The fact is, however, that so far we have been concerned with problems for which the Second Law of Motion is expressed *implicitly* in the energy equation. This point may be appreciated if we think for a moment of how the energy equation is deduced for a purely mechanical system. The starting point is Newton's Second Law, that the force acting on a body is equal to the rate of change of momentum in the direction of the force, i.e.

$$F = \frac{d(mC)}{dt} \tag{18.23}$$

Equation (18.23) is the simplest form of *momentum equation.*

If a body of constant mass m is moved a distance dx by the force F, we can write

$$F \, dx = m\left(\frac{dC}{dt}\right) dx$$

And since $dx = C \, dt$, this becomes

$$F \, dx = mC \, dC$$

which on integration yields

$$\int_1^2 F \, dx = \frac{m}{2}(C_2^2 - C_1^2)$$

The LHS can be integrated directly if there exists a function of x, which we may denote by P, such that $dP/dx = -F$. We then have

$$\int_1^2 -dP = \frac{m}{2}(C_2^2 - C_1^2)$$

or

$$P_1 + \tfrac{1}{2}mC_1^2 = P_2 + \tfrac{1}{2}mC_2^2 \tag{18.24}$$

In these circumstances there is a quantity $(P + mC^2/2)$ which remains constant during the motion; it is called the energy of the body. $mC^2/2$ is the kinetic energy and P the potential energy. If the force is simply that due to gravity,

$F = \text{constant} = -mg$, and the change in potential energy is

$$P_2 - P_1 = mg(x_2 - x_1)$$

Or again, if the force is the restoring force of an extended spring, $F = -kx$ where k is the spring stiffness, and

$$P_2 - P_1 = \frac{k}{2}(x_2^2 - x_1^2)$$

The integrated equation (18.24), which is an equation of mechanical energy, is equivalent to the equation of momentum and the two are interchangeable. It is often more convenient to use the energy equation because it relates scalar quantities; the momentum equation, on the other hand, relates vector quantities.

The simplest energy equation for a purely mechanical system is only another form of the momentum equation because it has been deduced from it without further reference to empirical data. But this energy equation applies only to frictionless systems. Friction forces are not simple functions of position (i.e. we cannot write $dP/dx = -F$), and they involve the transformation of mechanical forms of energy into other quite different forms (e.g. internal energy) with which classical mechanics is not concerned. A more comprehensive energy equation can be formulated only when the additional generalisation of the First Law of Thermodynamics has been introduced. Then the energy equation rests upon its own empirical ground and applies to any system whether frictionless or not and whether adiabatic or not; it is no longer simply another form of the momentum equation. We should not be surprised, however, if the energy and momentum equations appear to be identical when friction forces are assumed to be absent and the process is adiabatic. Conversely, when these conditions are *not* fulfilled, we can usefully employ both the general energy equation *and* the momentum equation, because they are no longer identical but express different fundamental principles.

It is now necessary to apply Newton's Second Law of Motion to fluid flow. The deduction of the most general form of this momentum equation is left to texts on fluid dynamics; we shall restrict our attention to one-dimensional steady flow. Heat may be transferred to the fluid provided that it changes the fluid properties uniformly across the cross-section of flow.

Consider the open system between planes 1 and 2 in Fig. 18.10. In time dt the mass between 1 and 2 plus the mass equal to dm moves to the right. Newton's law states that the vector sum ΣF of all the external forces acting on

Fig. 18.10
Force on a duct due to fluid flow

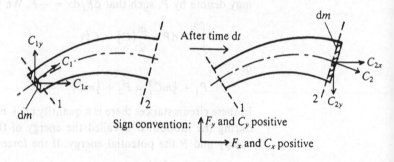

Sign convention: F_y and C_y positive
F_x and C_x positive

Fig. 18.11
Pressure forces on an
element of a straight duct

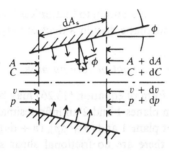

the mass is equal to the rate of change of momentum of the mass. Assuming there are no components of the vector quantities of force, velocity and momentum in a direction perpendicular to the plane of the paper, and resolving in the x and y directions, we obtain

$$\Sigma F_x = \frac{1}{dt}\{(M_{12x} + C_{2x}\,dm) - (M_{12x} + C_{1x}\,dm)\}$$

$$\Sigma F_y = \frac{1}{dt}\{(M_{12y} + C_{2y}\,dm) - (M_{12y} + C_{1y}\,dm)\}$$

M_{12x} and M_{12y} are the vector components of the total momentum of the fluid within the boundary of the open system, and for steady flow they do not change with time. Moreover, dm/dt is the rate of mass flow, which we denote simply by $\dot{m}$. We therefore have as the momentum equation

$$\Sigma F_x = \dot{m}(C_{2x} - C_{1x}) \quad \text{and} \quad \Sigma F_y = \dot{m}(C_{2y} - C_{1y}) \tag{18.25}$$

From the continuity equation, $\dot{m}$ is given by

$$\dot{m} = \frac{A_1 C_1}{v_1} = \frac{A_2 C_2}{v_2}$$

For our purpose in this chapter it is sufficient to consider only a straight duct, as in Fig. 18.11. The resultant of all forces in the y-direction is then zero, so that the momentum equation reduces to

$$\Sigma F = \dot{m}(C_2 - C_1) \tag{18.26}$$

The term ΣF includes all externally impressed forces on the mass of fluid between planes 1 and 2 which affect the change of momentum. It may include (a) gravitational forces; (b) hydrostatic forces, due to p_1 and p_2 acting on the areas A_1 and A_2, and due to the pressure exerted by the wall on the fluid; and (c) frictional forces due to the shear stress at the wall.* We may ignore gravitational forces in any application we shall consider in this book, just as we have already done when applying the energy equation. Equation (18.26) will now be applied to three simple cases in turn: (1) isentropic flow in a duct of

---

* The only logical way of allowing for friction in a one-dimensional treatment is to assume that all the friction is concentrated at the wall. In the real flow, friction between the layers of fluid results in a non-uniform distribution of properties at right angles to the flow and the flow cannot, strictly speaking, be visualised as 'one-dimensional' at all.

varying area; (2) heat addition to frictionless flow in a duct of constant area; and (3) irreversible adiabatic flow in a duct of varying area.

18.3.1 Isentropic flow in a duct of varying area

The differential form of equation (18.26) may be obtained by applying it to an element between planes 1 and 2 an infinitesimal distance apart. The properties are p, v, C etc. at plane 1 and $(p + dp)$, $(v + dv)$, $(C + dC)$ etc. at plane 2. With isentropic flow there are no frictional shear stresses so that the only forces affecting the flow are the pressure forces shown in Fig. 18.11. These are the pressure forces pA and $(p + dp)(A + dA)$ at each end of the element, and the reaction on the fluid from the hydrostatic pressure along the wall. The average force normal to the surface of the wall is $(p + dp/2)\,dA_s$, where dA_s is the surface area. It is only the component of this force in the axial direction which contributes to the change in momentum, and this is

$$\left(p + \frac{dp}{2}\right)dA_s \sin\phi = \left(p + \frac{dp}{2}\right)dA$$

Equation (18.26) in differential form is therefore

$$pA - (p + dp)(A + dA) + \left(p + \frac{dp}{2}\right)dA = \dot{m}\,dC$$

Neglecting second-order terms, and remembering that $\dot{m}$ is equal to AC/v, this reduces to

$$A\,dp + \left(\frac{AC}{v}\right)dC = 0 \tag{18.27}$$

or alternatively,

$$v\,dp + C\,dC = 0 \tag{18.28}$$

Equation (18.28) is the same as the energy equation applied to isentropic flow, i.e. equation (18.5). Thus, as expected for adiabatic frictionless flow, the momentum and energy equations are identical. This is the reason why the momentum equation did not appear explicitly in the analysis given in section 18.1.

18.3.2 Heat addition to frictionless flow in a duct of constant area

The case now to be considered approximates to the process in the combustion chamber of a turbojet engine.* Since the flow is not adiabatic, the energy and momentum equations will not be identical, and it is easy to show that the flow cannot be completely described without using both equations.

---

* Although there is a considerable amount of friction in an actual chamber, arising from the use of baffles to stabilise the flame, it is usual to take this into account separately by assuming that all the friction occurs prior to the combustion which is here simulated by an addition of heat.

When the fluid is a perfect gas, the energy equation is

$$\dot{Q} = \dot{m}\{c_p(T_2 - T_1) + \tfrac{1}{2}(C_2^2 - C_1^2)\}$$

Owing to the increase of temperature, and therefore of specific volume, the velocity will increase in a duct of constant area, i.e. $C_2 > C_1$. Without knowing the change of pressure, this increase of velocity cannot be predicted, and the energy equation is evidently not sufficient to enable Q to be calculated for a given temperature rise or vice versa.

The differential form of the momentum equation for frictionless flow has already been deduced as equation (18.27), i.e.

$$A\,dp + \left(\frac{AC}{v}\right)dC = 0$$

In this case both A and (AC/v) are constant, so that the equation can be integrated directly to give

$$(p_2 - p_1) = -\frac{C_1}{v_1}(C_2 - C_1) \tag{18.29}$$

This equation, together with the energy equation, the equation of state and the continuity equation, provide four equations which can be solved for the four unknowns. That is, if $\dot{Q}$ and the initial conditions are known, p_2, T_2, v_2 and C_2 can be predicted; or when T_2 and the initial conditions are given, $\dot{Q}$, p_2, v_2 and C_2 can be found.

The calculation is too lengthy to be elaborated here, but the foregoing outline suffices to show that the momentum equation is essential for the solution of this type of problem. Furthermore, it also shows clearly that the heat addition to a fluid in a constant area duct cannot be achieved without a drop of pressure. It is apparent from the momentum equation that $p_2 = p_1$ only if $C_2 = C_1$. To achieve this it would be necessary to use a divergent duct, or a duct of such large cross-sectional area that changes in velocity are negligible.

18.3.3 Irreversible adiabatic flow in a duct of varying area

When the effect of friction is considered, the frictional force due to the shear stress along the wall of the duct must be included in the momentum equation. With reference to Fig. 18.12, and denoting the shear stress by τ, the force due

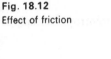

Fig. 18.12
Effect of friction

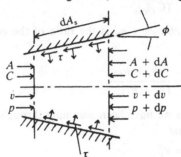

to friction is $\tau \, dA_s$. The component in the axial direction opposing motion is therefore

$$\tau \, dA_s \cos \phi = \tau \left(\frac{dA}{\sin \phi} \right) \cos \phi$$

Including this force in equation (18.27), we have

$$- A \, dp - \tau \, dA \cot \phi = \frac{AC}{v} dC$$

or

$$v \, dp + C \, dC + \frac{\tau v}{A} \cot \phi \, dA = 0 \qquad (18.30)$$

Equation (18.30) is evidently different from the energy equation for adiabatic flow, which is

$$dh + C \, dC = 0$$

The two equations become identical when $\tau = 0$ because then the process also becomes isentropic and dh is equal to $v \, dp$.

τ can be determined by experiment, but it is found to be a function of the velocity and turbulence of the fluid and the surface roughness of the duct (see section 22.1). It is therefore not a constant and varies along the duct. If the variation of τ along the duct is known, equation (18.30) can be used in conjunction with the energy equation, the equation of state and the continuity equation to predict the state of the fluid at any point in the duct. Although such a procedure is sometimes illuminating (see Ref. 18), it is very laborious. For practical purposes, e.g. when designing nozzles, it is usual to take account of friction by introducing empirical coefficients which can be used directly in conjunction with calculations based on the assumption of isentropic flow. Three such coefficients are in common use in nozzle design and they are defined as follows.

When the primary interest is in the exit velocity produced by the nozzle, it is usual to use either a velocity coefficient or a nozzle efficiency. The *velocity coefficient* k_C is defined as the ratio of the actual exit velocity to that calculated for the same pressure ratio on the assumption of isentropic flow, i.e.

$$k_C = \frac{C_2}{(C_2)_{\text{isen}}}$$

The *nozzle efficiency* η_N is the ratio of the actual to the isentropic enthalpy drop, i.e.

$$\eta_N = \frac{h_1 - h_2}{(h_1 - h_2)_{\text{isen}}}$$

If $C_1 \approx 0$, as we have been assuming throughout our discussion of nozzles, it is evident that

$$\eta_N = k_C^2$$

Fig. 18.13
Nozzle profiles

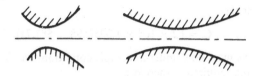

When the primary interest lies in the mass flow passed by the nozzle, a *coefficient of discharge* is used, defined by

$$k_D = \frac{\dot{m}}{\dot{m}_{\text{isen}}}$$

Nozzles with straight axes usually have efficiencies ranging from 94 to 99 per cent, whereas those with curved axes, as used in turbines, have efficiencies ranging from 90 to 95 per cent. The efficiency depends largely upon the profile of the nozzle. According to a one-dimensional isentropic treatment, there is nothing to choose between the two nozzles shown in Fig. 18.13. In practice the shorter nozzle, having the smaller surface area swept by the fluid, incurs less friction loss provided the included angle of the divergent part does not exceed 30 degrees.

The use of a coefficient of discharge and a nozzle efficiency in the design of a convergent-divergent nozzle is illustrated by the following example.

Example 18.3   A nozzle is required to pass an air flow of 1.5 kg/s. The inlet conditions are zero velocity, pressure 3.5 bar and temperature 425 °C; the air is to be expanded to 1.4 bar. Determine the throat area required if the coefficient of discharge is assumed to be 0.98.
      Also calculate the exit velocity and exit area if the nozzle efficiency is assumed to be 95 per cent.

The critical pressure ratio under isentropic conditions is

$$\frac{p_c}{p_1} = \left(\frac{2}{\gamma + 1}\right)^{\gamma/(\gamma-1)} = \left(\frac{2}{2.4}\right)^{1.4/0.4} = 0.528$$

Since the overall pressure ratio is 0.4, a convergent-divergent nozzle will be required for complete expansion within the nozzle. The conditions at the throat with isentropic flow will be

$$p_t = p_c = 0.528 \times 3.5 = 1.848 \text{ bar}$$

$$T_t = \frac{2}{\gamma + 1} T_1 = \frac{2 \times 698}{2.4} = 581.7 \text{ K}$$

$$v_t = \frac{RT_t}{p_t} = \frac{0.287 \times 581.7}{100 \times 1.848} = 0.903 \text{ m}^3/\text{kg}$$

The corresponding velocity at the throat may be found directly from the energy equation instead of using (18.17), i.e.

$$\tfrac{1}{2}C_t^2 = c_p(T_1 - T_t)$$

439

Hence

$$C_t = \{2 \times 10^3 \times 1.005(698 - 581.7)\}^{1/2} = 483.5 \, \text{m/s}$$

The mass flow under isentropic conditions would be $(1.5/0.98)$ kg/s. The throat area required is therefore

$$A_t = \frac{\dot{m}v_t}{C_t} = \frac{1.5 \times 0.903}{0.98 \times 483.5} [\text{m}^2] = 28.6 \, \text{cm}^2$$

If the expansion were isentropic, the final temperature would be

$$T_2' = T_1\left(\frac{p_2}{p_1}\right)^{(\gamma-1)/\gamma} = 698\left(\frac{1.4}{3.5}\right)^{0.4/1.4} = 537 \, \text{K}$$

Assuming a nozzle efficiency of 0.95, the actual final temperature will be given by

$$0.95 = \frac{T_1 - T_2}{T_1 - T_2'} = \frac{698 - T_2}{698 - 537}$$

from which $T_2 = 545$ K. The exit velocity will therefore be

$$C_2 = \{2 \times 10^3 \times 1.005(698 - 545)\}^{1/2} = 554.6 \, \text{m/s}$$

Also,

$$v_2 = \frac{RT_2}{p_2} = \frac{0.287 \times 545}{100 \times 1.4} = 1.117 \, \text{m}^3/\text{kg}$$

and hence the exit area required is

$$A_2 = \frac{\dot{m}v_2}{C_2} = \frac{1.5 \times 1.117}{554.6} [\text{m}^2] = 30.2 \, \text{cm}^2$$

Summary

The fundamental principles which may be used in the solution of problems of one-dimensional steady flow are

(1) First Law of Thermodynamics;
(2) Second Law of Thermodynamics;
(3) Conservation of Mass;
(4) Newton's Second Law of Motion.

In addition we have the Equation of State, or its equivalent in tables of properties.
  Only four equations are necessary to determine the flow. When the flow is reversible and adiabatic we may make direct use of a consequence of the Second Law of Thermodynamics, i.e. that the entropy is constant. Under these conditions, separate consideration of Newton's Second Law is superfluous because the momentum and energy equations are identical. When the flow is either irreversible or non-adiabatic we cannot make direct use of the consequences of the Second Law of Thermodynamics, but we can then use Newton's Second Law of Motion.
  We have only carried out analyses for very simple cases—and not all of these

have been carried to completion owing to the length of the calculation. It is not surprising that more sophisticated methods are used in the proper study of gas dynamics. For example, in order to obtain the simple expressions of nozzle flow, (18.10) to (18.16), we had to assume a negligible inlet velocity. In fact equally simple expressions can be obtained when the inlet velocity is finite once the concepts of *stagnation* (or *total*) temperature and pressure are introduced. The velocity term is then taken into account implicitly rather than explicitly. Where velocity terms must occur explicitly, much simplification of the equations is possible if the velocity is expressed as a fraction of the local sonic velocity; this ratio is known as the *Mach number*. The use of such concepts is essential if manageable equations are to be obtained when dealing simultaneously with changes of area, heat addition and friction (see Ref. 11). Gas dynamic concepts have not been introduced here because they would have obscured the fundamental links between thermodynamics and gas dynamics which it has been our object to present.

18.4 Jet propulsion engines

As a final example of the use of the momentum equation we shall discuss briefly the nature of *propulsive work* produced by aircraft power plant. When an aircraft is flying horizontally at a constant speed C_A, the drag of the aircraft must be balanced by an equal and opposite thrust F_N produced by the power plant. The rate of work done is then equal to the product $F_N C_A$, and this is known as the propulsive work (strictly 'power'). Any estimation of this quantity must involve an application of the momentum equation since we are concerned directly with forces.

Propulsion engines fall into two distinct classes: those which make use of atmospheric air as the main propulsive fluid, and those which carry their own propulsive fluid. The latter are known as rocket motors and will be considered separately. For a full treatment of jet propulsion see Ref. 23.

18.4.1 Propulsion engines using atmospheric air

All propulsion engines consist of one or more of the three components depicted in Fig. 18.14, namely a diffuser, a source of energy and a propelling nozzle. No diffuser or nozzle is used in the aircraft piston engine, and the energy source consists of a piston engine producing mechanical work which is used to drive

Fig. 18.14
Schematic representation
of a propulsion engine

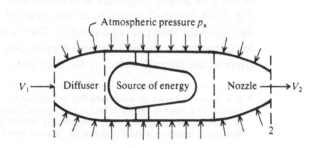

441

a propeller. All three components are used in a *turbojet* engine, and in this case the energy source comprises a compressor, a combustion chamber and a turbine. No net work is produced by the turbine, but some of the energy available in the gases leaving the turbine is used in the propelling nozzle to produce a high-speed jet. At very high aircraft speeds sufficient pressure rise is obtained in the diffuser alone and there is no need for a compressor and therefore for the turbine which drives it. This leads to the idea of the *ramjet* engine, consisting simply of a diffuser, a combustion chamber and a propelling nozzle. Owing to the direct dependence of pressure rise upon aircraft speed, the ramjet propelled vehicle must be given an initial velocity before the engine can function. Moreover, pressures sufficiently high for good efficiency can be obtained only at supersonic speeds, when the pressure rise across shock waves at the inlet can be utilised.

In all these forms of power plant the thrust is produced by accelerating a mass of air and increasing its momentum in a rearward direction. The net reaction upon the aircraft is the useful thrust F_N. An expression for F_N can be obtained by considering the momentum equation. In what follows it will be assumed that the mass flow of propulsive fluid is constant between inlet and outlet of the engine, i.e. that the mass of fuel added is negligible. The exhaust gases leaving a piston engine provide only a minute part of the total propulsive fluid and the assumption is obviously permissible in this instance. It is also valid for a turbojet engine because the fuel/air ratios used are small, but it is not such a good approximation in the case of a ramjet engine where the fuel/air ratios are approximately stoichiometric.

The momentum equation (18.26) states that

$$\Sigma F = \dot{m}(C_2 - C_1)$$

When deriving this equation we were considering flow through a stationary duct; the velocities relative to such a duct are absolute velocities (i.e. relative to the earth) and consequently they have been denoted by the symbol C. We are here considering a duct possessing motion relative to the earth, but if the duct is moving with a *uniform* velocity the equation is still valid.* The velocities in the equation can be regarded as either absolute velocities or velocities relative to the duct. Velocities relative to a moving duct will always be denoted by V. The momentum equation can therefore also be written as

$$\Sigma F = \dot{m}(V_2 - V_1) \tag{18.31}$$

and it is this form which we shall use in what follows. Subscripts 1 and 2 will be used to denote properties at the inlet and outlet, referring once again to Fig. 18.14. We shall denote by R' the resultant of all the forces exerted *by the duct* upon the fluid passing through it. These comprise the hydrostatic pressure forces normal to the wall, and the friction forces along the wall (where 'wall' refers to the internal surface of the duct and the external surface of any body

---

* It is shown in books on mechanics that any dynamical equation based on Newton's Laws of Motion, and which is known to hold in one frame of reference, must also hold in any other frame of reference that moves with a uniform velocity relative to the first. Any such frame in which a Newtonian equation is valid is termed an 'inertial frame'.

attached to the duct and immersed in the stream). From the discussion of ΣF in the previous section it will be evident that ΣF is equal to R' plus the net pressure force $(p_1 A_1 - p_2 A_2)$. The momentum equation can therefore be written as

$$R' + (p_1 A_1 - p_2 A_2) = \dot{m}(V_2 - V_1)$$

From Newton's Third Law of Motion, the net force exerted by the fluid *on the duct*, R say, must be equal and opposite to R', i.e. $R = -R'$. So far we have always considered forces to be positive if they act in the direction for which the fluid velocity is taken as positive. When discussing propulsive forces, it is more convenient *to change the sign convention and treat the forces as positive in the direction of motion of the aircraft*. If we denote by F_T the force exerted by the fluid on the duct which produces a thrust in the direction of motion of the aircraft, then $F_T = -R = R'$. The momentum equation can therefore be written as

$$F_T + (p_1 A_1 - p_2 A_2) = \dot{m}(V_2 - V_1)$$

and hence*

$$F_T = (p_2 A_2 + \dot{m}V_2) - (p_1 A_1 + \dot{m}V_1)$$

Although F_T is the total force exerted by the propulsive fluid upon the duct, it is not the net force exerted by the duct upon the aircraft. There are pressure forces acting on the external surface of the duct which are not balanced unless A_2 is equal to A_1. The external pressure is the atmospheric pressure p_a, and the net external force assisting the motion of the duct is therefore $p_a(A_1 - A_2)$. The net thrust F_N which the power plant exerts upon the aircraft is found by adding this external force to F_T. There will be other external forces due to friction on the outside of the duct, but these are normally included in the drag of the aircraft as a whole. It follows that the net thrust is given by

$$F_N = (p_2 A_2 + \dot{m}V_2) - (p_1 A_1 + \dot{m}V_1) + p_a(A_1 - A_2) \qquad (18.32)$$

Under certain conditions (18.32) can be reduced to a simpler form. When the aircraft is flying at subsonic speeds, p_1 is equal to p_a, and V_1 is equal in magnitude to the aircraft speed C_A. (These equalities do not hold at supersonic speeds because of the effect of shock waves at the inlet.) With these modifications, and writing V_j (jet velocity relative to the aircraft) for V_2, equation (18.32) appears as

$$F_N = \dot{m}(V_j - C_A) + A_2(p_2 - p_a) \qquad (18.33)$$

The first term on the RHS of (18.33) is called the *momentum thrust* and the second the *pressure thrust*. The pressure thrust is in some cases zero. For example, when the propulsive jet is produced by a propeller the downstream pressure is atmospheric, i.e. $p_2 = p_a$. Or again, the propelling nozzle of a turbojet engine is a simple converging nozzle; p_2 will therefore be equal to p_a when the pressure

---

* In gas dynamics the quantity $(pA + mV)$ at any plane in the flow is known as the *stream thrust* at that plane.

Fig. 18.15
Propulsion engines

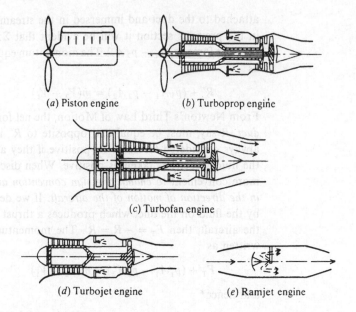

(a) Piston engine   (b) Turboprop engine

(c) Turbofan engine

(d) Turbojet engine   (e) Ramjet engine

ratio (outlet/inlet) is greater than the critical pressure ratio (section 18.1.2). In such circumstances the thrust is simply

$$F_N = \dot{m}(V_J - C_A) \tag{18.34}$$

From the simple expression (18.34), it is obvious that the same thrust can be achieved by using either an engine producing a high-velocity jet of low mass flow (turbojet), or one which produces a low-velocity jet of high mass flow (propeller). The choice can be shown to depend upon the aircraft speed, as follows. The energy supplied by the fuel is used in two ways: (a) in producing the propulsive power $F_N C_A$, and (b) in producing a jet having an absolute kinetic energy of $\dot{m}(V_J - C_A)^2/2$. The latter represents a waste of energy, although it cannot be made zero without at the same time reducing the thrust to zero. If the wasted kinetic energy in the jet is to be small, however, $(V_J - C_A)$ must not be too great, i.e. we require a high-speed jet for a fast aircraft and a low-speed jet for a slow aircraft.

Such considerations as these have led to the development of the range of power plant shown diagrammatically in Fig. 18.15. Proceeding from (a) to (e), the propulsive jet decreases in mass flow and increases in velocity. (a) represents the piston engine and propeller. (b) is a turboprop engine, where the low-velocity jet from the propeller is combined with the high-velocity jet from the turbine engine. In (c), the turbofan (or by-pass) engine, the propeller is replaced by a fan giving a jet of smaller mass flow but of higher velocity. (d) is the simple turbojet and (e) the ramjet.

18.4.2   Rocket motors

There is one remaining type of propulstion unit to consider, which is in a class by itself—namely the *rocket motor*. It is distinguished from the other means of

Fig. 18.16
A liquid-fuelled rocket motor

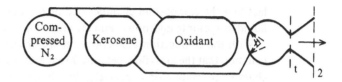

propulsion by the fact that it makes no use of the atmosphere but carries its own oxidant. For this reason it is the only power plant suitable for use at very high altitudes or in outer space.

The rocket motor consists essentially of a combustion chamber and propelling nozzle. For short durations, such as those involved in temporary thrust boosting or starting a ram-jet propelled vehicle, the most economical rocket is obtained by using solid fuel. For longer durations a liquid fuel (e.g. kerosene) and liquid oxidant (e.g. nitric acid or hydrogen peroxide) are always preferred. In what follows we shall adopt rocket practice and use the term 'fuel' to include the oxidant; enthalpies of combustion, for example, are always quoted per unit mass of reacting material which the rocket must carry. The fuel is either fed into the combustion chamber by mechanical pumps, or forced in by compressed nitrogen carried in a separate container as indicated in Fig. 18.16. Since it is possible to operate a rocket combustion chamber at relatively high pressures— 20 bar or more—very high jet velocities and large thrusts can be obtained.

To make full use of the large pressure drop across the propelling nozzle, a convergent-divergent nozzle is always employed. It will be operating in the choked condition and the mass flow passed by the nozzle (equal to the mass flow of fuel) is therefore given by equation (18.21), namely

$$\dot{m} = A_t p_1 \left\{ \frac{\gamma}{RT_1} \left(\frac{2}{\gamma + 1} \right)^{(\gamma + 1)/(\gamma - 1)} \right\}^{1/2}$$

This is assuming isentropic expansion and that the combustion gases behave as a perfect gas. The values of γ and the combustion temperature T_1 are more or less fixed by the properties of the reactants employed, i.e. by the enthalpy of combustion and specific heats. A rough estimate of T_1 can be obtained by treating the combustion as a constant pressure, adiabatic process. Due account must be taken of dissociation, however, because approximately stoichiometric mixtures are used and the temperatures are very high—in the region of 2800 K. This type of calculation has been described in section 15.7. One of the unknowns is the extent to which the reaction still continues during the expansion of the nozzle. The real expansion must lie between two extremes which can be calculated on the basis of two assumptions, both starting from chemical equilibrium having been reached in the combustion chamber. (a) As the gases expand in the nozzle, chemical equilibrium is obtained at each section, corresponding to the temperature and pressure at that section, implying that recombination proceeds along the nozzle. Or (b) no further reaction takes place as the gases cool during the expansion in the nozzle (so-called 'frozen flow'), because there is no time available during the fast flow for chemical equilibrium to establish itself. The calculations are further complicated by the

445

fact that the combustion chamber and nozzle must be cooled—usually by the liquid fuel prior to injection—and the process is therefore not strictly adiabatic.

With the combustion temperature more or less fixed, it is evident from the equation that the mass flow per unit throat area is a function only of combustion chamber pressure—or, conversely, that the combustion pressure is fixed by the rate at which fuel is fed into the chamber. The maximum permissible pressure is determined by the high-temperature strength of the materials used in the construction of the chamber.

The main factors affecting the performance of the rocket motor are apparent from the expression for the thrust produced. The working fluid has no initial momentum relative to the rocket, and V_1, p_1 and A_1 are zero in the momentum equation (18.32). The net thrust is therefore

$$F_N = \dot{m}V_2 + A_2(p_2 - p_a)$$

If the nozzle is designed for complete expansion from the combustion pressure to p_a, the pressure thrust is zero and the thrust is simply

$$F_N = \dot{m}V_2$$

The exit velocity V_2 is given by equation (18.17), and with complete expansion the pressure ratio can be denoted by p_a/p_1, so that

$$V_2 = \left[\frac{2\gamma}{1-\gamma} RT_1 \left\{ \left(\frac{p_a}{p_1} \right)^{(\gamma-1)/\gamma} - 1 \right\} \right]^{1/2}$$

Combining this equation with the mass flow equation, we have the thrust per unit throat area as

$$\frac{F_N}{A_t} = p_1\gamma \left[\frac{2}{\gamma-1} \left(\frac{2}{\gamma+1} \right)^{(\gamma+1)/(\gamma-1)} \left\{ 1 - \left(\frac{p_a}{p_1} \right)^{(\gamma-1)/\gamma} \right\} \right]^{1/2} \qquad (18.35)$$

Equation (18.35) shows that for a given nozzle (A_t) and given reactants (γ), the thrust at any altitude (p_a) is a function only of the combustion pressure p_1, i.e. of the rate of fuel supply. The thrust is not dependent upon the combustion temperature, except in so far as γ depends slightly upon this quantity.

The thrust itself is not, however, the most important criterion of the performance of a rocket. Such a large proportion of the total mass of a rocket comprises fuel, and fuel containers, that it is the thrust per unit flow of fuel which really matters. This quantity, called the *specific impulse I*, can be found by combining the mass flow and thrust equations to give

$$I = \frac{F_N}{\dot{m}} = \left[RT_1 \frac{2\gamma}{\gamma-1} \left\{ 1 - \left(\frac{p_a}{p_1} \right)^{(\gamma-1)/\gamma} \right\} \right]^{1/2} \qquad (18.36)$$

From this expression it may be seen that a high combustion temperature is necessary for good performance. Remembering that the gas constant for the expanding products is equal to $\tilde{R}/\tilde{m}$, where $\tilde{R}$ is the molar gas constant and $\tilde{m}$ is the molar mass, it is also apparent that it is desirable to choose a fuel which yields a product of low molar mass. It is in fact a high value of the ratio of

$T_1/\tilde{m}$ which is important when considering the choice of fuel. In general, fuels having a high hydrogen content prove to be the best, enabling high specific impulses to be obtained without the use of excessively high combustion temperatures.

In arriving at equations (18.35) and (18.36) we supposed that the gases are expanded to ambient pressure in the nozzle, and therefore that the pressure thrust is zero. When operating at high altitudes this is not practicable, because complete expansion would require a nozzle having a very large exit/throat area ratio (and in space it would be infinite). This in turn implies a long nozzle with considerable friction loss. Theoretically, with isentropic expansion, the thrust can be shown to be a maximum with complete expansion; the reduction in momentum thrust as a result of using a smaller area ratio is never entirely compensated by the additional pressure thrust due to p_2 being greater than p_a. This is not necessarily true when friction is taken into account because the theoretical jet velocity, and hence momentum thrust, are not achieved. A considerable departure from the optimum nozzle area ratio can in fact be permitted without much loss of thrust. Equations (18.35) and (18.36) may be expanded to include the pressure thrust term, but it is easier to work from first principles as indicated in the following example.

Example 18.4 A rocket nozzle has an exit/throat area ratio of 3:1. Assuming that the expansion is isentropic, estimate the thrust per unit throat area and the specific impulse, when the combustion temperature is 3000 K, the combustion pressure is 20 bar, and atmospheric pressure is 1 bar. Assume that the gases have a molar mass of 33.5 kg/kmol and that γ is 1.2.

The mass flow per unit throat area from equation (18.21) is

$$\frac{\dot{m}}{A_t} = p_1 \left\{ \frac{\gamma}{RT_1} \left(\frac{2}{\gamma+1} \right)^{(\gamma+1)/(\gamma-1)} \right\}^{1/2}$$

Now the specific gas constant is

$$R = \frac{\tilde{R}}{\tilde{m}} = \frac{8.3145 \left[\dfrac{kJ}{kmol\ K} \right]}{33.5 \left[\dfrac{kg}{kmol} \right]} = 0.248\ kJ/kg\ K$$

and hence

$$\frac{\dot{m}}{A_t} = 20[bar] \times 10^5 \left[\frac{N/m^2}{bar} \right]$$

$$\times \left\{ \frac{1.2}{0.248 \left[\dfrac{kJ}{kg\ K} \right] \times 10^3 \left[\dfrac{J\ or\ N\,m}{kJ} \right] \times 3000[K]} \left(\frac{2}{2.2} \right)^{2.2/0.2} \right\}^{1/2}$$

$$= 1504 \left[\frac{N\,kg}{m^5} \times \frac{kg\,m/s^2}{N} \right]^{1/2} = 1504\ kg/s\ m^2$$

The pressure in the plane of the exit p_2 will be greater than atmospheric pressure and its value is determined by the area ratio. A simple equation for p_2 in terms of known quantities cannot be formulated, but the following graphical method may be adopted:

$$\frac{\dot{m}}{A_1} = \frac{A_2 V_2}{A_1 v_2} = \frac{3V_2}{v_2}$$

(NB: Here V is relative velocity and v specific volume.) V_2 may be found directly from the energy equation which, with V_1 equal to zero, yields

$$V_2 = \{2c_p(T_1 - T_2)\}^{1/2}$$

Since $c_p = \gamma R/(\gamma - 1) = 1.488\ \text{kJ/kg K}$,

$$V_2 = \left\{2 \times 1488\left[\frac{J}{\text{kg K}}\right](3000[K] - T_2)\right\}^{1/2}$$

$$= 54.55\left[\frac{m}{s\ K^{1/2}}\right](3000[K] - T_2)^{1/2}$$

Also, v_2 can be found in terms of T_2 from

$$v_2 = \frac{RT_2}{p_2} = \frac{RT_2(T_1/T_2)^{\gamma/(\gamma-)}}{p_1}$$

$$= \frac{248\left[\dfrac{J}{\text{kg K}}\right]T_2\left(\dfrac{3000[K]}{T_2}\right)^{1.2/0.2}}{20 \times 10^5\left[\dfrac{N}{m^2}\right]}$$

$$= 0.000\,124\left[\frac{m^3}{\text{kg K}}\right]T_2\left(\frac{3000[K]}{T_2}\right)^6$$

Substituting for V_2 and v_2 in the expression for the mass flow per unit throat area $(\dot{m}/A_1)$, we have

$$1504\left[\frac{\text{kg}}{s\,m^2}\right] = \frac{3 \times 54.55\left[\dfrac{m}{s\,K^{1/2}}\right](3000[K] - T_2)^{1/2}}{0.000\,124\left[\dfrac{m^3}{\text{kg K}}\right]T_2\left(\dfrac{3000[K]}{T_2}\right)^6}$$

$$0.001\,14\frac{T_2}{[K]}\left(\frac{3000}{T_2/[K]}\right)^6 = \left(3000 - \frac{T_2}{[K]}\right)^{1/2}$$

Evaluating each side of the equation for a series of values of $T_2/[K]$ and plotting the results, we arrive at the solution $T_2 = 1906\ \text{K}$. Hence

$$V_2 = 54.55\left[\frac{m}{s\,K^{1/2}}\right](3000[K] - 1906[K])^{1/2} = 1804\ \text{m/s}$$

$$p_2 = \frac{20[\text{bar}]}{(3000/1906)^6} = 1.315\ \text{bar}$$

The thrust per unit throat area is therefore

$$\frac{F_N}{A_t} = \frac{\dot{m}}{A_t} V_2 + \frac{A_2}{A_t}(p_2 - p_a)$$

$$= \left\{1504\left[\frac{kg}{s\,m^2}\right] \times 1804\left[\frac{m}{s}\right]\right\} + \{3 \times 10^5(1.315 - 1.0)\}\left[\frac{N}{m^2}\right]$$

$$= (2.713 + 0.095) \times 10^6\left[\frac{N}{m^2}\right] = 2.808 \times 10^6 \, N/m^2$$

The specific impulse is then given by

$$I = \frac{F_N/A_t}{\dot{m}/A_t} = \frac{2808[kN/m^2]}{1504[kg/s\,m^2]} = 1.87 \, kN \text{ per } kg/s$$

19

Rotary Expanders and Compressors

This chapter describes the way in which work is transferred in rotary expanders and compressors. The former are always referred to as turbines. In a turbine the working fluid enters at a high pressure and acquires increased kinetic energy as it expands to a lower pressure in a ring of fixed nozzles. The stream of fluid then undergoes a change of momentum as it flows through passages between blades attached to the rotor, and the component in a direction tangential to the circle of rotation produces the output torque at the shaft.

This series of events is reversed in the rotary compressor. Input torque from some external source imparts a change of momentum to the working fluid passing between the rotor blades. Having acquired an increased velocity, the fluid then slows down with an accompanying rise of pressure while flowing through a ring of fixed diffusers.

There are two main types of turbine and rotary compressor, distinguished by whether the flow through the machine is in the axial or the radial direction. Accordingly, this chapter may be divided into four main sections, dealing respectively with the axial-flow turbine, the axial-flow compressor, the radial-flow turbine and the radial-flow compressor. In all these machines the fluid undergoes a continuous steady-flow process and the speed of flow is very high. For this reason comparatively small machines can handle large mass flows and large work transfers, and the processes can be assumed to be adiabatic.

It is worth emphasising here that although the Roots blower and the vane pump are rotary compressors, they are both positive-displacement machines and as such have been described in Chapter 16. In a positive-displacement compressor the fluid is prevented from flowing back in the direction of the pressure gradient by solid surfaces. No such positive control of the flow exists in the compressors considered in this chapter, where compression is produced by the processes of acceleration and subsequent diffusion.

19.1 Momentum principles applied to flow through a rotor

Before dealing with the four types of rotary machine, it is helpful to consider the general case of steady flow through passages in a rotor when the absolute

Fig. 19.1

Flow through a rotor

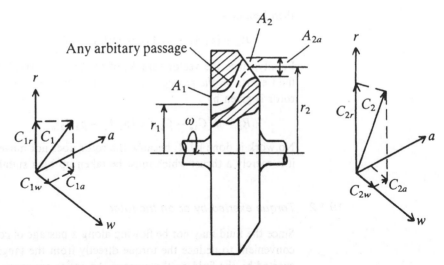

Any arbitary passage

velocity of the fluid has components in the axial, radial and tangential directions. The axial and radial components will be denoted by subscripts a and r, and the tangential component, commonly called the *whirl velocity*, by subscript w. For simplicity we shall assume that the flow is 'one-dimensional', i.e. that the fluid enters the rotor with uniform properties through an area A_1 at a mean radius r_1, and leaves with uniform properties through an area A_2 at a mean radius r_2. The passages joining the inlet and outlet areas may be curved, and the area change (i.e. whether the passages are convergent or divergent) is governed by the velocity and pressure changes which the fluid is required to undergo in the rotor. With the aid of Fig. 19.1 we shall consider the forces produced when a fluid flows at a steady rate $\dot{m}$ through a passage in the rotor.

19.1.1   Axial thrust on the rotor

We have seen in section 18.3 that the vector sum of all the external forces acting on the fluid in a passage is equal to the rate of change of momentum between the inlet and outlet sections (equation (18.25)). Applying this result to the axial components of the forces and velocities, we have

$$\Sigma F_a = \dot{m}(C_{2a} - C_{1a})$$

Forces are always taken as positive in the direction in which the velocity is treated as positive. The vector sum ΣF_a may be split into two parts: (a) the sum R'_a of the pressure forces and friction shear forces which the passage wall exerts on the fluid; and (b) the net hydrostatic pressure force $(p_1 A_1 - p_2 A_2)_a$ which the fluid exerts over the inlet and outlet areas in the axial direction.* The equation

---

* A word of warning is necessary about the general validity of the momentum equation which we are now applying to a curved passage in a rotor. We have always tacitly assumed, and will continue to do so, that any shear forces along the planes 1 and 2 at inlet and outlet are negligible. Although there are no such forces across planes at right angles to the flow in the straight ducts considered in Chapter 18, they will be present at the inlet and outlet of a curved passage, in a rotor when there is a component of velocity along the plane. In such cases our steady-flow energy equation is also not strictly true because, since the rotor is moving, these shear forces will result in energy transfers which would have to be included in the work term $\dot{W}$.

then becomes

$$R'_a + (p_1 A_1 - p_2 A_2)_a = \dot{m}(C_{2a} - C_{1a})$$

Finally, since the vector sum R_a of the pressure and friction forces which the fluid exerts *on the passage wall* must be equal to $-R'_a$, the axial force on the rotor is given by

$$R_a = \dot{m}(C_{1a} - C_{2a}) + (p_1 A_1 - p_2 A_2)_a \tag{19.1}$$

No work is done by R_a because the rotor does not move in the axial direction; it is merely a thrust which must be taken up by a suitable thrust bearing.

19.1.2   Torque exerted by or on the rotor

Since the fluid may not be flowing along a passage of constant radius, it is not convenient to deduce the torque directly from the tangential (or whirl) forces exerted by the fluid on the passage. An easier approach is provided by the use of the concept of *angular momentum*, i.e. moment of momentum. The principle of angular momentum is commonly stated in mechanics as follows: *the rate of change of angular momentum of a system of particles about a fixed point is equal to the sum of the moments of the external forces about that point.* The sum of these moments is the torque applied to the system undergoing the change of momentum. To apply the principle of angular momentum to the flow through a rotor, the usual argument adopted for dealing with open systems can be used.

Consider a steady-flow system consisting of the mass of fluid in the rotor passage together with an elemental mass δm which is about to enter the rotor through A_1. In time δt this elemental mass enters, and an equal mass δm leaves through A_2. For steady flow, the angular momentum of the fluid within the passage does not change with time. The whole change in angular momentum during time δt is therefore equal to the difference between the angular momentum of the mass δm at inlet and outlet, namely

$$\delta m(r_2 C_{2w} - r_1 C_{1w})$$

and the rate of change of angular momentum becomes

$$\frac{\delta m}{\delta t}(r_2 C_{2w} - r_1 C_{1w})$$

This must be equal to the moment about the axis of all the external forces applied *by the rotor to the fluid*, and this is the torque T which must be applied to drive the rotor if the machine were a compressor. In the limit, $\delta m/\delta t$ is the rate of mass flow $\dot{m}$, so that

$$T = \dot{m}(r_2 C_{2w} - r_1 C_{1w}) \tag{19.2}$$

If the rotor is moving with a uniform angular velocity ω, the rate of work done *by the rotor on the fluid* is

$$\dot{W} = \omega T = \dot{m}\omega(r_2 C_{2w} - r_1 C_{1w})$$

If we write $U_1 (= \omega r_1)$ and $U_2 (= \omega r_2)$ for the rotor velocities at the inlet and outlet section, this equation reduces to

$$\dot{W} = \dot{m}(U_2 C_{2w} - U_1 C_{1w}) \tag{19.3}$$

This would be the power *input* required to drive the machine.

When the machine is a turbine, the power *output* is produced at the expense of the angular momentum of the fluid, so that $C_{2w} < C_{1w}$ and $\dot{W}$ is negative in accordance with our sign convention. The expression for the torque (19.2) would also yield a negative value, implying that the torque would be exerted *by* the fluid *on* the rotor.

Finally, for a truly axial-flow machine, where $r_2 = r_1 = r$, we can write $U = U_1 = U_2$ and equation (19.3) simplifies to

$$\dot{W} = \dot{m}U(C_{2w} - C_{1w}) \tag{19.4}$$

U is the rotor blade velocity (ωr) at the mid-height of the blades, i.e. at the mean radius of the annulus.

Little need be said about the radial component of the fluid velocity. Normally the fluid enters and leaves the rotor through annuli, so that the flow is symmetrically disposed about the rotor axis and a change in the radial component of velocity has no net effect upon the rotor. If the flow is not symmetrical about the axis of rotation a net radial force may have to be taken up by the shaft bearings, but no work is done by this force.

19.2 Axial-flow turbines

When the design of turbines is being considered, it is usual to drop the thermodynamic sign convention and treat the work output as a positive quantity. In what follows, we shall write the equations in such a way that they yield positive values for W or $\dot{W}$ so that they will then be in a form familiar to turbine designers. To avoid contradicting our sign convention, however, we will use the modulus sign, although a turbine designer would find this unnecessary. Equations (19.3) and (19.4) will therefore be written as

$$|\dot{W}| = \dot{m}(U_1 C_{1w} - U_2 C_{2w}) \tag{19.3a}$$

$$|\dot{W}| = \dot{m}U(C_{1w} - C_{2w}) \tag{19.4a}$$

An axial-flow turbine consists of one or more *stages*, each stage comprising one annulus of fixed *stator blades* followed by one of moving *rotor blades* as in Fig. 19.2a. Usually the total pressure drop across the stage is divided between the stator and rotor blade rows as illustrated in Fig. 19.2b. The division is normally expressed, not in terms of pressure drops, but in terms of enthalpy drops. The criterion used is the *degree of reaction* Λ, defined as

$$\Lambda = \frac{\text{enthalpy drop in rotor blades}}{\text{enthalpy drop in stage}} = \frac{h_1 - h_2}{h_0 - h_2} \tag{19.5}$$

The two most common values of Λ used are 0 and 0.5 (or 50 per cent). When the degree of reaction is zero, all the stage pressure drop occurs in the stator

Fig. 19.2
An axial-flow turbine
stage

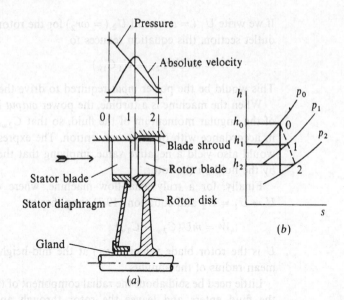

(b)

blades (which are then often referred to as *nozzle blades*) and the stage is called an *impulse stage*. In a 50 per cent reaction design the pressure ratios across the stator and rotor blades are approximately equal. This will be referred to here simply as a *reaction stage* because we shall not be considering the use of other values of Λ.

The mode of action of the turbine can best be studied by following the path of the fluid through a single stage at the mean radius of the annulus, as in Fig. 19.3. We shall adopt the practice, now commonly used for both turbines and compressors, of measuring all blade and fluid flow angles from the axial direction. The fluid enters the stage with velocity C_0 at pressure p_0 and is expanded to p_1 in the stator blades. It leaves these blades with a velocity C_1, in a direction

Fig. 19.3
Velocity triangles for a
turbine stage

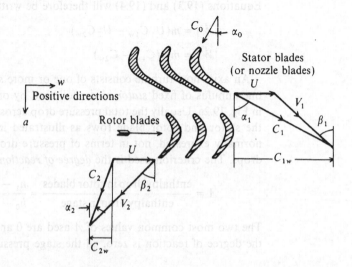

Fig. 19.4
Velocity diagrams of a
turbine stage

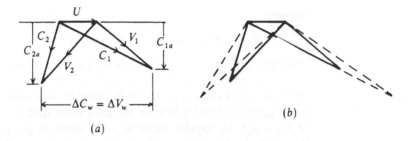

(a)

(b)

making an angle α_1 with the axial direction. C_1 must satisfy the energy equation

$$\tfrac{1}{2}(C_1^2 - C_0^2) = h_0 - h_1 \tag{19.6}$$

The velocity of the fluid relative to the moving blades can be found by subtracting vectorially the blade speed U. This is easily accomplished by drawing the inlet velocity triangle. To avoid a multiplicity of indices, relative velocities will be denoted by V, and the relative velocity at inlet to the rotor blades is therefore V_1. V_1 makes an angle β_1 with the axial direction, and if the fluid is to flow smoothly into the blade passages without undue disturbance, the inlet angle of the blades must be made approximately equal to β_1. If the outlet angle of the rotor blades is β_2, the direction of the relative velocity at outlet V_2 will also be approximately β_2. Applying the energy equation to the flow *relative to the rotor blades*, it follows that

$$\tfrac{1}{2}(V_2^2 - V_1^2) = h_1 - h_2 \tag{19.7}$$

because no work is done in the frame of reference of the moving blades. V_2 must satisfy this equation. Vectorial addition of the blade speed then gives the absolute velocity C_2 and the direction α_2. Usually, if this is one stage of a multistage turbine, C_2 will be made equal to C_0 and α_2 equal to α_0; the fluid can then pass on to another similar stage.

Equation (19.4a) gives the rate of work done, i.e.

$$|\dot{W}| = \dot{m}U(C_{1w} - C_{2w}) = \dot{m}U\Delta C_w$$

Note that the whirl component of the absolute outlet velocity C_{2w} is negative in the case depicted in Fig. 19.3. It is usually convenient to combine the inlet and outlet velocity triangles to give the velocity diagram of Fig. 19.4a. It is then easy to see that the algebraic difference of C_{1w} and C_{2w} is equal to the algebraic difference of the whirl components of the relative velocities at inlet and outlet. Thus*

$$|\dot{W}| = \dot{m}U\Delta C_w = \dot{m}U\Delta V_w \tag{19.8}$$

The axial thrust can be obtained from equation (19.1). For an axial-flow stage the areas A_1 and A_2 are normal to the axial direction, and consequently (19.1)

---

* The interchangeability of ΔC_w and ΔV_w is to be expected because, as we have already pointed out in section 18.4.1, the momentum equation upon which (19.8) is based applies in any inertial frame of reference and we are here treating the rotating blade passages as if they are moving linearly with a uniform absolute velocity U.

becomes

$$R_a = \dot{m}(C_{1a} - C_{2a}) + (p_1 A_1 - p_2 A_2) \tag{19.9}$$

Evidently the term $\dot{m}(C_{1a} - C_{2a})$ is negative for the particular case shown in Fig. 19.4a. It must be pointed out that equation (19.9) does not necessarily give the total thrust exerted on the shaft bearings. In addition to R_a there may be a net pressure thrust acting on the solid rotor disk, of area A_d say, equal to $A_d(p_1 - p_2)$. In impulse turbines p_2 is equal to p_1, and if $A_1 = A_2$ as in Fig. 19.2, the thrust due to the pressure terms is zero. Thus only small thrust bearings are required. To reduce the thrust in multistage reaction turbines, the fluid is sometimes introduced at the mid-point of the casing and allowed to expand in opposite axial directions; the machine is then called a *double-flow turbine*.

As an alternative to equation (19.8), an expression for the work done can be found in terms of the fluid velocities by eliminating the enthalpy term from the energy equation. Thus, applying the energy equation between planes 1 and 2 of Fig. 19.2a, we have

$$|\dot{W}| = \dot{m}\{(h_1 - h_2) + \tfrac{1}{2}(C_1^2 - C_2^2)\}$$

Absolute velocities are used here (i.e. velocities relative to the turbine casing) so that the work term must be included. No work is done in the stator row and $\dot{W}$ is therefore the rate of work done in the stage. Using (19.7), the enthalpy term can be eliminated to give

$$|\dot{W}| = \frac{\dot{m}}{2}\{(C_1^2 - C_2^2) + (V_2^2 - V_1^2)\} \tag{19.10}$$

Equation (19.10) can be shown to be identical with (19.8) by considering the geometry of the velocity triangles. Thus

$$C_1^2 = V_1^2 + U^2 + 2V_1 U \sin \beta_1$$
$$C_2^2 = V_2^2 + U^2 - 2V_2 U \sin \beta_2$$

Subtracting,

$$C_1^2 - C_2^2 = V_1^2 - V_2^2 + 2U(V_1 \sin \beta_1 + V_2 \sin \beta_2)$$

But

$$\Delta V_w = V_1 \sin \beta_1 + V_2 \sin \beta_2$$

and therefore

$$|\dot{W}| = \dot{m}U\Delta V_w = \frac{\dot{m}}{2}\{(C_1^2 - C_2^2) + (V_2^2 - V_1^2)\}$$

The agreement between the two derivations is not surprising because the energy equation contains implicitly the laws of motion. Once the thermodynamic properties are eliminated, the energy equation should yield the same result as an equation derived from purely mechanical considerations.

So far we have concentrated on what happens in an individual stage, and we must now briefly consider the turbine as a whole. The chief aim in the design of a turbine is to utilise the available isentropic enthalpy drop with the least possible friction loss and in the smallest number of stages. It should be clear from equation (19.8) that the work done per stage increases with the blade speed U, but consideration of the centrifugal stresses in the rotating parts leads to a maximum permissible blade speed. With the blade speed fixed, an attempt to use a small number of stages (and hence a large enthalpy drop per stage) may mean that a smaller fraction of the enthalpy drop is converted into work and that a larger fraction remains as kinetic energy in the stream leaving the rotor blades. This should be clear from Fig. 19.4b. Furthermore, high fluid velocities lead to large friction losses. A useful criterion which indicates the effectiveness of energy abstraction in a stage is the *diagram efficiency* η_d (sometimes called the *utilisation factor*). This is defined as

$$\eta_d = \frac{\text{work calculated from velocity diagram}}{\text{energy available to rotor blades}} \tag{19.11}$$

The denominator is the kinetic energy at inlet to the rotor blades, $\dot{m}C_1^2/2$, plus the energy $\dot{m}(V_2^2 - V_1^2)/2$ made available by any expansion in the rotor. From equation (19.10) it is apparent that the difference between the denominator and the numerator is the rejected kinetic energy $\dot{m}C_2^2/2$.

It must be emphasised that although a low diagram efficiency indicates the probability of large friction losses, $(1 - \eta_d)$ does not itself necessarily represent a loss. This is because the kinetic energy leaving one stage can be used in the following state. The total work done by an expansion in a multistage turbine can be found by summing the individual stage outputs. That is, per unit mass flow we have

$$|\dot{W}_{12}| = (h_1 - h_2) + \tfrac{1}{2}(C_1^2 - C_2^2)$$
$$|\dot{W}_{23}| = (h_2 - h_3) + \tfrac{1}{2}(C_2^2 - C_3^2)$$
$$\vdots$$
$$|\dot{W}_{n,n+1}| = (h_n - h_{n+1}) + \tfrac{1}{2}(c_n^2 - C_{n+1}^2)$$
$$\sum|\dot{W}| = (h_1 - h_{n+1}) + \tfrac{1}{2}(C_1^2 - C_{n+1}^2)$$

Here subscripts 12, 23 etc. refer to the inlet and outlet of each complete stage. Evidently the interstage velocities are irrelevant except in so far as they affect the friction losses.

Even the kinetic energy at outlet from the last stage, or *leaving loss*, can be utilised to some extent by fitting a diffuser (usually in the form of a volute) to the turbine exhaust. The effect of the diffuser is to increase the pressure drop across the turbine as illustrated in Fig. 19.5. In the figure the diffusion process is depicted as being isentropic, but in practice friction only permits part of the leaving loss to be recovered in this way.

The various relations derived in the foregoing paragraphs will now be applied to particular stage designs.

Fig. 19.5
Effect of a diffuser at
turbine exit

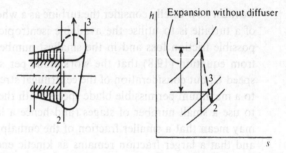

19.2.1 *Impulse stage*

In an impulse stage, where nominally all the enthalpy drop occurs in the stator blade row, it is usual to refer to these blades as *nozzle blades* or simply as *nozzles*. With no enthalpy drop across the rotor blades, there would be no change in relative velocity of the fluid as it passes through the rotor blade passages. In the absence of friction there would also be no change in pressure or specific volume across the rotor blades, and the continuity equation then requires the area at right angles to the direction of flow to be the same at inlet and outlet. With reference to Fig. 19.6, these areas are $l_1 np \cos \beta_1$ at inlet and $l_2 np \cos \beta_2$ at outlet; n is the number of blades in the row, p is the pitch, and l is the height of the blade. The simplest method of obtaining equal areas is to maintain the blade height constant and make β_2 equal to β_1. If this is done the velocity diagram for the impulse stage* appears as in Fig. 19.6. In practice, friction will occur in the passages, and if the blade passages have equal inlet and outlet areas there will be a small pressure and enthalpy drop resulting in a slight acceleration of the fluid relative to the blades.† In the following analysis friction in the rotor blade passages will be neglected.

Expressions for the work done by the stage and the diagram efficiency can be found as follows. With reference to Fig. 19.6, for the case where $V_2 = V_1$ and $\beta_2 = \beta_1$, evidently

$$\Delta V_w = 2V_1 \sin \beta_1 = 2(C_1 \sin \alpha_1 - U)$$

Hence

$$|\dot{W}| = \dot{m} U \Delta V_w = 2\dot{m} U (C_1 \sin \alpha_1 - U) \tag{19.12}$$

With an impulse stage the only energy available to the rotor blades is $\dot{m} C_1^2 / 2$. The diagram efficiency is therefore

$$\eta_d = \frac{2\dot{m} U (C_1 \sin \alpha_1 - U)}{\dot{m} C_1^2 / 2} = 4 \frac{U}{C_1} \left(\sin \alpha_1 - \frac{U}{C_1} \right) \tag{19.13}$$

The ratio U/C_1 is called the *blade speed ratio*.

---

* In steam turbine practice it is customary to refer to a single-stage impulse turbine as a de Laval turbine, and a turbine consisting of a number of such stages in series as a Rateau turbine.
† This effect of friction is not obvious, but all that can be done here is to refer the reader to the well-known Fanno lines of fluid mechanics.

Fig. 19.6
Impulse stage

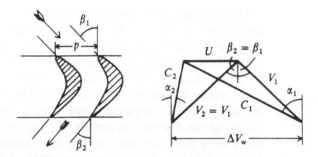

Other things being equal, equation (19.12) indicates that the work output increases with increase in nozzle outlet angle α_1. An increase in α_1, however, implies a reduced axial velocity ($C_1 \cos \alpha_1$) and hence an increase in annulus area if the same mass flow is to be passed through the stage. The nozzle blade surface area over which the fluid flows is therefore increased, and this in turn implies an increase in nozzle friction loss. Considerations of this kind lead to the use of nozzle outlet angles of between 60 and 75 degrees. If α_1 is assumed to be fixed, equation (19.13) can be differentiated with respect to the blade speed ratio, and the result can be equated to zero to find the value of U/C_1 which yields a maximum value of η_d. Thus

$$\frac{d(\eta_d)}{d(U/C_1)} = 4 \sin \alpha_1 - 8 \frac{U}{C_1}$$

which equals zero when

$$\frac{U}{C_1} = \frac{\sin \alpha_1}{2} \tag{19.14}$$

It will be seen by inspection of the velocity diagram that this optimum blade speed ratio corresponds to the case where the outlet velocity is axial, i.e. when the outlet kinetic energy is a minimum. Substituting (19.14) in (19.13) we have

$$(\eta_d)_{max} = \sin^2 \alpha_1 \tag{19.15}$$

Similarly, the power output at optimum blade speed ratio becomes

$$|\dot{W}| = 2\dot{m}U^2 \tag{19.16}$$

The variation of η_d with U/C_1 is shown in Fig. 19.7.

Fig. 19.7
Variation of η_d with blade
speed ratio for an impulse
stage

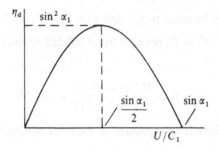

The maximum permissible blade speed that can be used depends upon the temperature of the working fluid, the strength of the heat-resisting alloys available, and the life required of the turbine; blade speeds of about 250 m/s are common, but speeds as high as 370 m/s are sometimes used. When the rotational speed at which the turbine is required to operate is low, the blade speed is often chosen well below the permissible limit. It is then determined by the need to use a well-proportioned annulus; too high a blade speed at low rotational speed implies an annulus of large mean diameter and small height (for a given mass flow and therefore fixed annulus area). This might involve the use of unduly short blades, particularly at the high-pressure end of the turbine where the specific volume of the fluid is small. Irrespective of how the blade speed is determined, once it is fixed equation (19.14) can be used to determine C_1, and hence the stage enthalpy drop or number of stages for a given overall enthalpy drop. This procedure is illustrated by the following example.

Example 19.1 A multistage gas turbine is to be designed with impulse stages, and is to operate with an inlet pressure and temperature of 6 bar and 900 K, and an outlet pressure of 1 bar. The isentropic efficiency of the turbine is likely to be 85 per cent. All the stages are to have a nozzle outlet angle of 75 degrees, equal inlet and outlet rotor blade angles, a mean blade speed of 250 m/s, and equal inlet and outlet gas velocities. Estimate the number of stages required. Assume $c_p = 1.15 \, \text{kJ/kg K}$ and $\gamma = 1.333$.

The final temperature, assuming isentropic expansion, is

$$T' = \frac{900}{(6/1)^{0.333/1.333}} = 575 \text{ K}$$

Hence the actual overall temperature drop is

$$0.85(900 - 575) = 276.3 \text{ K}$$

The energy equation for the flow through any nozzle row is

$$\tfrac{1}{2}(C_1^2 + C_0^2) = c_p(T_0 - T_1)$$

If the optimum blade speed ratio is to be used, C_1 is given by

$$C_1 = \frac{2U}{\sin \alpha_1} = \frac{2 \times 250}{0.966} = 517.6 \text{ m/s}$$

C_0 is to be equal to C_2, and with $\beta_2 = \beta_1$ we have

$$C_2 = C_1 \cos \alpha_1 = 517.6 \times 0.259 = 134.1 \text{ m/s}$$

Hence

$$T_0 - T_1 = \frac{517.6^2 - 134.1^2}{2 \times 10^3 \times 1.15} = 108.7 \text{ K}$$

Since there is no expansion in the rotor blades, $(T_0 - T_1)$ will also be the stage temperature drop, and therefore the number of stages becomes

$$\frac{276.3}{108.7} = 2.54$$

Evidently three stages are required. The blade speed ratio used will be greater than the optimum, and the required expansion will be obtained with slightly lower gas velocities.

19.2.2 Velocity-compounded impulse stage

Before considering reaction designs it is necessary to mention an important modification to the simple impulse stage. Sometimes it is desirable to carry out a large enthalpy drop in one stage, in which case the fluid velocities are very high and, owing to the blade speed limitation, the U/C_1 ratio is low and the work output is consequently a low fraction of the available enthalpy drop. The work output can be increased by *velocity compounding*, even though still using a low blade speed ratio. The method is illustrated in Fig. 19.8, which shows a *two-row velocity-compounded stage*. A velocity-compounded stage is known as a *Curtis stage*.

The flow through the nozzles and the first moving row is similar to the flow through a simple impulse stage, except that the ratio U/C_1 is much smaller. The fluid leaves the first row of rotor blades with a high velocity C_2 at an angle α_2 and enters a row of fixed guide blades having an inlet angle α_2. No further expansion takes place and these blades merely turn the stream into the direction required for entry to a second row of rotor blades, i.e. C_3 equals C_2. The guide blades are often made symmetrical, with the outlet angle α_3 equal to the inlet angle α_2, and the blade height will then be the same at inlet and outlet to give

Fig. 19.8
Velocity-compounded
impulse stage

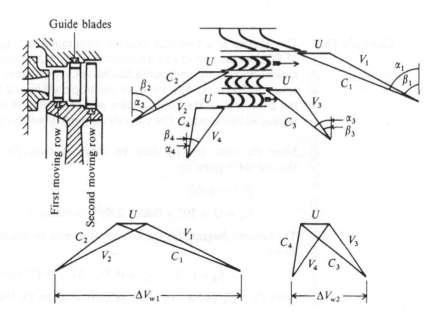

Guide blades

equality of areas. The geometry of the velocity triangles then fixes the magnitude V_3 and direction β_3 of the relative velocity at inlet to the second moving row. If these blades are also symmetrical, β_4 is equal to β_3 and V_4 is equal to V_3. The velocity diagrams are then determined, and the work done is

$$|\dot{W}| = \dot{m}U(\Delta V_{w1} + \Delta V_{w2}) \tag{19.17}$$

where subscripts 1 and 2 refer to the first and second rows of moving blades.

With the foregoing assumptions about symmetrical moving and guide blades, and unchanged relative velocities in the moving and guide blade passages, it is easy to show that for a given value of α_1 the diagram efficiency is a maximum when

$$\frac{U}{C_1} = \frac{\sin \alpha_1}{4} \tag{19.18}$$

The leaving velocity C_4 is then axial. It can also be shown that with this optimum value of U/C_1 the diagram efficiency is the same as for the simple impulse stage, i.e.

$$(\eta_d)_{max} = \sin^2 \alpha_1$$

but that the work done becomes

$$|\dot{W}| = 6\dot{m}U^2 + 2\dot{m}U^2 = 8\dot{m}U^2 \tag{19.19}$$

Thus, for any given blade speed, a two-row stage can utilise four times the enthalpy drop of a simple impulse stage without any reduction in diagram efficiency. The velocities are of course high in the nozzles and first rotor row, and friction losses may be rather large. One important use of a velocity-compounded stage is mentioned in section 19.2.4.

Example 19.2 The nozzles of a two-row velocity-compounded stage have outlet angles of 68 degrees and utilise an isentropic enthalpy drop of 200 kJ per kg of steam. All moving and guide blades are symmetrical, and the mean blade speed is 150 m/s. Assuming an isentropic efficiency for the nozzles of 90 per cent, find all the blade angles and calculate the specific power output produced by the stage. The velocity at inlet to the stage can be neglected.

Since the inlet velocity may be assumed zero, the outlet velocity from the nozzles is given by

$$\tfrac{1}{2}C_1^2 = \eta_N \Delta h'$$

$$C_1 = (2 \times 10^3 \times 0.90 \times 200)^{1/2} = 600 \text{ m/s}$$

The velocity diagram for the first row can now be drawn as in Fig. 19.9, from which

$$\beta_1 = \beta_2 = 61.0°, \quad \alpha_2 = 48.7°, \quad \Delta V_{w1} = 812 \text{ m/s}$$

With $C_3 = C_2$ and $\alpha_3 = \alpha_2$, the velocity diagram for the second row can also

Fig. 19.9

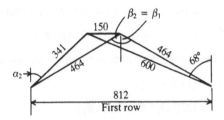
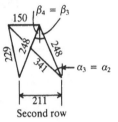

First row

Second row

be drawn, from which

$$\beta_3 = \beta_4 = 25.2°, \quad \Delta V_{w2} = 211 \text{ m/s}$$

The specific power, i.e. the work output per kg/s of steam, is therefore

$$|\dot{W}| = U(\Delta V_{w1} + \Delta V_{w2}) = \frac{150(812 + 211)}{10^3} = 153.5 \text{ kW}$$

Note that even with the comparatively low blade speed used in the foregoing example, the relative velocity at entry to the first row of rotor blades is very high. If it is too near the local velocity of sound in the fluid, losses will be incurred by the formation of shock waves in the blade passages. For this reason the two-row impulse stage is not suitable for use with high blade speeds—and for this reason also, three-row stages, which have an even lower optimum U/C_1 ratio, are seldom used. It is worth noting that sonic velocity, given by $\{-v^2(\partial p/\partial v)_s\}^{1/2}$ in general or $(\gamma R T)^{1/2}$ for a perfect gas (see section 18.1.1), is higher at the high-pressure end of an expansion. It follows that higher fluid velocities relative to the blade are permissible in the first few stages of a multistage turbine and therefore that this might be where a two-row impulse stage can be used without incurring losses from shock waves. We shall see in section 19.2.4 that there are in fact good reasons for choosing this type of stage for the high-pressure end of a turbine.

19.2.3   Reaction stage

Before considering the special case of 50 per cent reaction, it is convenient to derive a general expression for the degree of reaction in terms of the main variables. This is most easily done when the velocities at inlet and outlet of the stage are equal and when the axial velocity remains constant throughout the stage. Both these conditions are commonly used in reaction designs because they enable the same blade shapes to be used in successive stages.

In general the degree of reaction is

$$\Lambda = \frac{h_1 - h_2}{h_0 - h_2}$$

Since the velocities are to be the same at inlet and outlet of the stage, the energy equation, per unit mass flow, reduces to

$$|\dot{W}| = h_0 - h_2$$

Therefore from equation (19.8), and using the nomenclature of Fig. 19.3,

$$h_0 - h_2 = U\Delta V_w = UC_a(\tan \beta_1 + \tan \beta_2)$$

Also, applying the energy equation to the flow relative to the rotor blades,

$$h_1 - h_2 = \tfrac{1}{2}(V_2^2 - V_1^2)$$
$$= \tfrac{1}{2}C_a^2(\sec^2 \beta_2 - \sec^2 \beta_1)$$
$$= \tfrac{1}{2}C_a^2(\tan^2 \beta_2 - \tan^2 \beta_1)$$

It follows that

$$\Lambda = \frac{C_a}{2U}(\tan \beta_2 - \tan \beta_1) \qquad (19.20)$$

Putting $\Lambda = 0$ in (19.20) yields the impulse stage with $\beta_1 = \beta_2$, and putting $\Lambda = 0.5$ we have the reaction stage with

$$\frac{U}{C_a} = \tan \beta_2 - \tan \beta_1 \qquad (19.21)$$

From the geometry of the velocity triangles we also have the equation

$$U = C_a(\tan \alpha_1' - \tan \beta_1) = C_a(\tan \beta_2 - \tan \alpha_2)$$

Comparing this with (19.21) we get

$$\alpha_1 = \beta_2 \quad \text{and} \quad \alpha_2 = \beta_1$$

Also, from the initial assumptions that $C_2 = C_0$ and $C_a = C_0 \cos \alpha_0 = C_2 \cos \alpha_2$, it follows that

$$\alpha_2 = \alpha_0$$

Evidently, for a 50 per cent reaction design the stator and rotor blades have the same shape, and the velocity diagram is symmetrical as shown in Fig. 19.10a. (Note that the rotor blades also act as nozzles in a reaction design. This is the reason why the first row of blades is referred to as a stator row rather than a nozzle row.)

The optimum blade speed ratio for the reaction stage can be found as follows. From the symmetry of Fig. 19.10a,

$$\Delta V_w = 2C_1 \sin \alpha_1 - U$$

Fig. 19.10
Velocity diagrams for a
reaction stage

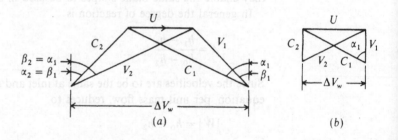

$$\beta_2 = \alpha_1$$
$$\alpha_2 = \beta_1$$

(a)

(b)

and therefore, per unit mass flow,

$$|\dot{W}| = U\Delta V_w = U(2C_1 \sin \alpha_1 - U) \tag{19.22}$$

Since there is an enthalpy drop in the rotor blades, the energy available to the rotor blades per unit mass flow is

$$\frac{C_1^2}{2} + \frac{(V_2^2 - V_1^2)}{2}.$$

And since $V_2 = C_1$ this becomes

$$C_1^2 - \tfrac{1}{2}V_1^2$$

Furthermore,

$$V_1^2 = C_1^2 + U^2 - 2C_1 U \sin \alpha_1$$

and therefore the energy available is

$$\tfrac{1}{2}(C_1^2 - U^2 + 2C_1 U \sin \alpha_1)$$

It follows that

$$
\begin{aligned}
\eta_d &= \frac{2U(2C_1 \sin \alpha_1 - U)}{(C_1^2 - U^2 + 2C_1 U \sin \alpha_1)} \\[2mm]
&= \frac{2\dfrac{U}{C_1}\left(2 \sin \alpha_1 - \dfrac{U}{C_1}\right)}{1 - \left(\dfrac{U}{C_1}\right)^2 + 2\left(\dfrac{U}{C_1}\right) \sin \alpha_1}
\end{aligned}
\tag{19.23}
$$

Differentiating (19.23) with respect to U/C_1 and equating to zero we have the optimum blade speed ratio given by

$$\frac{U}{C_1} = \sin \alpha_1 \tag{19.24}$$

When the optimum blade speed ratio is used, the velocity diagram appears as in Fig. 19.10b.

Substituting (19.24) in (19.22), the work done for a rate of flow $\dot{m}$ becomes

$$|\dot{W}| = \dot{m}U^2 \tag{19.25}$$

and substituting (19.24) in (19.23) yields

$$(\eta_d)_{max} = \frac{2 \sin^2 \alpha_1}{1 + \sin^2 \alpha_1} \tag{19.26}$$

Fig. 19.11 shows the variation of diagram efficiency with U/C_1 for the three types of stage described. The significance of these curves will be discussed in the next subsection.

Fig. 19.11
Comparison of η_d for
different types of stage

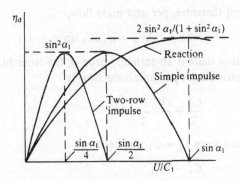

19.2.4   Multistage turbines and internal losses

The overall enthalpy drop across a turbine, particularly in steam turbine plant, is usually great enough to require the use of a large number of stages in series. As many as fifty stages may be required. Assuming that optimum blade speed ratios are used in each case, the power output per stage for the three types considered has been shown to be

Two-row impulse: $8 \dot{m} U^2$

Simple impulse: $2 \dot{m} U^2$

Reaction: $\dot{m} U^2$

It might therefore be supposed that it is advantageous to use a succession of two-row impulse stages, since this would result in the least number of blade rows for a given overall enthalpy drop. However, it is also important to utilise the given isentropic enthalpy drop with the minimum loss, and when losses are taken into account the order of merit is not so obvious.

The losses in a turbine may be divided conveniently into two groups. There will be *external losses* due to bearing friction and the power required to drive auxiliaries. These losses will be similar for all types of turbine and will not be considered here. The second and major group, the *internal losses*, may be dealt with under two heads as follows.

Blading friction losses
The fluid friction in the nozzle and rotor blade passages results in the actual enthalpy drop being less than the isentropic enthalpy drop. These friction losses are proportional to the square of the average relative velocity through the blading, and the surface area of blading swept by the fluid; they also depend on the nature of the flow. In general, for the same surface area and average relative velocity, the friction incurred by flow in a curved passage is less when the flow is accelerating, as in reaction blading, than it is when the velocity is substantially constant as in impulse blading. The reason for this is as follows. Most of the friction occurs in a boundary layer where there is a steep velocity gradient, and it is much less in a laminar boundary layer than in a turbulent

Fig. 19.12
Comparative velocity
diagrams, using optimum
U/C_1 ratios and same
values of U and α_1

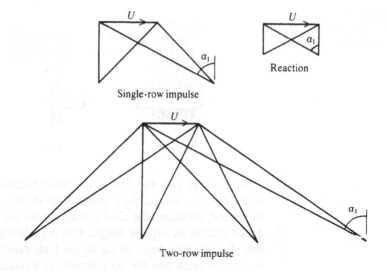

Single-row impulse

Reaction

Two-row impulse

boundary layer.* The boundary layer on a blade is normally turbulent over the concave surface, but on the convex surface it is initially laminar and only becomes turbulent at some distance from the leading edge. The effect of having a falling pressure gradient in the direction of flow is to cause the desirable laminar condition to prevail over a great part of the blade surface.

A comparison of the velocity diagrams for the three types of stage (Fig. 19.12) shows that the average velocity through the stator and rotor blading is less for the reaction stage than for either of the others. This fact, coupled with the beneficial pressure gradient across the reaction rotor blades, is sufficient to outweigh the effect of the greater surface area incurred by the larger number of stages in a reaction design. The net result is that friction losses are least in a multistage reaction turbine.

Leakage losses
Turbine rotor blading is carried either on a series of disks or on a drum, as shown in Figs 19.13a and b. Because clearance is needed between the moving and stationary parts, some fluid passes through the turbine without doing its full complement of work on the blading. Losses incurred in this way are called leakage losses and, since they involve a form of throttling, they contribute to the irreversible increase of entropy which occurs during the expansion.

The leakage flow area between the stator diaphragm and the rotor shaft in Fig. 19.13a is obviously much less than that between the stator tips and the rotor drum in Fig. 19.13b. The disk construction is therefore always used for impulse stages, because the pressure difference across a stator row is comparatively large. On the other hand, the drum construction is usually preferred for reaction stages where the pressure drop across a stator row is not so great, because this type of construction does avoid the inevitable friction loss incurred by any disk spinning in a fluid.

---

* The concept of a boundary layer is described in section 22.1.

Fig. 19.13
Disk and drum
construction

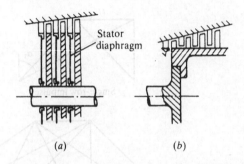

Stator
diaphragm

(a)   (b)

The leakage past the tips of the rotor blades will clearly be greater in a
reaction stage, owing to the pressure drop which is absent in any impulse design.
In general, therefore, the total leakage losses are rather greater in a reaction
design than in an impulse design. This is particularly true at the high-pressure
end of a turbine where, owing to the high density of fluid, the annulus area
required is small and the tip clearance is a relatively large proportion of the
blade height.

Summing up, we have seen that there are two main sources of loss to consider:

(a) Blading friction losses, which are least for a reaction design
(b) Leakage losses, which are least for an impulse design.

A glance at the expansion on a $p-v$ diagram (Fig. 19.14) will emphasise the
fact that when the work is divided equally between the stages (i.e. when
approximately equal stage pressure *ratios* are used), the pressure *differences*
causing leakage are greatest at the high-pressure end of a turbine. Furthermore,
these pressure differences are particularly large in turbines of high pressure ratio
(inlet/outlet). As a general rule, the leakage losses predominate over the friction
losses at the high-pressure end of high pressure-ratio turbines (e.g. most steam
turbines), whereas at the low-pressure end, or throughout low pressure-ratio
turbines (e.g. gas turbines), the friction losses predominate.

Taken together, the points made in the previous paragraph explain why
reaction blading is invariably used for gas turbines, and why steam turbines
normally have impulse stages at the high-pressure end. The choice of stages in
steam turbines varies widely with the range of steam conditions employed and
the relative importance of capital cost and turbine efficiency. Generally speaking,
turbine isentropic efficiency is the primary consideration because, apart from

Fig. 19.14
Pressure differences

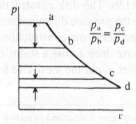

$\dfrac{p_a}{p_b} = \dfrac{p_c}{p_d}$

the saving in fuel, a lower steam consumption implies a smaller boiler and condenser which together account for the largest fraction of the capital cost of the whole plant. In high pressure-ratio steam turbines it is usual to use at least two turbines in series: a high-pressure turbine with impulse stages followed by a low-pressure reaction turbine. The first impulse stage is commonly a two-row velocity-compounded design, because with the pressures and superheats used in modern plant it is important to achieve a large enthalpy drop in the first row of nozzles. Not only does this avoid exposing the turbine casing and rotor to the extreme steam conditions, but it also appreciably increases the volume flow before the steam reaches the first row of rotor blades. Without this increase in volume the blades might otherwise be too small for good efficiency. Even with an initial two-row impulse stage, it is sometimes necessary to use *partial admission* to avoid too small a blade height; the required flow area is obtained with a reasonable annulus height by blanking off sectors of the row of nozzles. It is of interest to note that the power output of steam turbines is commonly controlled by varying the inlet area in this way.

After this brief discussion of the sources of loss in a turbine, it can now be explained why small turbines (i.e. turbines of low mass flow and small work output) have poorer efficiencies than large turbines. When the blades are very small, both the fluid friction loss and the leakage loss become a large proportion of the work done: the former because the boundary layer occupies a relatively large portion of the passage, and the latter because clearances between stationary and moving parts cannot be reduced proportionately.

We opened this subsection with a comparison of the three types of stage on the basis of number of stages required, and went on to show that, when losses are considered, reaction designs are usually preferred in spite of the relatively large number of stages they involve. The position as regards number of stages is not quite as poor as our simple analysis has indicated, however, because the optimum blade speed ratio need not necessarily be used. Fig. 19.11 indicates that the curve of diagram efficiency for a reaction stage is fairly flat near the optimum U/C_1 ratio, and it is possible to use a lower value of U/C_1 (i.e. a larger enthalpy drop per stage) without an appreciable loss in efficiency. It must be remembered, however, that the diagram efficiency is only a rough guide to the probable susceptibility of a stage to friction losses, and the true optimum blade speed ratio for maximum *isentropic* efficiency ($\Delta h/\Delta h_{\text{isen}}$) is not necessarily the nominal optimum value we have been deducing. The true optimum can only be found from a more complete analysis which makes use of friction data obtained from tests on rows of blades in 'cascade tunnels'.* Although this cannot be entered into here, we shall consider qualitatively the likely effect of using higher and lower values of the U/C_1 ratio in a reaction stage.

Fig. 19.15 shows the velocity diagrams for blade speed ratios less than, equal to and greater than the nominal optimum value. The blade speed U and the stator blade outlet angle α_1 have been assumed the same in each case. It will

---

* The type of analysis used for gas turbines can be found in Ref. 13.

Fig. 19.15
Reaction stage with low
and high values of U/C_1
(same U and α_1)

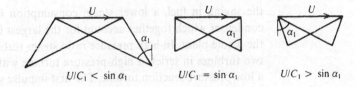

$U/C_1 < \sin \alpha_1$ $U/C_1 = \sin \alpha_1$ $U/C_1 > \sin \alpha_1$

be seen that the use of a low U/C_1 ratio involves

(a) Higher fluid velocities.

(b) Decrease in surface area swept by the fluid.

The surface area is reduced both because of the smaller number of stages required, and because the higher axial velocity implies that a smaller annulus area is required to pass the given mass flow. Item (b) partially offsets (a) but, since the friction is proportional to the square of the fluid velocity, item (a) predominates and there is a decrease in isentropic efficiency of the stage.

The use of a high U/C_1 ratio involves

(a) Lower fluid velocities.

(b) Increase in surface area, owing to the greater number of stages and lower axial velocity.

In this case there may even be a slight rise in isentropic efficiency as the U/C_1 ratio is increased from the nominal optimum value, and the eventual fall in efficiency is more gradual. Fig. 19.16 shows a typical curve of isentropic efficiency versus U/C_1 ratio. It follows that a rather greater sacrifice in efficiency may be incurred by attempting to use a smaller number of stages (i.e. lower U/C_1 ratio) than might be supposed from simple consideration of the variation in diagram efficiency.

To close this discussion of losses, one form of loss peculiar to steam turbines must be mentioned. It was suggested in section 11.3 that it is undesirable for much of the expansion to occur in the wet region. It seems that liquid in the steam flow appears in three places, namely as a film running along the casing, as a fine mist suspended in the steam, and as a film on the surface of the stator blades (a liquid film does not form on the rotor blades because any moisture is flung off by centrifugal effects). The film on the stator blades detaches itself in relatively large droplets at velocities well below the mean velocity of the vapour, although sufficiently high to cause erosion damage at the leading edges

Fig. 19.16
Isentropic efficiency of
reaction stage

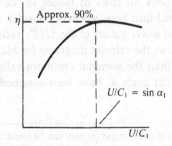

Approx. 90%

η

$U/C_1 = \sin \alpha_1$

U/C_1

Fig. 19.17
Effect of a wet vapour

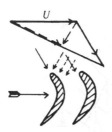

of the rotor blades, as indicated by the dashed arrows in Fig. 19.17. The turbine efficiency is also reduced. An annular collecting slot in the casing is often used to reduce erosion, but clearly this does not remove the moisture which does the damage. More recently, slots in the trailing edges of hollow stator blades through which the liquid film is sucked away have been tried on an experimental scale (see Ref. 20). Provided that the liquid from the trailing edge can be removed, the 0.88 lower limit for dryness fraction suggested in section 11.3 might not represent the absolute limit it has been thought to be.

19.2.5 *Stage efficiency, overall efficiency, reheat factor and polytropic efficiency*

Both the isentropic efficiency of a stage, and the overall isentropic efficiency of a turbine, can be defined in various ways depending on whether it is desired to take account of the whole, or a particular part, of the losses incurred. We have seen that the work done on the blading is less than can be expected from the isentropic enthalpy drop because of blading friction loss and leakage loss. Both these forms of loss increase the entropy of the expanding fluid and lead to a reduced actual enthalpy drop. Before the work done on the blading reaches the shaft, some of it will be dissipated in overcoming the disk friction loss when disk construction is employed. This loss also contributes to the increase in entropy and the reduction in enthalpy drop. All these internal losses affect the state of the fluid flowing through the stage or turbine. Efficiencies defined in terms of the internal work delivered *to* the shaft are called *internal efficiencies*. Finally, the work delivered *by* the shaft, or *shaft work*, is even smaller by reason of the external losses (e.g. bearing friction) which do not affect the state of the fluid; efficiencies based upon the shaft work may be called *external efficiencies*. We shall here be concerned solely with the internal efficiency of a stage or turbine.

The internal work done during the expansion of unit mass flow from state 1 to state 2 is

$$|\dot{W}| = (h_1 - h_2) + \tfrac{1}{2}(C_1^2 - C_2^2)$$

In a multistage turbine the interstage velocities are equal, or nearly so, and for our purposes we can simply write

$$|\dot{W}| = (h_1 - h_2) = \Delta h$$

The internal work is a maximum when the expansion between the given pressures is isentropic, i.e.

$$|\dot{W}|_{\mathrm{max}} = (h_1 - h_2') = \Delta h'$$

Fig. 19.18
The reheat factor

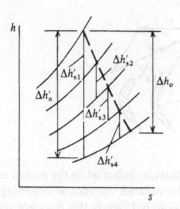

Defining the efficiency always as $|\dot{W}|/|\dot{W}|_{max}$, we arrive at the following definitions of the isentropic efficiency of a stage η_s and overall isentropic efficiency of a turbine η_o:

$$\eta_s = \frac{\Delta h_s}{\Delta h_s'} \quad \text{and} \quad \eta_o = \frac{\Delta h_o}{\Delta h_o'}$$

The following argument may be used to show that η_o is always greater than η_s. For simplicity, we shall consider a four-stage turbine with each stage having the same efficiency η_s. The expansion is shown on an h–s diagram in Fig. 19.18. The dashed curve indicates the average state of the fluid during the actual expansion; in steam turbine practice it is called the *line of condition*. The total work can be expressed either in terms of the overall isentropic enthalpy drop as

$$\eta_o \Delta h_o'$$

or in terms of the isentropic stage enthalpy drops as

$$\eta_s(\Delta h_{s1}' + \Delta h_{s2}' + \Delta h_{s3}' + \Delta h_{s4}') = \eta_s \Sigma \Delta h_s'$$

Equating these expressions, we have

$$\eta_o = \eta_s \frac{\Sigma \Delta h_s'}{\Delta h_o'} = \eta_s \mathscr{R} \tag{19.27}$$

$\Sigma \Delta h_s'$, called the *cumulative enthalpy drop*, is evidently greater than $\Delta h_o'$, because the vertical height between any pair of constant pressure lines increases with increase of entropy. The ratio $\mathscr{R}$ of the cumulative enthalpy drop to the isentropic enthalpy drop is called the *reheat factor*, and it is always greater than unity.

The physical interpretation of this result is that the internal losses in any stage (except the last) are partially recoverable in subsequent stages owing to the 'reheating' effect of friction. It follows that it is more important to use high-efficiency stages at the low-pressure end of a turbine than at the high-pressure end. It should also be evident from the foregoing analysis that the difference between η_o and η_s increases as the overall pressure ratio of the turbine is increased. For this reason, turbines of high pressure ratio tend to be more efficient than those of low pressure ratio.

Example 19.3   Twelve successive stages of a reaction steam turbine have blades with effective inlet and outlet angles of 10° and 70° respectively. The mean diameter of the blade rows is 1.2 m and the speed of rotation is 3000 rev/min. If the axial velocity is constant throughout the stages, estimate the specific enthalpy drop per stage.

The steam inlet conditions are 10 bar and 250 °C, and the outlet pressure is 0.2 bar. Assuming a reheat factor of 1.04, estimate the stage efficiency (defined without reference to the kinetic energy term).

Determine the approximate blade height at the outlet of the sixth stage, if the twelve stages are to develop 7500 kW. Assume the line of condition to be straight on the *h*–*s* diagram.

The mean blade speed is

$$U = \pi dN = \frac{\pi \times 1.2 \times 3000}{60} = 188.5 \text{ m/s}$$

The velocity diagram can now be drawn to scale as in Fig. 19.19a, or the required velocities can be calculated as follows:

$$\frac{V_1}{\sin 20} = \frac{U}{\sin 60} \quad \text{hence} \quad V_1 = 74.4 \text{ m/s}$$

From symmetry,

$$\Delta V_w = U + 2V_1 \sin 10 = 214.3 \text{ m/s}$$

Therefore

$$|W| = U\Delta V_w = \frac{188.5 \times 214.3}{10^3} = 40.4 \text{ kJ/kg}$$

Since there is no change of kinetic energy between inlet and outlet, the specific enthalpy drop per stage must also be 40.4 kJ/kg.

The actual enthalpy drop for the 12 stages is 12 × 40.4 = 48.4 kJ/kg. Using the *h*–*s* chart for steam, as illustrated in Fig. 19.19b, the initial enthalpy is found to be 2944 kJ/kg, and after isentropic expansion to 0.2 bar the enthalpy is 2281 kJ/kg, i.e. there is an isentropic drop of 663 kJ/kg. The overall efficiency

Fig. 19.19

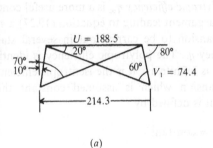

$U = 188.5$
20°   80°
70°
10°   60° $V_1 = 74.4$
—214.3—

(a)

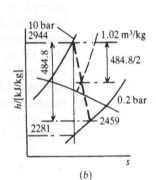

10 bar
2944   1.02 m³/kg
484.8/2
484.8
0.2 bar
2459
2281

h/[kJ/kg]

s

(b)

is therefore

$$\eta_o = \frac{484.8}{663} = 0.731$$

If the reheat factor is 1.04, the stage efficiency must be

$$\eta_s = \frac{0.731}{1.04} = 0.703$$

The assumed line of condition can be located on the $h-s$ diagram since the actual final enthalpy is $2944 - 484.8 = 2459 \, \text{kJ/kg}$. After the sixth stage, half of the actual enthalpy drop has occurred, i.e. the enthalpy is $2944 - 242.4 = 2702 \, \text{kJ/kg}$. At this point the steam is still superheated and the pressure is 1.75 bar. By interpolation in the tables at this pressure and $h = 2702 \, \text{kJ/kg}$, the specific volume is found to be $v = 1.02 \, \text{m}^3/\text{kg}$. The power output required is 7500 kW (or kJ/s), so that the mass flow of steam must be

$$\frac{7500}{484.8} = 15.47 \, \text{kg/s}$$

The axial velocity, from the velocity diagram, is

$$V_{1a} = V_1 \cos 10 = 73.27 \, \text{m/s}$$

and therefore the annulus area required is

$$A = \frac{\dot{m}v}{V_{1a}} = \frac{15.47 \times 1.02}{73.27} = 0.215 \, \text{m}^2$$

If the mean diameter is d and the blade height l,

$$A = \pi d l$$

and hence

$$l = \frac{0.215}{\pi \times 1.2} = 0.0570 \, \text{m} = 5.70 \, \text{cm}$$

We have seen that the overall isentropic efficiency of a turbine increases as the overall pressure ratio (p_1/p_2) increases. When carrying out a series of cycle calculations to determine the optimum pressure ratio, as in section 12.2 for example, it is clearly misleading to assume a constant value for the overall turbine efficiency η_o over the range of pressure ratio. For such purposes the *small-stage* or *polytropic efficiency* η_∞ is a more useful concept. It can be arrived at by taking the argument leading to equation (19.27) a step further. There we assumed the expansion to be carried out in several stages, each having the isentropic efficiency η_s. The polytropic efficiency is identical with η_s when the number of stages is infinite, i.e. it is the isentropic efficiency of an infinitesimal step in the expansion which is assumed constant throughout the whole expansion. Thus it is defined by

$$\eta_\infty = \frac{dh}{dh'} = \text{constant} \tag{19.28}$$

where $-dh$ and $-dh'$ are respectively the actual and isentropic enthalpy drops over the pressure drop $-dp$. That the relation between η_∞ and η_o is simple when the fluid is a perfect gas can be shown as follows. For an isentropic expansion we have $T/p^{(\gamma-1)/\gamma} = $ constant, which on differentiation becomes

$$\frac{dT'}{T} = \frac{\gamma - 1}{\gamma}\frac{dp}{p}$$

Combining this with (19.28), and remembering that for a perfect gas $dh = c_p\, dT$ and $dh' = c_p\, dT'$, we get

$$\frac{dT}{T} = \eta_\infty \frac{\gamma - 1}{\gamma}\frac{dp}{p}$$

and on integration, η_∞ being constant by definition,

$$\frac{T_2}{T_1} = \left(\frac{p_2}{p_1}\right)^{\eta_\infty(\gamma-1)/\gamma} \tag{19.29}$$

Finally, from the definition of η_o we have

$$\eta_o = \frac{T_1 - T_2}{T_1 - T'_2} = \frac{1 - (T_2/T_1)}{1 - (T'_2/T_1)} = \frac{1 - (p_2/p_1)^{\eta_\infty(\gamma-1)/\gamma}}{1 - (p_2/p_1)^{(\gamma-1)/\gamma}} \tag{19.30}$$

This equation enables the variation of η_o with pressure ratio to be determined for any given value of η_∞.

Note that if we write

$$\eta_\infty(\gamma - 1)/\gamma = (n - 1)/n$$

equation (19.29) is the relation between p and T for a polytropic process undergone by a perfect gas. Thus the definition of η_∞ implies the assumption that this non-isentropic process is polytropic, and hence the origin of the term 'polytropic efficiency'. Note also that the concepts of polytropic efficiency and reheat factor are alternative ways of accounting for the 'reheating' effect of friction; the former has been found the more useful for gas turbine calculations and the latter for steam turbine calculations.

19.3 Axial-flow compressors

We have already noted in the introduction to this chapter that, from the point of view of the exchange of energy between the fluid and the rotor, the compressor can be regarded as a reversed turbine. An axial compressor stage is therefore always thought of as a row of rotor blades followed by a row of stator blades, as in Fig. 19.20a. The velocity triangles are usually depicted as in Fig. 19.20b. The processes undergone by the fluid as it passes through the stage at the mean diameter of the annulus are as follows.

The fluid approaches the rotor blades with absolute velocity C_0 at an angle α_0. The relative velocity at inlet V_0 is obtained by vectorial subtraction of the blade speed U. If V_0 is found to be in the direction β_0, the rotor blade inlet

Fig. 19.20
An axial-flow compressor
stage

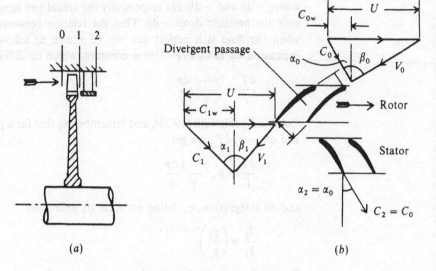

(a)

(b)

angle must also be approximately equal to β_0 for the fluid to flow over the blade without interference. The rotor blade passage is made divergent and the flow is diffused, the fluid leaving with a reduced relative velocity V_1 at an angle β_1. Vectorial addition of the blade speed gives the absolute velocity C_1 at outlet from the rotor and its direction α_1; C_1 is larger than C_0 owing to the work done on the fluid by the rotor. The inlet angle of the stator blade is made approximately equal to α_1, and the fluid is diffused in the stator passage. The velocity is reduced to C_2, and the stream leaves in the direction α_2. If the fluid is to leave the stage in a condition suitable for entry to another similar stage, C_2 and α_2 must be made equal to C_0 and α_0.

The work done in the stage, given by equation (19.4) but with the notation of Fig. 19.20, is

$$\dot{W} = \dot{m}U(C_{1w} - C_{0w})$$

It is evident from the velocity triangles that this is a positive quantity, in agreement with our sign convention for work. If the two velocity triangles are combined as in Fig. 19.21a it is convenient to write the equation as

$$\dot{W} = \dot{m}U\Delta C_w \tag{19.31}$$

where ΔC_w is $(C_{1w} - C_{0w})$.

Fig. 19.21
Velocity diagrams for a
compressor stage

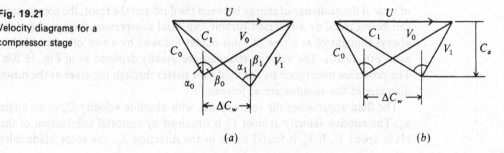

(a)

(b)

In the stage just described, some increase of enthalpy, and therefore of pressure, is obtained in both rotor and stator rows. The concept of degree of reaction is also useful here, and for compressors it is defined as the ratio of the enthalpy rise in the rotor to the enthalpy rise in the stage, i.e.

$$\Lambda = \frac{h_1 - h_0}{h_2 - h_0}$$

The losses associated with fluid friction and blade tip clearance are found to be a minimum when the pressure rise is approximately equally divided between the rotor and the stator, and therefore a 50 per cent reaction design is normally used. By a similar analysis to that employed in section 19.2.3, it can be shown that with equal inlet and outlet velocities, and a constant axial velocity through the stage, 50 per cent reaction implies that the rotor and stator blades are identical in shape, i.e.

$$\beta_0 = \alpha_1 \quad \text{and} \quad \beta_1 = \alpha_0$$

The velocity diagram is then symmetrical as in Fig. 19.21b. This is the only type of stage design that will be considered here.

When a value for the isentropic efficiency is available, the stage pressure ratio can be deduced as follows. Since axial compressors are used exclusively for compressing gases (normally air), the perfect gas relations may be introduced. With equal inlet and outlet velocities, the steady-flow energy equation applied to the whole stage is simply

$$\dot{W} = \dot{m} c_p (T_2 - T_0)$$

and hence

$$c_p(T_2 - T_0) = U \Delta C_w \tag{19.32}$$

If the isentropic efficiency of the stage η_s is defined as the ratio of the isentropic temperature rise $(T'_2 - T_0)$ to the actual temperature rise $(T_2 - T_0)$, we have

$$(T'_2 - T_0) = \eta_s(T_2 - T_0)$$

$$\frac{T'_2}{T_0} = 1 + \eta_s \frac{(T_2 - T_0)}{T_0}$$

Consequently,

$$\frac{p_2}{p_0} = \left(\frac{T'_2}{T_0}\right)^{\gamma/(\gamma-1)} = \left\{1 + \eta_s \frac{(T_2 - T_0)}{T_0}\right\}^{\gamma/(\gamma-1)} \tag{19.33}$$

Substituting equation (19.32) in (19.33) we get finally

$$\frac{p_2}{p_0} = \left(1 + \eta_s \frac{U \Delta C_w}{c_p T_0}\right)^{\gamma/(\gamma-1)} \tag{19.34}$$

Equation (19.33) may also be used to obtain the overall pressure ratio of a multistage compressor if the overall isentropic efficiency is substituted for η_s and the subscripts 0 and 2 refer to the inlet and outlet of the whole compressor.

Fig. 19.22
Polytropic efficiency

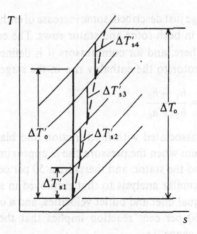

The overall temperature rise is the sum of the stage temperature rises, and if the same work is done in each of N stages it is simply $N \Delta T$. By a similar argument to that used when deducing the reheat factor for turbines, in conjunction with Fig. 19.22, it is easy to show that the overall isentropic efficiency of a compressor is *less* than the stage efficiency, and that this difference increases as the pressure ratio of a compressor is increased by adding more stages. The concept of polytropic efficiency is useful here also; for a compression it is defined as

$$\eta_{\infty} = \frac{dh'}{dh}$$

For a perfect gas, by repeating the argument used in deriving equation (19.29), we have the actual outlet temperature given by

$$\frac{T_2}{T_1} = \left(\frac{p_2}{p_1}\right)^{(\gamma - 1)/\gamma\eta_{\infty}}$$

We must now discuss briefly the factors which limit the pressure rise that can be obtained efficiently in one stage. Before doing so it is necessary to emphasise the essential difference between a compressor and a turbine, namely that the flow in the rotor and stator passages of a compressor is diffusing, whereas it is accelerating in a turbine (Fig. 19.23). It is always more difficult to arrange for an efficient deceleration of flow than for an efficient acceleration. In a diffusion process there is a natural tendency for the fluid to break away from the wall of the diverging passage, reverse its direction, and flow back in the direction of the falling pressure gradient. This will occur if the rate of divergence of the passage is too great, and the tendency is particularly marked when the passage is curved. The difference between the nature of the flow in a compressor and a turbine has a number of important consequences. First, the blade design is much more critical in a compressor. Whereas turbine blade profiles can be constructed quite satisfactorily of circular arcs and straight lines, compressor blades must be of aerodynamic shape, i.e. of aerofoil section. A less obvious

Fig. 19.23
Comparison of turbine and compressor blades

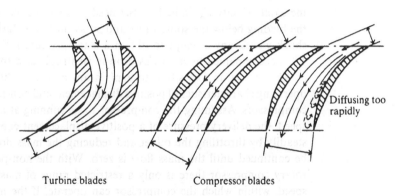

Diffusing too rapidly

Turbine blades   Compressor blades

consequence is that the work done in a compressor stage cannot actually be estimated from equation (19.31) as it stands. The result of trying to induce a flow in a direction opposing the pressure gradient is that the axial velocity distribution across the annulus settles down after the first few stages into the peaky profile shown in Fig. 19.24. The effect of this is that the one-dimensional treatment of this chapter is not nearly so adequate for compressors as it is for turbines, and the work done on unit mass of fluid depends to a greater extent than in a turbine on the radius at which the fluid is flowing through the annulus. In order to obtain an estimate of the average work done from one-dimensional considerations it has been found necessary to multiply equation (19.31) by an empirical coefficient, called the *work done factor*. A typical value, except for the first few stages where it is nearer unity, is 0.86.

The work done factor expresses a limitation upon the work that can be put into a stage. It should not be confused with the isentropic efficiency, which indicates how much of this actual work is usefully employed in raising the pressure and how much is dissipated by friction. The other most important factor limiting the work which can be put into a stage is the permissible rate of divergence of the blade passage. Fig. 19.23 shows that this will be a function of the angle through which the fluid is deflected, i.e. $(\beta_0 - \beta_1)$ for the rotor and $(\alpha_1 - \alpha_2)$ for the stator. For the 50 per cent reaction design we are considering, equation (19.31) can be expressed as

$$\dot{W} = \dot{m} U C_a (\tan \beta_0 - \tan \beta_1)$$

In this form it is clear that a limitation on $(\beta_0 - \beta_1)$ is reflected in a limitation on the work that can be put into a stage, and hence on the pressure ratio that can be obtained. With the blade speed limited by stressing considerations, and

Fig. 19.24
Axial velocity distributions

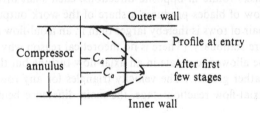

Compressor annulus

Outer wall

Profile at entry

C_a

C_a

After first few stages

Inner wall

479

the axial velocity C_a limited by the need to keep the gas velocities relative to the blading below the sonic value and so avoid losses due to the formation of shock waves, any attempt to obtain a stage pressure ratio much in excess of 1.2 is accompanied by a serious drop in isentropic efficiency.

We are now in a position to explain an important difference between the operating characteristics of positive displacement and non-positive displacement compressors. Assuming the compressor to be running at a constant rotational speed, the delivery pressure of a positive displacement compressor is increased steadily by throttling the outlet and reducing the mass flow. This process can be continued until the mass flow is zero. With the non-positive displacement rotary compressor there is only a restricted range of mass flow, at any given speed, within which the compressor can operate. If the mass flow is reduced beyond a certain point, the directions of the velocities relative to the blading are so widely different from the blade angles that the flow breaks down completely. The compressor is then said to *surge*. Even within the restricted range of operation the efficiency varies considerably, and it can only be maintained at a high value by varying the rotational speed and mass flow simultaneously in such a way that the velocity triangles maintain the same shape.

19.4   Radial-flow turbines

The axial-flow turbine is nearly always preferred to its radial-flow counterpart. There are, however, a few special applications for which the radial-flow turbine is sometimes used and it deserves a brief mention here. There are two possibilities to be considered: outward flow and inward flow.

19.4.1   *Outward-flow turbines*

When the pressure ratio is large, as with steam turbines, it is essential to use outward radial flow rather than inward radial flow. This is because the increase in volume as the expansion proceeds can be partly accommodated by the increase in flow area associated with increase in diameter.

The Ljungström steam turbine is the only commercial outward-flow turbine. Briefly, it consists of concentric rows of blades, similar in shape to those of an axial-flow reaction turbine, attached to the opposing faces of two rotor disks, as in Fig. 19.25. The axial cross-section of the rotor exhibits a flow path of a convergent-divergent character. At first the increase in flow area with diameter is rather greater than is required to accommodate the increase in volume flow, but later the reverse applies and the blades must be increased in length. The disks rotate in opposite directions, each shaft driving a generator. Thus each row of blades produces a share of the work output, and the work output per pair of rows is thereby larger than in an axial-flow machine where half the rows are stationary. (There is no theoretical reason why the 'stator' rows should not be allowed to rotate in an axial-flow turbine but the mechanical difficulties are rather greater.) The velocity triangles for any row are similar to those for an axial-flow reaction stage, the main difference being that the blade velocity is

Fig. 19.25
Rotor for a Ljungström
turbine

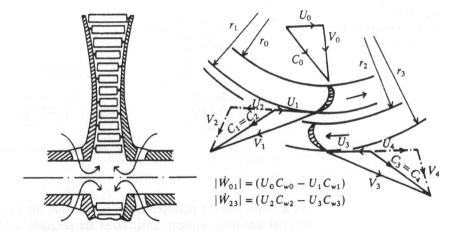

$$|\dot{W}_{01}| = (U_0 C_{w0} - U_1 C_{w1})$$
$$|\dot{W}_{23}| = (U_2 C_{w2} - U_3 C_{w3})$$

greater at outlet than at inlet. The work done on any blade row is found from the rate of change of angular momentum in the usual way, using equation (19.3a).

The Ljungström turbine has the advantage that it is very short in length, and this reduces the difficulties due to differential expansion on starting. It can in fact be started from cold in a matter of minutes, and it is this feature which made it popular as a power plant for 'stand-by' or 'peak-load' electrical generation—a requirement now frequently fulfilled by gas turbine sets.

19.4.2   *Inward-flow turbines*

When the turbine pressure ratio is comparatively small, as in gas turbine plant, it is possible to obtain the required increase in flow area with an inward-flow arrangement such as that shown in Fig. 19.26. This type of turbine is similar to the Francis hydraulic turbine. The gas enters the turbine via a volute and flows through a row of fixed nozzles situated around the periphery of the rotor. The high-velocity stream then flows inward between vanes attached to the side

Fig. 19.26
Inward radial-flow turbine

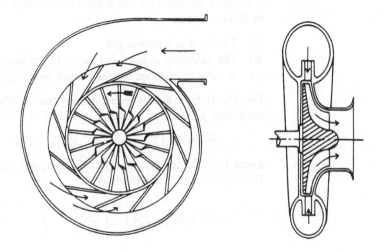

Fig. 19.27
Velocity triangles for an
inward-flow turbine

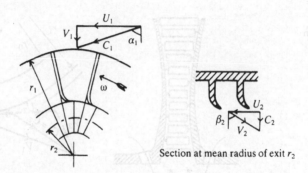

Section at mean radius of exit r_2

of the rotor, and the passages are so shaped that the flow finally exhausts in
an axial direction. Straight radial vanes are generally used, partly for ease of
manufacture, but mainly because centrifugal forces would produce undesirable
bending stresses in curved vanes.

With radial vanes, the velocity of the gas relative to the rotor at entry must
be in the radial direction if the gas is to enter the passages smoothly. The inlet
velocity triangle therefore appears as in Fig. 19.27. For a given rotor tip speed
U_1, nozzle angle α_1 and absolute velocity C_1, the relative velocity will be V_1.
The whirl component of the absolute velocity C_{1w} is equal to U_1. A cross-section
through the 'eye' of the rotor, at the mean radius of the exit annulus, is also
shown in Fig. 19.27. If the outlet velocity C_2 is to be truly axial, the outlet
velocity triangle shows that the relative velocity V_2 must make an angle β_2 with
the axial direction. The rotor vanes must therefore be bent into this direction
at the exit. Since there is no angular momentum at the outlet, equation (19.3a)
becomes simply

$$|\dot{W}| = \dot{m}U_1 C_{1w}$$

And since C_{1w} is equal to U_1, this reduces to

$$|\dot{W}| = \dot{m}U_1^2 \qquad (19.35)$$

A simple expression for the pressure ratio required to produce this work can
be deduced when

(a) The fluid is a perfect gas
(b) The velocities at inlet and outlet of the turbine are equal
(c) A value is assumed for the overall isentropic efficiency of the turbine η_o

The steady-flow energy equation applied to the whole turbine, with inlet
conditions denoted by subscript 0, is then

$$|\dot{W}| = \dot{m}c_p(T_0 - T_2) = \dot{m}c_p\eta_o(T_0 - T_2')$$

where T_2' is the temperature after an isentropic expansion to the final pressure.
This equation can be written as

$$|\dot{W}| = \dot{m}c_p\eta_o T_0\left\{1 - \left(\frac{p_2}{p_0}\right)^{(\gamma-1)/\gamma}\right\}$$

Fig. 19.28
Two-stage radial turbine

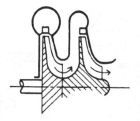

Equating this to (19.35) we have

$$\frac{p_2}{p_0} = \left(1 - \frac{U_1^2}{\eta_o c_p T_0}\right)^{\gamma/(\gamma-1)} \tag{19.36}$$

The permissible rotor tip speed depends upon the gas temperature; it is not likely to be much greater than 460 m/s when the gas inlet temperature is 1200 K. Using these values of U_1 and T_0, an isentropic efficiency of 85 per cent, and typical values of c_p and γ for combustion gases of 1.15 kJ/kg K and 1.333, the pressure ratio becomes

$$\frac{p_2}{p_0} = \left(1 - \frac{460^2}{10^3 \times 1.15 \times 0.85 \times 1200}\right)^{1.333/0.333} = \frac{1}{2.22}$$

It is apparent that if inlet/outlet pressure ratios of much more than 2 are required, more than one stage is necessary. Unfortunately the ducting arrangements necessary for compounding radial turbines involve a rather tortuous flow path, as illustrated in Fig. 19.28. The additional friction loss associated with this does not arise in axial-flow machines where the multiplication of stages presents no problem. For this reason the axial-flow turbine is always preferred when the pressure ratio is such that more than one radial stage would be required. Even when only low pressure-ratio turbines of the two types are compared, the axial machine normally has the higher efficiency. A radial design only becomes competitive for small turbines of low mass flow because then, as was pointed out in section 19.2.4, the axial-flow turbine becomes very inefficient.

19.5   Radial-flow compressors

Although the inward radial-flow turbine has so far been little used, its opposite number, the centrifugal compressor, has been used extensively both in small sizes as superchargers and in large sizes as compressors for gas turbine plant. Centrifugal compressors have lower isentropic efficiencies than axial compressors, but other compensating advantages have proved to be important for some applications.

In appearance the centrifugal compressor is very similar to the radial turbine shown in Fig. 19.26. The rotor, or *impeller*, is driven in the opposite direction, so increasing the angular momentum of the fluid (normally air). There is also a pressure rise due to centrifugal effects. The fluid leaves the impeller with a

Fig. 19.29
Velocity triangles for a
centrifugal compressor

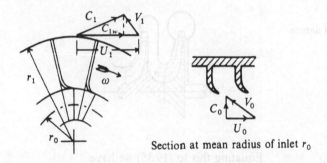

Section at mean radius of inlet r_0

high velocity and flows through fixed diffuser passages in which the remaining
pressure rise is obtained.

The velocity triangles at the inlet and outlet of the impeller are shown in
Fig. 19.29, for the normal case where the absolute inlet velocity is axial. Ideally
the fluid should be ejected from the periphery of the impeller at such a velocity
that the whirl component C_{1w} is equal to the impeller tip speed U_1. Owing to
the inertia of the air trapped between the impeller vanes, C_{1w} is always less
than U_1, the difference depending upon the number of vanes. The power input,
from equation (19.3), is

$$\dot{W} = \dot{m} U_1 C_{1w}$$

Introducing the overall isentropic efficiency, and assuming equal inlet and outlet
velocities for the compressor as a whole, the energy equation becomes

$$\dot{W} = \dot{m} \frac{c_p}{\eta_o}(T_2' - T_0)$$

Hence the pressure ratio is given by

$$\frac{p_2}{p_0} = \left(\frac{T_2'}{T_0}\right)^{\gamma/(\gamma-1)} = \left(1 + \frac{T_2' - T_0}{T_0}\right)^{\gamma/(\gamma-1)}$$

$$= \left(1 + \frac{\eta_o U_1 C_{1w}}{c_p T_0}\right)^{\gamma/(\gamma-1)} \tag{19.37}$$

For an air compressor, the maximum permissible peripheral speed would be
about 460 m/s because, although not subject to high temperatures, the impeller
is normally made of light alloy. With the usual number of impeller vanes, C_{1w}
is about $0.9\,U_1$. Using these figures, together with $c_p = 1.005\,\text{kJ/kg K}$, $\gamma = 1.4$,
$T_0 = 288\,\text{K}$ and $\eta_o = 0.8$, the pressure ratio becomes

$$\frac{p_2}{p_0} = \left(1 + \frac{0.8 \times 0.9 \times 460^2}{10^3 \times 1.005 \times 288}\right)^{1.4/0.4} = 4.39$$

Impellers made from titanium permit higher tip speeds to be used, and pressure
ratios of between 6 and 7 are then possible. As with radial turbines, the losses
associated with compounding usually mean that the axial-flow machine is
preferred when more than one radial stage would be required. Centrifugal
compressors producing pressure ratios much greater than 6 are therefore not

used when high efficiency and low weight are important requirements. When size and weight are unimportant, a high efficiency can be obtained from multistage radial compressors if intercoolers are fitted between the stages.

This chapter provides the briefest possible introduction to the study of rotary expanders and compressors. A more detailed introduction, but one which still employs an integrated approach to the subject of turbo-machinery as a whole, is provided by Ref. 6. For more practical details the reader must turn to specialised books on each type of machine, such as Ref. 1 for gas turbines and Ref. 2 for axial-flow turbines.

20

Direct Conversion

Often the production of mechanical work from a source of energy is merely an intermediate step in the production of electricity. It might be expected that if this intermediate step were eliminated the conversion of chemical or nuclear energy into electrical energy could be made with smaller and lighter equipment or perhaps with greater efficiency. Devices for *direct conversion* which are receiving most attention at present can be classified as follows:

(1) Thermionic converters
(2) Thermoelectric converters
(3) Photovoltaic generators
(4) Magnetohydrodynamic generators
(5) Fuel cells

It is much too early to say which of these has the greatest potential for development or what are the applications for which each type is most suited. Broadly, the first three are likely to be suitable as sources of auxiliary power, the fourth for large-scale power generation and the fifth for medium power outputs such as are required for road vehicles.

The theories on which the design of these systems are based are likewise at an early stage of development. An understanding of them demands a knowledge of thermodynamics, electromagnetics, fluid mechanics and solid-state physics which is beyond the scope of this book.* All we shall attempt here is a brief description of the main features of each type of device, with an indication of the points at which thermodynamics plays a part in the theory. It is hoped that this introduction to the topic will stimulate interest and encourage the engineering student to pay greater attention to supporting science courses. Such is the pace of change that subjects of study which are now peripheral may well become central in his or her lifetime.

The performance of four of the devices listed above is limited by thermodynamic considerations, as will be apparent later. Thermionic and thermoelectric converters are heat engines, even if unconventional forms,

---

* Ref. 24 is recommended as an attempt to present a coherent introduction to the subject of direct conversion in a single volume, as opposed to books, comprising collections of papers by specialists.

in which electrons acting as the 'working fluid' can be said to be taken through a cycle. The maximum efficiency of such converters is therefore limited to the Carnot value $(T_1 - T_2)/T_1$, based on the temperatures of the source and sink between which they are operating. On the other hand, magnetohydrodynamic generators and fuel cells are essentially open systems, drawing on steady supplies of reactants at ambient conditions which ideally could leave as products at ambient conditions. The ambient conditions can in practice be taken to be the standard state $(p^\ominus, T_0)$, and the work output is therefore limited to the maximum work of reaction as explained in section 17.5 (and is also equal to the change in Gibbs function $\Delta g_0^\ominus$ as shown in section 7.9.3). Photovoltaic generators are the exception, because here electromagnetic radiation is converted directly to electricity without the intermediate step of a conversion to heat or a chemical reaction.

It is worth pointing out that the laws of thermodynamics, and the energy equation $Q + W = \Delta U$, apply to more complex systems than those with which this book is primarily concerned. For example, they apply equally to systems involving electric and magnetic effects. The concept of work has to be widened, however, to embrace other than mere mechanical work, and more than two properties may have to be specified to fix the state of the system. Consider for example a system comprising an electrolytic cell, with an external circuit through which flows a quantity of electricity or charge $\delta \mathscr{Z}$ impelled by a potential difference $\mathscr{V}$. If the external circuit consists of a simple resistance, the energy flow $\mathscr{V} \delta \mathscr{Z}$ will be dissipated as ohmic heating; this is analogous to the situation where mechanical work done by a system is dissipated by friction. But in principle it is possible to pass $\delta \mathscr{Z}$ through a perfect electric motor (i.e. one with no copper, iron and windage losses) which will do mechanical work equal to $\mathscr{V} \delta \mathscr{Z}$. Any mode of energy transfer *which can in principle be converted into mechanical work without loss* can be included in the work term of the energy equation. W then becomes a symbol for a more generalised concept of thermodynamic work. If the operation of the electrolytic cell involves the liberation of gases, there may be work transfer due to a change in volume also. Thus for a reversible cell the energy equation could be written as

$$dQ = dU + p\,dV + \mathscr{V}\,d\mathscr{Z}$$

It would be found that in this case the internal energy U is a function of three properties, e.g. p, T and $\mathscr{V}$. Before turning to books on direct conversion such as Ref. 24, the student will find it helpful to obtain this kind of background material from Ref. 8 of Part I.

20.1 Thermionic converters

Thermionic devices make use of the fact that when a metal plate is heated some of the free electrons are emitted from the surface. The distribution of energy among the free electrons, and the binding forces which exist at the surface, are such that only the faster moving electrons are emitted. The number emitted

Fig. 20.1
A diode converter

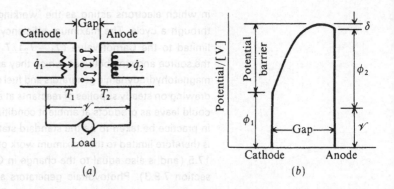

(a)

(b)

increases when the general energy level is raised by increasing the temperature of the metal.

The simplest form of thermionic device is the vacuum diode shown in Fig. 20.1, in which two opposing plates are maintained at different temperatures T_1 and T_2. Since the current density (A/m^2) emitted from the surface is a function of temperature, there will be a net flow of electrons from the high-temperature electrode (cathode) to the low-temperature electrode (anode), returning to the cathode via an external circuit. The retarding potential barrier which the electrons leaving the cathode must overcome is illustrated in Fig. 20.1b as $(\delta + \phi_2 + \mathscr{V} - \phi_1)$. ϕ_1 and ϕ_2 are the potential barriers for electrons within the material of the cathode and anode respectively; in solid-state physics ϕ is referred to as the *work function* of the material, and its value varies greatly with the state of the metal surface. δ is the retarding potential due to the cloud of electrons in the space between the electrodes, and is called the *space charge barrier*. $\mathscr{V}$ is the output voltage. Using electromagnetic theory to calculate the number of electrons per unit area which have sufficient energy to overcome the barrier, a relation may be deduced for the net current density $\mathscr{I}$ from cathode to anode in terms of ϕ, δ, $\mathscr{V}$ and the temperatures T_1 and T_2. The net power output is then $\mathscr{I}\mathscr{V}$ per unit area of emissive surface.

It is possible to apply the steady-flow energy equation to an open system containing the cathode, with inlet and outlet planes across the conductor leading to the cathode and the space between the electrodes. The rate of heat flow $\dot{q}_1$ required to maintain unit area of cathode at T_1 is equal to the algebraic sum of the energy of the electrons flowing across the gap and in the conducting lead, the thermal radiation from the plate, and the conduction of heat in the lead. An expression can thereby be obtained for $\dot{q}_1$, and hence finally for the efficiency of conversion $\mathscr{I}\mathscr{V}/\dot{q}_1$.

With present-day materials, reasonable efficiencies can be achieved only if the space charge barrier δ is kept to a minimum. And with a vacuum diode this can be done only by maintaining a very small gap between the electrodes (< 0.025 mm), which is difficult at the high temperatures required ($T_1 > 1600$ K). Another approach is to introduce an ionising agent into the gap to neutralise the space charge. It is expected that, with further development, power densities of up to 300 kW/m^2 will be achieved with an efficiency of about 15 per cent.

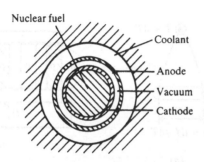

If we view the system with its external leads and load as a whole, we can see that the electrons pass through a cycle of states while heat is supplied and rejected at the cathode and anode respectively. The maximum efficiency is therefore limited to $(T_1 - T_2)/T_1$. As there are no highly stressed parts, very high temperatures can be used. But the inevitably high rate of irreversible heat transfer by radiation to the anode prohibits the use of large temperature *differences* and the efficiency obtainable cannot be very high. Thermionic converters are likely to be used either as a source of auxiliary power in space applications, where small size and low weight are important, or as 'topping' devices in conjunction with conventional power plant to make use of the hitherto unused temperature drop between available combustion temperatures and permissible boiler operating temperatures. In the latter case, the electrons would be the high-temperature working fluid in a binary cycle. Experiments are proceeding on these lines in the nuclear power field, by incorporating the converter into nuclear fuel elements as shown in Fig. 20.2. The tubular sheath around the fuel rod is the cathode, and the coolant, which is the heat source for the conventional power plant, flows along the outside of the tubular anode.

20.2   Thermoelectric converters

When the junctions of a loop of two wires of dissimilar metal are maintained at different temperatures, an electric current is produced in the circuit; this is the net result of the Peltier and Seebeck effects. The open-circuit potential difference produced, per unit temperature difference between the junctions, is called the *Seebeck coefficient* or *thermoelectric power* α (see Fig. 20.3a). With pairs of ordinary metals the value of α is only of the order of a few μV/K; this is adequate for use as thermocouples but much too low to be of interest for direct conversion. The development of semiconductors, however, which have thermoelectric powers in the region of mV/K, has now made thermoelectric converters a practical possibility. Useful power outputs can be obtained by connecting a large number of pairs in series.

The Seebeck effect in metals is due to the diffusion of electrons along the temperature gradient from the hot to the cold junction. If this is greater in one metal than the other there will be a net flow of electrons around the circuit. In semiconductors the rate of diffusion is much greater, and furthermore the effect in each limb of the pair can be *additive* for the following reason. In some types

Fig. 20.3
Thermoelectric converter

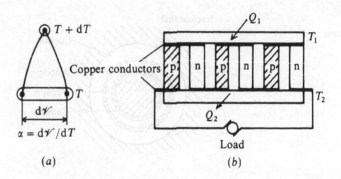

$\alpha = d\mathscr{V}/dT$

(a) (b)

of semiconductor the charge carriers are electrons as in ordinary metals; these are referred to as n-type materials. But in others, p-type materials, the charge carriers are positive and can be regarded as 'holes' vacated by electrons. The current produced in a pair of n- and p-type materials is in effect equal to the sum of the rates of diffusion of negative and positive charge carriers.

A high thermoelectric power α is not the only criterion of importance in the choice of material for a thermoelectric converter. Fig. 20.3b shows a typical arrangement with hot junctions at T_1 and cold junctions at T_2. It should be clear that a low thermal conductivity k is necessary to keep the heat flow by conduction across the elements to a minimum, and a low electrical resistivity ρ is required to reduce the internal ohmic ($\mathscr{I}^2\mathscr{R}$) losses. Semiconductors are also good in these respects, because they are essentially materials of low thermal and electrical conductivity with the latter alone improved by the addition of impurities. α, k and ρ are temperature dependent and, when arriving at what is called the *figure of merit M* for a pair of n- and p-type materials, it has been found convenient to include the temperature range which it is intended to employ. The figure of merit commonly used is

$$M = \frac{\alpha^2 (T_1 + T_2)}{k\rho} \frac{}{2} \qquad (20.1)$$

The thermoelectric converter is like the thermionic variety in that it is a heat engine with a flow of charge carriers as the working fluid. The maximum possible efficiency is therefore $(T_1 - T_2)/T_1$. This could be achieved only if the figure of merit were infinite, i.e. if there were no irreversibilities due to thermal conduction or ohmic loss between the hot and cold junctions. A thermodynamic analysis can be used to show that the practical ideal efficiency of conversion for a given value of M is given by

$$\eta = \frac{T_1 - T_2}{T_1} \frac{(1 + M)^{1/2} - 1}{(1 + M)^{1/2} + (T_2/T_1)} \qquad (20.2)$$

A not very rigorous derivation of this equation can be found in Ref. 24. Since we are here dealing with essentially irreversible processes, the relatively new science of irreversible thermodynamics is necessary for a rigorous treatment (see the chapter by Hatsopoulos and Keenan in Ref. 25). With present-day materials, M is about unity and T_1 and T_2 might be about 600 °C and 200 °C respectively. The corresponding ideal efficiency from equation (20.2) is thus about 10 per cent. Various losses not taken into account in deriving (20.2), such as those due to thermal contact resistance between the elements and the heat source and sink, result in actual efficiencies being nearer 5 per cent.

Unless new semiconductor materials can be developed which are capable of operating at high temperatures, thermoelectric converters are likely to be used as 'bottomers' rather than 'toppers' in binary cycles. They are especially suitable for waste heat recovery, perhaps using the exhaust gases of gas turbines as a source of heat, or the heat generated by a radioactive source as in the American Snap III generator designed for space applications. Thermoelectric generators using paraffin heating have been used in the USSR as a power source for radio receivers in rural areas. Thermoelectric devices can also be run in reverse; by supplying a current from an external source they act as refrigerators. The coefficient of performance is quite low, about 0.6, but the simplicity of the device makes it useful for some applications.

20.3 Photovoltaic generators

Electricity can be produced directly by exposing $p-n$ junctions to electromagnetic radiation. The conversion is due to quantum interactions between individual photons of radiation and the electronic structure of the cell material, which take place when the photon energy ($= hc/\lambda$) exceeds a certain threshold value (h is Planck's constant, c the velocity of light and λ the wavelength). The two most important types of energy source are (a) radioactive materials, which yield radiations of very short wavelength ($\approx 10^{-12}$ m), and (b) sunlight whose wavelength ranges around 10^{-6} m. Photovoltaic cells designed to use sunlight have received the most attention.

Photovoltaic effects in a solid were first observed in 1877 by Adams and Day who worked with selenium. The work led to the development of photographic exposure meters, but they convert no more than 0.8 per cent of the incident radiation into electrical energy. With the introduction of n- and p-type semiconductors in the 1950s, conversion efficiencies of about 6 per cent were obtained and it was possible to think of using photovoltaic cells as a power source. Efficiencies of 15 per cent are now obtained with silicon $p-n$ junctions.

Energy is produced by photons of radiation, creating free electrons and holes. To achieve a high efficiency it is necessary to produce electron–hole pairs very close to the p–n interface. Those far from the junction recombine without contributing to the cell's output. Furthermore, the internal resistance must be small. For these reasons cells consist of a very thin layer ($\approx 10^{-3}$ mm thick) of n-type material on a wafer of p-type material (≈ 0.5 mm thick). Unwanted surface recombination of electron–hole pairs is minimised by chemically etching the surface of the cell to leave it in a highly polished state, and reflection losses are reduced by using antireflection coatings. By considering the various losses inherent in the collecting and conversion processes, it can be shown by solid-state theory as in Ref. 24 that the theoretical maximum efficiency of a silicon cell is about 20 per cent, and with other possible materials such as gallium arsenide or cadmium telluride it is about 25 per cent. At present the actual efficiency of cells made of the theoretically better materials is lower than that of silicon cells.

Because the source of energy is free, the factor limiting the use of photovoltaic cells as a power source is not so' much the conversion efficiency as the high cost of production. So far this has limited their use largely to space applications, such as communication satellites, where the cost of the cells is a small proportion of the total cost of the system. Now that costs are falling towards a more commercial level, the efficiency has become more important because it determines the number of solar cells (still costly) required for a given power. output. The power produced per unit surface area of cell might be increased by concentrating the radiation with lenses or reflectors. Unfortunately the conversion efficiency of present materials is reduced as the temperature of the cell increases, so that the net effect is small. Cooling the cell is no answer; the result would simply be a thermoelectric system. Another possibility is the construction of multilayer cells of different materials, matching their electronic characteristics to the energy spectra of the radiation in such a way that a greater proportion of the wavelength range can be used. Efficiencies of over 30 per cent might then be possible.

20.4   Magnetohydrodynamic generators

Strictly speaking, it is doubtful whether the magnetohydrodynamic (MHD) generator can be called a direct conversion device; certainly there is no direct conversion of heat into electrical energy as in thermionic and thermoelectric converters. A gas at high pressure and temperature is still required as in conventional plant, but instead of using this via a turbine to drive metallic conductors through a magnetic field as in a conventional generator, the gas itself acts as a moving conductor (see Fig. 20.4). At very high temperatures a gas is ionised and the degree of ionisation can be enhanced by 'seeding' the gas with a small quantity of another substance such as caesium or potassium. Such ionised gases are referred to as plasmas. This conducting fluid is accelerated in a nozzle and passed at high velocity through a rectangular duct across which a magnetic field is applied at right angles to the direction of flow. An *EMF* is thereby generated in the fluid, which can be utilised by placing electrodes along the sides of the duct.

The flow in the duct is governed by the momentum and energy equations,

Fig. 20.4
Magnetohydro-dynamic duct *vis-à-vis* the conventional generator

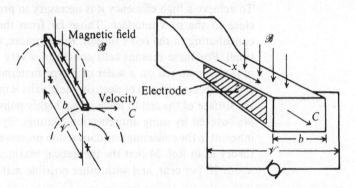

which in this case must include electrical force and energy terms. A simple derivation of these equations for one-dimensional frictionless adiabatic flow is given in Ref. 24, where they are shown to be:

$$\text{Momentum equation:}\qquad v\frac{dp}{dx} + C\frac{dC}{dx} = -v\mathcal{J}\mathcal{B}$$

$$\text{Energy equation:}\qquad \frac{C}{v}\frac{d}{dx}(h + \tfrac{1}{2}C^2) = -\frac{\mathcal{J}\mathcal{V}}{b}$$

Here $\mathcal{B}$ is the magnetic flux density, $\mathcal{V}$ the potential difference across the electrodes, b the distance between electrodes, and $\mathcal{J}$ the current density given by

$$\mathcal{J} = \sigma\left(\frac{\mathcal{V}}{b} - C\mathcal{B}\right)$$

where σ is the electrical conductivity of the fluid. From these equations it is possible to deduce such useful performance criteria as the rate at which enthalpy is converted into electrical energy, the ratio of actual to isentropic enthalpy drop, and the power produced per unit volume of duct. It can be shown that the last of these, the power density, is proportional to $\sigma C^2 \mathcal{B}^2$. The velocity of flow C is much higher than the speed at which a solid conductor can be rotated in a conventional generator, and this partially offsets the inherent disadvantage that σ (even for a seeded gas at 3000 K) is only about 100 $(\Omega\,\text{m})^{-1}$ compared with 10^7 $(\Omega\,\text{m})^{-1}$ for solid copper.

The overall efficiency will depend on the way in which the MHD duct is incorporated in the complete plant. Because sufficient ionisation can be achieved only at temperatures of 2500 °C or greater, the MHD generator is essentially a high-temperature device. Furthermore, the temperature must still be very high at outlet from the duct, so that to obtain a reasonable overall efficiency it must be used as a 'topper' in conjunction with a conventional cycle. A typical open-cycle scheme is shown in Fig. 20.5; it would be possible to use a completely closed cycle if the combustion chamber was replaced by a nuclear reactor, but the temperatures required for adequate ionisation are well beyond those at present possible in reactors. Considering the open-cycle plant shown, the MHD

Fig. 20.5
Possible MHD generator plant

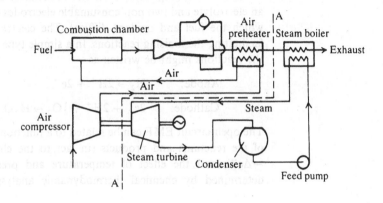

portion to the left of the dashed line A–A is an open system for which the efficiency might be expressed as

$$\frac{|\text{net electrical work}| - |\text{compressor work}|}{-\Delta h_0}$$

The net electrical output is the gross output less the power supplied to the electromagnetics producing the field $\mathcal{B}$, and Δh_0 is the enthalpy of combustion. (Those who have studied section 7.9.3 will appreciate that the denominator should strictly be the change in Gibbs function $-\Delta g_0^\ominus$.) For the plant as a whole, the numerator becomes the net electrical output, including that from the steam cycle, minus the feed pump work.

The major sources of loss are fluid friction, heat loss through the walls of the duct, and internal electrical resistance. These losses can be made a small fraction of the output only by using large ducts and high flow rates. It appears that the MHD generator is unlikely to be used for powers below the megawatt range. This is a case where little useful experimental work can be done on a small scale and thus development costs are very high. Several pilot plants have been built in the Soviet Union, and 1000 MW commercial units are now being designed using superconducting magnets and natural gas as the fuel.

20.5 Fuel cells

A fuel cell is a practical method of achieving a near reversible chemical reaction in which there is a conversion of chemical energy into electrical energy without even the intermediate step of conversion into random molecular energy (i.e. sensible internal energy). Thus, whereas the thermionic and thermoelectric forms of direct converter are essentially heat engines and subject to the Carnot limitation on efficiency, the fuel cell is not. Theoretically, the maximum work of a chemical reaction discussed in section 17.5 (and section 7.9.3) could be made available as electrical energy. The development of such a device, if capable of operating with hydrocarbon fuels or cheap derivatives such as carbon monoxide, would be a great step forward in the efficient utilisation of fuel resources.

The fuel cell (Fig. 20.6) is an electrochemical device consisting basically of an electrolyte and two non-consumable electrodes (often porous plates through which the fuel and oxidant diffuse). The electrodes play a catalytic role in facilitating the ionising reactions. In a simple type of hydrogen-oxygen fuel cell the reactions might be written as

Anode: $\quad H_2 \rightarrow 2H^+ + 2e^-$

Cathode: $\quad 2e^- + 2H^+ + \tfrac{1}{2}O_2 \rightarrow H_2O$

The open-circuit EMF can be related to a function of the enthalpy and entropy of the reactants and products (in fact to the change in the Gibbs function $-\Delta g_0^\ominus$), and the effect of temperature and pressure on the EMF can be determined by chemical thermodynamic analysis (see Ref. 26). The ideal

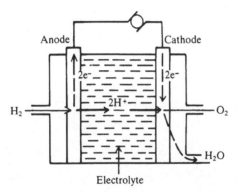

maximum work for the reaction is not made available in practice because of internal losses. These include inhibiting effects due to absorption of molecules on the surface of the electrodes, uneven concentration of the electrolyte when current is flowing, changes in the conductivity of the electrolyte near the electrodes, and ohmic heating ($\mathscr{I}^2\mathscr{R}$ loss) due to the resistance of the electrolyte. Depending on the fuel and oxidant employed, the EMF produced is between 0.5 V and 1.5 V, and any required output voltage can be obtained by connecting cells in series as in the ordinary electric battery. Current densities of up to 400 A/m^2 have been achieved.

Before about 1960, research in this field had been done by only a few individuals and mostly on the hydrogen-oxygen cell. The picture has been transformed since then, and now a large number of laboratories and research teams are actively engaged in this development. The result has been not only a marked increase in performance—in power density and efficiency—but also such a bewildering variety of types of cell that classification is difficult. Attempts have been made to classify them on the basis of operating temperature or pressure, and type of electrolyte, fuel, oxidant or electrode, but no neat picture has emerged. There is little doubt that fuel cells will find a place for special military and space applications, but whether they will come into more general use depends on finding means of using cheap fuel and extending their working life.

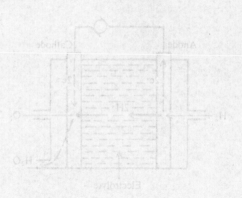

Part IV

Heat Transfer

Introduction

Heat is energy in transition under the motive force of a temperature difference, and the study of heat transfer deals with the rate at which such energy is transferred. When discussing thermodynamic processes, time is never considered a limiting factor, and ideal processes can be conceived during which heat is transferred by virtue of an infinitesimally small temperature difference. In actual processes some of the available temperature drop, which might be used for the production of work, must be sacrificed to ensure that the required quantity of heat is transferred in a reasonable time across a surface of reasonable size. Two types of problem are frequently of interest; the first, met in the design of boilers and heat exchangers, is concerned with the promotion of the required rate of heat transfer with the minimum possible surface area and temperature difference; the other is concerned with the prevention of heat transfer, i.e. with thermal insulation.

Three modes of heat transfer may be distinguished, but the fact that a temperature difference is necessary is common to all. One mode of heat transfer is that of *conduction*, discussed in Chapter 21, in which energy is transferred on a molecular scale with no movement of macroscopic portions of matter relative to one another. Fourier's law forms the basis of all calculations of heat transfer by conduction.

A second mode of heat transfer occurs when temperature differences exist between a fluid and a solid boundary. Here the redistribution of energy is partly due to conduction and partly due to transport of enthalpy by the motion of the fluid itself. Such motion can be due to a pump, as in the case of a fluid passing through the tubes of a heat exchanger, and this mode of heat transfer is called *forced convection*. On the other hand, the motion may be entirely due to density gradients in the fluid, caused by the temperature gradients—as when a stove heats the air in a room—and this is called *free* or *natural convection*. Convection is far more difficult to analyse than conduction because it is a combined problem of heat flow and fluid flow. The rate of heat transfer is influenced by all the fluid properties that can affect both heat and fluid flow, such as velocity, thermal conductivity, viscosity, density and thermal expansion. In finding an exact solution to any particular problem, it is essential to satisfy the equation of motion (Newton's Second Law), the equation of energy and the equation of continuity of flow, in addition to Fourier's law. The differential equations governing convection are complicated and exact solutions can be given in only a few simple cases. Some approximate analytical methods are given in Chapter 22, together with a description of an empirical approach using dimensional analysis.

The third mode of heat transfer is *radiation*, and this mode does not depend upon the existence of an intervening medium. All matter at temperatures above absolute zero emits energy in the form of electromagnetic waves. Gases at low pressure emit waves of particular frequencies only, which are the natural frequencies of vibration of the gas molecules. In gases at high pressure, or liquids and solids, the molecular vibrations are more damped, and the emission of energy is over wide frequency bands. It is impossible here to go into the mechanism of radiation, and from the engineer's point of view it is usually sufficient to know the total quantities of energy emitted and absorbed by matter at various temperatures. The calculation of radiation heat transfer, discussed in Chapter 23, is based mainly on the Stefan-Boltzmann, Kirchhoff, and Lambert Laws.

Often all three forms of heat transfer are involved simultaneously. It is then usual to calculate the rate of heat transfer by each mode separately, adding the separate effects to provide an estimate of the total rate of heat transfer. In this way a complex problem can be resolved, and the relative importance of the various modes of heat transfer can be assessed. A few simple examples are given in Chapter 24. The final result may not be exact, however, because a certain amount of interaction usually exists between the different modes.

In the study of heat transfer it is usual to talk about the flow of heat, and of heat being contained in a material, as if heat were something tangible. Although in thermodynamics we permit outselves to talk loosely about the flow of heat, we are always careful to distinguish between the energy in transition (heat) and the energy residing in the material (internal energy). This distinction is necessary because the change in internal energy can be due to either work or heat crossing the boundary of a system. Normally this distinction is unnecessary in heat transfer because we are considering processes during which the change in internal energy is due solely to a flow of heat, and we are not concerned with transformations of one form of energy into another. In heat transfer problems involving flowing fluids, some of the kinetic energy is transformed into random molecular energy by viscous forces, and greater care is needed in the use of the term 'heat'. Nevertheless, for low velocities of flow the quantities of kinetic energy involved are usually small compared with the rate at which heat is transferred to or from the fluid, so that again no harm is done by the loose usage of the term. In high-speed flow, however, when the dissipation of kinetic energy into random molecular energy may be considerable, the thermodynamic view of the concept of heat must be retained.

21

Conduction

When temperature differences are present in any matter, heat flows from the hot to the cold regions until the temperatures are equalised. This occurs even when the movement of macroscopic portions of matter is prevented as in solids. The actual mechanism is complicated, but a brief explanation is as follows.

In solids the conduction of heat is partly due to the impact of adjacent molecules vibrating about their mean positions, and partly due to internal radiation. When the solid is a metal, there are also large numbers of mobile electrons which can easily move through the matter, passing from one atom to another, and they contribute to the redistribution of energy in the metal. Indeed the contribution of the mobile electrons predominates in metals, thus explaining the relation which is found to exist between the thermal and electrical conductivity of such materials.[*]

In liquids, single molecules may make large excursions with frequent collisions, even when large-scale motion (convection) of the fluid is completely suppressed, and such movement assists the conduction of heat. Although the mobility of individual molecules is even greater in gases, the conductivity is appreciably lower than that of liquids and solids owing to the relatively long 'mean free path' in gases and hence the comparatively infrequent impact between the molecules.

The detailed analysis of the mechanism of conduction is not discussed in this chapter. The first sections deal with Fourier's law of conduction, and its application to one-dimensional steady-flow problems. The general equation for unsteady three-dimensional heat flow is then derived. In the course of introducing relaxation methods, a two-dimensional steady-flow problem is solved. Finally, one-dimensional unsteady (transient) problems are considered with the aid of a numerical method.

For a brief discussion of the status of Fourier's law, vis-à-vis the laws of thermodynamics, the reader may turn to the end of section 6.7.

21.1 Fourier's law of heat conduction

Fourier's law of conduction is based on the empirical observation of one-dimensional steady heat flow through a solid. *One-dimensional* flow implies that

---

[*] A fairly easy but comprehensive modern explanation is given by J. D. Eshelby in Ref. 35, p. 267.

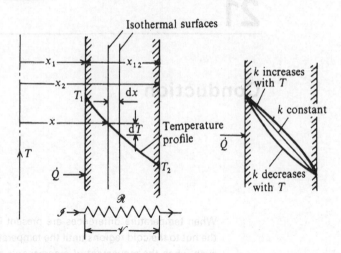

Fig. 21.1
One-dimensional steady
heat conduction through
a plane-parallel wall

the temperature is uniform over surfaces perpendicular to the direction x of heat conduction (Fig. 21.1a), and such surfaces are called *isothermal* surfaces. *Steady flow* implies that the temperature at any point does not vary with time. It follows from considerations of continuity that in one-dimensional steady flow the rate of heat flow through successive surfaces is constant.

Consider a plane layer of thickness dx, with one face maintained at a temperature T and the other at $(T + dT)$. The rate of heat flow $\dot{Q}$ is found to be proportional to the area of flow A and to the temperature difference of dT across the layer, and inversely proportional to the thickness dx. This is Fourier's law, and it can be expressed by the equation

$$\dot{Q} = -kA\left(\frac{dT}{dx}\right) \tag{21.1}$$

The constant of proportionality k is called the *thermal conductivity* of the material. The negative sign indicates that the heat flow is positive in the direction of temperature fall while treating k as a positive quantity.

Steady one-dimensional conduction demands that $\dot{Q}$ be constant through successive layers of the wall; if this were not so, the temperature in any layer dx with unequal inflow and outflow would vary with time. It follows that $\dot{Q}$ is not a function of x. Equation (21.1) therefore implies that if k is constant then (dT/dx) must also be constant, and thus the temperature profile is linear. Equation (21.1) can be integrated between limits x_1 and x_2, to enable the heat flow to be expressed in terms of the surface temperatures T_1 and T_2 by

$$\dot{Q} = -kA\frac{T_2 - T_1}{x_{12}} \tag{21.2}$$

When $\dot{Q}$ is in kW (or kJ/s), A in m^2, and the temperature gradient (dT/dx) in K/m, the units of k become kW/m K. Fig. 21.2 indicates that more convenient numbers are obtained if k is expressed in W/m K, and this smaller unit will often be used.

Fig. 21.2
Some values of thermal
conductivity $k/[W/m\,K]$

$T/[K]$	250	300	400	500	600	800
Aluminium	208	202	209	222	234	277
Copper	393	386	377	372	367	357
Steel (0.5% C)	57	55	52	48	45	38
Glass		0.8–1.1				
Building brick		0.35–0.7				
Concrete		0.9–1.4				
Asbestos		0.163	0.194	0.206		
Mercury, liquid	7.5	8.1	9.4	10.7	12.8	13.7
Sodium, liquid	135 (sol.)	135 (sol.)	86	80	74	6.3
Water (sat.)	2.22 (ice)	0.614	0.687	0.642		
Steam (sat.)		0.0184	0.0275	0.0432		
Steam (low p)		0.0188	0.0266	0.0357	0.0463	0.0708
Hydrogen	0.0156	0.182	0.228	0.272	0.315	0.402
Air	0.0223	0.0262	0.0337	0.0404	0.0466	0.0577
Carbon dioxide	0.0129	0.0166	0.0246	0.0335	0.0431	0.0560

Fig. 21.2 gives some representative values of thermal conductivity for various materials, and it will be seen that the thermal conductivity varies with temperature. However, if the temperature difference $(T_2 - T_1)$ between the outside faces of the slab in Fig. 21.1a is small, a mean value of k may be chosen and assumed constant. When the temperature difference across the slab is large, due account must be taken of the variation of thermal conductivity with temperature. Typical temperature profiles for variable conductivities are shown in Fig. 21.1b. Unless otherwise stated, k will be assumed constant, but the method of calculating the heat transfer when k is a function of temperature is illustrated in the following example.

Example 21.1 The conductivity of a plane-parallel wall is not constant, but can be expressed with sufficient accuracy as a linear function of temperature, $k = aT + b$. Show that equation (21.2) can be used to calculate the rate of heat flow, if the arithmetic mean of the conductivities k_1 and k_2, at the temperatures T_1 and T_2 respectively, is substituted for k.

Considering unit area of wall, and writing $\dot{q} = \dot{Q}/A$, equation (21.1) becomes

$$\dot{q} = -k\left(\frac{dT}{dx}\right) = -(aT + b)\left(\frac{dT}{dx}\right)$$

For one-dimensional steady flow $\dot{q}$ is independent of x and hence, by integration between x_1 and x_2 (Fig. 21.1a), we have

$$\dot{q}(x_2 - x_1) = -\frac{a}{2}(T_2^2 - T_1^2) - b(T_2 - T_1)$$

or

$$\dot{q} = -\left\{\frac{a}{2}(T_2 + T_1) + b\right\}\frac{T_2 - T_1}{x_{12}}$$

But the mean conductivity is

$$\frac{k_2 + k_1}{2} = \frac{(aT_2 + b) + (aT_1 + b)}{2} = \left\{\frac{a'}{2}(T_2 - T_1) + b\right\}$$

and hence equation (21.2) can be applied in the manner suggested.

That there is some similarity between the flow of heat and that of electricity becomes apparent when equation (21.2) is compared with Ohm's law, $\mathscr{I} = \mathscr{V}/\mathscr{R}$. The temperature difference, responsible for the heat conduction, plays an analogous part to the potential difference or voltage $\mathscr{V}$ in the conduction of electricity. The current $\mathscr{I}$ can then be compared to the heat flow per unit area $\dot{q}$, and the resistance $\mathscr{R}$ to the value of x_{12}/k (see Fig. 21.1a). The practical value of this *electrical analogy* will become clear in the next section.

21.2 One-dimensional steady conduction through a composite wall

A wall built up of three different materials is shown in Fig. 21.3. The surface temperatures of the wall are T_1 and T_4, and the temperatures of the interfaces are T_2 and T_3. For steady flow through the wall, the heat flow through successive slabs must be the same for reasons of continuity, and hence

$$\dot{q} = -k_{12}\frac{T_2 - T_1}{x_{12}} = -k_{23}\frac{T_3 - T_2}{x_{23}} = -k_{34}\frac{T_4 - T_3}{x_{34}} \qquad (21.3)$$

It follows from (21.3) that

$$-(T_2 - T_1) - (T_3 - T_2) - (T_4 - T_3) = -(T_4 - T_1)$$

$$= \dot{q}\left(\frac{x_{12}}{k_{12}} + \frac{x_{23}}{k_{23}} + \frac{x_{34}}{k_{34}}\right) \qquad (21.4)$$

Fig. 21.3
Heat conduction through
a composite wall

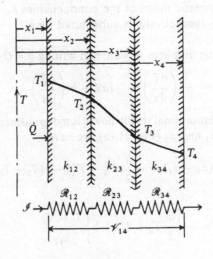

For the complete wall as a whole we can write

$$\dot{q} = -U(T_4 - T_1) \tag{21.5}$$

where U is an *overall heat transfer coefficient* for the wall, defined by (21.5). It follows from (21.4) and (21.5) that

$$\frac{1}{U} = \frac{x_{12}}{k_{12}} + \frac{x_{23}}{k_{23}} + \frac{x_{34}}{k_{34}}$$

or in general for any number of layers

$$\frac{1}{U} = \sum \frac{\Delta x}{k} \tag{21.6}$$

Here $1/U$ is the overall resistance to heat flow, and it is equal to the sum of the individual resistances x_{12}/k_{12} etc. in *series*. This might be expected from the electrical analogy illustrated in Fig. 21.3. The approach by way of equations (21.5) and (21.6) makes it possible to find the heat flow through a composite wall in terms of the surface temperatures, without calculating the interface temperatures. We have assumed, however, that there is no contact resistance between the layers; poor contact will lead to a temperature discontinuity at the interfaces and may result in a marked reduction in the rate of heat transfer because of the very low conductivity of air.

Frequently it is required to calculate the heat flow through a wall separating two fluids of known temperature, when the surface temperatures of the wall are unknown. A typical temperature distribution in a fluid near a wall is shown in Fig. 21.4. Most of the temperature drop occurs very near the wall in a relatively stagnant boundary layer which adheres to the wall. Some distance from the wall the heat transfer is assisted by convection, and the temperature drop becomes more gradual until in practice it vanishes completely. The heat flow in the fluid boundary layer could theoretically be calculated from Fourier's law

$$\dot{q} = -k_f \left(\frac{dT}{dx} \right)_w \tag{21.7}$$

where $(dT/dx)_w$ is the temperature gradient in *the fluid* immediately adjacent to the wall, and k_f is the thermal conductivity of the fluid film at the wall. But

Fig. 21.4
Temperature profile in a
fluid boundary layer

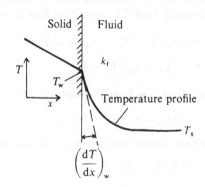

$(dT/dx)_w$ is a quantity which cannot easily be measured in practice, and it is more usual to express the heat flow from the wall to a fluid by an equation of the form

$$\dot{q} = -\alpha_c(T_s - T_w) \tag{21.8}$$

where α_c is a *convection heat transfer coefficient* or *film coefficient*, and T_s is the uniform fluid temperature so..ie distance from the wall, referred to as the *free-stream temperature*. To make the sign convention and general appearance of equation (21.8) consistent with that of Fourier's equation (21.7), we have introduced the negative sign in (21.8). The temperature change $(T_s - T_w)$ in the x-direction must always be written in the correct order to make $\dot{q}$ positive in the direction of temperature fall. Comparing (21.7) and (21.8), it is evidently possible to think of a stagnant fluid layer of thickness $\delta = k_f/\alpha_c$ which has the same resistance to heat flow as the actual fluid. *The heat flow calculated from (21.8) includes the combined effects of conduction and convection in the fluid, and the two cannot be separated.* The value of α_c is difficult to calculate, and methods of evaluating it will be considered in Chapter 22. It is a function of numerous variables, such as the fluid viscosity and density and the fluid velocity relative to the wall; it is *not* a physical constant valid for a particular fluid under all conditions of convective heat transfer. For the time being it will merely be assumed that α_c can be found.

In addition to heat transfer by convection from the wall surface to its surroundings, the wall may also lose or gain heat by radiation. It is again convenient to express this heat transfer by the equation

$$\dot{q} = -\alpha_r(T_s - T_w) \tag{21.9}$$

where α_r is a *radiation heat transfer coefficient*. In this case T_s is the temperature of the *surface* with which the wall is exchanging heat by radiation. α_r is a function of several variables, such as the temperatures, emissivities and absorptivities of the radiating surfaces. The evaluation of α_r is considered in Chapter 23, and here it is merely assumed that its value can be found.

Let us now consider a composite wall which separates two fluids at temperatures T_a and T_b (Fig. 21.5). For simplicity, it is assumed that the surfaces with which the wall is exchanging heat by radiation have the same temperature as the intervening fluid. The total heat flow to the wall is given by

$$\dot{q} = -\alpha_{ca}(T_1 - T_a) - \alpha_{ra}(T_1 - T_a)$$
$$= -(\alpha_{ca} + \alpha_{ra})(T_1 - T_a) \tag{21.10}$$

Similarly the heat flow from the wall is

$$\dot{q} = -(\alpha_{cb} + \alpha_{rb})(T_b - T_4) \tag{21.11}$$

An overall heat transfer coefficient U can now be defined by

$$\dot{q} = -U(T_b - T_a) \tag{21.12}$$

Fig. 21.5
Heat exchange between
two fluids through a
composite wall

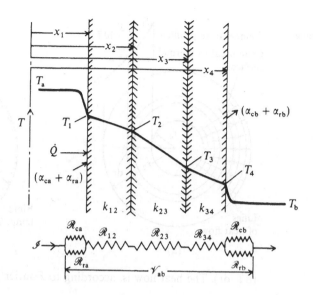

It then follows from (21.3), (21.10), (21.11) and (21.12) that

$$\frac{1}{U} = \frac{1}{\alpha_{ca} + \alpha_{ra}} + \frac{x_{12}}{k_{12}} + \frac{x_{23}}{k_{23}} + \frac{x_{34}}{k_{34}} + \frac{1}{\alpha_{cb} + \alpha_{rb}}$$

or in general

$$\frac{1}{U} = \sum \frac{1}{\alpha_c + \alpha_r} + \sum \frac{\Delta x}{k} \tag{21.13}$$

Again considering the electrical analogy, the overall resistance to heat flow $1/U$ is equal to the sum of the individual resistances $1/(\alpha_{ca} + \alpha_{ra})$, x_{12}/k_{12} etc. Here $1/\alpha_{ca}$ and $1/\alpha_{ra}$ are two resistances in *parallel*.

21.3 Radial steady conduction through the wall of a tube

When the inner and outer surfaces of a long tube are each at a uniform temperature, heat flows radially through the tube wall. Owing to symmetry, any cylindrical surface concentric with the axis of the tube is an isothermal surface, and the direction of heat flow is normal to such a surface. To calculate the steady rate of conduction through the wall, it will be found convenient to consider unit length of tube rather than unit surface area. Continuity considerations indicate that the radial heat flow per unit length of the tube through successive layers must be constant if the flow is steady. Thus, since the area of successive layers increases with radius, the temperature gradient must decrease with radius. The temperature distribution will therefore appear as in Fig. 21.6a.

Consider any elemental cylindrical tube of thickness dr. The area of flow per unit length of tube is $2\pi r$, and the temperature gradient normal to this tube is

Fig. 21.6

Radial flow through a
thick tube and a
composite tube

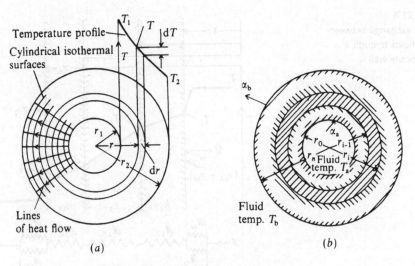

(a)

(b)

$(\mathrm{d}T/\mathrm{d}r)$. The heat flow is, according to Fourier's law,

$$\dot{Q} = -k2\pi r\left(\frac{\mathrm{d}T}{\mathrm{d}r}\right)$$

Hence, since $\dot{Q}$ is independent of r, we obtain by integration

$$\dot{Q}\ln\frac{r_2}{r_1} = -2\pi k(T_2 - T_1)$$

and thus the heat flow *per unit length of tube* is

$$\dot{Q} = -\frac{2\pi k(T_2 - T_1)}{\ln(r_2/r_1)} \tag{21.14}$$

Considering a compound tube of n concentric layers, with fluid flowing through it and around it (Fig. 21.6b), it is possible to derive an expression for the overall heat transfer coefficient *per unit length of tube U'*, analogous to equation (21.13) for the plane parallel wall. If T_a and T_b are the temperatures of the fluids inside and outside the wall respectively, the rate of heat flow per unit length of tube is

$$\dot{Q} = -U'(T_b - T_a)$$

And using the same argument as in the previous section for deriving (21.13), it may be shown that U' is given by the expression

$$\frac{1}{U'} = \frac{1}{2\pi r_0\alpha_a} + \sum_{i=1}^{n}\frac{\ln(r_i/r_{i-1})}{2\pi k_i} + \frac{1}{2\pi r_n\alpha_b} \tag{21.15}$$

Here α_a and α_b are the respective total surface heat transfer coefficients, i.e. $(\alpha_{ca} + \alpha_{ra})$ and $(\alpha_{cb} + \alpha_{rb})$.*

---

* It will be apparent after reading Chapter 23 that, unless the internal fluid is radiating, α_{ra} must be zero.

In the case of a single thin tube of thickness Δx, for which the inner and outer radii are nearly equal, (21.15) reduces to

$$\frac{1}{U'} = \frac{1}{2\pi r \alpha_a} + \frac{\Delta x}{2\pi r k} + \frac{1}{2\pi r \alpha_b}$$

Hence the overall heat transfer coefficient *per unit area* of tube wall is

$$\frac{1}{U} = \frac{1}{\alpha_a} + \frac{\Delta x}{k} + \frac{1}{\alpha_b}$$

which is identical with the expression for a flat plate.

21.4 The differential equation of three-dimensional conduction

In the previous sections only one-dimensional steady conduction has been considered, i.e. when the temperature only varies in the direction of heat flow and is uniform over any plane surface normal to the direction of flow. To calculate the heat flow through a conductor of any arbitrary shape, it will be shown that the problem reduces to one of finding the temperature distribution in the conductor, and once this is known the problem is effectively solved. A three-dimensional equation will be derived which is applicable to both steady and unsteady conduction. In subsequent sections it will be applied first to steady and then to unsteady conduction. 'Steady' implies that the temperature at any point does not change with time.

Consider a solid body having a plan view of the shape shown in Fig. 21.7. To get a picture of the temperature distribution, points of equal temperature can be joined to form *isothermal surfaces* (Fig. 21.7 shows these only in two dimensions). The picture of the temperature distribution is called the *temperature field*.

Here we shall consider only materials which are homogeneous and isotropic:

Fig. 21.7
Heat flow in the corner of a wall

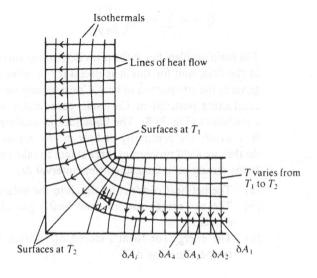

Isothermals

Lines of heat flow

Surfaces at T_1

T varies from T_1 to T_2

Surfaces at T_2

δA_i δA_4 δA_3 δA_2 δA_1

509

homogeneous because their density, specific heat and thermal conductivity are the same everywhere in the temperature field; isotropic because the thermal conductivity at any point is the same in all directions. For such materials the flow of heat is in the direction of maximum temperature gradient, i.e. at right angles to the isothermal surfaces. The *lines of heat flow*, which therefore cut the isothermal surfaces orthogonally, are also shown in Fig. 21.7.

Consider any elemental area dA; the heat flow through this element during a time interval dt is given by Fourier's law as

$$dQ = -k\,dA\left(\frac{\partial T}{\partial n}\right)dt$$

or the rate of heat flow is given by

$$d\dot{Q} = -k\,dA\left(\frac{\partial T}{\partial n}\right) \qquad (21.16)$$

where $(\partial T/\partial n)$ is the temperature gradient *normal* to dA. The following procedure may be adopted for calculating the total rate of heat flow through the conductor once the temperature distribution, or *temperature field*, is known. An isothermal surface is selected and divided into elemental areas δA_1, δA_2 etc., and the normal gradient is found for each element. For steady flow, any isothermal surface may be chosen because the total rate of heat flow is the same for all such surfaces. Thus the rate of heat flow through dA_1 is

$$\delta\dot{Q}_1 = -k\,\delta A_1\left(\frac{\partial T}{\partial n}\right)_1$$

where $(\partial T/\partial n)_1$ is the temperature gradient normal to the isothermal surface at δA_1. The total rate of heat flow through the material can be found by integrating this equation over the whole area A of the isothermal surface, and hence

$$\dot{Q} = -\sum_{i=1}^{n} k\,\delta A_i\left(\frac{\partial T}{\partial n}\right)_i \qquad (21.17)$$

The main problem lies in the prior determination of the temperature distribution in the field, and for this it is necessary to solve the differential equation that governs the conduction of heat. Consider any volume element $(dx\,dy\,dz)$ of the conducting material in Cartesian coordinates with its edges parallel to the coordinates (Fig. 21.8). The basic idea in establishing the differential equation is to satisfy the continuity of flow in any region of the temperature fluid. To do this, we shall proceed in three stages to take account of the following energy terms during an infinitesimal time interval dt:

(a) The net heat conduction dQ_c into the volume element
(b) The net energy (or 'internal heat') generation dQ_g within the volume element
(c) The energy (or 'heat') stored dQ_s within the element as a result of a temperature rise dT.

Fig. 21.8
Derivation of the
differential equation of
conduction

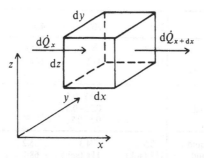

All three can be positive or negative, but energy conservation demands that

$$dQ_s = dQ_c + dQ_g$$

Let us proceed by first thinking of the volume element $(dx\,dy\,dz)$ in steady flow without internal heat generation. The heat inflow must be equal to the heat outflow, otherwise the temperature of the element will change with time. The rate of heat inflow through the left-hand face $(dy\,dz)$, i.e. in the x-direction, is

$$d\dot{Q}_x = -k(dy\,dz)\left(\frac{\partial T}{\partial x}\right)$$

and the outflow from the right-hand face $(dy\,dz)$ is

$$d\dot{Q}_{x+dx} = -k(dy\,dz)\frac{\partial}{\partial x}\left\{T + \left(\frac{\partial T}{\partial x}\right)dx\right\}$$

$$= -k(dy\,dz)\left\{\left(\frac{\partial T}{\partial x}\right) + \left(\frac{\partial^2 T}{\partial x^2}\right)dx\right\}$$

Similar equations can be written down for the y- and z-directions. The net rate of heat inflow by conduction is thus

$$d\dot{Q}_c = (d\dot{Q}_x - d\dot{Q}_{x+dx}) + (d\dot{Q}_y - d\dot{Q}_{y+dy}) + (d\dot{Q}_z - d\dot{Q}_{z+dz})$$

$$= k(dx\,dy\,dz)\left(\frac{\partial^2 T}{\partial x^2} + \frac{\partial^2 T}{\partial y^2} + \frac{\partial^2 T}{\partial z^2}\right)$$

For steady flow $d\dot{Q}_c = 0$, hence

$$\frac{\partial^2 T}{\partial x^2} + \frac{\partial^2 T}{\partial y^2} + \frac{\partial^2 T}{\partial z^2} = 0 \qquad\qquad (21.18)$$

There may be energy generating sources inside the conducting material as the result, for example, of nuclear fission, or of a flow of electric current and the ohmic heating of the material. If $\dot{q}_g$ is the rate of the heat generated per unit volume, the total rate of heat generated in the volume element $(dx\,dy\,dz)$ is

$$d\dot{Q}_g = \dot{q}_g(dx\,dy\,dz)$$

For steady flow with internal energy generation, $d\dot{Q}_c + d\dot{Q}_g = 0$ and hence

$$k(dx\,dy\,dz)\left(\frac{\partial^2 T}{\partial x^2} + \frac{\partial^2 T}{\partial y^2} + \frac{\partial^2 T}{\partial z^2}\right) + \dot{q}_g(dx\,dy\,dz) = 0$$

Fig. 21.9
Some values of thermal
diffusivity

$$\kappa = \frac{k/\rho c_p}{10^{-6}\,[\text{m}^2/\text{s}]}$$

T/[K]	250	300	400	500	600	800
Aluminium	96.5	93.7	97.0	103	107	128
Copper	114	112	107	103	99.4	94.2
Steel (0.5% C)		15				
Glass		0.35–0.5				
Building brick		0.25–0.5				
Concrete		0.5–0.8				
Mercury liquid	3.9	4.3	5.2	6.0	7.3	8.0
Sodium liquid	117 (sol.)	114 (sol.)	68	68	66	60
Water (sat.)	1.24 (ice)	0.147	0.172	0.165		
Steam (sat.)		382	9.39	0.962		
Steam (1 atm)			25.2	41.5	62.7	120
H_2 (1 atm)	113	155	257	382	529	892
Air (1 atm)	15.7	22.2	37.6	55.6	75.4	119.1
CO_2 (1 atm)	7.60	11.0	19.5	30.8	44.8	71.5

or

$$\frac{\partial^2 T}{\partial x^2} + \frac{\partial^2 y}{\partial y^2} + \frac{\partial^2 T}{\partial z^2} + \frac{\dot{q}_g}{k} = 0 \tag{21.19}$$

The term $\dot{q}_g$ may be a function of position, i.e. $\dot{q}_g = f(x, y, z)$, but for steady flow it cannot be a function of time.

Finally, in unsteady conduction, energy may be stored by (or drained from) the element. If the temperature of the element rises at a rate of $(\partial T/\partial t)$, the rate of energy storage* amounts to

$$d\dot{Q}_s = (\text{heat capacity})\left(\frac{\partial T}{\partial t}\right)$$

$$= \rho c_p (dx\,dy\,dz)\left(\frac{\partial T}{\partial t}\right) = \left(\frac{\rho c_p}{k}\right) k(dx\,dy\,dz)\left(\frac{\partial T}{\partial t}\right)$$

An energy balance then prescribes that

$$d\dot{Q}_s = d\dot{Q}_c + d\dot{Q}_g$$

and hence

$$\frac{1}{\kappa}\left(\frac{\partial T}{\partial t}\right) = \frac{\partial^2 T}{\partial x^2} + \frac{\partial^2 T}{\partial y^2} + \frac{\partial^2 T}{\partial z^2} + \frac{\dot{q}_g}{k} \tag{21.20}$$

where $\kappa = k/\rho c_p$ is a dimensional group called the *thermal diffusivity* of the material; the dimensions are $[\text{length}]^2/[\text{time}]$ and typical values are given in Fig. 21.9. We shall meet κ again, not only in unsteady conduction but also in convection.

---

* It is more correct to say that the net inflow of heat is equal to the increase of internal energy of the layer plus the work done against adjacent layers in expansion or contraction. If the pressure in the wall and outside is constant, the relevant specific heat capacity is c_p as used here.

Equation (21.20) is normally referred to as the *general conduction equation* in Cartesian coordinates. It is not completely general, however, because it is restricted to isotropic and homogeneous materials as explained at the beginning of this section. Analytical solutions of equation (21.20) are possible only for relatively simple shapes of conductors. The following example of steady one-dimensional heat flow with internal heat generation illustrates how the boundary conditions are applied to the solution of the differential equation.

Example 21.2   An electric current of 34 000 A flows along a flat steel plate 1.25 cm thick and 10 cm wide. The temperature of one surface of the plate is 80 °C and that of the other is 95 °C. Find the temperature distribution across the plate, and the value and position of the maximum temperature. Also calculate the total amount of heat generated per metre length of plate and the flow of heat from each surface of the plate. The end effects along the short sides of the plate may be neglected, i.e. it may be assumed that no heat flows across these surfaces. It may also be assumed that the ohmic heating is generated uniformly across the section. The resistivity of the steel is $\rho = 12 \times 10^{-6}$ ohm cm, and its thermal conductivity is $k = 54$ W/m K.

This is essentially a one-dimensional problem with uniform heat generation throughout the conductor. The governing differential equation is

$$\frac{\partial^2 t}{\partial x^2} + \frac{q_g}{k} = 0$$

The heat generated per unit volume $\dot{q}_g$ is ρi^2, where i is the current density given by

$$i = \frac{34\,000\,[\text{A}]}{1.25 \times 10\,[\text{cm}^2]} = 2720\text{ A/cm}^2$$

Hence

$$\dot{q}_g = \rho i^2 = 12 \times 10^{-6}\,[\Omega\,\text{cm}] \times 2720^2\,[\text{A}^2/\text{cm}^4] = 88\,780\text{ kW/m}^3$$

The differential equation therefore becomes

$$\frac{\partial^2 T}{\partial x^2} + \frac{88\,78\,[\text{kW/m}^3]}{0.054\,[\text{kW/m K}]} = 0 \quad \text{or} \quad \frac{\partial^2 T}{\partial x^2} + 1\,664\,000\,[\text{K/m}^2] = 0$$

Integrating this equation, we obtain

$$T = -822\,000\,[\text{K/m}^2]x^2 + Ax + B$$

where A and B are constants to be determined from the boundary conditions.
Choosing the origin of the x-coordinate at the 95 °C surface of the plate (Fig. 21.10), we can write for $x = 0$ m

$$95\,°\text{C} = B$$

and for $x = 0.0125$ m

$$80\,[°\text{C}] = -822\,000(0.0125)^2\,[\text{K}] + A(0.0125)\,[\text{m}] + B$$

Fig. 21.10

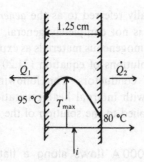

Hence the equation for the temperature variation with x becomes*

$$T = -822\,000[\text{K/m}^2]x^2 + 9075[\text{K/m}]x + 95[°\text{C}]$$

The temperature distribution is therefore parabolic. Differentiating with respect to x and equating to zero, we find the position of the maximum temperature, i.e.

$$\frac{dT}{dx} = -1\,644\,000[\text{K/m}^2]x + 9075[\text{K/m}] = 0$$

and

$$x = 0.005\,52\,\text{m} = 0.552\,\text{cm}$$

The value of the maximum temperature is

$$T_{max} = \{-822\,000(0.005\,52)^2 + 9075(0.005\,52) + 95\}[°\text{C}]$$

$$= 120°\text{C}$$

The heat flow *from* the plate across the 95 °C surface *per metre length* of bar is

$$\dot{Q}_1 = kA\left(\frac{dT}{dx}\right)_{x=0} = \left\{0.054 \times \frac{10 \times 1}{100} \times 9075\right\}[\text{kW}]$$

$$= 49.0\,\text{kW or kJ/s}$$

The heat flow *from* the plate across the 80 °C surface is

$$\dot{Q}_2 = -kA\left(\frac{dT}{dx}\right)_{x=0.0125}$$

$$= \left\{-0.054 \times \frac{10 \times 1}{100}(-11\,480)\right\}[\text{kW}] = 62.0\,\text{kW or kJ/s}$$

The sum of $\dot{Q}_1$ and $\dot{Q}_2$ which is equal to 111 kW must be equal to the total heat generated per unit length of plate by ohmic heating, i.e. $\dot{q}_g$ (volume/metre length). Thus

$$\dot{Q}_g = 88\,780[\text{kW/m}^3] \times (1 \times 0.0125 \times 0.1)[\text{m}^3] = 111\,\text{kW}$$

---

* Here it is clear from the context that T is a Celsius temperature. The equation involves the addition of two increments of temperature *change*, correctly expressed in K, to the boundary condition given as a Celsius temperature.

In the next section a numerical method of solution is introduced which can be applied to complicated shapes, and this method is applied to a two-dimensional example. A good survey of mathematical methods used for the solution of conduction problems is given in Ref. 10.

One other approach is via the electrical analogy. It is essentially an experimental approach, but it is easier to arrange for a flow of electricity than for a flow of heat, and to measure potential differences and currents rather than temperature differences and heat flows. The method makes use of the fact that the steady flow of electricity in a three-dimensional conductor is governed by the equation

$$\frac{\partial^2 \mathscr{V}}{\partial x^2} + \frac{\partial^2 \mathscr{V}}{\partial y^2} + \frac{\partial^2 \mathscr{V}}{\partial z^2} = 0$$

where $\mathscr{V}$ is the potential distribution $\mathscr{V} = f(x, y, z)$ throughout the conductor. This equation is clearly similar to equation (21.19). The current $\delta\mathscr{I}_1$ flowing through any elemental area δA_1 in a direction normal to δA_1 is

$$\delta\mathscr{I}_1 = -\frac{1}{\rho}\delta A_1\left(\frac{\partial \mathscr{V}}{\partial n}\right)_1$$

where ρ is the resistivity of the material. Summing over the whole of an isopotential surface, the total current is given by

$$\mathscr{I} = -\sum_{i=1}^{n}\frac{1}{\rho}\delta A_i\left(\frac{\partial \mathscr{V}}{\partial n}\right)_i$$

which is similar to equation (21.17). Thus potentials can be related to temperatures, and currents to heat flows.

Thinking of the two-dimensional corner of Fig. 21.7, a simple electrical analogue can be produced from a sheet of metallised paper of uniform and relatively high resistivity, cut to the appropriate shape, with copper strips placed along the boundaries. The low resistivity of the copper strips ensures that any voltages $\mathscr{V}_1$ and $\mathscr{V}_2$ applied to them will be uniform and analogous to the isothermal boundaries T_1 and T_2. The potential at any point in the field can be measured by a simple probe and voltmeter, and the corresponding temperature found from

$$\frac{T}{T_1 - T_2} = \frac{\mathscr{V}}{\mathscr{V}_1 - \mathscr{V}_2}$$

Once the temperature distribution has been obtained, the heat flow can be calculated using equation (21.17). More sophisticated analogues, capable of handling three-dimensional problems, can be built using an electrolytic solution in a tank with conducting sides of appropriate shape. For a detailed treatment the reader can turn to Ref. 40.

515

21.5 Numerical solution of two-dimensional steady conduction

It has been explained in the previous section that the solution of a multi-dimensional conduction problem consists essentially of finding the temperature distribution in the conducting material. This involves the solution of the differential equation (21.20), which may be extremely difficult except for a few simple shapes.* To solve this equation it is necessary to know the boundary conditions of the temperature field, e.g. the temperature distribution at the edge of the region considered, and the distribution of the internal heat sources if any. It can be proved (Ref. 9) that, for any given shape and boundary conditions, there is only the one solution to (21.20), i.e. there is only one possible temperature distribution.

This section describes an approximate numerical method for solving two-dimensional steady conduction problems. For such problems equation (21.20) reduces to

$$\frac{\partial^2 T}{\partial x^2} + \frac{\partial^2 T}{\partial y^2} + \frac{\dot{q}_g}{k} = 0 \qquad (21.21)$$

The object of the numerical method is to find values of the temperature in the conducting material at a limited number of points. It is most convenient to cover the region considered by a square net, and to find the temperature at the mesh points (Fig. 21.11). Whereas a general analytic solution gives the values of the temperature everywhere in the field as a function $T = \phi(x, y)$, the numerical method merely finds numerical values of the temperature at the mesh

Fig. 21.11
Relaxation method applied to two-dimensional conduction

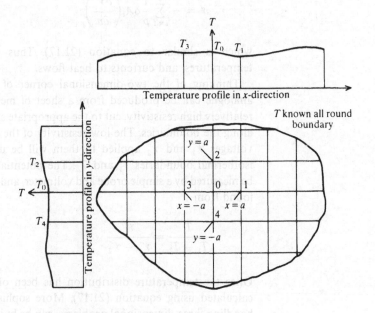

* For analytical methods see Refs 3 and 19.

points selected. Temperatures at other points can then be found by some method of interpolation.

It is possible to view the temperature field as a temperature surface or a relief map in the three-dimensional Cartesian coordinates (x, y, T); the variation of T in the x- and y-directions may be visualised by taking sections through the surface in these directions. Taking any mesh point 0 as the origin of the coordinates, it is often possible to express the variation of temperature T in each of the x- and y-directions by a power series, i.e.

$$T = b_0 + b_1 x + b_2 x^2 + b_3 x^3 + \ldots]_{y = \text{constant}}$$

$$T = c_0 + c_1 y + c_2 y^2 + c_3 y^3 + \ldots]_{x = \text{constant}}$$

This can always be done when T varies continuously in the field. By means of Maclaurin's theorem it is possible to express the value of T at any distance x from 0 in terms of differential coefficients of $T = \phi(x)$ at $x = 0$. Thus

$$T_0 = b_0$$

$$\left(\frac{\partial T}{\partial x} \right)_0 = 1 b_1$$

$$\left(\frac{\partial^2 T}{\partial x^2} \right)_0 = 1 \times 2 b_2$$

$$\left(\frac{\partial^3 T}{\partial x^3} \right)_0 = 1 \times 2 \times 3 b_3 \quad \text{and so on}$$

And the variation of T in the x-direction can be written as

$$T = T_0 + \left(\frac{\partial T}{\partial x} \right)_0 \frac{x}{1!} + \left(\frac{\partial^2 T}{\partial x^2} \right)_0 \frac{x^2}{2!} + \left(\frac{\partial^3 T}{\partial x^3} \right)_0 \frac{x^2}{3!} + \ldots$$

The values of the temperature at the mesh points 1 and 3, at distances $x = a$ and $x = -a$ from 0 respectively, are therefore given by

$$T_1 = T_0 + \left(\frac{\partial T}{\partial x} \right)_0 \frac{a}{1!} + \left(\frac{\partial^2 T}{\partial x^2} \right)_0 \frac{a^2}{2!} + \left(\frac{\partial^3 T}{\partial x^3} \right)_0 \frac{a^3}{3!} + \ldots$$

and

$$T_3 = T_0 - \left(\frac{\partial T}{\partial x} \right)_0 \frac{a}{1!} + \left(\frac{\partial^2 T}{\partial x^2} \right)_0 \frac{a^2}{2!} - \left(\frac{\partial^3 T}{\partial x^3} \right)_0 \frac{a^3}{3!} + \ldots$$

Hence, neglecting fourth-power and higher terms,

$$T_1 + T_3 = 2T_0 + a^2 \left(\frac{\partial^2 T}{\partial x^2} \right)_0 \tag{21.22}$$

This approximation can be made if the chosen mesh width a is sufficiently small; it will be explained in Example 21.3 how it is possible to tell when a is small enough for the fourth-power term to be negligible.

Fig. 21.12
The conducting rod
analogy

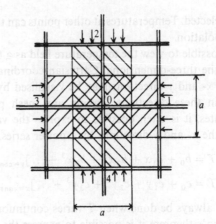

By similar reasoning it can be shown that

$$T_2 + T_4 = 2T_0 + a^2\left(\frac{\partial^2 T}{\partial y^2}\right)_0 \tag{21.23}$$

where T_2 and T_4 are the temperatures at the mesh points 2 and 4 respectively. Substituting (21.22) and (21.23) in (21.21), we get

$$\left(\frac{\partial^2 T}{\partial x^2}\right)_0 + \left(\frac{\partial^2 T}{\partial y^2}\right)_0 + \frac{\dot{q}_g}{k} = \frac{T_1 + T_2 + T_3 + T_4 - 4T_0}{a^2} + \frac{\dot{q}_g}{k} = 0 \tag{21.24}$$

The finite difference relation (21.24) can also be deduced in a somewhat easier way. The homogeneous conducting material can be imagined to be replaced by conducting rods connecting the mesh points (Fig. 21.12), and the conductivity of the rods is chosen to be equivalent to the conductivity of the shaded region. Considering *unit depth of material* (i.e. perpendicular to the paper), the flow through the rod from mesh point 1 to 0 is

$$\dot{Q}_1 = -k(1 \times a)\frac{T_0 - T_1}{a} = -k(T_0 - T_1)$$

The total flow towards the mesh point 0 from 1, 2, 3, 4 is therefore

$$\dot{Q} = \dot{Q}_1 + \dot{Q}_2 + \dot{Q}_3 + \dot{Q}_4$$
$$= -k(T_0 - T_1) - k(T_0 - T_2) - k(T_0 - T_3) - k(T_0 - T_4)$$
$$= k(T_1 + T_2 + T_3 + T_4 - 4T_0)$$

If the heat generated per unit volume is $\dot{q}_g$, the equivalent heat that is generated at each mesh point is $\dot{q}_g a^2$. With steady flow, for reasons of continuity, it follows that

$$k(T_1 + T_2 + T_3 + T_4 - 4T_0) + \dot{q}_g a^2 = 0$$

which is equivalent to (21.24).

An equation of the form (21.24) can be written down for each mesh point in the field. Thus the differential equation, which must be satisfied everywhere in the field, can be replaced by a finite difference relation which must be satisfied at a finite number of points in the field. The accuracy of the numerical solution depends on the density of the mesh chosen.

In principle, to obtain a numerical solution it is necessary to write down a linear equation corresponding to (21.24) for each mesh point, and the solution of the differential equation is thus reduced to a solution of a finite number of linear simultaneous equations. In practice the solution of these equations by conventional methods is not feasible, because the large number of simultaneous equations would result in considerable labour. When several problems of the same type are to be solved, it is probably worth writing a computer program, making use of matrices. For the occasional problem, or for checking a program, a convenient procedure of successive approximation by the *relaxation method* can be used: this method is best explained by a numerical example.

Example 21.3 The temperature of one side of a long 18 cm thick wall is 100 °C, and of the other is 400 °C. Metal ribs, 48 cm apart, project 6 cm into the high-temperature side. The conductivity of the ribs is very high compared with the conductivity of the wall, so that their temperature may be assumed to be 400 °C. Calculate the steady rate of heat flow through each 48 cm segment of the wall, and also find the heat flow if the ribs were omitted.

A typical segment covered with a 6 cm square mesh is drawn in Fig. 21.13. To solve the problem, the boundary conditions all round the segment must be known. The upper part of the figure shows the approximate shape of the isothermals, and it is evident that it is reasonable to assume that at sections 1–1 and 3–3 the temperature gradient perpendicular to the wall is constant. The boundary values of temperature around the segment are thus fully determined, and are underlined.

The next step in the solution is to guess the temperatures at all the mesh points. Although the process of successive approximation will finally provide the best answer obtainable with the coarse mesh chosen, a reasonably close estimate will of course shorten the procedure. By a rough process of interpolation it is possible to select a reasonable set of temperatures, and their values are shown in the top left-hand quadrants at each mesh point. Owing to the symmetry of the segment about section 2–2, only half of it need be considered.

The finite difference relation (21.24) must be satisfied at each mesh point. Checking this at point b, for example, we find that

$$T_c + 100 + T_a + T_f - 4T_b = 220 + 100 + 200 + 310 - (4 \times 205) = 10$$

The error, of magnitude 10, is called the *residual* at point b, and it is entered into the top right-hand quadrant at the mesh point. Similarly all other residuals are found and entered in corresponding positions. The object of the process of relaxation is to modify all the guessed temperature values until the residuals have vanished, i.e. until all the residuals are 'relaxed'.

The alterations to the initial guesses are written above the temperatures, and one alteration is carried out at a time. The procedure is to start with the mesh point which has the numerically largest residual, i.e. point d. It is clear from the finite difference relation (21.24) that if we increase the value of the

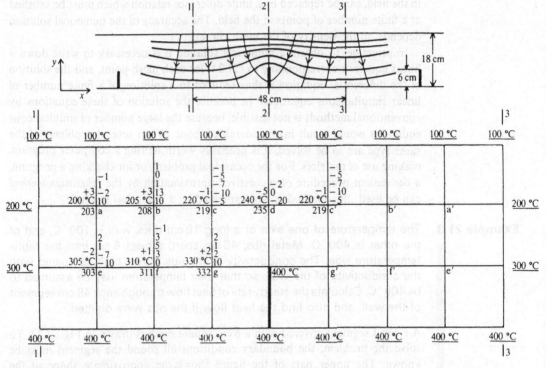

18 cm

6 cm

|← 48 cm →|

y↑
x

|1 |2 |3 | | | | | | | |3

100 °C	100 °C	100 °C	100 °C	100 °C	100 °C	100 °C	100 °C	100 °C	100 °C
	−1 1	1 0	−1 −5 −7	−2	−1 −5 −7				
	+3 −2	+3 13	−1 −10	−5 0 −20	−1 −10				
200 °C	200 °C 10	205 °C 10	220 °C −5	240 °C −20	220 °C −5				**200 °C**
	203 a	208 b	219 c	235 d	219 c′	b′	a′		
	2	3 5	2 1						
	−2 −7	+1 3	+2 2						
300 °C	305 °C −10	310 °C 0	330 °C 10	400 °C		g′	f′	e′	**300 °C**
	303 e	311 f	332 g						
400 °C	400 °C	400 °C	400 °C	400 °C	400 °C	400 °C	400 °C	400 °C	**400 °C**

|1 | | | | | | | | |3

Fig. 21.13 Relaxation of the 6 cm mesh

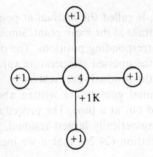

temperature by 1 K at a mesh point, we alter the residual by −4 at that point. Also, applying (21.24) to the four neighbouring points, we see that their residuals are altered as a result of this change by +1 each. The basic operation of +1 K applied to any mesh point is expressed by the *relaxation operator* of Fig. 21.14. To eliminate the residual at point d, we must change the temperature by −20/4 = −5 K. The residual 0 is entered at d, and the residuals at c and c′ are changed from −5 to −10. As the other two neighbouring points of d are fixed boundary temperatures, i.e. 100 °C and 400 °C, no alteration is made at these points. From the new set of residuals, again the largest is selected and the procedure is repeated. The relaxation is continued in the order shown in the table given below. It should be noted that when T_c is altered by −1 K, the residual at d is changed by −2 and not by −1; we have to consider point c′

at the same time for reasons of symmetry. It will also be noted that to avoid fractional changes in temperature, we do not always reduce the residuals to zero in any one operation. To avoid fractional temperatures in the final solution, the residuals are not completely relaxed, but their algebraic sum for the whole segment should be made as near zero as possible. The changes in temperature are added to the initial guesses at each mesh point, and the algebraic sum is located in the bottom left-hand quadrant. (There is only one change of temperature at each mesh point in this example, but in other cases more than one change at some of the points may be necessary before the mesh is relaxed.)

Residual at	a	b	c, c'	d	e	f	g
Initial set of residuals	10	10	−5	−20	−10	0	10
Operation:							
(1) −5 K at d			−10	0			
(2) +3 K at a	−2	13			−7		
(3) +3 K at b	1	1	−7			3	
(4) +2 K at g			−5			5	2
(5) −2 K at e	−1				1	3	
(6) −1 K at c		0	−1	−2			1
(7) +1 K at f		1			2	−1	2
Sum of final set of residuals = 0	−1	1	−1	−2	2	−1	2

To calculate the heat flow through the wall, we may make use of the 'conducting rod' analogy described previously. Thus the heat flow from b to the wall surface (per metre height of wall, perpendicular to the paper) is $-k(100[°C] - T_b)$. Hence the total outflow from the section, taking account of its symmetry, is

$$\dot{Q}_{out} = k(200 - 100) + 2k(203 - 100) + 2k(208 - 100)$$
$$+ 2k(219 - 100) + k(235 - 100) = 895[K]k$$

To check, we may calculate the inflow from the hot face, which is

$$\dot{Q}_{in} = k(400 - 300) + 2k(400 - 303) + 2k(400 - 311)$$
$$+ 4k(400 - 332) + k(400 - 235) = 909[K]k$$

The $4k$ term arises because of the contribution from the metal rib to points g and g'. We may take as the answer the average value

$$\dot{Q} = \frac{\dot{Q}_{in} + \dot{Q}_{out}}{2} = \frac{909k + 895k}{2} = 902[K]k$$

In order to check whether the mesh is sufficiently fine, i.e. that a is small enough for the fourth-power term to be neglected in the Maclaurin expansion, the process must be repeated with a finer mesh. If the new temperatures differ only slightly from the old values, the mesh is sufficiently fine; otherwise we must proceed to an even finer mesh. Labour is saved if the original points are

Fig. 21.15
Relaxation of the
$6/\sqrt{2}$ cm mesh

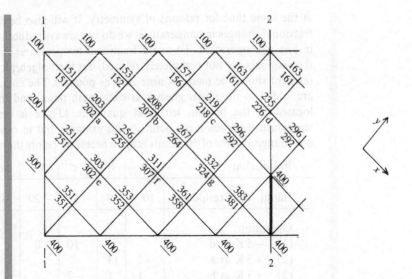

featured in the new mesh, and we may choose one of $6/\sqrt{2}$ cm width, as shown in Fig. 21.15. The values of temperature at a, b, c, d, e, f, g are taken from the previous solution, and the values of the new points are found by interpolation. It follows from the derivation of equation (21.21) that the rotation of the coordinates (termed 'transformation') has no effect on this differential equation, and hence the same finite difference relation applies.

After relaxing, we find that T_d undergoes the largest change, i.e. from 235 °C to 226 °C. Recalculating the average heat flow, we find that

$$\tfrac{1}{2}(\dot{Q}_{in} + \dot{Q}_{out}) = \tfrac{1}{2}(862k + 880k) = 871\,[\text{K}]\,k$$

Using a mesh of 3 cm, T_d becomes 225 °C, and the average heat flow

$$\tfrac{1}{2}(\dot{Q}_{in} + \dot{Q}_{out}) = \tfrac{1}{2}(875k + 877k) = 876\,[\text{K}]\,k$$

Thus, by progressively choosing a finer mesh, we can converge as close to an accurate solution as we wish. Without the ribs the heat flow through a 48 cm segment of the wall would be

$$\dot{Q} = -k\frac{0.48 \times 1(100 - 400)}{0.18} = 800\,[\text{K}]\,k$$

If it is impossible to fit a square net accurately into the boundary of the region considered, there may be mesh points near the boundary with links shorter than a (Fig. 21.16). It can be shown that the difference relation to be satisfied for such a point is

$$\frac{2T_1}{\xi(1 + \xi)} + \frac{2T_2}{\eta(1 + \eta)} + \frac{2T_3}{(1 + \xi)} + \frac{2T_4}{(1 + \eta)} - 2T_0\left(\frac{1}{\xi} + \frac{1}{\eta}\right) + \frac{\dot{q}_g a^2}{k} = 0 \quad (21.25)$$

There are numerous tricks by means of which the process of relaxation may be shortened. For these and more complicated types of problem, the reader is referred to Ref. 1.

Fig. 21.16
A mesh point near an
irregular boundary

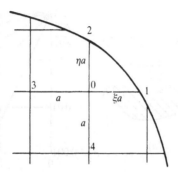

The 'random' selection of the largest absolute residual in the relaxation process is suitable for hand calculations because this leads to rapid convergence. When a computer is available, such a procedure would not be appropriate and a line-by-line iteration process is preferable. The residuals in a line are eliminated by solving the linear equations pertaining to that line assuming that the temperature values in the two adjacent lines are 'correct'. The procedure involves sweeping repeatedly line by line through the region until the required accuracy is attained. It is helpful to sweep in the direction of lesser temperature gradients to achieve rapid convergence. Ref. 43 describes one such computer-based procedure in some detail.

At the end of section 21.4 we saw how a simple electrical analogue can be constructed to provide a solution to the two-dimensional form of equation (21.19). Often it is preferable to have, not an analogue providing a 'continuous' solution, but one which is equivalent to the 'lumped' approximation represented by Fig. 21.11 or the conducting rod picture of Fig. 21.12. A mesh of resistances connecting junctions 0, 1, 2, 3, 4 etc. can be used, and voltage and current measurements obtained from this provide an equivalent to the approximate numerical solution. The advantage of a lumped circuit is that 'heat sources' can be easily incorporated, and unsteady flow can be simulated by inserting capacitances at the mesh points (Ref. 29).

21.6 Unsteady conduction

It is frequently of interest to know the heat flow through a solid when the flow is not steady, e.g. through the wall of a furnace that is being heated or cooled, or through the cylinder wall of an internal-combustion engine. To calculate the heat flow under these conditions it is again first necessary to find the temperature distribution in the solid; in this case, however, the distribution varies continuously with time. We shall consider two simple cases of some practical importance.

21.6.1 The quenching of a billet

When a metal billet of uniform temperature T is suddenly plunged into a large liquid bath of temperature T_s, the internal resistance to heat flow is often small

Fig. 21.17
The quenching of a billet

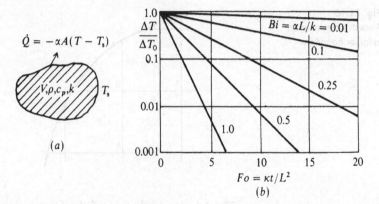

$$\dot{Q} = -\alpha A(T - T_s)$$

$V, \rho, c_p, k \qquad T_s$

(a)

(b)

compared with the resistance between the billet surface and the fluid. This may be the case in the quenching of small steel components during heat treatment. It is then reasonable to assume that the temperature T, though changing with time t, is nevertheless uniform throughout the billet at any instant.

Let the billet in Fig. 21.17a have a volume V, surface area A, density ρ and specific heat capacity c_p, and let us assume that the surface heat transfer coefficient between the billet and the liquid is constant and equal to α. Further, we may treat the bath as large enough for its temperature to be substantially constant at T_s. The energy lost by the billet during a time interval dt is equal to the heat transferred to the liquid, and can be expressed by the equation

$$dQ = \rho c_p V \frac{dT}{dt} = -\alpha A(T - T_s)$$

or, if we write $\Delta T = T - T_s$,

$$\frac{d(\Delta T)}{\Delta T} = -\frac{\alpha A}{\rho c_p V} dt$$

This equation can be integrated, and with boundary conditions $\Delta T = \Delta T_0 = T_0 - T_s$ at $t_0 = 0$ the result is

$$\ln \frac{\Delta T}{\Delta T_0} = -\frac{\alpha A t}{\rho c_p V} \quad \text{or} \quad \frac{\Delta T}{\Delta T_0} = \exp\{-(\alpha A t / \rho c_p V)\}$$

It will be noted that the solution depends on the shape of the billet only in so far as this determines the ratio of volume to surface area V/A, and this ratio is a linear dimension which we shall denote by L. Introducing L and the thermal conductivity k for the billet in the manner shown below, and writing the thermal diffusivity κ for the group $k/\rho c_p$, the index can be written as

$$\frac{\alpha A t}{\rho c_p V} = \left(\frac{\alpha}{k}\frac{V}{A}\right)\left\{\frac{k}{\rho c_p}\left(\frac{A}{V}\right)^2 t\right\} = \left(\frac{\alpha L}{k}\right)\left(\frac{\kappa t}{L^2}\right) = (Bi)(Fo)$$

and hence

$$\frac{\Delta T}{\Delta T_0} = \exp\{-(Bi)(Fo)\} \tag{21.26}$$

The solution for this simple case can be expressed in terms of two dimensionless groups—the *Biot number* $Bi = \alpha L/k$ and the *Fourier number* $Fo = \kappa t/L^2$—which are also important parameters in more complicated situations of unsteady conduction. These groups require further comment.

Bi is a measure of the relative resistance to heat flow of the inside of the solid to that of the adjacent fluid. A low Biot number implies that most of the resistance is in the fluid boundary layer; a high Biot number implies that most of the resistance is within the solid. The solution for the billet given by equation (21.26) applies only to relatively low values of Bi because of the initial assumption made about the internal resistance. It is important to note that Bi differs from the Nusselt number $Nu = \alpha L/k$, which we shall meet in the study of convection, in that Nu contains the *fluid* conductivity.

Fo represents a dimensionless time-scale. It contains the dimensional group $\kappa = k/\rho c_p$, called the thermal diffusivity of the material, which we have already met when deriving the differential equation of three-dimensional conduction in section 21.4.

The solution (21.26) for the billet can be represented in a simple graphical way, by plotting $\Delta T/\Delta T_0$ on a logarithmic scale against a linear scale of Fo. Lines of constant Bi radiate from $\Delta T/\Delta T_0 = 1$ as shown in Fig. 21.17b.

When the internal resistance of the billet is not negligible, the temperature history becomes a function of the spatial coordinates also. To establish the temperature field as a function of time it is necessary to solve the differential equation of unsteady three-dimensional conduction, equation (21.20). A solution for the temperature field then takes the form

$$\frac{\Delta T}{\Delta T_0} = f\left(Bi, Fo, \frac{x}{L}, \frac{y}{L}, \frac{z}{L} \right)$$

where L is any suitably chosen linear dimension of the solid (not necessarily V/A as in the present case). Solutions have been obtained for a large variety of shapes for the initial conditions considered here, namely a uniform initial temperature in the solid which is then subjected to a step change of ambient temperature. When presented graphically, such solutions appear very much like Fig. 21.17b, except that each point (x, y, z) within the solid requires a separate chart. For example, considering the radial-symmetrical case of a sphere,

$$\frac{\Delta T}{\Delta T_0} = f\left(Bi, Fo, \frac{r}{r_0} \right)$$

where r_0 is the outer radius of the sphere; a separate chart is needed for each value of $0 < r < r_0$ of interest. Typical charts of this kind can be found in Refs 41 and 42.

21.6.2 Numerical solution of unsteady one-dimensional conduction

In section 21.6.1 we presented a solution for the case where T is not a function of position. We shall now proceed with the more general case where T varies with position and also consider more difficult boundary conditions; but we

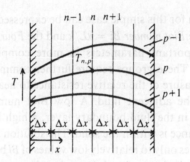

Fig. 21.18
Unsteady one-dimensional
conduction

shall restrict ourselves to one-dimensional flow. A numerical method will be
used to obtain the solution, first when the boundary condition is given in the
form of a prescribed temperature variation of the solid surface, and then when
it is given as a variation of ambient fluid temperature coupled with a known,
but not necessarily constant, surface heat transfer coefficient.

Before the numerical method can be outlined, it is necessary to adapt the
differential equation (21.20) derived in section 21.4 to one-dimensional conduction.
This is done simply by dropping the y and z terms. Moreover, we shall restrict
ourselves in what follows to conduction without internal heat generation. The
governing equation then becomes

$$\frac{\partial T}{\partial t} = \kappa \left(\frac{\partial^2 T}{\partial x^2} \right) \tag{21.27}$$

The next step is to develop a finite difference relation which can be used to
determine the temperature at a discrete number of sections, such as $n - 1$, n,
$n + 1$, separated by equal space intervals Δx as in Fig. 21.18. Since the
temperature at these planes varies with time, it is necessary to find values at
successive instants of time, $p - 1$, p, $p + 1$, which are conveniently separated
by equal time intervals Δt. Thus each temperature will be denoted by two
subscripts; $T_{n,p}$, for example, means the temperature in the wall at section n at
the instant p. By making use of equation (21.22), the differential coefficient
$(\partial^2 T / \partial x^2)$ in equation (21.27) can be replaced by

$$\left(\frac{\partial^2 T}{\partial x^2} \right)_{n,p} = \frac{T_{n+1,p} + T_{n-1,p} - 2T_{n,p}}{\Delta x^2} \tag{21.28}$$

The differential coefficient $(\partial T / \partial t)$ can be written*

$$\left(\frac{\partial T}{\partial t} \right)_{n,p} = \frac{T_{n,p+1} - T_{n,p}}{\Delta t} \tag{21.29}$$

It follows that equation (21.27), applied to section n at time p, can be replaced

---

* It may appear more obvious to replace $(\partial T / \partial t)_{n,p}$ by a 'time-centred' finite difference ratio over
the period, $(\partial T / \partial t)_{n,p} = (T_{n,p+1} - T_{n,p-1})/2\Delta t$, but it is found that solutions involving this
approximation become unstable in the sense briefly explained after Example 21.4.

by the finite difference relation

$$T_{n,p+1} - T_{n,p} = \frac{\kappa \Delta t}{\Delta x^2}(T_{n+1,p} + T_{n-1,p} - 2T_{n,p}) \tag{21.30}$$

$\kappa \Delta t / \Delta x^2$ will be recognised as a Fourier number similar to that encountered in section 21.6.1, and equation (21.30) can thus be written as

$$T_{n,p+1} = (Fo)\left\{T_{n+1,p} + T_{n-1,p} + \left(\frac{1}{Fo} - 2\right)T_{n,p}\right\} \tag{21.31}$$

Although the Fourier number Fo can be given any desired value by appropriate choice of Δt and Δx, we shall see later that not all values are acceptable. Taking typical values of Fo used in practice, we obtain

$$\text{For } Fo = \tfrac{1}{2}: \qquad T_{n,p+1} = \tfrac{1}{2}(T_{n+1,p} + T_{n-1,p}) \tag{21.31a}$$

$$\text{For } Fo = \tfrac{1}{3}: \qquad T_{n,p+1} = \tfrac{1}{3}(T_{n+1,p} + T_{n-1,p} + T_{n,p}) \tag{21.31b}$$

$$\text{For } Fo = \tfrac{1}{4}: \qquad T_{n,p+1} = \tfrac{1}{4}(T_{n+1,p} + T_{n-1,p} + 2T_{n,p}) \tag{21.31c}$$

Such equations can be seen to give the 'future' temperature $T_{n,p+1}$ as a weighted average of the 'present' temperatures at planes $n-1$, n, $n+1$.

In order to find a solution of equation (21.27), whether analytically or via equation (21.30), boundary conditions must be specified. It is essential to know (a) the temperature distribution through the wall at some time t_0, and (b) the variation of temperature with time at two boundary planes. A simple example, where the temperature distribution is initially uniform, will show how the computation might be set out for desk calculation.

Example 21.4 A wall is 25 cm thick and initially, at $t = 0$, the temperature is uniform throughout at 100 °C. One surface is maintained at 100 °C, while the other increases linearly with time to 700 °C in two hours. Determine the temperature distribution at the end of this period if the thermal diffusivity of the material is $0.52 \times 10^{-6} \, \text{m}^2/\text{s}$.

We will choose five space intervals, so that $\Delta x = 0.05 \, \text{m}$. Then if Fo is to be $\tfrac{1}{4}$ say, the time interval will be

$$\Delta t = \frac{Fo \Delta x^2}{\kappa} = \frac{\tfrac{1}{4} \times 0.05^2}{0.52 \times 10^{-6} \times 3600} = 0.334 \, \text{h}$$

In this example, with $Fo = \tfrac{1}{4}$, six time increments of Δt fit almost exactly into a 2 h period. If this were not so it would be possible to use a value of Fo not exactly equal to a round figure, but a better way would be to calculate the temperatures just before and just after the required time and interpolate the temperatures obtaining at that time.

Applying equation (21.31c) we get the results shown in the table (the boundary conditions being in bold type); the equation for $T_{2,1\frac{1}{3}}$, for example, is

$$T_{2,1\frac{1}{3}} = \tfrac{1}{4}\{101.6 + 207.8 + (2 \times 118.7)\} = 136.7 \, ^\circ\text{C}$$

The final line of figures gives the desired temperature distribution.

Hours	T_0	T_1	T_2	T_3	T_4	T_5
0	100	100	100	100	100	100
$\frac{1}{3}$	200	100	100	100	100	100
$\frac{2}{3}$	300	125	100	100	100	100
1	400	162.5	106.2	100	100	100
$1\frac{1}{3}$	500	207.8	118.7	101.6	100	100
$1\frac{2}{3}$	600	258.6	136.7	105.5	100.4	100
2	700	313.4	159.4	112.0	101.6	100

The rates of heat flow through planes $n-1$, n, $n+1$ are not equal (and vary with time) as a result of the storage of energy in the material between the planes. But once the temperature distributions have been obtained, the amount of heat flowing through some plane n during a time interval Δt can be estimated from the average temperature gradient $(\partial T/\partial x)_n$ at that section during this time interval, i.e.

$$Q_n = -kA\left(\frac{\partial T}{\partial x}\right)_n \Delta t \tag{21.32}$$

The average temperature gradient for calculating Q_n during the time interval Δt, from p to $p+1$, would be

$$\left(\frac{\partial T}{\partial x}\right)_{n,p+\frac{1}{2}} = \frac{1}{4\Delta x}\{(T_{n+1,p} + T_{n+1,p+1}) - (T_{n-1,p} + T_{n-1,p+1})\} \tag{21.33}$$

The question arises whether Fo can be chosen arbitrarily, i.e. whether Δx and Δt can be chosen independently. If it can, this would imply that the coefficient $\{(1/Fo) - 2\}$ of the temperature $T_{n,p}$ in equation (21.31) can assume negative values, namely when $Fo > \frac{1}{2}$. In fact a choice of $Fo > \frac{1}{2}$ would imply, from equation (21.31), that the higher the value of $T_{n,p}$ the lower will be the resulting value of $T_{n,p+1}$; it can be shown by the following argument that this may lead to difficulties vis-à-vis the Law of Conservation of Energy. Let us assume that at a given instant p the distribution of temperature is as in Fig. 21.19. Referring to equation (21.30), the longer the chosen time interval Δt and therefore the higher the value of Fo, other things being equal, the higher will be the rise $(T_{n,p+1} - T_{n,p})$. Provided T_{n+1} and T_{n-1} do not change during Δt, the maximum permissible rise of $T_{n,p+1}$ is to point A, because then the inflow of heat to section

Fig. 21.19
Criterion for Fo

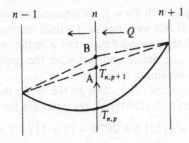

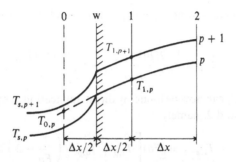

Fig. 21.20
Varying fluid temperature as a boundary condition

n is exactly balanced by the outflow. This can be seen to correspond to a value of $Fo = \frac{1}{2}$, equation (21.31a). Inspection of the temperature gradients shows that a rise to point B, obtained by making $Fo > \frac{1}{2}$, would imply that an increase of temperature is obtained with a heat outflow from section n which is larger than the heat inflow, and this clearly contradicts the Law of Conservation of Energy. Of course $Fo = \frac{1}{2}$ does not represent an absolute limiting criterion—because T_{n+1} and T_{n-1} will themselves change during Δt and, depending upon whether they rise or fall, the criterion could in principle be somewhat larger or smaller than $Fo = \frac{1}{2}$. Nevertheless, because the method finds $T_{n,p+1}$ in terms of temperatures at instant p, neglecting what happens to T_{n+1} and T_{n-1} during Δt, the relevant criterion for self-consistency of the method is

$$Fo \leqslant \tfrac{1}{2} \tag{21.34}$$

Satisfying (21.34) serves a further purpose: it also ensures that the solution is stable (i.e. that the temperature profiles do not diverge from or increasingly oscillate about the exact solution). This is because the criterion for stability is in fact usually less stringent than (21.34).*

We may now turn to an extension of the method to cover the more practical case where the temperature variation of a fluid adjacent to the wall is known, rather than the temperature variation of the wall surface. In such circumstances we also require a knowledge of the heat transfer coefficient α between surface and fluid. Referring to Fig. 21.20, we may make use of the condition of continuity of heat flow at the wall surface w by writing for unit area

$$-k\left(\frac{\partial T}{\partial x}\right)_{w,p} = -\alpha(T_{w,p} - T_{s,p}) \tag{21.35}$$

where $T_{s,p}$ is the bulk fluid temperature at time p. This condition is best applied by subdividing the wall as shown, namely with plane 1 a distance $\Delta x/2$ in from the surface. (The temperature gradients are greater near the surface and a narrower space interval here leads to greater accuracy.) The introduction of an imaginary extension of the wall to plane 0 in the fluid, also a distance $\Delta x/2$ from the surface, then enables us to satisfy equation (21.35) by writing

$$k\frac{T_{1,p} - T_{0,p}}{\Delta x} = \alpha(T_{w,p} - T_{s,p}) \tag{21.36}$$

---

* For a discussion of criteria of stability of such solutions the reader may turn to Refs 22, 25 or 19.

Further, putting $t_w = (T_1 + T_0)/2$ and $Bi = \alpha \Delta x/k$, algebraic manipulation yields

$$t_{0,p} = \left\{ \frac{2(Bi)}{2 + (Bi)} \right\} T_{s,p} + \left\{ \frac{2 - (Bi)}{2 + (Bi)} \right\} T_{1,p} \tag{21.37}$$

$T_{1,p+1}$ can now be found by direct application of equation (21.31) to the sections 0, 1 and 2, namely

$$T_{1,p+1} = (Fo)\left[T_{2,p} + T_{0,p} + \left(\frac{1}{Fo} - 2 \right) T_{1,p} \right]$$

which, on substituting for $T_{0,p}$ from (21.37), becomes

$$T_{1,p+1} = (Fo)\left[t_{2,p} + \frac{2(Bi)}{2 + (Bi)} T_{s,p} + \left\{ \frac{1}{Fo} - \frac{2 + 3(Bi)}{2 + (Bi)} \right\} T_{1,p} \right] \tag{21.38}$$

In this case we avoid a negative coefficient of $T_{1,p}$ by making

$$Fo \leqslant \frac{2 + (Bi)}{2 + 3(Bi)} \tag{21.39}$$

This is less stringent than $Fo \leqslant \frac{1}{2}$ provided that $Bi \leqslant 2$, and the Biot number can always be made less than 2 by a suitable choice of Δx. Note that equation (21.38) is only required for calculating values of T_1; values of T_2, T_3 etc. will be obtained from the appropriate form of equation (21.31) in the manner illustrated in Example 21.4.

When the heat transfer between fluid and wall is required over a period, we may make use of the right-hand side of equation (21.35). Thus

$$q = - \sum_{t=0}^{p} \Delta t\alpha(T_{w,p} - T_{s,p}) \tag{21.40}$$

For this purpose we shall require values of T_w, and these can be found by substituting equation (21.37) in the expression $T_{w,p} = (T_{1,p} + T_{0,p})/2$ to yield

$$T_{w,p} = \frac{2T_{1,p} + (Bi) T_{s,p}}{2 + (Bi)} \tag{21.41}$$

It is necessary to use the average values of T_w and T_s during each period when applying equation (21.40). The following example will make this clear.

Example 21.5 Let the wall in Example 21.4 separate two fluids, one fluid remaining at 100 °C while the other rises to 700 °C in 2 hours. The film coefficient on each side may be assumed constant and equal to 0.32 kW/m² K, and the conductivity of the wall material is 8.7×10^{-4} kW/m K. Estimate the heat flow into and out of the wall, and the energy stored in the wall, during the 2 hour period per square metre of wall surface.

If we make the same choice of Δx as before, the Biot number becomes

$$Bi = \frac{\alpha \Delta x}{k} = \frac{0.32 \times 0.05}{8.7 \times 10^{-4}} = 18.4$$

This is greater than 2, but $\{2 + (Bi)\}/\{2 + 3(Bi)\} = 0.357$, so that a Δt of $\frac{1}{3}$ h, and hence the value of $Fo = \frac{1}{4}$ used before, will satisfy criterion (21.39). The numerical equations required for the computation of the temperature distribution are therefore as follows:

(a) Equation (21.31c) for values of T_2, T_3, T_4.
(b) For T_1 and T_5, from equation (21.38),

$$T_{1,p+1} = \tfrac{1}{4}(T_{2,p} + 1.80T_{s1,p} + 1.20T_{1,p})$$

$$T_{5,p+1} = \tfrac{1}{4}(T_{4,p} + 1.80T_{s2,p} + 1.20T_{5,p})$$

The coefficients have been evaluated to two decimal places; when rounding off, note that the sum of the coefficients must equal $1/\bar{Fo}$, i.e. $1 + 1.80 + 1.20 = 4$.

(c) For T_{w1} and T_{w2}, from equation (21.41),

$$T_{w1,p} = \frac{2T_{1,p} + 18.4T_{s1,p}}{20.4}$$

$$T_{w2,p} = \frac{2T_{5,p} + 18.4T_{s2,p}}{20.4}$$

The table gives the results; the columns headed T_{w1} and T_{w2} are completed after the temperatures at the other planes have been computed. Finally, the relevant average values during the time intervals and in the space intervals have been shown in parentheses.

Hours	T_{s1}	T_{w1}	T_1	T_2	T_3	T_4	T_5	T_{w2}	T_{s2}
0	100	100	100	100	100	100	100	100	100
	(150)	(145)							
$\frac{1}{3}$	200	190	100	100	100	100	100	100	100
	(250)	(238)							
$\frac{2}{3}$	300	285	145	100	100	100	100	100	100
	(350)	(333)							
1	400	381	204	111	100	100	100	100	100
	(450)	(429)							
$1\frac{1}{3}$	500	477	269	132	103	100	100	100	100
	(550)	(526)							
$1\frac{2}{3}$	600	574	339	159	110	101	100	100	100
	(650)	(623)							
2	700	672	412	192	120	103	100	100	100
			(542)	(302)	(156)	(112)	(102)	(100)	

The heat inflow to the wall per unit area is, from equation (21.40),

$$q = \tfrac{1}{3} \times 3600 \times 0.32(5 + 12 + 17 + 21 + 24 + 27) = 40\,700 \text{ kJ/m}^2$$

$(T_{w2} - T_{s2})$ is zero throughout the period, so that there is no heat outflow and the energy stored in the wall must also be 40 700 kJ/m^2. This can be checked by adding the quantities of energy stored in the three elements of width Δx and the two elements of widths $\Delta x/2$ according to the equation

$$q_{stored} = \Sigma \rho c_p \Delta x (T_{n,p} - T_{n,0})$$

$$\rho c_p = \frac{k}{\kappa} = \frac{8.7 \times 10^{-4}}{0.52 \times 10^{-6}} = 1673 \text{ kJ/m}^3 \text{ K}$$

$$q_{stored} = 1673 \left[\frac{0.05}{2}(542 - 100) + 0.05\{(302 - 100) \right.$$

$$+ (156 - 100) + (112 - 100) + (102 - 100)\}$$

$$\left. + \frac{0.05}{2}(100 - 100) \right] = 41\,200 \text{ kJ/m}^2$$

The discrepancy between the results is only about 1 per cent, which is an indication that the numerical results are self-consistent and correct. The agreement is not proof that the solution is close to the exact solution; to establish this it is necessary to proceed in stages with smaller space and time intervals until no marked change in the numerical values occurs, taking care that at each stage criteria (21.34) and (21.39) are satisfied. Alternatively, methods are available which enable the errors in the finite difference approximation to be estimated: see Refs 22 and 25.

It should be clear from the foregoing how the treatment can be modified when the film coefficient is not constant but varies with time. The Biot number will then also carry the subscript p, namely Bi_p, and the coefficients in equation (21.38) will be numerically different for each time interval. One possible reason why α might be a function of time is that the fluid velocity varies with time; or again, in free convection, it would vary as the temperature difference $(T_w - T_s)$ changed. For extensions of the method to cover other boundary conditions, such as those associated with composite walls, the reader can turn to Refs 15 and 25.

Finally, it should be noted that the conditions in the examples given here are such that the required restriction on Fo can be met with reasonable values of Δx and Δt. In other circumstances it may be that it can be met only by using too few space and time intervals for accuracy, or such a large number of intervals that the computation is unduly lengthy. Other forms of finite difference relation can be used which overcome such difficulties, and Ref. 25 deals with this point also.

22

Convection

The study of heat transfer by convection is concerned with the calculation of rates of heat exchange between fluids and solid boundaries. It was pointed out in the Introduction to Part IV that the solution of the differential equations that govern the transfer of heat by convection usually presents considerable mathematical difficulties, and exact solutions can rarely be obtained. This chapter is confined to a description of methods giving approximate solutions to some simple but important cases of steady heat flow.

It is known from experience that the main resistance to heat flow from a wall to a fluid is in a comparatively thin boundary layer adjacent to the wall. The first method of calculating rates of heat transfer presented here makes use of the hydrodynamic concept of a *velocity boundary layer* and the analogous thermal concept of a *temperature boundary layer*. The object of this procedure is to find the value of the temperature gradient $(dT/dy)_0$ in the fluid in the immediate vicinity of the wall. It is assumed that the fluid at the wall adheres to it, and therefore that the heat flow at the wall is by conduction and not by convection, i.e.

$$\dot{Q} = -kA\left(\frac{dT}{dy}\right)_0$$

The second method presented is like the first in that it studies the behaviour of the boundary layer. It makes use of the similarity, first pointed out by Reynolds, between the mechanism of fluid friction in the boundary layer (i.e. the transfer of fluid momentum to the wall) and the transfer of heat by convection. When this analogy is valid, rates of heat transfer can be predicted from the measurement of the shear stress between a fluid and a wall.

The third method is concerned with model testing, used to obtain information in a form which is applicable to similar systems of any scale. It is based on the principle of dynamic similarity, and employs the method of dimensional analysis for the correlation of empirical data.

It was pointed out in section 21.2 (equation (21.8)) that it is customary in engineering to express rates of heat transfer between a fluid and a wall by a relation of the form

$$\dot{Q} = -\alpha A (T_s - T_w)$$

where α is a *convection* or *film* heat transfer coefficient. (The subscript c on α_c can be dispensed with in this chapter since we shall not be referring here to the equivalent radiation coefficient α_r.) It must be remembered that α is not a physical constant of the fluid. α is a function of all the parameters that affect the heat flow, such as viscosity and velocity, and it may even depend on A and $(T_s - T_w)$ because $\dot{Q}$ does not necessarily vary linearly with these variables. The results of the three methods of approach just outlined are usually expressed in terms of the coefficient α, and the problem of finding $\dot{Q}$ is simply transferred to the evaluation of α.

Before the methods of determining α can be discussed, it is necessary to present some facts about the properties of the velocity boundary layer which is formed when a fluid flows past a flat plate, or through a cylindrical tube. No attempt is made here to derive the results quoted, and for their derivation the reader is referred to books on fluid dynamics such as Ref. 18.

22.1 Some results of simple boundary layer theory

The flow of fluids in the vicinity of solid surfaces is discussed briefly in this section. Attention is focused on the velocity distribution near a wall and the shear stress between fluid and wall, both of which are of interest in the study of convection heat transfer. There are two main types of flow. In *laminar* or *streamline* flow, fluid elements move in continuous paths, or streamlines, without mixing with the fluid in adjacent paths. In *turbulent* flow, eddy motion of small fluid elements is superimposed on the main flow; the velocities of individual elements fluctuate in the direction of flow and perpendicular to it, and so result in the mixing of the fluid.

Two cases are described here, namely two-dimensional flow parallel to a flat plate, and flow through a cylindrical tube. Historically, the flow in tubes was studied first, and many of the results were applied later to flow past flat plates. A more logical presentation is possible, however, if the flat plate is considered first, and this order is adopted here. The equations presented apply to liquids, or to gases flowing with velocities sufficiently low for compressibility effects to be negligible.

22.1.1 *Flow of fluid over a flat plate*

When a fluid flows with a free stream velocity U_s over a flat plate, it is assumed that the fluid velocity adjacent to the surface is zero, i.e. that there is no slip between fluid and surface.* At increasing distances perpendicular to the plate, the stream velocity approaches the free stream velocity U_s asymptotically. In

---

* This assumption is far from accurate for gases at very low pressures. See R. M. Drake and E. D. Kane in Ref. 35, p. 117, and Ref. 6, Chapter 10.

Fig. 22.1
Growth of a laminar
boundary layer

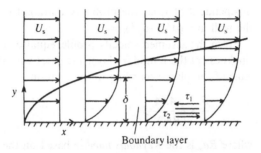

Boundary layer

fluid dynamics it is usual to divide the flow region artificially into two parts. The region adjacent to the wall, in which the velocity varies from U_s at some distance δ to zero at the wall, is called the *boundary layer*. The other region, called the *free stream*, lies outside the boundary layer, and there the velocity is assumed to be equal to U_s everywhere.

If the flow of the fluid approaching the leading edge of the plate is laminar, a laminar boundary layer of thickness δ builds up on the plate (Fig. 22.1). At the edge of the plate δ is zero, and it increases gradualiy with the distance x. The shear stress τ at any point in the fluid in an x–z plane is proportional to the velocity gradient (dU/dy) at that point. The constant of proportionality is called the *dynamic viscosity* μ of the fluid, so that

$$\tau = \mu\left(\frac{dU}{dy}\right) \tag{22.1a}$$

Or, in terms of the *kinematic viscosity* ν,

$$\tau = \rho\nu\left(\frac{dU}{dy}\right) \tag{22.1b}$$

Thus the shear stress is zero outside the boundary layer, and increases to a maximum value at the wall where the velocity gradient is greatest. Equation (22.1a) is sometimes known as *Newton's law of viscosity*.

The velocity profile in the laminar boundary layer at some distance x from the leading edge can be approximately described by a cubic parabola, i.e.

$$\frac{U}{U_s} = \frac{3}{2}\left(\frac{y}{\delta}\right) - \frac{1}{2}\left(\frac{y}{\delta}\right)^3 \tag{22.2}$$

It can be seen that this equation satisfies the following conditions:

(a) $U = 0$ at the wall, where $y = 0$.
(b) $U = U_s$ at the edge of the boundary layer, where $y = \delta$.
(c) $(dU/dy)_\delta = 0$ at $y = \delta$.
(d)   The curvature of the velocity profile at the wall $(d^2U/dy^2)_0 = 0$.

Condition (d) must be satisfied for the following reason. In the immediate proximity of the wall, velocities and accelerations are small, and the only forces acting on the fluid layers are viscous shear stresses. Hence, for dynamic equilibrium of the layer at the wall (Fig. 22.1), $\tau_1 = \tau_2$ and $(dU/dy)_{y \simeq 0}$ is independent of y, i.e. the profile is a straight line in the immediate vicinity of the wall and $(d^2 U/dy^2)_0 = 0$.

From the assumed velocity profile, equation (22.2), it can be shown that the thickness of the boundary layer increases with the distance x from the leading edge of the plate according to the relation

$$\frac{\delta}{x} = \frac{4.64}{(Re_x)^{1/2}} \tag{22.3}$$

where Re_x is the *Reynolds number* based on the distance x, i.e.

$$Re_x = \frac{\rho U_s x}{\mu} \tag{22.4}$$

The shear stress τ_w at the wall is usually expressed in terms of the dynamic head of the free stream as follows:

$$\tau_w = f\frac{\rho U_s^2}{2} \tag{22.5}$$

where f is a dimensionless *friction factor*, which is a function of the Reynolds number.* τ_w must also be equal to $\mu(dU/dy)_0$, according to equation (22.1a), so that an expression for f can be derived from (22.2), (22.3) and (22.5). The local friction factor f_x at x is then found to be[†]

$$f_x = \frac{0.664}{(Re_x)^{1/2}} \tag{22.6}$$

It is essential to distinguish between the local factor f_x and the average factor f over the length x which can be found by integration. Considering unit width of plate, the total drag force on the length x is

$$\int_0^x f_x \frac{\rho U_s^2}{2} dx$$

This is equal to $f(\rho U_s^2/2)x$, by definition of the average factor f, and hence it can be shown that

$$f = \frac{1.328}{(Re_x)^{1/2}} = 2f_x \tag{22.7}$$

Beyond a certain critical distance x_{cr} from the leading edge, the flow loses its laminar character, eddies develop, and the flow becomes fully turbulent after a transition region (Fig. 22.2). The critical distance, in terms of the Reynolds

---

* Several friction factors, which not only differ in name but are also defined as multiples of f used here, can be found in the literature; caution is necessary when using equations involving such factors.

[†] The expression actually quoted here has been obtained from the accurate expression for the velocity profile of the boundary layer. If (22.2) is used, the numerator becomes 0.647.

ig. 22.2
ransition of laminar
oundary layer into a
urbulent boundary layer

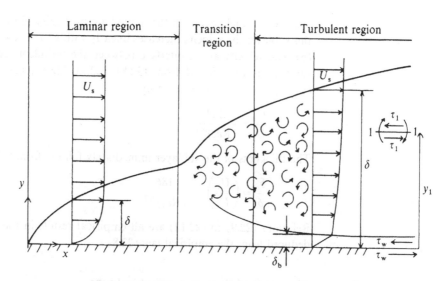

number, has been found from experiment to be

$$Re_{cr} = 500\,000 \quad \text{i.e.} \quad x_{cr} = \frac{\mu}{\rho U_s} 500\,000$$

Although the critical distance x_{cr} may be considerably less than this if the free stream approaching the plate is turbulent, there is always at least a short distance at the nose of the plate over which there is a laminar boundary layer.

The friction factor for a turbulent boundary layer cannot be deduced theoretically, but it has been found experimentally to be given by

$$f_x = \frac{0.0592}{(Re_x)^{0.2}} \tag{22.8}$$

In turbulent flow the eddies act as macroscopic carriers of free stream momentum to the wall; in laminar flow the transfer of momentum is due solely to molecular carriers, i.e. viscous friction. It follows that the velocity gradient near the wall in a turbulent boundary layer is much steeper than in a laminar one. Prandtl has shown that equation (22.8) implies that the velocity profile in the turbulent boundary layer must follow a one-seventh power law, i.e.

$$\frac{U}{U_s} = \left(\frac{y}{\delta}\right)^{1/7} \tag{22.9}$$

The thickness of the turbulent boundary layer can then be shown to be given by

$$\frac{\delta}{x} = \frac{0.38}{(Re_x)^{0.2}} \tag{22.10}$$

The boundary layer condition (d), shown to be satisfied by the laminar velocity profile given by equation (22.2), must also be satisfied by the turbulent profile at the wall. But from equation (22.9) it is clear that $(d^2 U/dy^2)_0 \neq 0$ at the wall. This discrepancy need not cause concern because there is always a thin laminar sublayer of thickness δ_b in the immediate proximity of the wall (Fig. 22.2). In this sublayer the velocity increases linearly with y to satisfy boundary condition (d). The velocity at the interface between the turbulent layer and the laminar sublayer is then found from (22.8), (22.9), (22.10) and the linear relation $(U/U_b) = (y/\delta_b)$, to be given by

$$\frac{U_b}{U_s} = \frac{2.11}{(Re_x)^{0.1}} \qquad (22.11)$$

The thickness of the sublayer immediately follows from (22.9) to (22.11) as

$$\frac{\delta_b}{\delta} = \left(\frac{U_b}{U_s}\right)^7 = \frac{186}{(Re_x)^{0.7}} \qquad (22.12)$$

Relations (22.9) to (22.12) are all empirical results in the sense that they are deduced from the empirical law (22.8).

22.1.2 Flow of fluid through a cylindrical tube

When a fluid approaches a tube with a uniform velocity U_s, a boundary layer gradually builds up until it reaches the centre of the tube. The velocity profile is then said to be *fully developed*, and may be assumed not to vary down the tube. Although the velocity profile actually approaches its final shape only asymptotically, it has been found that for practical purposes it is fully developed in laminar flow at a distance l_e from the entrance of the tube (Fig. 22.3), where

$$\frac{l_e}{d} = 0.0288(Re_d) \qquad (22.13)$$

Distance l_e is called the *entrance* or *approach length*. The Reynolds number is defined by

$$Re_d = \frac{\rho U_m d}{\mu} \qquad (22.14)$$

Fig. 22.3
Establishment of a fully developed velocity profile in a tube

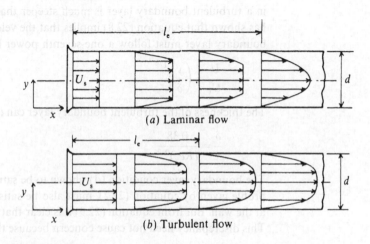

(a) Laminar flow

(b) Turbulent flow

i.e. it is calculated on the basis of the tube diameter d and the weighted mean velocity U_m. The *weighted mean velocity* at any cross-section is defined by the equation

$$\int_A \rho U \, dA = \rho U_m A \tag{22.15}$$

where $\rho U_m A$ is the total rate of mass flow through A. If the Reynolds number exceeds the critical value for flow through tubes (≈ 2300), the flow becomes turbulent in the approach length, and the velocity profile becomes fully established in a distance less than that predicted by (22.13). This is shown in Fig. 22.3b.

For fully developed laminar flow the velocity profile is parabolic, and is given by

$$\frac{U}{U_r} = 2\left(\frac{y}{r}\right) - \left(\frac{y}{r}\right)^2 \tag{22.16}$$

where r is the radius of the tube, U_r is the velocity at the axis of the tube, and U is the velocity at a distance y from the wall. It is often convenient to work in terms of the weighted mean velocity U_m, as defined by (22.15), because this value can be obtained from the mass flow which is often more easily measured than U_r. The value of the velocity for any annulus of width dy at radius $(r - y)$ may be found from (22.16), and if this is substituted in (22.15) we get

$$\int_0^r \rho U_r \left\{ 2\left(\frac{y}{r}\right) - \left(\frac{y}{r}\right)^2 \right\} 2\pi(r - y) \, dy = \rho U_m \pi r^2$$

This reduces to

$$\frac{U_m}{U_r} = 0.5 \tag{22.17}$$

If the shear stress τ_w at the wall is expressed in terms of the dynamic head of the fluid as follows

$$\tau_w = f \frac{\rho U_m^2}{2} \tag{22.18}$$

then by making use of equations (22.1a), (22.16) and (22.17) we get

$$f = \frac{16}{Re_d} \tag{22.19}$$

For fully developed turbulent flow the shear stress at the wall can also be expressed by (22.18), where

$$f = \frac{0.0791}{(Re_d)^{1/4}} \tag{22.20}$$

Equation (22.20) cannot be deduced theoretically; it is an experimental relation, called the *friction law of Blasius*, and it holds reasonably well up to Reynolds

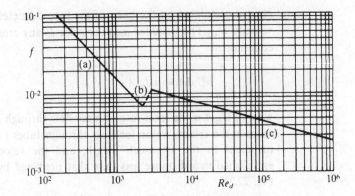

Fig. 22.4
Friction factor for a
smooth tube: (a) laminar
flow equation (22.19);
(b) transition range;
(c) turbulent flow
equation (22.20)

numbers of about 200 000 (Fig. 22.4). Prandtl has shown that, as an implication of (22.20), the velocity profile must follow a one-seventh power law, i.e.

$$\frac{U}{U_r} = \left(\frac{y}{r}\right)^{1/7}$$

(22.21)

This equation is similar to (22.9) for the flat plate, except that the boundary layer thickness δ is replaced by the radius r, and the free stream velocity U_s by the velocity at the axis U_r.

The weighted mean velocity for the turbulent velocity profile can be calculated from (22.15) and (22.21) as

$$\int_0^r \rho U_r \left(\frac{y}{r}\right)^{1/7} 2\pi(r - y)\,dy = \rho U_m \pi r^2$$

which reduces to

$$\frac{U_m}{U_r} = 0.817$$

(22.22)

As with the turbulent boundary layer near a flat plate, there is always a thin laminar sublayer at the tube wall. It can be shown that the velocity at the edge of the sublayer is given by

$$\frac{U_b}{U_r} = \frac{1.99}{(Re_d)^{1/8}}$$

(22.23)

and the thickness of the sublayer follows immediately from (22.21) and (22.23) as

$$\frac{\delta_b}{d} = \frac{1}{2}\left(\frac{U_b}{U_r}\right)^7 = \frac{61.8}{(Re_d)^{7/8}}$$

(22.24)

Like relations (22.9) to (22.12), the relations (22.21) to (22.24) are essentially empirical, because they have been deduced from an empirical friction law—the law of Blasius (22.20).

22.1.3   Shear stress due to eddy motion

So far we have only considered the magnitude of the shear stress *at the wall*, expressing the result in terms of the friction factor *f*. The analysis has been based on equation (22.1a), which was introduced when discussing laminar flow. Since even with turbulent flow there is always a laminar sublayer next to the wall, the question of the general validity of equation (22.1a) has not arisen. However, before we can discuss the analogy between the transfer of momentum and the transfer of heat (section 22.4), it is necessary to know something about the shear stress in regions where the flow is turbulent.

The shear stress in the turbulent boundary layer at section 1–1 in Fig. 22.2, a distance y_1 from the wall, is not given by equation (22.1a) because there is an exchange of mass across the surface 1–1 and the momentum is transferred by both macroscopic and molecular carriers. Owing to eddy motion, the fluid velocity fluctuates and the instantaneous velocity U_1 in the x-direction can be resolved into two components. If $\bar{U}_1$ represents the mean velocity of the fluid, and U_1' represents the instantaneous superimposed velocity fluctuation, then

$$U_1 = \bar{U}_1 + U_1' \tag{22.25}$$

Similarly, the instantaneous velocity in the y-direction can be written as

$$V_1 = \bar{V}_1 + V_1' \tag{22.26}$$

For steady flow $\bar{U}_1$ and $\bar{V}_1$ are constants and, although the values of U_1' and V_1' fluctuate, their mean values must be zero over a time Δt which is long compared with the period of fluctuation.

Now let an infinitesimal time interval d*t* be considered. The mass flow upward (positive) through unit area of surface 1–1 during time d*t* is $\rho V_1\,dt$; the momentum in the x-direction carried upward through this surface is $(\rho V_1\,dt)U_1$. The shear stress acting along 1–1 due to eddy motion only, $\tau_{\varepsilon1}$, must be equal to the *average rate* at which momentum is transported through unit surface area along 1–1, i.e.

$$\tau_{\varepsilon1} = \frac{\rho}{\Delta t}\int_0^t (U_1 V_1)\,dt$$

If this integral is positive, the net flow of momentum is upward, i.e. away from the wall, and if it is negative, the net flow of momentum is towards the wall. On substitution of (22.25) and (22.26) this becomes

$$\tau_{\varepsilon1} = \frac{\rho}{\Delta t}\int_0^t (\bar{U}_1 \bar{V}_1 + \bar{U}_1 V_1' + U_1' \bar{V}_1 + U_1' V_1')\,dt \tag{22.27}$$

But because the time averages of the fluctuating components of the velocities, U_1' and V_1', are both zero,

$$\frac{\rho}{\Delta t}\int_0^t (\bar{U}_1 V_1')\,dt = \frac{\rho \bar{U}_1}{\Delta t}\int_0^t V_1'\,dt = 0$$

$$\frac{\rho}{\Delta t}\int_0^t (U_1' \bar{V}_1)\,dt = \frac{\rho \bar{V}_1}{\Delta t}\int_0^t U_1'\,dt = 0$$

Therefore

$$\tau_{\varepsilon 1} = \frac{\rho}{\Delta t} \int_0^t (\bar{U}_1 \bar{V}_1 + U_1' V_1') \, dt$$

Now let us restrict the analysis to 'one-dimensional' flow, i.e. flow for which $\bar{V}_1 = 0$, although V_1' may still assume finite values. This restriction effectively covers the two cases which are considered here: for flow past a flat plate, the thickness of the turbulent boundary layer increases very slowly and therefore $\bar{V}_1$ is negligible; for fully developed flow through a tube, $\bar{V}_1$ must be exactly zero. With this restriction, then, the first term in the integral is also zero and (22.27) reduces to

$$\tau_{\varepsilon 1} = \frac{\rho}{\Delta t} \int_0^t (U_1' V_1') \, dt = \rho (U_1' V_1')_{\text{mean}} \qquad (22.28)$$

where $(U_1' V_1')_{\text{mean}}$ is the time average of the product $(U_1' V_1')$.

The question arises as to whether the time average of $(U_1' V_1')$ differs from zero. Although the time averages of U_1' and V_1' are individually zero, the answer to this question is not immediately obvious. Consider a positive V_1', i.e. an instantaneous flow upward through 1–1. As this flow arrives from a region which, *on the average*, has a velocity lower than $\bar{U}_1$, the fluid element arriving at 1–1 produces negative U_1' at 1–1; hence $(U_1' V_1')$ is, *on the average*, negative for positive V_1'. Now consider a negative V_1', i.e. an instantaneous flow downward through 1–1. As this flow arrives from a region in which, *on the average*, the velocity is greater than $\bar{U}_1$, the fluid element arriving at 1–1 produces a positive U_1' at 1–1; hence $(U_1' V_1')$ is, *on the average*, negative for negative V_1'. Thus, on the whole $(U_1' V_1')_{\text{mean}}$ is negative and not zero. This simplified picture indicates that there is a net flow of momentum towards the wall, resulting in a shear stress as indicated in Fig. 22.2. Thus the shear stress due to eddy motion at 1–1 is of the same sense as that due to viscous forces. To be able to sum these separate effects, we may write, by analogy with equation (22.1b),

$$\tau_{\varepsilon 1} = \rho \varepsilon_1 \left(\frac{d\bar{U}}{dy} \right)_1$$

where ε is called the *eddy diffusivity*. This quantity is defined by equating the two expressions for $\tau_{\varepsilon 1}$, i.e.

$$\tau_{\varepsilon 1} = -\rho (U_1' V_1')_{\text{mean}} = \rho \varepsilon_1 \left(\frac{d\bar{U}}{dy} \right)_1 \qquad (22.29)$$

The negative sign must be introduced if ε is to be a positive quantity like v, since $(d\bar{U}/dy)_1$ is always positive and we have just seen that $(U_1' V_1')_{\text{mean}}$ is always negative.

The total shear stress is the result of the viscous and eddy shear stresses, or in other words the flow of momentum towards the wall is due to a molecular diffusion of momentum *and* a macroscopic diffusion of momentum. Hence

$$\tau_1 = \rho v \left(\frac{d\bar{U}}{dy}\right)_1 + \rho \varepsilon_1 \left(\frac{d\bar{U}}{dy}\right)_1 = \rho(v + \varepsilon_1)\left(\frac{d\bar{U}}{dy}\right)_1 \tag{22.30}$$

It must be emphasised that the eddy diffusivity* is a function of the turbulence and it is not a property of the fluid, although the turbulence arises as a result of fluid viscosity. ε changes in value with the distance from the wall. In the sublayer where the flow is laminar and $V' = 0$, ε must be zero, but its value rapidly increases to many times the value of v in the turbulent layer. The following are some experimental values for the distance from the wall of a tube at which $\varepsilon = 10v$, for various Reynolds numbers. The distance from the wall is expressed as a fraction of the tube radius.

Re_d	4 000	10 000	100 000
y/r	0.23	0.10	0.01

To end this section summarising boundary layer theory, we must note certain restrictions on the application of the equations quoted. Relations (22.8), (22.11), (22.12) for a flat plate, and (22.20), (22.23), (22.24) for a tube, which apply to turbulent flow, are only valid if the surfaces are *hydraulically smooth*. The criterion of smoothness is that the unevenness of the surface must be less than $0.4\delta_b$. Since δ_b decreases with increase in flow velocity, smoothness is a particularly important factor at high velocities. Relations for rough surfaces will not be given here.

In the derivation of the relations given in this section, it has been assumed that there are no temperature gradients in the boundary layer. Since μ and ρ vary with temperature, temperature gradients in the fluid affect the validity of these relations. For fluid flow where the temperature difference between the *free stream temperature* T_s and the wall temperature T_w is not too great, all the equations can be used with reasonable accuracy if the fluid properties are evaluated at a *film temperature* T_f, where T_f is defined as

$$T_f = \frac{T_s + T_w}{2} \tag{22.31}$$

For flow through a tube, T_f is usually defined in terms of the *weighted mean temperature* T_m and the wall temperature T_w, i.e.

$$T_f = \frac{T_m + T_w}{2} \tag{22.32}$$

T_m, at any cross-section of the tube, is the temperature that the fluid would assume if it were thoroughly mixed, and is in fact the temperature often measured in experimental work.

Example 22.1 Air at 15 °C and 1 atm flows with a velocity of 8 m/s past a flat plate which is maintained at a uniform temperature of 115 °C. Calculate the thickness of the boundary layer 0.6 m from the leading edge, and estimate the position

---

* For a full discussion of the concept of eddy diffusivity see Ref. 18, Chapters 18 and 19.

of the point of transition to turbulent flow. Also calculate the total drag force on one side of the plate, per metre width of plate, over the first 0.6 m.

The film temperature T_f is $(15 + 115)/2 = 65\,°C$. At this temperature the density of air at atmospheric pressure is $\rho = 1.046\,\text{kg/m}^3$, and its viscosity is $\mu = 2.021 \times 10^{-5}\,\text{kg/m s}$ (see Ref. 14). Hence the Reynolds number 0.6 m from the leading edge is

$$Re_x = \frac{\rho U_s x}{\mu} = \frac{1.046 \times 8 \times 0.6}{2.021 \times 10^{-5}} = 248\,400$$

The thickness of the boundary layer at this point is therefore

$$\delta = \frac{4.64x}{(Re_x)^{1/2}} = \frac{4.64 \times 0.6}{248\,400^{1/2}} = 0.005\,59\,\text{m} = 0.559\,\text{cm}$$

The point of transition, assuming that the approaching air is initially laminar, will be at

$$x_{cr} = \frac{\mu}{\rho U_s}(Re_{cr}) = \frac{2.021 \times 10^{-5}}{1.046 \times 8} \times 500\,000 = 1.2\,\text{m}$$

The average friction factor is

$$f = \frac{1.328}{(Re_x)^{1/2}} = \frac{1.328}{248\,400^{1/2}} = 0.002\,66$$

The total drag force over the first 0.6 m, per metre width of plate, is therefore

$$\tau_w A = f\frac{\rho U_s^2}{2} A = 0.002\,66 \times \frac{1.046 \times 8^2}{2}(0.6 \times 1)$$

$$= 0.0534\,\text{kg m/s}^2\,\text{or N}$$

It is interesting to note how the velocity profile for laminar flow is distorted from its parabolic shape when the fluid flowing through a tube is cooled or heated. Curve a in Fig. 22.5 shows the simple parabolic profile in *isothermal flow*, i.e. for the limiting case of heat transfer by convection with $(T_w - T_m) \rightarrow 0$, when there are negligible temperature gradients in the fluid. When the fluid is heated $T_w > T_m$, and when it is cooled $T_w < T_m$. As the temperature is increased, the viscosity of a liquid decreases and the viscosity of a gas increases. Thus when a liquid is heated the viscosity at the wall is lower than at the axis, and the gradient at the wall is increased compared with the parabolic profile, as is

Fig. 22.5
Distortion of parabolic velocity profile in laminar flow through a tube

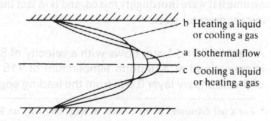

b Heating a liquid or cooling a gas

a Isothermal flow

c Cooling a liquid or heating a gas

shown by curve b. Curve b also serves to represent the velocity profile of a gas when it is cooled. Curve c shows the distortion of the profile for a liquid that is being cooled or a gas that is being heated.

In the following sections two simple cases are considered: the heating or cooling of a fluid flowing parallel to a plate; and the heating or cooling of a fluid flowing through a cylindrical tube with a fully established velocity profile. It will be assumed that the fluid is either a liquid or a gas and that the fluid properties are independent of temperature.

22.2 Forced convection in laminar flow over a flat plate

When a plate is heated or cooled to a uniform temperature T_w, starting at a distance x_a from the leading edge of the plate, temperature gradients are set up in the fluid (Fig. 22.6).* The temperature of the fluid immediately adjacent to the wall is T_w, and far away from it the fluid temperature is equal to the tree stream temperature T_s. It is possible to divide the fluid temperature field artificially into two regions. The region adjacent to the wall, in which the temperature varies from T_s to T_w, is called the *temperature boundary layer*. The other region lies outside the boundary layer, and there the temperature is assumed to be everywhere equal to the temperature T_s. Thus the concept of the temperature boundary layer is analogous to that of the velocity boundary layer.

At any section $x > x_a$ (Fig. 22.6) the profile of the temperature boundary layer may be expressed as a polynomial in y, and it may be assumed that a cubic parabola adequately describes the profile. Hence

$$T = T_w + ay + by^2 + cy^3$$

It is more convenient to work in terms of the temperature difference between fluid and wall. If we write θ for $(T - T_w)$, the expression becomes

$$\theta = ay + by^2 + cy^3 \tag{22.33}$$

Fig. 22.6
Development of the
temperature boundary
layer along a flat plate

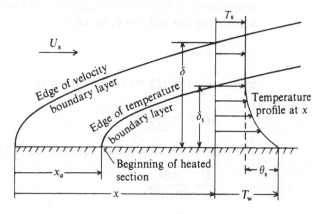

Beginning of heated section

---

* The method given in sections 22.2 and 22.3 was first developed and applied by G. Kroujiline (Ref. 27). The presentation in this chapter is based on the work of E. R. G. Eckert (Ref. 6, Chapter 7).

a, b and c can be found by applying the boundary conditions as follows. At the wall, where $y = 0$, the fluid layer is at rest and can have no velocity component perpendicular to the wall. Therefore at the wall the heat transfer is entirely by conduction and not by transport of fluid, i.e.

$$\dot{q}_w = -k\left(\frac{dT}{dy}\right)_0 = -k\left(\frac{d\theta}{dy}\right)_0 \tag{22.34}$$

where k is the thermal conductivity of the fluid. Hence from equation (22.34),

$$\left(\frac{d^2\theta}{dy^2}\right)_0 = 0 \quad \text{and therefore} \quad b = 0$$

If the thickness of the temperature boundary layer is denoted by δ_t, then the following further two boundary conditions must be satisfied at $y = \delta_t$:

$$\theta = \theta_s \quad \text{and} \quad \left(\frac{d\theta}{dy}\right)_{\delta_t} = 0$$

On substituting the three boundary conditions in the cubic parabola for the temperature profile (22.33), this becomes

$$\frac{\theta}{\theta_s} = \frac{3}{2}\left(\frac{y}{\delta_t}\right) - \frac{1}{2}\left(\frac{y}{\delta_t}\right)^3 \tag{22.35}$$

The rate of heat flow per unit area at the wall at section x can be calculated by finding the value of $(d\theta/dy)_0$ from equation (22.35). Substituting this value in equation (22.34), we have

$$\dot{q}_w = -k\frac{3}{2\delta_t}\theta_s \tag{22.36}$$

The value of δ_t in (22.36) is still unknown, and must be found before $\dot{q}_w$ can be calculated. It is convenient to introduce into this equation the ratio of the temperature boundary layer thickness δ_t to the velocity boundary layer thickness δ. Denoting this ratio by ψ, we have

$$\psi = \frac{\delta_t}{\delta} \tag{22.37}$$

so that equation (22.36) can be written as

$$\dot{q}_w = -\frac{3}{2\psi\delta}k\theta_s \tag{22.38}$$

The value of δ is known from equation (22.3), i.e.

$$\frac{\delta}{x} = \frac{4.64}{(Re_x)^{1/2}}$$

and hence

$$\dot{q}_w = -\frac{3}{2 \times 4.64\psi x}(Re_x)^{1/2}k\theta_s \tag{22.39}$$

Fig. 22.7
Derivation of heat flow
equation

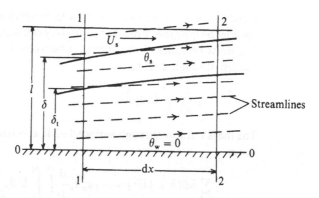

The problem is thus reduced to the determination of the value of ψ. It will be assumed initially that $\delta_t \leqslant \delta$, i.e. $\psi \leqslant 1$; this assumption will be justified later.

22.2.1 Derivation of the heat flow equation of the boundary layer

Consider a region near the surface of the plate of unit width perpendicular to the paper in the z-direction (Fig. 22.7). Let this region be bounded by two surfaces 1–1 and 2–2, a distance dx apart. The other surfaces limiting this region are the surface of the plate 0–0, and a surface 1–2 outside the edges of the temperature and velocity boundary layers a distance l away from the wall.

The continuity and energy equations can now be applied to this open system. The streamlines are of the form shown by the dashed lines in Fig. 22.7. For continuity of mass, the difference between the mass entering the region across plane 1–1 and the mass leaving across plane 2–2 is equal to the mass leaving across plane 1–2. Since no external work is done on or by the fluid passing through the region, the steady-flow energy equation states that the net rate of heat flow into the region must equal

$$\sum_{2-2} \delta\dot{m}(h + \tfrac{1}{2}U^2) + \sum_{1-2} \delta\dot{m}(h + \tfrac{1}{2}U^2) - \sum_{1-1} \delta\dot{m}(h + \tfrac{1}{2}U^2)$$

where $\delta\dot{m}$ is the mass entering or leaving per unit time with a specific enthalpy h and a specific kinetic energy $U^2/2$. We shall assume, in what follows, that the kinetic energy of the fluid is insignificant compared with the enthalpy; only in high-speed flow need the kinetic energy be taken into account.[*] Furthermore, since the fluids considered are either gases or liquids (i.e. flow without change of phase), we may substitute $c_p T$ for h because the enthalpy varies but little with pressure.

With these modifications, we have

$$\sum_{1-1} \delta\dot{m}(h + \tfrac{1}{2}U^2) = \rho c_p \int_0^l TU\,\mathrm{d}y$$

$$\sum_{2-2} \delta\dot{m}(h + \tfrac{1}{2}U^2) = \rho c_p \int_0^l TU\,\mathrm{d}y + \rho c_p \frac{\mathrm{d}}{\mathrm{d}x}\left(\int_0^l TU\,\mathrm{d}y\right)\mathrm{d}x$$

---

[*] See Introduction to Part IV, and Ref. 6, Chapter 10.

ρ and c_p are assumed not to vary with temperature, and are therefore written outside the integrals. From the continuity equation, the mass of the fluid leaving 1–2 must be equal to the difference between the inflow through 1–1 and the outflow through 2–2, i.e.

$$-\rho \frac{d}{x}\left(\int_0^l U \, dy \right) dx$$

The mass outflow through surface 1–2 is at a temperature T_s, since $l > \delta_t$, and hence

$$\sum_{1-2} \delta \dot{m}(h + \tfrac{1}{2}U^2) = -\rho c_p T_s \frac{d}{dx}\left(\int_0^l U \, dy \right) dx$$

Because the temperature gradient across 1–2 is zero, there can be no conduction of heat across this surface. Also, since the gradients $(d\theta/dx)$ across 1–1 and 2–2 are small compared with $(d\theta/dy)$, and since the heat conducted across these surfaces is negligible compared with the flow of energy due to transport of fluid across them, we can neglect any heat conduction across these two surfaces. We may assume therefore that the only heat which crosses the boundary of the region is that which flows across the wall surface 0–0. The rate of flow of heat into the region from the wall 0–0 is given by

$$d\dot{Q}_w = -k \, dx \left(\frac{d\theta}{dy} \right)_0$$

If the flow of heat is away from the wall, θ decreases with increase of y and hence the negative sign. For steady heat and fluid flow, the equation expressing the First Law becomes

$$-k \, dx \left(\frac{d\theta}{dy} \right)_0 = \rho c_p \frac{d}{dx}\left(\int_0^l T U \, dy \right) dx - \rho c_p T_s \frac{d}{dx}\left(\int_0^l U \, dy \right) dx$$

If κ is substituted for $k/\rho c_p$, and θ for $(T - T_w)$, this reduces to

$$\frac{d}{dx} \int_0^l (\theta_s - \theta) U \, dy = \kappa \left(\frac{d\theta}{dy} \right)_0 \tag{22.40}$$

κ is the *thermal diffusivity* of the fluid, first introduced in section 21.4. Equation (22.40) is called the *heat flow equation* of the boundary layer.

22.2.2 Solution of the heat flow equation

It is now possible to substitute the equations of the velocity and temperature profiles (22.2) and (22.35) in the heat flow equation. The right-hand side of (22.40) becomes

$$\kappa \left(\frac{d\theta}{dy} \right)_0 = \kappa \frac{3}{2\delta_t} \theta_s = \frac{3 \kappa \theta_s}{2 \psi \delta} \tag{22.41}$$

The left-hand side of (22.40) can be split into two integrals, i.e.

$$\int_0^l (\theta_s - \theta) U \, dy = \int_0^{\delta_t} (\theta_s - \theta) U \, dy + \int_{\delta_t}^l (\theta_s - \theta) U \, dy$$

The second integral, between limits $\delta_t > y > l$, must be zero, because between these limits $(\theta_s - \theta) = 0$. The integral in the left-hand side of (22.40) can therefore be written

$$\int_0^l (\theta_s - \theta) U \, dy = \theta_s U_s \int_0^{\delta_t} \left\{ 1 - \frac{3}{2}\left(\frac{y}{\delta_t}\right) + \frac{1}{2}\left(\frac{y}{\delta_t}\right)^3 \right\} \left\{ \frac{3}{2}\left(\frac{y}{\delta}\right) - \frac{1}{2}\left(\frac{y}{\delta}\right)^3 \right\} dy$$

$$= \theta_s U_s \delta \left(\frac{3}{20}\psi^2 - \frac{3}{280}\psi^4 \right) \approx \theta_s U_s \delta \frac{3}{20}\psi^2 \qquad (22.42)$$

Note that the ratio $\psi = \delta_t/\delta$ is less than 1, according to the assumption made at the beginning of this section, so that $3\psi^4/280 \ll 3\psi^2/20$ and can therefore be neglected.

Substituting (22.41) and (22.42) in the heat flow equation (22.40), this can now be rewritten as

$$\frac{3}{20}\theta_s U_s \frac{d}{dx}(\psi^2 \delta) = \frac{3}{2}\frac{\kappa \theta_s}{\psi \delta}$$

or

$$0.1 U_s \psi \delta \frac{d}{dx}(\psi^2 \delta) = \kappa$$

Hence

$$0.1 U_s \left(\psi^3 \delta \frac{d\delta}{dx} + 2\psi^2 \delta^2 \frac{d\psi}{dx} \right) = \kappa$$

The terms containing the velocity boundary thickness δ can be found from equation (22.3). Since

$$\frac{\delta}{x} = \frac{4.64}{(Re_x)^{1/2}}, \qquad \delta^2 = \frac{21.5 x \mu}{U_s \rho}, \qquad \delta \frac{d\delta}{dx} = 0.5 \frac{21.5 \mu}{U_s \rho}$$

The heat flow equation therefore becomes

$$0.1 U_s \left(\psi^3 0.5 \frac{21.5\mu}{U_s \rho} + 2\psi^2 \frac{21.5 x \mu}{U_s \rho} \frac{d\psi}{dx} \right) = \kappa$$

or

$$1.075 \left(\psi^3 + 4\psi^2 x \frac{d\psi}{dx} \right) = \frac{k}{\rho c_p \mu} \frac{\rho}{} = \frac{k}{c_p \mu}$$

The group $c_p \mu/k$ occurs frequently in convection theory and is called the *Prandtl number*; it is a dimensionless group involving three fluid properties, and is thus itself a property of the fluid. Writing Pr for $c_p \mu/k$, the heat flow equation reduces to

$$\psi^3 + \frac{4}{3}x\frac{d(\psi^3)}{dx} = \frac{1}{1.075(Pr)} \tag{22.43}$$

The differential equation (22.43) can now be solved for ψ. Dividing throughout by $4x^{1/4}/3$, the left-hand side of the equation is transformed into a perfect differential:

$$\frac{3}{4}\psi^3 x^{-1/4} + x^{3/4}\frac{d(\psi^3)}{dx} = \frac{3}{4}\frac{x^{-1/4}}{1.075(Pr)}$$

and hence

$$\frac{d(x^{3/4}\psi^3)}{dx} = \frac{3}{4}\frac{x^{-1/4}}{1.075(Pr)}$$

Integrating, we have

$$x^{3/4}\psi^3 = \frac{x^{3/4}}{1.075(Pr)} + C$$

and therefore

$$\psi^3 = \frac{1}{1.075(Pr)} + Cx^{-3/4}$$

The value of the constant C in the solution can be found from the boundary condition $\psi = 0$ when $x = x_a$; thus $C = -x_a^{3/4}/1.075(Pr)$. The solution is therefore

$$\psi = \frac{1}{\{1.075(Pr)\}^{1/3}}\left\{1 - \left(\frac{x_a}{x}\right)^{3/4}\right\}^{1/3} \tag{22.44}$$

The solution will now be restricted to the special case of a plate heated all along its length, i.e. when $x_a = 0$. In this case

$$\psi = \frac{1}{\{1.075(Pr)\}^{1/3}} \approx \frac{1}{(Pr)^{1/3}} \tag{22.45}$$

Thus when a plate is heated from the leading edge, the ratio of the thickness of the temperature and velocity boundary layers is constant along the length of the plate. If the value of ψ is now substituted in equation (22.39), the heat flow at section x is given by

$$\dot{q}_w = -\frac{3\{1.075(Pr)\}^{1/3}}{2 \times 4.64x}(Re_x)^{1/2}k\theta_s = -0.331(Pr)^{1/3}(Re_x)^{1/2}\frac{k\theta_s}{x}$$

An exact solution to this problem has yielded a similar answer, but with a numerical constant of 0.332.* The equation can now be divided by $k\theta_s/x$.

---

* The excellent agreement is fortuitous; the solution given here is approximate because the velocity and temperature profiles were described by cubic parabolas. In fact these profiles can only be described accurately by infinite series; see Ref. 18, Chapter 14.

Remembering also that the heat transfer or film coefficient α is defined by the equation

$$\dot{q}_w = -\alpha(T_s - T_w) = -\alpha\theta_s$$

the local heat transfer coefficient α_x at section x can be calculated from the relation

$$\frac{\alpha_x x}{k} = 0.332(Pr)^{1/3}(Re_x)^{1/2}$$

The group $\alpha_x x/k$ appears frequently in heat transfer equations and is called the *Nusselt number*. It will be denoted by Nu_x, the subscript x indicating that the value refers to a distance x from the leading edge of the plate. The Nusselt number is a dimensionless group, and is a measure of the rate of heat transfer by convection; it has here been shown that it can be expressed as a function of two dimensionless groups, the Reynolds number which describes the flow, and the Prandtl number which is a property of the fluid. Thus

$$Nu_x = 0.332(Pr)^{1/3}(Re_x)^{1/2} \tag{22.46}$$

When the plate is heated from the leading edge over a length l, the average value of α over the heated length is given by

$$\alpha = \frac{1}{l}\int_0^l \alpha_x\,dx$$

If the value of α_x given by (22.46) is substituted in the integral, this yields

$$\alpha = 2\alpha_l \quad \text{or} \quad Nu = 2(Nu_l) \tag{22.47}$$

where α_l and Nu_l are the local heat transfer coefficient and local Nusselt number respectively at $x = l$.

It remains to justify the assumption that $\psi = \delta_t/\delta \leqslant 1$. For this purpose let the most unfavourable case be considered, namely when the plate is heated over its entire length. Evidently the result expressed as equation (22.45) is an accord with the assumption provided that the Prandtl number for the fluid is equal to or greater than 1. This is so for most liquids except molten metals, as can be seen from Fig. 22.8. The special case of liquid metals is discussed briefly at the end of this section. The Prandtl number for gases and dry vapours varies only slightly, and lies between 0.65 and 1. A brief consideration of (22.42), which is the first equation affected by the assumption $\psi \leqslant 1$, shows that the error introduced by neglecting the fourth-power term is small even if ψ is slightly greater than unity. Thus the assumption can be justified even for gases and vapours. We may also infer from (22.45) and Fig. 22.8 that the thicknesses of the velocity and temperature boundary layers for gases are practically equal, whereas for a very viscous lubricating oil, for which $Pr = 1000$, say, δ_t is about $\delta/10$.

Owing to the length of the solution for the flat plate, it is worth retracing the

Fig.22.8
Typical values of Prandtl number $c_p \mu / k$

T/[K]	250	300	400	500	600	800
Hydrogen	0.713	0.706	0.690	0.675	0.661	0.633
Air	0.720	0.707	0.688	0.680	0.680	0.690
Carbon dioxide	0.773	0.763	0.737	0.703	0.686	0.694
Steam (low p)		0.93	0.94	0.95	0.93	0.89
Steam (sat.)		0.96	1.01	1.30		
Water (sat.)		5.81	1.34	0.85		
Ammonia (sat. liq.)	1.70	1.13				
Freon 12 (sat. liq.)	3.5	3.5				
Mercury, liquid	0.0353	0.0261	0.0173	0.0129	0.0095	0.0079
Sodium, liquid			0.0097	0.0069	0.0055	0.0046
Mineral oils		10–1000				

principal steps in the argument:

(a) The heat flow at the wall at a distance x from the leading edge of the plate is given by equation (22.34):

$$\dot{q}_w = -k\left(\frac{d\theta}{dy}\right)_0$$

It is therefore necessary to find the temperature profile at x, in the form $\theta = \phi(y)$.

(b) By introducing the concept of the temperature boundary layer of finite thickness δ_t, and by assuming that the functions $\theta = \phi(y)$ is a cubic parabola, the heat flow at the wall is found to be given by equation (22.36):

$$\dot{q}_w = -k\frac{3}{2\delta_t}\theta_s$$

but δ_t has still to be determined.

(c) The formation of the temperature boundary layer must depend upon the flow, and therefore upon the profile of the velocity boundary layer of thickness δ. Introducing the ratio $\psi = \delta_t/\delta$ and the value of δ in terms of Re_x into equation (22.36), we derive equation (22.39):

$$\dot{q}_w = -\frac{3}{2 \times 4.64\psi x}(Re_x)^{1/2}k\theta_s$$

This equation can be written in terms of the Nusselt number

$$Nu_x = \frac{3}{2 \times 4.64}\frac{Re_x}{\psi}$$

or in general terms

$$Nu_x = \phi(Re_x, \psi)$$

(d) Using the continuity and energy equations, we arrive at the heat flow equation of the boundary layer which enables the value of ψ to be expressed in terms of physical properties of the fluid and the distance x from the leading edge of the plate, i.e. from equation (22.44)

$$\psi = \phi\left(\frac{c_p \mu}{k}, \frac{x_a}{x}\right) = \phi\left(Pr, \frac{x_a}{x}\right)$$

When the plate is heated from the leading edge, ψ is independent of x, and from equation (22.45)

$$\psi = \phi(Pr)$$

Hence the final result for this latter case is given in the form

$$Nu_x = \phi(Re_x, Pr) \tag{22.48}$$

In the foregoing we have assumed that the fluid properties are constant, but in practice the properties vary with temperature. The procedure recommended at the end of section 22.1, of using property values at a 'film temperature', can normally be adopted with reasonable accuracy. For large temperature gradients this may not always be satisfactory, however, and this point will be discussed more fully in section 22.5.

Example 22.2

For the conditions given in Example 22.1, calculate the heat transfer coefficient 0.6 m from the leading edge of the plate. Hence calculate the rate of heat transfer from one side of the plate to the air, per metre width of plate, over the first 0.6 m.

From Ref. 14 Pr for air at $65\,^{\circ}\text{C}$ is 0.699, and from Example 22.1 Re_x is 248 400. Hence the local Nusselt number 0.6 m from the leading edge is

$$Nu_x = 0.332(Pr)^{1/3}(Re_x)^{1/2} = 0.332 \times 0.699^{1/3} \times 248\,400^{1/2} = 147$$

The conductivity of air at $65\,^{\circ}\text{C}$ is $k = 2.913 \times 10^{-5}\,\text{kW/m K}$. Hence the value of the local heat transfer coefficient is

$$\alpha_x = (Nu_x)\frac{k}{x} = 147 \times \frac{2.913 \times 10^{-5}}{0.6} = 0.007\,14\,\text{kJ/m}^2\,\text{s K}$$

The average heat transfer coefficient α over the length x is $2\alpha_x$, and hence the rate of heat transfer over the first 0.6 m, per metre width of plate, is

$$\dot{Q} = -\alpha A(T_s - T_w)$$

$$= -(2 \times 0.007\,14)(0.6 \times 1)(5 - 115) = 0.857\,\text{kJ/s or kW}$$

22.2.3 Solution applicable to liquid metals

Finally, we must see how the solution presented here can be modified to be valid for liquid metals. Such substances have become of increasing importance in recent years as heat transfer media in nuclear reactors. The point at which we can expect the analysis to be incorrect for liquid metals is where it is assumed that $\delta_t < \delta$ because, although equation (22.45) is no longer strictly applicable, it suggests qualitatively that $\delta_t > \delta$ when $Pr < 1$. Let us re-examine equation (22.40) in conjunction with Fig. 22.7 and the assumption that $\delta_t > \delta$.

The integral on the left-hand side of (22.40) can be split into three parts, namely

$$\int_0^l (\theta_s - \theta)U\,dy = \int_0^\delta (\theta_s - \theta)U\,dy + \int_\delta^{\delta_t} (\theta_s - \theta)U\,dy + \int_{\delta_t}^l (\theta_s - \theta)U\,dy$$

Following the argument at the beginning of section 22.2.2, the third integral must be zero. Also, U in the second integral is constant and equal to U_s, because the limits of integration lie outside the velocity boundary layer. Further simplification can be achieved by assuming that for liquid metals, which have very low values of Pr, $\delta \ll \delta_t$. We can then ignore the first integral and write finally

$$\int_0^l (\theta_s - \theta)U\,dy \approx U_s \int_0^{\delta_t} (\theta_s - \theta)\,dy \qquad (22.49)$$

This approximation is tantamount to assuming that the velocity is uniform and equal to U_s from the wall surface; this represents an idealised type of flow often referred to as *slug flow*. The heat flow equation now becomes

$$U_s \frac{d}{dx} \int_0^{\delta_t} (\theta_s - \theta)\,dy = \kappa \left(\frac{d\theta}{dy}\right)_0$$

and on substituting equation (22.35) for θ it is easy to show that integration yields

$$\frac{\delta_t}{x} = \left\{ \frac{8}{(Re_x)(Pr)} \right\}^{1/2} \qquad (22.50)$$

Substitution of this expression for δ_t in (22.36) then gives

$$Nu_x = 0.530\{(Re_x)(Pr)\}^{1/2} \qquad (22.51)$$

The product $(Re_x)(Pr)$ is a dimensionless group called the *Péclet number Pe*, and it is an important parameter in liquid metal convection.

An exact solution to the problem, when the plate is heated to a uniform temperature, gives

$$Nu_x = 0.487(Pe)^{1/2} \quad \text{when} \quad Pr = 0.03$$
$$Nu_x = 0.516(Pe)^{1/2} \quad \text{when} \quad Pr = 0.01$$
$$Nu_x = 0.526(Pe)^{1/2} \quad \text{when} \quad Pr = 0.006$$

To check that our assumption of $\delta \ll \delta_t$ is reasonable, we may find an expression for $\psi = \delta_t/\delta$ by combining equations (22.3) and (22.50) to give

$$\psi = \frac{0.609}{(Pr)^{1/2}} \qquad (22.52)$$

This is of the same form as equation (22.45), i.e. $\psi = f(Pr)$, and for a typical liquid metal of $Pr = 0.01$ it yields a value of $\psi = 6$. Thus the approximation of slug flow appears not unreasonable.

The approximate solution for liquid metals is based on the heat flow equation

(22.40), which itself may not always be valid for such substances. It will be remembered that when deriving (22.40) the temperature gradient $d\theta/dx$ was assumed small compared with $d\theta/dy$, enabling us to ignore any conduction across planes 1–1 and 2–2 in Fig. 22.7. For liquid metals, conduction in the direction of flow may not always be negligible, particularly at low values of Re_x and therefore of Pe. On the other hand, the approximate solution is valid some way into the turbulent flow region, where the one-seventh power velocity profile is closer to the slug flow model, because eddy mixing has relatively little effect on heat transfer over and above the contribution from the high thermal conductivity of the liquid metal.

22.3 Forced convection in fully-developed laminar flow through a tube

The problem of calculating the value of the heat transfer coefficient in fully-developed laminar flow in a tube is considerably easier than the problem of the flat plate dealt with in the previous section. The reason is that, once the flow is fully established, the fluid can have no velocity components normal to the wall anywhere in the cross-section, otherwise successive velocity profiles would not be identical (Fig. 22.9). There is no divergence of the streamlines away from the wall as in Fig. 22.7, and the flow of energy in the radial direction must therefore be entirely by conduction.

It will be assumed, as for the flow past a flat plate, that conduction in an axial direction can be neglected, i.e. that anywhere in the fluid $(\partial T/\partial x) \ll (\partial T/\partial y)$, and therefore in the axial direction the energy transport is entirely by convection. It will also be assumed that the properties of the fluid are independent of temperature, or that the temperature difference between fluid and wall is sufficiently small for such variations to be neglected. This last assumption implies that the velocity profile is parabolic, i.e. that equation (22.16) is valid:

$$\frac{U}{U_r} = 2\left(\frac{y}{r}\right) - \left(\frac{y}{r}\right)^2$$

As with the flat plate, the temperature profile may again be approximately expressed by a cubic parabola (Fig. 22.9)

$$T = T_w + ay + by^2 + cy^3$$

g. 22.9
lly developed flow
rough a tube

Identical velocity profiles

Geometrically similar temperature profiles

Effectively stagnant layer

555

or, working in terms of the temperature difference $\theta = T - T_w$,

$$\theta = ay + by^2 + cy^3 \qquad (22.53)$$

Consider a length l of the cylinder. The rate of radial conduction at any radius $(r - y)$ is given by

$$\dot{Q} = -k2\pi(r - y)l\left(\frac{d\theta}{dy}\right)$$

In the immediate vicinity of the wall the fluid layers are effectively stagnant, and there is little convection in the axial direction. The only heat flow is by conduction in the radial direction. To satisfy continuity of heat flow, this implies that as $y \to 0$, $\dot{Q}$ becomes independent of y, i.e. $\dot{Q}_1 = \dot{Q}_w$ in Fig. 22.9. Hence near the wall, by differentiating the previous equation with $\dot{Q}$ treated as constant,

$$\left(\frac{d^2\theta}{dy^2}\right) = -\frac{\dot{Q}}{2\pi kl(r - y)^2} = \frac{1}{(r - y)}\left(\frac{d\theta}{dy}\right)$$

And therefore when $y = 0$ we have the first boundary condition,

$$\left(\frac{d^2\theta}{dy^2}\right)_0 = \frac{1}{r}\left(\frac{d\theta}{dy}\right)_0$$

Applying this boundary condition to (22.53), we get

$$\left(\frac{d\theta}{dy}\right)_0 = a = r\left(\frac{d^2\theta}{dy^2}\right)_0 = r2b$$

Two further boundary conditions can be stated at the axis of the tube where $y = r$:

$$\theta = \theta_r, \text{ and from symmetry, } (d\theta/dy)_r = 0$$

Applying these two boundary conditions to (22.53), it follows that

$$\theta_r = ar + br^2 + 3cr^2$$

$$\left(\frac{d\theta}{dy}\right)_r = 0 = \dot{a} + 2br + 3cr^2$$

The constants a, b, c can now be found from the three boundary conditions, and on substituting their values in (22.53) the equation becomes

$$\frac{\theta}{\theta_r} = \frac{6}{5}\left(\frac{y}{r}\right) + \frac{3}{5}\left(\frac{y}{r}\right)^2 - \frac{4}{5}\left(\frac{y}{r}\right)^3 \qquad (22.54)$$

The rate of heat flow per unit area at the wall is

$$\dot{q}_w = -k\left(\frac{d\theta}{dy}\right)_0 = -\frac{6}{5}k\frac{\theta_r}{r} = -\alpha_r(T_r - T_w)$$

and therefore the Nusselt number based on the temperature difference between axis and wall $(T_r - T_w) = \theta_r$ is

$$(Nu_d)_r = \frac{\alpha_r d}{k} = 2.4 \tag{22.55}$$

Subscript r refers to the fluid temperature used in the definition of α, and subscript d to the characteristic linear dimension. It must be emphasised that this result is the Nusselt number at any section x once the flow has become fully developed, and thus the local and average values are the same in this region.

It is more convenient to work in terms of a temperature difference $\theta_m = (T_m - T_w)$, where T_m is the weighted mean temperature of the fluid, since T_m is usually the temperature measured in practice. By definition, T_m at any cross-section of the tube is the temperature that the fluid would assume if it were thoroughly mixed. By considering a strip dy at radius $(r - y)$, T_m is thus defined by the equation

$$\int_0^r \rho c_p U T 2\pi (r - y)\, dy = \rho c_p U_m T_m \pi r^2$$

The product $\rho U_m \pi r^2 = \rho U_m A$ is given by equation (22.15), and hence

$$\int_0^r \rho c_p U T 2\pi (r - y)\, dy = c_p T_m \int_0^r \rho U 2\pi (r - y)\, dy$$

$U = \phi(y)$ is given by (22.16), and $T = \phi(y)$ by (22.54). Again treating the properties ρ and c_p as constant, and working in terms of θ instead of T, we get

$$\rho c_p 2\pi \int_0^r U_r \left\{ 2\left(\frac{y}{r}\right) - \left(\frac{y}{r}\right)^2 \right\} \theta_r \left\{ \frac{6}{5}\left(\frac{y}{r}\right) + \frac{3}{5}\left(\frac{y}{r}\right)^2 - \frac{4}{5}\left(\frac{y}{r}\right)^3 \right\}(r - y)\, dy$$

$$= \rho c_p 2\pi \theta_m \int_0^r U_r \left\{ 2\left(\frac{y}{r}\right) - \left(\frac{y}{r}\right)^2 \right\}(r - y)\, dy$$

Hence

$$\theta_m = \frac{102}{175}\theta_r = 0.583\theta_r$$

The heat transfer coefficient at the wall can now be defined in terms of θ_m, i.e.

$$\dot{q}_w = -\alpha(T_m - T_w) = -\alpha\theta_m$$

The Nusselt number, defined in terms of α based on θ_m, then becomes

$$Nu_d = \frac{\alpha d}{k} = (Nu_d)_r \frac{\theta_r}{\theta_m} = \frac{2.4}{0.583} = 4.12 \tag{22.56}$$

The method given here is only approximate because it is based on an assumed particular temperature profile, namely a cubic parabola. An exact solution to the problem of fully developed flow also leads to the result $Nu_d = $ constant, but the value of the constant depends upon a thermal boundary condition along the wall of the tube which did not have to be stipulated in the preceding approximate method. Two alternative boundary conditions of considerable interest are (a) constant wall temperature T_w, and (b) constant heat flux $\dot{q}_w$ which is equivalent to constant temperature gradient at the wall $(dT/dy)_0$. Boundary condition (a), which may be approached in practice with a tube heated on the outside by a condensing vapour, leads to the result

$$Nu_d = 3.65$$

Boundary condition (b) can be approached with a tube which is heated by an electric current passing through it, and in this case

$$Nu_d = 4.36$$

The approximate constant of 4.12 therefore falls between the two exact results and is in reasonable agreement with both.

The calculation of the heat transfer in the entrance section of a tube is considerably more complicated than that for fully developed flow. In addition to distinguishing between different thermal boundary conditions along the tube wall, it is necessary to consider whether at the beginning of the heated section the velocity profile is already developed or whether it is developing simultaneously with the temperature profile, i.e. whether there is an unheated entrance length or not. Whatever case is considered, the value of the temperature gradient at the wall is infinite at the beginning of the heated section and $Nu_d = \infty$. Along the tube the Nusselt number falls and approaches the appropriate constant value asymptotically. A rough rule is that the local Nu_d effectively reaches the asymptotic value when $l/d = 0.05(Re)(Pr)$. This means that with a fluid of high Pr, like a viscous mineral oil, the entrance length can be very long: laminar flow conditions are quite likely to be encountered with such fluids.

As has been pointed out in Section 22.1, and illustrated in Fig. 22.5, the velocity profile in fully developed flow is not parabolic because of the dependence of viscosity on temperature. Since the temperature profile is a function of the velocity profile, the former will also be changed and even the foregoing accurate solutions are only valid for 'isothermal flow', i.e. for the limiting case of heat transfer by convection as $\theta_m \to 0$. It may also be noted that, with a finite temperature difference between fluid and wall, the velocity profile may be further distorted by *free* convection currents superimposed on the flow in the tube; this is only significant in large-diameter tubes at low Reynolds numbers.

It will be appreciated that a full treatment of heat transfer in laminar flow in a tube, including the effects of an entrance length, different thermal boundary conditions, variable properties and free convection, is very complex. For further details the reader is referred to Ref. 6.

22.4 Forced convection in turbulent flow and the Reynolds analogy

So far it has not been possible to produce a complete analytical solution for heat transfer by forced convection when the flow is turbulent. It was suggested by Reynolds, however, that there exists a similarity between heat and momentum transfer in forced convection, and that it should be possible to predict rates of

Fig. 22.10
Relation between heat
flow and shear stress in a
boundary layer

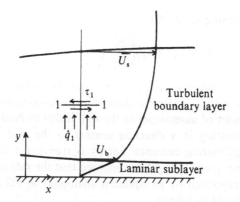

heat transfer from hydrodynamic measurements, e.g. from the measurement of viscous drag or shear stress on a surface.* The reason for this similarity is as follows.

Consider a fluid flowing over a wall as in Fig. 22.10. Along any section such as 1–1 there is a viscous shear stress due to a molecular momentum transfer given by

$$\tau_{v1} = \mu \left(\frac{dU}{dy} \right)_1 = \rho v \left(\frac{dU}{dy} \right)_1$$

There is also heat flow by molecular conduction through 1–1, given by

$$\dot{q}_{\kappa 1} = -k \left(\frac{dT}{dy} \right)_1 = -\rho c_p \kappa \left(\frac{dT}{dy} \right)_1$$

The similarity between the foregoing equations is apparent. When considering turbulent flow it is necessary to show that there is also a similarity between the equation expressing the shear stress due to eddy motion, and the equation expressing the heat flow due to eddy motion.

In section 22.1 we resolved the local instantaneous velocity components U_1, V_1 at 1–1 into mean velocity components $\bar{U}_1$, $\bar{V}_1$ and superimposed fluctuation components U'_1, V'_1. Thus we wrote equations (22.25) and (22.26) respectively as

$$U_1 = \bar{U}_1 + U'_1 \quad \text{and} \quad V_1 = \bar{V}_1 + V'_1$$

By assuming $\bar{V}_1$ to be negligible, it was then shown that, in addition to the viscous shear stress, there must be a shear stress due to eddy motion across 1–1 given by (22.29), namely

$$\tau_{\varepsilon 1} = -\rho (U'_1 V'_1)_{\text{mean}} = \rho \varepsilon_1 \left(\frac{d\bar{U}}{dy} \right)_1$$

The eddy diffusivity ε is a function of the local velocity fluctuations, i.e. it is a quantity depending on the amount of turbulence. The total shear stress is,

---

* Ref. 21. Also see Ref. 10, Chapter 24.

according to (22.30),

$$\tau_1 = \rho(v + \varepsilon_1)\left(\frac{d\bar{U}}{dy}\right)_1$$

It is stated in section 22.1, and must be emphasised again here, that for steady flow with $\bar{V}_1$ negligible there is no *net* mass transfer through 1–1, and that the transfer of momentum to the wall is due to fluid elements of various velocities fluctuating in a direction normal to the wall, exchanging momentum with neighbouring elements. Energy is transferred through the fluid by a similar process, and it might be supposed that the rate of transfer via eddy motion can be expressed by an equation analogous to (22.29); such an equation can be deduced as follows.

Let the temperature of the wall be higher than the temperature of the free stream. The instantaneous temperature T_1 at 1–1 fluctuates, owing to the occasional arrival of hot eddies from below and cold eddies from above, and we may thus write

$$T_1 = \bar{T}_1 + T_1' \tag{22.57}$$

The mass flow per unit area across surface 1–1, during a time interval dt, is $\rho V_1 \, dt$, and the transport of energy across unit area is thus $(\rho V_1 \, dt)c_p T_1$. Considering a period Δt, which is long compared with the period of velocity fluctuations, the average rate of heat flow may be found by integration as

$$\dot{q}_{\varepsilon 1} = \frac{1}{\Delta t}\int_0^t \rho c_p V_1 T_1 \, dt$$

By substituting the values of V_1 and T_1 from (22.26) and (22.57) in the integral, we obtain

$$\dot{q}_{\varepsilon 1} = \frac{\rho c_p}{\Delta t}\int_0^t (\bar{V}_1 \bar{T}_1 + \bar{V}_1 T_1' + V_1' \bar{T}_1 + V_1' T_1') \, dt$$

For steady flow the time averages of the velocity and temperature fluctuations are zero, i.e.

$$\int_0^t \bar{V}_1 T_1' \, dt = \bar{V}_1 \int_0^t dt = 0$$

$$\int_0^t V_1' \bar{T}_1 \, dt = \bar{T}_1 \int_0^t V_1' \, dt = 0$$

Further, as has been explained, $\bar{V}_1$ is zero or nearly so for the cases we are considering. Hence

$$\int_0^t \bar{V}_1 \bar{T}_1 \, dt = 0$$

Thus the heat transfer per unit area at 1–1 is

$$\dot{q}_{\varepsilon 1} = \frac{\rho c_p}{\Delta t}\int_0^t (V_1' T_1') \, dt = \rho c_p (V_1' T_1')_{\text{mean}} \tag{22.58}$$

where $(V_1' \, T_1')_{mean}$ stands for the time average of the product of the instantaneous velocity fluctuation V_1' and the temperature fluctuation T_1'. This equation is similar to (22.28),

$$\tau_{t1} = \rho(U_1' \, V_1')_{mean}$$

which relates the shear stress to the product of the instantaneous velocity fluctuation components.

The energy flow across 1–1 may be written, by analogy with Fourier's law, as

$$\dot{q}_{t1} = -\rho c_p \varepsilon_{H1} \left(\frac{d\bar{T}}{dy} \right)_1$$

where ε_H is an *eddy diffusivity for heat flow*, defined by

$$\dot{q}_{t1} = \rho c_p (V_1' \, T_1')_{mean} = -\rho c_p \varepsilon_{H1} \left(\frac{d\bar{T}}{dy} \right)_1 \qquad (22.59)$$

Two principal questions relating to the value of $(V_1' \, T_1')_{mean}$, and therefore to ε_H, remain to be answered.

First, is the time average of the product $(V_1' \, T_1')$ different from zero? Although the time averages of V_1' and T_1' are individually zero, the answer to this question is not immediately obvious. Consider a positive V_1', i.e. an instantaneous flow upward through 1–1. As this flow arrives from a region which, *on the average*, is hotter than 1–1, $(V_1' \, T_1')$ is, *on the average*, positive for positive V_1'. Now consider a negative V_1', i.e. an instantaneous flow downward through 1–1. As this flow arrives from a region which, *on the average*, is colder than 1–1, $(V_1' \, T_1')$ is again, *on the average*, positive. Thus on the whole $(V_1' \, T_1')_{mean}$ is greater than zero, except in a region of no temperature gradient where T' must always be zero, or in a region of laminar flow where V' must also be zero. As $(d\bar{T}/dy)$ must be negative according to the adopted sign convention of positive heat flow into the fluid from the wall, the negative sign has been introduced into (22.59) to define ε_H as a positive quantity. The total heat flow through 1–1, which is a result of a molecular energy flow and an energy flow due to eddy motion, is therefore

$$\dot{q}_1 = -k \left(\frac{d\bar{T}}{dy} \right)_1 - \rho c_p \varepsilon_{H1} \left(\frac{d\bar{T}}{dy} \right)_1$$

or

$$\dot{q}_1 = -\rho c_p (\kappa + \varepsilon_{H1}) \left(\frac{d\bar{T}}{dy} \right)_1 \qquad (22.60)$$

where κ is the *thermal diffusivity* of the fluid.

The second question of fundamental importance is whether the eddy diffusivity for heat flow, as defined by (22.59), is numerically equal to the eddy diffusivity for momentum transfer, as defined by (22.29). Although an eddy moving across the stream tends to assume the temperature and momentum of the new layer into which it moves, if it returns to its original layer immediately it will not necessarily have assumed the momentum and temperature of its new surroundings completely. The values of ε and ε_H depend on the speed of adaptability of an eddy, and that need not be the same for momentum as it is for temperature. H. Reichardt* investigated the problem in some detail, and concluded that the eddy diffusivities for momentum transfer and heat transfer are not necessarily equal, although they are nearly equal for turbulent flow through tubes and over flat plates. For simplicity we shall assume here that the same value ε can be used in equations (22.29) and (22.59), and these equations thus serve as starting points for our similarity considerations between heat transfer and friction. It is necessary to state here again, however, that the value of ε varies from point to point in a turbulent fluid, although no assumption need be made about the variation of its value with the coordinates (x, y).

22.4.1 The simple Reynolds analogy

We now require to find the relation between the heat flow $\dot{q}_w$ and the shear stress τ_w at the wall, and for this purpose equations (22.30) and (22.60) may be rewritten in the following form:

$$dU = \frac{\tau \, dy}{\rho(v + \varepsilon)} \tag{22.61}$$

$$dT = -\frac{\dot{q} \, dy}{\rho c_p(\kappa + \varepsilon)} \tag{22.62}$$

We have dropped the bar over U and T in (22.61) and (22.62) because only mean values are required in what follows and there is no need to retain this distinguishing mark. If it is required to find the relation between shear stress and heat flow in terms of some convenient reference velocities and temperatures, it is first necessary to integrate these equations between limits of y corresponding to the required reference planes. Usually the velocities and temperatures in the free stream and at the wall are the values known. Thus by integration we obtain

$$U_s - U_w = U_s = \int_0^l \frac{\tau \, dy}{\rho(v + \varepsilon)} \tag{22.63}$$

$$t_s - t_w = \theta_s = -\int_0^l \frac{\dot{q} \, dy}{\rho c_p(\kappa + \varepsilon)} \tag{22.64}$$

The upper limit of the integral $y = l$ is chosen in the free stream, i.e. l is larger than both δ and δ_t.

To evaluate the integrals it is of course necessary to know how τ, $\dot{q}$ and ε vary with the distance from the wall y. For the purpose of comparing $\dot{q}_w$ and τ_w, however, this is not necessary. The analysis will be restricted initially to fluids whose kinematic viscosity and thermal diffusivity are equal, i.e. when

$$v = \kappa \quad \text{or} \quad \frac{\mu}{\rho} = \frac{k}{\rho c_p}$$

---

* Ref. 28. Also see S. E. Isakoff and Th. B. Drew, and G. I. Taylor, in Ref. 35, pp. 405 and 193. For a good discussion of the concept of eddy diffusivity in turbulent heat transfer theory, see Ref. 20.

The Prandtl number of the fluids considered is therefore

$$Pr = \frac{c_p \mu}{k} = 1$$

It follows that whatever may be the variation of ε with y, $(v + \varepsilon)$ and $(\kappa + \varepsilon)$ are equal and therefore vary in the same way with y. Further, it is an experimental fact, which can be justified by theoretical considerations (Ref. 28), that the heat flow normal to the wall and the shear stress τ along surfaces parallel to the wall vary in an approximately similar way with y. This is a particularly reasonable assumption for flow over plates and *turbulent* flow through cylindrical tubes. The assumption implies that in general

$$\frac{\dot{q}_1}{\tau_1} = \frac{\dot{q}_w}{\tau_w} \neq \phi(y)$$

Dividing (22.64) by (22.63), and ignoring the negative sign which arises from the sign convention adopted for τ and $\dot{q}$, we have

$$\frac{\theta_s}{U_s} = \frac{\int_0^l \dfrac{\dot{q}\,dy}{\rho c_p(\kappa + \varepsilon)}}{\int_0^l \dfrac{\tau\,dy}{\rho(v + \varepsilon)}} = \frac{\dot{q}_w}{\tau_w c_p} \frac{\int_0^l \dfrac{\tau\,dy}{(\kappa + \varepsilon)}}{\int_0^l \dfrac{\tau\,dy}{(v + \varepsilon)}}$$

and hence

$$\frac{\dot{q}_w}{\tau_w c_p} = \frac{\theta_s}{U_s} \tag{22.65}$$

This relation is called the *Reynolds analogy*. It gives the ratio of the local rate of heat transfer to the local shear stress at the solid boundary.

Let the flow over a flat plate be considered first. Equation (22.65) can be used as it stands, and for smooth plates τ_w can be found from (22.5) and (22.8). It is convenient to put (22.65) into non-dimensional form: first we rewrite it as

$$\frac{\dot{q}_w}{\theta_s} = \frac{\tau_w}{U_s} c_p$$

and then by suitable multiplications and divisions of both sides of the equation we get

$$\frac{\dot{q}_w x}{\theta_s k} = \frac{\tau_w}{\rho U_s^2} \frac{\rho U_s x}{\mu} \frac{c_p \mu}{k}$$

where x is the distance from the leading edge of the plate. This equation can now be rewritten as

$$Nu_x = \frac{f_x}{2}(Re_x)(Pr)$$

where f_x is the local friction factor defined by (22.5). As this relation has been derived on the assumption that the Prandtl number of the fluid is 1, we finally obtain for the local Nusselt number

$$Nu_x = \frac{f_x}{2}(Re_x) \tag{22.66}$$

Since f_x is merely a function of Reynolds number (equation (22.6)), we arrive at the same form of result as that obtained for the laminar flow of fluids having a Prandtl number of unity, i.e. that the Nusselt number is a function of Reynolds number, equation (22.48).

Usually we are interested to find the average Nusselt number, and not its local value. In this case we can calculate, or find from experiment directly, the average shear stress on the plate; this average value can then be used in (22.65) to find the average rate of heat flow over the plate, and hence the average Nusselt number can be deduced.

To apply the Reynolds analogy to flow through tubes, (22.63) and (22.64) must be considered afresh, although the only modification required is in the upper limit of the integrals. There is no 'free stream', and the appropriate reference section is the tube axis, where $y = r$. Equation (22.65), when applied to flow through a tube, thus becomes

$$\frac{\dot{q}_w}{\tau_w c_p} = \frac{\theta_r}{U_r}$$

If the upper limit applied to the integrals in equations (22.63) and (22.64) is merely y, where the temperature difference is θ and the velocity is U, the equivalent of (22.65) becomes

$$\frac{\dot{q}_w}{\tau_w c_p} = \frac{\theta}{U}$$

Since $(\dot{q}_w/\tau_w c_p)$ is independent of y, this equation implies that the temperature and velocity profiles are geometrically similar. It can be shown that $\theta_m/U_m \approx \theta_r/U_r$, and the ratio of the weighted mean temperature and velocity may be used instead of the ratio of their values at the axis. The Reynolds relation for turbulent flow in tubes then becomes

$$\frac{\dot{q}_w}{\tau_w c_p} = \frac{\theta_m}{U_m} \tag{22.67}$$

This can again be put into non-dimensional form, as

$$\frac{\dot{q}_w d}{\theta_m k} = \frac{\tau_w}{\rho U_m^2} \frac{\rho U_m d c_p \mu}{\mu} \frac{c_p \mu}{k}$$

and hence, as the Prandtl number has been assumed to be unity, at any section x

$$Nu_d = \frac{f}{2}(Re_d) \tag{22.68}$$

τ_w (or f) can be found from measurements of the pressure drop, as in the following example, or for smooth tubes it can be found from the friction law of Blasius, equation (22.20).

Example 22.3 At some section of a cooled tube, having an inner diameter of 5 cm, air is at 150 °C and 1 atm and flows with a velocity of 8 m/s. The surface temperature of the tube is maintained at 40 °C. If the static pressure drop per metre length of tube is 1.6×10^{-4} bar, calculate approximately the temperature drop of the air over the next metre of tube.

Instead of working out the shear stress and heat transfer per unit surface area of tube, it is more convenient to evaluate them for a *surface area corresponding to unit length of tube*. The shear force on the wall per metre length of tube, F_w, is therefore

$$F_w = \tau_w \pi d l = \Delta p l \pi \left(\frac{d}{2}\right)^2$$

$$= 1.6 \times 10^{-4}\left[\frac{\text{bar}}{\text{m}}\right] \times 10^5\left[\frac{\text{N/m}^2}{\text{bar}}\right] \times 1[\text{m}] \times \pi 0.025^2[\text{m}^2] = 0.0314\,\text{N}$$

As a first approximation we may assume that for air $Pr = 1$, i.e. that the Reynolds relation (22.67) can be applied. Hence the rate of heat transfer per metre length of tube, $\dot{Q}_w$, is

$$\dot{Q}_w = \dot{q}_w \pi d l = \frac{F_w c_p \theta_m}{U_m}$$

$$= \frac{0.0314\left[\text{N or}\dfrac{\text{kg m}}{\text{s}^2}\right] \times 1.017\left[\dfrac{\text{kJ}}{\text{kg K}}\right] \times \dfrac{\theta_m}{[\text{K}]}[\text{K}]}{8\left[\dfrac{\text{m}}{\text{s}}\right]}$$

$$= 0.003\,99\,\frac{\theta_m}{[\text{K}]}\,\text{kJ/s (or kW)}$$

Here c_p has been taken from Ref. 14 at $T_1 = 150 °C$ (Fig. 22.11); when T_2 has been found a more accurate result can be obtained by repeating the calculation with c_p evaluated at $(T_1 + T_2)/2$.

The average value of θ_m over the metre length is

$$\theta_m = \left(\frac{150 + T_2/[°C]}{2} - 40\right)\text{K}$$

Fig. 22.11

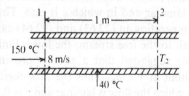

565

Hence

$$\dot{Q}_w = 0.003\,99\left(\frac{150 + T_2/[°C]}{2} - 40\right) kJ/s$$

From an energy balance, this must also be equal to the enthalpy drop of the air in cooling from 150°C to T_2, and hence

$$\dot{Q}_w = \rho c_p U_m \frac{\pi d^2}{4}(150°C - T_2)$$

Although the velocity U_m falls along the tube and ρ rises, owing to the cooling of the air, for a duct of constant cross-sectional area the product ρU_m remains constant. Thus ρU_m may be evaluated from the known conditions at section 1, and hence

$$\dot{Q}_w = 0.8373 \times 1.017 \times 8 \times \frac{\pi}{4} \times 0.05^2 \times (150 - T_2/[°C])\,kJ/s$$

$$= 0.0134(150 - T_2/[°C])\,kJ/s$$

Eliminating $\dot{Q}_w$ from this and the previous equation, we get

$$0.003\,99\left(\frac{150 + T_2/[°C]}{2} - 40\right) = 0.0314(150 - T_2/[°C])$$

and hence $T_2 = 121°C$. Therefore the temperature drop of the air over the metre length is

$$150°C - T_2 = 29\,K$$

22.4.2 The Prandtl-Taylor modification of the Reynolds analogy

We have seen how eddy motion in a boundary layer promotes momentum transfer (resulting in shear stresses) and heat transfer, and we have drawn attention to the similarity between these two processes. Thence, by making certain assumptions which could not be adequately justified here, we derived the relation (22.65) between the shear stress and the heat flow at a solid boundary. This simple relation, called the Reynolds analogy, was derived for fluids of $Pr = 1$, i.e. for cases where $v = \kappa$. Now the assumption essential to the argument is that $(v + \varepsilon) = (\kappa + \varepsilon)$ at any distance from the wall. In a region of high turbulence this equality is still valid, even if $v \neq \kappa$, because normally in such a region $\varepsilon \gg \kappa$ or v. (An important exception is when the fluid is a liquid metal: see the end of this section.) But though the flow at some distance from the wall may be highly turbulent, there is a sublayer of thickness δ_b adjacent to the wall in which the flow is laminar and in which ε is zero. Thus when considering a fluid of $Pr \neq 1$, the integration in (22.63) and (22.64) cannot be carried out in one step from the wall to the free stream; the lower limit must be $y > \delta_b$.

Prandtl and Taylor suggested that a good approximation is obtained by choosing the lower limit at $y = \delta_b$. Thus the flow region is divided into two parts: the sublayer in which the flow is laminar and $\varepsilon = 0$, and the region outside the sublayer in which ε is considered large enough for the assumption of $(v + \varepsilon) = (\kappa + \varepsilon)$ to be valid even when $Pr \neq 1$ (Fig. 22.10).

Consider the flow over a flat plate first. By changing the limits of the integrals in (22.63) and (22.64) to $y = \delta_b$ and $y = l$, we obtain

$$U_s - U_b = \int_{\delta_b}^{l} \frac{\tau \, dy}{\rho(v + \varepsilon)} \tag{22.69}$$

$$T_s - T_b = -\int_{\delta_b}^{l} \frac{\dot{q} \, dy}{\rho c_p (\kappa + \varepsilon)} \tag{22.70}$$

Dividing (22.70) by (22.69), and making the same assumptions as before about the expressions under the integrals, we obtain

$$\frac{\dot{q}_b}{\tau_b c_p} = \frac{T_s - T_b}{U_s - U_b} = \frac{\theta_s - \theta_b}{U_s - U_b} \tag{22.71}$$

For the laminar sublayer, in which the velocity gradient is constant (see section 22.1.1), the shear stress is given by

$$\tau_w = \tau_b = \mu \left(\frac{dU}{dy} \right) = \mu \frac{U_b}{\delta_b} \tag{22.72}$$

The heat flow through the thin sublayer is by conduction only, and thus the temperature gradient through this layer must also be constant. Hence

$$\dot{q}_w = \dot{q}_b = -k \left(\frac{dT}{dy} \right) = -k \frac{T_b - T_w}{\delta_b} = -k \frac{\theta_b}{\delta_b} \tag{22.73}$$

Dividing (22.73) by (22.72), and ignoring the negative sign as before, we get

$$\frac{\dot{q}_w}{\tau_w} = \frac{\dot{q}_b}{\tau_b} = \frac{k}{\mu} \frac{\theta_b}{U_b} \tag{22.74}$$

Eliminating θ_b from (22.71) and (22.74), the following relation is obtained:

$$\frac{\dot{q}_w}{\tau_w c_p} = \frac{\theta_s}{U_s} \frac{1}{1 + \frac{U_b}{U_s}(Pr - 1)} \tag{22.75}$$

This relation is the *Prandtl-Taylor modification of the Reynolds analogy*, and it reduces to (22.65) when $Pr = 1$. The ratio of the velocities U_b/U_s for smooth plates can be taken from (22.11), and (22.75) can be put in non-dimensional form in the same way as (22.65). The relation finally obtained is

$$Nu_x = \frac{f_x}{2} \frac{(Re_x)(Pr)}{1 + 2.11(Re_x)^{-0.1}(Pr - 1)} \tag{22.76}$$

When considering turbulent flow through a tube, the integration of (22.69) and (22.70) must be carried out between limits of $y = \delta_b$ and $y = r$. This procedure yields the relation

$$\frac{\dot{q}_w}{\tau_w c_p} = \frac{\theta_r}{U_r} \frac{1}{1 + \dfrac{U_b}{U_r}(Pr - 1)}$$

The velocity and temperature profiles in the laminar sublayer are linear according to (22.72) and (22.73), and are therefore geometrically similar. When the limits in equations (22.69) and (22.70) are δ_b and y, the equivalent of (22.71) becomes

$$\frac{\theta - \theta_b}{U - U_b} = \frac{\dot{q}_b}{\tau_b c_p}$$

As $\dot{q}_b / \tau_b c_p$ is independent of y, this equation implies that the velocity and temperature profiles are also geometrically similar in the turbulent layer. This result was obtained before when considering a fluid of $Pr = 1$. Again $\theta_m / U_m \approx \theta_r / U_r$, and the ratio of the weighted mean temperature and velocity may be used in the foregoing equation instead of the ratio of their values at the axis. The modified Reynolds relation thus becomes

$$\frac{\dot{q}_w}{\tau_w c_p} = \frac{\theta_m}{U_m} \frac{1}{1 + \dfrac{U_b}{U_r}(Pr - 1)} \tag{22.77}$$

For fully developed flow in smooth tubes the ratio U_b / U_r is found from (22.23), and putting (22.77) into non-dimensional form we get finally

$$Nu_d = \frac{f}{2} \frac{(Re_d)(Pr)}{1 + 1.99(Re_d)^{-1/8}(Pr - 1)} \tag{22.78}$$

Again f can be found from measurements of the pressure drop, or for smooth tubes from (22.20) where it is expressed in terms of Re_d. Equations (22.76) and (22.78) show that for forced convection the Nusselt number is a function of the Reynolds and Prandtl numbers.

It is worth noting that the dimensionless combination $Nu/\{(Re)(Pr)\}$ is often used as an alternative for Nu when presenting heat transfer data; it is called the *Stanton number St* and is equal to $\alpha / c_p \rho U$. Equation (22.78) can then be written as

$$St = \frac{f}{2} \frac{1}{1 + 1.99(Re_d)^{-1/8}(Pr - 1)}$$

It should also be apparent that the simple Reynolds analogy then becomes $St = f/2$. The main reason why the concept of the Stanton number has found favour lies in the ease with which it is obtained from experimental data. For example, from the energy balance on a heated or a cooled fluid in a tube we can write

$$\alpha \pi d l \theta_m = \rho U \frac{\pi d^2}{4} c_p (T_2 - T_1)$$

or

$$\frac{\alpha}{c_p \rho U} = St = \frac{d\,(T_2 - T_1)}{4l} \frac{}{\theta_m}$$

Thus St can be obtained directly from the tube dimensions and temperature measurements without reference to fluid properties.

Example 22.4   Recalculate Example 22.3 taking the correct Prandtl number for air. (Property values used in the solution are taken from Ref. 14.)

At the mean film temperature $T_f = (136 + 40)/2 = 88\,°C$, Pr for air is 0.695. Thus for air the modified relation by Prandtl and Taylor should be used. It is first necessary to calculate the ratio U_b/U_r, and, assuming that the tube is smooth and the flow fully developed, this ratio is given by equation (22.23), namely

$$\frac{U_b}{U_r} = \frac{1.99}{(Re_d)^{1/8}}$$

The Reynolds number is $Re_d = \rho U_m d/\mu$. Since the product ρU_m remains constant, it may be evaluated for the conditions at section 1 (Fig. 22.11). The viscosity μ at T_f is $2.122 \times 10^{-5}\,kg/m\,s$. Hence

$$Re_d = \frac{0.8373 \times 8 \times 0.05}{2.122 \times 10^{-5}} = 15\,780$$

$$\frac{U_b}{U_r} = \frac{1.99}{(15\,780)^{1/8}} = 0.594$$

The rate of heat flow per metre length of tube is therefore

$$\dot{Q}_w = \frac{F_w c_p}{U_m\left\{1 + \dfrac{U_b}{U_r}(Pr - 1)\right\}}\theta_m = \frac{0.0314 \times 1.017}{8\{1 + 0.594(0.695 - 1)\}}\left(\frac{150 + T_2}{2} - 40\right)$$

$$= 0.004\,88\left(\frac{150 + T_2}{2} - 40\right)kJ/s$$

From the energy balance, this must again be equal to

$$\dot{Q}_w = \rho c_p U_m \frac{\pi d^2}{4}(150 - T_2) = 0.0134(150 - T_2)\,kJ/s$$

Eliminating $\dot{Q}_w$ from this and the previous equation, we get

$$0.004\,88\left(\frac{150 + T_2}{2} - 40\right) = 0.0134(150 - T_2)$$

and hence $T_2 = 116\,°C$. Therefore the temperature drop of the air over the metre length is

$$150\,°C - 116\,°C = 34\,K$$

which is about one-sixth greater than the result obtained by assuming $Pr = 1$.

Fig. 22.12

Effect of Prandtl number
on the temperature profile

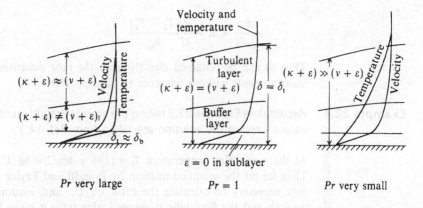

Velocity and
temperature

$(\kappa + \varepsilon) \approx (v + \varepsilon)$

$(\kappa + \varepsilon) \neq (v + \varepsilon)_1$

Velocity

Temperature

$\delta_t \approx \delta_b$

Pr very large

Turbulent
layer

$(\kappa + \varepsilon) = (v + \varepsilon)$

Buffer
layer

$\varepsilon = 0$ in sublayer

Pr = 1

$(\kappa + \varepsilon) \gg (v + \varepsilon)$

$\delta = \delta_t$

Temperature

Velocity

Pr very small

The Prandtl-Taylor modification of the Reynolds analogy permits the calculation of heat transfer data from friction data for fluids having Prandtl numbers from about 0.5 to 2. The limited range of application of this modification is due to the choice of $y = \delta_b$ as the lower limit of the integration of (22.63) and (22.64); the assumption that outside the sublayer $\varepsilon \gg v$ or κ is not accurate, and the larger the Prandtl number the larger is the error introduced by assuming that $(\kappa + \varepsilon) = (v + \varepsilon)$. Von Kármán improved on the Prandtl-Taylor approach by considering three layers, namely the laminar sublayer, the fully turbulent boundary layer, and a *buffer layer* between in which ε, v and κ are all of the same order of magnitude. Only in the fully turbulent region, outside the buffer layer, can it normally be assumed that $\varepsilon \gg v$ or κ.

Extreme conditions exist when the Prandtl number of a fluid is very high, e.g. several thousand as for a very viscous oil, or when it is very low, e.g. of the order of 0.01 as for a liquid metal. Fig. 22.12 illustrates the simple case of $Pr = 1$ side by side with these two extremes, for flow over a flat plate. For the case of $Pr = 1$ the velocity and temperature profiles are identical. We have already seen that this is so for laminar flow, i.e. equation (22.45) with Pr put equal to 1 yields $\delta_t = \delta$; this, together with the similarity of equations (22.2) and (22.35), means that the boundary layers are identical. It can be shown that this identity is also true for a turbulent boundary layer when $Pr = 1$.

When Pr is very large (i.e. when k is very small) δ_t is much smaller than δ (as in laminar flow, equation (22.45)) and the temperature boundary layer may lie almost entirely in the laminar sublayer of thickness δ_b. When δ_b is known, $\dot{q}_w$ can simply be calculated from (22.73) by putting $T_b = T_s$; alternatively it is possible to obtain a fair estimate of δ_b from experimental values of $\dot{q}_w$. Thus turbulence, and the value of ε, will have little effect on the temperature profile, but will merely affect the velocity profile.

When Pr is very small, as for liquid metals, the molecular diffusivity κ $(= k/\rho c_p)$ is relatively large and may predominate over the eddy diffusivity ε even when turbulence is extreme, i.e. even when $\varepsilon \gg v$. In other words, the effective conductivity $\rho c_p (\kappa + \varepsilon) \approx \rho c_p \kappa$ is fairly constant throughout the boundary layer, even though the effective viscosity $\rho(v + \varepsilon)$ may vary appreciably. Under such conditions the temperature gradient varies only slightly through the boundary layer, and again turbulence and ε play a small part in determining the temperature profile, which in fact extends beyond the edge of the velocity boundary layer. With fully developed flow in a tube, the boundary layer reaches the axis, and it is not difficult to predict the rate of turbulent convection. Since the effect of ε on the heat transfer is small, the rate of turbulent convection should be governed by a relation similar to that for laminar flow, i.e. $Nu_d = $ constant; the constant will not be quite the same as in equation (22.56) because the velocity profile is very different and therefore the temperature profile will also be altered slightly. A fair estimate of this constant for turbulent flow can be obtained from a slug flow model for which U is uniform across the tube, but in which the radial conductivity is put equal to $\rho c_p \kappa$, i.e. k. In fact it has been found that for liquid metals Nu_d rises only moderately over a wide range of Re_d well into the turbulent regime, and only extreme turbulence raises Nu_d significantly.

The analogy between heat and momentum transfer has been developed to cover the whole range of possible Prandtl numbers, and for the most general theories the reader is referred to Ref. 10, pp. 500–21, and Refs 31 and 36. The problem of liquid metals is treated specifically in Ref. 38.

The Reynolds analogy can be applied only if it may be assumed that the eddy diffusivity for momentum transfer is about equal to the eddy diffusivity for heat transfer. As already pointed out, this is a valid assumption for the boundary layer in a tube or near a flat plate. It does not apply, for example, in the turbulent wake formed when a fluid flows across a cylinder, and the analogy cannot be applied to find the rate of heat transfer in such cases. In general it may be said that the Reynolds analogy applies when the drag forces on a surface are due to *skin friction* alone, but not when some of the drag is due to flow separation from the surface as occurs in the flow round a cylinder or, to take a more interesting example, near the outlet of a cascade of axial-flow compressor blades.*

22.5   The principles of dynamic similarity and dimensional analysis applied to forced convection

We have seen that analytical solutions to the problem of heat transfer by forced convection can be found for laminar flow, although they are difficult even for simple geometric shapes. The Reynolds analogy provides a semi-analytical approach to turbulent convection problems, but this has also a limited range of application. The direct measurement of heat transfer coefficients is still the main approach to many problems concerning forced convection, and this section describes the method by which this empirical information can be correlated systematically so that a few experiments can produce results suitable for general application.

Initially we shall assume that the physical properties of the fluid do not vary with temperature; later the effect of such variation is discussed in some detail. Certain generalisations, which are not proved here, can be made about the

---

* Ref 32, p. 247.

Fig. 22.13
The principle of similarity
in forced convection

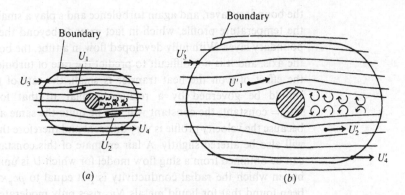

(a)   (b)

patterns of fluid and heat flow in forced convection, and these generalisations follow from the study of the complete set of differential equations (not given here) that describe forced convection.* Consider two regions, each within a specified *boundary* enclosing a solid body and a fluid around it. As an example we may think of two cylinders and limited regions around them in which fluids flow; these regions are referred to as the *fields* (Fig. 22.13). The two fields can easily be imagined to be similar in the sense that:

(a) The bodies and boundaries are geometrically similar.

(b) The velocity distributions around the boundaries are similar (in magnitude, direction and turbulence pattern).

(c) The temperature distributions around the boundaries are similar.

Once (a), (b) and (c) are satisfied, it is possible to prove that the following statements are valid for both laminar and turbulent flow:

(i) The velocity distributions *within* the fields will be similar when the Reynolds numbers $(\rho U l/\mu)$ are the same for both fields.

(ii) The temperature distributions *within* the fields will be similar when, in addition to condition (i), the Prandtl numbers $(c_p \mu/k)$ are the same for both fluids.

(iii) When (i) and (ii) are satisfied, then the Nusselt numbers (hl/k) for corresponding surface elements will be the same for both solid bodies, and hence the average Nusselt numbers will be the same for both surfaces.

When the Reynolds numbers are the same and the Prandtl numbers are the same, for both fields, the fields are said to be *dynamically* or *physically similar* from the point of view of forced convection heat transfer. Conditions of similarity (a), (b) and (c) by themselves do not ensure complete similarity.

These conclusions may be summarised by writing

$$Nu = \phi(Re, Pr) \tag{22.79}$$

i.e. the heat transfer expressed in terms of the Nusselt number *Nu*, for any particular geometrical arrangement, can be expressed as a function of the Reynolds number *Re* and the Prandtl number *Pr*. The general deduction (22.79),

---

* Ref. 10, Chapter 23, and Ref. 18, Chapter 14.

although not proved so far, is in general agreement with the particular solutions obtained in the preceding sections.

When comparing the Reynolds numbers in the two fields, any pair of reference velocities such as U_1, U'_1 or U_2, U'_2 can be chosen (Fig. 22.13), provided that the velocities are in corresponding positions in the two fields. The same remark applies to the choice of the linear dimension l in the Reynolds number and the Nusselt number; thus either the cylinder diameter or the cylinder radius may be chosen in the example considered.

It follows that empirical data, which have been obtained at certain Reynolds and Prandtl numbers for a certain geometrical arrangement of surfaces and flow, may be extended to geometrically similar arrangements under dynamically similar conditions. For instance, data can be obtained for large-scale heat exchangers from experiments on small-scale apparatus.

Example 22.5 The film coefficient for toluene, flowing at a speed of 2.6 ft/s through a pipe of 0.5 inch bore, is to be found. The average temperature of the toluene flowing through the pipe is 86 °F, and its properties at this temperature, expressed in British (ft lb h R) units, are:

Specific heat c_p:	0.41 Btu/lb R
Viscosity μ:	1.23 lb/ft h
Thermal conductivity k:	0.0859 Btu/ft h R
Density ρ:	55.6 lb/ft^3

It is desired to obtain the information from experiments carried out with water flowing through a pipe of 2 cm bore. Specify the conditions of the experiment from which the information is to be obtained, i.e. the temperature and velocity of the water, in SI units.

Also, if the film coefficient for water found from the correct experiment is 3.61 kW/m^2 K, what is the value for toluene under the above conditions?

The Reynolds number and the Prandtl number respectively must be the same for the water experiment as for the toluene. For toluene,

$$Pr = \frac{c_p \mu}{k} = \frac{0.41 \times 1.23}{0.0859} = 5.87$$

$$Re_d = \frac{\rho U d}{\mu} = \frac{55.6(2.6 \times 3600)(0.5/12)}{1.23} = 17\,630$$

Previously we have assumed that the fluid properties do not vary with temperature. The conclusions reached so far in this section will be assumed correct, provided the temperature differences in the fluid are not too great, even if the properties are functions of temperature. All non-dimensional groups must then be evaluated at the mean fluid temperature. The Prandtl number is a property of the fluid, and is therefore dependent on temperature. The Reynolds number depends on the fluid properties ρ and μ and on the fluid velocity U. It is therefore first necessary to specify the correct temperature for the experiment, so that it can be carried out at the right Prandtl number. The Reynolds number can then be adjusted by a suitable selection of the velocity U.

Since the properties of water vary but little with pressure, the values for saturated water in Ref. 14 may be used. The relevant values are:

$T/[^\circ C]$	20	25	30	35
Pr	6.95	6.09	5.39	4.80
$c_p/[\text{kJ/kg K}]$	4.183	4.181	4.179	4.178
$\mu/10^{-6}[\text{kg/m s}]$	1002	890	797	718
$k/10^{-6}[\text{kW/m K}]$	603	611	618	625
$v/[\text{m}^3/\text{kg}]$	0.001	0.001	0.001	0.001

By interpolation, the correct average temperature for the Prandtl numbers to be the same is therefore 26.6 °C. To find U,

$$Re_d = 17\,630 = \frac{1000 \times 0.02U/[\text{m/s}]}{861 \times 10^{-6}}$$

and hence $U = 0.759\,\text{m/s}$.

The Nusselt number for the water experiment was found to be

$$Nu_d = \frac{\alpha d}{k} = \frac{3.61 \times 0.02}{613 \times 10^{-6}} = 118$$

Hence the film coefficient for toluene is given by

$$\frac{\alpha(0.5/12)}{0.0859} = 118 \quad \text{or} \quad \alpha = 243\,\text{Btu/ft}^2\,\text{h R} \quad (= 1.38\,\text{kW/m}^2\,\text{K})$$

In order to arrive at the general form of the solution given by (22.79), it is not necessary to derive the complete set of differential equations governing forced convection; (22.79) can be obtained by *dimensional analysis* using the method of indices.* The disadvantage of this method is that it is necessary to know from previous experience all the variables on which the heat transfer depends before the analysis can be commenced.

The dimensional analysis which follows will be devoted to finding the form of an expression for the heat transfer coefficient α defined by

$$\alpha = -\frac{\dot{q}}{T_s - T_w} = -\frac{\dot{q}}{\theta_s}$$

in terms of all the variables that affect the heat transfer. From the previous sections it is clear that the variables that may affect α in forced convection are

viscosity	μ
density	ρ
thermal conductivity	k
specific heat capacity	c_p
temperature (relative to wall)	θ
fluid velocity	U
characteristic linear dimension	l

Since the solution to be obtained is to apply to geometrically similar surfaces, it is sufficient to include among the variables a single dimension l which is characteristic of the field considered. For the example illustrated in Fig. 22.13,

* Refs 4 and 12.

the cylinder diameter d is one possible choice. In general, we can write

$$\alpha = \phi(\mu, \rho, k, c_p, \theta, U, l) \tag{22.80}$$

The terms in any physical equation must always be dimensionally homogeneous, and such equations can always be expanded into a sum of a finite or an infinite number of terms. For example, equation (22.80) can be written

$$\alpha = A\mu^{a_1}\rho^{a_2}k^{a_3}c_p^{a_4}\theta^{a_5}U^{a_6}l^{a_7} + B\mu^{b_1}\rho^{b_2}k^{b_3}c_p^{b_4}\theta^{b_5}U^{b_6}l^{b_7} + \ldots \tag{22.81}$$

in which each term has the same dimensions as α.

In the function considered there are eight variables, and Buckingham's Π theorem states that if the least number of independent fundamental units is n, then the function can be reduced to one involving $(8 - n)$ non-dimensional groups. Equation (22.79) suggests, however, that the solution can be expressed in terms of three non-dimensional groups. This requires some explanation since it implies the use of five fundamental units instead of the three (mass, length, time) usually accepted.*

Thermodynamics suggests that the units of heat are the same as those of mechanical energy, i.e. $(\text{mass})(\text{length})^2/(\text{time})^2$. When considering phenomena including transformations of energy, it would be impossible to treat heat as a fundamental unit. However, it was pointed out in the Introduction to Part IV that in many practical heat transfer processes, rates of energy transformation are small compared with rates of energy transfer. In this field of study, therefore, heat may usually be regarded as a fundamental unit. For similar reasons temperature may be regarded as fundamental. Temperature occurs in products such as $\alpha\theta$, $k\theta$ and $c_p\theta$. Such products always have the dimensions of heat, and temperature does not appear explicitly in their units. It is therefore of no consequence what dimensions are given to θ, and for the purpose of the present analysis it may be regarded as a fundamental unit. The dimensions of α, k and c_p are then fixed by this choice. We shall discuss later the results of an analysis in which heat is assigned the dimensions of energy and is not regarded as fundamental.

It is now possible to tabulate the units of the eight variables, each number in the table indicating the dimension of each fundamental unit:

	mass	length	time	heat	temperature
α	0	-2	-1	1	-1
μ	1	-1	-1	0	0
ρ	1	-3	0	0	0
k	0	-1	-1	1	-1
c_p	-1	0	0	1	-1
θ	0	0	0	0	1
U	0	1	-1	0	0
l	0	1	0	0	0

* Dimension is the power of a fundamental unit in a derived unit. For example, the gravitational acceleration g has the units $(\text{length})/(\text{time})^2$; the dimensions of length are 1, those of time -2, and those of mass 0 (see Appendix A, section A.1).

Five linear simultaneous equations can be written down for each term in (22.81), which must be satisfied if the function of α is to be dimensionally homogeneous. Considering the first term,

$$
\begin{aligned}
\text{mass:} && 0 &= a_1 + a_2 - a_4 \\
\text{length:} && -2 &= -a_1 - 3a_2 - a_3 + a_6 + a_7 \\
\text{time:} && -1 &= -a_1 - a_3 - a_6 \\
\text{heat:} && 1 &= a_3 + a_4 \\
\text{temperature:} && -1 &= -a_3 - a_4 + a_5
\end{aligned}
$$

There are seven unknowns in these equations, and a solution can only be obtained in terms of two of the unknowns which can be arbitrarily chosen. On their choice, however, will depend the actual non-dimensional groups obtained. It is desirable to separate the effect of velocity into one group, and to do this it is necessary to solve in terms of the index a_6 of U. The other variable which it is convenient to keep in one group is c_p, and therefore the solution should be obtained also in terms of a_4. Finding the values of a_1, a_2, a_3, a_5, a_7 in terms of a_4 and a_6, the following are obtained:

$$
\begin{aligned}
a_1 &= a_4 - a_6 \\
a_2 &= a_6 \\
a_3 &= 1 - a_4 \\
a_5 &= 0 \\
a_7 &= a_6 - 1
\end{aligned}
$$

Similarly the values of b_1, b_2, b_3, b_5, b_7 can be found in terms of b_4 and b_6. Equation (22.81) then becomes

$$
\alpha = A \frac{k}{l} \left(\frac{\rho U l}{\mu} \right)^{a_6} \left(\frac{c_p \mu}{k} \right)^{a_4} + B \frac{k}{l} \left(\frac{\rho U l}{\mu} \right)^{b_6} \left(\frac{c_p \mu}{k} \right)^{b_4} + \ldots
$$

or

$$
Nu = A(Re)^{a_6}(Pr)^{a_4} + B(Re)^{b_6}(Pr)^{b_4} + \ldots \tag{22.82}
$$

The coefficients $A, B, \ldots$ and the indices $a_4, a_6, b_4, b_6, \ldots$ are constants which must be found experimentally for any particular geometric arrangement of the heat transfer surfaces and flow.

If this analysis is carried out in a similar way, but with heat given the dimensions of energy, we arrive at a relation between four non-dimensional groups, i.e. Nu, Re, Pr and the additional group $U^2/c_p\theta$. It is worth looking into the significance of the last group a little more closely. In the analysis it is not essential to take the temperature θ relative to the surface, but the absolute temperature T can be taken instead; the group $U^2/c_p T$, called the *Eckert number*, is then obtained. When the fluid is a gas this group has a well-known significance. By dividing the group by the pure number $(\gamma - 1)$ its character is unchanged, and it then becomes equal to $U^2/\gamma RT$. This will be recognised as the square of the *Mach number* of a perfect gas, and we know from experiments with high-speed gas flow that the Mach number has a considerable effect on the heat transfer. This is to be expected because large amounts of kinetic energy are dissipated

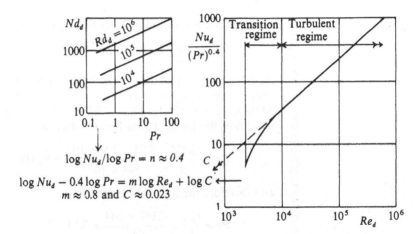

Fig. 22.14
Forced convection in fully
developed flow through a
ube

by viscous friction in the boundary layer. At low velocities, when the dissipation of kinetic energy is negligible, the influence of the Eckert number is small and the analysis presented here is valid.

It has been found that for many common configurations the experimental results fall on a single curve if they are plotted in an appropriate way. One procedure is illustiaicd in Fig. 22.14 for flow through a tube. First of all, $\log(Nu_d)$ is plotted against $\log(Pr)$ for several values of Re_d, and it is found that approximately straight lines are obtained with a slope n which is nearly the same for all Reynolds numbers in the turbulent regime. Then by plotting $\log\{(Nu_d)/(Pr)^n\}$ against $\log(Re_d)$, a single curve is obtained. For a limited range of Reynolds number this plot is also found to be a straight line, of slope m say, and the Nusselt number can then be expressed by the relation

$$Nu_d = C(Re_d)^m (Pr)^n \qquad (22.83)$$

The values of C and m for the appropriate range of Re_d can easily be taken from the logarithmic plot. Equation (22.83) implies that in practice only the first term in the series of equation (22.82) need be used for a limited range of Reynolds number.

The advantages of presenting heat transfer data in terms of non-dimensional groups are several. Mainly, this method of presentation allows empirical data to be applied to a wide range of physical conditions by application of the principle of dynamic similarity, and requires few experiments to cover a wide range of fluid properties. Also, considerable savings can be made by carrying out experiments on small-scale apparatus instead of full-scale plant. Lastly, data presented in non-dimensional form are suitable for use in any consistent system of units, whether metric or British, and the likelihood of errors arising from confusing the units of the large number of variables involved is minimised.

Example 22.6   Calculate the heat transfer coefficient for water flowing through a 2 cm diameter tube with a velocity of 2.5 m/s. The average temperature of the water is 50 °C, and the surface temperature of the tube is slightly below this temperature. For turbulent flow through tubes,

$$Nu_d = 0.023(Re_d)^{0.8}(Pr)^{0.4}$$

As the surface temperature of the tube differs only slightly from the mean bulk temperature of the water, all properties may be taken at the latter temperature. At 50 °C, $c_p = 4.182$ kJ/kg K, $k = 643 \times 10^{-6}$ kW/m K, $\mu = 544 \times 10^{-6}$ kg/m s, $\rho = 1/v = 988$ kg/m³ (from Ref. 14). Hence

$$Re_d = \frac{\rho U d}{\mu} = \frac{9.88 \times 2.5 \times 0.02}{544 \times 10^{-6}} = 90\,800$$

and therefore the flow is turbulent. Also

$$Pr = \frac{c_p \mu}{k} = \frac{4.182 \times 544}{643} = 3.54$$

and hence the Nusselt number is

$$Nu_d = 0.023(90\,800)^{0.8}(3.54)^{0.4} = 353$$

The heat transfer coefficient becomes

$$\alpha = \frac{k}{d} Nu_d = \frac{643 \times 10^{-6}}{0.02} 353 = 11.35 \text{ kW/m}^2 \text{ K}$$

Dimensional analysis has shown that the relative temperature θ does not appear in the solution (22.82). When the fluid properties are not constant, but vary with temperature, it may not always be possible to correlate experimental data by this equation satisfactorily. Such lack of correlation would be apparent by a scatter of experimental points on logarithmic plots such as Fig. 22.14, and the scatter would be particularly noticeable for points obtained from experiments with large temperature differences.

Nusselt has shown* that if the variation of properties with temperature can be written as functions of the *absolute* temperatures in the form

$$\mu = \mu_0 \left(\frac{T}{T_0}\right)^a, \quad \rho = \rho_0 \left(\frac{T}{T_0}\right)^b, \quad k = k_0 \left(\frac{T}{T_0}\right)^c, \quad c_p = c_{p0} \left(\frac{T}{T_0}\right)^d \tag{22.84}$$

where μ_0, ρ_0, k_0 and c_{p0} are property values at some reference temperature T_0, then (22.82) can be modified to include such variations of properties by simply adding a non-dimensional group (T_w/T_s). Hence

$$Nu = \phi \left(Re, Pr, \frac{T_w}{T_s} \right)$$

which for the limiting case of 'isothermal flow' reduces to (22.79). Frequently we can write

$$Nu = C(Re)^m (Pr)^n \left(\frac{T_w}{T_s}\right)^p \tag{22.85}$$

* Ref. 23 and Ref. 10, pp. 496–9.

The ratio (T_w/T_s) is truly non-dimensional, because the ratio of the absolute temperatures is the same on any scale of temperature. Nusselt's method gives particularly good results with gases, as their property variations are well represented by equations (22.84) over a wide range of temperature. For liquids (22.84) can usually be applied over a moderate range of temperature only, and an equation of the form (22.85) is required for each range of temperature.

Other methods than that of Nusselt are often used to allow for variations of fluid properties with temperature. A common procedure is to use an equation of the form of (22.83), and to evaluate the properties used in the Nusselt, Reynolds and Prandtl numbers at a film temperature T_f, this being defined as

$$T_f = \frac{T_b + T_w}{2} \tag{22.86}$$

T_b is the temperature of the bulk of the fluid; it is equal to the free stream temperature T_s for flow over a flat plate, and to the weighted mean temperature T_m for flow through a tube (see (22.31) and (22.32)). When the film temperature is not uniform over the whole surface (it may vary from entrance to exit of a tube), the properties are often evaluated at the arithmetic mean of the inlet and outlet film temperatures.

A word of warning: when using any published equation of the form of (22.83) to obtain a value of α, it is necessary to know how the original experimental correlation was obtained, i.e. how Nu, Re and Pr have been calculated when producing the curves from which C, m and n have been deduced. Some experimenters find it best to correlate data with all or some of the fluid properties taken at the bulk temperature rather than at the film temperature. Thus to find the heat transfer coefficient from an expression of the form (22.83), it is essential to find out first what reference temperatures have been used in deducing C, m and n, and then substitute values of properties corresponding to these temperatures. References 2, 13 and 29 are good sources of empirical correlations.

Example 22.7   Air at atmospheric pressure and a temperature of 90 °C flows with a velocity of 8 m/s *across* a 2.5 cm diameter tube. The tube is maintained at a temperature of 650 °C. Calculate the rate of heat transfer per metre length of tube. For air, the rate of heat transfer can be calculated from the relation

$$Nu_d = C(Re_d)^n \left(\frac{T_w}{T_s}\right)^{n/4}$$

For Reynolds numbers between 40 and 4000, $C = 0.600$ and $n = 0.466$. This empirical relation has been formulated with the fluid properties taken at the film temperature.

The film temperature is $T_f = (90 + 650)/2 = 370$ °C, and from Ref. 14 we find that at this temperature $k = 4.913 \times 10^{-5}$ kW/m K and $v = 5.75 \times 10^{-5}$ m²/s. The Reynolds number is given by

$$Re_d = \frac{Ud}{v} = \frac{8 \times 0.025}{5.75 \times 10^{-5}} = 3480$$

and the ratio of the absolute surface temperature to the free stream temperature by

$$\frac{T_w}{T_s} = \frac{923}{363} = 2.54$$

Hence the Nusselt number is

$$Nu_d = 0.600 \times 3480^{0.466} \times 2.54^{0.1165} = 29.9$$

and the film coefficient is

$$\alpha = \frac{k}{d} Nu_d = \frac{4.913 \times 10^{-5}}{0.025} 29.9 = 0.0588 \,\text{kW/m}^2\,\text{K}$$

The rate of heat transfer per metre length of tube is

$$\dot{Q} = -\alpha A (T_s - T_w) = -0.0588(\pi \times 0.025 \times 1)(90 - 650) = 2.59 \,\text{kW}$$

22.6 Heat transfer from a vertical wall by free convection

When a temperature difference is established between a wall and a stationary fluid, the fluid adjacent to the wall will move upward if the wall temperature is higher than that of the fluid, and downward if the wall temperature is lower. The cause of the movement is the temperature gradient itself. This sets up density gradients in the fluid resulting in *buoyancy forces* and free convection currents. The rate of heat transfer depends mainly on the fluid motion, and this is very largely governed by a balance between buoyancy and viscous forces; inertia forces play only a small part in free convection.

Consider any fluid element at a temperature θ above the surrounding fluid; the density ρ of this element is smaller than the density ρ_s of the bulk of the fluid, and it is given by $\rho = \rho_s/(1 + \beta\theta)$, where β is the coefficient of cubical expansion. The velocity of this element is a function of the buoyancy force acting on it, which for unit volume is

$$(\rho_s - \rho)g = \beta g \rho \theta \tag{22.87}$$

It follows that in a solution for the rate of heat transfer by free convection, the group of variables $\beta g \rho \theta$ may be expected to appear. In this section the concepts of the velocity and temperature boundary layers are applied to find an analytical solution for the rate of heat transfer from a vertical wall to a fluid, *when the flow is laminar*.

A velocity and a temperature boundary layer will build up at the wall, as shown in Fig. 22.15. The temperature gradually varies from T_w at the wall to T_s at the edge of the temperature boundary layer where $y = \delta_t$. The velocity gradually varies from zero at the wall to some maximum value in the velocity boundary layer, and then to zero at the edge of this boundary layer where $y = \delta$. It has been found from experiment and confirmed by theory that the thickness of the velocity and temperature boundary layers are about equal (except for very viscous fluids). This is to be expected, since the fluid will tend to rise only in the region where the temperature of the fluid is increased. It is

Fig. 22.15
Free laminar convection
near a heated vertical wall

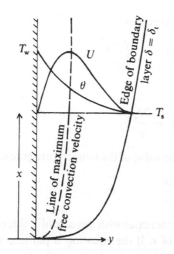

beyond the scope of this book to derive the value of δ, and the result[*] is simply quoted here as

$$\frac{\delta}{x} = 3.93(Pr)^{-1/2}\left(Pr + \frac{20}{21}\right)^{1/4}(Gr_x)^{-1/4} \tag{22.88}$$

Here x is the height above the bottom of the heated wall. Gr_x is a dimensionless group called the *Grashof number*, and it is equal to

$$Gr_x = \frac{\beta g \rho^2 x^3 \theta}{\mu^2} \tag{22.89}$$

The heat flow at the wall at x is

$$\dot{q}_w = -k\left(\frac{d\theta}{dy}\right)_0 = -\alpha_x \theta_s \tag{22.90}$$

where α_x is the local heat transfer coefficient at x. To find α_x it is first necessary to find the temperature gradient $(d\theta/dy)_0$ at the wall. Following the procedure adopted in section 22.2, first the temperature profile is expressed in terms of a polynomial in y, and then the temperature gradient is deduced from the polynomial. Let the temperature profile be approximated by a quadratic parabola

$$T - T_w = \theta = ay + by^2 \tag{22.91}$$

To find the values of the constants a and b, the following boundary conditions may be used:

$$\theta = \theta_s \quad \text{when} \quad y = \delta$$

$$\left(\frac{d\theta}{dy}\right) = 0 \quad \text{when} \quad y = \delta$$

---

[*] The equation was derived independently by E. R. G. Eckert and H. B. Squire, and details can be found in Refs 6 and 29.

Hence (22.91) becomes

$$\frac{\theta}{\theta_s} = 2\left(\frac{y}{\delta}\right) - \left(\frac{y}{\delta}\right)^2 \tag{22.92}$$

and therefore

$$\left(\frac{d\theta}{dy}\right)_0 = \frac{2\theta_s}{\delta}$$

Substituting the value of the temperature gradient $(d\theta/dy)_0$ in (22.90), we obtain

$$\alpha_x = \frac{2k}{\delta}$$

Since δ clearly increases with increase of x, this equation implies that α_x decreases with increase of x. If the equation is put into non-dimensional form, we have

$$Nu_x = \frac{\alpha_x x}{k} = 2\left(\frac{x}{\delta}\right) \tag{22.93}$$

The value of δ can be taken from (22.88), and hence

$$Nu_x = 0.509(Pr)^{1/2}\left(Pr + \frac{20}{21}\right)^{-1/4}(Gr_x)^{1/4} \tag{22.94}$$

In general terms $Nu_x = \phi(Pr, Gr_x)$, suggesting that the Grashof number plays a part in free convection analogous to the part played by the Reynolds number in forced convection.

It is usually of interest to know the average of α over a height l, and this can easily be found by integration. If α is this average value, and α_l is the value at height l, then

$$\alpha = \frac{1}{l}\int_0^l \alpha_x \, dx$$

If α_x is found from (22.94) and substituted in the integral, we find that

$$\alpha = \frac{4}{3}\alpha_l \quad \text{or} \quad Nu = \frac{4}{3}(Nu_l) \tag{22.95}$$

For air, as well as for many other gases, $Pr \approx 0.70$. Substituting this value in (22.94), the relation for the local Nusselt number simplifies to

$$Nu_x = 0.376(Gr_x)^{1/4} \tag{22.96}$$

It has been shown in Ref. 26 that a horizontal cylinder of diameter d has the same average heat transfer coefficient as a vertical plate of height $l = 2.76d$. Using this result, the expression for the average Nusselt number of the cylinder becomes

$$Nu_d = 0.527(Pr)^{1/2}\left(Pr + \frac{20}{21}\right)^{-1/4}(Gr_d)^{1/4} \tag{22.97}$$

where d is the characteristic dimension used in the Nusselt and Grashof numbers. When $Pr = 0.70$, this reduces to

$$Nu_d = 0.389(Gr_d)^{1/4} \tag{22.98}$$

In forced convection the Reynolds number is a criterion of whether the flow is laminar or turbulent. The critical Reynolds number above which the flow is turbulent depends on the geometric configuration; thus for flow through tubes the critical value of Re_d is about 2300, and for flow over a plate the critical value of Re_x is about 500 000 (see section 22.1). In free convection the product $(Gr)(Pr)$ serves as a criterion of turbulence, the exact value depending on the geometric configuration. For a vertical plate the flow becomes turbulent when $(Gr_x)(Pr)$ is about 10^9. The product $(Gr)(Pr)$ itself is a non-dimensional group called the *Rayleigh number Ra*.

Analytical solutions for free convection problems are usually difficult and even impossible when the flow is turbulent. As in forced convection, the principle of similarity and the method of dimensional analysis are widely used for the systematic correlation of empirical data. In the following section the method of indices is applied to the dimensional analysis of free convection.

22.7 The principles of dynamic similarity and dimensional analysis applied to free convection

At the beginning of the previous section it was shown that the group of variables $\beta g \rho \theta$ plays an important part in the phenomenon of free convection, and it must therefore be included amongst the variables considered in the dimensional analysis. As θ and ρ appear already in the list of variables in section 22.5, only the product βg need be added to that list; the units of βg are (length)/(temperature)(time)^2. The velocity U, on the other hand, which is a controlling factor in forced convection, can be omitted from the list for our present purpose. It is true that in free convection the fluid attains some velocity, and this affects the rate of heat transfer, but the free convection velocity is not an *independent* variable. Thus the final list of relevant variables is given by

$$\alpha = \phi(\mu, \rho, k, c_p, \theta, \beta g, l) \tag{22.99}$$

Carrying out a dimensional analysis in the manner described in section 22.5, the functional relation can be reduced to

$$Nu = A(Gr)^{a_1}(Pr)^{a_2} + B(Gr)^{b_1}(Pr)^{b_2} + \ldots \tag{22.100}$$

$A, B, \ldots, a_1, a_2, b_1, b_2, \ldots$ are constants which must be found by experiment for any particular configuration of which the characteristic dimension is l. The value of θ in the Grashof number $Gr (= \beta g \rho^2 l^3 \theta / \mu^2)$ must always be measured in a certain reference position for the purpose of consistent correlation. It is usual to take θ as the temperature of the undisturbed fluid relative to the surface, i.e. $\theta = (T_s - T_w)$.

Once again the experimental results may be plotted on logarithmic scales. There are theoretical reasons (see Ref. 23) why the indices of Pr and Gr in

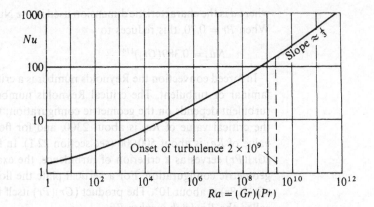

Fig. 22.16
Free convection from a
vertical wall

(22.100) should be equal in laminar convection (for any configuration), and in this case we can write that

$$Nu = \phi\{(Gr)(Pr)\} = \phi\left(\frac{\beta g \rho^2 l^3 \theta}{\mu^2} \frac{c_p \mu}{k}\right)$$

When convection is fully turbulent, theory suggests that

$$Nu = \phi\{(Gr)(Pr)^2\} = \phi\left(\frac{\beta g \rho^2 l^3 \theta}{\mu^2} \frac{c_p^2 \mu^2}{k^2}\right)$$

Note that μ cancels in the latter case, implying that the heat transfer becomes independent of the viscous stresses in the fluid. Under normal conditions fully developed turbulence exists, if at all, only over part of the heated surface. It is therefore common to correlate experimental results for Nu with $(Gr)(Pr)$, although sometimes a better correlation can be obtained with $(Gr)(Pr)^n$ where $1 < n < 2$. When experimental values are plotted with $\log(Nu)$ as the ordinate and $\log\{(Gr)(Pr)\}$ as the abscissa, the plot for free convection from a wall appears as shown in Fig. 22.16. For a limited range of $(Gr)(Pr)$ it is possible to express the Nusselt number Nu by the relation

$$Nu = C\{(Gr)(Pr)\}^m \tag{22.101}$$

and the values of C and m can be taken from the logarithmic plot for the appropriate range.

It is interesting to note that for free convection from a vertical wall the slope of the curve in Fig. 22.16, and therefore the index m, become equal to 1/3 when $(Gr)(Pr)$ is greater than 2×10^9. This is in the range of turbulent convection, as has been explained in section 22.6. Since l appears in the Grashof number to the power of 3, and in the Nusselt number to the power of 1, α_x in the turbulent range is not a function of height. Thus α_x decreases in value as the boundary layer thickens over the lower section of the wall, where the flow is laminar, and then increases fairly suddenly to assume a constant value above a certain height where the flow is turbulent.

To allow for the variation of property values with temperature, the procedures

. 22.17
nplified equations for
e convection heat
nsfer coefficients in air
atmospheric pressure

	Average $\alpha/[\mathrm{W/m^2 K}]$	
	Laminar or transition	Turbulent
Vertical plate, or cylinder of large diameter, of height l	$10^4 < Gr < 10^9$ $1.42\{(\theta/l)/[\mathrm{K/m}]\}^{1/4}$	$10^9 < Gr < 10^{12}$ $1.31(\theta/[\mathrm{K}])^{1/3}$
Horizontal cylinder of diameter d	$10^4 < Gr < 10^9$ $1.32\{(\theta/d)/[\mathrm{K/m}]\}^{1/4}$	$10^9 < Gr < 10^{12}$ $1.25(\theta/[\mathrm{K}])^{1/3}$
Square plate $l \times l$: heated plate facing up, or cooled plate facing down	$10^5 < Gr < 2 \times 10^7$ $1.32\{(\theta/l)/[\mathrm{K/m}]\}^{1/4}$	$2 \times 10^7 < Gr < 3 \times 10^{10}$ $1.52(\theta/[\mathrm{K}])^{1/3}$
Square plate $l \times l$: cooled plate facing up, or heated plate facing down	$3 \times 10^5 < Gr < 3 \times 10^{10}$ $0.59\{(\theta/l)/[\mathrm{K/m}]\}^{1/4}$	

recommended at the end of section 22.5 may be used. Most commonly, property values at the film temperature are used in the dimensionless groups. Simplified formulae for free convection for both the laminar and the turbulent range can be given for air at or near atmospheric pressure; those for the more important configurations are summarised in Fig. 22.17.

Inspection of the Grashof number Gr shows that the gravitational acceleration g appears in this group, in addition to the properties of the fluid, the linear dimension l and the temperature difference θ. Full turbulence in free convection can be produced by increasing g and thereby the value of Gr. An effective increase in g always occurs in a vessel rotating at high speed, owing to centripetal acceleration. A hollow gas turbine blade internally cooled by a liquid is a practical example (Ref. 39).

There are instances when heat is transferred by combined free and forced convection, but few experimental data are available. We have already mentioned that free convection may play a significant part in forced convection at low Reynolds numbers. If the dimensional analysis is carried out to allow for both modes of convection, by including the variables U and βg simultaneously, the following relation is obtained:

$$Nu = \phi(Re, Gr, Pr) \tag{22.102}$$

22.8   Convection with change of phase

Some of the most important industrial processes involving transfers of heat occur when the fluid changes its phase during the process, i.e. when it evaporates or condenses. As these processes usually take place at approximately constant pressure, the temperature of the bulk of the fluid can be assumed to be constant. Condensation and evaporation are now considered in turn.

Fig. 22.18
Formation of a
condensate film on a
vertical wall

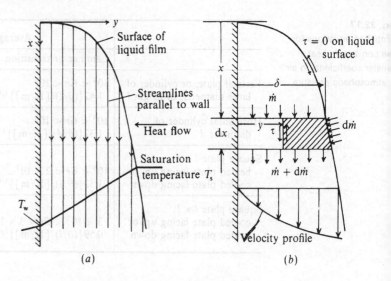

(a)   (b)

22.8.1   Condensation of a vapour on a vertical surface

In 1916 Nusselt* presented a method for predicting the rate of heat transfer
from a vapour condensing in a laminar film and running down a vertical surface
of uniform temperature, and this method is presented here (Fig. 22.18). One
assumption made is that the vapour which flows parallel to the surface, whether
up or down, flows so slowly that its drag on the condensed liquid film can be
neglected. A further assumption is that the motion of any liquid element in the
condensed film is governed solely by a balance of the gravity and viscous forces
acting on the element; hydrostatic pressure forces and inertia forces are therefore
neglected.

The condensing film has zero thickness at the top of the wall, and it thickens
as additional condensate settles on the vapour–liquid interface while the film
flows down the wall. Because the thickening is almost entirely due to this process
and not to a retardation of the liquid in the falling film, the streamlines can be
assumed to be vertical as indicated in Fig. 22.18a and the flow can be treated
as laminar. The temperature of the interface is the saturation temperature T_s
corresponding to the vapour pressure, and the wall temperature T_w must lie
below T_s for condensation to occur. Inside the film, therefore, the temperature
and enthalpy of the bulk of the condensate must be below the saturation values.
It follows that no heat can flow from the film towards the vapour, and all the
heat transfer, resulting from the liberation of energy from the vapour condensing
on the liquid film, is towards the wall. Also this heat transfer must be entirely
by conduction because the streamlines are vertical. The temperature gradient
in the film is therefore constant, assuming no variation of the liquid conductivity
with temperature within the film. Considering unit width of wall, as in
Fig. 22.18b, the rate of heat flow towards the wall through a strip of height dx

* Ref. 24. For an excellent survey on recent work see A. P. Colburn in Ref. 35, pp. 1–11.

is therefore

$$d\dot{Q} = -k \, dx \frac{T_w - T_s}{\delta} = -\alpha_x \, dx (T_w - T_s) = -\alpha_x \, dx \, \theta_s \qquad (22.103)$$

Thus

$$\alpha_x = \frac{k}{\delta}$$

and putting this in non-dimensional form,

$$Nu_x = \frac{\alpha_x x}{k} = \frac{x}{\delta} \qquad (22.104)$$

To find the local heat transfer coefficient α_x, or the corresponding Nusselt number Nu_x, it is first necessary to find the film thickness δ.

Consider the equilibrium of the shaded element of the strip dx; it is assumed that the velocity of such an element is governed by the balance of the shear force and the gravity force acting on it. Hence

$$\tau \, dx = \mu \left(\frac{dU}{dy} \right) dx = (\delta - y) \, dx \, \rho g$$

or

$$dU = \frac{\rho g}{\mu} (\delta - y) \, dy$$

Integrating this expression between $y = 0$ and y we find the velocity at y, and thus we find the velocity distribution through the film to be

$$U = \frac{\rho g}{\mu} \left(\delta y - \frac{y^2}{2} \right) \qquad (22.105)$$

The amount of liquid flowing through a cross-section of the film of unit width and thickness δ, at a distance x from the top of the plate, is

$$\dot{m} = \int_0^\delta \rho U \, dy = \frac{\rho^2 g}{\mu} \int_0^\delta \left(\delta y - \frac{y^2}{2} \right) dy = \frac{\rho^2 g \delta^3}{3\mu} \qquad (22.106)$$

The outflow through a section $(x + dx)$ from the top of the plate is $(\dot{m} + d\dot{m})$, and therefore the amount condensing on the film over the height dx is

$$(\dot{m} + d\dot{m}) - \dot{m} = d\dot{m} = \frac{\rho^2 g \delta^2}{\mu} d\delta$$

The heat conducted through the film is equal to the latent enthalpy given up by the condensing mass $d\dot{m}$. Strictly speaking, the heat conducted into the wall is slightly greater than this; some sensible enthalpy must be transferred also, because the average temperature of the film is below the saturation temperature as indicated in Fig. 22.18a. However, we shall in the first instance ignore the effect of this subcooling. The rate of heat transfer across the film is then given by

$$d\dot{Q} = h_{fg}\,d\dot{m} = h_{fg}\frac{\rho^2 g\delta^2}{\mu}\,d\delta \tag{22.107}$$

From (22.103) and (22.107),

$$d\dot{Q} = k\,dx\frac{\theta_s}{\theta} = h_{fg}\frac{\rho^2 g\delta^2}{\mu}\,d\delta$$

By integration between the limits $x = 0$, where $\delta = 0$, and x, we find the film thickness δ at section x as

$$\delta^4 = \frac{4\mu k\theta_s x}{h_{fg}\rho^2 g} \tag{22.108}$$

Substituting (22.108) in (22.104), the Nusselt number at section x is found to be

$$Nu_x = \left(\frac{h_{fg}\rho^2 gx^3}{4\mu k\theta_s}\right)^{1/4} \tag{22.109}$$

The group of the variables in (22.109) is dimensionless, but it has not yet been given a name. When the plate is inclined at an angle ϕ to the vertical, equation (22.109) can be applied if $g\cos\phi$ is substituted for g.

It is frequently of interest to know the average value of the heat transfer coefficient α or the average Nusselt number Nu over a height l, and these will be derived in two ways. First, we can do this by integration, namely

$$\alpha = \frac{1}{l}\int_0^l \alpha_x\,dx = \frac{4}{3}\alpha_l \quad \text{or} \quad Nu = \frac{4}{3}(Nu_l) \tag{22.110}$$

where α_l and Nu_l are the terminal values at $x = l$. The second way is based on equation (22.106) which can be used to calculate $\dot{m}_l$, the total drainage of condensate at $x = l$. The total quantity of heat transferred, neglecting subcooling, is $\dot{m}_l h_{fg}$, and the average heat transfer coefficient is

$$\alpha = \frac{\dot{m}_l h_{fg}}{\theta_s l} = \frac{\rho^2 g h_{fg}\delta_l^3}{3\mu\theta_s l} \tag{22.111}$$

Substitution of δ_l from equation (22.108) yields the same result as equation (22.110).

In deriving equation (22.107) we neglected the effect of subcooling, and this is permissible for steam. It has been shown (Ref. 34) that for laminar film condensation the equations derived so far are valid when a fictitious value h'_{fg} is used, defined by

$$h'_{fg} = h_{fg}\left(1 + \frac{3}{8}\frac{c_p\theta_s}{h_{fg}}\right) \tag{22.112}$$

The ratio $c_p\theta_s/h_{fg}$ is a dimensionless group called the *Jakob* or *phase-change number*, which represents a ratio of sensible to latent enthalpy. With steam condensing at 1 atm and a wall temperature of 60 °C, for example, we would have

$$h'_{fg} = 2256.7\left(1 + \frac{3}{8}\frac{4.198 \times 40}{2256.7}\right) kJ/kg = 2256.7 \times 1.028 \ kJ/kg$$

Thus the heat transferred is increased by less than 3 per cent by the subcooling.

How should we deal with temperature dependence of properties? The only property which is significantly affected by this is the liquid dynamic viscosity μ. It has been found that the reciprocal of μ for steam and other liquids is approximately linearly proportional to the liquid absolute temperature T over a wide range of T. Making use of this approximation, it can be shown (Ref. 34) that property values are best taken at a reference temperature T_r, where

$$T_r = T_s - \tfrac{3}{4}\theta_s \tag{22.113}$$

i.e. at a temperature corresponding to a distance $(1/4)\delta$ from the wall.

Nusselt has shown* that a horizontal cylinder of diameter d has the same average heat transfer coefficient as a vertical plate of height $l = 2.85d$. Therefore from (22.109) and (22.110) the expression for the average Nusselt number of a horizontal cylinder becomes

$$Nu_d = 1.03\left(\frac{h_{fg}\rho^2 gd^3}{4\mu k\theta_s}\right)^{1/4} \tag{22.114}$$

The rate of condensation has in some instances been observed to be considerably higher, and in others lower, than the theory of Nusselt would suggest. There are three principal reasons why it is sometimes higher. First, when the vapour velocity is high, the drag exerted on the film surface will reduce the film thickness and increase its velocity, resulting in an overall increase in the rate of heat transfer (see Ref. 34). Secondly, after a certain distance down the wall the rate of condensate flow $\dot{m}$ may exceed a critical value above which the film becomes rippled and turbulent. This critical value is governed by a film Reynolds number (usually defined as $4\dot{m}/\mu$), and this in turn is affected by the magnitude of the vapour drag on the film. Thirdly, when the fluid is water vapour it sometimes condenses as droplets on the surface and not as a continuous film. Clean steam condensing on a clean surface always condenses *filmwise*, but any contaminants produce patchy dropwise condensation as shown at the top of Fig. 22.19a. This does not normally increase the rate of heat transfer. There are surface coatings, however, that alter the surface tension so that the droplet surfaces make an acute angle with the wall as shown in the lower part of the figure. Such droplets soon become heavy enough to run down, sweeping up smaller droplets on the way. It is this form of condensation which is usually denoted by the term *dropwise*, and it leads to very high heat transfer coefficients. It has been found that certain organic compounds on the cooled surface promote this desirable form of condensation; so too do coatings of some precious metals such as gold, although they are too expensive for normal industrial use. Unfortunately, the organic compounds have proved unstable in the presence

---

* Ref. 10, pp. 667–73.

Fig. 22.19
Effects of (a) dropwise
condensation and (b) the
presence of a gas

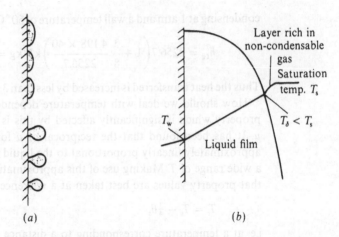

Layer rich in
non-condensable
gas
Saturation
temp. T_s

T_w

$T_\delta < T_s$

Liquid film

(a)   (b)

of oxygen, and shutting down a condenser therefore destroys their effectiveness. The surface area of a condenser designed for dropwise condensation would be much too small were the condensation to revert to the filmwise mode and, so far, intentional dropwise promotion has proved to be impractical.

One important cause of a lower rate of heat transfer is the presence of non-condensable gases in the vapour; air, for example, is often present in steam condensers. Owing to the condensation of the steam on the water film, the steam–air mixture in the vicinity of the film is relatively richer in air content than the bulk of the mixture. This results in the formation of a non-condensable gas boundary layer of high thermal resistance on the liquid film (Fig. 22.19b) and the condensing steam must diffuse through the gas layer. The liquid–vapour interface temperature is then below the saturation temperature of the bulk of the vapour, and it is instead the saturation temperature corresponding to the *partial* pressure of the steam at the interface. The temperature gradient available for conduction through the liquid film is therefore less than it is in the absence of air. This is an additional reason why it is so important to exclude non-condensable gases from condensers (see section 14.4).

Example 22.8   Steam at a pressure of 0.065 bar condenses on a vertical plate 0.6 m square. If the surface temperature of the plate is maintained at 14 °C, estimate the rate of condensation taking the effect of subcooling into account.

The latent enthalpy h_{fg} of steam at 0.065 bar is 2412 kJ/kg and the saturation temperature is 37.7 °C. The appropriate reference temperature for the properties of the liquid film, according to equation (22.113), is

$$T_r = 37.7[°C] - \left\{\frac{3}{4}(37.7 - 14)\right\}[K] = 19.925 °C \approx 20 °C$$

The relevant properties, from Ref. 14, are

$$c_p = 4.183 \text{ kJ/kg K}, \qquad \rho = 998 \text{ kg/m}^3$$

$$\mu = 1002 \times 10^{-6} \text{ kg/m s}, \qquad k = 603 \times 10^{-6} \text{ kW/m K}$$

and the effective enthalpy, from equation (22.112), is

$$h'_{fg} = 2412\left\{1 + \frac{3}{8}\frac{4.183(37.7 - 14)}{2412}\right\} = 2449 \text{ kJ/kg}$$

The terminal Nusselt number at $x = l$ is

$$Nu_l = \left(\frac{h_{fg}\rho^2 gl^3}{4\mu k\theta_s}\right)^{1/4}$$

$$= \left\{\frac{2449 \times 998^2 \times 9.81 \times 0.6^3}{4 \times 1002 \times 10^{-6} \times 603 \times 10^{-6}(37.7 - 14)}\right\}^{1/4}$$

$$= 3082$$

and the average heat transfer coefficient α, which is equal to 4/3 times the coefficient at $x = l$, is therefore

$$\alpha = \frac{4}{3}\frac{k}{l}(Nu_l) = \frac{4}{3}\frac{603 \times 10^{-6}}{0.6} 3082 = 4.13 \text{ kW/m}^2 \text{ K}$$

The total rate of heat transfer is

$$\dot{Q} = -\alpha A(T_w - T_s) = -4.13 \times 0.6^2(14 - 37.7) = 35.2 \text{ kW}$$

and the rate of condensation is

$$\dot{m}_l = \frac{\dot{Q}}{h'_{fg}} = \frac{35.2}{2449} = 0.0144 \text{ kg/s}$$

22.8.2 Boiling of liquids

Analysis of heat transfer to boiling liquids is difficult and theories are still incomplete. All that we shall attempt here is a qualitative description of the process to outline the factors governing the rate of heat transfer. The phenomena which occur in *forced-flow boiling* differ from those in *pool boiling*, and it will be necessary to discuss these separately.

Pool boiling

We speak of pool boiling when a large volume of liquid is heated by a submerged surface and the motion is caused by free convection currents stimulated by agitation of the rising vapour bubbles. Let us imagine an experiment in which a liquid is being heated over a hot plate. The heat flux $\dot{q}$ is gradually increased while the corresponding temperature difference θ between surface and bulk of the liquid is recorded. Different regimes may be distinguished.

At very low heat flux no boiling occurs, movement of the liquid is by simple *free convection*, and phase change takes place only as evaporation at the free surface of the liquid. In this regime (A–B in Fig. 22.20) the heat flux is approximately proportional to $\theta^{4/3}$; see the turbulent data in Fig. 22.17, from which $\alpha(= \dot{q}/\theta) \propto \theta^{1/3}$.

Increased heat flux will result in vapour bubble formation at the hot surface

Fig. 22.20
Regimes of pool boiling

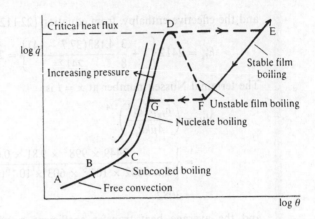

even though the bulk of the liquid may still be below saturation temperature. The bubbles which form in the hot boundary layer condense as they rise into the colder liquid, and ultimate phase change is still by evaporation at the free surface. Bubble agitation in this *subcooled boiling* regime is insignificant, so that there is little change in the slope of the $\dot{q}-\theta$ curve (B–C in Fig. 22.20).

A further increase in $\dot{q}$ leads to *nucleate boiling*, where the bulk of the fluid is at saturation temperature. Strictly speaking it is slightly above the saturation temperature as indicated in Fig. 22.21, for a reason which will be apparent later. In this regime, large numbers of bubbles form on the hot surface and travel through the bulk of the liquid to emerge at the free surface. The resulting increased agitation markedly improves the heat transfer, as shown by a steep rise of the $\dot{q}-\theta$ curve C–D.

A point is reached when the bubbles become so large and numerous that liquid has difficulty in flowing back to the heating surface as the bubbles rise. When this *critical heat flux* is reached (D), the surface suddenly becomes insulated by a continuous vapour blanket and there is a sudden jump in heating surface temperature (E). With water at atmospheric pressure, θ might be about 25 K at D and more than 1000 K at E. It will be appreciated that there is a real danger of a heating surface failing or melting when the critical heat flux is reached. The condition of sudden vapour blanketing is referred to as *burn-out*, even though with suitable materials physical burn-out need not occur.

When the heating surface can withstand higher temperatures, it is possible

Fig. 22.21
Temperature profile in a liquid boiling on a horizontal plate

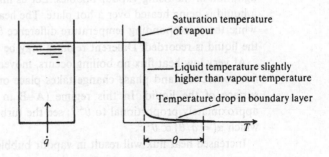

to increase $\dot{q}$ further and the regime is then referred to as *stable film boiling*. Heat transfer is by conduction and radiation across the vapour film, with the latter playing an increasingly important role at these large values of θ.

If now the heat flux is reduced below the value at E, the conditions do not jump back to those at D but follow a path to F. At this point the vapour film suddenly collapses and conditions revert to those at point G on the nucleate boiling curve. We may ask whether it is possible to maintain surface temperatures corresponding to values of θ between D and F. It is impossible when the surface is heated in such a way that $\dot{q}$ is the independent variable, e.g. when the heat flux is being controlled as with an electric heater. It is possible, however, when it is the surface temperature which is controlled, as when a condensing fluid at variable pressure is used to provide the necessary heat flux. The dashed curve F–D represents an unstable region where the vapour blanket alternately collapses and reforms.

The heat flux near D may be extremely high (for water at 1 atm it is about 1500 kW/m^2) and, because θ is small, the corresponding heat transfer coefficient is very large. It is therefore of interest to be able to operate as close as possible to D without running the risk of burn-out. Various semi-empirical relations have been proposed which enable the critical flux to be predicted (see Refs 6 and 5).

One of the difficulties in developing a satisfactory theory of boiling is the lack of complete understanding of how vapour bubbles are formed. Also, once a bubble is formed it is difficult to analyse its motion and that of the surrounding liquid: particularly when there is interference between and coalescence of numerous bubbles. The latter problem is one of fluid mechanics which we shall not consider here, but we will look briefly at the mechanism of bubble formation.

Let us consider a spherical vapour bubble of radius r in thermodynamic equilibrium with liquid at pressure p_1, as in Fig. 22.22a. If σ is the surface tension and p_v the vapour pressure in the bubble, a force balance on an equatorial plane gives

$$(p_v - p_1)\pi r^2 = \sigma 2\pi r \quad \text{or} \quad (p_v - p_1) = \frac{2\sigma}{r} \tag{22.115}$$

It is clear that a finite pressure difference must exist between the vapour and the liquid. Since at equilibrium the liquid temperature T_1 equals the vapour temperature T_v, it follows that the liquid must be superheated with respect to the liquid pressure (except for $r = \infty$ when the phase interface is plane). This is the cause of the superheat illustrated in Fig. 22.21.

Fig. 22.22
Bubble formation

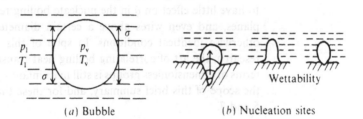

(a) Bubble (b) Nucleation sites

Equation (22.115) suggests that for an infinitesimal bubble the excess pressure required is infinite, and therefore that bubbles cannot form in the first place. Such extrapolation from the continuum to the molecular level is of doubtful validity. Nevertheless, with pure gas-free liquids on very smooth heating surfaces it is possible to maintain very high degrees of liquid superheat (e.g. 50 K for water at atmospheric pressure). This is an unstable situation leading to sudden explosive bulk boiling or 'bumping', subsequent desuperheating, and cyclic repetition of the process. In practice, dissolved gases, or even vapour trapped in surface roughness cavities, provide nucleation sites from which bubbles can grow with little initial superheat, as in Fig. 22.22b. Clearly the surface's roughness geometry will be important; so too will its wettability because of its effect on the surface tension between the liquid and the solid surface.

The conditions under which a bubble can exist and grow can be investigated further by applying the Clausius-Clapeyron equation (7.47). Thus

$$\frac{h_{fg}}{T_{sat} v_{fg}} = \frac{dp}{dT_{sat}} \approx \frac{p_v - p_l}{T_v - T_{sat}}$$

where T_{sat} is the saturation temperature at p_l. Combining this with (22.115) we have

$$T_v - T_{sat} = \frac{2\sigma T_{sat} v_{fg}}{h_{fg}} \times \frac{1}{r} \qquad (22.116)$$

Remembering that $T_v = T_l$ for equilibrium, equation (22.116) yields the equilibrium bubble radius for a given liquid superheat ($T_l - T_{sat}$). When not in equilibrium, if ($T_l - T_{sat}$) is greater than ($T_v - T_{sat}$) the bubble will grow by further evaporation, whereas if it is less the bubble will collapse. Conditions normally exist within the hot liquid boundary layer for a bubble to grow, although subsequently it may shrink or collapse as it travels through cooler liquid to the free surface.

The surface tension σ decreases with increase in pressure (or T_{sat}), and a glance at steam tables will show that the other part of the coefficient of $1/r$ in equation (22.116) also decreases with increase in pressure. It follows that, for the formation of bubbles of given r, less liquid superheat is required with increased pressure. Because a given surface provides nucleation sites of a given size, the temperature difference θ required to any value of $\dot{q}$ can be expected to fall with increase in pressure in the nucleate boiling regime. This tendency is indicated in Fig. 22.20.

Overall heating surface geometry (as distinct from surface roughness) seems to have little effect on $\dot{q}$ in the nucleate boiling regime; vertical and horizontal planes, and even wires above a certain diameter, give similar results under otherwise identical conditions. In spite of this advantage and much recent research, the art of correlating boiling heat transfer data for different fluids in terms of dimensionless groups is still in its infancy. Such correlations are beyond the scope of this brief summary, and for these the reader must turn to Refs 6, 5 and 7.

Forced-flow boiling

The nature of boiling in forced flow is similar to pool boiling in many respects, the most important difference being in the cause of burn-out. For simplicity we shall concentrate here on describing what happens in a vertical once-through boiler tube. Because there is a mixture of liquid and vapour, the flow cannot be symmetrical in a horizontal tube, and the vertical case provides a simpler picture. In a once-through tube, liquid below or at saturation point enters at the bottom, gradually evaporates until a dry or superheated vapour leaves at the top, and no water is recirculated from the exit to the entry: in such a tube the whole range of possible dryness fractions and regimes of boiling can be observed.

Before describing the various regimes it is first necessary to deal briefly with the nature of two-phase flow. This depends mainly on the volume ratio of vapour to liquid, although transition from one type of flow to another at any given ratio will also depend on the velocity of flow. When the quantity of liquid predominates, the vapour flows as dispersed bubbles in the liquid as shown in Fig. 22.23a. With increased vapour content, large vapour slugs tend to form of more or less stable size (Fig. 22.23b). Even higher vapour content results in annular flow (Fig. 22.23c), with a thin liquid film on the wall and a vapour core. The liquid film is usually rippled, with liquid droplets blown from the wave crests into the vapour core, so that annular flow is only a rough description. At even higher ratios of vapour to liquid the film may disappear and the liquid flows entirely as a suspended mist (Fig. 22.23d).

We can now describe what happens in a vertical tube with a constant heat flux along its length, and with a liquid below saturation temperature entering at the bottom, as in Fig. 22.24. The first section A is a region in which no boiling occurs and heat flow is governed by normal forced convection. In section B the bulk of the liquid is still below saturation, but bubbles form at the wall and collapse as they move inward. Section C covers the regime of simple nucleate boiling, and when the vapour content increases further this changes into the slug flow of section D with nucleation sites in the film on the wall. Further evaporation causes the flow to change to annular flow with suspended mist in section E. At first the film is thick with nucleation sites within

Fig. 22.23
Regimes of two-phase
flow

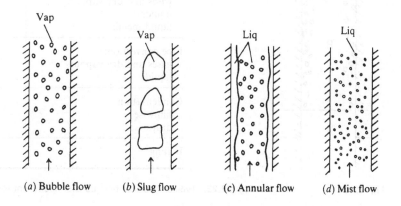

(a) Bubble flow   (b) Slug flow   (c) Annular flow   (d) Mist flow

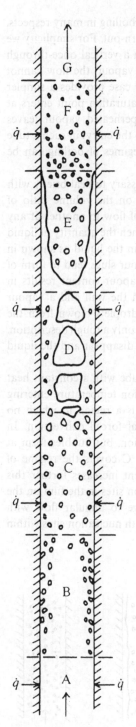

Fig. 22.24

the film, but as it thins out evaporation is confined to the free surface of the annular film and the heat is transferred through the film by simple conduction. Eventually, when the film has completely evaporated at the end of section E, there is a sudden jump in wall temperature because of the very poor heat transfer coefficient at the unwetted wall. The temperature rise at 'dry-out' may cause tube failure. (This jump will not, of course, be present when the wall temperature is maintained constant instead of $\dot{q}$.) Dry-out differs from burn-out caused by vapour blanketing in pool boiling; the latter type of phenomenon can also occur in forced flow, at section C, if the heat flux is sufficiently high. The dryness fraction at the point of dry-out is not unity because of the suspended mist. Evaporation continues in section F, heat being transferred by radiation from the wall, now at a high temperature, and by convection of the superheated vapour surrounding the mist. Finally the mist disappears and the vapour is superheated in section G.

Forced-flow boiling has received considerable attention because of the problems encountered in the design of boiling water nuclear reactors. It is necessary not only to be able to predict and avoid dry-out, but also to know the distribution of vapour/liquid ratio along the tube because this affects neutron absorption. The knowledge gained is now being applied to conventional boiler plant, where less critical conditions have provided little incentive to research in this field in the past. Ref. 7 provides a good survey of forced-flow boiling.

We will conclude the chapter by describing some special methods of increasing rates of convective heat transfer. Before doing so, however, it will be as well to have in mind the order of magnitude of the value of the film coefficient in normal convective situations. The table of Fig. 22.25 should give the reader a picture of the comparative rates of heat transfer to be expected with the various modes of convection discussed so far in this chapter.

	$\alpha/[\text{kW/m}^2\,\text{K}]$
Forced convection:	
gases and dry vapours	0.01–1
liquids	0.1–10
liquid metals	5–40
Free convection:	
gases and dry vapours	0.0005–1
liquids	0.05–3
Condensation:	
filmwise	0.5–30
dropwise	20–500
Boiling	0.5–20

Fig. 22.25 Typical values of heat transfer coefficient for different modes of convection

22.9 Heat transfer enhancement

There are many situations where the benefits obtained from an increase in the rate of heat transfer are very considerable. Some benefits are obvious, such as the reduction in size of large costly boilers, condensers and heat exchangers. Others are less obvious, such as the reduction in weight of an oil cooler for an aircraft engine, or because enhancement enables heat to be removed from equipment of restricted surface area. It is usual to speak of *active* and *passive* methods of enhancement. Active methods include fast-flowing streams of very high Reynolds number, and the application of high-voltage electric fields to increase convection in certain kinds of fluid. The most common type of passive method is the use of fins which, because of their importance, are discussed in some detail in section 24.3. Here we will confine ourselves to describing briefly three other passive methods which can be very effective in special circumstances:

(a) *fluidised beds*, which are particularly useful when the components to be heated or cooled must not be wetted and the provision of a high-speed gas stream is inconvenient or uneconomic;

(b) *special-geometry condenser surfaces*, which improve the already high heat transfer rate even further by thinning down the condensate film;

(c) *heat pipes*, which utilise combined evaporation and condensation to produce high conductivity 'rods' capable of removing heat from relatively inaccessible locations.

22.9.1 Fluidised beds

Fig. 22.26a shows a simple form of fluidised bed. A gas is blown through a porous plate at a rate just sufficient to keep a bed of sand-sized particles in suspension. The walls are heated (or cooled) to an appropriate temperature. The particles move about rapidly at random, and there is little opportunity for any insulating boundary layer to form on any solid surface in contact with the bed. Consequently the heat transfer coefficient between the containing walls

Fig. 22.26
Fluidised beds

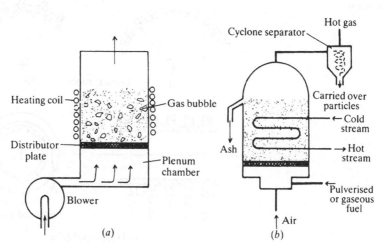

and the bed, or between the bed and any surface immersed in it, is very high: it is comparable with that achieved in a gas flow of large Reynolds number. Furthermore, the temperature and heat transfer coefficient are uniform throughout the bed. Electrically heated and water-cooled fluidised beds have been used for such varied purposes as determining the thermal characteristics of electronic components, and the thermal-shock testing of materials for gas turbines. It is easy to devise a mechanism whereby items can be automatically plunged into, and withdrawn from, the bed with any desired cycle time.

Fluidised beds have a potentially much more important use as part of a combustion system for burning low-quality fuels (Fig. 22.26b). The bed can be seeded with particles of material for absorbing sulphur oxides and other environmentally-harmful products of combustion. Energy can be extracted very effectively by immersing heat-exchanger tubing in the bed. Corrosion and erosion of such tubing at combustion temperatures is the main problem to be solved if fluidised bed combustion is to achieve its full commercial potential. A good introduction to fluidised bed technology, with useful references to specialised aspects, is provided by Ref. 16.

22.9.2   Special-geometry condenser surfaces

In section 22.8.1 we derived a theory which predicts the rate at which a laminar condensate film drains under the force of gravity down an isothermal plane surface. This theory is equally applicable when the condensate runs down outside a vertical tube. Strictly speaking, surface-tension forces should be incorporated in the analysis when the vapour–liquid interface is curved, but the effect is negligible when the curvature is uniform as with a circular tube (Fig. 22.27a). Surface-tension effects become significant, however, when the curvature is

Fig. 22.27
Special geometries for condenser tubes

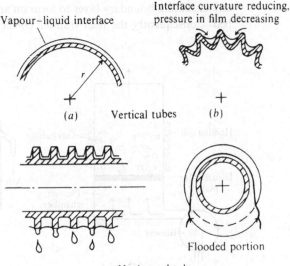

Vapour–liquid interface

Interface curvature reducing, pressure in film decreasing

r

(a)   Vertical tubes   (b)

Flooded portion

(c) Horizontal tube

non-uniform and there are local radii of curvature comparable in magnitude to the thickness of the condensate film. Use is made of this in the *Gregorig tube*.

In his classical paper (Ref. 45) Gregorig proposed the use of a vertical tube having the profile shown in Fig. 22.27b. He showed that the change from a high curvature on the peaks to smaller curvature in the valleys results in a lateral flow of condensate towards the valleys. Such flow is the outcome of pressure gradients towards the valleys caused by surface-tension effects. The peaks are thereby almost denuded of condensate, resulting in extremely high local heat fluxes. The valleys act as vertical drainage channels. Such tubes become progressively less effective towards the bottom as the valleys fill and eventually flood, and there is therefore a certain height, for given overall conditions, beyond which longer tubes should not be used. Gregorig tubing has been used successfully in desalination plant, reducing substantially the required surface area and hence capital cost.

Enhancement of condensation rate has also been achieved with horizontal tubes having circular fins. Not only do the fins increase the surface area in the usual way, but the spaces between the fins act as drainage channels with surface-tension effects again playing a major role. The lower parts of the periphery tend to flood, as illustrated in Fig. 22.27c, retaining condensate and making them ineffective; but the increased effectiveness of the upper parts more than compensates for this. The performance of finned tubing depends not only on the properties of the condensate film, but also on the fin material, spacing and height, so chosen as to maximise the thinly covered upper parts and minimise the flooded lower parts. A good survey of the performance of finned condenser tubing is provided by Ref. 46.

22.9.3 Heat pipes

In outward appearance, a heat pipe is simply a conducting rod. It has an unusually high conductivity, however, because it makes use of the high heat transfer coefficients associated with change of phase (see Fig. 22.25). The device consists essentially of a metal tube lined with a wick, and filled with a liquid and vapour in equilibrium as illustrated in Fig. 22.28. Liquid is evaporated at the hot end of the tube, and vapour flows up the centre to the cold end where it is condensed. The liquid is absorbed by the wick and returned to the hot end by capillary forces. The rate of heat transfer is an order of magnitude greater than is possible with a solid rod or simple fins.

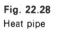

Fig. 22.28
Heat pipe

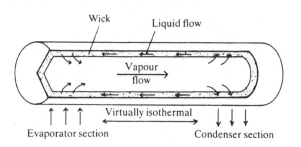

Heat pipes can be curved, and they have proved useful for conducting heat away from a confined space in awkward locations as in assemblies of electronic components. Much research has been carried out to find the best form of inner surface, wick material and fluid, for various ranges of temperature and special applications. Ref. 8 describes some of this work.

23

Radiation

The laws governing the transfer of heat by radiation are presented in this chapter. First the laws of emission of energy from black and grey surfaces are described. Then methods of calculating energy exchanges between black and grey surfaces at different temperatures are given, assuming that the intervening gas does not absorb any of the radiation. Finally, the radiation from gases and flames is discussed briefly in general terms.

23.1 The laws of black-body radiation

When radiation impinges on matter it may be totally or partially reflected, transmitted through it, or absorbed. The ratio of reflected to total incident energy is called the *reflectivity* ρ of the material; the ratio of transmitted to total incident energy is called the *transmissivity* τ; and the ratio of absorbed to total incident energy is called the *absorptivity* α. Therefore

$$\rho + \tau + \alpha = 1 \tag{23.1}$$

Practically all solid materials used in engineering are opaque to thermal radiation (even glass is only transparent to a fairly narrow range of wavelengths), and thermal radiation is in fact either reflected or absorbed within a very shallow depth of matter. Thus, for solids, it is possible to write

$$\rho + \alpha = 1 \tag{23.2}$$

When radiation is absorbed by a material, it normally increases the random molecular energy and therefore the temperature of the absorbing material. In this way radiation can be said to result in 'heat transfer', although this need not always be the case. Sometimes the energy absorbed is converted into other forms as, for example, when visible radiation falls on a photoelectric cell and some of it is transformed into electrical energy. With ordinary materials such effects are usually insignificant, and they are not considered here.

A material whose absorptivity is 1, i.e. one which absorbs all the radiant energy of whatever frequency incident upon it, is called a *black body*. The laws of radiation for a black body are of fundamental importance, and they are

Fig. 23.1

Spatial distribution of
energy emitted from a
surface element dA

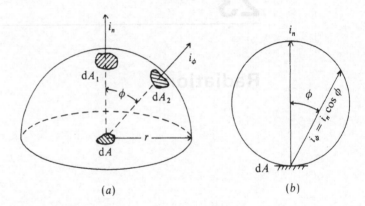

(a)   (b)

comparatively simple. This section is devoted to a presentation* of these laws
and to a discussion of some of their implications.

It is an experimental fact that unit surface area of a black body emits more
energy by radiation than unit area of any other body at the same temperature.
(This fact is also a consequence of Kirchhoff's law which is introduced in
section 23.2.) The total energy emitted per unit time by unit area of a black
surface is proportional to the fourth power of the absolute temperature T. This
relation is expressed by the *Stefan-Boltzmann law*

$$\dot{q}_b = \sigma T^4 \tag{23.3}$$

σ is called the Stefan-Boltzmann constant; it is equal to $56.7 \times 10^{-12}\ \text{kW/m}^2\ \text{K}^4$.
The subscript b will be used to denote black-body radiation.

The 'composition' of radiant energy is non-uniform in two respects. First, a
surface element does not radiate energy with equal intensity in all directions.
Secondly, the radiation emitted consists of electromagnetic waves of various
wavelengths and the energy is not distributed uniformly over the whole range
of wavelengths. These two aspects of radiation will now be considered in turn.

The spatial distribution of energy emission from an element can be represented
in the following way. The total flow of energy $d\dot{Q}_b$ from an element dA, given
by $(\dot{q}_b\, dA)$, can be imagined to flow through a hemisphere of radius r, as in
Fig. 23.1a. Consider the surface elements dA_1 and dA_2 on this hemisphere, dA_1
lying on the normal to dA, and dA_2 on a line making an angle ϕ with the
normal. The solid angle subtended by dA_1 at dA is $d\omega_n = dA_1/r^2$, and by dA_2
is $d\omega_\phi = dA_2/r^2$. The solid angle subtended by the whole hemisphere at dA is
$2\pi r^2/r^2 = 2\pi$ steradians.

Let the rate of flow of energy through dA_1 be $d\dot{Q}_{bn}$ and through dA_2 be
$d\dot{Q}_{b\phi}$. Then we shall write

$$d\dot{Q}_{bn} = i_n\, d\omega_n\, dA \tag{23.4}$$

$$d\dot{Q}_{b\phi} = i_\phi\, d\omega_\phi\, dA \tag{23.5}$$

---

* For further discussion and formal proofs see Ref. 10.

Fig. 23.2
Normal intensity of
radiation i_n

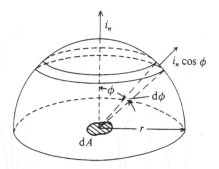

where i_n is the *intensity of radiation* in the normal direction and i_ϕ is the intensity
of radiation in the ϕ-direction. i_n and i_ϕ are defined by (23.4) and (23.5)
respectively. The spatial distribution of i_ϕ is expressed by *Lambert's cosine law*

$$i_\phi = i_n \cos \phi \tag{23.6}$$

Lambert's law is illustrated graphically in polar coordinates in Fig. 23.1b. It
follows from (23.5) and (23.6) that in general

$$d\dot{Q}_{b\phi} = i_n \cos \phi \, d\omega \, dA \tag{23.7}$$

for any surface element that subtends an angle $d\omega$ at dA.

To find an expression for i_n in terms of the temperature of the emitting surface,
consider a strip on the hemisphere at an angle ϕ to the normal, the strip
subtending an angle $d\phi$ at dA (Fig. 23.2). The solid angle subtended by this
strip at dA is

$$d\omega = \frac{2\pi r \sin \phi (r \, d\phi)}{r^2} = 2\pi \sin \phi \, d\phi$$

and thus the radiation passing through this strip is given by (23.7) as

$$d\dot{Q}_{b\phi} = i_n 2\pi \sin \phi \cos \phi \, d\phi \, dA$$

The total radiation from dA passing through the hemisphere per unit time is

$$\dot{Q}_b = i_n 2\pi \, dA \int_0^{\pi/2} \sin \phi \cos \phi \, d\phi = i_n 2\pi \, \delta A \int_0^{\pi/2} \tfrac{1}{2} \sin 2\phi \, d\phi = i_n \pi \, dA$$

But $\dot{Q}_b$ is also given by (23.3) as

$$\dot{Q}_b = \sigma T^4 \, dA$$

It therefore follows that

$$i_n = \frac{\sigma T^4}{\pi} \tag{23.8}$$

This equation, giving the intensity of normal black radiation, is a consequence
of the Stefan-Boltzmann law and Lambert's law.

Energy emitted in the form of radiation (i.e. electromagnetic waves) from a
black surface is not emitted at one frequency only, but over a wide and

Fig. 23.3

Planck's law of the
variation of
monochromatic emissive
power with wavelength

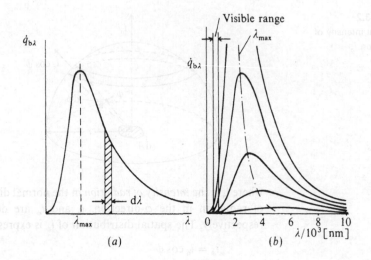

(a) (b)

continuous range of frequencies. The wavelength λ of each wave emitted into vacuum, and for all practical purposes into air, is related to the wave frequency v by the simple expression

$$v\lambda = c \tag{23.9}$$

where c is the velocity of propagation of the wave, 3×10^8 m/s.*

Consider the energy emitted within a limited range of wavelengths $d\lambda$. The total amount of energy $d\dot{q}_b$ emitted per unit time and unit area from a black surface within the *waveband* $d\lambda$ can be written as

$$d\dot{q}_b = \dot{q}_{b\lambda}\,d\lambda \tag{23.10}$$

where $\dot{q}_{b\lambda}$, called the *monochromatic emissive power*, is defined by this equation. The spectral distribution of $\dot{q}_{b\lambda}$, i.e. its variation over all wavelengths, is given by *Planck's law*

$$\dot{q}_{b\lambda} = \frac{c_1\lambda^{-5}}{e^{c_2/\lambda T} - 1} \tag{23.11}$$

where c_1 and c_2 are constants, equal to 37.4×10^{-20} kW m^2 and $0.014\,39$ m K respectively. $\dot{q}_{b\lambda}$ is evidently a function of the surface temperature T. A typical distribution curve for a given value of T is shown in Fig. 23.3a. The total energy emitted per unit time and unit area of black surface is given by the area under the curve, which must in turn be equal to the energy emission found from the Stefan-Boltzmann law (23.3). Thus

$$\dot{q}_b = \int_0^\infty \dot{q}_{b\lambda}\,d\lambda = \sigma T^4 \tag{23.12}$$

---

* The 17th CGPM (1983) *defined* the velocity of light as being exactly equal to 299 792 458 m/s. This definition, taken together with the SI definition of the unit of time, the second, provides the SI base unit of length, the metre.

The higher the temperature T, the larger is the proportion of energy emitted at the shorter wavelengths, and also the shorter is the wavelength λ_{max} for the peak value of $\dot{q}_{b\lambda}$. Fig. 23.3b shows $\dot{q}_{b\lambda}$ distribution curves for various temperatures, clearly showing the shift of λ_{max} to shorter wavelengths with increased temperature. The position of the maximum of $\dot{q}_{b\lambda}$ in the waveband is expressed by *Wien's displacement law*, which states that λ_{max} is inversely proportional to the absolute temperature T, i.e.

$$\lambda_{max} T = 0.002\,90 \text{ m K} \tag{23.13}$$

Equation (23.13) can be derived by differentiation of (23.11). It is interesting to note that at the temperature of the sun's surface (≈ 6000 K), λ_{max} is in the visible range of wavelengths, i.e. 400 nm to 800 nm, and about 40 per cent of the energy is emitted in this range. At the average temperature of the tungsten filament of an incandescent lamp (≈ 2800 K), only about 10 per cent of the energy is emitted in the visible range; thus the incandescent lamp is more efficient as a heat source than as a light source.

It must be emphasised that all the foregoing laws are concerned with black-body radiation because their derivation (not given here) is based on the assumption that the body is capable of absorbing completely any radiation incident upon it.

Example 23.1   The temperature of a black surface, 0.2 m^2 in area, is $540\,°C$. Calculate the total rate of energy emission, the intensity of normal radiation, and the wavelength of maximum monochromatic emissive power.

From the Stefan-Boltzmann law (23.3), it follows that

$$\dot{Q} = \sigma T^4 A = 56.7 \left(\frac{813}{1000} \right)^4 0.2 = 4.95 \text{ kW}$$

From (23.8), the intensity of normal black radiation is

$$i_n = \frac{\sigma T^4}{\pi} = \frac{56.7}{\pi} \left(\frac{813}{1000} \right)^4 = 7.88 \text{ kW/m}^2 \text{ steradian}$$

From Wien's law (23.13), it follows that

$$\lambda_{max} = \frac{0.0029}{T} = \frac{0.0029}{813} = 3.57 \times 10^{-6} \text{ m}$$

23.2   Kirchhoff's law and grey-body radiation

No real material emits and absorbs radiation according to the laws of the black body, and only a few, such as lamp-black and platinum-black, approach the black-body condition closely. (It is shown later in this section how an effectively 'black surface' can be obtained for use when checking the laws of black-body radiation experimentally.) Although the laws governing radiation from real bodies are complicated and will not be discussed here, there is another type of 'ideal' body to which many materials approximate in practice and for which the laws of radiation are simple modifications of the black-body laws. Before introducing this second 'ideal' body it is necessary to enunciate an important principle known as Kirchhoff's law.

Kirchhoff's law relates the *absorptivity* and the *emissivity* of a body. Before stating the law it is first necessary to extend the notion of absorptivity α given at the beginning of the previous section, and to introduce the concept of 'emissivity'. The capacity of a body to absorb thermal radiation is not the same for all wavelengths and all angles of incidence: the *monochromatic absorptivity* at any wavelength λ and angle of incidence ϕ is defined as the ratio of the energy absorbed in the waveband $d\lambda$ through the solid angle $d\omega$ to the total incident energy within that waveband and solid angle. Generally it is found that the absorptivity so defined is a function not only of λ and ϕ but also of the surface temperature T, i.e.

$$\alpha_{\lambda\phi T} = f(\lambda, \phi, T) \tag{23.14}$$

The *total hemispherical emissivity* ε, or simply the *emissivity* ε, is defined as the ratio of the total energy $\dot{q}$ emitted by a surface to the total energy $\dot{q}_b$ emitted by a black surface at the same temperature. Thus

$$\varepsilon = \left(\frac{\dot{q}}{\dot{q}_b}\right)_T \tag{23.15}$$

As with the absorptivity, the emissivity is not the same at all wavelengths and angles of emission. We may define the *monochromatic emissivity* at any wavelength λ and angle of emission ϕ as the ratio of the energy emitted in the waveband $d\lambda$ through the solid angle $d\omega$ to the energy that would be emitted by a black surface at the same temperature over $d\lambda$ and through $d\omega$. Generally it is found that the emissivity defined in this way is a function of λ, ϕ and the surface temperature T, i.e.

$$\varepsilon_{\lambda\phi T} = f(\lambda, \phi, T) \tag{23.16}$$

A material whose monochromatic emissivity is not constant, but varies with wavelength, angle of incidence or surface temperature, is called a *selective emitter*. A typical distribution curve of monochromatic emissive power $\dot{q}_\lambda$ for a body whose monochromatic emissivity varies with wavelength is shown in Fig. 23.4a. The distribution curve for a black surface at the same temperature is included for comparison.

We are now in a position to state *Kirchhoff's law: the monochromatic emissivity of a surface 1 at T_1 is equal to its monochromatic absorptivity for radiation received from a surface 2 at the same temperature $T_2 = T_1$.* This law may be expressed symbolically as

$$\varepsilon_{\lambda\phi} = \phi_{\lambda\phi}]_{T_1 = T_2} \tag{23.17}$$

Kirchhoff's law is true for any wavelength λ and angle ϕ, and it is therefore also true for the average values, i.e. total hemispherical values, of α and ε. For simplicity we shall give a proof only for these average values.

Fig. 23.4
Selective and grey
emission

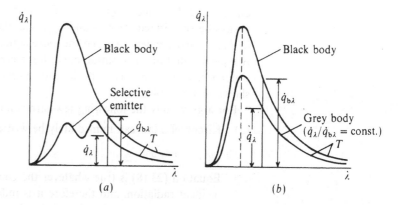

(a)   (b)

Consider a convex black body of area A_1 at temperature T_1 in a black
enclosure of the same uniform temperature T_1 (Fig. 23.5). The energy emitted
by this body is $\sigma T_1^4 A_1$. This must be equal to the energy radiated by the
enclosure that impinges on the body A_1, if the system is to maintain thermal
equilibrium. Now suppose the black body is replaced by a non-black body of
emissivity ε_1, but otherwise of exactly the same shape and temperature as the
body it replaces. The radiation falling on A_1 will still be equal to $\sigma T_1^4 A_1$, some
of which is absorbed while the remainder is reflected into the black enclosure.
The radiation emitted by A_1 is reduced to $\varepsilon_1 \sigma T_1^4 A_1$ and, by definition of α,
the energy absorbed is $\alpha_1 \sigma T_1^4 A_1$. For the temperature of the body to remain
the same, it must absorb as much radiation as it emits. Thus the absorptivity
α_1 of the non-black body A_1 must be equal to its emissivity ε_1, which proves
Kirchhoff's law.

It is important to emphasise that Kirchhoff's law does *not* apply to selective
emitters when $T_1 \neq T_2$, the deviation increasing with the difference in temperature
between the surfaces exchanging energy. If it did apply, there would be no point
in painting the roof of a house white in the tropics; this is an advantage only
because white paint has a low value of α for the sun's high-temperature radiation
(of mainly short wavelength), while having a high value of ε for its own
low-temperature radiation (of mainly very long wavelength). The laws of energy
exchange for selective emitters are difficult, and for these the reader is referred
to Refs 10 and 17.

For many purposes it is sufficiently accurate to assume that materials are
non-selective emitters. A body whose monochromatic emissivity does not depend

Fig. 23.5
Proof of Kirchhoff's law

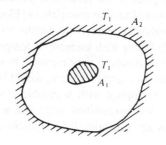

on λ, ϕ and T is called a *grey body*. For such a body the symbols ε and α can always be substituted for $\varepsilon_{\lambda\phi T}$ and $\alpha_{\lambda\phi T}$, e.g. the emissivity at any wavelength $(\dot{q}_\lambda/\dot{q}_{b\lambda})$ is independent of λ and therefore equals the average emissivity $(\dot{q}/\dot{q}_b)$. A typical radiation distribution curve for a grey body is shown in Fig. 23.4b, where it may be compared with the corresponding curve for a selective emitter shown in Fig. 23.4a.

For a grey body the following laws are valid:

(a) Kirchhoff's law can immediately be written in the simpler form

$$\varepsilon = \alpha \tag{23.18}$$

Equation (23.18) is true whatever the composition by wavelength of the incident radiation, and therefore it is independent of the temperature of the surface from which the radiation is received.

(b) The Stefan-Boltzmann law applies with $(\varepsilon\sigma)$ replacing the constant σ, i.e.

$$\dot{q} = \varepsilon\dot{q}_b = \varepsilon\sigma T^4 \tag{23.19}$$

(This equation is in a sense also true for a selective emitter, but then ε is a complicated function of T and not a constant.)

(c) Lambert's cosine law applies unchanged, i.e.

$$i_\phi = i_n \cos\phi \tag{23.20}$$

The only difference between a grey body and a black body with respect to this law is that i_n is smaller than i_{bn}. The distribution of i with ϕ is unchanged because for a grey body ε does not vary with ϕ.

(d) It follows from (b) and (c) that the relation for the normal intensity of radiation equivalent to (23.8) is

$$i_n = \frac{\varepsilon\sigma T^4}{\pi} \tag{23.21}$$

In the following sections we shall only consider energy exchanges between black or grey bodies, but it must be remembered that great care must be taken in applying grey-body rules, particularly when temperature differences are large. We shall also assume that any intervening gas does not absorb or emit radiation. This assumption is permissible if the gas is air, but when the gas contains appreciable amounts of carbon dioxide or water vapour, as it does in furnaces, the assumption is not admissible (see section 23.5).

Some selected values of emissivities are tabulated in Fig. 23.6. For real bodies ε is a function of λ, ϕ and T, but only the normal values ε_n, averaged over all wavelengths, are given in the table. It is possible to make a few generalisations about the behaviour of various materials. (a) Electrical non-conductors (including non-metallic liquids) have emissivities mostly above 0.8 at ordinary temperatures, the value usually falling with increase of temperature. The ratios of their total hemispherical emissivities to their normal emissivities $\varepsilon/\varepsilon_n$ fall within the range 0.95 to 1, whereas for a grey body $\varepsilon/\varepsilon_n$ would be unity; nevertheless, Lambert's cosine law can be applied with negligible error. (b) Clean, polished metallic solids have very low emissivities, often below 0.10 at room temperature, but their emissivities are substantially proportional to the absolute temperature.

Fig. 23.6
Normal emissivities ε_n for various materials

$T/[K]$	300	500	800
Aluminium: polished	0.04	0.04	0.06
oxidised	0.09	0.12	0.17
Chromium polished	0.08	0.17	0.27
Copper: polished	0.02	0.02	0.03
oxidised	0.56	0.61	0.83
Steel: polished	0.07	0.10	0.14
oxidised	0.79	0.79	0.79
Mercury liquid	0.10		
Silver polished	0.02	0.02	0.03
Tungsten: polished	0.04	0.06	0.08
filament	0.32	0.32	0.32
White paint	0.96	0.91	0.71
Lampblack paint	0.96	0.97	0.97
Asbestos paper	0.93	0.94	0.94
Quartz glass	0.93	0.89	0.68
Plaster	0.92	0.92	
Building brick	0.93		
Water (and ice)	0.96		

They are, on the whole, selective emitters. The ratios of total hemispherical emissivities to their normal emissivities $\varepsilon/\varepsilon_n$ lie between 1.1 and 1.3, and Lambert's cosine law can be applied with moderate accuracy only. (c) Oxidised or greasy metal surfaces have emissivities which are several times higher than those of clean metal surfaces.

Evidently the emissivity ε of a body is a property of surface finish as well as of the material itself. Fig. 23.7a explains why a matt surface is 'blacker' than a smooth or specular surface. Owing to surface irregularities, any ray striking a matt surface is not likely to be reflected away from the surface after one incidence only, but is likely to suffer multiple reflections first. The irregularities in the surface act as 'hollow spaces' of high absorptivity. Consequently it follows from Kirchhoff's law that the emissivity of a matt surface is also higher than that of a polished surface made of the same material.

Although there is no perfectly black material, it can now be seen how a small surface which emits 'black radiation' can be obtained. Consider a hollow sphere with a relatively small aperture δA, the inner surface of which is at a uniform temperature (Fig. 23.7b). Any ray entering the aperture δA is partly absorbed

Fig. 23.7
a) Effect of surface finish on emissivity;
b) the 'perfect' black body

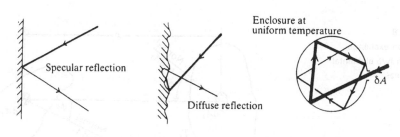

Specular reflection

Diffuse reflection

Enclosure at uniform temperature

δA

(a) Surface effects

(b) 'Perfect' black body

and partly reflected. The reflected ray, considerably reduced in intensity compared with the incident ray, is again partly absorbed and partly reflected on a second incidence, and so on for successive reflections. Owing to the smallness of the aperture it is improbable that any appreciable amount of reflected radiant energy escapes through it. This means that the surface element δA is effectively black for incident radiation, whatever the wavelength. According to Kirchhoff's law, however, the emissivity of δA must be equal to its absorptivity, and therefore δA will emit black radiation corresponding to the inner surface temperature of the sphere.

23.3 Radiation exchange between two black surfaces

When two surfaces can 'see' one another, each absorbs some of the radiation emitted by the other. If the surfaces are at different temperatures, the net result is an energy flow from the hotter to the colder body. Let us consider two surface elements of areas dA_1 and dA_2 on two *black* bodies at temperatures T_1 and T_2 respectively (Fig. 23.8). The two surface elements are a distance x apart, and their normals are inclined at angles ϕ_1 and ϕ_2 respectively to the line x joining them. The energy exchange can be calculated in the following way.

Element dA_2 subtends a solid angle $d\omega_1 = dA_2 \cos\phi_2/x^2$ at dA_1. The intensity of radiation from dA_1 in the x-direction is $i_1 = i_{n1} \cos\phi_1$, and therefore the radiation incident upon and absorbed by dA_2 is

$$d\dot{Q}_{b1} = i_1\, d\omega_1\, dA_1$$

$$= \frac{i_{n1} \cos\phi_1 \cos\phi_2\, dA_1\, dA_2}{x^2} \tag{23.22}$$

Element dA_1 subtends a solid angle $d\omega_2 = dA_1 \cos\phi_1/x^2$ at dA_2. Therefore the radiation emitted by dA_2 and absorbed by dA_1 is

$$d\dot{Q}_{b2} = i_2\, d\omega_2\, dA_2$$

$$= \frac{i_{n2} \cos\phi_1 \cos\phi_2\, dA_1\, dA_2}{x^2} \tag{23.23}$$

But the normal intensity of black-body radiation is given by the relation (23.8) as $i_n = \sigma T^4/\pi$, and hence the exchange of radiation between the two surface

Fig. 23.8
Radiation exchange between two elemental black areas

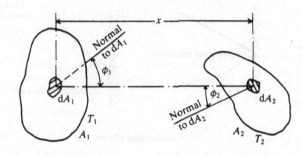

elements is

$$dQ_b = d\dot{Q}_{b2} - d\dot{Q}_{b1} = \frac{\sigma \cos\phi_1 \cos\phi_2 \, dA_1 \, dA_2}{\pi x^2}(T_2^4 - T_1^4) \qquad (23.24)$$

The solution of any particular problem of heat exchange between black bodies depends upon whether the double integration of equation (23.24) can be carried out. When the surfaces are small compared with their distance apart, fairly flat, and uniform in temperature, an approximate solution can be obtained without integration by substituting areas A_1 and A_2 in (23.24), together with the approximate values of ϕ_1 and ϕ_2. This is illustrated in the following example, together with a method involving a single integration.

Example 23.2   A circular disk of 3 m diameter is exposed to radiation escaping from a furnace through an opening of 0.1 m² area. The disk is parallel and coaxial with the opening, and is placed 5 m away from it. The opening may be assumed to radiate as a black body at 1540 °C. Calculate the rate at which energy from the opening falls on the disk.

First approximate solution
To obtain a very approximate solution, it is assumed that the areas of both opening and disk are small. The energy falling on the disk A_2 (Fig. 23.9) is given by combining (23.22) and (23.8):

$$\dot{Q}_{b1} = \frac{i_{n1} \cos\phi_1 \cos\phi_2 A_1 A_2}{x^2} = \frac{\sigma \cos\phi_1 \cos\phi_2 A_1 A_2}{\pi x^2} T_1^4$$

A_1 is 0.1 m², and $A_2 = \pi 3^2/4 = 7.07$ m². For $\cos\phi_1$ and $\cos\phi_2$ we may write 1 as an approximation, although some surface elements see one another at considerable inclinations. Thus

$$\dot{Q}_{b1} = \frac{56.7 \times 1 \times 1 \times 0.1 \times 7.07}{\pi 5^2}\left(\frac{1813}{1000}\right)^4 = 5.51 \text{ kW}$$

Fig. 23.9

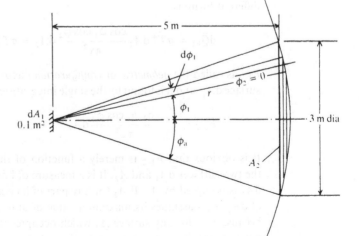

Second approximate solution

In this solution it is still assumed that the opening A_1 is small, but the area of the disk is divided into elemental areas; the energy falling on each area is calculated separately, and the sum total is found by a single integration. Instead of calculating the energy falling on the disk, it is easier to calculate the energy falling on the cap of the sphere seen by the opening within the half-angle $\phi_a = \tan^{-1}(1.5/5) = 16.7°$. Consider a strip on the sphere at an angle ϕ_1, subtending an angle $d\phi_1$ at dA_1. The area of the strip is

$$dA_2 = 2\pi r \sin \phi_1 (r \, d\phi_1) = 2\pi r^2 \sin \phi_1 \, d\phi_1$$

and the energy falling on this strip is

$$d\dot{Q}_{b1} = \frac{\sigma \cos \phi_1 \cos 0 A_1 2\pi r^2 \sin \phi_1 \, d\phi_1}{\pi r^2} T_1^4$$

$$= \sigma A_1 T_1^4 2 \sin \phi_1 \cos \phi_1 \, d\phi_1 = \sigma A_1 T_1^4 \sin 2\phi_1 \, d\phi_1$$

The total energy falling on the cap of the sphere, and therefore on the disk, is

$$\dot{Q}_{b1} = \int_0^{\phi_a} \sigma A_1 T_1^4 \sin 2\phi_1 \, d\phi_1 = -\sigma A_1 T_1^4 \left[\frac{1}{2} \cos 2\phi_1 \right]_0^{\phi_a}$$

$$= -56.7 \times 0.1 \left(\frac{1813}{1000} \right)^4 \frac{1}{2} (0.835 - 1) = 5.05 \text{ kW}$$

This answer is 8 per cent lower than the one given by the first approximation. To obtain an exact answer it is necessary to divide both disk and opening into elemental areas, and find the value of $\dot{Q}_{b1}$ by a double integration. This, though feasible, would be extremely laborious and the change in the answer would be very small in this particular case.

When the foregoing approximate solution is not permissible, the following procedure may be adopted. Equation (23.22) can be rewritten in a slightly different form as

$$d\dot{Q}_{b1} = \sigma T_1^4 \, dA_1 \frac{\cos \phi_1 \cos \phi_2}{\pi x^2} dA_2 = \sigma T_1^4 \, dA_1 \, dF_{1-2}$$

F_{1-2} is called the *geometric* or *configuration factor* of surface A_2 with respect to surface dA_1, and it is found by the single integration of dF_{1-2} over the area A_2, i.e.

$$F_{1-2} = \int_{A_2} \frac{\cos \phi_1 \cos \phi_2}{\pi x^2} dA_2 \tag{23.25}$$

It is obvious that F_{1-2} is merely a function of the geometric configuration of the two surfaces dA_1 and A_2. It is a measure of how much of the field of view of dA_1 is occupied by A_2. If A_2 (or any part of it) occupies the whole field of view of dA_1, F_{1-2} assumes its maximum value of unity; this can be easily visualised because F_{1-2} for any surface A_2 which occupies the whole field of view of dA_1 must be the same as F_{1-2} for a hemisphere A_2 surrounding dA_1. For a hemisphere

A_2, equation (23.25) can be integrated (this is similar to the integration for the cap of the sphere in Example 23.2) to give

$$F_{1-2} = \int_0^{\pi/2} \frac{\cos \phi_1 \cos 0}{\pi r^2} 2\pi r^2 \sin \phi_1 \, d\phi_1 = 1$$

Equation (23.23) can be rewritten in a similar form, i.e.

$$d\dot{Q}_{b2} = \sigma T_2^4 \, dA_1 \frac{\cos \phi_1 \cos \phi_2}{\pi x^2} dA_2 = \sigma T_2^4 \, dA_1 \, dF_{1-2}$$

Hence the net radiation exchange between dA_1 and dA_2 follows as

$$d\dot{Q}_b = d\dot{Q}_{b2} - d\dot{Q}_{b1} = \sigma(T_2^4 - T_1^4) \, dA_1 \, dF_{1-2} \qquad (23.26)$$

This equation is equivalent to (23.24).

In order to find the total energy exchange between A_1 and A_2, it is necessary to divide surface A_1 into a number of small, equal, surface elements dA_1 and to find the geometric factor of surface A_2 with respect to each of these elements. This can sometimes be done analytically, or else a numerical step-by-step method or a graphical method may be employed.* It is then possible to find an arithmetic mean value F'_{1-2} of the individual values of F_{1-2} for all the elements on A_1, and the total energy exchange is finally obtained from

$$\dot{Q}_b = \sigma(T_2^4 - T_1^4)A_1 F'_{1-2} \qquad (23.27)$$

The procedure for finding $\dot{Q}_b$ can be reversed by writing (23.24) in the form

$$d\dot{Q}_b = \sigma(T_2^4 - T_1^4) \, dA_2 \, dF_{2-1}$$

where F_{2-1} is the geometric factor of surface A_1 with respect to dA_2, given by

$$F_{2-1} = \int_{A_1} \frac{\cos \phi_1 \cos \phi_2}{\pi x^2} dA_1 \qquad (23.28)$$

An average geometric factor F'_{2-1} for equal elemental areas dA_2 can then be found in the same way as F'_{1-2}, and the total energy exchange can then be found from

$$\dot{Q}_b = \sigma(T_2^4 - T_1^4)A_2 F'_{2-1} \qquad (23.29)$$

The two procedures outlined above merely represent ways of integrating (23.24) and they differ only in the order of integration. Since A_1 and A_2 are independent variables, $\dot{Q}_b$ must be independent of the order of integration, and it therefore follows from (23.27) and (23.29) that

$$A_1 F'_{1-2} = A_2 F'_{2-1} \qquad (23.30)$$

Sometimes it is easier to follow one order of integration rather than another, and consideration should be given to this choice before a solution is attempted.

A particularly common case of radiant energy exchange is the one where

---

* See Ref. 6, Chapter 14. A useful compilation of configuration factors for a range of geometries can be found in Ref. 37.

Fig. 23.10
Radiation exchange
between a black body
and a black enclosure

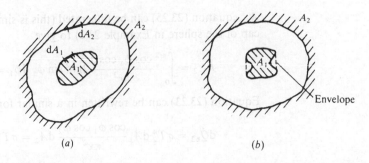

(a) (b)

area A_2 completely encloses area A_1. Let it first be assumed that A_1 consists of convex and flat surfaces only as in Fig. 23.10a, so that no two surface elements of A_1 can see one another. Now consider an element dA_2 on A_2; the geometric factor of A_1 with respect to dA_2 is less than unity because A_1 does not occupy the whole field of view of dA_2. Now consider any element dA_1 on A_1; the geometric factor of A_2 with respect to dA_1 must be unity, because the whole field of view of dA_1 is occupied by A_2. Hence the average geometric factor F'_{1-2} is equal to 1, and the radiation exchange follows from (23.27) as

$$\dot{Q}_b = \sigma(T_2^4 - T_1^4)A_1 \qquad (23.31)$$

It also follows from (23.30) that $F'_{2-1} = A_1/A_2$.

Equation (23.31) can also be deduced by a different argument. A_1 emits energy equal to $\sigma T_1^4 A_1$. A_2 emits energy $\sigma T_2^4 A_2$, but only $\sigma T_2^4 A_1$ falls on A_1, the rest being reabsorbed by A_2. If this were not so, the net energy exchange would not be zero when $T_2 = T_1$, as it must be when the system is in equilibrium. This argument assumes that the spatial distribution of energy emission from A_2 is the same at all temperatures, i.e. whether $T_2 = T_1$ or $T_2 \neq T_1$, and the assumption is valid because Lambert's law implies that the spatial distribution of radiation does not vary with temperature. Hence in general

$$\dot{Q}_b = \sigma T_2^4 A_1 - \sigma T_1^4 A_1 = \sigma(T_2^4 - T_1^4)A_1$$

which is in agreement with (23.31).

When the area A_1 has concave elements as in Fig. 23.10b, so that parts of A_1 can see one another, less than $\sigma T_1^4 A_1$ escapes into the enclosure. However, when any concave portion δA_1 can be sealed by a plane surface of area $\delta A'_1$ (e.g. a cavity with a circular perimeter on a sphere or any dent on a plane), it is not difficult to show by considering the thermal equilibrium of this element that what escapes the cavity must be equal to $\sigma T_1^4 \delta A'_1$. Thus in such cases the envelope area can be used instead of A_1 in equation (23.31). The calculation is much more difficult when a cavity cannot be sealed by a plane surface, but in many cases equation (23.31) with A_1 taken as the minimum possible envelope area provides a good approximation to the exact answer. An extreme case where this approximation would lead to a completely erroneous result is a sphere with a long rod projecting from it.

Equation (23.31) can easily be extended to the case when A_1 is grey, and although the behaviour of grey bodies in general is left to the next section, we may consider the simple case of a grey body in a black enclosure here. We have seen that when A_1 is black, the radiation emitted by A_1 and absorbed by A_2 is $\sigma T_1^4 A_1$, and the radiation emitted by A_2 and absorbed by A_1 is $\sigma T_2^4 A_1$. Let A_1 now be replaced by an identical body of temperature T_1, but of emissivity ε_1. The radiation emitted by A_1 is $\varepsilon_1 \sigma T_1^4 A_1$, and it is all absorbed by the black enclosure. The radiation emitted by A_2 and falling on A_1 is still equal to $\sigma T_2^4 A_1$, but only a fraction ε_1 is absorbed (since $\alpha_1 = \varepsilon_1$). The reflected radiation is then reabsorbed by the black enclosure. Thus the net energy exchange is

$$\dot{Q} = \varepsilon_1 \sigma T_2^4 A_1 - \varepsilon_1 \sigma T_1^4 A_1 = \varepsilon_1 \sigma (T_2^4 - T_1^4) A_1 \qquad (23.32)$$

Equation (23.32) can also be used if the enclosure is not black but grey, provided the enclosure A_2 is very large compared with the body A_1. The radiation emitted by A_1 is $\varepsilon_1 \sigma T_1^4 A_1$, and all of this is absorbed by the enclosure even though it is not black, because any reflected radiation is finally absorbed by A_2 after multiple reflections and only a negligible fraction falls again on A_1. This would not be so if the body and enclosure were of comparable size. Since the relatively large enclosure is *effectively* black as far as absorption is concerned, Kirchhoff's law implies that it must be black as far as emission is concerned. Equation (23.32) can thus be applied to a grey body in either a black, or a relatively large, enclosure.

Except for the simple case of radiation exchange between a grey body and an enclosure, the treatment of grey-body radiation is usually difficult. This is chiefly due to the fact that it is necessary to consider the effect of reflected energy, as will be apparent from the next section.

23.4   Radiation exchange between two grey surfaces

In order to illustrate the method of finding the heat exchange when reflected radiation is significant, it is best to choose an example in which the geometric factor presents no additional difficulty, i.e. when $F_{1-2} = F_{2-1} = 1$, and therefore $A_1 = A_2$ from (23.30). A case that satisfies this condition is that of two very large parallel plates of area A, whose distance apart is small compared with the size of the plates so that the radiation escaping at their edges is negligible. Another case is that of two concentric bodies which are a small distance apart compared with their dimensions, so that their areas are effectively equal (Fig. 23.11).

Fig. 23.11
Radiation exchange
between two grey
surfaces with a geometric
factor of unity, i.e. $A_1 = A_2$

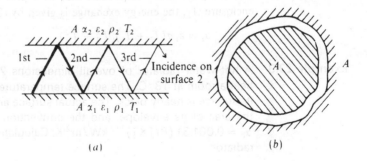

Consider the radiation emitted by the grey surface 1; it is equal to $\varepsilon_1 \sigma T_1^4 A$. The amount absorbed by the grey surface 2 is $\alpha_2(\varepsilon_1 \sigma T_1^4 A) = \varepsilon_1 \varepsilon_2 \sigma T_1^4 A$ (since $\varepsilon = \alpha$). The amount reflected by surface 2 is $\rho_2(\varepsilon_1 \sigma T_1^4 A)$, of which surface 1 absorbs $\alpha_1 \rho_2(\varepsilon_1 \sigma T_1^4 A)$ and reflects $\rho_1 \rho_2(\varepsilon_1 \sigma T_1^4 A)$. With the second incidence on surface 2, this surface absorbs $\alpha_2 \rho_1 \rho_2(\varepsilon_1 \sigma T_1^4 A) = \rho_1 \rho_2(\varepsilon_1 \varepsilon_2 \sigma T_1^4 A)$. Similarly it can be shown that on a third incidence, after a further reflection from surface 1, surface 2 absorbs $\rho_1^2 \rho_2^2(\varepsilon_1 \varepsilon_2 \sigma T_1^4 A)$, and so on. The net amount of energy leaving surface 1 and being absorbed by surface 2 is therefore given by the series

$$\dot{Q}_1 = \varepsilon_1 \varepsilon_2 \sigma T_1^4 A \{1 + (\rho_1 \rho_2) + (\rho_1 \rho_2)^2 + \ldots\}$$

Similarly it can be shown that of the energy $\varepsilon_2 \sigma T_2^4 A$ radiated by surface 2, a net amount

$$\dot{Q}_2 = \varepsilon_1 \varepsilon_2 \sigma T_2^4 A \{1 + (\rho_1 \rho_2) + (\rho_1 \rho_2)^2 + \ldots\}$$

is absorbed by surface 1. The energy exchange is therefore

$$\dot{Q} = \dot{Q}_2 - \dot{Q}_1 = \varepsilon_1 \varepsilon_2 \sigma (T_2^4 - T_1^4) A \{1 + (\rho_1 \rho_2) + (\rho_1 \rho_2)^2 + \ldots\}$$

The series in brackets is converging, because $\rho_1 \rho_2 < 1$, and the sum of the terms is $1/(1 - \rho_1 \rho_2)$. The net energy exchange is therefore

$$\dot{Q} = \frac{\varepsilon_1 \varepsilon_2}{1 - \rho_1 \rho_2} \sigma (T_2^4 - T_1^4) A$$

Remembering that $\rho = (1 - \alpha) = (1 - \varepsilon)$, this becomes

$$\dot{Q} = \frac{\varepsilon_1 \varepsilon_2}{1 - (1 - \varepsilon_1)(1 - \varepsilon_2)} \sigma (T_2^4 - T_1^4) A$$

$$= \frac{1}{(1/\varepsilon_1) + (1/\varepsilon_2) - 1} \sigma (T_2^4 - T_1^4) A \qquad (23.33)$$

When ε_1 and ε_2 are equal to 1, this reduces to the corresponding expression for black-body radiation (23.31).

When convection and radiation transfer from a surface are considered simultaneously, as in section 21.2, it is convenient to be able to express the radiation heat transfer in terms of a heat transfer coefficient α_r which is defined by equation (21.9), i.e.

$$\dot{Q} = \alpha_r A_1 (T_2 - T_1)$$

For the particularly important case of a grey body A_1 in a black or large enclosure A_2, the energy exchange is given by (23.32), and hence

$$\alpha_r = \varepsilon_1 \sigma (T_2 + T_1)(T_2^2 + T_1^2) \qquad (23.34)$$

Example 23.3 A hot water radiator of overall dimensions 2 m × 1 m × 0.2 m is used to heat a room at 18 °C. The surface temperature of the radiator is 60 °C, and its surface is nearly black. The actual surface area of the radiator is 2.5 times the area of its envelope, and the convection heat transfer coefficient is $\alpha_c = 0.001\,31\,(\theta/[\mathrm{K}])^{1/3}\,\mathrm{kW/m^2\,K}$. Calculate the rate of heat loss from the radiator.

As the surface of the radiator is nearly black, the area of the envelope A_e may be assumed to radiate as a black body. The area of the envelope is

$$A_e = 2\{(2 \times 1) + (2 \times 0.2) + (1 \times 0.2)\} = 5.2 \, \text{m}^2$$

The effective radiation heat transfer coefficient is given by putting $\varepsilon_1 = 1$ in equation (23.34) as

$$\alpha_r = 56.7 \times 10^{-12}(291 + 333)(291^2 + 333^2) = 0.006\,92 \, \text{kW/m}^2 \, \text{K}$$

The convection heat transfer is from the whole radiator surface, which is $2.5A_e$, and the convection heat transfer coefficient is

$$\alpha_c = 0.001\,31(60 - 18)^{1/3} = 0.004\,55 \, \text{kW/m}^2 \, \text{K}$$

The total rate of heat loss is

$$\dot{Q} = \alpha_r A_e \theta + \alpha_c 2.5A_e \theta = (\alpha_r + 2.5\alpha_c)A_e \theta$$
$$= \{0.006\,92 + (2.5 \times 0.004\,55)\}5.2(60 - 18) = 4.0 \, \text{kW}$$

When the geometric factor is not unity, and the surfaces exchanging energy by radiation are grey, the calculations are usually very difficult. *Radiation network analysis* is the name given to a particularly powerful method of handling problems of grey-body exchange. The reader is referred to Ref. 44 for a complete exposition, but the principle of the method can be simply stated. Two new terms are introduced, *irradiation* $\dot{G}$ and *radiosity* $\dot{J}$, where

$\dot{G}$ = total radiation incident on unit area of surface per unit time

$\dot{J}$ = total radiation leaving unit area of surface per unit time

The radiosity is the sum of the energy emitted and the energy reflected, i.e. $\dot{J} = \varepsilon \dot{q}_b + \rho \dot{G}$. But $\rho = 1 - \alpha = 1 - \varepsilon$, so that

$$\dot{J} = \varepsilon \dot{q}_b + (1 - \varepsilon)\dot{G} \quad \text{or} \quad \dot{G} = (\dot{J} - \varepsilon \dot{q}_b)/(1 - \varepsilon)$$

The net energy leaving a surface is then

$$\dot{Q} = A(\dot{J} - \dot{G}) = A\{\dot{J} - (\dot{J} - \varepsilon \dot{q}_b)/(1 - \varepsilon)\} = \frac{\dot{q}_b - \dot{J}}{(1 - \varepsilon)/\varepsilon A} \qquad (23.35)$$

If we now interpret $(\dot{q}_b - \dot{J})$ as a potential, driving energy away from a surface through a 'surface resistance' $(1 - \varepsilon)/\varepsilon A$, the equation can be represented by Fig. 23.12a. The surface resistance is zero for a black body (i.e. when $\varepsilon = 1$).

Now consider radiation exchange between any pair of surfaces 1 and 2 having areas A_1 and A_2. The energy leaving 1 which falls on 2 is $\dot{J}_1 A_1 F_{1-2}$, and that which leaves 2 and falls on 1 is $\dot{J}_2 A_2 F_{2-1}$. The net exchange, remembering that

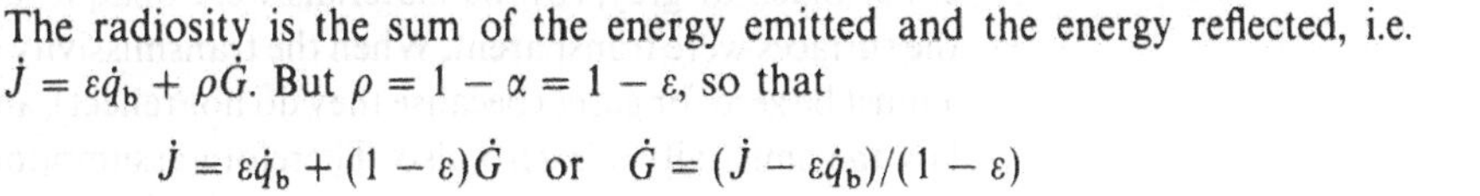

Fig. 23.12
Principles of radiation
network analysis

(a) (b) (c)

617

$A_1 F_{1-2} = A_2 F_{2-1}$, is therefore

$$\dot{Q} = A F_{1-2}(\dot{J}_1 - \dot{J}_2) = \frac{(\dot{J}_1 - \dot{J}_2)}{1/A_1 F_{1-2}} \qquad (23.36)$$

Treating $(\dot{J}_1 - \dot{J}_2)$ as a potential, and $1/A_1 F_{1-2}$ as a 'space resistance', this equation is represented by Fig. 23.12b. The complete radiation network for the problem then appears as the series of resistances in Fig. 23.12c, so that we can immediately write

$$\dot{Q} = \frac{\dot{q}_{b1} - \dot{q}_{b2}}{\{(1 - \varepsilon_1)/\varepsilon_1 A_1\} + \{1/A_1 F_{1-2}\} + \{(1 - \varepsilon_2)/\varepsilon_2 A_2\}} \qquad (23.37)$$

where $(\dot{q}_{b1} - \dot{q}_{b2})$ is simply $\sigma(T_1^4 - T_2^4)$.

When more complicated situations arise, such as when more than two surfaces are involved, or when there is an intervening medium having a transmissivity less than unity, the electrical network becomes quite elaborate. The solution is relatively straightforward, however, using the principles of electrical network theory—such as Kirchhoff's current law, which states that the net current entering a junction in the network is zero.

23.5 Radiation from gases and flames

The quantitative calculations of radiation from gases and flames is beyond the scope of this book, but a few general points can be made here.

Previous sections have dealt with the calculation of energy exchange between solid surfaces. The assumptions made were that (a) the radiating materials were either black or grey, (b) the materials were opaque, and (c) any gases between the surfaces were transparent. When the transmissivity τ is unity, the absorptivity α must be zero for gases (because they do not reflect), and hence from Kirchhoff's law the emissivity ε is zero also. Therefore assumption (c) implies that the gas takes no part in the energy exchange. Air is effectively transparent, as are other diatomic and monatomic gases. Water vapour and carbon dioxide are the main gases met in industrial processes which are imperfect transmitters and radiate to an appreciable extent. However, even these gases only affect radiation exchange significantly if the volume of radiating gas is of considerable thickness. This is due to the fact that gases emit and absorb 'in depth'; the energy is not merely emitted or absorbed by the surface of a gas volume, and successive layers of the gas take part in the process of radiation. With solids, only a few molecular layers near the surface are involved. When the intervening gases do play a significant part in the transfer of heat, the treatment is difficult because gases are highly selective emitters and hence cannot be considered grey. One important case, where the volume of gas certainly has 'depth', is the atmosphere. The concentration of carbon dioxide is increasing due to mankind's use of fossil fuels, and this may significantly decrease the atmosphere's transmissivity for low-temperature radiation. There is concern that this will in turn lead to an increase in the general ambient temperature level—the so-called 'greenhouse effect'.

Flames are hot volumes of gas in which chemical reactions are taking place. The radiation from flames is due to two sources. First, some radiation, manifested by a faint blue colour, arises from the reacting gases; such radiation is usually low of intensity. Secondly, when flames are obtained from the combustion of hydrocarbons, solid incandescent carbon particles appear in the combustion region as intermediate products of the combustion process. Ash particles may also be suspended in the flame. Such particles radiate as solid bodies, giving flames their yellow colour, and provide the major contribution to the radiation heat transfer. The radiation from flames can be calculated only if the density and distribution of the suspended solid matter are known. In practice, for a flame with substantial amounts of suspended matter, a reasonable approximation is obtained by assuming the flame to be black.

A yellow flame, rich in suspended solid particles, is called a *luminous flame*, and a blue flame, poor in suspended particles, a *non-luminous flame*. Though a non-luminous flame may be appreciably hotter than a luminous one (the latter indicating incomplete combustion), a luminous flame may be more efficient because it more readily transfers its energy to other bodies by radiation. In gas fires used for space heating, the jets of non-luminous flame are partly surrounded by mantles of refractory material so that these mantles, when heated, make the radiation from the fire more effective.

Further information and useful empirical data on radiation from gases and flames can be found in Refs 13 and 17.

24

Combined Modes of Heat Transfer

Many problems in which conduction, convection and radiation occur simultaneously can be treated with the aid of an overall heat transfer coefficient in the manner suggested in section 21.2. The overall coefficient can be found once the relevant expressions for the individual heat transfer coefficients have been obtained. In this chapter we shall present examples involving this method of approach.

It was noted in the Introduction to Part IV that although the simple addition of the separate effects is often permissible, it does not always provide an exact solution. Under some conditions there is a significant interaction between the different modes. For example, when a liquid flows over a heated plate the radiation emitted by the plate is absorbed gradually by successive layers of fluid: this alters the temperature and velocity profiles in the boundary layer, and hence also the convection heat transfer. It is difficult to allow for such interaction and it is normally neglected in practical calculations.

24.1 The heat exchanger

One of the most common examples of heat exchange is the heat transfer from one fluid to another when the fluids are separated by a solid wall. The apparatus in which this type of process occurs is called a *heat exchanger*. In a heat exchanger the temperature of the fluids along the surface of the wall is rarely uniform. To predict the rate of heat transfer, it is necessary to know the overall heat transfer coefficient U for the wall and fluid boundary layers. The calculation is simplified if U can be assumed independent of the distance along the heat exchanger, and if a mean temperature difference $\Delta\bar{T}$ between the fluids can be found such that the rate of heat transfer can be expressed by the equation

$$\dot{Q} = UA\Delta\bar{T} \tag{24.1}$$

The assumption that the overall heat transfer coefficient does not vary along the heat exchanger is never strictly true, but it may be a good approximation if at least one of the fluids is a gas. For a gas, the film coefficient is fairly constant over the whole surface because it depends on properties which do not vary appreciably over moderate ranges of temperature. Furthermore, the

g. 24.1
e parallel-flow and
unter-flow heat
changer

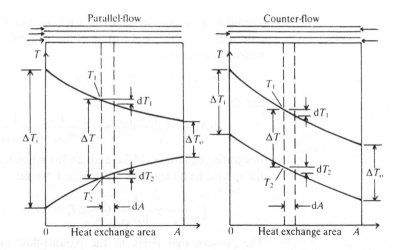

resistance of the gas film is considerably greater than that of the metal wall or the liquid film, and the value of the gas film resistance effectively determines the value of the overall heat transfer coefficient U.

Only the two simplest forms of heat exchanger are considered here in any detail, and initially we shall assume that neither fluid changes phase. Fig. 24.1 shows diagrammatically a *parallel-flow* and a *counter-flow* heat exchanger, together with typical axial temperature distributions for the fluids flowing through the passages. The temperature distribution is plotted against heat exchange area, i.e. against the area of the surface that separates the two fluids. The purpose of the following analysis is to find a suitable mean temperature difference $\Delta \bar{T}$ for use when calculating the total rate of heat exchange for a parallel-flow or a counter-flow heat exchanger from equation (24.1).

The rate of heat transfer through any short section of heat exchanger tube of surface area dA is

$$d\dot{Q} = U\, dA(T_1 - T_2) = U\, dA\, \Delta T \tag{24.2}$$

Consider the parallel-flow heat exchanger first. While flowing over this section the hot fluid cools, and the cold fluid is heated, in the direction of increasing area. Assuming that no heat is lost to the surroundings, the heat exchange must also be equal to the magnitude of the enthalpy change of each of the two fluids, namely

$$d\dot{Q} = -\dot{m}_1\, dh_1 = +\dot{m}_2\, dh_2$$

where $\dot{m}_1$ and $\dot{m}_2$ are the rates of mass flow of the hot, or primary, and of the cold, or secondary, fluids respectively. In terms of specific heat capacities c_{p1} and c_{p2} this can be written as

$$d\dot{Q} = -\dot{m}_1 c_{p1}\, dT_1 = +\dot{m}_2 c_{p2}\, dT_2$$

Hence

$$d(\Delta T) = d(T_1 - T_2) = dT_1 - dT_2 = -\left(\frac{1}{\dot{m}_1 c_{p1}} + \frac{1}{\dot{m}_2 c_{p2}}\right) d\dot{Q} \tag{24.3a}$$

Considering the counter-flow heat exchanger unit, it can be seen that the only difference is that the temperature of the cold fluid decreases in the direction of increasing area. Hence

$$d\dot{Q} = -\dot{m}_1 c_{p1}\, dT_1 = -\dot{m}_2 c_{p2}\, dT_2$$

and thus

$$d(\Delta T) = dT_1 - dT_2 = -\left(\frac{1}{\dot{m}_1 c_{p1}} - \frac{1}{\dot{m}_2 c_{p2}}\right) d\dot{Q} \qquad (24.3b)$$

Integrating equations (24.3a) and (24.3b) between inlet i and outlet o, assuming the specific heat capacities are constant, we get

$$-\left(\frac{1}{\dot{m}_1 c_{p1}} \pm \frac{1}{\dot{m}_2 c_{p2}}\right)\dot{Q} = \Delta T_o - \Delta T_i \qquad (24.4)$$

The positive sign refers to the parallel-flow exchanger, and the negative sign to the counter-flow type. Also, substituting for $d\dot{Q}$ in equation (24.3a,b) from (24.2), we obtain

$$-\left(\frac{1}{\dot{m}_1 c_{p1}} \pm \frac{1}{\dot{m}_2 c_{p2}}\right)U\, dA = \frac{d(\Delta T)}{\Delta T}$$

By integration between inlet i and outlet o, since U is assumed constant, this becomes

$$-\left(\frac{1}{\dot{m}_1 c_{p1}} \pm \frac{1}{\dot{m}_2 c_{p2}}\right)UA = \ln\frac{\Delta T_o}{\Delta T_i} \qquad (24.5)$$

Finally, dividing (24.4) by (24.5), we obtain

$$\dot{Q} = UA\frac{\Delta T_o - \Delta T_i}{\ln(\Delta T_o/\Delta T_i)} \qquad (24.6)$$

Comparing (24.6) with (24.1), it is clear that the required mean temperature difference is

$$\Delta \bar{T}_{\ln} = \frac{\Delta T_o - \Delta T_i}{\ln(\Delta T_o/\Delta T_i)} \qquad (24.7)$$

This is called the *logarithmic mean temperature difference*, denoted by the subscript ln, and the expression is the same for both types of heat exchanger.

Example 24.1 Ethylene glycol flows at a rate of 0.5 kg/s through a thin-walled copper tube of diameter $d_1 = 1.25$ cm; water flows at 0.375 kg/s in the opposite direction through the annular space formed by this tube and a tube of diameter $d_2 = 2$ cm. The ethylene glycol, which enters at 100°C, is required to leave at 60°C, while the water enters at 10°C. Calculate the length of tube required. Also calculate the length of tube required if the water were flowing in the same direction as the ethylene glycol. The following empirical correlations are applicable: for turbulent flow through a tube

$$Nu_d = 0.023\,(Re_d)^{0.8}\,(Pr)^{0.4} \qquad (24.8)$$

and for turbulent flow through an annulus

$$\frac{\alpha}{c_p \rho C}(= St) = 0.023\,(Re_{d'})^{-0.2}\,(Pr)^{-2/3} \tag{24.9}$$

with all properties taken at bulk temperature. (C in this example denotes velocity.) In (24.9) $Re_{d'}$ is based on the equivalent diameter

$$d' = \frac{4\,(\text{cross-section area})}{\text{wetted circumference}} = \frac{4\pi\,(d_2^2 - d_1^2)}{4\pi\,(d_2 + d_1)} = (d_2 - d_1)$$

The product ρC, which appears in the Reynolds and Stanton numbers, must be constant for each fluid along the tube and equal to $\dot{m}/A$. Thus for ethylene glycol

$$\rho C = \frac{0.5 \times 4}{\pi (0.0125)^2} = 4070 \text{ kg/m}^2 \text{ s}$$

and for water

$$\rho C = \frac{0.375 \times 4}{\pi\{(0.02)^2 - (0.0125)^2\}} = 1960 \text{ kg/m}^2 \text{ s}$$

Calculation of film coefficient for ethylene glycol α_e
The relevant properties and dimensionless groups are set out below, for the bulk temperature at inlet and outlet, and for the mean bulk temperature.

	60 °C	80 °C	100 °C
$c_p/[\text{kJ/kg K}]$	2.56	2.65	2.74
$\mu/10^{-4}[\text{kg/m s}]$	51.7	32.1	21.4
$k/10^{-4}[\text{kW/m K}]$	2.60	2.61	2.63
$Pr = c_p\mu/k$	50.9	32.6	22.3
$(Pr)^{0.4}$	4.82	4.03	3.46
$Re_d = \rho C d/\mu$	9 840	15 800	23 800
$(Re_d)^{0.8}$	1 560	2 280	3 170
Nu_d from (24.8)	173	211	252
$\alpha_e/[\text{kW/m}^2 \text{ K}]$	3.60	4.41	5.30

Calculation of film coefficient for water α_w
The outlet temperature of the water is found from an energy balance, assuming no heat losses to the surroundings. Thus

$$\dot{m}_1 c_{p1}(T_{1i} - T_{1o}) = \dot{m}_2 c_{p2}(T_{2o} - T_{2i})$$

and substituting the values from the data

$$0.5 \times 2.65(100 - 60) = 0.375 \times 4.18(T_{2o}/[°C] - 10) = 53.0 \text{ kW}$$

Hence $T_{2o} = 43.8\,°C$, and the mean bulk temperature can be taken as 27 °C. The properties and dimensionless groups are set out below, as for ethylene glycol.

	10 °C	27 °C	44 °C
$c_p/[\text{kJ/kg K}]$	4.19	4.18	4.18
$\mu/10^{-4}[\text{kg/m s}]$	13.0	8.53	6.05
$k/10^{-4}[\text{kW/m K}]$	5.87	6.14	6.37
$Pr = c_p\mu/k$	9.29	5.81	3.97
$(Pr)^{2/3}$	4.42	3.23	2.51
$Re_{d'} = \rho C(d_2 - d_1)/\mu$	11 300	17 200	24 300
$(Re_{d'})^{0.2}$	6.47	7.03	7.54
$\alpha_w/[\text{kW/m}^2\,\text{K}]$ from (24.9)	6.61	8.30	9.96

Calculation of tube length for counter flow
The resistance of the thin copper tube separating the two fluids can be neglected in comparison with the film resistance. The overall heat transfer coefficient U at any section along the tube is therefore given by

$$\frac{1}{U} = \frac{1}{\alpha_e} + \frac{1}{\alpha_w}$$

At the ethylene glycol inlet (or water outlet) we therefore have

$$\frac{1}{U_i} = \frac{1}{(\alpha_e)_{100}} + \frac{1}{(\alpha_w)_{44}} = \frac{1}{5.30} + \frac{1}{9.96} \quad \text{or} \quad U_i = 3.46\,\text{kW/m}^2\,\text{K}$$

Similarly, at the ethylene glycol outlet (or water inlet) we have

$$\frac{1}{U_o} = \frac{1}{3.60} + \frac{1}{6.61} \quad \text{or} \quad U_o = 2.33\,\text{kW/m}^2\,\text{K}$$

Evidently U is by no means constant along the heat exchanger surface, which is the assumption upon which equations (24.1) and (24.7) are based. These equations will yield an approximate solution, however, if an average value of U is used, i.e. if we take $U = (3.46 + 2.33)/2 = 2.90\,\text{kW/m}^2\,\text{K}$.

The logarithmic mean temperature difference, using the notation of Fig. 24.1, is

$$\Delta \bar{T}_{\text{ln}} = \frac{\Delta T_o - \Delta T_i}{\ln(\Delta T_o/\Delta T_i)} = \frac{(60 - 10) - (100 - 43.8)}{\ln\{(60 - 10)/(100 - 43.8)\}} = 53.1\,\text{K}$$

Hence, from (24.1), the required tube length l is given by

$$\dot{Q} = U(\pi d_1 l)\Delta \bar{T}_{\text{ln}}$$

$$l = \frac{53.0}{2.90 \times \pi \times 0.0125 \times 53.1} \approx 8.8\,\text{m}$$

Calculation of tube length for parallel flow
In this case we have, at the ethylene glycol inlet (and water inlet),

$$\frac{1}{U_i} = \frac{1}{5.30} + \frac{1}{6.61} \quad \text{or} \quad U_i = 2.94\,\text{kW/m}^2\,\text{K}$$

And at the outlet

$$\frac{1}{3.60} + \frac{1}{9.96} \quad \text{or} \quad U_o = 2.64 \, \text{kW/m}^2 \, \text{K}$$

The average value of U is therefore 2.79 kW/m² K. Hence

$$\Delta \bar{T}_{\ln} = \frac{(60 - 43.8) - (100 - 10)}{\ln\{(60 - 43.8)/(100 - 10)\}} = 43.0 \, \text{K}$$

$$l = \frac{53.0}{2.79 \times \pi \times 0.0125 \times 43.0} \approx 11.2 \, \text{m}$$

NB: For various reasons explained in the following paragraphs, this solution is only approximate. It is more usual to adopt the quicker method of obtaining an average U from α_e and α_w at the mean bulk temperatures of 80 °C and 27 °C respectively. The reader can easily verify that virtually the same lengths are obtained. The method of obtaining U used in this example is preferable, however, because it entails finding the extreme values of the Reynolds number. Hence it is possible to see whether the flow is laminar or turbulent, and thereby verify whether the appropriate equations for α are being used.

Example 24.1 shows that although the expression for the logarithmic mean temperature difference is the same for both types of heat exchanger, its value is higher for the counter-flow type. Thus for given mass flows and temperature changes, the counter-flow heat exchanger requires less surface area than its parallel-flow equivalent. The difference is most marked if the heat capacity $\dot{m}c_p$ of the two fluids is the same. When the heat capacity of one fluid is infinite, as occurs in a heat exchanger with one fluid condensing or evaporating, the merits of these two types are equal. This is evident from Fig. 24.2, since the logarithmic mean temperature difference is obviously independent of the direction of flow of fluid 1.

In Example 24.1 it was assumed that the resistance of the metal tube separating the two fluids is negligible compared with the resistances of the two fluid boundary layers. This is usually true when the metal wall is very clean, but with many fluids deposits gradually build up on the wall. If such deposits are likely to be formed, it is necessary to allow for their resistance, and this is usually done by means of 'fouling factors'. The allowance made depends upon the nature of the fluid (e.g. whether hard, soft, or distilled water is used), and

Fig. 24.2
Heat exchanger with one fluid condensing over the whole area

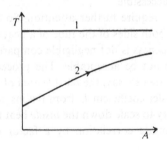

[24.1]

Fig. 24.3

Cross-flow heat exchanger, showing typical temperature distributions at inlet and outlet

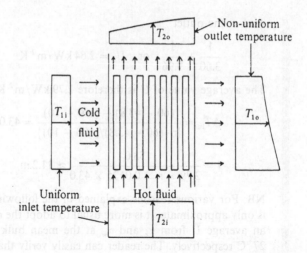

also on the frequency with which the heat exchanger can be put out of commission for cleaning. A fouling factor is usually quoted as a resistance to be added to the 'clean' overall resistance $1/U$.

In some problems it is not permissible to take an average value of U and to assume that it is constant over the whole area of the heat exchanger; this is the case when the temperature range through which a fluid is heated or cooled is very large. A more accurate equation for $\dot{Q}$ can be derived by assuming that U varies linearly with temperature through the heat exchanger, from U_i at inlet to U_o at outlet. It can then be shown that the rate of heat transfer is given by

$$\dot{Q} = A\,\frac{U_i \Delta T_o - U_o \Delta T_i}{\ln(U_i \Delta T_o / U_o \Delta T_i)} \tag{24.10}$$

In view of the relative inaccuracy of the empirical equations from which the film coefficients are obtained, and the uncertainty about entrance length and fouling effects, the simpler analysis is usually adequate.

The *cross-flow* heat exchanger, illustrated in Fig. 24.3, occupies a position intermediate between the parallel-flow and counter-flow types. The analysis for finding the mean temperature difference is more complicated in this case, and the reader is referred to more advanced texts (Refs 11 and 33). Typical temperature distributions at inlet and outlet are shown in the figure. The cross-flow exchanger, although less economic in size than the counter-flow type, is sometimes preferred when it makes the layout of ducts and piping more convenient and accessible.

Two problems require further attention. So far we have assumed that the surface areas on both sides of the tube of a heat exchanger are the same. When the tube wall thickness is not negligible compared with its mean diameter, this assumption may not be acceptable. The procedure then is to refer the heat transfer per unit area to, say, the *outside* area of the tube. When calculating the overall heat transfer coefficient U from the inside, wall and outside resistances, it is then necessary to scale down the *inside* heat transfer coefficient α_{in} obtained from the appropriate correlation by a factor of d_{in}/d_{out}, so that the inside

g. 24.4
ell-and-tube
xed-flow heat
changer

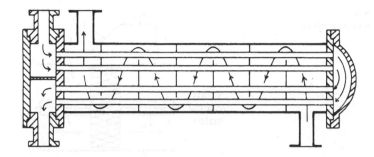

resistance becomes $d_{out}/\alpha_{in}d_{in}$. (Any inside fouling factor must be modified in a similar manner.) The wall resistance, which from section 21.3 is $\ln(d_{out}/d_{in})2\pi k$ per unit *length* of tube, must be multiplied by πd_{out} to provide the resistance $d_{out}\ln(d_{out}/d_{in})/2k$ per unit outside area.

The second problem relates to the independent variables which are known in the heat exchanger specification. In Example 24.1 both inlet temperatures and one outlet temperature were known, and the second outlet temperature was obtained from an energy balance. It was then possible to deduce the unknown surface area. Sometimes, however, we have a heat exchanger of known area for which the unknown outlet temperature of both fluids must be estimated. Or perhaps the outlet temperatures are known at the design point but estimates of these temperatures are required when conditions such as flow rates are changed. The method of Example 24.1 is not well suited to such calculations because it would involve a tedious procedure of trial and error. An alternative procedure using the concept of *number-of-transfer units*, and referred to as the NTU method, leads to the values of outlet temperature directly. Ref. 33 provides a good presentation of this method.

Many heat exchangers do not fall into any of the simple categories mentioned. Fig. 24.4 shows a typical shell-and-tube heat exchanger with parallel-, cross- and counter-flow paths; such an exchanger is usually referred to as a *mixed-flow* type. Rather than carry out the analysis from first principles, designers usually refer to published curves of mean temperature difference for the principal types of mixed-flow heat exchanger.*

The heat exchangers discussed so far are sometimes called *recuperators*. In this type, heat flows steadily and continuously from one fluid to another through a containing wall. An entirely different type of heat exchanger, in which the flow of heat is intermittent, is known as a *regenerator*. In the regenerator a matrix of metal comes into contact alternately with the hot and the cold fluid, first absorbing energy for a time, and then rejecting it. In the design shown in Fig. 24.5 the matrix is rotating, the hot fluid flowing through the top half and the cold fluid through the bottom half of the matrix (see Ref. 33). The flow passages are suitably sealed from each other. In other types, the fluids are passed alternately through two stationary matrices by opening and closing valves. Rotary regenerators are suitable only when the pressures of the two streams

---

* T. Tinker in Ref. 35, pp. 89–116, and Refs 2 and 11.

Fig. 24.5
A rotating regenerator

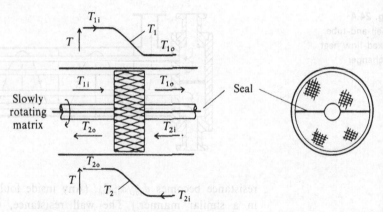

are not very different: air preheating in boiler plant as discussed in section 11.6 is one such application.

24.2 Heat flow through a wall

When a wall separates two fluids of known temperature, it was shown in section 21.2 that the heat flow through the wall can be calculated from equations (21.12) and (21.13). These equations require a knowledge of the surface coefficients, which we have seen depend upon the temperature of the wall surfaces. Because the wall temperatures are unknown and the coefficients are not simple functions of these temperatures, there is in fact no direct easy way of calculating the heat flow. The simplest method is to guess these temperatures, and proceed by a method of successive approximation. The procedure is best illustrated by a numerical example.

Example 24.2 A brick wall of conductivity $k = 6.92 \times 10^{-4}$ kW/m K, and of thickness 23 cm, separates two rooms of height 4 m. The mean temperature of the air and other surfaces with which the wall is exchanging heat on the left is 65 °C, and on the right is 10 °C (Fig. 24.6). Estimate the heat flow per m^2 of wall area.

Let us assume initially that the surface temperatures of the wall are $T_1 = 55$ °C on the left, and $T_2 = 20$ °C on the right. The free convection heat transfer coefficients can be found from the appropriate equation in Fig. 22.17. To

Fig. 24.6

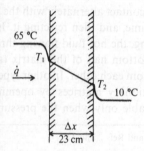

decide whether the laminar or turbulent equation is applicable we must make a rough estimate of Gr. We shall calculate its value midway up the wall, and take the properties of air at an average value of the two room temperatures, namely $\frac{1}{2}(10 + 65)\,°C \approx 310\,K$. Hence $\beta = (1/T) = (1/310)\,K^{-1}$ and $v = 1.66 \times 10^{-5}\,m^2/s$. Thus

$$Gr = \frac{\beta g x^3 \theta}{v^2} = \frac{(1/310) \times 9.81 \times 2^3 \times 10}{(1.66 \times 10^{-5})^2} \approx 9.2 \times 10^9$$

The flow is evidently turbulent over most of the wall and there is no need to make more precise estimates of Gr for the two sides of the wall separately. The appropriate free-convection equation from Fig. 22.17 is $\alpha_c = 0.001\,31(\theta/[K])^{1/3}\,kW/m^2\,K$. For our guess of the surface temperatures,

$$\alpha_{c1} = \alpha_{c2} = 0.001\,31(65 - 55)^{1/3} = 0.001\,31(20 - 10)^{1/3}$$

$$= 0.002\,82\,kW/m^2\,K$$

From Fig. 23.6 the normal emissivity ε_n for brick is 0.93. We pointed out in section 23.2 that $\varepsilon/\varepsilon_n$ is $0.95 \rightarrow 1$ for this kind of material. Hence the total hemispherical emissivity $\varepsilon \approx 0.9$. The radiation heat transfer coefficient to the left of the wall, from (23.34), is

$$\alpha_{r1} = 0.9 \times 56.7 \times 10^{-12}(338 + 328)(338^2 + 328^2)$$

$$= 0.007\,54\,kW/m^2\,K$$

On the right, the radiation coefficient is

$$\alpha_{r2} = 0.9 \times 56.7 \times 10^{-12}(293 + 283)(293^2 + 283^2)$$

$$= 0.004\,88\,kW/m^2\,K$$

The overall heat transfer coefficient, given by equation (21.13), is

$$\frac{1}{U} = \frac{1}{\alpha_{c1} + \alpha_{r1}} + \frac{\Delta x}{k} + \frac{1}{\alpha_{c2} + \alpha_{r2}}$$

$$= \frac{1}{0.002\,82 + 0.007\,54} + \frac{0.23}{6.92 \times 10^{-4}} + \frac{1}{0.002\,82 + 0.004\,88}$$

$$= 559\,\frac{m^2\,K}{kW}$$

$$U = 0.001\,79\,kW/m^2\,K$$

To check the accuracy of our original guess of T_1 and T_2, we can apply the equation of continuity. For steady flow,

$$\dot{q} = -U(10 - 65) = 0.001\,79 \times 55 = 0.0985\,kW/m^2$$

$$= -(\alpha_{c1} + \alpha_{r1})(T_1 - 65) = -0.010\,36(T_1 - 65)$$

$$= -(\alpha_{c2} + \alpha_{r2})(10 - T_2) = -0.007\,70(10 - T_2)$$

These equations yield

$$T_1 = 55.5\,°C \quad \text{and} \quad T_2 = 22.8\,°C$$

The procedure can now be repeated with the new values of the surface temperatures. This second approximation gives the following results:

$$\alpha_{c1} = 0.002\,77 \text{ kW/m}^2\,\text{K}, \qquad \alpha_{c2} = 0.003\,06 \text{ kW/m}^2\,\text{K}$$

$$\alpha_{r1} = 0.007\,56 \text{ kW/m}^2\,\text{K}, \qquad \alpha_{r2} = 0.004\,95 \text{ kW/m}^2\,\text{K}$$

$$U = 0.001\,81 \text{ kW/m}^2\,\text{K}, \qquad \dot{q} = 0.0996 \text{ kW/m}^2$$

$$T_1 = 55.4\,°\text{C}, \qquad\qquad T_2 = 22.4\,°\text{C}$$

It is evident from the last values of $\dot{q}$, T_1 and T_2 that a further approximation is unnecessary, and the required heat flow is therefore 0.0996 kW/m².

24.3 Heat flow through a fin

When heat has to be exchanged between a surface and a fluid, the effective area is often increased by fins projecting from the surface, as in air-cooled petrol engines or in finned-tube heat exchangers. Most of the resistance to heat flow is usually in the fluid boundary layer adjacent to the surface, and this may be materially reduced by an increase in surface area; the increase in wall resistance due to the additional fin material is normally relatively small. Here we shall consider in detail only prismatic fins projecting from a plane surface. By a *prismatic fin* we mean a projection having a cross-section, taken parallel to the plane surface, which has an area and a perimeter constant along its length. For example, referring to the rectangular fin shown in Fig. 24.7a, neither $A = 2bl$ nor $P = 2(l + 2b)$ is a function of x. The cross-section may, however, have an arbitrary and even irregular shape, as shown in Fig. 24.7b.

The heat flow pattern, i.e. heat flow lines and isothermals, for a slender rectangular fin ($2b \ll h$ and l) is shown in the left-hand fin of Fig. 24.7a. We shall adopt a major simplification in the theory by assuming that the lines of flow are parallel to the flanks of the fin, implying plane isothermals. The case

Fig. 24.7
Heat flow through a cooling fin

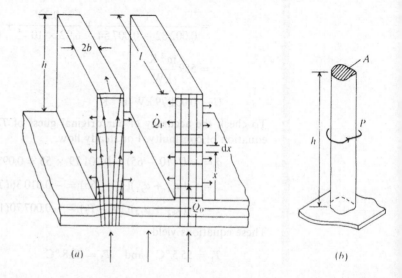

(a) (b)

then reduces to a 'one-dimensional' problem as shown in the right-hand fin. We shall further assume that the combined convection and radiation heat transfer coefficient α is constant over the fin surface, i.e. $\alpha \neq f(x)$.

It will be remembered from section 21.4 that the initial step in any conduction problem is to find the temperature distribution in the conductor. This will involve the derivation of a differential equation, the solution of which, in this simple case, provides the one-dimensional temperature distribution $T = f(x)$. The heat transfer from the flanks of the fin $\dot{Q}_F$ can then be found from

$$\dot{Q}_F = \int_0^h \alpha P(T - T_s)\, dx \tag{24.11}$$

where T_s is the free stream-temperature of the adjacent fluid. This heat loss must be equal to the heat conducted into the fin at its root, given by

$$\dot{Q}_0 (= \dot{Q}_F) = -kA\left(\frac{dT}{dx}\right)_0 \tag{24.12}$$

where the subscript 0 refers to $x = 0$. It is usually easier to calculate the heat loss from (24.12) than (24.11).

24.3.1   The solution of the differential equation for a prismatic fin

The one-dimensional differential equation for the prismatic fin can be derived from first principles, but here we shall adopt the more direct route of using the steady one-dimensional version of the general conduction equation (21.20), namely

$$\frac{d^2 T}{dx^2} + \frac{\dot{q}_g}{k} = 0 \tag{24.13}$$

Because of the assumption of one-dimensional heat flow, we may regard the transfer of heat from the flanks as negative heat generation, and therefore write

$$\dot{q}_g(A\, dx) = -\alpha(P\, dx)(T - T_s) \tag{24.14}$$

Writing $\theta = T - T_s$, we can rearrange the differential equation to yield

$$\frac{d^2\theta}{dx^2} - m^2\theta = 0 \tag{24.15}$$

where $m = (\alpha P/kA)^{1/2}$. The general solution of (24.15) is

$$\theta = Me^{mx} + Ne^{-mx} \tag{24.16}$$

The values of the constants of integration M and N can be found from the boundary conditions. At the root, where $x = 0$, the fin temperature is T_0 say, and hence

$$\theta_0 = T_0 - T_s = M + N \tag{24.17}$$

The heat loss from the tip of a slender fin is very small compared with that from the flanks, and can often be neglected. If so, we have a second boundary condition, namely when $x = h$:

$$\dot{Q}_h = -2kbl\left(\frac{d\theta}{dx}\right)_h = 0$$

and hence

$$\left(\frac{d\theta}{dx}\right)_h = 0 \tag{24.18}$$

Differentiating (24.16) therefore, and putting $x = h$,

$$Mme^{mh} + Nme^{-mh} = 0 \tag{24.19}$$

The constants of integration are found from (24.17) and (24.19) as

$$M = \theta_0 \frac{e^{-mh}}{e^{mh} + e^{-mh}} \quad \text{and} \quad N = \theta_0 \frac{e^{mh}}{e^{mh} + e^{-mh}} \tag{24.20}$$

Substituting these values in (24.16), we get the solution for the temperature profile along the fin as

$$\theta = \theta_0 \frac{e^{m(h-x)} + e^{-m(h-x)}}{e^{mh} + e^{-mh}} = \theta_0 \frac{\cosh m(h-x)}{\cosh mh} \tag{24.21}$$

For steady conduction, the heat flow from the fin surface is equal to the heat flow through the base of the fin, as already indicated by equation (24.12). Thus the solution for the heat flow is

$$\dot{Q}_0 = -kA\left(\frac{d\theta}{dx}\right) = mkA\theta_0 \frac{\sinh m(h-x)}{\cosh mh}\Big]_{x=0}$$

$$= mkA\theta_0 \tanh mh \tag{24.22}$$

The temperature excess $\theta_h (= T_h - T_s)$ at the tip of the fin, putting $x = h$ in (24.21), is

$$\theta_h = \frac{\theta_0}{\cosh mh} \tag{24.23}$$

An approximate correction for the small heat loss from the tip can be found, using this value of θ_h, from

$$\dot{Q}_{\text{tip}} = \alpha A \theta_h \tag{24.24}$$

When applying this fin theory it is usually a simple matter to arrive at a suitable expression for the parameter m. For example, for a cylindrical fin of diameter d,

$$m = \left(\frac{\alpha \pi d}{k\pi d^2/4}\right)^{1/2} = \left(\frac{4\alpha}{kd}\right)^{1/2} \tag{24.25}$$

and for the slender rectangular fin, for which $2b \ll l$,

$$m = \left[\frac{\alpha 2(l + 2b)}{k(2bl)}\right]^{1/2} \approx \left(\frac{\alpha}{kb}\right)^{1/2} \tag{24.26}$$

Equation (24.22) can sometimes be used with acceptable accuracy for thin circular fins, of thickness $2b$ and height h, on a tube. The condition is that h is much smaller than the diameter of the tube, as with an air-cooled engine cylinder for example. Only then can the tube be treated approximately as a plane surface. When h is comparable with the tube diameter, the differential equation must be derived from first principles using polar coordinates and the solution involves Bessel functions.

A particularly difficult problem in applying fin theory is that of obtaining a realistic value of the combined convection and radiation heat transfer coefficient $\alpha = (\alpha_c + \alpha_r)$. In practice α will not be constant but will vary along the height of the fin, and an appropriate mean value must be estimated. Such a value will depend on the fluid properties, on the nature of the convection (whether free or forced), on the fin geometry, and in particular on the fin spacing. When fin spacing is reduced, the boundary layers on adjacent fins may interact and α_c may drop off dramatically. The radiation coefficient α_r will be less affected by geometry, and an upper limit is provided by the equivalent of black-body radiation from the envelope area.

It is interesting to note that, as in other conduction problems with a boundary condition given in terms of a surface heat transfer coefficient (e.g. section 21.6), the solution for the fin contains implicitly a Biot number Bi. Thus, if we denote by L the ratio of solid cross-section area to perimeter, then

$$mh = \left(\frac{\alpha L}{k}\right)^{1/2} \frac{h}{L} = (Bi)^{1/2} \frac{h}{L} \qquad (24.27)$$

A typical application of the solution for a prismatic fin is provided by a thermometer pocket immersed in a fluid stream as shown in Fig. 24.8. Evidently the thermometer will indicate a temperature T_h somewhere between T_s and T_0. The following numerical example illustrates the order of error that may be involved when using this method of temperature measurement.

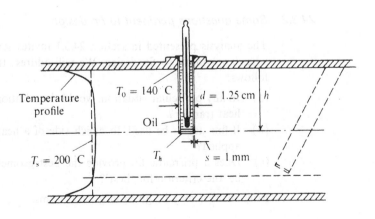

Fig. 24.8
The thermometer pocket

Example 24.3 Superheated steam at a mean temperature $T_g = 200\,°C$ flows through a 10 cm diameter pipe. A brass pocket dips radially into the pipe with its closed end on the centre line, and the root of the pocket is at $T_0 = 140\,°C$. The diameter of the pocket is $d = 1.25$ cm and its wall thickness is $s = 1$ mm. The conductivity k for brass is 0.112 kW/m K, and it is estimated that the combined convection and radiation heat transfer coefficient α for the pocket surface is 0.397 kW/m^2 K. Predict the thermometer reading T_h. Assume that the thermometer reads the temperature of the bottom plate of the pocket, and that conduction in the axial direction through the thermometer stem and surrounding oil is negligible compared with the conduction along the pocket wall (Fig. 24.8).

The temperature at the end of the pocket is given by putting $x = h$ in (24.18), i.e.

$$T_h - T_s = (T_0 - T_s)\frac{\cosh m(h - h)}{\cosh mh} = -\frac{60\,[\mathrm{K}]}{\cosh mh}$$

The effective cross-sectional area to be used in (24.20) is approximately equal to πds, and the circumference of the rod is πd. Hence

$$m = \left(\frac{\alpha \pi d}{k\pi ds}\right)^{1/2} = \left(\frac{\alpha}{ks}\right)^{1/2} = \left(\frac{0.397}{0.112 \times 0.001}\right)^{1/2} = 59.5\ \mathrm{m}^{-1}$$

Since

$$\cosh mh = \cosh(59.5 \times 0.05) \approx 9.87$$

$$T_h - T_s = -\frac{60}{9.87} = -7.1\ \mathrm{K} \quad \text{or} \quad T_h = 193.9\,°C$$

Clearly the error can be reduced by lagging the pipe to increase T_0, and also by increasing the product (mh). (a) m can be increased by using a thinner tube, or by using a metal of lower conductivity. If the conductivity is reduced excessively, however, the radial resistance to heat flow increases to such an extent that the temperature distribution is no longer 'one-dimensional' and the foregoing treatment is not applicable. (b) h may be increased by inclining the pocket and letting it project beyond the pipe axis as shown by the dashed pocket in Fig. 24.8: the tip should of course remain clear of the boundary layer near the wall.

24.3.2 Some questions pertinent to fin design

The analysis presented in section 24.3.1 invites several questions to be asked when applying it to fin design. We will address three such question in what follows:

(a) In any particular situation, would the addition of fins increase the rate of heat transfer?

(b) If fins are to be used, to which side of a heat exchanger should they be applied?

(c) Does a prismatic fin provide the best geometry, and what is, or should be, the criterion for 'best'?

Brief answers may be given in general terms.

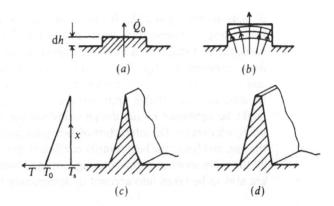

Addition of fins

The beneficial effect of increased surface area provided by fins is counteracted by increased wall resistance due to the additional material. Consider a flat surface on which a fin of infinitesimal height dh is attached, as in Fig. 24.9a. The fin will be beneficial if

$$\left(\frac{d\dot{Q}_0}{dh}\right) > 0 \quad \text{at } h = 0$$

but the increase in wall resistance will more than outweigh the effect of increased area if

$$\left(\frac{d\dot{Q}_0}{dh}\right) < 0 \quad \text{at } h = 0$$

The expression for Q_0 given by equation (24.22) cannot be used when applying this criterion, because it applies only to slender fins for which the approximations of one-dimensional treatment and zero tip loss are valid. An accurate two-dimensional analysis, where the heat flow lines and isothermals are as in Fig. 24.9b, yields the result that the heat transfer from a plane surface is always increased by some prismatic fin area when Bi is less than 0.2, where $Bi = A/kP$. In fact this is the case in most practical situations for both free and forced convection unless the fluid is a liquid metal.

Position of fins

We often meet situations when the heat transfer coefficients for the two sides of a wall are not equal, and such inequality may be particularly pronounced when one fluid is a gas and the other a liquid. It is easy to show that the intuitive feeling that it is more beneficial to add fins to the side having the lower heat transfer coefficient (e.g. the gas side) is correct. It must be remembered, however, that with heat exchangers the rate of heat transfer is not the only criterion of effectiveness; sometimes the pressure drop is important, and fins increase this.

Optimum geometry

A prismatic fin is not the best geometry when 'best' means the minimum amount of material for a given $\dot{Q}_0$. It can be shown that a tapering fin which gives a linear drop of temperature from root to tip uses the least material. On this basis, the best shape for a fin of rectangular cross-section is one having curved flanks tapering to a tip of zero width, as in Fig. 24.9c. For reasons of strength and cost of manufacture the trapezoidal profile of Fig. 24.9d would normally be used as a reasonable approximation. Other geometrical parameters that might be optimised in any design study are the aspect ratio ($h/2b_0$) and the pitch/width ratio. The interaction of these parameters with the fluid flow between the fins, and hence the heat transfer coefficient, makes this a complex problem— all the more so when manufacturing costs and running costs of the installation are also to be taken into account in determining the 'best' design of fin.

24.4 Thermocouple in a gas stream

When a thermocouple is used to measure the local temperature T_g of a hot gas flowing through a pipe of lower temperature T_w, the thermocouple indicates a temperature T_p, such that $T_w < T_p < T_g$ (Fig. 24.10). The exact value of T_p is determined by a balance of heat transfers to and from the couple junction. The junction gains heat by convection (assuming that radiation from the gas stream is negligible), and it losses heat by radiation to the wall and by conduction along the wire. The conduction loss can often be neglected if fine-gauge wire is used, particularly if the wire is laid along an isothermal for some distance before it is taken out of the pipe radially, as shown in the figure. The energy balance between the convection gain and radiation loss can then be written as

$$\alpha_c A(T_g - T_p) = \alpha_r A(T_p - T_w)$$

and hence the true gas temperature T_g can be written in terms of the thermocouple reading T_p and a correction term as

$$T_g = T_p + (T_p - T_w)\frac{\alpha_r}{\alpha_c} \qquad (24.28)$$

Fig. 24.10
Different types of thermocouple

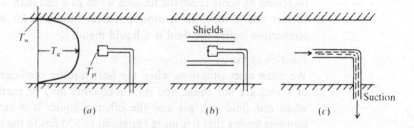

(a) (b) (c)

Example 24.4   Air at atmospheric pressure flows over a thermocouple junction with a velocity of 3 m/s. The temperature of the pipe wall is $T_w = 670$ K, and the couple indicates an air temperature of $T_p = 850$ K. The couple is butt welded, as shown in Fig. 24.10a, and its diameter at the junction is $d = 1.2$ mm. The emissivity of the wire is $\varepsilon = 0.2$. For the flow across wires, the convection heat transfer can be found from

$$Nu_d = 0.5(Re_d)^{0.5} \qquad (24.29)$$

Calculate the true temperature of the air.

As we do not know the exact air temperature, we may use its property values at 850 K, which are (from Ref. 14)

$$k = 6.03 \times 10^{-5}\,\text{kW/m}^2\,\text{K} \quad \text{and} \quad v = 9.06 \times 10^{-5}\,\text{m}^2/\text{s}$$

The heat transfer to the wire by convection can be found from

$$Nu_d = 0.5\left\{\frac{3 \times 0.0012}{9.06 \times 10^{-5}}\right\}^{0.5} = 3.15$$

and hence

$$\alpha_c = \frac{k}{d}(Nu_d) = \frac{6.03 \times 10^{-5}}{0.0012} \times 3.15 = 0.158\,\text{kW/m}^2\,\text{K}$$

The radiation heat transfer coefficient is, from equation (23.34),

$$\alpha_r = 0.2 \times 56.7 \times 10^{-12}(850 + 670)(850^2 + 670^2) = 0.0202\,\text{kW/m}^2\,\text{K}$$

Hence the true air temperature according to (24.28) is

$$T_g = 850 + (850 - 670)\frac{0.0202}{0.158} = 873\,\text{K}$$

Since the temperature range between couple and air is only 23 K, it is immaterial whether the properties in (24.29) are evaluated at the bulk, film or couple temperature.

From (24.28) it can be seen that the accuracy of the thermocouple reading can be improved by the following methods:

(a) By reducing α_r. This can be achieved by shielding the junction with one or more concentric shields, as is shown in Fig. 24.10b. The shields assume temperatures intermediate between T_w and T_p, and thus reduce the radiation loss.

(b) By increasing α_c. This can be done by using finer wire because, from (24.29), $\alpha_c \propto (1/d)^{0.5}$. It is also possible to increase α_c by increasing the gas velocity over the junction. The thermocouple wire can be surrounded by a tube through which some gas from the main stream is sucked at a high velocity (Fig. 24.10c). Such an instrument is called a suction pyrometer.

The simple analysis given in this section is only applicable when the velocity of the gas stream is low, i.e. not more than about 50 m/s. When a thermocouple is placed in a gas stream, the gas is brought to rest at the 'stagnation point' of the junction and the loss of kinetic energy appears as a local rise in pressure and temperature. This effect is appreciable with high gas velocities, and special designs of thermocouple have to be used (see Ref. 30 for example).

Appendix A

Dimensions and Units

A.1 Introduction

Even though the principles of thermodynamics be well understood, difficulties may be encountered when solving numerical problems because of the different systems of units in which data in the literature have been expressed in the past. The purpose of this appendix is to make clear what is involved in the concept of a system of units, and to compare the SI (Système International d'Unités) with older systems. References for further reading on these topics are recommended in section A.5.

First it should be appreciated that the measurement of a physical quantity, such as a length l, is accomplished by comparing it with some standard measure of the quantity, l_u say. Measurements are ratios such as $l_1/l_u, l_2/l_u,\ldots$ and are thus pure numbers. When l_u is elevated to a universal standard of comparison it is called a *unit*. Similar considerations apply to derived quantities such as velocity and pressure which are measured in terms of *derived* units such as m/s and N/m^2 (or Pa) respectively; they are derived from *base units* of mass, length, time etc. It follows that a physical quantity can be regarded as a product of a pure number and a unit, i.e.

$$\text{physical quantity} = \text{number} \times \text{unit} \qquad (A.1)$$

This is a widely accepted convention, and it follows that *neither the physical quantity nor the symbol used to denote it should imply a particular choice of unit*. Thus if we write

$$l_1 = l_2 \qquad (A.2)$$

we imply that the two lengths are equal in an absolute sense irrespective of the system of measurement employed. One must, of course, use the same units for similar quantities when applying any such physical equation, i.e. the units used must be *consistent*.

Operations on equations involving physical quantities, units and numerical values should follow the ordinary rules of algebra. For example, to convert a length measured in feet to one in metres the following simple procedure can be used. The conversion relation 1 ft = 0.3048 m can be written

$$1 = \frac{0.3048\,\text{m}}{1\,\text{ft}}$$

Then if $l_1 = 7$ ft we may multiply by unity without affecting the equation, and so write

$$l_1 = 7\,\text{ft} \times \frac{0.3048\,\text{m}}{1\,\text{ft}} = 2.1336\,\text{m} \qquad (A.3)$$

The convention implied by equation (A.1) leads to another recommended practice which is adopted in this book. The numerical values along the coordinate of a graph, or entered in a table, can be regarded as pure numbers. When so regarded, it follows that the correct coordinate label or column heading should be the ratio of the physical quantity (or its symbol) and the unit. For example,

$$\text{for length} \frac{l}{[m]} \quad \text{and} \quad \text{for pressure} \frac{p}{[N/m^2]}$$

If the numerical values have been divided by a power of 10, say by 10^5, the label should be divided similarly. Thus a point on a pressure coordinate read off as 4.5 and labelled as

$$\frac{p}{10^5[N/m]}$$

means that

$$\frac{p}{10^5[N/m^2]} = 4.5 \quad \text{or} \quad p = 4.5 \times 10^5 \frac{N}{m^2}$$

No ambiguity can arise as to whether 10^5 or 10^{-5} is intended in the last expression when the ordinary rules of algebra are applied in this way.

The requirement of consistency is more far-reaching than implied by equation (A.2). A physical equation will normally involve several terms such as

$$P_1 + P_2 + P_3 + \ldots = 0$$

where $P_1, P_2, P_3, \ldots$ may be base or derived quantities. It is not sufficient that consistent units be used; in addition, all Ps must be of the same *kind*. It is nonsense to write $8\,m/s + 6\,s = \ldots$ because a velocity cannot be added to a time. To make clear what is meant by the 'same kind of physical quantity' it is necessary to introduce the idea of a *fundamental Unit*, such as mass **M**, length **L**, time **T**, and the idea of *dimension*, which is the power of a fundamental Unit in a *derived Unit*. For example, velocity has the derived Unit LT^{-1}, comprising the fundamental Units **L** and **T** of dimensions 1 and -1 respectively. *All meaningful physical equations must be dimensionally homogeneous.* In other words, the dimensions of the fundamental Units must be the same for each term in a physical equation. The equation $8\,m/s + 6\,s = \ldots$ is not dimensionally homogeneous, and is therefore meaningless, because the dimensions of the fundamental Units $[\mathbf{M, L, T}]$ for the first term are $[0, 1, -1]$, whereas for the second term they are $[0, 0, 1]$.

It should be appreciated that we have now used the word 'unit' in two different senses: first to denote a *measure* of a quantity, and secondly to denote a *kind* of quantity. This usage is confusing, and in this appendix we employ a capital letter when using the word in the second sense.

Summarising the points made so far:

(a) All physical equations are dimensionally homogeneous and should be written in such a way that they are correct whatever consistent system of units is employed (but see a further restriction regarding *coherence* below).

(b) Mathematical manipulation of physical quantities and units must follow the ordinary rules of algebra.

(c) A physical symbol should not be used to represent only the numerical part of a physical quantity; for example, 'a tube length of $l\,m$' is incorrect phraseology because from equation (A.1) it evidently contains a square power of the length dimension. If a need arises to denote the numerical part by a symbol, this can be done using a suitably modified symbol, but the recommended practice is to use explicitly the ratio (physical quantity/ unity), e.g. $l/[m]$.

A.2   SI and coherence

The units in terms of which all derived units in any system are expressed are called base units. Their choice is arbitrary and dictated by convenience. SI employs seven base units, namely metre (m), kilogram (kg), second (s), ampere (A), kelvin (K), mole (mol) and candela (cd). Let us consider the derived physical quantity of velocity, defined in terms of distance s and time t as

$$v = k\frac{s}{t}$$

where k is a numerical coefficient. In coherent systems, coefficients such as k are made equal to unity, and it immediately follows that the unity of velocity is m/s. This apparently simple idea is particularly important in the definition of force which stems from Newton's Second Law of Motion.

$$f \propto ma \quad \text{or} \quad f = kma \tag{A.4}$$

where f is the force, m the mass and a the acceleration. SI differs from many older systems of units in that, being coherent, it makes k equal to unity and thus (A.4) can be written

$$f = ma \tag{A.5}$$

With a coherent system it follows that when the units of any two of the quantities in (A.5) are chosen, the unit of the third is fixed. In SI the kilogram (kg) is chosen as the unit of mass, and 1 m/s^2 as the unit of acceleration. The unit of force, the newton (N), is then defined by equation (A.5) as

$$1[N] = 1[kg] \times 1[m/s^2] \tag{A.6}$$

Similarly, on the cm-g-s system we have the dyne defined by

$$1[dyne] = 1[g] \times 1[cm/s^2] \tag{A.7}$$

The difficulty arises when a non-coherent system of units is employed, i.e. when the units of all three quantities in equation (A.5) are chosen independently of one another. We can then no longer put $k = 1$ in equation (A.4). In the past, European engineers used a unit of force called the kilogram-force (written kgf) which is defined as the gravitational force on a mass of 1 kg, i.e. the weight of 1 kg. Since the conventionally accepted gravitational acceleration is

$$g_n = 9.806\,65 \text{ m/s}^2 \approx 9.81 \text{ m/s}^2$$

we have from equation (A.4)

$$1[kgf] = k \times 1[kg] \times 9.81[m/s^2] \tag{A.8}$$

which yields

$$k = \frac{1}{9.81}\left[\frac{s^2 \text{ kgf}}{\text{kg m}}\right] \quad \text{or} \quad \frac{1}{9.81}\left[\frac{\text{kgf}}{N}\right] \tag{A.9}$$

Using the non-coherent m-kgf-kg-s system of units, the physical equation equivalent to (A.4), expressing the Second Law of Motion, thus becomes

$$f = \frac{1}{9.81}\left[\frac{s^2 \text{ kgf}}{\text{kg m}}\right]ma \tag{A.10}$$

Rearranging (A.10) we have

$$\frac{f}{[\text{kgf}]} = \frac{1}{9.81}\frac{m}{[\text{kg}]}\frac{a}{[m/s^2]} \tag{A.11}$$

In (A.11) the 9.81 is merely a dimensionless constant relating two quantities of the same kind, namely the kgf unit of force and the $kg\,m/s^2$ (or N) unit of force, just as the 0.3048 is a constant relating the metre to the foot in equation (A.3). If we denote by primed symbols the numerical parts of each physical quantity, equation (A.11) can also be written as

$$f' = \frac{1}{9.81} m'a' \tag{A.12}$$

together with the statement that f' is in kgf, m' is in kg and a' is in m/s^2. Both (A.11) and (A.12) can be seen to be different ways of writing a purely *numerical equation*. In the past, equations (A.10), (A.11) and (A.12) have often simply been written as

$$f = \frac{1}{9.81} ma$$

followed by the specification that f is in kgf, m in kg and a in m/s^2. This is bad practice because it disregards the convention contained in (A.1) and leaves it to the reader to decide from the context whether the symbols stand for physical quantities or pure numbers.

Although not used in this book, it is worth mentioning another coherent metric system—the m-kgf-s system—in which k in equation (A.4) is again equal to unity and the kgf is retained as the unit of force. The unit of mass, sometimes referred to as the *technical unit of mass*, is then defined by equation (A.5), i.e.

$$1[\text{kgf}] = 1[\text{technical unit of mass}] \times 1[\text{m}/\text{s}^2] \tag{A.13}$$

Comparing this with equation (A.8) when $k = 1$, it follows that

$$1[\text{technical unit of mass}] = 9.81[\text{kg}] \tag{A.14}$$

Here 9.81 is a dimensionless conversion factor between two mass units, arbitrarily chosen to be *numerically* equal to the conventional value of the gravitational acceleration g_n. Some writers use the symbol g_0 when referring to this number.

As an example of how coherent and non-coherent systems are used in conjunction with a physical equation, we may consider a simple mechanical energy equation expressing the fact that when a body undergoes a change of position and velocity in a field of force, the decrease of potential energy is equal to the increase in kinetic energy. For example, in the vicinity of the earth, where the force can be regarded as independent of position, the physical equation is

$$f(z_1 - z_2) = \tfrac{1}{2} m(C_2^2 - C_1^2) \tag{A.15}$$

where f is the force of gravity acting on a body of mass m as it moves from one height z_1 to another z_2, and C is the velocity of the body (f is equal to mg in this particular case). The equation is dimensionally homogeneous, each term having the derived Unit of energy ML^2T^{-2}. On the coherent m-kg-s system the equivalent numerical equation is

$$\frac{f}{[\text{N}]} \frac{(z_1 - z_2)}{[\text{m}]} = \frac{1}{2} \frac{m}{[\text{kg}]} \frac{(C_2^2 - C_1^2)}{[\text{m}^2/\text{s}^2]} \tag{A.16}$$

or

$$f'(z_1' - z_2') = \tfrac{1}{2} m'(C_2'^2 - C_1'^2) \tag{A.17}$$

However, when the non-coherent m-kgf-kg-s system is used, the physical equation equivalent to (A.15) becomes

$$f(z_1 - z_2) = \frac{1}{9.81}\left[\frac{s^2\,kgf}{kg\,m}\right]\frac{1}{2}m(C_2^2 - C_1^2) \tag{A.18}$$

Substituting numerical values of f', z', m' and C' into this equation yields

$$f'[kgf](z_1' - z_2')[m] = \frac{1}{9.81}\left[\frac{s^2\,kgf}{kg\,m}\right]\frac{1}{2}m'[kg](C_2'^2 - C_1'^2)\left[\frac{m^2}{s^2}\right] \tag{A.19}$$

This makes it possible to check that the units on both sides of the equation do indeed balance.

Referring back to point (a) at the end of section A.1, it can now be stated that *all physical equations in this book are written in such a way that they are correct whatever consistent and coherent system of units is employed.*

Minor modifications to the pure and coherent SI have been found convenient, such as the use of the kilojoule (kJ) instead of the joule (J) for the unit of energy, and the bar for $10^5\,N/m^2$ (or Pa) as the unit of pressure. Although these changes are merely a matter of size of unit which is still decimally related to the coherently derived unit, they can occasionally lead to difficulties. Where dimensional checks are helpful, they have been set out in the manner of equation (A.19); particular attention is drawn to equation (8.5) and Examples 10.1, 10.7, 18.4 and 22.3. Where in the course of a numerical solution there is no obvious difficulty with units, it is unnecessary to be so rigorous. For example, in Example 9.1a we have written

$$Q = m(u_2 - u_1) = 0.6014(1457 - 2711) = -754\,kJ$$

It would have been pedantic to write

$$Q = m(u_2 - u_1) = 0.6014[kg](1457[kJ/kg] - 2711[kJ/kg]) = -754\,kJ$$

The old British systems of units are analogous to the metric systems already described, with the coherent ft-lb-s system parallel to the SI, and the non-coherent ft-lbf-lb-s system parallel to the m-kgf-kf-s system. The coherent ft-lbf-s system, with the slug as the unit of mass, is parallel to the m-kgf-s system with its technical unit of mass. Remembering that the conventional value of g is

$$g_n = 9.806\,65\,\frac{m}{s^2}\frac{1\,ft}{0.3048\,m} = 32.1740\,\frac{ft}{s^2} \approx 32.2\,\frac{ft}{s^2}$$

we can write down the British equivalents of equations (A.6), (A.8), (A.9), (A.13) and (A.14) as follows:

$$1[poundal(pdl)] = 1[pound(lb)] \times 1[ft/s^2] \tag{A.6B}$$

$$1[pound\text{-}force(lbf)] = k \times 1[pound(lb)] \times 1[ft/s^2] \tag{A.8B}$$

$$k = \frac{1}{32.2}\left[\frac{s^2\,lbf}{lb\,ft}\right] \quad or \quad \frac{1}{32.2}\left[\frac{lbf}{pdl}\right] \tag{A.9B}$$

$$1[pound\text{-}force(lbf)] = 1[slug] \times 1[ft/s^2] \tag{A.13B}$$

$$1[slug] = 32.2[lb] \tag{A.14B}$$

Fig. A.1 concluding this appendix summarises the more important SI units used in this book and their usual metric-technical and British equivalents. It is worth pointing out that although SI is not unique in being coherent, it is unique in that its unit of mechanical power is *identical* with its unit of electrical power, namely

$$1\,W(= 1\,J/s = 1\,N\,m/s) = 1[ampere(A)] \times 1[volt(V)] \tag{A.20}$$

This identity leads to numerous simplifications in many branches of engineering and physics.

A.3 The unit symbol for temperature: K or °C?

A generally accepted principle is that each unit should be represented by one, and only one, unit symbol. A second principle is that the unit symbol should *not* be used to explain the meaning of the physical quantity. Where such explanation is necessary, it should be attached to the physical quantity or the symbol representing it; this could be done by adding a subscript or superscript to the symbol. For example, when performing experiments it is often necessary to distinguish between absolute and gauge pressure, and this could be done by writing

$$p_a = 5 \times 10^5 \, \text{N/m}^2 \quad \text{and} \quad p_g = 4 \times 10^5 \, \text{N/m}^2$$

We would be incorrect if we attached particulars to the unit by writing

$$p = 5 \times 10^5 \, \text{N/m}^2 \, \text{abs} \quad \text{and} \quad p = 4 \times 10^5 \, \text{N/m}^2 \, \text{gauge}$$

Similarly, we should *not* indicate a height 5000 m above sea level as

$$z = 5000 \, \text{sea-m or m}_{sea}$$

and a height above another datum, say a plateau at 2000 m above sea level, as

$$z = 3000 \, \text{pla-m or m}_{pla}$$

In both cases we should measure in metres, m, and indicate the datum by writing z_{sea} or z_{pla}.

At this point the observant student will realise that the unit symbols for temperature are anomalous. In principle we should denote an absolute temperature, a temperature difference, and a temperature measured from the Celsius datum of $T = 273.15$ K, all by the unit symbol K. For historical reasons, however, the last is always denoted by °C. For example, an absolute temperature of 298.15 K is equivalent to a Celsius temperature of 25°C. Thus °C is not a pure unit symbol, but doubles up as a *datum indicator* as well. It would have been preferable had we adopted the usage of, say, attaching a subscript C to the symbol T to indicate a Celsius temperature and writing in this case $T_C = 25$ K. The traditional practice, however, has been to write either $T = 25\,°C$ or $t = 25\,°C$. In the worked examples where Celsius temperatures are referred to, we have used the first form for the fourth edition; this leaves t free to denote time. In all physical equations T must refer to absolute temperature, as should be self-evident from the derivation of the equations.

Two dilemmas arise out of the anomaly. First, which unit symbol should be used for the *difference* between the Celsius temperatures? We should, and we do, write

$$\Delta T = T_2 - T_1 = 56\,°C - 34\,°C = 22 \, \text{K}$$

The unit symbol °C should *not* be attached to the 22 because 22 is not a temperature relative to the Celsius datum.

The second dilemma concerns the cancellation of K and °C when multiplying and dividing quantities whose units involve those of temperature. As a simple example, imagine constructing a specific enthalpy table for air with h_0 taken as zero at $T_0 = 10\,°C$. At any other temperature, $h = c_p(T - T_0)$. Thus if $c_p = 1.005 \, \text{kJ/kg K}$ and $T = 50\,°C$,

$$h = 1.005 \frac{\text{kJ}}{\text{kg K}} \times (50\,°C - 10\,°C)$$

Can we cancel K with °C to arrive at the normal unit for h, namely kJ/kg? The answer is yes because, *in its function as a unit designator*, °C = K. In this case it is obvious from what we have said about temperature differences, because $(50\,°C - 10\,°C) = 40$ K.

A.4 Amount-of-substance and molar quantities

Since 1971 the mole unit has been defined in terms of a quantity called the 'amount of substance' (see section 8.5.2). The name was introduced because, when dealing with physical quantities, we normally have a name for the *concept* of the quantity which is separate from the name of the *unit*. Thus we distinguish the 'mass' and its unit the 'kilogram' (or some accepted multiple). Furthermore, the name of the concept should *not* imply a particular unit, as used to be the case when speaking of the 'number of moles (or kmol) of X' instead of the 'amount of substance of X'. Unfortunately it was not possible to agree on a succinct English name (as *Stoffmenge* in German, for example) and this has given rise to two linguistic difficulties.

First, there is the obvious confusion of the noun 'amount of substance' with the corresponding ordinary English phrase (cf. amount of money). Instead of relying on the context to indicate which is meant, we have chosen to hyphenate the name, viz. amount-of-substance. We hope this will become the accepted practice in due course.

Secondly, there is the difficulty of what to do when wishing to use the concept in adjectival form. When the concept has a simple name like 'mass' it is acceptable to use it adjectivally (strictly as an adjectival noun), as in 'mass velocity' or 'mass concentration'. Even in this case, however, it has been considered preferable to use a separate adjective 'specific' to mean 'per unit mass', as in specific volume, specific enthalpy etc. It would be impossibly clumsy to use a noun like amount-of-substance adjectivally, and it has reluctantly been accepted to use 'molar' as the adjective—molar volume, molar enthalpy and so on—meaning 'per unit amount-of-substance'. We say 'reluctantly' because the adjective might be thought to imply that the *unit* is the mole. There is no such implication and the unit could be any acceptable multiple of the mole. It so happens that molar quantities in this book are normally in units per kmol (m^3/kmol, kJ/kmol etc.).

A.5 Further reading

The following publications are particularly authoritative and useful:

For a detailed description of SI:
  The International System of Units (HMSO, 1986).

For an explanation of the relation between, and use of, physical quantities, units and numerical values:
  Quantities, Units and Symbols. A report by the Symbols Committee of the Royal Society (1975).
  ISO 31/0-1981 *General Principles Concerning Quantities, Units and Symbols* (International Standardization Organization, 1981). Also published as BS 5775: Part 0: 1982 *Specification for Quantities, Units and Symbols* (British Standards Institution, London, 1982).
  MAYHEW, Y. R. 'Conventions and nomenclature for physical quantities, units, numbers and mathematics', in *Heat Exchanger Design Handbook* (Hemisphere, 1989).

For conversion factors between various systems of units:
  BS 350: Part 1: 1974 *Conversion Factors and Tables* (British Standards Institution, London, 1974).

Fig. A.1
Relations between metric and British systems of units

Physical quantity	Metric units: SI	Metric units: m-kgf-kg-s	Metric units: m-kgf-s	British units: ft-lb-s	British units: ft-lbf-lb-s	British units: ft-lbf-s
Length[1]	**m**	**m**		**ft**	**ft**	
Mass	**kg**	**kg**	kg × 9.806 65 [eq. A.14]	**lb**	**lb**	slug = lb × 32.1740 [eq. A.14B]
Time	**s**	**s**		**s**	**s**	
Temperature (see section A.3)	**K**	**K**		**R**	**R**	
Specific volume	$\frac{m^3}{kg}$	$\frac{m^3}{kg}$	$\frac{m^3}{(kg \times 9.806\,65)}$	$\frac{ft^3}{lb}$	$\frac{ft^3}{lb}$	$\frac{ft^3}{(lb \times 32.1740)}$
Force	N [eq. A.6]	**kgf**		pdl [eq. A.6B]	**lbf**	
Pressure[2]	Pa(= 1 N/m^2) *or* bar (= 10^5 N/m^2)	kgf/cm^2		pdl/ft^2	lbf/ft^2	
Energy[3]	J(= 1 N m) *or* kJ(= 10^3 J)	*mechanical*: kgf m; *thermal*: kcal (≈ 427 kgf m)		ft pdl	*mechanical*: ft lbf; *thermal*: Btu(≈ 778 ft lbf)	
Rate of energy flow	W(= 1 J/s) *or* kW(= 10^3 J/s)	*mechanical*: kgf m/s *or* metric hp(= 75 kgf m/s); *heat*: kcal/s		ft pdl/s	*mechanical*: ft lbf/s *or* British hp(= 550 ft lbf/s); *heat*: Btu/s	

1 The base units of each system are in bold type.
2 This book sometimes uses the *standard atmosphere* (atm) defined by

$$1 \text{ atm} = 1.013\,25 \text{ bar} = 101\,325 \text{ N/m}^2$$

The kgf/cm^2 is also called the *technical atmosphere* and it is usually denoted by 'at'. It is worth noting that

$$1 \text{ atm} \approx 760 \text{ mm Hg} \qquad 1 \text{ bar} \approx 750 \text{ mm Hg} \qquad 1 \text{ at} \approx 736 \text{ mm Hg}$$

3 For definitions of the calorimetric units kcal and Btu see section 1.3 and the footnote in section 2.3.

Appendix B

Problems

The following problems are numbered by chapter. Answers have been obtained using the abridged tables of properties of Ref. 17 in Part II. For air, unless otherwise stated, the approximate composition and specific heat capacity data given on p. 26 of those tables have been used. More generally, when the variation of c_p with temperature is significant, mean values are always used based on the value at the mean temperature.

As a solutions manual is now available, students should heed the health warning at the end of the Prologue to this book.

7.1 Derive the Maxwell relation

$$\left(\frac{\partial T}{\partial v}\right)_s = -\left(\frac{\partial p}{\partial s}\right)_v$$

Using this and the relation

$$\left(\frac{\partial x}{\partial y}\right)_z \left(\frac{\partial y}{\partial z}\right)_x \left(\frac{\partial z}{\partial x}\right)_y = -1$$

derive the three remaining Maxwell relations.

7.2 Show that

$$\left(\frac{\partial \beta}{\partial p}\right)_T = -\left(\frac{\partial \kappa}{\partial T}\right)_p$$

The compressibility of a substance varies linearly with temperature at constant pressure, according to the law $\kappa = A + BT$. Show that the change in the coefficient of expansion during an isothermal process is given by

$$\beta_2 - \beta_1 = -B(p_2 - p_1)$$

7.3 c_p for a particular substance is found to be independent of pressure and to vary with temperature according to the equation $c_p = a + bT + cT^2$, where a, b and c are constants. Derive an expression for the true mean c_p for the range T_1 to T_2. Show that the difference between this mean value and the arithmetic mean of c_p at T_1 and T_2 is equal to $-c(T_2 - T_1)^2/6$.

7.4 The Clausius equation of state is $p(v - b) = RT$. For a substance obeying this equation, find expressions for β and κ in terms of p and v. Also, given the relation $c_p = T(\partial s/\partial T)_p$, show that c_p can be a function only of T.

7.5 The Dieterici equation of state is $p(v - b)e^{a/vRT} = RT$, where a, b and R are constants. Find an expression for the coefficient of cubical expansion, and show that this approximates to the value of β for a perfect gas when T and v are large.

7.6 Show that the difference between the specific heat capacities of a van der Waals gas is given by

$$c_p - c_v = R\frac{1}{1 - 2a(v - b)^2/RTv^3}$$

The general expression $c_p - c_v = \beta^2 Tv/\kappa$ need not be derived.

7.7 Show that the slope on the $h-s$ diagram is equal to

(a) T along a constant pressure line
(b) $T - (1/\beta)$ along an isothermal
(c) $T + \{(c_p - c_v)/c_v\beta\}$ along a constant volume line.

The general relations $c_p - c_v = \beta^2 Tv/\kappa$ and $c_v = T(\partial s/\partial T)_v$ need not be derived.

7.8 Starting with the functions $g = h - Ts$ and $h = u + pv$, show that

$$\left(\frac{\partial s}{\partial p}\right)_T = -\left(\frac{\partial v}{\partial T}\right)_p \quad \text{and} \quad c_p = T\left(\frac{\partial s}{\partial T}\right)_p$$

Hence show that

$$ds = \frac{c_p\,dT}{T} - \left(\frac{\partial v}{\partial T}\right)_p dp$$

Derive expressions for the change of entropy during an isothermal compression from p_1 to p_2 at temperature T, (a) for a perfect gas, and (b) for a gas obeying the law

$$pv = RT + \left(b - \frac{a}{RT^2}\right)p$$

7.9 Given that

$$ds = \frac{c_p\,dT}{T} - \left(\frac{\partial v}{\partial T}\right)_p dp = \frac{c_v\,dT}{T} + \left(\frac{\partial p}{\partial T}\right)_v dv$$

show that

$$c_p - c_v = T\left(\frac{\partial v}{\partial T}\right)_p\left(\frac{\partial p}{\partial T}\right)_v$$

Hence show that for a perfect gas the difference between c_p and c_v is R, and that for a gas having the characteristic equation

$$pv = RT + \left(b - \frac{a}{RT^2}\right)p$$

the difference is approximately $R + (4ap/RT^3)$.

7.10 Derive the following thermodynamic relations:

$$c_p = T\left(\frac{\partial s}{\partial T}\right)_p \quad \text{and} \quad c_v = T\left(\frac{\partial s}{\partial T}\right)_v$$

Show that on a p–v diagram the ratio of the slope of the isentropic through a point to the slope of an isothermal through the same point is equal to the ratio c_p/c_v.

7.11 Deduce the thermodynamic relations

(i) $\left(\dfrac{\partial h}{\partial p}\right)_T = v - T\left(\dfrac{\partial v}{\partial T}\right)_p = -c_p\left(\dfrac{\partial T}{\partial p}\right)_h$

(ii) $\left(\dfrac{\partial u}{\partial v}\right)_T = T\left(\dfrac{\partial p}{\partial T}\right)_v - p$

Any Maxwell relation used need not be derived. With the aid of equation (ii), show that

$$\left(\frac{\partial u}{\partial p}\right)_T = -T\left(\frac{\partial v}{\partial T}\right)_p - p\left(\frac{\partial v}{\partial p}\right)_T$$

The quantity $c_p(\partial T/\partial p)_h$ is known as the Joule-Thomson cooling effect. Show that this cooling effect is equal to $(3C/T^2) - b$ for a gas having the equation of state

$$(v - b) = \frac{RT}{p} - \frac{C}{T^2}$$

Finally, show that in general the cooling effect can be accounted for by a combination of a departure from Joule's law $[(\partial u/\partial p)_T = 0]$ and a departure from Boyle's law $[(\partial pv/\partial p)_T = 0]$, and check this by determining these two partial differential coefficients for the foregoing gas. Hence explain why, under certain conditions, a throttling process can be accompanied by a rise of temperature.

7.12 Show that the Joule coefficient $(\partial T/\partial v)_u$ and the Joule-Thomson coefficient $(\partial T/\partial p)_h$ are given respectively by

$$\left(\frac{\partial T}{\partial v}\right)_u = \frac{1}{c_v}\left\{p - T\left(\frac{\partial p}{\partial T}\right)_v\right\} \quad \text{and} \quad \left(\frac{\partial T}{\partial p}\right)_h = -\frac{1}{c_p}\left\{v - T\left(\frac{\partial v}{\partial T}\right)_p\right\}$$

Any Maxwell relations used need not be derived. What would happen in an adiabatic steady-flow throttling process with negligible change of kinetic energy if (i) $v/T < (\partial v/\partial T)_p$, and (ii) $v/T > (\partial v/\partial T)_p$? What is the practical significance of a changeover from (i) to (ii) for a real gas?

Show that for a gas which obeys the equation of state $pv = RT$, both coefficients are zero. The equation of state of a real gas can be put in a form

$$pv = RT + Bp + Cp^2 + Dp^3 + \dots$$

where $B, C, D, \dots$ are functions of temperature only. The table gives values of B for nitrogen and, provided that the pressure is not too high, the series can be terminated at Bp. Plot B against T and hence deduce the temperature at which (a) the behaviour of nitrogen approximates the equation of state of a perfect gas, and (b) the temperature at which the changeover $v/T \lessgtr (\partial v/\partial T)_p$ occurs.

$T/[\text{K}]$	200	300	400	500	600	700	800	900
$B/10^{-3}[\text{m}^3/\text{kg}]$	-1.242	-0.162	$+0.325$	$+0.599$	$+0.762$	$+0.880$	$+0.955$	$+1.011$

Finally show that, at least over the temperature range considered, the Joule coefficient for nitrogen at moderate pressure must always be negative. Give a physical reason why this conclusion about the sign of the Joule coefficient should apply to all gases under any conditions.

[(a) 325 K (b) 620 K]

7.13 Given that

$$c_v = T\left(\frac{\partial s}{\partial T}\right)_v \quad \text{and} \quad c_p = T\left(\frac{\partial s}{\partial T}\right)_p$$

and writing $s = s(T, v)$, make use of any Maxwell relation to show that

$$c_p - c_v = T\left(\frac{\partial p}{\partial T}\right)_v\left(\frac{\partial v}{\partial T}\right)_p$$

Within a certain range of p and T, superheated steam behaves such that c_p and pv/T ($= R'$ say) are functions only of entropy. Show, by obtaining an expression for c_v in terms of c_p, R' and s, that c_v must also be a function only of entropy.

Making use of the given equation for c_p, show that $c_p = T(\partial v/\partial T)_p(\partial p/\partial T)_s$. Thence show that for the steam referred to above, an isentropic process is a true polytropic, i.e. that $p/T^n = $ constant, and that

$$n = \frac{c_p}{R' + c_p(dR'/ds)}$$

Finally, if the characteristic equation of the steam is found to be $pv = RT - Ap/T^3$ (where R and A are constants), and c_p at zero pressure is found to vary linearly with T, determine an expression for c_p as a function of p and T.

[$c_p = 12Ap/T^4 + B + CT$]

7.14 Show that

$$\left(\frac{\partial c_p}{\partial p}\right)_T = -T\left(\frac{\partial^2 v}{\partial T^2}\right)_p \quad \text{and} \quad ds = c_p\frac{dT}{dp} - \left(\frac{\partial v}{\partial T}\right)_p dp$$

There is no need to derive any Maxwell relation used. Hence, find expressions for c_p, s, h and u, for a gas having the characteristic equation

$$v = \frac{RT}{p} + a - \frac{b}{T^3}$$

where R, a, b are constants. c_p at zero pressure has a constant value of c_{p0}, and s and h are arbitrarily chosen to be zero at the state defined by p_1 and T_1.

7.15 The specific volume of liquid water is $0.001\,000\,2$ m^3/kg and that of ice is $0.001\,091$ m^3/kg, at $0.01\,°C$. The latent heat of fusion of ice at this temperature is 333.5 kJ/kg. Making use of the Clausius-Clapeyron equation, calculate the rate of change of melting point of ice with pressure in K/bar.

[$-0.007\,44$ K/bar]

7.16 An empirical relation between saturation vapour pressure and saturation temperature for mercury is

$$\log_{10}\frac{p}{\text{[bar]}} = 7.0323 - \frac{3276.6}{T/\text{[K]}} - 0.6520\log_{10}\frac{T}{\text{[K]}}$$

Using the Clausius-Clapeyron equation, calculate the specific volume v_g of saturated mercury vapour at 0.1 bar. The specific volume of saturated mercury liquid v_f may be neglected, and the latent enthalpy of vaporisation at 0.1 bar is 294.54 kJ/kg.

[2.140 m³/kg]

9.1 1 kg of air can be expanded between two states as it does 20 kJ of work on the surroundings and receives 16 kJ of heat. A second kind of expansion can be found between the same initial and final states which requires a heat input of only 9 kJ. What is the change of internal energy in the first expansion, and what is the work done by the air in the second expansion?

[−4 kJ, −13 kJ]

9.2 A closed system receives 168.7 kJ of heat at constant volume. It then rejects 177 kJ of heat while it has 40 kJ of work done on it at constant pressure. If an adiabatic process can be found which will restore it to its initial state, how much work will be done by the system during that process? If the value of the internal energy in the initial state is arbitrarily put equal to zero, find the internal energies at the other two states.

[−31.7 kJ; 168.7 kJ, 31.7 kJ]

9.3 1800 kJ of heat is transferred to 1 m³ of air at 14 bar and 200 °C. Find (a) the final temperature and pressure if the volume remains constant, and (b) the final temperature and volume if the pressure remains constant. After which process has the internal energy of the air the greater value?

When the air is then expanded isothermally to a pressure of 7 bar, what is the final volume in each case? ·

[(a) 445 °C, 21.3 bar, 3.04 m³ (b) 375 °C, 1.37 m³, 2.74 m³]

9.4 0.75 kg of air has a pressure of 3 bar and a temperature of 125 °C. After it has received 900 kJ of heat at constant volume, find the final temperature and pressure. If the air then expands adiabatically doing 915 kJ of work, (a) by how much is its internal energy changed during the expansions, and (b) is the value lower or higher than before the heating process?

[1796 °C, 15.6 bar; (a) −915 kJ, (b) lower]

9.5 1 kg of gas expands reversibly and adiabatically, its temperature falling·from 240 °C to 115 °C while its volume is doubled. The gas does 90 kJ of work in the process. Find the values of c_v and c_p, and the molar mass of the gas.

[0.72 kJ/kg K, 1.01 kJ/kg K; 28.7 kg/kmol]

9.6 State the characteristics of (i) an isothermal and (ii) an adiabatic expansion.

A bicycle pump which has a stroke of 20 cm is used to force air into a tyre against a pressure of 4 bar. What length of stroke will be swept through before air begins to enter the tyre when the piston is pushed in (a) slowly and (b) quickly? Assume that the atmospheric pressure is 1 bar.

[(a) 15 cm (b) 12.57 cm]

9.7 A certain mass of gas expanding reversibly at constant pressure does 5 kJ of work. Calculate the quantity of heat which must be transmitted to the gas, and how much of this heat is used to raise the internal energy of the gas. Assume only that the gas is perfect and that $\gamma = 1.66$.

[12.58 kJ, 7.58 kJ]

9.8 A cylinder of 8 cm internal diameter is fitted with a piston loaded by a coil spring of stiffness 140 N/cm of compression. The cylinder contains 0.0005 m³ of air at 15 °C and

3 bar. Find the amount of heat which must be supplied for the piston to move a distance
of 4 cm.

[0.417 kJ]

9.9 Starting from the non-flow energy equation, show that the specific heat capacity c_n of
a perfect gas may be expressed by

$$c_n = \left(\frac{\gamma - n}{1 - n}\right)c_v$$

where $c_n = dQ/dT$ in a reversible polytropic process.

9.10 During the reversible expansion of 0.23 kg of air in a cylinder, it was found that the rate
of heat supply per unit *fall* of temperature was constant and equal to 0.114 kJ/K. Show
that the law of expansion must have been of the form $Tv^x = $ constant, where x is a
constant, and find the index of polytropic expansion. Also, find the work done if the
drop in temperature is 50 K.

[1.236, −13.97 kJ]

9.11 0.3 m^3 of air at 26 °C and 1 bar is compressed reversibly and polytropically to 0.07 m^3.
Find the final pressure and temperature, the work done, the changes in internal energy
and enthalpy, and the heat transferred, when the index of compression has the values
0.9, 1.0, 1.4, 1.5. This should be treated as an exercise in methodical computation.

[For $n = 1.5$: 8.87 bar, 346 °C, 64.0 kJ, 80.3 kJ, 112.3 kJ, 16.3 kJ]

9.12 A quantity of air occupying a volume of 1 m^3 at 4 bar and 150 °C is allowed to expand
isentropically to 1 bar. Its enthalpy is then raised by 70 kJ by heating at constant pressure.
What is the total work done during this process?

If the process is to be replaced by a reversible polytropic expansion which will result
in the same final state being reached, what index of expansion is required? Will the
work done be greater or less in magnitude than in the original process?

[−346 kJ; 1.305, greater]

9.13 A certain mass of carbon dioxide is contained in a vessel of 0.5 m^3 capacity, at an
atmospheric temperature of 15 °C and a pressure of 20 bar. A valve is opened momentarily
and the pressure immediately falls to 10 bar. Some time later the temperature of the
remaining gas is again atmospheric and the pressure is found to be 11.78 bar. By making
suitable assumptions, estimate the value of γ for the gas.

Find also the change in internal energy undergone by the mass of gas remaining in
the vessel (a) during the first part of the process, and (b) during the whole process.

[1.303; (a) −290 kJ (b) 0]

9.14 Imagine two curves intersecting at some point on a p–v diagram. The curves are to
represent reversible processes undergone by a perfect gas; one is an adiabatic process
and the other an isothermal process. Show that the ratio of the slope of the adiabatic
curve to the slope of the isothermal curve, at the point of intersection, is equal to γ.

A gas having a value of γ equal to 1.66 is expanded reversibly from the same initial
state (a) isothermally and (b) adiabatically, such that the pressure ratio is 5 in each
case. Calculate the ratio of the work done during (a) to the work done during (b).

[2.25]

9.15 6 kg of air expands reversibly from a pressure of 13 bar to 1.3 bar, the index of expansion being 1.2. Find from first principles the change in entropy of the air, and sketch the process on the $T-s$ diagram.

[1.652 kJ/K]

9.16 The initial state of a perfect gas is defined by T_1 and v_1, and the final state by T_3 and v_3. Find the change of entropy per unit mass along any three different reversible paths connecting these states (each consisting of two consecutive processes), and show that the same result is obtained in each case.

9.17 Explain briefly why reversibility is used as a criterion of an ideal process, illustrating your answer by referring to the irreversibility of heat transfer across a finite temperature difference.

1 kg of air undergoes a Joule free expansion from a volume of $1 m^3$ to a volume of $8 m^3$. What is the change in entropy (a) of the air and (b) of the surroundings? Had the process been a reversible isothermal expansion between the same two states, what would these changes of entropy have been? Hence compare the net change of entropy of the 'universe' in the two cases, and comment on the result.

[(a) 0.597 kJ/K (b) 0 in first part; (a) 0.597 kJ/K (b) −0.597 kJ/K in second]

9.18 Show from first principles that, for a perfect gas with constant specific heat capacities expanding polytropically (i.e. according to the law pv^n = constant) in a non-flow process, the change of entropy can be expressed by

$$s_2 - s_1 = \frac{n - \gamma}{\gamma - 1} \frac{R}{n} \ln \frac{p_2}{p_1}$$

Gaseous methane is compressed polytropically by a piston from 25 °C and 0.80 bar to a pressure of 5.0 bar. Assuming an index of compression of 1.2, calculate the change of entropy and work done, per unit mass of gas. The relative molecular mass of methane is 16 and $\gamma = 1.30$. Explain which of the answers depends upon an assumption that the process is (a) reversible and (b) non-flow.

[−0.265 kJ/kg K, 276 kJ/kg]

9.19 A quantity of carbon dioxide ($\tilde{m} = 44 kg/kmol$) having a mass of 0.5 kg expands reversibly and polytropically in a cylinder while the temperature falls from 500 °C to 100 °C. The index of expansion is 1.20, and c_v for carbon dioxide over the temperature range can be taken as 0.871 kJ/kg K. For the carbon dioxide, calculate the heat transferred and the change of entropy. What must have been the change of entropy of the surroundings?

If the previously described frictionless process were still the same, but the heat had been transferred to the boundary of the cylinder from a reservoir at a constant temperature at 530 °C, what would then have been the changes in entropy of the carbon dioxide in the cylinder and of the surroundings? Explain the significance of the results by referring to the principle of increasing entropy.

[14.8 kJ, 0.02696 kJ/K, −0.02696 kJ/kg; 0.02696 kJ/K, −0.01843 kJ/kg]

9.20 A thermally insulated vessel is divided into two parts by a conducting wall. One part of the vessel contains 3 kg of a gas having a molar mass $\tilde{m} = 40 kg/kmol$ and a ratio of specific heat capacities $\gamma = 5/3$, the initial temperature being 20 °C. The other part contains 2 kg of the same gas, initially at −10 °C. Calculate the change of entropy of the total contents of the vessel during the process in which heat transfer across the dividing wall causes a state of thermal equilibrium to be reached.

[0.02166 kJ/K]

9.21 The partial evaporation of 1 kg of saturated water at 7 bar is accompanied by the transfer of 100 kJ of work. Find the dryness fraction of the steam formed, and the increase in internal energy of the fluid during the change of phase.

[0.526, 987 kJ]

9.22 A mass of 1.5 kg of water at 30 bar and 200 °C is expanded reversibly and isothermally behind a piston to form steam at a lower pressure. The heat transferred during the process is 3750 kJ. Determine the final pressure and the work done during the expansion, and sketch the process on a T–s diagram. Assume that the properties of compressed water are independent of pressure.

Explain briefly why the concept of entropy had to be used in the solution, whereas this would not have been so had the substance been a perfect gas.

[1.6 bar, −1042 kJ]

9.23 A vertical insulated cylinder of 0.1 m² cross-sectional area contains 0.92 kg of water at 15 °C, and a piston resting on the water exerts a constant pressure of 7 bar. An electric heater forms the bottom of the cylinder and communicates heat to the water at the rate of 0.5 kW. Calculate the time taken by the piston to rise through a distance of 1.3 m.

[52.5 min]

9.24 A mass of 0.12 kg of steam initially saturated at 10 bar expands reversibly in a cylinder until the pressure is 1 bar. The volume is then found to be 0.17 m³. Assuming that the process is polytropic, find the index of expansion and the heat transferred during the process. Find also the change of entropy and sketch the process on the T–s diagram.

[1.16, −10.4 kJ, −0.0264 kJ/K]

9.25 Steam at 16 bar, dryness fraction 0.95, expands reversibly in a cylinder until the pressure is 3 bar. Calculate the final specific volume and the final temperature of the steam, given that the expansion follows the law pv = constant.

Using the same initial data as before for the steam, calculate the heat that would have been supplied per unit mass had the expansion been isothermal.

If the working substance were helium (of molar mass $\tilde{m}$ = 4 kg/kmol) at the same initial temperature as the steam, and expanding between the same pressures, calculate the final specific volume and temperature (a) when the expansion is of the form pv = constant and (b) when the expansion is isothermal.

[0.6267 m³/kg, 145.7 °C; 522 kJ; 3.29 m³/kg, 201.4 °C]

9.26 A mass of 1 kg of steam, at a pressure and temperature of 15 bar and 500 °C, expands reversibly and polytropically to a final state of 4 bar and 200 °C by displacing a piston in a cylinder. Calculate the polytropic index, the work done and the heat transferred.

In an unresisted adiabatic expansion, 1 kg of steam expands from the same initial state to the same final volume as in the previous expansion. Show by interpolation between appropriate pressures, or in any other way, that the final pressure will be about 6.6 bar. Also calculate the quantity of heat that must then be transferred at constant volume for the pressure to drop to 4 bar.

[1.6093, −228 kJ/kg, −244 kJ/kg; −472 kJ/kg]

9.27 A vessel having a capacity of 0.6 m³ contains steam at 15 bar and 250 °C. Steam is blown off until the pressure drops to 4 bar, after which the valve is closed and the vessel is cooled until the pressure is 3 bar. Assuming that the expansion of the gas remaining in the vessel is isentropic during blow-off, calculate (a) the mass of steam blown off, (b) the dryness of the steam in the vessel after cooling, and (c) the heat transferred during the cooling process.

[2.601 kg, 0.736, −625 kJ]

9.28 2 kg of steam is initially at a pressure of 3 bar. The initial dryness fraction is such that when the steam has been heated at constant volume to 4 bar it is saturated. After this heating process the steam is compressed isentropically to 10 bar. Find the final temperature, and the heat and work transfers. Sketch the process on the $T-s$ and $p-v$ diagrams.

[243.7 °C, 960 kJ, 292 kJ]

9.29 Steam is expanded isentropically from a pressure $p_1 = 8$ bar to $p_2 = 0.8$ bar. Assuming that the expansion can be described approximately by a polytropic law $pv^n = $ constant, find the average values of n for the expansion over this pressure range when the initial values of dryness fraction x_1 are 1.0, 0.9, 0.8 and 0.7. Hence plot n against x_1 and deduce an equation for n of the form $n = a + bx_1$, where a and b are constants.

[$1.035 + 0.1x_1$]

9.30 Superheated steam at a temperature of 275.6 °C and a pressure of 4 bar is compressed reversibly and isothermally in a non-flow process until it attains a saturated liquid state. Calculate the work done per unit mass of steam in both of the following ways: (i) from the equation $W_{12} = \Delta u_{12} - Q_{12}$, using property values in the initial and final states; (ii) from the equation $W_{12} = -\int_1^2 p \, dv$, assuming that the compression in the superheat region follows a polytropic path.

Explain any discrepancy in the answers obtained.

[881 kJ/kg, 841 kJ/kg]

10.1 Air enters a centrifugal compressor at 1.05 bar and 15 °C, and leaves at 2 bar and 97 °C. The mass flow is 50 kg/min. What power is actually required to drive the compressor, and what would be the power required for the same pressure ratio if the compression had been frictionless? What is the rate of increase of enthalpy due to friction?

[68.7 kW, 48.6 kW, 20.1 kW]

10.2 An air flow of 8 kg/min enters a nozzle with a negligible velocity and expands from a pressure of 4 bar to 2.2 bar. The temperature falls from 900 °C to 750 °C in the process. Find the velocity of the air as it leaves the nozzle, the velocity which would have been reached had the expansions been frictionless, and the nozzle efficiency.

Indicate briefly, with the aid of a sketch of the $T-s$ diagram, two ways in which the rate of change of entropy during the real expansion may be calculated, and find the change of entropy per minute by one of these methods.

[549 m/s, 608 m/s, 0.815; 0.268 kJ/K min]

10.3 Air is flowing through a well-lagged duct. At some section A the pressure and temperature are 1.5 bar and 187 °C, and at some distance along the duct at section B the pressure and temperature are 1.3 bar and 160 °C. In which direction is the air flowing?

[from B to A]

10.4 Air, at the rate of 18 kg/s, enters a turbine at 800 °C with a velocity of 100 m/s. The air expands adiabatically, but not isentropically, as it passes through the turbine, and leaves with a velocity of 150 m/s. It then passes through a diffuser wherein the velocity is reduced to a negligible value and the pressure is increased to 1.01 bar. The air is exhausted to atmosphere at this pressure. If the process in the diffuser can be assumed to be isentropic, and the turbine produces 3600 kW, find the pressure of the air between the turbine and the diffuser.

Say, by referring to a sketch of the process on the $T-s$ diagram, why you think a diffuser is added to the turbine.

[0.966 bar]

10.5 A centrifugal compressor delivers 9 kg of air per second at a pressure ratio of 4. The inlet pressure and temperature of the air are 1.01 bar and 15 °C, and the outlet temperature is 177 °C. If the velocity of the air at inlet to the compressor is 120 m/s and at outlet is 60 m/s, find the power absorbed by the compressor.

The compressed air is heated at constant pressure and allowed to expand in a nozzle to 1.01 bar. Neglecting any change in velocity between compressor outlet and nozzle inlet, find the rate of heat transfer necessary for a velocity of 760 m/s to be produced at the nozzle exit. Assume that the expansion in the nozzle is isentropic.

[1417 kW, 3826 kW]

10.6 Air at 0.83 bar and 5 °C enters the intake (i.e. diffuser) of a jet engine with a velocity of 270 m/s. The air decelerates reversibly in the intake to a negligible velocity before entering the compressor. Calculate the pressure of the air at inlet to the compressor (a) if the process can be assumed adiabatic and (b) if heat is transferred at such a rate that the temperature remains at 5 °C throughout the process.

[(a) 1.27 bar (b) 1.31 bar]

10.7 Say briefly why 'enthalpy' is a useful concept when dealing with open systems.

Air at atmospheric pressure and 15 °C enters a duct with a velocity of 270 m/s. The duct at first diverges so that the velocity of the air is reduced to a negligible value, and the pressure and temperature are consequently increased. The air then passes into a length of duct where heat is supplied at constant pressure, raising the temperature still further to 1000 °C. At this temperature, and still with negligible velocity, the air enters a nozzle wherein it expands to atmospheric pressure. Assuming that the processes in the diffuser and nozzle are isentropic, find the heat supplied per unit mass flow, and the velocity of the air leaving the nozzle.

[953 kJ/kg, 534 m/s]

10.8 A diffuser reduces the velocity of an air stream from 300 m/s to 30 m/s. If the inlet pressure and temperature are 1.01 bar and 315 °C and the diffuser efficiency is 90 per cent, determine the outlet pressure. Find also the outlet area required for the diffuser to pass a mass flow of 9 kg/s.

[1.271 bar, 0.428 m^2]

10.9 A large foundry hall has to be supplied with a total of 10 kg/s of fresh air through eight square grilles placed around its perimeter, the pressure and temperature in the exit plane of each grille being 1.02 bar and 4 °C. Air outside the foundry, at 1.01 bar and 16 °C, is drawn into a common inlet duct 0.800 m × 0.800 m square. After entering the duct the air passes through a fan which requires 7 kW, and then flows through a bank of refrigerated tubes. The duct then divides into eight branches, leading to the exit grilles at the perimeter of the hall. The fan raises the pressure of the air sufficiently to overcome pressure losses over the cooling tubes and in the ducting, and to provide the velocity head at the exits from the grilles.

Calculate the heat that has to be transferred to the cooling tubes. You may assume that acoustic cladding around the ducting also insulates it thermally, and that the change of kinetic energy across the system is negligible for the purpose of the energy equation.

Calculate the velocity of the air in the square inlet duct, and the dimensions of each outlet duct if the outlet velocity is not to exceed 14 m/s. State clearly any assumptions you wish to make, and show that the neglect of the kinetic energy term in the energy equation was justified.

[− 127.6 kW; 12.83 m/s, 0.26 m]

10.10 Oxygen ($\dot{m} = 32$ kg/kmol, $c_p = 0.927$ kJ/kg K) enters a pipe of 8 mm diameter at a rate of 0.0173 kg/s, and at a pressure of 2 bar and a temperature of 85 °C. It flows adiabatically, but not reversibly, to a point in the pipe where its pressure has dropped to 1.3 bar and its temperature is 69 °C. Over the following section of the pipe, heat is removed without significant change of pressure such that the original entropy is restored. Calculate the rate at which heat is transferred through the pipe wall in this part of the process and sketch a T–s diagram showing the whole process.

Check, using the steady-flow energy equation, that the information about the first section is self-consistent.

[− 0.465 kW]

10.11 The dryness fraction of steam is to be determined by passing a sample first through a separating calorimeter, which merely separates some of the liquid physically from the vapour, and then through a throttling calorimeter. The following results have been noted:

Steam main pressure	10 bar
Pressure after throttle	1 bar
Temperature after throttle	128 °C
Mass collected in separator	0.86 kg
Mass collected after throttling	11.6 kg

Find the dryness fraction of the sample.

What is the minimum dryness fraction of steam at 10 bar that could be measured when using the throttling calorimeter alone with an outlet pressure of 1 bar?

[0.91, 0.95]

10.12 Steam enters a turbine with a negligible velocity at 40 bar and 410 °C. It leaves the turbine with a high velocity through a pipe of 0.16 m² cross-sectional area where the pressure is 0.14 bar and the dryness fraction is 0.93. The turbine output is 2000 kW. Deduce an equation for the outlet velocity and verify that it is approximately 156 m/s. Finally, show that the expansion in the turbine is irreversible.

10.13 A turbine is normally supplied with steam at 40 bar and 300 °C, but to accommodate a reduction in load the steam has been throttled to 7 bar before it enters the turbine. Determine the percentage reduction in power output, assuming that the turbine exhaust pressure remains unchanged at 0.34 bar and that the turbine isentropic efficiency and mass flow remain unchanged.

Why would you expect the mass flow, in practice, to fall as a result of throttling?

[32.4 per cent]

10.14 At some point in a geothermal borehole, the hot water is sufficiently depressurised to begin to turn into steam: the fluid is then saturated water at a pressure of 44 bar. From this point to the wellhead the expansion in the borehole can be considered isentropic, and at the wellhead the pressure is 15 bar. Determine the dryness fraction at the wellhead.

Two possible ways of using this steam are to be compared:

(a)   The water is separated from the mixture at the wellhead pressure, and dry saturated steam is expanded isentropically in a turbine to a condenser pressure of 0.12 bar.

(b) The wet steam at the wellhead is throttled to a pressure of 10 bar before the separation process is carried out, and the dry steam component is then expanded in the turbine as before.

Sketch the processes on a T–s diagram, and calculate the work done per kg of wet borehole steam for each of the two schemes. Comment on the result.

[0.1293; (a) −94.5 kJ/kg (b) −111.13 kJ/kg]

10.15 Dry saturated steam at 34 bar is supplied to a turbine and expands isentropically through it to 3 bar. One-third of the steam at entry is branched off, throttled adiabatically to 3 bar, and then allowed to mix with the turbine exhaust steam in a mixing chamber. Determine the final state of the steam leaving the chamber, neglecting changes of kinetic energy.

Calculate the relative values of the cross-sectional areas of the pipes leading into and out of the mixing chamber, such that changes in velocity across the chamber are to be zero.

Calculate the amount of heat transferred per unit mass of mixture to condense it at constant pressure and cool it to a temperature of 30 °C.

[h = 2518 kJ/kg, x = 0.9043; 1/0.6185/0.4058; −2392 kJ/kg]

10.16 What assumptions are usually made when calculating the overall changes in properties that occur across a throttle valve?

Steam at 20 bar flows through a throttle valve into a water-cooled tube. The pressure and temperature at a point between the valve and the cooled section are 1.5 bar and 150 °C. Calculate the dryness fraction of the steam at inlet to the valve. Estimate also the quantity of heat that must be transferred in the cooled tube, per kg of steam, for the final dryness fraction to be the same as before throttling. Assume that the pressure drop in the water-cooled section is 0.5 bar and that the change in velocity is negligible.

If the tube is of constant diameter, and the velocity of the steam is 100 m/s at entry to the cooled section, what effect would the change in velocity have on the rate of heat transfer, expressed as a percentage of the previous estimate?

[0.9862, 129 kJ/kg; 2.7 per cent]

10.17 Wet steam at a pressure of 40 bar flows through a steam main. A sample is drawn off at the rate of 17.4 kg/h and is passed over an electric heating element placed in the draw-off pipe. Electric energy is dissipated at a rate of 1.16 kW and the pressure of the sample drops to 38 bar. The sample is then throttled to 1 bar and is found to be at a temperature of 140 °C. Calculate the dryness fraction of the steam in the main, and also the value just before throttling. Illustrate your solution by appropriate diagrams, and explain clearly any assumptions made in the solution.

The electric supply is disconnected. Determine the dryness fraction before throttling, and the thermodynamic state of the sample after throttling.

[0.8343, 0.9740; 0.8352, 0.9300]

10.18 A lagged vessel of 1.4 m³ capacity is full of steam at a pressure of 14 bar and 0.85 dryness fraction. Water at 15 °C is injected under a constant head of 150 m. How much water will it be necessary to inject to reduce the pressure in the vessel to 7 bar, and what will be the final dryness fraction?

[14.9 kg, 0.196]

10.19 A compressed air bottle, containing air at 34 bar and 15 °C, is to be used to drive a small turbine as an emergency starter for an engine. The turbine is required to produce an average output of 4 kW for a period of 30 seconds. Assuming that the expansion is isentropic, that the pressure in the bottle is allowed to fall to 3.4 bar during the process, and that the turbine exhausts to atmosphere at 1.01 bar, determine the necessary capacity of the bottle.

[0.029 m³]

11.1 A steam turbine plane operates on the Rankine cycle with a boiler pressure of 50 bar and a condenser pressure of 0.14 bar. The steam leaves the boiler at 400 °C. Draw up a complete energy balance for the ideal plant, including the feed pump term, and find the cycle efficiency, work ratio and specific steam consumption. Sketch the cycle on the T–s diagram. Show how the cycle would appear if the processes in the turbine and feed pump were not reversible, and hence explain why the cycle efficiency would be lower in practice.

[0.352, 0.995, 3.44 kg/kW h]

11.2 Neglecting the feed pump term, compare the Rankine cycle efficiency of a high-pressure steam plant operating at 80 bar with that of a low-pressure plant at 40 bar. In both cases the maximum temperature is 400 °C and the condenser pressure is 0.07 bar. Explain your results briefly.

Also find the ratio of the capacities of the condensing plant (i.e. ratios of heat rejection), assuming that the turbines are to produce the same power.

[0.391, 0.364; 0.893 (HP/LP)]

11.3 A steam turbine plant is throttle governed and operates with a boiler pressure and temperature of 40 bar and 350 °C, and a condenser pressure of 0.2 bar. The isentropic efficiency of the turbine may be assumed constant at 0.80 for all operating conditions. Plot curves showing the variation of cycle efficiency and specific steam consumption with turbine inlet pressure, as the steam is throttled from 40 bar to 10 bar. The h–s chart should be used, and the feed pump term may be neglected.

p	40	30	20	10	bar
η	0.261	0.249	0.232	0.203	
SSC	4.85	5.08	5.45	6.23	kg/kW h

11.4 A reheat cycle, using steam, works between pressures of 140 bar and 0.040 bar. The steam is superheated at 500 °C on entry to the turbine, and after expansion to a dryness fraction of 0.950 it is reheated to 450 °C before completing its expansion to the condenser pressure. Find the reheat pressure and cycle efficiency, assuming an isentropic efficiency of 0.87 in each turbine and in the feed pump. (A process of successive approximations must be used to find the reheat pressure, and this is most quickly done on an h–s chart.)

[4 bar, 0.383]

11.5 A steam turbine is supplied with steam at 40 bar and 450 °C, and exhausts at 0.035 bar. Neglecting the feed pump term, find the ideal Rankine cycle efficiency of the plant. Compare this with the ideal efficiency which could be obtained if regenerative feed heating were employed, assuming the use of open heaters and (a) one bleeding point at 3 bar, (b) three bleeding points at 15, 3 and 0.5 bar.

[0.390; (a) (0.1804 kg) 0.414 (b) (0.1059 kg, 0.0913 kg, 0.0196 kg) 0.429]

11.6 Calculate the efficiency of a regenerative cycle using a single feed water heater, neglecting the feed pump term. The steam leaves the boiler at 30 bar superheated to 450 °C, and the condenser pressure is 0.035 bar. The heater is of the *closed* type, and the bled steam is flashed into the condenser.

[(bleeding pressure 2.7 bar, 0.165 kg) 0.401]

11.7 A steam turbine plant works between the limits of 20 bar and 300 °C, and 0.035 bar. Compare the following three schemes:

   (a) A simple Rankine cycle

   (b) A reheat cycle, with the steam reheated to 300 °C at the pressure where it becomes saturated

   (c) A regenerative cycle, with one bleed point (open heater) at the pressure where the steam becomes saturated.

Assume in all cases that the isentropic *stage* efficiency of the turbines is 0.71. For each scheme find the cycle efficiency, the work done, the heat rejected per kg of steam leaving the boiler, and the final dryness fraction. (NB: To solve the problem it is necessary to draw the line of condition on the *h–s* diagram; see section 19.2.5. In drawing the line, select about ten stages of about equal work output for the complete expansion; the exact number chosen will not affect the position of the line of condition significantly, provided that the number is not too small.)

$$\begin{bmatrix} \text{(a)} & 0.260, & 756 \text{ kJ/kg}, & 2157 \text{ kJ/kg}, & 0.885 \\ \text{(b)} & 0.268, & 874 \text{ kJ/kg}, & 2392 \text{ kJ/kg}, & 0.981 \\ \text{(c)} & 0.275, & 684 \text{ kJ/kg}, & 1808 \text{ kJ/kg}, & 0.885 \end{bmatrix}$$

11.8 A steam turbine plant operates with a boiler pressure and temperature of 60 bar and 550 °C, and a condenser pressure of 0.08 bar. At a point in the expansion where the pressure is 14 bar, a portion of the steam is bled off and passed to a closed feed-water heater. A further portion is bled off when the pressure is 2.5 bar and this is fed to an open feed-water heater. The open heater also receives steam flashed (i.e. throttled) from the closed heater. The overall isentropic efficiency of the turbine is 0.85, and the line of condition is straight on the *h–s* diagram.

Draw a line diagram of the circuit, showing the essential components, and sketch the cycle on a *T–s* diagram. Calculate the external heat supply, and the mass of steam bled off to each heater, per kilogram of water entering the boiler. Ignore the feed pump work and make the usual idealising assumptions about the feed heaters.

An open feed heater is often incorporated to de-aerate the steam. Explain briefly why it is desirable to keep the amount of air in a steam condenser to a minimum.

[2710 kJ/kg; 0.1106 kg, 0.1190 kg]

11.9 Saturated steam at 30 bar enters a high-pressure turbine and expands isentropically to a pressure at which its dryness fraction is 0.841. At this pressure the moisture is extracted and returned to the boiler via a feed pump. The remainder, assumed to be dry steam, is expanded isentropically to 0.04 bar in a low-pressure turbine, and the condensate is returned to the boiler via a second feed pump. Calculate the ideal cycle efficiency, taking into account the feed pump terms.

Calculate the cycle efficiency when the isentropic efficiency of each turbine and feed pump is 0.80. What is then the dryness fraction at the exit of each turbine? Compare results with those of Example 11.3.

[0.357; 0.291, 0.880, 0.871]

11.10 Calculate the cycle efficiency of the ideal binary vapour cycle depicted in Fig. 11.31. It is seen that the steam cycle operates between pressures of 30 bar and 0.04 bar, and uses a superheat temperature of 450 °C. The mercury cycle works between pressures of 14 bar and 0.1 bar, the mercury entering the turbine in a dry saturated condition. The mercury condenser acts as the steam boiler, with the feed water being preheated and the steam superheated by the combustion gases of the mercury boiler. The feed pump terms can be neglected.

[0.518]

11.11 The turbine of a steam power plant operating on the Rankine cycle is supplied with superheated steam at 40 bar and 500 °C. Condensation is at 1.2 bar, and the condenser waste heat is transferred during the day as process heat. At night the process heat is not required and the heat is transferred to a Rankine cycle plant designed to utilise low-grade heat by employing R134a as the working fluid. This cycle operates without superheat at an upper saturation temperature of 90 °C; coolant is available which allows condensation to take place at 20 °C. The steady electric output from the steam plant is 10 000 kW, and this is supplied partly to the factory and partly to the national grid according to requirements. The power output from the R134a plant, during the periods when it is operating, goes into the grid.

Assuming no heat losses, neglecting feed pump work, and assuming isentropic expansion in the turbines of both cycles, calculate the power output and cycle efficiency of the R134a power plant.

[−4016 kW, 0.156]

11.12 A factory requires 2250 kW from its electric motors for driving machinery, 15 000 kW of heat at a temperature of 139 °C from process steam. Two alternative schemes are considered:

(a) The power is taken from the main electricity grid with an overall thermal efficiency from fuel to motors of 20 per cent. The process steam is raised in a special boiler plant with an overall efficiency of 80 per cent.

(b) The power is generated in the factory's steam power plant; the initial steam conditions are 27 bar and 320 °C, and the condenser temperature is 29 °C. The overall efficiency from turbine rotor output to electric motor output is 70 per cent; the internal isentropic efficiency of the turbine is 80 per cent; the boiler efficiency is 85 per cent. Process steam is obtained by bleeding off the required amount of steam from the appropriate intermediate stage of the turbine. Assume a straight line of condition for the turbine on the h–s diagram.

Estimate the relative merits of the two schemes from the point of view of fuel economy.

[scheme (b) 19.0 per cent saving over scheme (a)]

11.13 The figure depicts a steam plant in which steam at a pressure of 35 bar and a temperature of 370 °C expands at a rate $\dot{m}$ through a high-pressure turbine, and at a lower rate

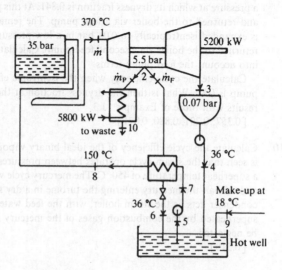

through a low-pressure turbine, to provide a total power output of 5200 kW. At a pressure of 5.5 bar, steam at a rate of $\dot{m}_P$ is extracted and fed to a process heat exchanger which provides 5800 kW of heat at saturation temperature, the extracted condensed steam then going to waste; a further quantity $\dot{m}_F$ is taken through a closed feed heater to the hot well at 36 °C. The condensate at 0.07 bar is pumped from the condenser into the hot well at 36 °C, and make-up water enters the hot well at 18 °C. The feed water is pumped from the hot well through the feed heater into the boiler at 150 °C.

Assume isentropic expansion in both turbines, and neglect feed pump terms and heat losses from the plant. Set up energy equations for the two turbines, the process heat exchanger, the hot well and the feed heater, and hence determine $\dot{m}$, $\dot{m}_P$ and $\dot{m}_F$. Use the h–s chart wherever possible. Also sketch a T–s diagram, giving clear details of the compressed liquid region.

[$\dot{m} = 7.46$ kg/s, $\dot{m}_P = 2.80$ kg/s, $\dot{m}_F = 1.48$ kg/s]

11.14 It has been decided to operate a steam power station with a relatively high condenser pressure of 8 bar, so that the condenser cooling water can be used for a district heating scheme. The steam pressure and temperature at exit from the boiler plant are 100 bar and 600 °C. If 500×10^3 kW are required for district heating, calculate the rate of steam required to flow through the condenser. What would be the net power output from the plant? Assume that the plant operates on the ideal Rankine cycle, and include the feed pump work in your calculations.

The plant is part of a nuclear power station, and the heating fluid for the steam boiler is carbon dioxide gas. The gas, having a value of c_p equal to 1.14 kJ/kg K, enters the boiler at 620 °C and leaves at 310 °C with negligible change of kinetic energy. Calculate the rate of flow of carbon dioxide required.

[231.4 kg/s, 1693×10^3 kW; 1894 kg/s]

11.15 The following steam cycle is to be adopted for a nuclear power station to make the best use of the low-grade heat available from the reactor. Steam leaves the boiler at a rate of 200 kg/s, at 90 bar and 400 °C, and expands to 20 bar in a high-pressure turbine of 87 per cent isentropic efficiency. The steam exhausting from this turbine then mixes adiabatically with 140 kg/s of steam which leave a low-pressure section of the boiler at 20 bar in a dry saturated condition. The steam leaves the mixing chamber at 20 bar and expands in a low-pressure turbine of 90 per cent isentropic efficiency to a condenser pressure of 0.10 bar. Some steam is bled from this turbine at a point where the pressure is 4 bar, for use in an open feed heater.

Sketch the plant, and calculate the power output and cycle efficiency. Ignore the feed pump work and use the h–s chart where possible. A straight line of condition may be assumed for the low-pressure turbine.

[276.7 MW, 0.341]

11.16 To avoid having additional inlet and outlet pipes through the wall of the pressure vessel of pressurised-water nuclear reactors, it is usual to employ a steam-heated reheat cycle. Steam is bled from the boiler delivery main to reheat the steam leaving the high-pressure turbine before it enters the low-pressure turbine. The data for the cycle are as follows:

Boiler outlet condition: saturated steam at	60 bar
LP turbine inlet pressure	5 bar
Condenser pressure	0.05 bar
HP turbine isentropic efficiency	0.80 bar
LP turbine isentropic efficiency	0.87 bar
Reheat temperature	270 °C

The feed pump terms can be neglected, and it may be assumed that the bled steam leaves the reheater at a temperature equal to that at the high-pressure turbine exit. Determine the dryness fractions at the high- and low-pressure turbine exits, and the cycle efficiency.

Also determine these quantities if no reheating were used. (NB: The 0.05 bar line on the $h-s$ diagram will need to be extrapolated.)

Comment briefly on the results.

[0.853, 0.908, 0.313; 0.853, 0.741, 0.322]

12.1 In a gas turbine plant, air is compressed from 1.01 bar and 15 °C through a pressure ratio of 4. It is then heated to 650 °C in a combustion chamber, and expanded back to atmospheric pressure. Calculate the cycle efficiency and work ratio if a perfect heat exchanger is employed. The isentropic efficiencies of the turbine and compressor are 0.85 and 0.80 respectively.

[0.319, 0.319]

12.2 In a gas turbine plant, air is compressed through a pressure ratio of 6 from 15 °C. It is then heated to the maximum permissible temperature of 750 °C and expanded in two stages each of expansion ratio $\sqrt{6}$, the air being reheated between the stages to 750 °C. A heat exchanger allows the heating of the compressed air through 75 per cent of the maximum range possible. Calculate the cycle efficiency, the work ratio and the net work output per kg of air. The isentropic efficiencies of the compressor and turbine are 0.80 and 0.85 respectively.

[0.324, 0.385, 152 kJ/kg]

12.3 In a gas turbine plant, air at 10 °C and 1.01 bar is compressed through a pressure ratio of 4. In a heat exchanger and combustion chamber the air is heated to 700 °C while its pressure drops 0.14 bar. After expansion through the turbine the air passes through the heat exchanger which cools the air through 75 per cent of the maximum range possible, while the pressure drops 0.14 bar; the air is finally exhausted to atmosphere. The isentropic efficiency of the compressor is 0.80, and that of the turbine 0.85. Calculate the efficiency of the plant.

[0.228]

12.4 In a gas turbine, air at 15 °C is compressed from 1.01 bar through a pressure ratio of 6, after which it is heated to a temperature of 750 °C. It is then expanded in a turbine to atmospheric pressure. Assume the following:

Isentropic efficiency of compressor	0.80
Isentropic efficiency of turbine	0.85
c_p in compressor	1.005 kJ/kg K
c_p in combustion chamber and turbine	1.130 kJ/kg K
Pressure loss in combustion chamber	0.14 bar
Gas constant for products	same as for air

Calculate the cycle efficiency and work ratio.

[0.204, 0.320]

12.5 A closed-cycle gas turbine plant consists of a compressor, a heat exchanger, a heater, a two-stage turbine with reheater, and a cooler. The maximum and minimum pressures and temperatures in the cycle are 30 bar and 570 °C, and 7.5 bar and 15 °C. The pressure in the reheater is 15 bar. Sketch the layout of the plant and indicate pressures and temperatures between the components if (a) the heat exchanger is used, (b) the heat exchanger is by-passed. Calculate the ideal cycle efficiencies and work ratios in both cases. The gas used in the circuit is helium, which has a molar mass of 4 kg/kmol and $c_v = 1.5R$.

[(a) 0.478, 0.478 (b) 0.359, 0.478]

12.6 In an air-standard cycle, heat is supplied at constant volume to raise the temperature of the air from T_1 to T_2. The air then expands isentropically until its temperature falls to T_1; and after this it is returned to its original state by a reversible isothermal compression. Show that the cycle efficiency is

$$\eta = 1 - \frac{T_1}{(T_2 - T_1)} \ln \frac{T_2}{T_1}$$

Calculate the efficiency when the pressure rises from 10 bar to 35 bar during the supply of heat.

Explain briefly (a) why you would expect the efficiency of this cycle to be less than the Carnot efficiency, and (b) why this cycle would not be used in practice.

[0.498]

12.7 An air-standard cycle consists of the following processes: isentropic compression from 15 °C, 1.01 bar through a compression ratio of 5; heat addition at constant volume of 2600 kJ/kg; isentropic expansion to the initial volume; heat rejection at constant volume. Sketch the cycle on p–v and T–s diagrams, and calculate its ideal efficiency, mean effective pressure and peak pressure.

[0.475, 18.9 bar, 73.0 bar]

12.8 The cycle in problem 12.7 is modified so that the heat is added (a) at constant pressure, (b) half at constant volume and half at constant pressure. The compression ratio is increased so as to allow the same peak pressure as before. Sketch the two cycles on p–v and T–s diagrams, and calculate their ideal efficiencies and mean effective pressures.

[(a) $r_v = 21.3$, 0.593, 19.8 bar (b) $r_v = 8.37$, 0.552, 19.9 bar]

12.9 In a Carnot cycle, 1 kg of air is compressed isothermally from 1.0 bar to 4.0 bar, the temperature being 10 °C. The maximum temperature reached in the cycle is 400 °C. Find the efficiency and mean effective pressure of the cycle.

[0.579, 1.96 bar]

12.10 Compare the net work outputs of a Carnot cycle and an Ericsson cycle. The following conditions are common to both cycles: air is the working fluid; the maximum and minimum temperatures are 800 °C and 60 °C; and the ratio of the maximum volume to the minimum volume is 25.

Explain briefly why the use of a perfect regenerator can bring the efficiency of the Ericsson cycle up to the Carnot efficiency, whereas it cannot do this for the Joule cycle.

[62.8 kJ/kg, 435 kJ/kg]

12.11 An ideal heat engine cycle consists of the following processes: air initially at 1.01 bar and 15 °C is compressed to 20 bar according to the law $pv^{1.2} = $ constant; heated at constant pressure until the temperature is 800 °C; expanded isentropically to its initial volume; and finally cooled at constant volume until the pressure is again 1.01 bar. Find the efficiency and work ratio of the cycle. If the efficiency ratio is 0.7, what is the efficiency of the engine?

Say briefly: (a) why the efficiency of the ideal cycle is less than that of a Carnot cycle operating between reservoirs at 800 °C and 15 °C, and (b) why the actual efficiencies of engines operating on these two cycles might not be so different.

[0.465, 0.512, 0.326]

13.1 A vapour compression refrigerator using R134a works between temperature limits of −5 °C and 40 °C. The refrigerant leaves the compressor dry saturated. Calculate the refrigeration effect and coefficient of performance if (a) the refrigerant leaves the condenser saturated, and (b) the refrigerant is subcooled to 20 °C before entering the throttle valve.

[(a) 131.2 kJ/kg, 4.54 (b) 163.1 kJ/kg, 5.65]

13.2 In a refrigerator, R134a is compressed isentropically from a saturated state at −5 °C to a pressure of 11.59 bar. The refrigerant is then cooled at constant pressure to 25 °C, and is throttled down to a temperature of −5 °C at which it is evaporated. Determine the temperature and enthalpy after compression in two ways: (a) by using the columns in the tables and (b) by assuming that the specific heat capacity of the superheated vapour is $c_p = 1.153$ kJ/kg K. Sketch the cycle on T–s and p–h diagrams and calculate the coefficient of performance by each method.

[(a) 4.94 (b) 4.95]

13.3 The working fluid in a heat pump installation is ammonia. The ammonia, after evaporation to a dry saturated state at 2 °C, is compressed to a pressure of 12.37 bar at which it is cooled and condensed to a saturated liquid state. It then passes through a throttle valve and returns to the evaporator. Sketch the cycle on T–s and p–h diagrams and calculate the coefficient of performance, assuming that the isentropic efficiency of compression is 0.85.

Describe briefly the mode of operation of an absorption refrigerator, and discuss its advantages and disadvantages *vis-à-vis* the compression type.

[7.80]

13.4 Background heating for a house is provided by a heat pump which, by virtue of its refrigeration capacity, also services a cold room used as a larder. The heating required is 2.5 kW, which is provided by hot water circulating through the heat pump condenser, and the evaporator takes its heat from the cold room. The heat pump/refrigerator uses Refrigerant 134a and operates with a condenser pressure of 23.6 bar and an evaporator pressure of 2.43 bar. The refrigerant enters the compressor, which has an isentropic efficiency of 0.85, with 5 K superheat, and enters the throttle valve as a saturated liquid. Calculate the mass flow of refrigerant and the rate of heat extraction from the cold room.

The heat pump is driven by an electric motor of 0.90 efficiency. Calculate the thermal advantage of the plant as a heat pump over that of direct heating by electricity. Finally, if electricity is produced from primary fuel with an efficiency of 0.35, what is the overall thermal advantage over that of heating the house by primary fuel?

[0.0174 kg/s, 1.508 kW; 2.27, 0.794]

13.5 An ammonia refrigerator works between the temperature limits of −4 °C and 26 °C. After isentropic compression the refrigerant leaves the compressor saturated and is subcooled to 18 °C. Calculate the coefficient of performance. Illustrate the cycle on T–s and p–h diagrams. (Use the values given below only.)

T [°C]	p [bar]	h_f [kJ/kg]	h_{fg} [kJ/kg]	h_g [kJ/kg]	s_f [kJ/kg K]	s_g [kJ/kg K]
−4	3.691	162.8	—	—	0.647	—
26	10.34	303.7	1162.8	—	1.140	—

For liquid ammonia, $c_p = 4.78$ kJ/kg K.

[8.62]

13.6   A heat pump using ammonia as a working fluid operates between temperature limits of 4 °C and 50 °C (saturated temperature in condenser). If the working fluid enters the compressor saturated, and is condensed to a saturated liquid, calculate the coefficient of performance of the ideal cycle.

If the heat pump is driven by a steam turbine, with inlet conditions 40 bar and 300 °C, calculate the ideal advantage of the combined turbine and heat pump over a direct heater to supply heat at 50 °C. Assume that (a) the turbine condenser works at 29 °C, and (b) the turbine condenser works at 50 °C and the rejected heat is used. In either case a heat source at over 300 °C is available.

[5.95; (a) 2.19 (b) 2.66]

13.7   Water is drawn from a river at 7 °C and has to be heated to 64 °C. Calculate the advantage of using the heat pump plant described below over direct heating of the water. Assume that a heat source above 450 °C is available.

   (a) R134a heat pump: compressor driven by steam turbine; condenser temperature 60 °C and evaporator temperature –5 °C; R134a enters compressor as saturated vapour and enters throttle valve as saturated liquid.

   (b) Steam turbine plant: steam pressure and temperature leaving boiler 30 bar and 450 °C respectively; condenser temperature 76 °C.

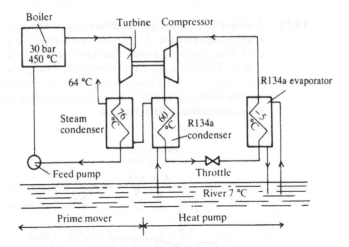

Take 100 per cent isentropic efficiencies for turbine and compressor, and neglect all heat losses. The water drawn from the river passes first through the refrigerant condenser and then through the steam condenser.

[1.81]

13.8   Refrigerant 134a is to be the working fluid in a vapour-compression heat pump plant which is to heat circulating water for a central heating system. The plant is to be used to extract heat from a sewage system, and the compressor is to be driven by an oil engine having an overall thermal efficiency of 40 per cent. Further heat, equivalent to 40 per cent of the calorific value of the oil engine fuel, is to be recovered by passing the circulating water through the engine cylinder cooling jacket and through a heat exchanger in the exhaust system of the engine. To keep the evaporator to a reasonable size, the temperature difference between sewage, at a mean temperature of 15 °C, and Refrigerant 134a is to be 10 K. The refrigerant enters the compressor dry saturated, and after isentropic compression it is desuperheated, condensed and subcooled to 40 °C at a pressure of 13.17 bar. The circulating water enters the plant at 30°C. Calculate the minimum mass flow of water per unit mass flow of refrigerant, if the temperature difference at any pinch point which may occur is to be at least 6 K.

Also calculate the total amount of heat which will be transferred to the circulating water, per unit mass flow of water, and the water temperature at exit from the plant. Sketch the plant, a T–s diagram for the refrigerant, and a T–H diagram for the refrigerant and the circulating water.

[2.86 kg of H_2O per kg of R134a; 70.0 kJ, 46.8 °C]

13.9 An ammonia refrigeration cycle works between a condenser saturation temperature of 50°C and an evaporator temperature of −50°C. The liquid entering the throttle valve is saturated. The vapour entering the compressor has an entropy of 5.365 kJ/kg K, i.e. it will reach saturation at −2°C. Calculate the refrigeration effect and the coefficient of performance.

The cycle is modified as shown in Fig. 13.5. The temperature in the flash chamber is −2°C, and the saturated vapour bled off is mixed with the saturated vapour leaving the first-stage compressor. Calculate the correct amount to be bled, the refrigeration effect, and the coefficient of performance, all quantities to be based on 1 kg passing through the condenser.

[774.2 kJ/kg, 1.58; 0.197 kg, 822.4 kJ/kg, 1.86]

13.10 A refrigerator, operating on ammonia, is shown diagrammatically in the figure. Saturated liquid at a temperature of −30 °C flows at station 1 and saturated liquid at a temperature of 10 °C at stations 3, 4 and 7. Saturated vapour flows at station 5, at a temperature of −30 °C. There are no pressure losses except through the spray nozzle. The flash chamber, compressor and liquid pump are all adiabatic and the last two both operate with an isentropic efficiency of 0.80. The specific volume of liquid ammonia, which can be regarded as incompressible, is 0.0015 m³/kg.

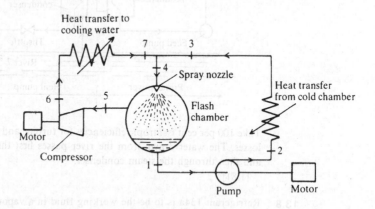

Determine the coefficient of performance, and the mass flow rate of ammonia through the liquid pump for a refrigeration effect of 10 kW.

[3.97, 0.0549 kg/s]

14.1 The analysis of air by volume, and values of c_p at 300 K and the molar masses for the constituents, are given below. Find the molar mass and gas constant for air, and the values of c_p and c_v at 300 K.

	N_2	O_2	Ar	CO_2
V_i/V	0.7809	0.2095	0.0093	0.0003
$\tilde{m}_i/[\text{kg/kmol}]$	28.013	31.999	39.948	44.010
$c_p/[\text{kJ/kg K}]$	1.040	0.918	0.520	0.846

[28.96 kg/kmol, 0.2871 kJ/kg K, 1.005 kJ/kg K, 0.718 kJ/kg K]

14.2 A mixture of 6 kg of oxygen and 9 kg of nitrogen has a pressure of 3 bar and a temperature of 20 °C. Determine for the mixture: (a) the mole fraction of each component, (b) the molar mass, (c) the specific gas constant, (d) the volume and density, and (e) the partial pressures and partial volumes.

[(a) 0.368, 0.632 (b) 29.48 kg/kmol (c) 0.282 kJ/kg K (d) 4.13 m³, 3.63 kg/m³ (e) 1.10 bar, 1.90 bar; 1.52 m³, 2.61 m³]

14.3 A mixture of 2 kg of hydrogen and 4 kg of nitrogen is compressed in a cylinder so that the temperature rises from 22 °C to 150 °C. The mean values of c_p over this temperature range for the constituents are 14.45 (H_2) and 1.041 (N_2) kJ/kg K. Assuming that the process is reversible and that the polytropic index of compression is 1.2, find the heat transferred during the process. Find also the change in entropy of each constituent and of the mixture.

[−3065 kJ; −7.563 kJ/K (H_2), −1.068 kJ/K (N_2), −8.631 kJ/K (mixture)]

14.4 The products of combustion of a fuel have the following composition by volume: N_2 0.77, CO_2 0.13, O_2 0.10. How much heat must be transferred, per kg of mixture, to cool the gas from 820 °C to 100 °C in steady flow at constant velocity? The average molar heat capacities at constant pressure of the constituents, over this temperature range, are N_2 31.08, CO_2 50.51, O_2 33.38 kJ/kmol K.

[−799 kJ]

14.5 A vessel contains 1 kmol of oxygen and 2 kmol of nitrogen, each at 100 °C and 2 bar but separated by a wall. Calculate the total entropy of the system assuming that the entropy of each gas is zero at 0 °C and 1 atm.

If the separating wall is removed so that the two gases can mix freely, calculate the final temperature and entropy of the mixture. Assume that there is no heat exchange with the surroundings, that the volume of the vessel is unchanged by the removal of the partition, and that $\gamma = 1.40$ for oxygen and nitrogen.

[10.29 kJ/K; 100 °C, 26.16 kJ/K]

14.6 The figure illustrates an idealised machine for mixing gases reversibly. A volume V_1 of gas A is contained to the left of a piston which is permeable only to this gas, and a volume V_2 of gas B is contained to the right of a second piston permeable only to gas B. Both gases are at pressure p and temperature T, and initially the pistons are only an infinitesimal distance apart. To accomplish the mixing the pistons are allowed to move apart slowly, and the temperature of the surroundings is not allowed to differ by more than an infinitesimal amount from T. Show that the gases can be mixed reversibly

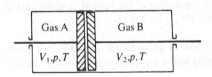

Gas A   Gas B

V_1, p, T V_2, p, T

in this manner and that the work done is given by

$$W = pV_2 \ln \frac{V_1 + V_2}{V_2} + pV_1 \ln \frac{V_1 + V_2}{V_1}$$

$$= \tilde{R}T \left(n_2 \ln \frac{n_1 + n_2}{n_2} + n_1 \ln \frac{n_1 + n_2}{n_1} \right)$$

Also express the partial pressures of the gases in the mixture in terms of p, V_1 and V_2.

14.7 Use the semipermeable membrane concept to derive an expression for the increase in entropy which occurs when perfect gases, which are initially at the same pressure, are mixed isothermally.

Calculate the minimum work required to separate $1\,m^3$ of atmospheric air (assumed to be 0.21 O_2 and 0.79 N_2 by volume) at 1 bar and 15 °C into oxygen and nitrogen each at 1 bar and 15 °C. Calculate also the minimum work required to produce the same quantity of oxygen at 1 bar and 15 °C when the nitrogen remains in the atmosphere.

[51.39 kJ, 32.77 kJ]

14.8 A closed vessel of $0.3\,m^3$ capacity contains dry air at 1 bar and 31.0 °C. Water is allowed to drip into the vessel until the air is saturated. Find the mass of water added and the resultant pressure in the vessel, assuming that the temperature remains at 31.0 °C.

If the contents of the vessel are then raised to 65 °C and more water is admitted until the air is again saturated, what will be the total pressure in the vessel?

[0.009 63 kg, 1.045 bar; 1.362 bar]

14.9 A closed vessel of $0.3\,m^3$ contains $0.06\,m^3$ of water, the remaining volume being occupied by a mixture and air and water vapour. The pressure in the vessel is 1 bar and the temperature 29.0 °C. Heat is then supplied to raise the temperature to 138.9 °C. Calculate the mass of water evaporated, the final pressure in the vessel and the amount of heat that must have been transferred. Use accurate values of v_f from p. 10 of the tables. (Note that although some of the water evaporates, the volume of vapour actually decreases because of the thermal expansion of the liquid remaining.)

[0.4434 kg, 4.83 bar, 28 560 kJ]

14.10 Air, just saturated with water vapour at 17.5 °C and at a total pressure of 1 bar, is compressed reversibly and isothermally in a cylinder to a total pressure of 2 bar. Assuming that the volume of any water present can be neglected, determine the change in entropy of the mixture per kg of dry air.

[−0.2561 kJ/K]

14.11 A turbine, having an isentropic efficiency of 0.85, operates with a mass flow of 15 kg/s of combustion products which expand from 1000 K and 3 bar to 1 bar. The composition of the products by volume and the mean values of c_p of the constituents are as follows:

	N_2	CO_2	H_2O
V_i/V	0.70	0.12	0.18
$c_p/[kJ/kg\,K]$	1.146	1.204	2.217

Calculate the output of the turbine, and the rate of increase of entropy of the gases.

[−3655 kW, 0.814 kW/K]

14.12 A steady flow of water containing air is at a temperature of 70 °C, and it is de-aerated by spraying into a large thermally insulated vessel which is maintained at a pressure of

0.21 bar. Some of the water evaporates and a mixture of air and water vapour is pumped out of the bottom of the vessel. If the temperature within the vessel is 60 °C, determine the proportion of the water entering the vessel which is pumped out with the air.

[0.0178]

14.13   Wet steam enters a condenser at 0.07 bar and is condensed at the rate of 2200 kg/h. If the air leakage is 12 kg/h, and the temperature of both condensate and air extracted is 35 °C, find the mass of water vapour carried away by the air pump per hour. The partial pressure of the air at entry to the condenser may be neglected.

If the rate of flow and temperature rise of the cooling water are 800 kg/min and 20 K respectively, calculate the dryness fraction of the steam at inlet to the condenser.

[30.6 kg/h, 0.764]

14.14   The temperature of the windows in a house on a day in winter is 5 °C. When the temperature in the room is 23 °C, and the barometric pressure is 74.88 cm Hg, what would be the maximum relative humidity that could be maintained in the room without condensation on the window panes? Under these conditions find the partial pressures of the water vapour and air, the specific humidity, and the density of the mixture.

[31.05 per cent; 0.008 72 bar, 0.9896 bar, 0.005 48, 1.172 kg/m^3]

14.15   Air at a rate of 20 kg/min, and at 1.012 bar, 30 °C and 80 per cent relative humidity, enters a mixing chamber and mixes adiabatically with 8 kg/min of dry air at 1.012 bar and 5 °C. The mixture leaves the chamber at 0.97 bar. Determine the temperature, and the specific and relative humidities, of the mixture leaving the chamber.

[23.0 °C, 0.0153, 82.9 per cent]

14.16   A fan takes in dry air at 10 °C and 1.013 bar at a rate of 2.3 kg/s and blows it into a humidifying duct of 0.070 m^2 cross-sectional area. The fan produces a pressure rise of 0.011 bar with an isentropic efficiency of 0.65. Water at 10 °C is sprayed into the duct and the air–water mixture, after heating, leaves dry saturated at 1.021 bar and 75 °C. Calculate (a) the fan work, neglecting compressibility; (b) the amount of water sprayed into the duct; (c) the heat supplied, neglecting kinetic energy changes in the energy equation; and (d) the velocity of the air at exit.

[3.12 kW, 0.8678 kg/s, 2398 kW, 51.64 m/s]

14.17   A volume of 60 m^3 of moist air is passed through a heating chamber per minute. It enters at 1 bar and 13 °C, with a relative humidity of 80 per cent, and leaves at 24 °C without change of pressure. Determine the final relative humidity of the air and the rate of heat transfer to the air.

[0.402, 807 kJ/min]

14.18   A fan discharges 300 m^3 of moist air per minute at 36 °C, 1.10 bar and 92 per cent relative humidity. Find the specific humidity of the mixture, and the mass of water vapour and dry air passing through the fan per minute.

The moist air is passed over refrigerator coils in order to dehumidify it, and leaves the refrigerator chamber with a pressure and temperature of 0.98 bar and 7 °C. The condensate also leaves the chamber at 7 °C. Determine the final specific humidity of the mixture, the mass of water condensing on the cooling coils per minute, and the rate of heat transfer to the cooling coils.

[0.0325, 11.49 kg/min, 353.6 kg/min; 0.00642, 9.22 kg/min, −33 820 kJ/min]

14.19 Turbine condenser cooling water is sprayed at a rate of 1000 kg/min into a natural-draught cooling tower at a temperature of 26 °C, and the water returns to the condenser at 12 °C. Air is drawn into the tower at 15 °C, with a relative humidity of 55 per cent, and leaves the tower saturated at 24 °C. Calculate the mass flow of moist air into the tower and the rate of loss of cooling water by evaporation. It may be assumed that the total pressure throughout the tower is 1 atm.

[1411 kg/min, 18.31 kg/min]

14.20 Water from a condensing plant is cooled in a forced-draught cooling tower. The draught is produced by a fan absorbing 4 kW as it induces an air flow of 110 m³/min at atmospheric conditions of 0.98 bar, 17 °C and relative humidity 60 per cent. The air leaves the tower saturated and at a temperature of 30 °C. If the temperature of the water entering the tower is 50 °C and the rate of flow from the tower is 80 kg/min, find the temperature of the water leaving the tower and the rate of flow of water entering the tower.

[27.2 °C, 82.65 kg/min]

15.1 A gaseous fuel has the following volumetric composition: CH_4 0.38, H_2 0.26, N_2 0.06, CO 0.26, CO_2 0.04. Find the stoichiometric air/fuel ratio by volume and the corresponding wet and dry volumetric analyses of the products of combustion.

[4.86; CO_2 0.121, H_2O 0.182, N_2 0.697; CO_2 0.1845, N_2 0.8515]

15.2 Ethyl alcohol has the chemical formula C_2H_6O. Calculate the stoichiometric air/fuel ratio by mass and the corresponding wet volumetric analysis of the products of combustion.

Determine also the wet volumetric analysis of the products when 10 per cent excess air is supplied with the fuel.

[8.96; CO_2 0.123, H_2O 0.184, N_2 0.693; CO_2 0.113, H_2O 0.169, O_2 0.017, N_2 0.701]

15.3 Find the stoichiometric air/fuel ratio by mass for benzene (C_6H_6). In an engine test using benzene the air/fuel ratio was observed to be 12. Estimate the wet gravimetric composition of the exhaust gases.

[13.2; CO_2 0.201, CO 0.038, H_2O 0.053, N_2 0.708]

15.4 The composition by mass of a fuel oil is 0.857 carbon, 0.142 hydrogen and 0.001 incombustibles. Find the stoichiometric air/fuel ratio. If the dry exhaust gas analysis is found to be CO_2 0.1229, N_2 0.8395 and O_2 0.0376 by volume, determine the actual air/fuel ratio used.

[14.68; 17.82 by carbon balance]

15.5 In an engine test the dry volumetric analysis of the products was CO_2 0.0527, O_2 0.1338 and N_2 0.8135. Assuming that the fuel is a pure hydrocarbon and that it is completely burnt, estimate the ratio of carbon to hydrogen in the fuel by mass, and the air/fuel ratio by mass.

[5.33; 39.6]

15.6 The dry volumetric analysis of the flue gases during a boiler trial showed CO_2 0.062, O_2 0.139 and N_2 0.799. The ultimate analysis of the coal used was: C 0.80, H 0.055, O 0.065, ash 0.08. Determine the excess air per kg of coal.

[20.6 kg by carbon balance]

15.7 Find the net and gross calorific values at constant pressure per kg of *mixture* at 25 °C, for stoichiometric mixtures of (a) air and benzene vapour (C_6H_6), and (b) air and octane vapour (C_8H_{18}). The enthalpies of combustion at 25 °C are $-3\,169\,540$ kJ/kmol of C_6H_6, and $-5\,116\,180$ kJ/kmol of C_8H_{18}; both figures are for the case where the water in the products is in the vapour phase.

[(a) 2861 kJ/kg, 2981 kJ/kg; (b) 2796 kJ/kg, 3012 kJ/kg]

15.8 A mixture, having a volumetric analysis of CO_2 0.10, CO 0.40 and air 0.50, is contained in a vessel of fixed capacity at a temperature of 0 °C. When the mixture is exploded by a spark, estimate (a) the gravimetric composition of the products, and (b) the temperature they would reach, assuming that no dissociation takes place, that the process is adiabatic, and that the specific heat capacities of the gases are constant. Take $c_v/[$kJ/kg K$]$ as 1.045 (CO_2), 0.888 (CO), 0.830 (O_2) and 0.870 (N_2), and the *enthalpy* of combustion of CO at 25 °C as $-10\,107$ kJ/kg.

[CO_2 0.4543, CO 0.1773, N_2 0.3684; 2069 °C]

15.9 A cylinder contains a stoichiometric mixture of gaseous ethylene (C_2H_4) and air. The mixture occupies a volume of 14 litre and the pressure and temperature are 3.3 bar and 90 °C. The enthalpy of combustion of gaseous ethylene at 25 °C is $-47\,250$ kJ/kg when all the water in the products is in the vapour phase. Determine the heat transferred when complete combustion takes place at constant pressure and the final temperature is 280 °C. The appropriate mean specific heat capacities may be taken from tables.

Find also the temperature to which the products must be cooled for the water vapour to begin to condense. Assume that the total pressure in the cylinder remains constant at 3.3 bar.

[-123.1 kJ, 77.7 °C]

15.10 Octane vapour (C_8H_{18}) at 25 °C is supplied to a combustion chamber with air at 25 °C. The combustion takes place adiabatically in steady flow, the velocities are negligible and no work is transferred. Assuming complete combustion, determine the air/fuel ratio by mass if the products temperature is to be 790 °C. Use appropriate mean specific heat capacities taken from tables. The enthalpy of combustion of octane vapour at 25 °C is $-5\,116\,180$ kJ/kmol when all the water in the products is in the vapour phase.

[51.9]

15.11 The amounts-of-substance of products of combustion of a hydrocarbon fuel and air, when at 1 bar pressure and a certain temperature are, in kmol,

$$9.01\,CO_2 + 2.99\,CO + 5.72\,H_2O + 0.28\,H_2 + 1.635\,O_2 + 56.4\,N_2$$

Determine the equilibrium constants for the reactions

$$CO + \tfrac{1}{2}O_2 \rightleftharpoons CO_2 \quad \text{and} \quad H_2 + \tfrac{1}{2}O_2 \rightleftharpoons H_2O$$

Finally, set up the simultaneous equations necessary for determining the amounts-of-substance of products when the mixture of products is compressed to 10 bar without change of temperature.

[20.55, 139.3]

15.12 A stoichiometric mixture of hydrogen and air, initially at 25 °C, is burnt under steady-flow adiabatic conditions. It is found from a products analysis that 6 per cent of the hydrogen is unburnt owing to dissociation. Using the enthalpy of reaction for hydrogen given in the tables, and the appropriate energy equation, calculate the products temperature. Specific heat capacities of products at a guessed mean temperature of 1200 K may be used.

Finally, making use of the dissociation constant data ($\ln K^{\ominus}$) in the tables for the reaction $H_2 + \frac{1}{2}O_2 \rightarrow H_2O$, calculate the pressure under which combustion must have taken place.

[2416 K, 0.366 bar]

15.13 A mixture of carbon monoxide and air has 20 per cent more carbon monoxide than would be required for a stoichiometric mixture. It is compressed to a temperature and pressure of 550 K and 10 bar, and combustion then occurs at constant volume. If no heat is transferred to the surroundings, show that the temperature reached will be about 2975 K. The following data may be used:

At 2975 K the equilibrium constant is $K^\ominus = \dfrac{(p_{CO_2})(p^\ominus)^{1/2}}{(p_{CO})(p_{O_2})^{1/2}} = 3.346$

The internal energy of combustion of CO at 550 K is $-281\,310$ kJ/kmol. The internal energies of the relevant gases are:

	CO	CO$_2$	O$_2$	N$_2$	
550 K	2877	6116	3119	2838	[kJ/kmol]
2975 K	67878	126570	72369	67079	[kJ/kmol]

15.14 Heptane (C_7H_{16}) is burnt with 10 per cent less than the stoichiometric amount of air. Determine the amount-of-substance of each product per kilomole of heptane burnt when the products temperature is 2000 K. At this temperature the water–gas dissociation constant $(p_{H_2O})(p_{CO})/(p_{H_2})(p_{CO_2})$ is 4.527.

[$5.32CO_2 + 7.48H_2O + 1.68CO + 0.52H_2 + 37.24N_2$]

15.15 Recalculate Example 15.7, taking account of dissociation as outlined in section 15.7. Assume that the reaction takes place at a constant pressure of 4 bar. Start by guessing the final temperature (try initially $T = 2300$ K). Then proceed by a process of successive approximations to find the values of the six unknowns a, b, c, d, e and n. Finally check that the guess for T satisfies the energy equation. If it does not, repeat with another value of T.

[$T = 2310$ K, $d/n = 0.005\,582$, $a = 6.481\,17$ kmol, $b = 7.885\,83$ kmol, $c = 0.518\,83$ kmol, $d = 0.316\,50$ kmol, $e = 0.114\,17$ kmol, $n = 56.697\,45$ kmol; residual imbalance in energy equation ≈ -4500 kJ]

15.16 A vessel of volume 0.2 m^3 contains initially a stoichiometric mixture of gaseous C_2H_4O and oxygen at a temperature of 25 °C and a pressure of 1 bar. After complete combustion, the temperature is brought back to 25 °C.

(a) Construct the chemical equation.

(b) Determine the final pressure of the products.

(c) Determine the amount of water vapour in the products which condenses.

(d) Using the data of enthalpy of formation at 298 K given in the table below, calculate the enthalpy of reaction per kmol of C_2H_4O with the product water all in the liquid state.

(e) Calculate the magnitude of the heat transfer during the process.

Assume that all gaseous constituents behave as perfect gases and that the volume of liquid water is negligible compared with the volume of the vessel.

	CO$_2$(gas)	H$_2$O(gas)	H$_2$O(liq)	O$_2$(gas)	C$_2$H$_4$O(gas)
$\Delta\tilde{h}_f^\ominus$/[kJ/kmol]	$-393\,520$	$-241\,830$	$-285\,820$	0	$-52\,630$
$\tilde{m}$/[kg/kmol]	44	18	18	32	44

[(b) 0.603 09 bar (c) 0.078 392 kg or 0.004 355 1 kmol (d) $-1\,302\,330$ kJ (e) -2992 kJ]

16.1 Air is to be compressed through a pressure ratio of 10 from a pressure of 1 atm in one stage. Find the power required for a free air delivery of $3 \text{ m}^3/\text{min}$. Also find the rotational speed if the swept volume is 14.2 litre. The clearance volume is 6 per cent of the swept volume and $n = 1.3$ for compression and expansion.

[15.4 kW, 298 rev/min]

'6 2 Air is compressed in a reciprocating compressor from a pressure of 1 bar and a temperature of 15 °C to a pressure of 9 bar in one stage. The index of polytropic compression and expansion is 1.3 and the clearance volume is 4 per cent of the swept volume. Calculate the work done per kg of air delivered and the heat transferred during compression and expansion per kg of air.

[23.6 kJ, −57.4 kJ, 11.9 kJ]

16.3 A single-acting, two-stage air compressor runs at 300 rev/min and compresses $8.5 \text{ m}^3/\text{min}$, at 1 atm and 15 °C, to 40 bar. Calculate:

(a) The optimum pressure ratio for each stage.
(b) The theoretical power consumption of each stage if the compression in each cylinder is polytropic with $n = 1.3$ and intercooling is to a temperature of 15 °C.
(c) The quantities of heat rejected to the cylinder cooling jackets and in the intercooler.
(d) The swept volumes if the volumetric efficiencies of the low-pressure and high-pressure cylinders are 0.90 and 0.85.

[(a) 6.283 (b) 65.72 kW (c) 6.39 kW per cylinder, 26.88 kW (d) 0.0315 m^3, 0.0053 m^3]

16.4 A three-stage, single-acting compressor is required to compress 135 m^3 of free air per hour from 1 bar to 64 bar. Prove that with complete intercooling the stage pressure ratio should be equal to the cube root of the overall pressure ratio for the required power to be a minimum. Calculate the power needed in this case, assuming $n = 1.3$.

If the mean piston speed is to be 140 m/min, calculate the piston areas, neglecting clearance. State clearly any assumptions made.

[18.4 kW; 321 cm^2, 80.2 cm^2, 20.1 cm^2]

16.5 When a gas is compressed, the work done per unit mass flow may be given by

$$\text{(a)} \quad (h_2 - h_1) \quad \text{or} \quad \text{(b)} \quad \int_1^2 v \, dp$$

State precisely in which cases (a) and in which cases (b) can be applied.

Dry saturated steam at 1 bar is compressed isentropically to 7 bar. Calculate the work done using each of the above formulae, and explain any discrepancy in the results. (Use tables where necessary.)

[421 kJ/kg, 415 kJ/kg]

16.6 Derive an expression by which the indicated power of an engine can be found from an indicator card, the engine speed and the engine dimensions.

In a test on a vertical double-acting steam engine the following information was obtained:

area of indicator cards:	
out-stroke (top)	10.5 cm^2
in-stroke (bottom)	10.2 cm^2
length of indicator card	7.6 cm
spring constant	0.8 bar per cm
speed	120 rev/min

piston diameter	21.5 cm
piston rod diameter	3.7 cm
stroke	30.5 cm

Calculate the indicated power. If the mechanical efficiency of the engine is 80 per cent at the given load, find the torque developed.

[4.76 kW, 303 N m]

16.7 A single-acting steam engine has a swept volume of 50 litre and the cut-off occurs at 0.4 of the stroke. The steam in the main is saturated and at 13 bar, and the engine exhausts to a condenser at 0.7 bar. Neglecting the effects of clearance volume, and assuming that the expansion occurs according to $pV = $ constant, determine the percentage reduction in work output per machine cycle when the steam is throttled to 7 bar before it enters the steam chest. Find the isentropic efficiency for both the unthrottled and the throttled condition.

[49.7 per cent: 72.3 per cent, 67.5 per cent]

16.8 A reciprocating expander, supplied with air at 2 bar and 20 °C, is to develop 1 kW. Assuming reversible polytropic expansion to atmospheric pressure of 0.98 bar, with $n = 1.2$, calculate the mass flow of air required.

If the expander is designed to allow reversible expansion in the cylinder to 0 °C followed by a blow-down to atmosphere, calculate the quantity of air required to develop 1 kW. The effect of clearance volume may be neglected. Also estimate the maximum relative humidity of the supply if condensation must not occur before blow-down.

[1.062 kg/min; 1.088 kg/min, 40 per cent]

16.9 A rotary vane compressor has a free air delivery of 170 litre/min when it compresses air from 0.98 bar and 15 °C to 2.3 bar. Estimate the power required to drive the compressor when (a) the ports are so placed that there is no internal compression, (b) the ports are so placed that there is a 30 per cent reduction of volume before back-flow occurs. Assume adiabatic compression. What is the isentropic efficiency in each instance?

[(a) 0.373 kW, 0.718 (b) 0.285 kW, 0.938]

17.1 The stoichiometric mixture of compressed air and octane of Example 17.1 is burnt adiabatically at constant volume. Find the maximum temperature and pressure reached. Take the internal energy of combustion at 25 °C as $-5\,124\,800$ kJ/kmol of octane. After combustion the products are expanded isentropically to the original volume. Estimate the final temperature and pressure before blow-down. Neglect dissociation, but allow for variable specific heat capacities. Compare the results with those obtained assuming pure air with constant specific heat capacities throughout the problem.

[3056 K, 68.6 bar; 1893 K, 6.07 bar; 4620 K, 98.0 bar; 2121 K, 6.43 bar]

17.2 The equilibrium constant for the combustion equation $H_2 + \frac{1}{2}O_2 \rightleftharpoons H_2O(vap)$ is

$$K^{\ominus} = \frac{(p_{H_2O}(p^{\ominus})^{1/2}}{(p_{H_2})(p_{O_2})^{1/2}} = e^{92.207}$$

at 25 °C. Calculate the maximum work that can be derived from this reaction in surroundings at 25 °C, if the reactants are initially at a pressure of 10 bar and the products leave at the same pressure.

[231 340 kJ/kmol of H_2]

17.3 Calculate the maximum work that can be derived from a stoichiometric supply of air and CO, in surroundings at 25 °C, when: (a) the air and CO are supplied separately each at atmospheric pressure and the products leave as a mixture at atmospheric pressure; (b) the air and CO are supplied mixed at atmospheric pressure and the products leave mixed at atmospheric pressures. (This problem can be solved by visualising an appropriate van't Hoff box, similar to that discussed in sections 15.7.1 and 17.5 but with the addition of reversible mixing and unmixing processes achieved by the device described in problem 14.6.)

$$[(a) (257\,100 + 1577)\,kJ/kmol \text{ of } CO \text{ (b) } (257\,100 - 3516)\,kJ/\,kmol \text{ of } CO]$$

18.1 Steam expands isentropically in a nozzle to 1.5 bar. The initial pressure and temperature are 6 bar and 300°C, and the initial velocity is zero. Plot curves showing the variation with pressure along the nozzle of: cross-sectional area, mass flow per unit area, velocity and specific volume. Work from first principles and do not assume a value for the index of isentropic expansion.

18.2 A boiler generates 2000 kg of saturated steam per hour at 20 bar. Calculate the minimum free cross-sectional area required for a safety valve for the boiler.

$$[1.93\,cm^2]$$

18.3 Steam is applied to a nozzle at 11 bar and 0.95 dryness fraction, and expands isentropically to 1 bar. Assuming the law of expansion to be $pv^n = $ constant, determine the value of n from the initial and final conditions of the steam. Using this value, calculate the pressure and velocity of the steam at the throat of the nozzle, and the mass flow per unit throat area.

$$[1.1295, 6.36\,bar, 442\,m/s, 0.161\,kg/s\,cm^2]$$

18.4 Starting from the energy equation

$$c_p T_1 = c_p T_2 + \tfrac{1}{2} C_2^2$$

deduce equations (18.17) to (18.21) which describe the flow of a perfect gas through a nozzle when the initial velocity is zero.

18.5 A vessel of volume $0.28\,m^3$ is filled with 7 kg of air at a pressure of 20 bar. The vessel is punctured, the area of the leak being $1 \times 10^{-5}\,m^2$, and it may be assumed that the minimum area of the puncture is on the outside surface of the vessel. The pressure of the surrounding atmosphere is 1.01 bar. Calculate the pressure and mass of air in the vessel as the flow just ceases to be choked. The air within the vessel can be treated as expanding isentropically. Also calculate the initial rate of discharge when the vessel is first punctured, and the rate when choking just ceases. The choking mass flow per unit throat area can be taken from equation (18.21).

$$[1.912\,bar, 1.309\,kg; 0.0484\,kg/s \text{ and } 0.006\,47\,kg/s]$$

18.6 Helium at 6 bar and 90 °C expands isentropically through a convergent-divergent nozzle to 1 bar. Determine (a) the mass flow through a throat area of $3\,cm^2$; (b) the exit area required for complete expansion and the corresponding exit velocity. The molar mass of helium is 4 kg/kmol and $\gamma = 5/3$.

$$[(a) 9.03\,kg/min; (b) 3.99\,cm^2, 1390\,m/s]$$

18.7 A convergent-divergent nozzle, having an exit area twice the throat area, is designed to accept air with negligible velocity. Calculate the design value of the pressure ratio of the nozzle assuming isentropic flow. Say what happens when the downstream pressure falls below the design value.

$$[0.0939; 0.937 \text{ is also a solution, but what is its significance?}]$$

18.8 The pressure and temperature in the combustion chamber of a rocket motor are 24 bar and 2800 K. The nozzle is designed for complete expansion when the exit pressure is 1 bar. Find the exit/throat area ratio. Also, calculate the thrust per unit throat area when the rocket is operating in space where the surrounding pressure is zero. Assume isentropic expansion, and that for the expanding gases γ is 1.20 and the average molar mass is 33.5 kg/kmol.

[4.12, 3870 kN/m^2]

18.9 An ejector (jet compressor) is used to evacuate air from a tank where the pressure is 0.80 bar, with discharge to atmosphere. The pressure in the mixing chamber is 0.80 bar and the temperature after mixing is 47 °C. 1.8 kg of compressed air is used per kg of air pumped out of the tank. Calculate the efflux velocity V_2 required from the nozzle (see figure). Assume (a) a diffuser efficiency $(4 \rightarrow 5)$ of 0.70; (b) negligible velocity V_3 in the momentum balance for the mixing chamber; and (c) negligible exit velocity V_5 in the energy balance for the diffuser. Here diffuser efficiency is defined in terms of temperature rise rather than pressure rise, i.e. $\eta_D = (T'_5 - T_4)/(T_5 - T_4)$. Say why, for the ejector illustrated, assumption (b) is not necessary.

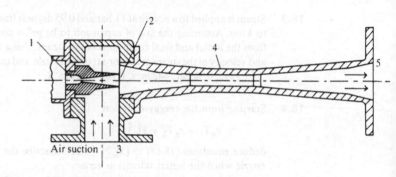

What is the pressure required for the compressed air at inlet to the nozzle to achieve the required velocity V_2? Assume isentropic expansion in the nozzle, and state any other simplifying assumptions you need to make.

[394 m/s, 1.70 bar]

18.10 Steam initially saturated at 10 bar expands isentropically to 4 bar. If the steam is supersaturated throughout the expansion, find the 'undercooling' in K at the end of the expansion, and the reduction in enthalpy drop due to supersaturation.

[50 K, 10 kJ/kg]

18.11 Saturated steam at 13 bar enters a convergent-divergent nozzle with negligible velocity. Determine the throat area required to pass a flow of 60 kg/min assuming that the steam expands isentropically in stable equilibrium. What will be the mass flow passed by this nozzle when the steam expands isentropically in a supersaturated condition?

[5.37 cm^2, 63.2 kg/min]

18.12 One method of determining the efficiency of a nozzle is to suspend it in such a way that the reactive force in the line of flow can be measured. In an experiment with a convergent-divergent steam nozzle the reactive force is found to be 360 N when initially dry saturated steam at 7 bar is expanded to 1 bar. The cross-sectional area of the throat is 4.5 cm^2 and the exit area is such that complete expansion is achieved under these conditions. Determine the efficiency of the nozzle, assuming that all the losses occur after the throat and that $n = 1.135$ for an isentropic expansion.

What will be the reactive force when the external pressure is reduced to 0.3 bar?

[0.946, 422 N]

18.13 In an experiment on a convergent-divergent steam nozzle having a throat area of 5 cm^2, the reaction in the line of flow is measured and found to be 0.613 kN. The steam enters dry saturated at 8 bar with negligible velocity, and the pressure in the exhaust chamber is 0.14 bar. Calculate the mass flow, and the isentropic efficiency to the nozzle, assuming that the expansion occurs under conditions of equilibrium with complete expansion in the nozzle.

Assuming that the isentropic efficiency remains unchanged, what would the reactive force have been had the steam expanded up to the throat in a supersaturated condition?

[0.585 kg/s, 0.891; 0.635 kN]

18.14 Air enters a duct of constant area with a pressure of 3.9 bar, a temperature of 120 °C, and a velocity of 100 m/s. Heat is transferred to the air at such a rate that at a second measuring station along the duct the pressure is 3.4 bar. If the flow were frictionless, what would be the temperature at this measuring section and the rate of heat transfer per unit mass flow?

[565 °C, 482 kJ/kg]

18.15 Carbon monoxide and oxygen in stoichiometric proportions react in a rocket combustion chamber, the temperature being 3000 K and the pressure 20 atm. Making use of the relevant equilibrium constant, calculate the fraction of CO which remains unburnt in the combustion chamber. Hence calculate the mean value of γ for the gas mixture in the chamber.

Assuming that the flow through the rocket nozzle is so fast that the products are 'frozen' in the equilibrium proportions which obtain in the combustion chamber, calculate the mass flow per unit throat area of nozzle. Specific heat capacity data at 3000 K may be used in the calculation.

[0.196 kmol per kmol of CO_2, 1.175; 1653 kg/m^2 s]

19.1 In a single-stage impulse turbine the nozzles discharge the fluid on to the blades at an angle of 65° to the axial direction, and the fluid leaves the blades with an absolute velocity at 300 m/s at an angle of 120° to the direction of motion of the blades. If the blades have equal inlet and outlet angles and there is no axial thrust, estimate the blade angle, the power produced per kg/s of fluid, and the diagram efficiency.

[53.7°, 144 kW, 0.762]

19.2 Steam at 7 bar and 300 °C expands to 3 bar in an impulse stage. The nozzle angle is 70°, the rotor blades have equal inlet and outlet angles, and the stage operates with the optimum blade speed ratio. Assuming that the isentropic efficiency of the nozzles is 0.9, and that the velocity at entry to the stage is negligible, deduce the blade angle used and the mass flow required for this stage to produce 75 kW.

[54°, 0.472 kg/s]

19.3 The fixed and moving blades in a two-row velocity-compounded impulse stage have equal inlet and outlet angles. Show that when the relative velocity is equal at inlet and outlet of each row, the optimum blade speed ratio is equal to $0.25 \sin \alpha_1$, where α_1 is the nozzle angle. Show also that the diagram efficiency is $\sin^2 \alpha_1$ when the optimum blade speed ratio is used.

19.4 Power for auxiliaries on a rocket motor is to be provided by a two-row velocity-compounded impulse stage. The pressure ratio across the turbine is 20 and the gases, having $\gamma = 1.25$ and $c_p = 2.38 \, \text{kJ/kg K}$, enter the turbine at 800 °C. The inlet and outlet angles of the rotor blades are 60° in each row. Assuming isentropic flow, negligible inlet velocity to the turbine, and an axial leaving velocity, find the blade speed, the power produced per kg/s of gas, and the diagram efficiency.

[400 m/s, 1122 kW, 0.976]

19.5 Steam is supplied to a turbine at 60 bar and 450 °C, and expands to 0.065 bar. The first one-fifth of the overall isentropic drop is to be absorbed in a two-row velocity-compounded impulse stage, the blade speed ratio being 0.22. The nozzle and guide blade outlet angles are 70°, and the blade angles at entry and exit of the first rotor row are equal.

The outlet blade angle of the second row is determined by the requirement that the axial thrust for the whole stage is to be zero. If the velocity coefficient of the nozzles is 0.98, and there is a 10 per cent drop in relative velocity in the fixed and moving blades, find the blade speed, and the blade angles for both fixed and moving blades.

[150.8 m/s, $\beta_1 = \beta_2 = 64.6°$, $\alpha_2 = 54.3°$, $\beta_3 = 54.3°$, $\beta_4 = 38.3°$]

19.6 When a reaction turbine runs at 3600 rev/min the steam consumption is 36 000 kg/h. The steam at a certain stage is at 0.34 bar with a dryness fraction of 0.95, and the stage develops 950 kW. The axial velocity of flow is constant and equal to 0.72 of the blade velocity, and the rotor and stator blades are of the same section having an outlet angle of 70°. Estimate the mean diameter of the annulus, and the blade height, at this point in the turbine.

[0.951 m, 11.5 cm]

19.7 Ten successive reaction stages of a gas turbine run at 30 rev/s and have the same mean diameter of 1.5 m. All blade sections have inlet and outlet angles of 0° and 70° respectively, and the axial velocity is constant. Estimate the power output for a mass flow of 55 kg/s.

At inlet to the turbine the pressure and temperature are 7 bar and 700 °C, and at outlet the pressure is 2.5 bar. Find the isentropic efficiency of the turbine, and the blade heights of the first and last rows. Take $c_p = 1.15 \, \text{kJ/kg K}$ and $\gamma = 1.333$ for the gas.

[11 000 kW; 0.789, 9.05 cm, 20.8 cm]

19.8 An impulse steam turbine operates with inlet conditions of 20 bar and 300 °C, and an outlet pressure of 2.6 bar. Suggest suitable interstage pressures if the pressure ratios of the stages are to be equal and simple convergent nozzles are to be used. Assuming that the isentropic efficiency of each stage is 0.7, draw the line of condition on the h–s diagram and find the overall isentropic efficiency and the reheat factor.

[0.721, 1.03]

19.9 A reaction turbine is supplied with steam at 15 bar and 250 °C and exhausts at 0.2 bar. Assuming that the stage efficiency is 0.75 and that the reheat factor is 1.04, find the specific steam consumption.

If the turbine develops 19 000 kW at 1200 rev/min, calculate the blade height and rotor drum diameter at a point in the turbine where the pressure is 1 bar. The stator and rotor blades are of the same section with an outlet angle of 70°, the blade speed ratio is 0.7, and the blade height is one-twelfth of the drum diameter. Assume that the line of condition is straight on the h–s diagram.

[6.46 kg/kW h; 15.0 cm, 1.80 m]

19.10 In a simple jet engine, air is compressed through a pressure ratio of 6, this ratio including intake diffusion. The aircraft is flying at an altitude of 10 000 m where the pressure is 0.2650 bar and the temperature is 223.3 K. Following combustion and expansion through the turbine, the gases are expanded in a propelling nozzle to the ambient pressure. Calculate the jet exit velocity assuming that

Polytropic efficiency of compression and expansion (including nozzle)	$\eta_\infty = 0.86$
Turbine inlet temperature	$= 950\,K$
For compressor	$\gamma = 1.400$
For turbine	$\gamma = 1.333$
Molar mass of air and combustion products	$\tilde{m} = 29.0\,kg/kmol$
Critical temperature ratio	$T_1/T_0 = 2/(1 + \gamma)$

Neglect pressure loss in combustion chamber and mass flow of fuel

Determine whether a convergent-divergent or merely a convergent propelling nozzle is required for complete expansion to ambient pressure.

[576 m/s; convergent-divergent nozzle]

19.11 It is required to provide a preliminary design for the nozzle blade ring of the first stage of an auxiliary turbine. The turbine is arranged in a double-flow casing, driving two feed pumps of a large power station, as shown in the figure. The turbine is to be supplied with low-pressure steam at 1 bar bled from the main turbine, with each half exhausting into the main power station condenser operating at 0.05 bar. The water from the wet bled steam is separated and then flashed back into the condenser, so that dry saturated steam is supplied to the turbine. The total power required from the auxiliary turbine is 5000 kW. Assuming isentropic expansion of the steam, calculate the mass flow of steam required by the turbine.

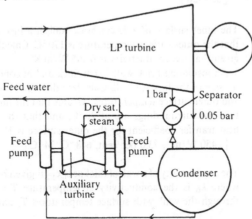

The first stage of the auxiliary turbine is to be a two-row impulse stage with an outlet pressure of 0.42 bar, and with a nozzle blade outlet angle of 70°. Calculate (i) the annulus area at exit from the ring, (ii) the blade height if the blade speed is to be 130 m/s and if the turbine is to rotate at 300 rev/min, and (iii) the total throat area of the nozzle blade ring.

Discuss some of the limitations and constraints that apply to the design of large LP steam turbines. Which of the constraints are eased by the feed pump drive arrangement adopted above?

[5.80 kg/s; 0.117 m², 0.045 m, 0.0375 m²]

19.12 An axial-flow compressor stage has equal inlet and outlet velocities at a constant axial velocity through the stage. Using the nomenclature of Fig. 19.21, show that the degree of reaction is given by

$$\Lambda = \frac{C_a}{2U}(\tan \beta_0 + \tan \beta_1)$$

Hence show that for 50 per cent reaction $\beta_0 = \alpha_1$ and $\beta_1 = \alpha_0 = \alpha_2$.

19.13 An axial-flow air compressor of 50 per cent reaction design has blades with inlet and outlet angles of 45° and 10° respectively. The compressor is to produce a pressure ratio of 6 with an overall isentropic efficiency of 0.85 when the inlet temperature is 40 °C. The blade speed and axial velocity are constant throughout the compressor. Assuming a value of 200 m/s for the blade speed, find the number of stages required when the work done factor is (a) unity, and (b) 0.89 for all stages.

[(a) 9 (b) 10]

19.14 A ten-stage axial-flow compressor provides an overall pressure ratio of 5 with an overall isentropic efficiency of 0.87, when the temperature of the air at inlet is 15 °C. The work is divided equally between the stages. A 50 per cent reaction design is used, with a blade speed of 220 m/s and a constant axial velocity through the compressor of 170 m/s. Estimate the blade angles.

[42.2°, 21.2°]

19.15 A centrifugal compressor produces a pressure ratio of 4 with an isentropic efficiency of 0.80, when running at 16 000 rev/min and inducing air at 15 °C in an axial direction. Assuming that the whirl velocity of the air leaving the impeller is 0.9 times the impeller tip speed, find the impeller tip diameter.

[52.8 cm]

21.1 The inner surface of a 23 cm brick wall of a furnace is kept at 820 °C, and it is found that the outer surface temperature is 170 °C. Calculate the heat loss per m ^{2} of wall area, given that the conductivity is 0.865 W/m K.

An insulating brick wall 23 cm thick and of conductivity 0.26 W/m K is added to the outside of the furnace wall. Calculate the reduction in heat loss, and the brick interface and outer surface temperatures. Assume that the inner surface temperature is unchanged, that the surroundings are at 20 °C, and that the combined convection and radiation heat transfer coefficient for the outer surface is 11.9 W/m² K.

[2450 W/m²; 73.6 per cent, 648 °C, 74 °C]

21.2 The conductivity of a wall of thickness x_{12} is given by the equation $k = k_0 + 2bT + 3cT^2$, where k_0 is the conductivity at temperature $T = 0$. Show that the steady heat flow through the wall, with surface temperatures T_1 and T_2, is given by

$$\dot{Q} = -\{k_0 + b(T_2 + T_1) + c(T_2^2 + T_2 T_1 + T_1^2)\}A\frac{(T_2 - T_1)}{x_{12}}$$

21.3 A double-glazed window, 1.4 m high and 2.3 m wide, consists of two layers of glass each 3 mm thick separated by an air gap 20 mm thick. The window is installed in the wall of a room in which the air temperature is maintained at 23 °C; the outer surface of the window is exposed to the atmosphere which is at a temperature of 2 °C. The surface heat transfer coefficient on the room-side surface of the window is 5.7 W/m² K and that on the outer surface is 9.1 W/m² K. The thermal conductivity of the glass is 0.76 W/m K.

(a) On the assumption that the air in the gap between the glass layers can be regarded

680

as a stationary layer of air of thermal conductivity 0.026 W/m K, calculate the heat transfer rate through the window, and the temperature of the room-side surface of the glass.

(b) Calculate the heat transfer rate for a similar sized window, with a single pane, assuming that all the remaining data are unchanged, and calculate the temperature of the room-side surface of the glass.

(c) Comment on the assumption in (a) about the air gap and explain how the resistance of the air gap would change if the thickness of the gap were to be changed.

[(a) 63 W, 19.6 °C; (b) 234 W, 10.3 °C]

21.4 Water at 65 °C flows through a 5 cm bore steel pipe 1 cm thick. The surroundings are at 20 °C. The pipe conductivity is 52 W/m K, and the surface heat transfer coefficients inside and outside are respectively 1136 W/m^2 K and 13 W/m^2 K. Calculate the heat loss per metre length of pipe and the surface temperatures.

An insulating layer 3 cm thick and of conductivity 0.17 W/m K is added to the outside of the pipe. Assuming the same inside heat transfer coefficient and an outside coefficient of 9.7 W/m^2 K, calculate the heat loss per metre length and the surface and interface temperatures.

[126.3 W/m, 64.29 °C, 64.18 °C; 53.7 W/m, 64.70 °C, 64.64 °C, 33.55 °C]

21.5 A pipe of outside diameter 9 cm is covered with two layers of insulating material each 3 cm thick, the conductivity of one material being four times that of the other. Show that the combined conductivity of the two layers is 28 per cent more when the better insulating material is put on the outside than when it is put on the inside.

21.6 A thin metal tube of radius r_1 is kept at a constant temperature T_1 and is lagged with a poor insulating material of conductivity k and external radius r. The temperature of the surroundings is T_2. Assuming a constant surface heat transfer coefficient α, find the radius r for maximum heat loss from the pipe. Explain the physical significance of the solutions you obtain.

[$r = k/\alpha$]

21.7 Heat is transferred from the inside of a hollow sphere having internal and external radii of r_1 and r_2 respectively. Show that the steady rate of heat conduction in terms of the surface temperatures is given by

$$\dot{Q} = -\frac{4\pi k r_2 r_1}{r_2 - r_1}(T_2 - T_1)$$

21.8 A hollow cylindrical copper bar, having internal and external diameters of 1.3 cm and 5 cm respectively, carries a current density of 5000 A/cm^2. Show that the radial temperature distribution in the bar is governed by the differential equation

$$\frac{d^2 T}{dr^2} + \frac{1}{r}\frac{dT}{dr} = -\frac{\dot{q}_g}{k}$$

The electrical resistivity ($\rho = 2 \times 10^{-6}\,\Omega\,\text{cm}$) and the thermal conductivity ($k = 381$ W/m K) may be assumed independent of temperature. Hence show that

$$T = -\frac{\dot{q}_g}{4k}r^2 + A \ln r + B$$

where A and B are constants of integration to be determined from the boundary conditions.

When the outer surface is maintained at 40 °C and no heat is removed through the central hole, find the position and value of the maximum temperature.

If the inner surface is cooled to 26 °C, with the outer still at 40 °C, find the position and value of the maximum temperature. Also calculate the heat removed internally and externally per m length of tube.

[55.4 °C at $r = 0.65$ cm; 41.9 °C at $r = 1.94$ cm; 52 200 W internally and 39 300 W externally]

21.9 A square chimney has internal and external dimensions of 0.6 m and 1.2 m respectively. The internal surface is at 260 °C and the external surface at 36 °C. Using the relaxation method, plot isothermal surfaces in the chimney wall, and calculate the heat loss per m height. The thermal conductivity of the brick is 0.88 W/m K.

[1900 W]

21.10 A rectangular aluminium bar of cross-section 6 cm × 8 cm carries a current density of 3354 A/cm². Find the temperature distribution throughout the cross-section, and hence calculate the heat lost to the surroundings per metre length of bar. The surface temperature of the bar is 40 °C.

Find the temperature distribution if the bar is hollow, 1 cm thick, and internally cooled to 50 °C. Assume that the total current carried and the external surface temperature are unchanged. Also calculate the total heat loss externally and internally per metre length of bar.

For aluminium: electrical resistivity = 4×10^{-6} Ω cm, $k = 225$ W/m K.

[maximum temperature 107 °C, 216 000 W/m; maximum temperature 56 °C, 432 000 W/m]

21.11 Derive equation (21.25).

21.12 Air at a temperature of 95 °C flows from a pipe. A thermocouple made of 0.9 mm diameter manganin-constantan wire, initially at room temperature of 15 °C, is moved suddenly into the hot air stream. Estimate the time interval after which the thermocouple indicates (a) 55 °C, (b) 94 °C. Neglect the effect of heat conduction away from the thermocouple junction and the effect of radiation, and assume the temperature to be uniform across the wire. The convection heat transfer coefficient between stream and wire can be taken as 0.11 kW/m² K. The following are average properties for manganin and constantan, which are nearly the same: $k = 0.026$ kW/m K, $c_p = 0.42$ kJ/kg K, $\rho = 8640$ kg/m³.

[(a) 5.2 s (b) 32.7 s]

21.13 In Example 21.5 the fluid on the hot side of the wall is maintained at 700 °C, after the heating-up period, for a further period of two hours. Plot a curve of rate of heat transfer to the wall against time from which the heating requirements for the whole four hours can be estimated.

[79 400 kJ/m²]

21.14 A 12 mm thick steel plate is in good thermal contact with a thick aluminium plate, both plates being initially at a uniform temperature of 100 °C. The outer surface 1 of the steel plate is suddenly raised to 600 °C and maintained at this temperature. How long will it take for the contact temperature T_c to reach 180 °C, and what will the temperature be at section 3 at that time?

Assume that at any internal section n the 'future' temperature $T_{n,p+1}$ is given by equation (21.31). Use the space subdivisions shown in the figure, a Fourier number

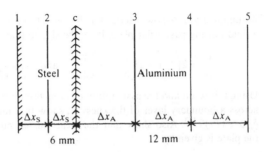

of $\frac{1}{2}$ in *one* of the materials, and first prove in any way you wish that for the contact plane

$$T_{c,p+1} = \frac{(Fo_S)(Fo_A)}{R(Fo_S) + Fo_A}\left\{2T_{2,p} + 2RT_{3,p} + \left(\frac{1}{Fo_S} + \frac{R}{Fo_A} - 2 - 2R\right)T_{c,p}\right\}$$

where $R = k_A \Delta x_S / k_S \Delta x_A$. For aluminium the conductivity $k_A = 235$ W/m K and the diffusivity $\kappa_A = 90 \times 10^{-6}$ m²/s; the values for steel are one-fifth and one-sixth of those for aluminium respectively.

[3.1 s, 130 °C]

22.1 Assuming a linear velocity distribution $U/U_s = y/\delta$ for the laminar boundary layer of a fluid flowing past a flat plate, it can be shown that the boundary layer thickness is given by

$$\delta/x = (12/Re_x)^{1/2}$$

Using this result and the assumption that the temperature distribution is linear across a boundary layer of thickness δ_t, show that, for a plate of uniform temperature, $\delta_t/\delta = (Pr)^{-1/3}$. Also show that the local Nusselt number at a distance x along the plate is given by

$$Nu_x = 12^{-1/2}(Re_x)^{1/2}(Pr)^{1/3}$$

22.2 Air at a temperature $T_a = 14\,°C$ and a pressure of 1 atm flows along both faces of a thin flat plate with a free stream velocity of $C = 30$ m/s, with the plate being maintained at a uniform temperature of $T_w = 90\,°C$. It has been shown theoretically that for laminar forced convection the heat transfer coefficient α_x at distance x from the leading edge of a plate is given by

$$\frac{\alpha_x x}{k} = 0.332(Pr)^{1/3}\left(\frac{\rho Cx}{\mu}\right)^{1/2}$$

For the flow to be laminar the value of the Reynolds number must not exceed 500 000. Estimate the longest distance x_{max} for this equation to hold, and calculate the rate of heat transfer per unit area at that distance. Use property values at a mean film temperature.

Prove that the average value α_m over the distance x is twice the value at x, and hence calculate the rate of heat transfer over the distance x_{max}, per unit width of plate.

Sketch how the velocity and temperature boundary layer thicknesses for air would change with x. Also show how these would vary if the fluid were (a) oil and (b) a liquid metal. Discuss the differences between the three fluids.

[0.301 m, 1.49 kW/m²; 1.78 kW]

22.3 Assuming a fourth-power series for the velocity profile of a laminar boundary layer of a fluid flowing past a flat plate, it can be shown that

$$\frac{U}{U_s} = 2\left(\frac{y}{\delta}\right) - 2\left(\frac{y}{\delta}\right)^3 + \left(\frac{y}{\delta}\right)^4 \quad \text{and} \quad \frac{\delta}{x} = \frac{5.84}{(Re_x)^{1/2}}$$

Using this result and the assumption of a fourth-power series for the temperature profile across a boundary layer of thickness δ_t, show that for a plate of uniform temperature $\delta_t/\delta \approx (Pr)^{-1/3}$. Also show that the local Nusselt number Nu_x at a distance x along the plate is given by

$$Nu_x = 0.343(Re_x)^{1/2}(Pr)^{1/3}$$

22.4 Given equation (22.46), derive equation (22.47).

22.5 Apply the heat flow equation of the boundary layer (22.40) to slug flow of a liquid metal along a plate of uniform temperature to find the thickness of the temperature boundary layer. θ would be the liquid metal temperature relative to the plate temperature. Assume that the temperature profile in the boundary layer can be described by an equation of the form

$$\theta = a\sin\left\{b\left(\frac{y}{\delta_t}\right) + c\right\}$$

where a, b and c are constants to be determined from the boundary conditions. Hence prove that the local Nusselt number Nu_x is given by

$$Nu_x = \left(\frac{\pi - 2}{4}\right)^{1/2}\{(Re_x)(Pr)\}^{1/2} = 0.534\{(Re_x)(Pr)\}^{1/2}$$

It can be shown that if the velocity profile can be approximated by an equation of the form

$$U = d\sin\left\{e\left(\frac{y}{\delta}\right) + f\right\}$$

where d, e and f are constants, then the velocity boundary layer thickness is given by

$$\frac{\delta}{x} = \left\{\frac{2\pi^2}{(4 - \pi)(Re_x)}\right\}^{1/2}$$

Show that for a liquid metal of $Pr = 0.01$ the temperature boundary layer thickness is approximately equal to 6δ.

22.6 Show that in fully developed flow in a tube the pressure drop is related to the friction factor by

$$\frac{\Delta p}{l} = \frac{4}{d}f\frac{\rho U_m^2}{2}$$

Explain why you would expect in the entrance region (a) the value of f to be larger than the value corresponding to fully developed flow, namely that given by equation (22.19) or (22.20); and (b) $\Delta p/l$ to be larger than that predicted from the above equation, even if the correct value of f were used.

22.7 Derive an expression for the ratio of heat transfer to power required to maintain the flow, in terms of the mean fluid velocity U_m and the mean temperature difference θ_m, for a tubular heat exchanger. Assume that the simple Reynolds analogy is valid. What deductions can you make from this expression?

$$[\dot{Q}/\dot{W} = c_p\theta_m/U_m^2]$$

22.8 It is proposed to use the modified Reynolds analogy (22.75) to predict the heat transfer from a cylinder rotating in still air with a turbulent boundary layer (critical $Re_d = \rho U_s d/\mu \approx 300$). Since U_s is the free stream velocity relative to the surface, U_s should be taken as the surface velocity of the cylinder. The shear stress for a rotating cylinder has been found to be

$$\tau_w = f\frac{\rho U_s^2}{2} \quad \text{where} \quad \frac{1}{\sqrt{f}} = -0.6 + 4.07\log_{10}\left(\frac{\sqrt{f}}{2}Re_d\right)$$

It has also been shown that for fluids with Pr not too different from unity, $U_b/U_s \approx 11.6\sqrt{(f/2)}$ in any turbulent boundary layer. Using these data, show that

$$Nu_d = \frac{f}{2}\frac{(Re_d)(Pr)}{1 + 11.6\sqrt{(f/2)}(Pr - 1)}$$

A 5 cm diameter cylinder rotates with a speed of 960 rev/min in air at 15 °C. Its surface temperature is 50 °C. Calculate the heat loss per metre length of cylinder.
[106.9 W]

22.9 Show by dimensional analysis that in forced convection $Nu = \phi(Re, Pr, U^2/c_pT)$, when frictional heating in the fluid cannot be neglected.

22.10 Air at 260 °C and 1 atm flows at 12 m/s through a thin metal tube of 2.5 cm diameter in surroundings at 15 °C. At what rate will the tube lose heat? What would be the percentage reduction in heat transfer if 2.5 cm of lagging of thermal conductivity 0.173 W/m K were put on the tube? The film coefficient inside the tube can be calculated from equation (24.8), and the combined convection and radiation coefficient from the metal and lagging can be taken as 18.7 W/m² K and 11.4 W/m² K respectively.
[246.1 W per metre length of tube, 41.4 per cent]

22.11 Air at the rate of 0.3 m³/min, at 15 °C and 1 atm, is to be heated to 260 °C while flowing through a 2 cm diameter tube which is maintained at a temperature of 480 °C. Calculate the length of tube required. Find the film coefficient from equation (24.8), and take as the mean tube–air temperature difference the arithmetic mean of the difference at inlet and outlet.
[0.872 m]

22.12 Given equation (22.94), derive equation (22.95).

22.13 An electric convection heater consists of a vertical cylinder 7.5 cm diameter, 1.2 m long, enclosing an element of 100 W rating. Estimate the equilibrium surface temperature of the cylinder when placed in a room at 20 °C. The cylinder may be treated as a vertical flat wall; see equation (22.94). (Neglect radiation.)
[108 °C]

22.14 Air flows normal to the axis of a long cylinder of diameter d with a velocity u. The heat transfer coefficient α can be assumed to depend on the relation $\alpha d/k = f[Re, (T_w/T_s)]$ (the Prandtl number being effectively constant for air). Here T_w is the absolute temperature of the cylinder surface and T_s is that of the free stream. Property values should be taken at the mean temperature $\frac{1}{2}(T_w + T_s)$. It is necessary to estimate the heat loss from a 12 mm diameter pipe for which $T_w = 330$ K, when placed in an air stream for which $T_s = 220$ K, $u = 6$ m/s and the pressure is 0.55 bar. A model experiment is planned with an electrically heated wire of 1.25 mm diameter in air at 300 K at a pressure of 1 atm. Find the correct wire temperature and air velocity for the experiment such that conditions can be deemed to be dynamically similar.

Experiments with the wire give a value of $\alpha = 0.66$ kW/m^2 K. What value do you predict for the heat loss per unit length of 12 mm diameter pipe?

[450 K, 53.9 m/s; 0.217 kW/m]

22.15 A calorifier, containing water at 50 °C, consists of a vertical cylinder of 0.5 m diameter, 0.5 m high. The vertical surface of the cylinder is jacketed, and the annular jacket being supplied with dry saturated steam at 1 atm, and the condensate collecting at the bottom is allowed to drain off. Heat is transferred to the water from the tank surface by free convection, and the average heat transfer coefficient can be calculated from

$$Nu_l = 0.60\{(Gr_l)(Pr)\}^{1/4} \quad \text{when} \quad 10^4 < (Gr_l)(Pr) < 10^9$$
$$Nu_l = 0.11\{(Gr_l)(Pr)\}^{1/3} \quad \text{when} \quad 10^9 < (Gr_l)(Pr) < 10^{12}$$

Here $Gr_l = \beta g \rho^2 l^3 \theta / \mu^2$, in which the linear dimension l is the height of the cylinder, and θ is the temperature difference between the surface and the bulk of the water. The coefficient of cubic expansion β for water can be taken as 6×10^{-4} K^{-1}, and the other properties should be taken at the mean film temperature.

Calculate the rate of heat transfer to the water, and the rate of temperature rise of the water. Assume that the resistance to heat transfer between steam and the inner surface of the cylinder can be neglected, and justify this assumption. State other assumptions, if any, which you need to make.

[48.22 kW, 0.1185 K/s]

22.16 A tube of 2.5 cm diameter and surface temperature of 50 °C is losing heat by free convection to air at 15 °C. In order to estimate the heat loss, model tests with a wire heated electrically to 270 °C are to be carried out in compressed air at 15 °C. The wire is to be 0.25 cm in diameter. Calculate the pressure that would be required, assuming that $Nu = \phi\{(Gr)(Pr)\}$ with properties evaluated at the film temperature.

[24.0 bar]

22.17 A 2000 W immersion heater is placed in a 5 cm diameter sealed horizontal tube, and is used to heat water to 60 °C. If the surface temperature of the tube is not to exceed 95 °C, calculate the length of tube required. For free convection $Nu_d = 0.53\{(Gr_d)(Pr)\}^{1/4}$, with all properties taken at film temperature. The coefficient of cubical expansion of water may be taken as 6.21×10^{-4} K^{-1}

[0.355 m]

22.18 A flue insulated on the outside passes gases which, to all intents and purposes, have properties identical to those of air. The density of the gases in the flue is ρ and of the air outside is ρ_s, so that $(\rho_s - \rho) \approx \rho \beta \theta$. Assuming that the shear stress on the inside surface is given by equations (22.18) and (22.20), show that

$$Gr_d = 2 \times 0.0791(Re_d)^{7/4}$$

Calculate the velocity in a flue 6 cm in diameter when the inside gas temperature is 80 °C and the outside air temperature is 20 °C. Also, using the simple Reynolds analogy in the form $St = \frac{1}{2}f$, estimate the inside convection heat transfer coefficient.

[2.53 m/s, 10 W/m^2 K]

22.19   Given equation (22.109), derive equation (22.110).

22.20   An engineer has to develop a dry quenching method and wants to estimate from measurements the heat transfer coefficient α between a bed consisting of small solid particles, fluidised by air percolating through it, and hot solids plunged into the bed. This he does by plunging a stainless steel sphere of radius $r_e = 6$ mm, preheated to a temperature $T_0 = 400\,°C$, into a bed maintained at $T_a = 20\,°C$ by the air stream. A thermocouple made with thin wires is fixed to the sphere with its junction at the centre, and the temperature T is monitored by a temperature recorder. It is found that the sphere centre temperature falls from $400\,°C$ to $210\,°C$ after a time lapse of $t = 6.5$ s. Assuming that the sphere can be regarded as having 'infinite' thermal conductivity, calculate the surface heat transfer coefficient. The properties of stainless steel are listed below.

A co-worker expresses the view that this simple method may be inaccurate because the internal resistance of the sphere may not be negligible. Use an appropriate temperature response chart, $\theta/\theta_0 = f(Bi, Fo)$ (e.g. from Ref. 42 in Part IV), to verify whether the criticism is justified. Clearly explain with the aid of sketches how you use the chart and state any assumption you are making.

Density	$\rho = 8000 \text{ kg/m}^3$
Thermal conductivity	$k = 16 \text{ W/m K}$
Specific heat capacity	$c_p = 500 \text{ J/kg K}$
Thermal diffusivity	$\kappa = 4 \times 10^{-6} \text{ m}^2/\text{s}$

[853 W/m^2 K, 1067 W/m^2 K]

23.1   A gas fire consumes 1 m^3 of gas an hour, of calorific value 17 600 kJ/m^3. Its radiant surface, measuring 22 cm × 30 cm, has an effective 'black-body' temperature of 590 °C in surroundings at 20 °C. Calculate the radiant efficiency of the fire.

A plate of 900 cm^2 area is placed 3 m away from the fire: (a) along a normal to the fire and parallel to the fire; (b) along a direction at 50° to the normal and parallel to the fire; and (c) as (b) but perpendicular to the line joining the fire and the plate. For each position calculate the radiant energy falling on the plate.

[41.9 per cent; (a) 6.62 W (b) 2.74 W (c) 4.26 W]

23.2   An outside wall of a house consists of two brick walls separated by an air gap. Calculate the heat exchange by radiation across the gap when the inner surfaces are at 13 °C and 7 °C. The emissivity of both surfaces is 0.9.

A thin aluminium sheet of emissivity 0.1 is placed in the air gap. With the inner brick surface temperatures unchanged, estimate the radiation heat transfer across the gap.

[25.2 W/m^2, 1.525 W/m^2]

24.1   680 kg/h of oil flows through a thin-walled, 1 cm diameter tube of an oil cooler; 550 kg/h of water flows in the opposite direction through the annular space formed by this tube and a larger tube. The oil, which enters the cooler at 150 °C, is required to leave at 70 °C when the cooling water enters at 10 °C. Calculate the length of tube required. Also calculate the length of tube required if the water were flowing in the same direction as the oil. (The film coefficient between oil and tube is 2.3 kW/m^2 K, and between water and tube 5.7 kW/m^2 K. The specific heat capacity of the oil is 2.18 kJ/kg K.)

[8.73 m, 13.67 m]

24.2   Steam condenses on the outside of a thin 2.5 cm diameter copper tube, 5.5 m long, the steam pressure being 0.07 bar. Water flows through the tube at the rate of 1.2 m/s, entering at 12°C and leaving at 24°C. Calculate the heat transfer coefficient between steam and water. Assuming that the heat transfer coefficient between steam and tube is 17 kW/m² K, estimate the coefficient between water and tube.

[3.35 kW/m² K, 4.17 kW/m² K]

24.3 Water flows through an annular space 2 metres in length, formed by an insulated pipe of 80 mm inside diameter surrounding an inner tube of 60 mm outside diameter. The water is to be heated from 15°C to 75°C. The inner tube contains a uniformly wound electric heating element, and the electric input is so controlled that the surface temperature of the inner tube does not anywhere exceed 90°C. Calculate the power rating of the element, and the mass flow of water that can be heated, for the following two extreme cases:

(a) The thermal conductivity and thickness of the inner tube are such that the surface temperature is evened out by axial conduction along the tube.
(b) The thermal conductivity and thickness are such that axial conduction is negligible in the inner tube.

In both cases assume that the Nusselt number $\alpha d_e/k$ in the annulus is constant and equal to 5, where the equivalent diameter d_e is the difference between the outer and inner *diameters* of the annulus and k is evaluated at the mean bulk temperature of the water.

[2.245 kW, 0.008 95 kg/s; 0.904 kW, 0.003 61 kg/s]

24.4 A heat exchanger consists of ten 2 m length pipes of 2.5 cm bore and 2.9 cm outer diameter, each running inside concentric pipes. Hot oil at the rate of 900 kg/h and initially at 250°C passes counter-current to cold oil at the rate of 1350 kg/h and an initial temperature of 15°C. Assuming an average overall heat transfer coefficient of 170 W/m² K and a constant specific heat capacity of 1.68 kJ/kg K, calculate the outlet temperature of the oils.

[147.6°C, 83.3°C.]

24.5 Derive equation (24.10).

24.6 Carbon dioxide at a temperature of 500 K and a pressure of 1 atm flows with a velocity of 15 m/s across an electrically heated tube which has a diameter of 2.5 cm and is maintained at 1100 K. By experiment it has been found that for a tube in cross-flow

$$Nu_d = 0.26(Re_d)^{0.6}(Pr)^{0.3}$$

when the properties are evaluated at the film temperature. Calculate the rate of heat transfer by convection per metre length of tube. (Use the data on p. 15 of the tables.)

If the tube can be considered grey, of emissivity 0.8, estimate the total electric power required for the heating element per metre length of tube. State clearly any additional assumptions you make.

[5.1 kW, 10.1 kW]

24.7 Recalculate problem 21.1 ignoring the given colder surface temperature in the first part and the given heat transfer coefficient in the second. Take the free convection coefficient as $\alpha_c = 1.31(\theta/[K])^{1/3}$ W/m² K, the radiation coefficient from equation (23.34) with $\varepsilon = 0.8$, and the temperature of the surroundings as 20°C in both cases.

[2445 W/m²; 73.6 per cent, 648°C, 78°C]

24.8 Recalculate problem 21.4, ignoring the given outside surface heat transfer coefficient.

Take the free convection coefficient from Fig. 22.17, and the radiation coefficient from equation (23.34) with $\varepsilon = 0.8$.

$[Gr_d \approx 1.6 \times 10^6, 119.7 \, W/m, 64.33\,°C, 64.21\,°C; Gr_d \approx 3.9 \times 10^6, 52.7 \, W/m, 64.70\,°C, 64.65\,°C, 34.10\,°C]$

24.9 A large volume of air at $49\,°C$ is separated from another large volume of air at $15\,°C$ by a vertical 0.25 cm thick sheet of (a) aluminium of emissivity 0.1 and conductivity 173 W/m K, and (b) cardboard of emissivity 0.9 and conductivity 0.173 W/m K. The free convection heat transfer coefficient is given by $\alpha_c = 1.31(\theta[K])^{1/3} \, W/m^2 \, K$. Compare the overall heat transfer coefficients with the two materials.

$[(a) \ 2.006 \, W/m^2 \, K \ (b) \ 4.270 \, W/m^2 \, K]$

24.10 Show that the rate of heat transfer by steady conduction through a thick-walled spherical vessel is given by

$$\dot{Q} = \frac{4\pi k r_o r_i}{r_o - r_i}(T_i - T_o)$$

where subscripts i and o refer to the inner and outer surfaces.

A relatively thin steel spherical pressure vessel of radius 4 m is to be annealed by applying electrical heating elements to the inner surface. The outer surface is lagged with material of thickness 0.2 m and thermal conductivity 0.20 W/m K. The metal temperature is to be maintained at a temperature of $730\,°C$, while the lagged sphere loses heat by free convection to the surrounding atmosphere which is at $15\,°C$. The convection heat transfer coefficient from a sphere in air is given by

$$\frac{\alpha}{[W/m^2 \, K]} = 1.33\left(\frac{\theta/r}{[K/m]}\right)^{1/4}$$

where r is the radius and θ is the temperature difference between surface and atmosphere. Determine the outer surface temperature, and the electric power required for the annealing process. Why will this calculation underestimate the actual power required?

$[175\,°C, \ 117.2 \, kW]$

24.11 The inner surface of a 1 cm thick metal wall is maintained at a uniform temperature of $120\,°C$. The combined convection and radiation heat transfer coefficient from the outer surface to surroundings at $15\,°C$ is 57 W/m² K (irrespective of whether there are or are not fins on the surface). Estimate the heat flow through the wall for a strip 1 m long by 0.018 m wide (i) if no fins are attached to the surface, (ii) if rectangular 0.5 cm × 5 cm fins are spaced at 1.8 cm pitch on the outer surface. Take the metal to be (a) aluminium with $k = 225 \, W/m \, K$, (b) steel with $k = 54 \, W/m \, K$. Also estimate the fin root and tip temperatures.

(NB: This is an open-ended question. It would seem that a two-dimensional solution, e.g. by relaxation, needs to be obtained between the inner surface and the root of the fin. The labour involved would not be justified, and the following semi-intuitive approach could be adopted. Assume initially that the fin root temperature is $120\,°C$ and calculate, as a first approximation, the heat flow $\dot{Q}_0$ into the fin. Using this value and a pseudo-one-dimensional approach, estimate the temperature drop across the wall. The final answer obtained will depend on the sophistication adopted and the number of successive approximations used.)

$[(a) \ (i) \ 107.5 \, W \ (ii) \ 616 \, W, \ T_0 = 118\,°C, \ T_h = 106\,°C; \ (b) \ (i) \ 107.6 \, W \ (ii) \ 490 \, W, \ T_0 = 112.5\,°C, \ T_h = 77\,°C]$

24.12   When deriving equation (24.22) for heat flow through the root of a fin it was assumed that the heat flow from the tip of the fin was negligible, i.e. $(d\theta/dx)_h = 0$. If the fin is short this assumption is invalid, and the correct boundary condition for the tip of the fin is $-kA(d\theta/dx)_h = -\alpha A\theta_h$. With this boundary condition it can be shown that

$$\dot{Q}_0 = mkA\theta_0 \frac{(\alpha/mk) + \tanh mh}{1 + (\alpha/mk)\tanh mh}$$

By differentiation, show that fins will not increase the heat flow from the surface unless $1/\alpha > b/2k$.

24.13   The average convection heat transfer coefficient α for flow normal to the axis of a circular cylinder is to be found from an experiment with a metal ring in a low-velocity wind tunnel, where the free-stream velocity is 0.60 m/s. The air, at a temperature $T_a = 300$ K, flows parallel to the axis of the ring (see figure). The ring is made of 12 mm diameter copper rod having a thermal conductivity of 380 W/m K, and the mean diameter of the ring is 300 mm. At a section 0 the ring is heated to a steady temperature $T_0 = 350$ K, and the steady temperature at section 1 diametrically opposite is found to be $T_1 = 310$ K. Making use of fin theory, calculate the average value of α.

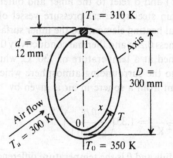

Assuming that the results can be correlated by the relation

$$Nu_d = C(Re_d)^{0.5}(Pr)^{0.3}$$

with all the properties taken at the free-stream temperature, calculate the value of the coefficient C.

$[27.2 \text{ W/m}^2 \text{ K}, 0.645]$

24.14   A copper tube T is pressed into a body B maintained at a temperature T_B and exposed to surroundings at a lower temperature T_s (see figure). The opening is sealed with a constantan foil F, to the centre of which is attached a thin copper wire W. T–F–W thus forms a back-to-back thermocouple capable of measuring the temperature difference between foil and rim centre. The foil, like the body, may be assumed to lose heat to the surroundings at a constant rate $\dot{q}$ per unit area. Neglecting any heat transfer by the wire and to or from the back of the foil, the heat transferred to the surroundings from the foil will be conducted radially inwards from the tube T and there will be an associated temperature drop $\Delta\theta$ from the periphery of the foil to the centre.

Prove that the radial temperature field in the foil is governed by the differential equation

$$\frac{d^2\theta}{dr^2} + \frac{1}{r}\frac{d\theta}{dr} - \frac{\dot{q}}{k\delta} = 0$$

where θ is the temperature measured relative to T_s.

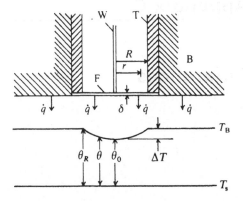

The solution to the differential equation is

$$\theta = \frac{\dot{q}}{4k\delta}r^2 + A \ln r + B$$

where A and B are arbitrary constants. By introducing suitable boundary conditions at $r = 0$ and $r = R$, show that the temperature distribution is given by

$$\theta = \theta_R - \frac{\dot{q}}{4k\delta}(R^2 - r^2)$$

and hence, with $\Delta T \ll \theta_R$,

$$\Delta T = \frac{\alpha \theta_R}{4k\delta}R^2$$

This device can be used to measure the heat loss from the surface only if ΔT is small compared with θ_R, otherwise $\dot{q}$ cannot be taken as uniform over the foil. Specify the thickness δ of the foil, of radius $R = 5$ mm and $k = 25$ W/m K, to give a drop ΔT of not more than 1.5 per cent of θ_R, assuming that the expected value of the surface heat transfer coefficient $\alpha = 7.5$ W/m² K.

[0.125 mm]

Appendix C

References

The books and papers mentioned in the text are arranged separately for the four parts. *Books*: the dates given refer to the latest known editions (not printings) at the time of going to press. *Periodicals*: bold figures refer to volumes, and ordinary figures to pages.

Part I

1 BRAITHWAITE R B *Scientific Explanation* (Cambridge University Press, 1953)
2 BRIDGMAN P W *The Nature of Thermodynamics* (Harvard University Press, 1941)
3 BRIDGMAN P W Condensed collection of thermodynamic formulas. *Mineralogy and Metallurgy, New York*, **7** (1926) 149
4 CARNOT S N L *Réflexions sur la puissance motrice du feu et sur les machines propres à developper cette puissance* (Bachelier, 1824), transl. Thurston, R. H. (American Society of Mechanical Engineers, 1943)
5 McGLASHAN M L *Chemical Thermodynamics* (Academic Press, 1979)
6 KEENAN J H *Thermodynamics* (Wiley, 1941)
7 PLANCK M *Treatise on Thermodynamics* transl. from 7th German edn (Longman, 1927)
8 ZEMANSKY M W and DITTMAN R *Heat and Thermodynamics* (McGraw-Hill, 1981)
9 GILLESPIE L J and COE J R The heat expansion of a gas of varying mass. *Journal of Chemical Physics* **1** (1933) 103–13
10 COOK S S Thermodynamics in the making. *Transactions of the NE Coast Institution of Engineers and Shipbuilders* **65** (1948–9) 65–84
11 HAYWOOD R W *Equilibrium Thermodynamics for Engineers and Scientists: Single Axiom Approach* (Krieger, 1990)
12 HORLOCK J H The rational efficiency of power plants with external combustion. *Thermodynamics and Fluid Mechanics Convention, Cambridge, April 1964, Proceedings of the Institution of Mechanical Engineers* **178**, Pt 3 I(v) (1963–4) 43–52
13 KOTAS T J *The Exergy Method of Thermal Plant Analysis* (Butterworth, 1985)

Part II

1 *NEL Steam Tables 1964* (HMSO, 1964)
2 CARNOT S N L *Réflexions sur la puissance motrice du feu et sur les machines propres à developper cette puissance* (Bachelier, 1824), transl. Thurston, R. H. (American Society of Mechanical Engineers, 1943)
3 COHEN H, ROGERS G F C and SARAVANAMUTTOO H I H *Gas Turbine Theory* (Longman, 1987)

692

4 BETT K E, ROWLINSON J S and SAVILLE G *Thermodynamics for Chemical Engineers* (Athlone Press, 1975)

5 JONES W *Air Condition Engineering* (Arnold, 1985)

6 CIBSE Psychrometric Chart (Chartered Institution of Building Service Engineers)

7 GOODGER E M *Combustion Calculations* (Macmillan, 1977)

8 GOODGER E M *Petroleum and Performance* (Butterworths, 1953)

9 HILSENRATH J et al. *Tables of Thermal Properties of Gases*, US National Bureau of Standards circular 564 (1955)

10 HODGE J *Cycles and Performance Estimation* (Butterworths, 1955)

11 THRELKELD J L *Thermal Environmental Engineering* (Prentice-Hall, 1970)

12 KEENAN J H and KAYE J *Gas Tables* (Wiley, 1948)

13 TIMMERHAUS, K D, and FLYNN, T M *Cryogenic Process Engineering* (Plenum, 1989)

14 KAUZMANN W *Kinetic Theory of Gases* (Benjamin, 1966)

15 LYDERSEN A L, GREENKORN R A and HOUGEN O A Generalised thermodynamic properties of fluids. University of Wisconsin, Engineering Experiment Station, report 4 (1955)

16 McADAMS W H *Heat Transmission* (Krieger, 1985)

17 ROGERS G F C and MAYHEW Y R *Thermodynamic and Transport Properties of Fluids—SI Units* (Basil Blackwell, 1995)

18 *Modern Power Station Practice*, 3 (Central Electricity Generating Board, 1963)

19 ROSE J W and COOPER J R *Technical Data on Fuel* (British National Committee, World Energy Conference, 1977)

20 ZEMANSKY M W and DITTMAN R *Heat and Thermodynamics* (McGraw-Hill, 1981)

21 JAKOB M Steam research in Europe and in America. *Engineering, London* **132** (1931) 143–6, 518–21, 550–1, 651–3, 684–6, 707–9, 744–6, 800–4

22 *Temperature: Its Measurement and Control in Science and Industry* American Institute of Physics, 1, **2** and 3 (Reinhold, 1941, 1955 and 1962), **4** (Instrument Society of America, 1972), **5** and 6 (American Institute of Physics, 1982 and 1992)

23 *Temperature Measurement* BS 1041 Parts 1, 2.1, 2.2, 3, 4, 5, 7 (British Standards Institution, various dates, some still in preparation)

24 WALKER G *Stirling Engines* (Oxford University Press, 1980)

25 *The International Temperature Scale of 1990* National Physical Laboratory (HMSO, 1990)

26 WITHERS J G Gas turbine combustion efficiency calculations. *Aircraft Engineering* **22** (1950) 218–22

27 *ASHRAE Handbook* (American Society of Heating, Refrigerating and Air-Conditioning Engineers, 1989)

28 *Proceedings of the United Nations Conference on New Sources of Energy* Rome, August 1961, **4–6**, Solar Energy (United Nations, 1964)

29 *CIBSE Guide Pt C 1–2* (Chartered Institution of Building Service Engineers, 1986)

30 STREHLOW R A *Combustion Fundamentals* (McGraw-Hill, 1984)

31 *Measurement of Humidity* National Physical Laboratory, Notes on Applied Science 4 (HMSO, 1970)

32 QUINN T J *Temperature* (Academic Press, 1990)

33 *Handbook of Chemistry and Physics* (Chemical Rubber Publishing Co., Cleveland, Ohio, revised frequently)

34 WEIR C D Optimisation of heater enthalpy rises in feed-heating trains. *Proceedings of the Institution of Mechanical Engineers* **174** (1960) 769–96

35 WOOTTON W R *Steam Cycles for Nuclear Power Plant* (Temple Press, 1958)

36 ROSSINI F D et al. *Selected Values of Chemical Thermodynamic Properties* US National Bureau of Standards circular 500 (1952)

WAGMAN D D *Selected Values of Chemical Thermodynamic Properties* US National Bureau of Standards technical note 270 (1965)

37 STULL D R and PROPHET H (eds) *Janaf Thermochemical Tables* (US Government Printing Office, 1971, supplements 1974, 1975, 1978)

38 District heating combined with electricity generation in the United Kingdom. *Department of the Environment Energy Paper* 20 (1977)

39 WILSON S S and RADWAN M S Appropriate thermodynamics for heat engine analysis and design. *International Journal of Mechanical Engineering Education* 5 (1977) 68–80

40 ROGERS G F C Limitations and uses of energy analysis. *Chartered Mechanical Engineer* September 1977, 48–51

41 *Process Integration* and *Application of Process Integration to Utilities, Combined Heat and Power, and Heat Pumps* 87030 (1988) and 89001 (1989) (ESDU International)

42 EASTOP T D and CROFT D R *Energy Efficiency* (Longman, 1990)

Part III

1 COHEN H, ROGERS G F C and SARAVANAMUTTOO H I H *Gas Turbine Theory* (Longman, 1987)

2 HORLOCK J H *Axial Flow Turbines: Fluid Mechanics and Thermodynamics* (Krieger, 1973)

3 HOTTEL H C, WILLIAMS G L and SATTERFIELD C N *Thermodynamic Charts for Combustion Processes* (Wiley, 1949)

4 RICARDO H R and HEMPSON J G G *The High-Speed Internal-Combustion Engine* (Blackie, 1968)

5 SHAPIRO A H *The Dynamics and Thermodynamics of Compressible Fluid Flow*, 1 (Wiley, 1953), 2 (Krieger, 1983)

6 SHEPHERD D G *Principles of Turbomachinery* (Collier-Macmillan, 1961)

7 GYARMATHY G and MEYER H Spontaneous condensation phenomena (in German). *VDI Forschungsheft* 508 (1965) 1–48

8 BINNIE A M and WOODS M W The pressure distribution in a convergent-divergent steam nozzle. *Proceedings of the Institution of Mechanical Engineers* 138 (1938) 229–66

9 LYSHOLM A J R A new rotary compressor. *Proceedings of the Institution of Mechanical Engineers* 150 (1943) 11–16

10 MILLER C D Relation between spark-ignition engine knock, detonation waves, and autoignition as shown by high-speed photography. National Advisory Committee on Aeronautics report 855 (1946)

11 LIEPMANN H W and ROSHKO A *Elements of Gas Dynamics* (Wiley, 1957)

12 SWAINE J Some design aspects of poppet-valve cylinder heads for spark-ignition liquid-cooled engines. *Proceedings of the Automobile Division, Institution of Mechanical Engineers* (1947–8) 51–9

13 AINLEY D G An approximate method for the estimation of the design point efficiency of axial flow turbines. Current Paper of the Aeronautical Research Council 30 (HMSO, 1950)

14 RICARDO H R Combustion in Diesel engines. *Proceedings of the Institution of Mechanical Engineers* 162 (1950) 145–8

15 Symposium on Superchargers and Supercharging, *Proceedings of the Automobile Division, Institution of Mechanical Engineers* (1956–7) 217–85

16 Third International Conference on Turbocharging and Turbochargers, Institution of Mechanical Engineers, no. 4 (1980)

17 KESTIN J and OWCZAREK J A The expression for work in a Roots blower. *Proceedings of the Institution of Mechanical Engineers* 1B (1952–3) 91–4

18 MAYHEW Y R and ROGERS G F C One-dimensional irreversible gas flow in nozzles. *Engineering, London* 175 (1953) 355–8

19 BROEZE J J *Combustion in Piston Engines* (Stam Press, 1963)

20 Symposium on Wet Steam, *Thermodynamics and Fluid Mechanics Convention, Liverpool, April 1966, Proceedings of the Institution of Mechanical Engineers* **180**, Pt 3J (1965–6)

21 HEYWOOD J B *Internal Combustion Engine Fundamentals* (McGraw-Hill, 1988)

22 ANSDALE R F N.S.U.-Wankel engine. *Automotive Engineer* **50** (1960) 166–76

23 HESSE W J and MUMFORD N V S *Jet Propulsion for Aerospace Applications* (Pitman, 1964)

24 ANGRIST S W *Direct Energy Conversion* (Allyn and Bacon, 1982)

25 KAYE J and WELSH J A (eds) *Direct Conversion of Heat to Electricity* (Wiley, 1960)

26 MITCHELL W *Fuel Cells* (Academic Press, 1963)

27 BENSON R S and WHITEHOUSE N D *Internal Combustion Engines* **1** and **2** (Pergamon, 1979)

Part IV

1 ALLEN D N DE G *Relaxation Methods in Engineering and Science* (McGraw-Hill, 1959)

2 *Heat Exchanger Design Handbook* (Hemisphere, regularly revised)

3 CARSLAW H S and JAEGER J C *Conduction of Heat in Solids* (Oxford University Press, 1959)

4 DUNCAN W J *Physical Similarity and Dimensional Analysis* (Edward Arnold, 1953)

5 ROHSENOW W M and HARTNETT J P (eds) *Handbook of Heat Transfer* (McGraw-Hill, 1973)

6 ECKERT E R G and DRAKE R M *Heat and Mass Transfer* (Krieger, 1981)

7 COLLIER J G *Convective Boiling and Condensation* (McGraw-Hill, 1981)

8 CHI S W *Heat Pipe Theory and Practice* (Hemisphere, 1976)

9 INGERSOLL L R, ZOBEL O J and INGERSOLL, A C *Heat Conduction* (University of Wisconsin Press, 1954)

10 JAKOB M *Heat Transfer* **1** (Wiley, 1949)

11 KERN D Q *Process Heat Transfer* (McGraw-Hill, 1950)

12 LANGHAAR H L *Dimensional Analysis and Theory of Models* (Krieger, 1979)

13 McADAMS W H *Heat Transmission* (Krieger, 1985)

14 ROGERS G F C and MAYHEW Y R *Thermodynamic and Transport Properties of Fluids— SI Units* (Basil Blackwell, 1995)

15 MAYHEW Y R Numerical method for unsteady one-dimensional conduction. *Bulletin of Mechanical Engineering Education* **3** (1964) 63–74

16 HOWARD J R *Fluidised Bed Technology: Principles and Applications* (Hilger, 1989)

17 WIEBELT J A *Engineering Radiation Heat Transfer* (Holt, Rinehart and Winston, 1966)

18 SCHLICHTING H *Boundary Layer Theory* (McGraw-Hill, 1979)

19 SCHNEIDER P J *Conduction Heat Transfer* (Addison-Wesley, 1955)

20 KESTIN J and RICHARDSON P D Heat transfer across turbulent incompressible boundary layers. *International Journal of Heat Mass Transfer* **6** (1963) 147–89

21 REYNOLDS O On the dynamical theory of incompressible viscous fluids and the determination of the criterion. *Philosophical Transactions of the Royal Society* **A186** (1895) 123–64

22 FOX L *Numerical Solution of Ordinary and Partial Differential Equations* (Pergamon, 1962)

23 NUSSELT W The fundamental law of heat transfer (in German). *Gesundheitsingenieur* **38** (1915) 477–82, 490–7

24 NUSSELT W The surface condensation of steam (in German). *Zeitschrift Verein deutscher Ingenieure* **60** (1916) 541–6, 569–75

25 *Modern Computing Methods* National Physical Laboratory, Notes on Applied Science 16 (HMSO, 1961)

26 HERMANN R Heat transfer by free convection from a horizontal cylinder in diatomic gases (in German). *VDI Forschungsheft* 379 (1936) 1–24

27 KROUJILINE G Investigation of the thermal boundary layer, and The theory of heat transmission by a circular cylinder in a transverse fluid flow (in French). *Technical Physics of the U.S.S.R.* 3 (1936) 183–94, 311–20

28 REICHARDT H Heat transfer through turbulent friction layers (in German). *Zeitschrift für angewandte Mathematik und Mechanik* 20 (1940) 297–328, transl.National Advisory Committee on Aeronautics technical memorandum 1047, Washington

29 LIENHARD J H *A Heat Transfer Textbook* (Prentice-Hall, 1981)

30 PROBERT R P and SINGHAM J R The measurement of gas temperatures in turbine engines. *Journal of Scientific Instruments* 23 (1946) 72–7

31 MARTINELLI R C Heat transfer to molten metals. *Transactions of the American Society of Mechanical Engineers* 69 (1947) 947–59

32 SMITH A G Heat flow in the gas turbine. *Proceedings of the Institution of Mechanical Engineers* 159 (1948) 245–54

33 KAYS W M and LONDON A L *Compact Heat Exchangers* (McGraw-Hill, 1964)

34 MAYHEW Y R, GRIFFITHS D J and PHILLIPS J W Effect of vapour drag on laminar film condensation on a vertical surface. *Thermodynamics and Fluid Mechanics Convention, Liverpool, April 1966, Proceedings of the Institution of Mechanical Engineers* 180, Pt 3J (1965–6) 280–7, 342–3

35 *Proceedings of the General Discussion on Heat Transfer London, September 1951, Institution of Mechanical Engineers*

36 SEBAN R A and SHIMAZAKI T T Heat transfer to a fluid flowing turbulently in a smooth pipe with walls at constant temperature. *Transactions of the American Society of Mechanical Engineers* 73 (1951) 803–9

37 HAMILTON D C and MORGAN W R Radiant-interchange configuration factors. *National Advisory Committee on Aeronautics technical note* 2836, Washington (1952)

38 *Liquid Metals Handbook* Atomic Energy Commission and Bureau of Ships, Department of the Navy, 2nd and 3rd edns (US Government Printing Office, 1952 and 1955)

39 COHEN H and BAYLEY F J Heat transfer problems of liquid-cooled gas-turbine blades. *Proceedings of the Institution of Mechanical Engineers* 169 (1955) 1063–74

40 KARPLUS W J *Analogue Simulation: Solutions of Field Problems* (McGraw-Hill, 1958)

41 HEISLER M P Temperature charts for induction and constant-temperature heating. *Transactions of the American Society of Mechanical Engineers* 69 (1947) 227–36

42 SCHNEIDER P J *Temperature Response Charts* (Wiley, 1963)

43 REECE G *Microcomputer Modelling by Finite Differences* (Macmillan, 1986)

44 HOLMAN J P *Heat Transfer* (McGraw-Hill, 1990)

45 GREGORIG R Film condensation on finely grooved surfaces with consideration of surface tension. *Zeitschift für angewandte Mathematik und Physik* 5 (1954) 36–49

46 MARTO P J An evaluation of film condensation on horizontal integral-fin tubes. *Transactions of the American Society of Mechanical Engineers* 110 (1988) 1287–1305

Appendix D

Nomenclature

The notation used in this book follows the recommendations of the references cited in Appendix A, section A.5. In particular, the selection of symbols and their styles—whether upright (roman) or sloping (italic)—is guided by certain principles:

(a) SI specifies the symbols to be used for *units* and that they be in upright type (e.g. kJ, m, kg).

(b) Upright type must also be used for mathematical functions and operators (e.g. sin, ln, Σ, Δ, d, e) and for chemical symbols (e.g. H_2O). The sign for a function, e.g. $y = f(x)$ or $\phi(x)$, is written in upright type. When the letter of a physical quantity is used to denote the function, e.g. internal energy $u = u(v, T)$, the sign of the function u is upright, whereas the physical quantity u, according to (c) below, is sloping.

(c) Symbols for *physical quantities* (mass m, pressure p) are always in sloping type, but no rigid rules for their selection can be formulated because of conflicting demands in different areas of science. The nomenclature we have chosen is presented here separately for the four parts of the book and represents a compromise between international recommendations for allied sciences.

(d) Letter subscripts and superscripts are generally in sloping type when derived from physical quantities (e.g. subscript p to denote constant pressure), but in upright type when representing abbreviations (e.g. m for mean, mech for mechanical). We have not followed this guideline when we felt clarity demanded otherwise.

Part I

A	area; non-flow exergy function
B	steady-flow exergy function
C	velocity
c_p	specific heat capacity at constant pressure
c_v	specific heat capacity at constant volume
E, e	internal energy, specific internal energy (in general)
f	specific Helmholtz function
G	Gibbs function

g	specific Gibbs function; gravitational acceleration
H, h	enthalpy, specific enthalpy
$\mathscr{J}$	Joule's equivalent
l	length
$m, \dot{m}$	mass, rate of mass flow
n	polytropic index
p	absolute pressure
$Q, \dot{Q}$	heat, rate of heat transfer (power)
R	gas constant
S, s	entropy, specific entropy
T	absolute thermodynamic temperature
U, u	internal energy, specific internal energy
V, v	volume, specific volume
$W, \dot{W}$	work, rate of work transfer (power)
z	height above datum

Greek symbols

β	coefficient of cubical expansion
η	efficiency
θ	temperature on any arbitrary scale
κ	compressibility
μ	Joule-Thomson coefficient

Part II

A	area
C	velocity
c	specific heat capacity
ΔG	Gibbs function of reaction
g	gravitational acceleration
H, h	enthalpy, specific enthalpy
ΔH	enthalpy of reaction
K	equilibrium constant
l	length
$m, \dot{m}$	mass, rate of mass flow
$\tilde{m}$	molar mass (per unit of amount-of-substance)
n	amount-of-substance; polytropic index
p, p_m	absolute pressure, mean effective pressure
$Q, \dot{Q}$	heat, rate of heat transfer (power)
R	specific gas constant
$\tilde{R}$	molar (universal) gas constant (per unit amount-of-substance)
r_c	cut-off ratio
r_p	pressure ratio
r_v	compression ratio
r_W	work ratio
S, s	entropy, specific entropy

T	thermodynamic temperature
U, u	internal energy, specific internal energy
ΔU	internal energy of reaction
V, v	volume, specific volume
$\tilde{v}$	molar volume (per unit amount-of-substance)
$W, \dot{W}$	work, rate of work transfer (power)
x	dryness fraction; mole fraction
Z	compressibility factor

Greek symbols

γ	the ratio c_p/c_v
η	efficiency
θ	temperature on any arbitrary scale
ϕ	relative humidity
ω	specific humidity (moisture content)

Subscripts

c	a property in the critical state
f	a property of the saturated liquid; a property of formation
g	a property of the saturated vapour
fg	a change of phase at constant pressure
i	a constituent in a mixture
P	the products of a chemical reaction
R	the reactants of a chemical reaction; a property in the reduced state

Superscripts

$\ominus$	a property of the standard pressure of $p^{\ominus} = 1$ bar
$\sim$	a property per unit amount-of-substance (i.e. a molar quantity; see section A.4)

Part III

A	area
a	area; velocity of sound
C	absolute velocity
c	specific heat capacity
d	diameter
F	force
g	gravitational acceleration
H, h	enthalpy, specific enthalpy
ΔH	enthalpy of reaction
I	specific impulse
K	equilibrium constant
k	indicator spring constant
k_C	nozzle velocity coefficient
k_D	coefficient of discharge

L	piston stroke
l	length
$m, \dot{m}$	mass, rate of mass flow
$\tilde{m}$	molar mass (per unit amount-of-substance)
N	machine cycles per unit time
n	polytropic index
P	potential energy
p, p_m	absolute pressure, mean effective pressure
$Q, \dot{Q}$	heat, rate of heat transfer (power)
R	gas constant; force
$\tilde{R}$	molar (universal) gas constant (per unit amount-of-substance)
$\mathscr{R}$	reheat factor
r	radius
r_p	pressure ratio
r_v	compression ratio
S, s	entropy, specific entropy
T	thermodynamic temperature
t	time
U	blade velocity
u	specific internal energy
V	volume; velocity relative to blade or duct
v	specific volume
$W, \dot{W}$	work, rate of work transfer (power)
x	dryness fraction

Greek symbols

α	angle of absolute velocity
β	angle of relative velocity
γ	the ratio c_p/c_v
η	efficiency
Λ	degree of reaction
τ	shear stress
ϕ	angle
ω	angular velocity

Subscripts

a	an axial component
c	a mass in a clearance volume
c	a critical value
f	a mass flowing through a machine
r	a radial component
t	a property at a throat
w	a whirl component

Superscripts

$\ominus$	a property at the standard pressure of $p^{\ominus} = 1$ bar

700

a property per unit amount-of-substance (i.e. a molar quantity; see section A.4)

Part IV

A	area
c_p	specific heat capacity at constant pressure
d	diameter
F	geometric or configuration factor
f	friction factor $(= 2\tau/\rho U^2)$
g	gravitational acceleration
H, h	enthalpy, specific enthalpy
h_{fg}	latent enthalpy of vaporisation
i	intensity of radiation
k	thermal conductivity
l	characteristic linear dimension; length
$m, \dot{m}$	mass, rate of mass flow
n	coordinate normal to a surface element
$Q, \dot{Q}$	heat, rate of heat transfer (power)
$\dot{q}$	rate of heat transfer per unit area (heat flux)
$\dot{q}_g$	rate of internal heat generation per unit volume
r	radius
T	thermodynamic temperature
t	time
U	velocity in x-direction; overall heat transfer coefficient
V	velocity in y-direction

Dimensionless groups

Bi	Biot number $(= \alpha l/k)$
Fo	Fourier number $(= \kappa t/l^2)$
Gr	Grashof number $(= \beta g \rho^2 l^3 \theta/\mu^2)$
Nu	Nusselt number $(= \alpha l/k)$
Pe	Péclet number $(= (Re)(Pr) = \rho U c_p l/k)$
Pr	Prandtl number $(= c_p \mu/k)$
Ra	Rayleigh number $(= (Gr)(Pr) = \beta g \rho^2 l^3 \theta c_p/\mu k)$
Re	Reynolds number $(= \rho U l/\mu)$
St	Stanton number $(= Nu/(Re)(Pr) = \alpha/\rho U c_p)$

Greek symbols

α	heat transfer coefficient; absorptivity
β	coefficient of cubical expansion
δ	thickness of boundary layer, of condensate film
ε	eddy diffusivity; emissivity
θ	temperature difference (relative to wall)
κ	thermal diffusivity $(= k/\rho c_p)$
λ	wavelength

μ	dynamic viscosity
v	kinetic viscosity ($= \mu/\rho$)
ρ	density; reflectivity
σ	Stefan-Boltzmann constant; surface tension
τ	shear stress; transmissivity
ϕ	angle
ψ	the ratio δ_t/δ
ω	solid angle

Subscripts

b	the edge of a sublayer; the bulk of a fluid; black-body radiation
c	convection
d	diameter
f	film
m	a mean value
r	the axis of a tube
r	radiation
s	the free stream
t	the temperature boundary layer
w	the wall
λ	the monochromatic value at a wavelength λ
ϕ	radiation at an angle ϕ

Index